Anaesthesia, Intensive Care and Perioperative Medicine A-Z

An Encyclopaedia of Principles and Practice

Sixth Edition

To
Gill, Emma and Abigail

to
Alison, Jonathan, Sophie and Alexander

and to
Pat, Ethan and Molly

Anaesthesia, Intensive Care and Perioperative Medicine A-Z

An Encyclopaedia of Principles and Practice

Sixth Edition

Steve M Yentis BSc MBBS FRCA MD MA
Consultant Anaesthetist, Chelsea and Westminster Hospital;
Honorary Reader, Imperial College London, UK

Nicholas P Hirsch MBBS FRCA FRCP FFICM
Retired Consultant Anaesthetist, The National Hospital for Neurology and Neurosurgery;
Honorary Senior Lecturer, The Institute of Neurology, London, UK

James K Ip BSc MBBS FRCA
Clinical Fellow in Anaesthesia, Great Ormond Street Hospital, London, UK

Original contributions by
Gary B Smith *BM FRCA FRCP*

ELSEVIER

EDINBURGH LONDON NEW YORK OXFORD PHILADELPHIA ST LOUIS SYDNEY TORONTO

ELSEVIER

First edition 1993
Second edition 2000
Third edition 2004
Fourth edition 2009
Fifth edition 2013
Sixth edition 2018

The right of Steve Yentis, Nicholas Hirsch and James Ip to be identified as authors of this work has been asserted by them in accordance with the Copyright, Designs and Patents Act 1988.

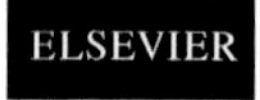

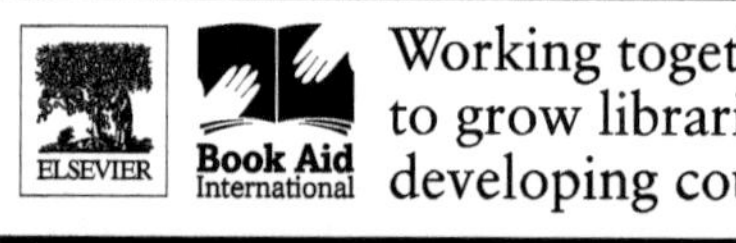

The publisher's policy is to use paper manufactured from sustainable forests

ISBN: 978-0-7020-7165-2

Printed in Great Britain

Last digit is the print number: 9 8 7 6 5 4 3 2

Content Strategists: Jeremy Bowes and Laurence Hunter
Content Development Specialist: Joshua Mearns
Project Manager: Julie Taylor
Design: Paula Catalano
Illustration Manager: Teresa McBryan
Marketing Manager: Deborah Watkins

Preface

In the 25 years since the publication of the first edition of our textbook, we have been delighted to find that 'the *A–Z*' has been adopted by both trainees and established practitioners alike. Whilst our original idea was to produce a readily accessible source of information for those sitting the Royal College of Anaesthetists' Fellowship examinations, it soon became obvious that the book appeals to a far wider readership. We hope that the *A–Z* will continue to be useful to all staff who help us care for patients on a daily basis, as well as to anaesthetists and intensivists of all grades.

As with previous new editions, each entry has been reviewed and, where appropriate, revised, and new ones inserted. We have also developed further the structured 'revision checklist' of entries, introduced in the 5th edition, that we hope will be useful to those preparing for examinations.

The difference between the list of entries in the first edition and those in the current one continues to increase, with a huge expansion of new entries and revision of existing ones. This change acknowledges the enormous breadth of information needed to satisfy the vast range of activities performed by our anaesthetic, intensive care, nursing and other colleagues, and also reflects the ever-changing field in which we work. With current consolidation of the role of anaesthetists as 'perioperative physicians', we have also developed and/or introduced entries that are particularly relevant to this aspect of our work, and emphasise this in the altered title of the book.

The publication of a textbook requires the support of a multitude of people. We are indebted to our colleagues, both junior and senior, who have gently criticised previous editions; their suggestions have been invaluable and have directly resulted in changes found in each new edition over the years. We are particularly grateful to Drs Helen Laycock and Harriet Wordsworth, Chelsea and Westminster Hospital/Imperial College, for advising on entries related to pain and pain management for this edition. We also thank the staff of Elsevier and their predecessors for their support during the life of this project. Finally, this is the second edition of the *A–Z* on which two of the original authors, SMY and NPH, have worked without the third, Gary Smith, though his contributions exist throughout the book in both the format and content of entries from previous editions. We are both delighted to continue to work with James Ip on this edition, having successfully done so on the previous one.

SMY
NPH
JKI

Explanatory notes

Arrangement of text

Entries are arranged alphabetically, with some related subjects grouped together to make coverage of one subject easier. For example, entries relating to tracheal intubation may be found under **I** as in **Intubation, awake**; **Intubation, blind nasal**, etc.

Cross-referencing

Bold type indicates a cross-reference. An abbreviation highlighted in bold type refers to an entry in its fully spelled form. For example, '**ALI** may occur …' refers to the entry **Acute lung injury**. Further instructions appear in italics.

References

Reference to a suitable article is provided at the foot of the entry where appropriate.

Proper names

Where possible, a short biographical note is provided at the foot of the entry when a person is mentioned. Dates of birth and death are given, or the date of description if these dates are unknown. No dates are given for contemporary names. Where more than one eponymous entry occurs, e.g., **Haldane apparatus** and **Haldane effect**, details are given under the first entry. The term 'anaesthetist' is used in the English sense, i.e., a medical practitioner who practises anaesthesia; the terms 'anesthesiologist' and 'anaesthesiologist' are not used.

Drugs

Individual drugs have entries where they have especial relevance to, or may by given by, the anaesthetist or intensivist. Where many different drugs exist within the same group, for example, β-adrenergic receptor antagonists, those which may be given intravenously have their own entry, whilst the others are described under the group description. The reader is referred back to entries describing drug groups and classes where appropriate.

Recommended International Nonproprietary Names (rINNs) and chemical names

Following work undertaken by the World Health Organization, European law requires the replacement of existing national drug nomenclature with rINNs. For most drugs, rINNs are identical to the British Approved Name (BAN). The Medicines Control Agency (UK) has proposed a two-stage process for the introduction of rINNs. For substances where the change is substantial, both names will appear on manufacturers' labels and leaflets for a number of years, with the rINN preceding the BAN on the drug label. For drugs where the change presents little hazard, the change will be immediate. For some drugs which do not appear in either of the above two categories, the British (or USP) name may still be used.

There are over 200 affected drugs, many of them no longer available. Affected drugs that are mentioned in this book (though not all of them have their own entries) are listed below—though please note that, in common with the British Pharmacopoeia, the terms 'adrenaline' and 'noradrenaline' will be used throughout the text in preference to 'epinephrine' and 'norepinephrine', respectively, because of their status as natural hormones. Thus (except for adrenaline and noradrenaline), the format for affected drugs is rINN (BAN), e.g., **Tetracaine hydrochloride** (Amethocaine). Non-BAN, non-rINN names are also provided for certain other drugs (for example, **Isoproterenol**, *see Isoprenaline*) to help direct non-UK readers or those unfamiliar with UK terminology.

Similarly, the International Union of Pure and Applied Chemistry (IUPAC) nomenclature of inorganic chemistry is used for consistency, even though some of the spelling (outside of drug names) is not widely used in UK English, e.g., sulfur/sulfate instead of sulphur/sulphate.

Examination revision checklist

At the front of the book is a checklist based on entries of particular relevance to examination candidates, which have been classified and listed alphabetically in order to support systematic study of examination topics according to the subject area.

continued over page

BAN	*rINN*
Adrenaline	Epinephrine
Amethocaine	Tetracaine
Amoxycillin	Amoxicillin
Amphetamine	Amfetamine
Amylobarbitone	Amobarbital
Beclomethasone	Beclometasone
Benzhexol	Trihexyphenidyl
Benztropine	Benzatropine
Busulphan	Busulfan
Cephazolin	Cefazolin
Cephradine	Cefradine
Cephramandole	Ceframandole
Chlormethiazole	Clomethiazole
Chlorpheniramine	Chlorphenamine
Corticotrophin	Corticotropin
Cyclosporin	Ciclosporin
Dicyclomine	Dicycloverine
Dothiepin	Dosulepin
Ethacrynic acid	Etacrynic acid
Ethamsylate	Etamsylate
Frusemide	Furosemide
Indomethacin	Indometacin
Lignocaine	Lidocaine
Methohexitone	Methohexital
Methylene blue	Methylthioninium chloride
Noradrenaline	Norepinephrine
Oxpentifylline	Pentoxifylline
Phenobarbitone	Phenobarbital
Sodium cromoglycate	Sodium cromoglicate
Sulphadiazine	Sulfadiazine
Sulphasalazine	Sulfasalazine
Tetracosactrin	Tetracosactide
Thiopentone	Thiopental
Tribavarin	Ribavarin
Trimeprazine	Alimemazine

Abbreviations

ACE inhibitors angiotensin converting enzyme inhibitors
ACTH adrenocorticotrophic hormone
ADP adenosine diphosphate
AF atrial fibrillation
AIDS acquired immune deficiency syndrome
ALI acute lung injury
APACHE acute physiology and chronic health evaluation
ASA American Society of Anesthesiologists
ASD atrial septal defect
ATP adenosine triphosphate
AV atrioventricular
bd twice daily
BP blood pressure
cAMP cyclic adenosine monophosphate
$CMRO_2$ cerebral metabolic rate for oxygen
CNS central nervous system
CO_2 carbon dioxide
COPD chronic obstructive pulmonary disease
CPAP continuous positive airway pressure
CPR cardiopulmonary resuscitation
CSE combined spinal–extradural
CSF cerebrospinal fluid
CT computed tomography
CVP central venous pressure
CVS cardiovascular system
CXR chest x-ray
DIC disseminated intravascular coagulation
DNA deoxyribonucleic acid
2,3-DPG 2,3-diphosphoglycerate
DVT deep vein thrombosis
ECF extracellular fluid
ECG electrocardiography
EDTA ethylenediaminetetraacetate
EEG electroencephalography
EMG electromyography
ENT ear, nose and throat
FEV_1 forced expiratory volume in 1 s
F_IO_2 fractional inspired concentration of oxygen
FRC functional residual capacity
FVC forced vital capacity
G gauge
GABA γ-aminobutyric acid
GFR glomerular filtration rate
GIT gastrointestinal tract
GTN glyceryl trinitrate
HCO_3^- bicarbonate
HDU high dependency unit
HIV human immunodeficiency virus
HLA human leucocyte antigen
5-HT 5-hydroxytryptamine
ICP intracranial pressure
ICU intensive care unit
IgA, IgG, etc. immunoglobulin A, G, etc.
im intramuscular
IMV intermittent mandatory ventilation
IPPV intermittent positive pressure ventilation
iv intravenous
IVRA intravenous regional anaesthesia
JVP jugular venous pressure
LM laryngeal mask
MAC minimal alveolar concentration
MAP mean arterial pressure
MH malignant hyperthermia
MI myocardial infarction
MODS multiple organ dysfunction syndrome
MRI magnetic resonance imaging
mw molecular weight
NAD(P) nicotinamide adenine dinucleotide (phosphate)
NHS National Health Service
NICE National Institute for Health and Care Excellence
NMDA *N*-methyl-D-aspartate
N_2O nitrous oxide
NSAID non-steroidal anti-inflammatory drug
O_2 oxygen
od once daily
ODA/P operating department assistant/practitioner
$P\text{CO}_2$ partial pressure of carbon dioxide
PE pulmonary embolus
PEEP positive end-expiratory pressure
$P\text{O}_2$ partial pressure of oxygen
PONV postoperative nausea and vomiting
pr per rectum
qds four times daily
RNA ribonucleic acid
RS respiratory system
SAD supraglottic airway device
sc subcutaneous
SIRS systemic inflammatory response syndrome
SLE systemic lupus erythematosus
SVP saturated vapour pressure
SVR systemic vascular resistance
SVT supraventricular tachycardia
TB tuberculosis
TBI traumatic brain injury
tds three times daily
TENS transcutaneous electrical nerve stimulation
THRIVE transnasal humidified rapid-insufflation ventilatory exchange
TIVA total intravenous anaesthesia
TPN total parenteral nutrition
TURP transurethral resection of prostate
UK United Kingdom
US(A) United States (of America)
VF ventricular fibrillation
$\dot{V}/\dot{Q}$ ventilation/perfusion
VSD ventricular septal defect
VT ventricular tachycardia

Examination revision checklist

This checklist has been compiled from entries of particular relevance to examination candidates, classified and listed alphabetically in order to support systematic study of examination topics. This list is not exhaustive, and, for clarity, entries that summarise a topic and incorporate multiple cross-references (e.g. Opioid analgesic drugs) have been included in preference to listing every relevant entry, e.g. Alfentanil, Fentanyl, Remifentanil, etc. The latter should still be referred to where appropriate, to gain relevant detail.

Checklist index:

PHYSIOLOGY

CARDIOVASCULAR

- Afterload.
- Albumin.
- Anaerobic threshold.
- Arterial blood pressure.
- Atrial natriuretic peptide.
- Autoregulation.
- Baroreceptor reflex.
- Baroreceptors.
- Blood.
- Blood flow.
- Blood groups.
- Blood volume.
- Capacitance vessels.
- Capillary refill time.
- Cardiac cycle.
- Cardiac output.
- Cardioinhibitory centre.
- Central venous pressure (CVP).
- Coagulation.
- Coronary blood flow.
- 2,3-Diphosphoglycerate (2,3-DPG).
- Ejection fraction.
- Exercise.
- Fetal haemoglobin.
- Fibrinolysis.
- Fluids, body.
- Haemoglobin (Hb).
- Haemorrhage.
- Heart rate.
- Hüfner constant.
- Hypotension.
- Insensible water loss.
- Left atrial pressure.
- Left ventricular end-diastolic pressure.
- Mixed venous blood.
- Myocardial contractility.
- Myocardial metabolism.
- Myoglobin.
- Oedema.
- Oncotic pressure
- Osmolality and osmolarity.
- Osmolar gap.
- Osmoreceptors.
- Osmosis.
- Osmotic pressure.
- Pacemaker cells.
- Perfusion pressure.
- Preload.
- Pulmonary artery pressure.
- Pulmonary circulation.
- Pulmonary vascular resistance.
- Pulse pressure.
- Right ventricular function.
- Sinus arrhythmia.
- Sinus bradycardia.
- Sinus rhythm.
- Sinus tachycardia.
- Starling forces.
- Starling's law (Frank–Starling law).
- Stroke volume.
- Stroke work.
- Systemic vascular resistance.
- Valsalva manoeuvre.
- Vasomotor centre.
- Venous return.
- Venous waveform.
- Vitamin K.

CELLULAR/MOLECULAR/METABOLISM

- Action potential.
- Active transport.
- Acute-phase response.
- Adenosine triphosphate and diphosphate.
- Adrenergic receptors.
- Basal metabolic rate.
- Calcium.
- Carbohydrates.
- Carbonic anhydrase.
- Catabolism.
- Catechol-*O*-methyl transferase (COMT).
- Complement.
- Cyclo-oxygenase (COX).
- Cytochrome oxidase system.
- Cytokines.
- Donnan effect (Gibbs–Donnan effect).
- Energy balance.
- Fats.

- G protein-coupled receptors.
- Glycolysis.
- Goldman constant-field equation.
- Histamine and histamine receptors.
- Homeostasis.
- 5-Hydroxytryptamine (5-HT, Serotonin).
- Immunoglobulins.
- Ketone bodies.
- Lactate.
- Magnesium.
- Membrane potential.
- Membranes.
- Metabolism.
- Methionine and methionine synthase.
- Monoamine oxidase (MAO).
- Muscle.
- Muscle contraction.
- Nernst equation.
- Nitrogen balance.
- Phosphate.
- Potassium.
- Prostaglandins.
- Second messenger.
- Sodium.
- Sodium/potassium pump.
- Tricarboxylic acid cycle.
- Vitamins.

ENDOCRINE/REPRODUCTIVE

- Adrenal gland.
- Calcitonin.
- Corticosteroids.
- Glucagon.
- Growth hormone.
- Insulin.
- Pituitary gland.
- Placenta.
- Pregnancy.
- Thyroid gland.
- Uterus.
- Vasopressin.

GASTROINTESTINAL

- Ammonia.
- Amylase.
- Biliary tract.
- Gastric contents.
- Gastric emptying.
- Liver.
- Lower oesophageal sphincter.
- Nutrition.
- Swallowing.
- Urea.
- Vomiting.

NERVOUS SYSTEM

- Acetylcholine.
- Acetylcholine receptors.
- Acetylcholinesterase.
- γ-Aminobutyric acid (GABA) receptors.
- Autonomic nervous system.
- Blood–brain barrier.
- Catecholamines.
- Cerebral blood flow.
- Cerebral metabolism.
- Cerebral perfusion pressure.
- Cerebrospinal fluid (CSF).
- Chemoreceptor trigger zone.
- Chemoreceptors.
- Dermatomes.
- Dopamine receptors.
- End-plate potentials.
- Evoked potentials.
- Gag reflex.
- Gate control theory of pain.
- Glutamate.
- Intracranial pressure (ICP).
- Memory.
- Monro–Kellie doctrine.
- Motor pathways.
- Motor unit.
- Muscle spindles.
- Myelin.
- *N*-Methyl-D-aspartate (NMDA) receptors.
- Nerve conduction.
- Neuromuscular junction.
- Neurone.
- Neurotransmitters.
- Nociception.
- Pain pathways.
- Parasympathetic nervous system.
- Pupil.
- Referred pain.
- Reflex arc.
- Refractory period.
- Sensory pathways.
- Sleep.
- Sympathetic nervous system.
- Synaptic transmission.
- 'Wind-up'.

RENAL

- Clearance.
- Clearance, free water.
- Creatinine clearance.
- Filtration fraction.
- Glomerular filtration rate (GFR).
- Juxtaglomerular apparatus.
- Kidney.
- Nephron.
- Renal blood flow.
- Renin/angiotensin system.
- Urine.

RESPIRATORY AND ACID/BASE

- Acid–base balance.
- Acidosis, metabolic.
- Acidosis, respiratory.
- Airway pressure.
- Airway resistance.
- Alkalosis, metabolic.
- Alkalosis, respiratory.
- Alveolar air equation.

- Alveolar–arterial oxygen difference.
- Alveolar gas transfer.
- Alveolar gases.
- Alveolar ventilation.
- Alveolus.
- Anion gap.
- Aortic bodies.
- Apnoea.
- Arteriovenous oxygen difference.
- Base.
- Base excess/deficit.
- Bicarbonate.
- Blood gas analyser.
- Blood gas interpretation.
- Bohr effect.
- Bohr equation.
- Breathing, control of.
- Breathing, work of.
- Buffers.
- Carbon dioxide (CO_2).
- Carbon dioxide dissociation curve.
- Carbon dioxide, end-tidal.
- Carbon dioxide transport.
- Carbon monoxide (CO).
- Carotid body.
- Chloride shift (Hamburger shift).
- Closing capacity.
- Compliance.
- Cough.
- Cyanosis.
- Davenport diagram.
- Dead space.
- Diffusing capacity (Transfer factor).
- Elastance.
- Fink effect.
- F_IO_2.
- Haldane effect.
- Henderson–Hasselbalch equation.
- Hering–Breuer reflex (Inflation reflex).
- Hydrogen ions (H^+).
- Hypoxia.
- Hypoxic pulmonary vasoconstriction.
- Intrapleural pressure.
- Laryngeal reflex.
- Lung.
- Lung volumes.
- Minute ventilation.
- Nitrogen washout.
- Oxygen cascade.
- Oxygen delivery.
- Oxygen extraction ratio.
- Oxygen flux.
- Oxygen saturation.
- Oxygen transport.
- Oxyhaemoglobin dissociation curve.
- Peak expiratory flow rate.
- pH.
- Pulmonary irritant receptors.
- Pulmonary stretch receptors.
- Respiratory muscles.
- Respiratory quotient.
- Respiratory symbols.
- Shunt.
- Shunt equation.
- Siggaard-Andersen nomogram.
- Standard bicarbonate.
- Strong ion difference.
- Surfactant.
- Venous admixture.
- Ventilation/perfusion mismatch.

CLINICAL ANATOMY

CARDIOVASCULAR SYSTEM

- Brachial artery.
- Carotid arteries.
- Coronary circulation.
- Femoral artery.
- Fetal circulation.
- Heart.
- Heart, conducting system.
- Jugular veins.
- Mediastinum.
- Pericardium.
- Venous drainage of arm.
- Venous drainage of leg.
- Vertebral arteries.

MUSCULOSKELETAL SYSTEM

- Cervical spine.
- Ribs.
- Skull.
- Temporomandibular joint.
- Vertebrae.

NERVOUS SYSTEM

- Brachial plexus.
- Brain.
- Cerebral circulation.
- Cranial nerves.
- Hypothalamus.
- Lumbar plexus.
- Meninges.
- Myotomes.
- Sacral plexus.
- Spinal cord.
- Spinal nerves.

RESPIRATORY SYSTEM

- Airway.
- Diaphragm.
- Intercostal spaces.
- Laryngeal nerves.
- Larynx.
- Nose.
- Pharynx.
- Phrenic nerves.
- Pleura.
- Tongue.
- Tracheobronchial tree.

SPECIAL ZONES

- Antecubital fossa.
- Epidural space.

- Femoral triangle.
- Neck, cross-sectional anatomy.
- Orbital cavity.
- Popliteal fossa.
- Sacral canal.
- Thoracic inlet.

PHARMACOLOGY

ANAESTHETIC AGENTS/SEDATIVES

- Anaesthesia, mechanism of.
- Concentration effect.
- Fluoride ions.
- Inhalational anaesthetic agents.
- Intravenous anaesthetic agents.
- Meyer–Overton rule.
- Minimal alveolar concentration (MAC).
- Second gas effect.

ANALGESICS

- Analgesic drugs.
- Capsaicin.
- Ethyl chloride.
- Non-steroidal anti-inflammatory drugs.
- Opioid analgesic drugs.
- Opioid receptor antagonists.
- Opioid receptors.

ANTI-INFECTIVES

- Antibacterial drugs.
- Antifungal drugs.
- Antimalarial drugs.
- Antituberculous drugs.
- Antiviral drugs.

BASIC PRINCIPLES

- Adverse drug reactions.
- Affinity.
- Agonist.
- Antagonist.
- Bioavailability.
- Dose–response curves.
- Drug development.
- Drug interactions.
- Efficacy.
- Enzyme induction/inhibition.
- Exponential process.
- Extraction ratio.
- First-pass metabolism.
- Half-life ($t_{1/2}$).
- Ionisation of drugs.
- Isomerism.
- Michaelis–Menten kinetics.
- Pharmacodynamics.
- Pharmacogenetics.
- Pharmacokinetics.
- pK.
- Potency.
- Prodrug.
- Protein-binding.
- Receptor theory.
- Tachyphylaxis.
- Target-controlled infusion (TCI).
- Therapeutic ratio/index.
- Time constant (τ).
- Volume of distribution (V_d).
- Washout curves.

CARDIOVASCULAR

- α-Adrenergic receptor agonists.
- α-Adrenergic receptor antagonists.
- β-Adrenergic receptor agonists.
- β-Adrenergic receptor antagonists.
- Antiarrhythmic drugs.
- Anticholinergic drugs.
- Antihypertensive drugs.
- Calcium channel blocking drugs.
- Calcium sensitisers.
- Cardiac glycosides.
- Diuretics.
- Inotropic drugs.
- Phosphodiesterase inhibitors.
- Statins.
- Sympathomimetic drugs.
- Vasodilator drugs.
- Vasopressor drugs.

ENDOCRINE/REPRODUCTIVE

- Carboprost.
- Contraceptives, oral.
- Corticosteroids.
- Desmopressin (DDAVP).
- Ergometrine maleate.
- Hormone replacement therapy.
- Hypoglycaemic drugs.
- Misoprostol.
- Oxytocin.
- Tocolytic drugs.

GASTROINTESTINAL

- Antacids.
- Antispasmodic drugs.
- Emetic drugs.
- H_2 receptor antagonists.
- Laxatives.
- Octreotide.
- Prokinetic drugs.
- Proton pump inhibitors.

HAEMATOLOGICAL

- Anticoagulant drugs.
- Antifibrinolytic drugs.
- Antiplatelet drugs.
- Cytotoxic drugs.
- Factor VIIa, recombinant
- Fibrinolytic drugs.
- Granulocyte colony-stimulating factor.
- Immunoglobulins, intravenous (IVIG).
- Immunosuppressive drugs.
- Protamine sulfate.

- Prothrombin complex concentrate.
- Thrombin inhibitors.

INTRAVENOUS FLUIDS

- Colloid.
- Colloid/crystalloid controversy.
- Crystalloid.
- Electrolyte.
- Intravenous fluid administration.
- Intravenous fluids.
- Tonicity.

LOCAL ANAESTHETICS

- EMLA cream.
- Local anaesthetic agents.
- Minimal blocking concentration (C_m).
- Minimal local anaesthetic concentration/dose/volume.

NEUROLOGICAL/PSYCHIATRIC

- Anticonvulsant drugs.
- Antidepressant drugs.
- Antiemetic drugs.
- Antihistamine drugs.
- Antiparkinsonian drugs.
- Antipsychotic drugs.
- Central anticholinergic syndrome.
- Dystonic reaction.
- Flumazenil.
- Nicotine.

NEUROMUSCULAR TRANSMISSION

- Acetylcholinesterase inhibitors.
- Cholinesterase, plasma.
- Denervation hypersensitivity.
- Depolarising neuromuscular blockade.
- Dibucaine number.
- Dual block (Phase II block).
- Hofmann degradation.
- Neuromuscular blocking drugs.
- Non-depolarising neuromuscular blockade.
- Priming principle.
- Recurarisation.
- Sugammadex sodium.

RESPIRATORY

- Bronchodilator drugs.
- Doxapram hydrochloride.
- Mucolytic drugs.

OTHER

- *N*-Acetylcysteine.
- Alcohols.
- Chemical weapons.
- Dantrolene sodium.
- Herbal medicines.
- Hyaluronidase.
- Lipid emulsion
- Magnesium sulfate.
- Propylene glycol.

PHYSICS AND MEASUREMENT

APPLIED PHYSICS AND CHEMISTRY

- Activation energy.
- Adiabatic change.
- Atmosphere.
- Avogadro's hypothesis.
- Bar.
- Beer–Lambert law.
- Bernoulli effect.
- Boiling point.
- Boyle's law.
- Calorie.
- Charge, electric.
- Charles' law.
- Coanda effect.
- Colligative properties of solutions.
- Critical pressure.
- Critical temperature.
- Critical velocity.
- Dalton's law.
- Density.
- Dew point.
- Diffusion.
- Doppler effect.
- Energy.
- Fick's law of diffusion.
- Flammability.
- Flow.
- Fluid.
- Force.
- Gas.
- Gas flow.
- Graham's law.
- Hagen–Poiseuille equation.
- Harmonics.
- Heat.
- Heat capacity.
- Henry's law.
- Humidity.
- Ideal gas law.
- Isotherms.
- Laplace's law.
- Laser surgery.
- Latent heat.
- Molarity.
- Normal solution.
- Ohm's law.
- Partial pressure.
- Partition coefficient.
- Pascal.
- Power (in Physics).
- Poynting effect.
- Pressure.
- Pseudocritical temperature.
- Radiation.
- Radioisotopes.
- Raoult's law.
- Resonance.
- Reynolds' number.

- Saturated vapour pressure (SVP).
- Solubility.
- Solubility coefficients.
- Specific gravity (Relative density).
- Starling resistor.
- Stoichiometric mixture.
- STP/STPD.
- Surface tension.
- Temperature measurement.
- Tension.
- Units, SI.
- Vapour.
- Venturi principle.
- Viscosity (η).
- Work.

CLINICAL MEASUREMENT

- Amplifiers.
- Arterial blood pressure measurement.
- Arterial cannulation.
- Arterial waveform.
- Becquerel.
- Bispectral index monitor.
- Body mass index (BMI).
- Calibration.
- Capnography.
- Carbon dioxide measurement.
- Cardiac output measurement.
- Cerebral function monitor.
- cgs system of units.
- Damping.
- Dilution techniques.
- End-tidal gas sampling.
- Fade.
- Fick principle.
- Flame ionisation detector.
- Flowmeters.
- Flow–volume loops.
- Gain, electrical.
- Gas analysis.
- Gas chromatography.
- Haldane apparatus.
- Hygrometer.
- Hysteresis.
- Impedance plethysmography.
- Isosbestic point.
- Korotkoff sounds.
- LiMON.
- Mass spectrometer.
- Monitoring.
- Neuromuscular blockade monitoring.
- Oscillotonometer.
- Oximetry.
- Oxygen measurement.
- Peak flowmeters.
- pH measurement.
- Phase shift.
- Plethysmography.
- Pneumotachograph.
- Pressure measurement.
- Pulse oximeter.
- Respirometer.
- Rotameter.
- Spectroscopy.
- Spirometer.
- Thromboelastography (TEG).
- Transducers.

ELECTRICITY

- Antistatic precautions.
- Capacitance.
- Conductance.
- Coulomb.
- Current.
- Current density.
- Defibrillation.
- Electrical symbols.
- Electrocution and electrical burns.
- Impedance, electrical.
- Inductance.
- Resistance.
- Volt.

STATISTICS

- Absolute risk reduction.
- Confidence intervals.
- Data.
- Degrees of freedom.
- Errors, statistical.
- Likelihood ratio.
- Mean.
- Median.
- Meta-analysis (Systematic review).
- Mode.
- Null hypothesis.
- Number needed to treat (NNT).
- Odds ratio.
- Percentile.
- Populations.
- Power (in Statistics).
- Predictive value.
- Probability (*P*).
- Randomisation.
- Receiver operating characteristic curves.
- Relative risk reduction.
- Samples, statistical.
- Sensitivity.
- Specificity.
- Standard deviation.
- Standard error of the mean.
- Statistical frequency distributions.
- Statistical significance.
- Statistical tests.
- Variance.

CLINICAL ANAESTHESIA

GENERAL TOPICS

- Altitude, high.
- Altitude, low.
- Anaesthesia, depth of.
- Anaesthesia, stages of.
- Anaesthetic morbidity and mortality.
- Anaesthetists' non-technical skills.

- Anaphylaxis.
- ASA physical status.
- Aspiration of gastric contents.
- Awareness.
- Bariatric surgery.
- Blood loss, perioperative.
- Bronchospasm.
- Carbon dioxide narcosis.
- Cardiac risk indices.
- Cardiopulmonary exercise testing.
- Cell salvage.
- Central venous cannulation.
- Confusion, postoperative.
- Consent for anaesthesia.
- Cricoid pressure (Sellick's manoeuvre).
- Cricothyroidotomy.
- Day-case surgery.
- Elderly, anaesthesia for.
- Electroconvulsive therapy.
- Emergence phenomena.
- Emergency surgery.
- Environmental impact of anaesthesia.
- Environmental safety of anaesthetists.
- Explosions and fires.
- Extubation, tracheal.
- Eye care.
- Fluid balance.
- Gas embolism.
- Heat loss, during anaesthesia.
- Hypotensive anaesthesia.
- Hypothermia.
- Hypoventilation.
- Hypovolaemia.
- Induction of anaesthesia.
- Induction, rapid sequence.
- Intubation, awake.
- Intubation, blind nasal.
- Intubation, complications of.
- Intubation, difficult.
- Intubation, failed.
- Intubation, fibreoptic.
- Intubation, oesophageal.
- Intubation, tracheal.
- Investigations, preoperative.
- Jehovah's Witnesses.
- Laparoscopy.
- Laryngoscopy.
- Laryngospasm.
- Liver transplantation.
- Malignant hyperthermia.
- Medicolegal aspects of anaesthesia.
- Nerve injury during anaesthesia.
- Obesity.
- Plastic surgery.
- Positioning of the patient.
- Postoperative analgesia.
- Postoperative cognitive dysfunction.
- Postoperative nausea and vomiting.
- Premedication.
- Preoperative assessment.
- Preoperative optimisation.
- Preoxygenation.
- Radiology, anaesthesia for.
- Recovery, enhanced.
- Recovery from anaesthesia.
- Regurgitation.
- Sedation.
- Seldinger technique.
- Shivering, postoperative.
- Smoking.
- Sore throat, postoperative.
- Stress response to surgery.
- Substance abuse.
- Teeth.
- Temperature regulation.
- Total intravenous anaesthesia (TIVA).
- Tourniquets.
- Transnasal humidified rapid-insufflation ventilator exchange (THRIVE).

CARDIOTHORACIC

- Cardiac surgery.
- Cardiopulmonary bypass.
- Heart transplantation.
- Lung transplantation.
- One-lung anaesthesia.
- Thoracic surgery.

ENT/MAXILLOFACIAL

- Airway obstruction.
- Bronchoscopy.
- Dental surgery.
- Ear, nose and throat surgery.
- Epistaxis.
- Facial trauma.
- Foreign body, inhaled.
- Injector techniques.
- Insufflation techniques.
- Ludwig's angina.
- Maxillofacial surgery.
- Stridor.
- Tonsil, bleeding.
- Trismus.

NEUROANAESTHESIA

- Head injury.
- Neurosurgery.
- Spinal surgery.

OBSTETRICS

- Amniotic fluid embolism.
- Antepartum haemorrhage.
- Aortocaval compression.
- Caesarean section.
- Confidential Enquiries into Maternal Deaths.
- Fetal monitoring.
- Fetus, effects of anaesthetic drugs on.
- HELLP syndrome.
- Obstetric analgesia and anaesthesia.
- Placenta praevia.
- Placental abruption.
- Postpartum haemorrhage.
- Pre-eclampsia.

OPHTHALMIC

- Eye, penetrating injury.
- Intraocular pressure.
- Oculocardiac reflex.
- Ophthalmic surgery.

ORTHOPAEDICS

- Bone cement implantation syndrome.
- Bone marrow harvest.
- Fat embolism.
- Fractured neck of femur.
- Kyphoscoliosis.
- Orthopaedic surgery.

PAEDIATRICS

- Apgar scoring system.
- Choanal atresia.
- Croup.
- Diaphragmatic herniae.
- Epiglottitis.
- Facial deformities, congenital.
- Gastroschisis and exomphalos.
- Necrotising enterocolitis.
- Neonate.
- Paediatric anaesthesia.
- Pyloric stenosis.
- Tracheo-oesophageal fistula.
- Transposition of the great arteries.

PAIN

- Acupuncture.
- Central pain.
- Coeliac plexus block.
- Complex regional pain syndrome.
- Gasserian ganglion block.
- Pain.
- Pain evaluation.
- Pain management.
- Pain, neuropathic.
- Patient-controlled analgesia.
- Phantom limb.
- Spinal cord stimulation.
- Stellate ganglion block.
- Sympathetic nerve blocks.
- Transcutaneous electrical nerve stimulation.
- Trigger points.

REGIONAL

- Adductor canal block.
- Ankle, nerve blocks.
- Blood patch, epidural.
- Brachial plexus block.
- Caudal analgesia.
- Cervical plexus block.
- Combined spinal–epidural anaesthesia.
- Dural tap.
- Epidural anaesthesia.
- Fascia iliaca compartment block.
- Femoral nerve block.
- Inguinal hernia field block.
- Intercostal nerve block.
- Interpleural analgesia.
- Intravenous regional anaesthesia.
- Knee, nerve blocks.
- Paravertebral block.
- Pecs block.
- Penile block.
- Peribulbar block.
- Post-dural puncture headache.
- Psoas compartment block.
- Rectus sheath block.
- Regional anaesthesia.
- Retrobulbar block.
- Sciatic nerve block.
- Serratus anterior plane block.
- Spinal anaesthesia.
- Sub-Tenon's block.
- Transversus abdominis plane block.
- Wrist, nerve blocks.

UROLOGY

- Extracorporeal shock wave lithotripsy.
- Renal transplantation.
- Transurethral resection of the prostate.
- TURP syndrome.
- Urinary retention.

VASCULAR

- Aortic aneurysm, abdominal.
- Aortic aneurysm, thoracic.
- Aortic dissection.
- Carotid endarterectomy.

CRITICAL CARE

GENERAL TOPICS

- Critical care.
- Imaging in intensive care.
- Lactic acidosis.
- Multiple organ dysfunction syndrome (MODS).
- Organ donation.
- Paediatric intensive care.
- Targeted temperature management.
- Transportation of critically ill patients.
- Withdrawal of treatment in ICU.

CARDIOVASCULAR

- Cardiogenic shock.
- Heparin-induced thrombocytopenia.
- Pulmonary artery catheterisation.
- Pulmonary capillary wedge pressure.
- Septic shock.
- Shock.

GASTROINTESTINAL

- Abdominal compartment syndrome.
- Glycaemic control in the ICU.
- Nutrition, enteral.
- Nutrition, total parenteral (TPN).
- Pancreatitis.

- Refeeding syndrome.
- Selective decontamination of the digestive tract.
- Stress ulcers.

NEUROLOGICAL

- Brainstem death.
- Cerebral hypoxic ischaemic injury.
- Cerebral protection/resuscitation.
- Coma.
- Confusion in the intensive care unit.
- Coning.
- Critical illness polyneuropathy.
- Guillain–Barré syndrome.
- Intracranial pressure monitoring.
- Sedation scoring systems.
- Spinal cord injury.
- Status epilepticus.
- Subarachnoid haemorrhage.
- Vegetative state.

ORGANISATIONAL

- APACHE scoring system.
- Care bundles.
- Intensive care follow-up.
- Intensive care unit.
- Mortality/survival prediction on intensive care unit.

RESPIRATORY

- Acute lung injury.
- Alveolar recruitment manoeuvre.
- Assisted ventilation.
- Barotrauma.
- Continuous positive airway pressure.
- Dynamic hyperinflation.
- Extracorporeal membrane oxygenation.
- High-frequency ventilation.
- Hypercapnia.
- Hypoxaemia.
- Inspiratory: expiratory ratio (I:E ratio).
- Intermittent positive pressure ventilation.
- Lung protection strategies.
- Non-invasive positive pressure ventilation.
- Pleural effusion.
- Pneumothorax.
- Respiratory failure.
- Respiratory muscle fatigue.
- Tracheostomy.
- Transfusion-related acute lung injury (TRALI)
- Ventilator-associated lung injury.
- Ventilator-associated pneumonia.
- Ventilators.
- Weaning from ventilators.

RESUSCITATION

- Advanced life support, adult.
- Basic life support, adult.
- Cardiac arrest.
- Cardiopulmonary resuscitation (CPR).
- Cardiopulmonary resuscitation, neonatal.
- Cardiopulmonary resuscitation, paediatric.
- Choking.
- Intraosseous fluid administration.
- Near-drowning.

TRAUMA

- Abdominal trauma.
- Burns.
- Chest trauma.
- Compartment syndromes.
- 'Golden hour'.
- Pelvic trauma.
- Peritoneal lavage.
- Rib fractures.
- Trauma.
- Traumatic brain injury.

EQUIPMENT

AIRWAY

- Airway exchange catheter.
- Airways.
- Cuffs, of tracheal tubes.
- Endobronchial tubes.
- Facemasks.
- Fibreoptic instruments.
- Intubation aids.
- Laryngeal mask (LM).
- Laryngoscope.
- Laryngoscope blades.
- Minitracheotomy.
- Oesophageal obturators and airways.
- Supraglottic airway device (SAD).
- Tracheal tubes.

BREATHING SYSTEMS

- Adjustable pressure-limiting valves.
- Anaesthetic breathing systems.
- Carbon dioxide absorption, in anaesthetic breathing systems.
- Circle systems.
- Coaxial anaesthetic breathing systems.
- Demand valves.
- Filters, breathing system.
- Heat–moisture exchanger (HME).
- Humidification.
- Nebulisers.
- Non-rebreathing valves.
- Reservoir bag.
- Scavenging.
- Self-inflating bags.
- Soda lime.
- Triservice apparatus.

GAS SUPPLY

- Air.
- Bodok seal.
- Cylinders.
- Filling ratio.
- Oxygen.
- Oxygen concentrator.

- Oxygen failure warning device.
- Pin index system.
- Piped gas supply.
- Pressure regulators.
- Vacuum insulated evaporator (VIE).

OTHER

- Anaesthetic machines.
- Blood filters.
- Checking of anaesthetic equipment.
- Contamination of anaesthetic equipment.
- Diathermy.
- Gauge.
- Luer connectors.
- Needles.
- Suction equipment.
- Syringes.
- Vaporisers.

MEDICINE

CARDIOLOGY

- Acute coronary syndromes.
- Aortic regurgitation.
- Aortic stenosis.
- Arrhythmias.
- Bundle branch block.
- Cardiac catheterisation.
- Cardiac enzymes.
- Cardiac failure.
- Cardiac pacing.
- Cardiac tamponade.
- Cardiomyopathy.
- Cardioversion, electrical.
- Congenital heart disease.
- Cor pulmonale.
- Defibrillators, implantable cardioverter.
- Echocardiography.
- Electrocardiography (ECG).
- Endocarditis, infective.
- Heart block.
- Hypertension.
- Ischaemic heart disease.
- Mitral regurgitation.
- Mitral stenosis.
- Myocardial ischaemia.
- Myocarditis.
- Percutaneous coronary intervention (PCI).
- Pericarditis.
- Prolonged Q–T syndromes.
- Pulmonary hypertension.
- Pulmonary oedema.
- Pulmonary valve lesions.
- Stokes–Adams attack.
- Torsades de pointes.
- Transoesophageal echocardiography.
- Tricuspid valve lesions.

DERMATOLOGY/MUSCULOSKELETAL/RHEUMATOLOGY

- Ankylosing spondylitis.
- Connective tissue diseases.
- Marfan's syndrome.
- Muscular dystrophies.
- Myotonic syndromes.
- Rheumatoid arthritis.
- Sarcoidosis.
- Stevens–Johnson syndrome.
- Systemic lupus erythematosus.
- Vasculitides.

ENDOCRINOLOGY

- Acromegaly.
- Adrenocortical insufficiency.
- Cushing's syndrome.
- Diabetes mellitus.
- Diabetic coma.
- Hyperaldosteronism.
- Hyperthyroidism
- Hypopituitarism.
- Hypothyroidism.
- Phaeochromocytoma.
- Sick euthyroid syndrome.
- Thyroid crisis.

GASTROENTEROLOGY

- Ascites.
- Carcinoid syndrome.
- Diarrhoea.
- Gastrointestinal haemorrhage.
- Gastro-oesophageal reflux.
- Hepatic failure.
- Hepatitis.
- Hiatus hernia.
- Liver function tests.

GENERAL

- Alcoholism.
- Anaemia.
- Decompression sickness.
- Deep vein thrombosis (DVT).
- Dehydration.
- Down's syndrome.
- Hypercalcaemia.
- Hyperglycaemia.
- Hyperkalaemia.
- Hypernatraemia.
- Hyperthermia.
- Hypocalcaemia.
- Hypoglycaemia.
- Hypokalaemia.
- Hypomagnesaemia.
- Hyponatraemia.
- Hypophosphataemia.
- Inborn errors of metabolism.
- Malignancy.
- Malnutrition.
- Porphyria.
- Pyrexia.
- Syndrome of inappropriate antidiuretic hormone secretion (SIADH).
- Systemic inflammatory response syndrome.
- Vasovagal syncope.

HAEMATOLOGY/IMMUNOLOGY

- Autoimmune disease.
- Blood compatibility testing.
- Blood products.
- Blood storage.
- Blood transfusion.
- Bone marrow transplantation.
- Coagulation disorders.
- Coagulation studies.
- Disseminated intravascular coagulation.
- Glucose-6-phosphate dehydrogenase deficiency.
- Haemoglobinopathies.
- Haemolysis.
- Haemophilia.
- Immunodeficiency.
- Latex allergy.
- Methaemoglobinaemia.
- Rhesus blood groups.
- Thrombocytopenia.
- Thrombotic thrombocytopenic purpura.
- Tumour lysis syndrome.
- von Willebrand's disease.

MICROBIOLOGY AND INFECTIOUS DISEASES

- Bacteria.
- Blood cultures.
- Catheter-related sepsis.
- Cellulitis.
- Clostridial infections.
- Human immunodeficiency viral (HIV) infection.
- Infection control.
- Influenza.
- Meningococcal disease.
- Necrotising fasciitis.
- Nosocomial infection.
- Notifiable diseases.
- Pseudomonas infections.
- Sepsis.
- Staphylococcal infections.
- Streptococcal infections.
- Tropical diseases.
- Tuberculosis (TB).

NEUROLOGY/PSYCHIATRY

- Amnesia.
- Anorexia nervosa.
- Anterior spinal artery syndrome.
- Autonomic hyperreflexia.
- Autonomic neuropathy.
- Cauda equina syndrome.
- Central pontine myelinolysis.
- Cerebral abscess.
- Cerebral ischaemia.
- Cerebral oedema.
- Cholinergic crisis.
- Coma scales.
- Convulsions.
- Demyelinating diseases.
- Electroencephalography (EEG).
- Electromyography (EMG).
- Encephalopathy.
- Epilepsy.
- Extradural (epidural) haemorrhage.
- Horner's syndrome.
- Hydrocephalus.
- Lumbar puncture.
- Meningitis.
- Migraine.
- Motor neurone disease.
- Motor neurone, lower.
- Motor neurone, upper.
- Myasthenia gravis.
- Neurofibromatosis.
- Neuroleptic malignant syndrome.
- Paralysis, acute.
- Parkinson's disease.
- Peripheral neuropathy.
- Post-traumatic stress disorder.
- Stroke.
- Subdural haemorrhage.
- Trigeminal neuralgia.

POISONING

- β-Adrenergic receptor antagonist poisoning.
- Alcohol poisoning.
- Barbiturate poisoning.
- Benzodiazepine poisoning.
- Carbon monoxide poisoning.
- Charcoal, activated.
- Chelating agents.
- Cocaine poisoning.
- Cyanide poisoning.
- Heavy metal poisoning.
- Iron poisoning.
- Opioid poisoning.
- Organophosphorus poisoning.
- Paracetamol poisoning.
- Paraquat poisoning.
- Poisoning and overdoses.
- Salicylate poisoning.
- Serotonin syndrome.
- Tricyclic antidepressant drug poisoning.

RENAL

- Acute kidney injury (AKI).
- Crush syndrome.
- Diabetes insipidus.
- Dialysis.
- Glomerulonephritis.
- Hepatorenal syndrome.
- Myoglobinuria.
- Oliguria.
- Renal failure.
- RIFLE criteria.

RESPIRATORY

- Aspiration pneumonitis.
- Asthma.
- Atelectasis.
- Bronchial carcinoma.
- Bronchiectasis.
- Bronchoalveolar lavage.

- Chest drainage.
- Chest infection.
- Chronic obstructive pulmonary disease.
- Cystic fibrosis.
- Dyspnoea.
- Forced expiration.
- Fowler's method.
- Helium.
- Hypocapnia.
- Lung function tests.
- Obstructive sleep apnoea.
- Oxygen, hyperbaric.
- Oxygen therapy.
- Oxygen toxicity.
- Pulmonary embolism (PE).
- Pulmonary fibrosis.

ORGANISATIONAL

- Advance decision.
- Clinical governance.
- Clinical trials.
- Coroner.
- COSHH regulations (Control of Substances Hazardous to Health).
- Critical incidents.
- Do not attempt resuscitation orders.
- Ethics.
- Incident, major.
- Mental Capacity Act 2005.
- National audit projects.
- Never events.
- Organ donation.
- Pollution.
- Recovery room.

RADIOLOGY

- Chest x-ray.
- Computed (axial) tomography (CT).
- Magnetic resonance imaging (MRI).
- Positron emission tomography (PET).
- Radioisotope scanning.
- Radiological contrast media.
- Ultrasound.

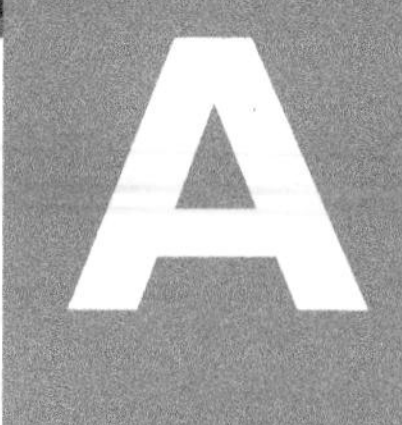

A severity characterisation of trauma (ASCOT). **Trauma scale** derived from the **Glasgow coma scale**, systolic BP, **revised trauma score**, **abbreviated injury scale** and age. A logistic regression equation provides a probability of mortality. Excludes patients with very poor or very good prognoses. Has been claimed to be superior to the **trauma revised injury severity score** system, although is more complex.

Champion HR, Copes WS, Sacco WJ, et al (1996). J Trauma; 40: 42–8

A–aDO_2, *see Alveolar–arterial oxygen difference*

ABA, *see American Board of Anesthesiology*

Abbott, Edward Gilbert, *see Morton, William*

Abbreviated injury scale (AIS). **Trauma scale** first described in 1971 and updated many times since. Comprises a classification of injuries with each given a six-digit code (the last indicating severity, with 1 = minor and 6 = fatal). The codes are linked to International Classification of Diseases codes, thus aiding standardisation of records. The anatomical profile is a refinement in which the locations of injuries are divided into four categories; the AIS scores are added and the square root taken to minimise the contribution of less severe injuries.

Gennarelli TA, Wodzin E (2006). Injury; 37: 1083–91

Abciximab. Monoclonal antibody used as an **antiplatelet drug** and adjunct to **aspirin** and **heparin** in high-risk patients undergoing **percutaneous coronary intervention**. Consists of Fab fragments of **immunoglobulin** directed against the glycoprotein IIb/IIIa receptor on the **platelet** surface. Inhibits platelet aggregation and thrombus formation; effects last 24–48 h after infusion. Careful consideration of risks and benefits should precede use because risk of bleeding is increased. Licensed for single use only.

- Dosage: initial loading of 250 µg/kg over 1 min iv, followed by iv infusion of 125 ng/kg/min (max 10 µg/min) 10–60 min (up to 24 h in unstable angina) before angioplasty with 125 µg/kg/min (up to 10 µg/min for 12 h afterwards).
- Side effects: bleeding, hypotension, nausea, bradycardia. Thrombocytopenia occurs rarely.

Abdominal compartment syndrome. Combination of increased **intra-abdominal pressure** (>12 mmHg [16 cmH_2O]) and organ dysfunction (e.g. following **abdominal trauma** or extensive surgery) resulting from haemorrhage or expansion of the **third space** fluid compartment. May also follow **liver transplantation**, **sepsis**, **burns** and acute **pancreatitis**. Intra-abdominal pressures above 15–18 mmHg (20–25 cmH_2O) may impair ventilation and be associated with reduced venous return, cardiac output, renal blood flow and urine output. Increased CVP may lead to raised ICP. Diagnosed by clinical features and intra-abdominal pressure measurement (performed via a bladder catheter or nasogastric tube, in combination with a water column manometer).

Management includes laparotomy ± Silastic material to cover the abdominal contents. **Paracentesis** may be effective if raised intra-abdominal pressure is due to accumulation of fluid, e.g. ascites. Full resuscitation must be performed before decompression as rapid release of pressure may result in sudden washout of inflammatory mediators from ischaemic tissues, causing acidosis and hypotension. Mortality of the syndrome is 25%–70%.

Kirkpatrick AW, Roberts DJ, De Waele J, et al (2013). Int Care Med; 39: 1190–206

See also, Compartment syndromes

Abdominal field block. Technique using 100–200 ml **local anaesthetic agent**, involving infiltration of the skin, subcutaneous tissues, abdominal muscles and fascia. Provides analgesia of the abdominal wall and anterior peritoneum, but not of the viscera. Now rarely used. **Rectus sheath block, transversus abdominis plane block, iliac crest block** and **inguinal hernia field block** are more specific blocks.

Abdominal sepsis, *see Intra-abdominal sepsis*

Abdominal trauma. May be blunt (e.g. road traffic accidents) or penetrating (e.g. stabbing, bullet wounds). Often carries a high morbidity and mortality because injuries may go undetected. Massive intra-abdominal blood loss or **abdominal compartment syndrome** may follow. The abdomen can be divided into three areas:
  - intrathoracic: protected by the bony thoracic cage. Contains the spleen, liver, stomach and **diaphragm**. Injury may be associated with **rib fractures**. The diaphragm may also be injured by blows to the lower abdomen (which impart pressure waves to the diaphragm) or by penetrating injuries of the chest.
  - true abdomen: contains the small and large bowel, bladder and, in the female, uterus, fallopian tubes and ovaries.
  - retroperitoneal: contains the kidneys, ureters, pancreas and duodenum. May result in massive blood loss from retroperitoneal venous injury.
- Management:
  - basic resuscitation as for **trauma** generally.
  - initial assessment: examination of the anterior abdominal wall, both flanks, back, buttocks, perineum (and in men, the urethral meatus) for bruises, lacerations, entry and exit wounds. Signs may be masked by unconsciousness, **spinal cord injury** or the effects of **alcohol** or drugs. Abdominal swelling usually indicates intra-abdominal haemorrhage; abdominal guarding or rigidity usually indicates visceral injury. Absence of bowel sounds may indicate intraperitoneal haemorrhage or peritoneal soiling with bowel contents. Colonic or rectal injuries may cause blood pr. A high

Table 1 Antigens and antibodies in ABO blood groups

Group	Incidence in UK (%)	Red cell antigen	Plasma antibody
A	42	A	Anti-B
B	8	B	Anti-A
AB	3	A and B	None
O	47	None	Anti-A and anti-B

index of suspicion is required for retroperitoneal injuries because examination is difficult.

- imaging: abdominal x-ray may reveal free gas under the diaphragm (erect or semi-erect; may also be visible on CXR) or laterally (lateral decubitus x-ray); other investigations include pelvic x-ray and urological radiology if indicated (e.g. iv urogram), **CT** and **MRI scanning** and **ultrasound**.
- **peritoneal lavage** is indicated in blunt abdominal trauma associated with:
  - altered pain response (**TBI**, spinal cord injury, drugs, etc.).
  - unexplained **hypovolaemia** following multiple trauma.
  - equivocal diagnostic findings.
- insertion of a nasogastric tube and urinary catheter (provided no urethral injury; a suprapubic catheter may be necessary).
- indications for laparotomy include penetrating injuries, obvious intra-abdominal haemorrhage, signs of bowel perforation or a positive peritoneal lavage.

Al-Mudhaffar M, Hormbrey P (2014). Br Med J; 348: g1140

See also, Pelvic trauma

ABO blood groups. Discovered in 1900 by Landsteiner in Vienna. Antigens may be present on red blood cells, with antibodies in the plasma (Table 1). The antibodies, mostly type-M **immunoglobulins**, develop within the first few months of life, presumably in response to naturally occurring antigens of similar structure to the blood antigens. Infusion of blood containing an ABO antigen into a patient who already has the corresponding antibody may lead to an adverse reaction; hence the description of group O individuals as universal donors, and of group AB individuals as universal recipients.

[Karl Landsteiner (1868–1943), Austrian-born US pathologist]

See also, Blood compatibility testing; Blood groups; Blood transfusion

ABPI, *see Ankle–Brachial Pressure Index*

Abruption, *see Antepartum haemorrhage*

Absolute risk reduction. Indicator of treatment effect in clinical trials, representing the decrease in risk of a given treatment compared with a control treatment, i.e., the inverse of the **number needed to treat**. For a reduction in incidence of events from a% to b%, it equals $(a - b)$%.

See also, Meta-analysis; Odds ratio; Relative risk reduction

Abuse of anaesthetic agents. May occur because of easy access to potent drugs by operating theatre or ICU staff. Anaesthetists are 2.5 times as likely to abuse agents than other physicians. **Opioid analgesic drugs** (especially **fentanyl**) are the most commonly abused agents, but others include **benzodiazepines**, **propofol** and **inhalational anaesthetic agents.** Abuse may be suggested by behavioural or mood changes or excessive and inappropriate requests for opioids. Main considerations include the safety of patients, counselling and psychiatric therapy for the abuser and legal aspects of drug abuse. May be associated with **alcoholism.**

Bryson EO, Silverstein JH (2008). Anesthesiology; 109: 905–17

See also, Misuse of Drugs Act; Sick doctor scheme; Substance abuse

Acarbose. Inhibitor of intestinal alpha glucosidases and pancreatic amylase; used in the treatment of **diabetes mellitus**, usually in combination with a **biguanide** or **sulfonylurea.** Delays digestion and absorption of starch and sucrose and has a small blood glucose-lowering effect.

See also, Meglitinides; Thiazolidinediones

Accessory nerve block. Performed for spasm of trapezius and sternomastoid muscles (there is no sensory component to the nerve). 5–10 ml **local anaesthetic agent** is injected 2 cm below the mastoid process into the sternomastoid muscle, through which the nerve runs.

Accident, major, *see Incident, major*

ACD, Acid–citrate–dextrose solution, *see Blood storage*

ACD-CPR, Active compression decompression CPR, *see Cardiac massage; Cardiopulmonary resuscitation*

ACE, Angiotensin converting enzyme, *see Renin/angiotensin system*

ACE anaesthetic mixture. Mixture of alcohol, chloroform and diethyl ether, in a ratio of 1:2:3 parts, suggested in 1860 as an alternative to chloroform alone. Popular into the 1900s as a means of reducing total dose and side effects of any one of the three drugs.

ACE inhibitors, *see Angiotensin converting enzyme inhibitors*

Acetaminophen, *see Paracetamol*

Acetazolamide. Carbonic anhydrase inhibitor. Reduces renal **bicarbonate** formation and hydrogen ion excretion at the proximal convoluted tubule, thereby inducing a metabolic **acidosis.** A weak **diuretic**, but rarely used as such. Also used to treat **glaucoma**, metabolic alkalosis, altitude sickness and childhood epilepsy. Useful in the treatment of severe **hyperphosphataemia** as it promotes urinary excretion of phosphate. May be used to lower **ICP** (e.g. in benign intracranial hypertension) by reducing **CSF** production. Has been used to alkalinise the urine in **tumour lysis syndrome** and to enhance excretion in drug intoxications, e.g. with salicylates.

- Dosage: 0.25–0.5 g orally/iv od/bd.

Acetylcholine (ACh). **Neurotransmitter**, the acetyl ester of choline (Fig. 1). Synthesised from acetylcoenzyme A and choline in **nerve** ending cytoplasm; the reaction is catalysed by choline acetyltransferase. Choline is actively

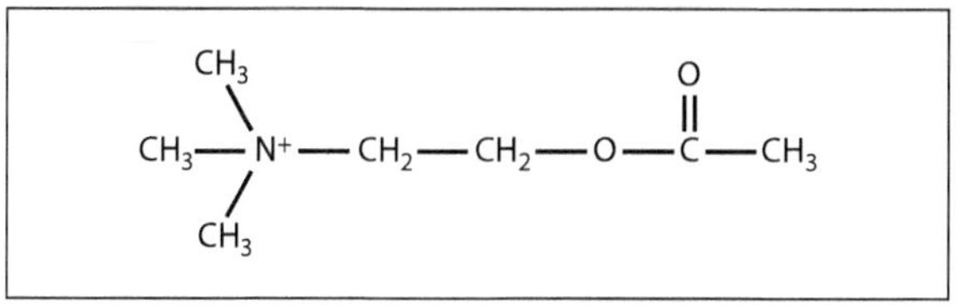

$$CH_3-N^+(CH_3)_2-CH_2-CH_2-O-C(=O)-CH_3$$

Fig. 1 Structure of acetylcholine

transported into the nerve and acetylcoenzyme A is formed in mitochondria. ACh is stored in vesicles.

- ACh is the transmitter at:
  - autonomic ganglia.
  - parasympathetic postganglionic nerve endings.
  - sympathetic postganglionic nerve endings at sweat glands and some muscle blood vessels.
  - the **neuromuscular junction**.
  - many parts of the CNS, where it has a prominent role in CNS plasticity (and therefore learning), attention and memory. Dysfunction of the CNS cholinergic system contributes to the memory disorder in Alzheimer's disease.

Actions may be broadly divided into either muscarinic or nicotinic, depending on the **acetylcholine receptors** involved. ACh is hydrolysed to choline and acetate by **acetylcholinesterase** on the postsynaptic membrane. Other esterases also exist, e.g. plasma **cholinesterase**.

[Alois Alzheimer (1864–1915), German neurologist and pathologist]

See also, Acetylcholine receptors; Neuromuscular transmission; Parasympathetic nervous system; Sympathetic nervous system; Synaptic transmission

Acetylcholine receptors. Transmembrane receptors activated by **acetylcholine** (ACh). Classified according to their relative sensitivity to **nicotine** or **muscarine** (Fig. 2a).

- Nicotinic receptors: ligand-gated ion channels present at numerous sites within the nervous system; notable examples include the **neuromuscular junction** (NMJ) and autonomic ganglia. Each receptor consists of five glycosylated protein subunits that project into the synaptic cleft. The adult receptor consists of 2 α, β, δ and ε units. The ε subunit is replaced by a γ subunit in the neonate. The subunits span the postsynaptic **membrane**, forming a cylinder around a central ion channel (Fig. 2b). The two α subunits of each receptor carry the binding sites for ACh. Occupation of these sites opens the ion channel, allowing cations (mainly sodium, potassium and calcium) to flow into the cell down their concentration gradients; this produces an excitatory postsynaptic potential. If these summate and exceed the threshold potential, an **action potential** is generated. Non-depolarising **neuromuscular blocking drugs** are reversible competitive antagonists of these receptors at the NMJ.
- Muscarinic receptors: **G protein-coupled receptors**, largely coupled to either **adenylate cyclase** or phospholipase C, via Gi and Gq proteins, respectively. Mediate postganglionic neurotransmission via parasympathetic neurones, as well as sympathetic outflow to sweat glands (Fig. 2a). Classified according to structural subtype, distribution and function:
  - M1: Gq-coupled; stomach (stimulates acid secretion) and brain (memory formation).
  - M2: Gi-coupled; heart; decreases heart rate, contractility and atrioventricular nodal conduction.

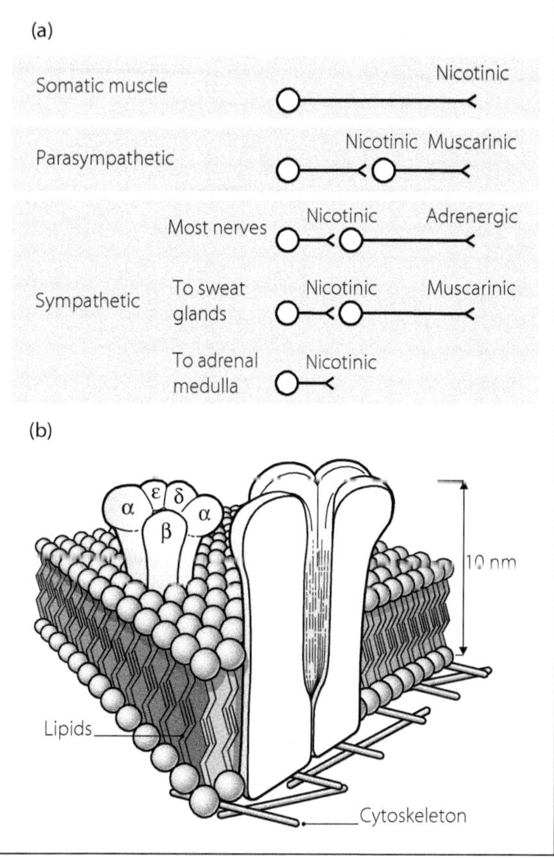

Fig. 2 (a) Types of acetylcholine receptors. (b) Structure of nicotinic acetylcholine receptor

  - M3: Gq-coupled; smooth muscle (increased tone, e.g. bronchiolar, intestinal), exocrine glands (stimulatory), brain (stimulatory at vomiting centre).
  - M4/5: brain and adrenal medulla.

Muscarinic receptor agonists include bethanechol, carbachol and pilocarpine (in the eye); antagonists include **hyoscine**, **atropine** and **ipratropium bromide**.

The activation threshold of muscarinic receptors is lower than that of nicotinic receptors. Injection of ACh or poisoning with **anticholinesterases** thus causes parasympathetic stimulation and sweating at lower doses, before having effects at autonomic ganglia and the NMJ at higher doses.

See also, Neuromuscular transmission; Parasympathetic nervous system; Sympathetic nervous system; Synaptic transmission

Acetylcholinesterase. **Enzyme** present at the synaptic membranes of cholinergic **synapses** and **neuromuscular junctions**. Also found in red blood cells and the placenta. Metabolises **acetylcholine** (ACh) to acetate and choline, thus terminating its action. Has a high catalytic activity, each molecule of acetylcholinesterase catalysing 25 000 molecules of ACh per second. The $N(CH_3)_3^+$ moeity of ACh binds to the anionic site of the enzyme, and the acetate end of ACh forms an intermediate bond at the esteratic site. Choline is liberated, and the intermediate substrate/enzyme complex is then hydrolysed to release acetate (Fig. 3).

See also, Acetylcholinesterase inhibitors; Neuromuscular transmission; Synaptic transmission

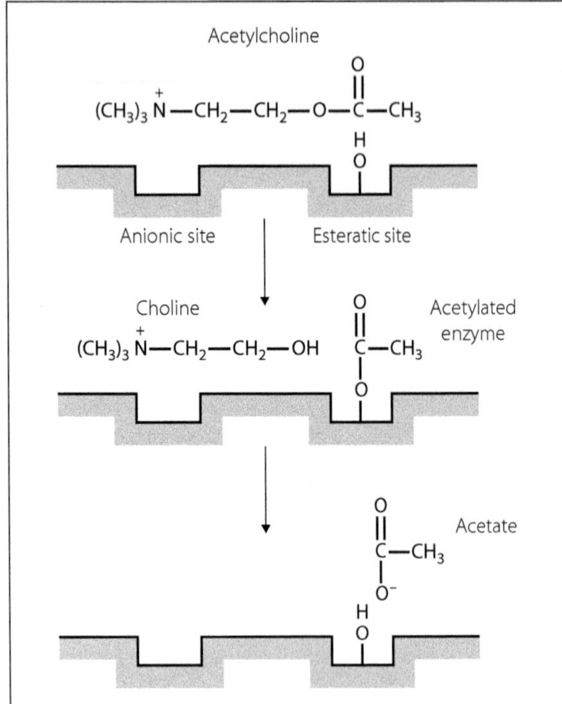

Fig. 3 Action of acetylcholinesterase

Acetylcholinesterase inhibitors. Substances that increase **acetylcholine** (ACh) concentrations by inhibiting **acetylcholinesterase** (AChE). Used clinically for their action at the **neuromuscular junction** in **myasthenia gravis** and in the reversal of **non-depolarising neuromuscular blockade**. Concurrent administration of an antimuscarinic agent, e.g. **atropine** or **glycopyrronium**, reduces unwanted effects of increased ACh concentrations at muscarinic receptors. Effects at ganglia are minimal at normal doses. Central effects may occur if the drug readily crosses the **blood–brain barrier**, e.g. **physostigmine** (used to treat the **central anticholinergic syndrome**).

Have also been used to treat tachyarrhythmias.

- Classified according to mechanism of action:
  - reversible competitive inhibitors: competitive inhibition at the anionic site of AChE prevents binding of ACh, e.g. **edrophonium, tetrahydroaminacrine.**
  - oxydiaphoretic (or 'acid-transferring') inhibitors: act as an alternative substrate for AChE, producing a more stable carbamylated enzyme complex. Subsequent hydrolysis of the complex and thus reactivation of the enzyme is slow. Examples:
    - **neostigmine**, physostigmine (few hours).
    - **pyridostigmine** (several hours).
    - **distigmine** (up to a day).
  - organophosphorus compounds: act by irreversibly phosphorylating the esteratic site of AChE; inhibition can last for weeks until new enzyme is synthesised. Examples include: **ecothiopate** (used for the treatment of glaucoma); parathion (an insecticide); sarin nerve gas (a chemical weapon).

Acetylcholinesterase inhibitors augment **depolarising neuromuscular blockade** and may cause depolarising blockade in overdose. They may also cause bradycardia, hypotension, agitation, miosis, increased GIT activity, sweating and salivation.

Centrally acting acetylcholinesterase inhibitors (e.g. donepezil, rivastigmine, galantamine) are used for symptomatic treatment of Alzheimer's dementia. Of anaesthetic relevance because of their side effects (including nausea, vomiting, fatigue, muscle cramps, increased creatine kinase, convulsions, bradycardia, confusion), enhancement of the actions of **suxamethonium**, and possible antagonism of non-depolarising **neuromuscular blocking drugs.**

[Alois Alzheimer (1864–1915), German neurologist and pathologist]

See also, Neuromuscular transmission; Organophosphorus poisoning

N-Acetylcysteine. Derivative of the naturally occurring **amino acid**, L-cysteine. A **free radical** scavenger, licensed as an antidote to **paracetamol poisoning.** Acts by restoring depleted hepatic stores of glutathione and providing an alternative substrate for a toxic metabolite of paracetamol. Also used as an ocular lubricant and to prevent nephropathy due to **radiological contrast media** in patients with reduced renal function.

Has been investigated for the treatment of fulminant **hepatic failure, MODS, ALI** and neuropsychiatric complications of **carbon monoxide poisoning**, as well as a possible role in protection against myocardial **reperfusion injury**. Also used as a mucolytic because of its ability to split disulfide bonds in mucus glycoprotein.

- Dosage:
  - paracetamol poisoning: 150 mg/kg (to a maximum of 12 g) in 200 ml 5% dextrose iv over 1 h, followed by 50 mg/kg in 500 ml dextrose over 4 h, then 100 mg/kg in 1 l dextrose over 16 h (maximum of 110 kg body weight used for obese patients).
  - to reduce viscosity of airway secretions: 200 mg 8 hourly, orally. May be delivered by nebuliser.
- Side effects: rashes, anaphylaxis. Has been associated with bronchospasm in asthmatics.

Achalasia. Disorder of oesophageal motility caused by idiopathic degeneration of nerve cells in the myenteric plexus or vagal nuclei. Results in dysphagia and oesophageal dilatation. A similar condition may result from American trypanosomal infection (Chagas' disease). **Aspiration pneumonitis** or repeated chest infections may occur. Treated by mechanical distension of the lower **oesophagus** or by surgery. Heller's cardiomyotomy (longitudinal myotomy leaving the mucosa intact) may be undertaken via abdominal or thoracic approaches. Preoperative respiratory assessment is essential. Patients are at high risk of aspirating oesophageal contents, and rapid sequence induction is indicated.

[Carlos Chagas (1879–1934), Brazilian physician; Ernst Heller (1877–1964), German surgeon]

See also, Aspiration of gastric contents; Induction, rapid sequence

Achondroplasia. Skeletal disorder, inherited as an autosomal dominant gene, although most cases arise by spontaneous mutation. Results in dwarfism, with a normal size trunk and shortened limbs. Flat face, bulging skull vault and spinal deformity may make tracheal intubation difficult, and the larynx may be smaller than normal. **Obstructive sleep apnoea** may occur. Foramen magnum and spinal canal stenoses may be present, the former resulting in cord compression on neck extension, the latter making neuraxial blockade difficult and reducing volume requirements for **epidural anaesthesia.**

Aciclovir. **Antiviral drug**; an analogue of nucleoside 2′-deoxyguanosine. Inhibits viral DNA polymerase; active against herpes viruses and used in the treatment of **encephalitis**, varicella zoster (chickenpox/shingles) and **postherpetic neuralgia**, and for prophylaxis and treatment of herpes infections in immunocompromised patients. Treatment should start at onset of infection; the drug does not eradicate the virus but may markedly attenuate the clinical infection.

- Dosage:
  - as topical cream, 5 times daily.
  - 200–800 mg orally, 2–5 times daily in adults.
  - 5–10 mg/kg iv tds, infused over 1 h.
- Side effects: rashes, GIT disturbances, hepatic and renal impairment, blood dyscrasias, headache, dizziness, severe local inflammation after iv use, confusion, convulsions, coma.

Acid. Species that acts as a proton (H^+) donor when in solution (Brønsted–Lowry definition).
[Johannes N Brønsted (1879–1947), Danish chemist; Thomas M Lowry (1874–1936), English chemist]
See also, Acid–base balance; Acidosis

Acidaemia. Arterial **pH** <7.35 or **hydrogen ion** concentration >45 nmol/l.
See also, Acid–base balance; Acidosis

Acid–base balance. Maintenance of stable **pH** in body fluids is necessary for normal **enzyme** activity, ion distribution and protein structure. Blood pH is normally maintained at 7.35–7.45 (**hydrogen ion** [H^+] concentration 35–45 nmol/l); intracellular pH changes with extracellular pH. During normal metabolism of neutral substances, organic acids are produced that generate hydrogen ions.

- Maintenance of pH depends on:
  - **buffers** in tissues and blood, which minimise changes in H^+ concentration.
  - regulation by kidneys and lungs; the kidneys excrete about 60–80 mmol and the lungs about 15 000–20 000 mmol H^+ per day.

Because of the relationship between CO_2, carbonic acid, **bicarbonate** (HCO_3^-) and H^+, and the ability to excrete CO_2 rapidly from the lungs, respiratory function is important in acid-base balance:

$$H_2O + CO_2 \rightleftharpoons H_2CO_3 \rightleftharpoons HCO_3^- + H^+$$

Thus hyper- and hypoventilation cause **alkalosis** and **acidosis**, respectively. Similarly, hyper- or hypoventilation may compensate for non-respiratory acidosis or alkalosis, respectively, by returning pH towards normal.

Sources of H^+ excreted via the kidneys include lactic acid from blood cells, muscle and brain, sulfuric acid from metabolism of sulfur-containing proteins, and acetoacetic acid from fatty acid metabolism.

- The kidney can compensate for acid–base disturbances in three ways:
  - by regulating the reabsorption of filtered HCO_3^- at the proximal convoluted tubule (normally 80%–90%):
    - filtered Na^+ is exchanged for H^+ across the tubule cell membrane.
    - filtered HCO_3^- and excreted H^+ form carbonic acid.
    - carbonic acid is converted to CO_2 and water by **carbonic anhydrase** on the cell membrane.
    - CO_2 and water diffuse into the cell and reform carbonic acid (catalysed again by carbonic anhydrase).
    - carbonic acid dissociates into HCO_3^- and H^+.
    - HCO_3^- passes into the blood; H^+ is exchanged for Na^+, etc.
  - by forming dihydrogen phosphate from monohydrogen phosphate in the distal tubule ($HPO_4^- + H^+ \rightarrow H_2PO_4^-$). The H^+ is supplied from carbonic acid, leaving HCO_3^-, which passes into the blood.
  - by combination of ammonia, passing out of the cells, with H^+, supplied as mentioned earlier. Resultant ammonium ions cannot pass back into the cells and are excreted.

In acid–base disorders, the primary change determines whether a disturbance is respiratory or metabolic. The direction of change in H^+ concentration determines acidosis or alkalosis. Renal and respiratory compensation act to restore normal pH, not reverse the primary change. For example, in the **Henderson–Hasselbalch equation**:

$$pH = pK_a + \log\frac{[HCO_3^-]}{[CO_2]}$$

adjustment of the HCO_3^-/CO_2 concentration ratio restores pH towards its normal value, e.g.:

- primary change: increased CO_2; leads to decreased pH (respiratory acidosis).
- compensation: HCO_3^- retention by kidneys; increased ammonium secretion, etc.

An alternative approach, suggested by Stewart in 1983, focuses on the **strong ion difference** to explain the underlying processes rather than the above 'traditional approach', which concentrates more on interpretation of measurements. It is based on the degree of dissociation of ions in solution, in particular the effects of strong ions and weak acids, and the role of bicarbonate as a marker of acid–base imbalance rather than a cause.
[Peter Stewart (1921–1993), Canadian physiologist]
See also, Acid; Base; Blood gas interpretation; Breathing, control of; Davenport diagram; Siggaard-Andersen nomogram

Acid–citrate–dextrose solution, *see Blood storage*

Acidosis. A process in which arterial **pH** <7.35 (or **hydrogen ion** >45 nmol/l), or would be <7.35 if there were no compensatory mechanisms of **acid–base balance**.
See also, Acidosis, metabolic; Acidosis, respiratory

Acidosis, metabolic. **Acidosis** due to metabolic causes, resulting in an inappropriately low **pH** for the measured arterial $P\text{CO}_2$.

- Caused by:
  - increased acid production:
    - **ketone bodies**, e.g. in **diabetes mellitus**.
    - **lactate**, e.g. in **shock**, **exercise**.
  - acid ingestion: e.g. **salicylate poisoning**.
  - failure to excrete **hydrogen ions** (H^+):
    - **renal failure**.
    - distal **renal tubular acidosis**.
    - **carbonic anhydrase** inhibitors.
  - excessive loss of **bicarbonate**:
    - diarrhoea.
    - gastrointestinal fistulae.
    - proximal renal tubular acidosis.
    - ureteroenterostomy.

- May be differentiated by the presence or absence of an **anion gap**:
  - anion gap metabolic acidosis occurs in renal failure, lactic acidosis, ketoacidosis, rhabdomyolysis and following ingestion of certain toxins (e.g. salicylates, methanol, ethylene glycol).
  - non-anion gap (hyperchloraemic) metabolic acidosis is caused by the administration of chloride-containing solutions (e.g. saline) in large volumes, amino acid solutions, diarrhoea, pancreatic fistulae, ileal loop procedures, after rapid correction of a chronically compensated respiratory alkalosis or renal tubular acidosis.
- Primary change: increased H^+/decreased bicarbonate.
- Compensation:
  - **hyperventilation**: plasma bicarbonate falls by about 1.3 mmol/l for every 1 kPa acute decrease in arterial $P\text{CO}_2$, which usually does not fall below 1.3–1.9 kPa (10–15 mmHg).
  - increased renal H^+ secretion.
- Effects:
  - hyperventilation (**Kussmaul breathing**).
  - confusion, weakness, coma.
  - cardiac depression.
  - **hyperkalaemia**.
- Treatment:
  - of underlying cause.
  - bicarbonate therapy is reserved for treatment of severe acidaemia (e.g. pH under 7.1) because of problems associated with its use. If bicarbonate is required, a formula for iv infusion is:

    $$\frac{\text{base excess} \times \text{body weight (kg)}}{3} \text{ mmol}$$

    Half this amount is given initially.
  - other rarely used agents include **sodium dichloroacetate**, **Carbicarb** (sodium bicarbonate and carbonate in equimolar concentrations) and THAM (**2-amino-2-hydroxymethyl-1,3-propanediol**).

Morris CG, Low J (2008). Anaesthesia; 63: 294–301 and 396–411

See also, Acidaemia; Acid–base balance

Acidosis, respiratory. Acidosis due to increased arterial $P\text{CO}_2$. Caused by alveolar **hypoventilation**.
- Primary change: increased arterial $P\text{CO}_2$.
- Compensation:
  - initial rise in plasma bicarbonate due to increased carbonic acid formation and dissociation.
  - increased acid secretion/bicarbonate retention by the kidneys. In acute hypercapnia, bicarbonate concentration increases by about 0.7 mmol/l per 1 kPa rise in arterial $P\text{CO}_2$. In chronic hypercapnia it increases by 2.6 mmol/l per 1 kPa.
- Effects: those of hypercapnia.
- Treatment: of underlying cause.

See also, Acidaemia; Acid–base balance

ACLS, *see Advanced Cardiac Life Support*

Acquired immune deficiency syndrome (AIDS), *see Human immunodeficiency viral infection*

Acromegaly. Disease caused by excessive **growth hormone** secretion after puberty; usually caused by a **pituitary** adenoma but ectopic secretion may also occur. Incidence is 6–8 per million population.
- Features:
  - enlarged jaw, tongue and larynx; widespread increase in soft tissue mass; enlarged feet and hands. Nerve entrapment may occur, e.g. carpal tunnel syndrome.
  - respiratory obstruction, including **obstructive sleep apnoea.**
  - tendency towards **diabetes mellitus**, **hypertension** and **cardiac failure** (may be due to **cardiomyopathy**). Thyroid and adrenal impairment may occur. Colorectal malignancy is more common.

Apart from the above diseases, acromegaly may present difficulties with tracheal intubation and maintenance of the airway.

Treatment is primarily pituitary surgery with or without subsequent radiotherapy. Some patients respond to bromocriptine or **somatostatin** analogues.

Nemergut EC, Dumont AS, Barry UT, Laws ER (2007). Anesth Analg; 101: 1170–81

ACS, *see Acute coronary syndromes*

ACT, Activated clotting time, *see Coagulation studies*

Acta Anaesthesiologica Scandinavica. Official journal of the Scandinavian Society of Anaesthesiology and Intensive Care Medicine, first published in 1957.

ACTH, *see Adrenocorticotrophic hormone*

Actin. One of the protein components of **muscle** (mw 43 000). In muscle, arranged into a double strand of thin filaments (F-actin) with globular 'beads' (G-actin), to which myosin binds, along their length. Present in all cells as microfilaments.

See also, Muscle contraction

Action potential. Sequential changes in **membrane potential** that result in the propagation of electrical impulses in excitable cells. Neuronal, myocardial and cardiac nodal action potentials have distinct characteristics, determined by their underlying ionic fluxes (Fig. 4).
- Neuronal action potential (Fig. 4a):
  - A: depolarisation of the membrane by 15 mV (threshold level).
  - B: rapid depolarisation to +40 mV.
  - C: repolarisation, rapid at first then slow.
  - D: hyperpolarisation.
  - E: return to the resting membrane potential.

Slow initial depolarisation causes opening of voltage-gated sodium channels (VGSCs) and influx of Na^+ into the cell, which causes further rapid depolarisation. Na^+ conductance then falls as the VGSCs enter an inactivated state. K^+ efflux via voltage-gated potassium channels occurs more slowly and helps bring about repolarisation. Normal ion distribution (and hence the resting membrane potential) is restored by the action of the **sodium/potassium pump**. The action potential is followed by a **refractory period**.
- Myocardial action potential (Fig. 4b):
  - phase 0: fast depolarisation and Na^+ influx via VGSCs.
  - phase 1: onset of repolarisation due to sodium channel closure.
  - phase 2: plateau due to Ca^{2+} influx via voltage-gated calcium channels (VGCCs).
  - phase 3: repolarisation and K^+ efflux.
  - phase 4: resting membrane potential.

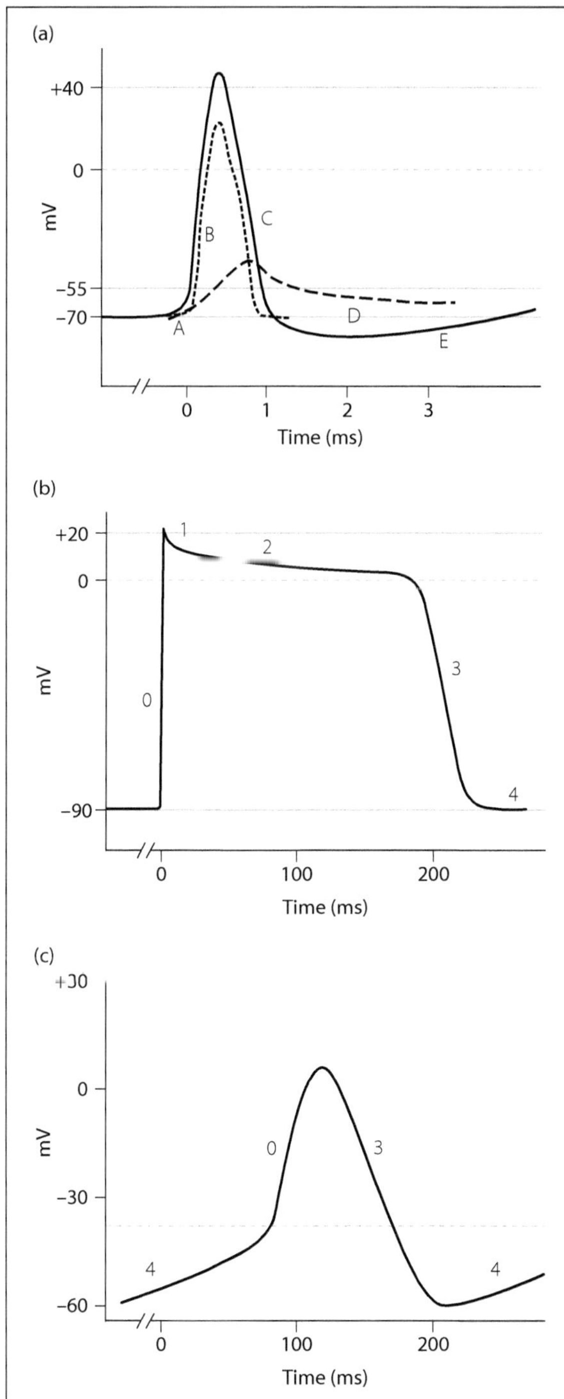

Fig. 4 (a) Nerve action potential *(solid)* showing changes in sodium *(dotted)* and potassium *(dashed)* conductance. (b) Cardiac action potential (see text). (c) Sinoatrial nodal action potential

The long plateau of phase 2 prolongs the refractory period, preventing tetanisation.

- Cardiac nodal action potential (Fig. 4c):
  - phase 4: slow spontaneous depolarisation (pacemaker potential) caused by a fall in K^+ efflux and slow Ca^{2+} influx via T-type VGCCs.
  - phase 0: depolarisation caused by opening of L-type VGCCs and Ca^{2+} influx.
  - phase 3: repolarisation caused by K^+ efflux.

Notably, there is no contribution by Na^+ flux to the action potential in **pacemaker cells.**

Cardiac excitability is modulated by autonomic inputs and antiarrythmic drugs via their effects on Na^+, K^+ and Ca^{2+} conductance.

See also, Nernst equation; Nerve conduction

Activated charcoal, *see Charcoal, activated*

Activated clotting time, *see Coagulation studies*

Activated protein C, *see Protein C*

Activation energy. Energy required to initiate a chemical reaction. For ignition of explosive mixtures of anaesthetic agents the energy may be provided by sparks, e.g. from electrical equipment or build-up of static electricity. Combustion of **cyclopropane** requires less activation energy than that of diethyl **ether.** Activation energy is less for mixtures with O_2 than with air, and least for **stoichiometric mixtures** of reactants.

See also, Explosions and fires

Active compression/decompression cardiopulmonary resuscitation, *see Cardiac massage; Cardiopulmonary resuscitation*

Active transport. Energy-requiring transport of particles across cell **membranes.** Protein 'pumps' within the membranes utilise energy (which is usually supplied by **ATP** metabolism) to move ions and molecules, often against concentration gradients. A typical example is the **sodium/potassium pump.**

Acupuncture. Use of fine **needles** (usually 30–33 G) to produce healing and pain relief. Originated in China thousands of years ago, and closely linked with the philosophy and practice of traditional Chinese medicine. Thus abnormalities in the flow of Qi (Chi: the life energy that circulates around the body along meridians, nourishing the internal organs) result in imbalance between Yin and Yang, the two polar opposites present in all aspects of the universe. Internal abnormalities may be diagnosed by pulse diagnosis (palpation of the radial arteries at different positions and depths). The appropriate organ is then treated by acupuncture at specific points on the skin, often along the meridian named after, and related to, that organ. Yin and Yang, and flow of Qi, are thus restored.

Modern Western acupuncture involves needle insertion at sites chosen for more 'scientific' reasons; e.g. around an affected area, at **trigger points** found nearby, or more proximally but within the appropriate **dermatome.** These may be combined with distant or local traditional points, although conclusive evidence for the existence of acupuncture points and meridians has never been shown. The needles may be left inserted and stimulated manually, electrically or thermally to increase intensity of stimulation. Pressure at acupuncture points (acupressure) may produce similar but less intense stimulation.

- Possible mechanisms:
  - local reflex pathways at spinal level.
  - closure of the 'gate' in the **gate control theory of pain.**
  - central release of **endorphins/enkephalins**, and possibly involvement of other **neurotransmitters.**
  - modulation of the 'memory' of pain.

Still used widely in China. Increasingly used in the West for chronic pain, musculoskeletal disorders, headache and migraine, and other disorders in which modern Western medicine has had little success. Claims that acupuncture may be employed alone to provide analgesia for surgery are now viewed with scepticism, although it has been used to provide analgesia and reduce **PONV**, e.g. 5 min stimulation at the point P6 (pericardium 6: 1–2 inches [2.5–5 cm] proximal to the distal wrist crease, between flexor carpi radialis and palmaris longus tendons).

Ernst E, Lee MS, Choi TY (2011). Pain; 152: 755–64

Acute coronary syndromes (ACS). Group of clinical conditions characterised by acute **myocardial ischaemia** and including unstable angina and **MI**; usually caused by acute thrombus formation within a coronary artery upon the exposed surface of a ruptured or eroded atheromatous plaque. May also occur due to coronary artery spasm, arteritis or sudden severe hypo- or hypertension.

- Classification:
  - **S–T segment** elevation MI (STEMI): ACS with S–T segment elevation on 12-lead **ECG**. Accounts for 40% of MI. Suggestive of total coronary artery occlusion. Consistently associated with elevated plasma biomarkers of myocardial damage. Immediate reperfusion therapy (*see later*) significantly improves outcomes. ACS with new-onset left **bundle branch block** (LBBB) or evidence of posterior infarction is included in this category for treatment purposes.
  - non-S–T segment elevation acute coronary syndromes (NSTEACS): suggestive of subtotal arterial occlusion. Immediate reperfusion therapy is not indicated, although early (within 24 h) **percutaneous coronary intervention** (PCI) may be considered in high-risk patients. Further subdivided into:
    - non-S–T segment elevation MI (NSTEMI); normal or non-specific changes on ECG, with elevated cardiac biomarkers.
    - unstable angina: ACS without elevated cardiac biomarkers.
- Clinical features:
  - pain as for **myocardial ischaemia**.
  - **arrhythmias**; **cardiac arrest** may occur.
  - anxiety, sweating, pallor, dyspnoea.
  - **hypertension** or **hypotension**.
  - **cardiac failure** and **cardiogenic shock**.

Severe infarction is usually associated with more severe symptoms and signs than unstable angina, although painless/silent infarction is also common.

- Differential diagnosis: pain and ECG changes may occur with lesions of:
  - heart/great vessels, e.g. **aortic dissection**, **pericarditis**.
  - lung, e.g. **PE**, **chest infection**.
  - oesophagus, e.g. spasm, inflammation, rupture.
  - abdominal organs, e.g. **peptic ulcer disease**, **pancreatitis**, **cholecystitis**.
- Investigations:
  - 12-lead ECG (*see Myocardial infarction for characteristic features of STEMI and their localisation by ECG pattern*). Bundle branch block may be evident. NSTEACS may coexist with a normal ECG or: S–T segment depression; S–T segment elevation insufficient to meet reperfusion therapy criteria (*see later*); T wave flattening or inversion; or biphasic T waves.
  - cardiac biomarkers:
    - **cardiac enzymes**: largely replaced by troponins.
    - cardiac troponins:
      - regulatory proteins involved in cardiac and skeletal **muscle contraction**.
      - composed of three subunits: C, T and I; plasma levels of the latter two are both specific and sensitive markers for myocardial damage.
      - levels may not rise until 6–8 h after onset of symptoms although more recent high-sensitivity assays of cardiac troponins may allow accurate diagnosis at 3 h.
      - levels peak at around 24 h, correlating with the extent of infarction, and may remain elevated for 7–10 days.
      - may be elevated in myocardial damage due to other causes, e.g. **myocarditis**, contusion and also other non-cardiac critical illness (e.g. **sepsis**, **renal failure**, PE), probably reflecting myocardial injury but in most cases not related to coronary artery disease. Likely benefit of NSTEMI treatment in these cases should be assessed on an individual patient basis.
  - **echocardiography**: may be used to assess regional and global ventricular function; regional wall motion abnormalities and loss of thickness suggest acute infarction. Also useful in diagnosing complications of MI (e.g. ventricular aneurysm, mitral regurgitation, mural thrombus).
- Immediate management of suspected ACS:
  - O_2 via facemask (only if evidence of **hypoxia** [S_pO_2 >94%], **pulmonary oedema** or ongoing ischaemia), cardiac monitoring, 12-lead ECG, iv access.
  - **aspirin** 300 mg orally.
  - analgesia (e.g. iv **morphine** in 2 mg increments).
  - sublingual **GTN**.
  - associated pulmonary oedema and arrhythmias should be treated in the usual way.
  - consideration for immediate reperfusion therapy if:
    - presentation <12 h after symptom onset, unrelieved by GTN.
    - S–T segment elevation >0.1 mV in two or more contiguous chest leads or two adjacent limb leads.
    - new-onset LBBB.
    - posterior infarction (dominant R wave and S–T depression in V_1–V_2 chest leads).
- Reperfusion strategies include:
  - pharmacological thrombolytic therapy: agents include **streptokinase**, **alteplase**, **tenecteplase** and **reteplase**. Survival benefit is reduced with increasing delay, and is negligible from 12 h after onset of symptoms. Administration of thrombolysis within 1 h of the patient calling for professional help is a national **audit** standard. Contraindications include active bleeding, recent trauma (including surgery and **CPR**), previous haemorrhagic **stroke**, uncontrolled hypertension and pregnancy.
  - primary PCI.
  - emergency **coronary artery bypass surgery**.

Thrombolysis is generally only preferred if primary PCI is unavailable or there would be delay of >90 min in delivering it and the presentation is within 3 h of symptom onset. Primary PCI is particularly superior if: there is **cardiogenic shock**; there are contraindications to thrombolysis; or the patient is at high risk of death (e.g. age >75, previous MI, extensive anterior infarct). Emergency surgery is generally reserved for those known to have disease uncorrectable by PCI or in whom primary PCI fails.

Patients not meeting criteria for immediate reperfusion (i.e., those with NSTEACS) are managed either invasively (PCI within 24 h plus **abciximab** iv) or conservatively (pharmacological management only). High-risk patients are most likely to benefit from invasive therapy.

- Pharmacological adjuncts include:
  - **clopidogrel** and low-molecular weight **heparin** (e.g. **enoxaparin**): should be given to all patients (in the absence of contraindications) with definite or strongly suspected ACS, in addition to aspirin. **Prasugrel** and **ticagrelor** are newer alternatives to clopidogrel, but the former is associated with increased risk of life-threatening bleeding.
  - GTN sublingually or by iv infusion if pain persists.
  - glycoprotein IIB/IIIa inhibitors (e.g. abciximab and **tirofiban**): beneficial in patients undergoing PCI, those at high risk of death, or both.
  - **β-adrenergic receptor antagonists**: reduce the rate of reinfarction and **VF** and should be commenced within 24 h if there are no contraindications, e.g. **heart block**, pulmonary oedema, hypotension. Those unable to receive β-blockers should receive one of the non-dihydropyridine **calcium channel blocking drugs** (e.g. **verapamil**).
  - **ACE inhibitors**: improve long-term survival after MI and should be commenced within 24 h, assuming no contraindications.
  - **magnesium** and **potassium** supplementation to maintain normal levels reduces the incidence of **arrhythmias**. Prophylactic administration of **anti-arrhythmic drugs** is no longer recommended.
  - implantable cardioverter defibrillators should be considered in patients following MI who have an ejection fraction <35%, and those with persisting ventricular arrhythmias

Timms A (2015). Br Med J; 351: h5153

See also, Defibrillators, implantable cardioverter

Acute cortical necrosis, *see Renal failure*

Acute crisis resource management, *see Crisis resource management*

Acute demyelinating encephalomyelopathy, *see Demyelinating diseases*

Acute kidney injury (AKI). Previously referred to as acute **renal failure**, describing a rapid deterioration (within 48 h) from baseline renal function; classified according to severity by the **RIFLE criteria**. An independent risk factor for in-hospital morbidity and mortality and a major cause of death in ICU, especially as part of **MODS**. May develop with or without pre-existing renal impairment. May follow any severe acute illness, dehydration, **trauma** or major surgery (especially involving the heart and great vessels), **hepatic failure**, obstetric emergencies, and any condition involving sustained hypotension. It is estimated that 20% of AKI is avoidable with good management.

- May be classified as:
  - prerenal: caused by renal hypoperfusion, e.g. **shock**, **hypovolaemia**, **cardiac failure**, renal artery stenosis.
  - renal: caused by renal disease:
    - glomerular, e.g.:
      - **glomerulonephritis**.
      - **diabetes mellitus**.
      - amyloid.
    - tubulointerstitial, e.g.:
      - acute tubular necrosis (ATN): accounts for 75% of hospital AKI. Caused by renal hypoperfusion or ischaemia and/or chemical toxicity, trauma or sepsis. Nephrotoxins include analgesics (e.g. chronic **aspirin** and **paracetamol** therapy), **NSAIDs, aminoglycosides, immunosuppressive drugs**, metformin, **radiological contrast media** and heavy metals. Usually (but not always) associated with **oliguria** (caused by tubular cell necrosis, tubular obstruction and cortical arteriolar vasoconstriction).
      - acute cortical necrosis: typically associated with **placental abruption**, **pre-eclampsia** and septic abortion, but also with factors causing ATN. Confirmed by renal biopsy. Usually irreversible.
      - tubulointerstitial nephritis/pyelonephritis.
      - polycystic renal disease.
      - tubular obstruction, e.g. in myeloma, **myoglobinuria**.
    - vascular, e.g. hypertension, connective tissue disease.
  - postrenal: caused by obstruction in the urinary tract, e.g. bladder tumour, prostatic hypertrophy.

Distinction between renal and pre- or postrenal failure is important because diagnosis guides treatment, and early intervention can prevent irreversible injury.

- Features:
  - oliguria/anuria.
  - **uraemia** and accumulation of other substances (e.g. drugs): nausea, vomiting, malaise, increased bleeding and susceptibility to infection, decreased healing.
  - reduced sodium and water excretion and **oedema**, **hypertension**, **hyperkalaemia**, **acidosis**.
- The following may aid diagnosis:
  - analysis of **urine**: e.g. tubular casts may be seen in ATN, myoglobinuria may be present.
  - plasma and urine indices (Table 2).
  - flushing of the urinary catheter using aseptic technique.
  - assessment of cardiac and volume status to exclude hypovolaemia.
  - a fluid challenge of, e.g. 200–300 ml increased urine output, may occur in incipient prerenal failure.

Table 2 Investigations used to differentiate between prerenal oliguria and acute kidney injury

Investigation	*Prerenal oliguria*	*Renal failure*
Specific gravity	>1.020	<1.010
Urine osmolality (mosmol/kg)	>500	<350
Urine sodium (mmol/l)	<20	>40
Urine/plasma osmolality ratio	>2	<1.1
Urine/plasma urea ratio	>20	<10
Urine/plasma creatinine ratio	>40	<20
Fractional sodium excretion (%)	<1	>1
Renal failure index	<1	>1

$$\text{Fractional sodium excretion} = \frac{\text{urine/plasma sodium ratio}}{\text{urea/plasma creatinine ratio}} \times 100\%$$

$$\text{and renal failure index} = \frac{\text{urine sodium}}{\text{urine/plasma creatinine ratio}}$$

  - diuretic administration, e.g. **furosemide** or **mannitol**: increased urine output may occur in incipient ATN but there is no evidence of a prophylactic or therapeutic effect; however, reduction in renal O_2 demand (furosemide) and scavenging of **free radicals** (mannitol) have been suggested as being theoretically beneficial.
  - renal **ultrasound** or biopsy.
- Management:
  - directed at the primary cause with optimisation of **renal blood flow**.
  - monitoring of weight, cardiovascular status, including JVP/CVP/pulmonary capillary wedge pressure as appropriate, urea and electrolytes, and acid–base status. Accurate recording of fluid balance is vital.
  - fluid restriction if appropriate, e.g. previous hour's urine output + 30 ml/h while oliguric.
  - **H_2 receptor antagonists** are commonly administered to reduce GIT haemorrhage.
  - treatment of hyperkalaemia.
  - monitoring of drug levels, as **clearance** may be reduced considerably.
  - various **dialysis** therapies.
  - adequate **nutrition**.

Goren O, Matot I (2015). Br J Anaesth; 115 (Suppl 2): ii3–14

Acute life-threatening events—recognition and treatment (ALERT). Multiprofessional course aimed at reducing the incidence of potentially avoidable **cardiac arrests** and admissions to **ICU**. Targeted especially at junior doctors and ward nurses. Sharing principles of many life-support training programmes (e.g. **ALS**, **ATLS**, **APLS**, **CCrISP**), its development embraces both **clinical governance** and multiprofessional education. Uses a structured and prioritised system of patient assessment and management to recognise and treat seriously ill patients or those at risk of deterioration.

Smith GB, Osgood VM, Crane S (2002). Resuscitation; 52: 281–6

See also, Early warning scores; Medical emergency team; Outreach team

Acute lung injury (ALI). Syndrome of pulmonary inflammation and increased pulmonary capillary permeability associated with a variety of clinical, radiological and physiological abnormalities that cannot be explained by, but may coexist with, left atrial or pulmonary capillary hypertension. Associated with **sepsis**, major **trauma**, **aspiration pneumonitis**, **blood transfusion**, **pancreatitis**, **cardiopulmonary bypass** and **fat embolism**. Onset is usually within 2–3 days of the precipitating illness or injury, although direct lung insults usually have a shorter latency. Acute respiratory distress syndrome (ARDS) is now regarded to be the most severe form of ALI, with a mortality of 30%–45%. Mortality is dependent on age (higher in the elderly), racial origin (higher in non-Caucasians) and aetiology (highest in sepsis-related ALI). The definitions of ALI and ARDS are increasingly being challenged and diagnostic criteria vary, but the 2012 Berlin definition has largely superseded that of the 1994 American-European Consensus Conference (AECC):

  - Major criterion: acute-onset arterial **hypoxaemia** resistant to **oxygen therapy** alone (P_aO_2/F_IO_2 <39.9 kPa [300 mmHg] for definition of ALI; <26.6 kPa [200 mmHg] for definition of moderate ARDS; <13.3 kPa [100 mmHg] for definition of severe ARDS), regardless of the level of ventilatory support.
  - Other features:
    - bilateral diffuse infiltrates seen on the CXR although it is often difficult to differentiate between ARDS and cardiogenic **pulmonary oedema**.
    - reduced respiratory **compliance** (≤40 ml/cm), lung volumes and increased **work of breathing**.
    - **$\dot{V}/\dot{Q}$ mismatch** with increased **shunt**.
    - increased **pulmonary vascular resistance** occurs in 25% of patients with severe ALI and is a risk factor for increased mortality.
    - **MODS** may occur and is a common cause of death.

  Measurement of **pulmonary wedge pressure** has been removed from the criteria.
- Pathophysiology: ALI results from damage to either the lung epithelium or endothelium. Two pathways of injury exist:
  - direct insult to lung, e.g. aspiration, **smoke inhalation**.
  - indirect result of an acute systemic inflammatory response involving both humoral (activation of **complement**, **coagulation** and **kinin** systems; release of mediators including **cytokines**, oxidants, **nitric oxide**) and cellular (neutrophils, macrophages and lymphocytes) components. Pulmonary infiltration by neutrophils leads to interstitial fibrosis, possibly because of damage caused by **free radicals**. Examples include sepsis, pancreatitis and fat embolism.

  Histopathological findings can be divided into three phases: exudative (oedema and haemorrhage); proliferative (organisation and repair); and fibrotic.
- Management involves prompt treatment of the underlying cause and supportive therapy:
  - general support: **nutrition**, **DVT** prophylaxis, prevention of nosocomial infection.
  - O_2 therapy, accepting S_pO_2 >90%. **CPAP** is often helpful as it improves **FRC**.
  - ventilatory support: **IPPV** may be necessary if CPAP is ineffective. **Lung protection strategies** improve survival in ARDS and consist of using low tidal volumes/inspiratory pressures (e.g. 4–6 ml/kg and $P_{Plateau}$ <30 cmH_2O) with moderate PEEP, tolerating a degree of respiratory acidosis (**permissive hypercapnia**). High-pressure recruitment manoeuvres and high PEEP are often beneficial in life-threatening hypoxaemia, but increase the risk of **barotrauma** and impaired cardiac output.

    Additional ventilatory strategies include **inverse ratio ventilation** (at **I:E ratios** of up to 4:1), **airway pressure release ventilation** and **high-frequency ventilation**. **Extracorporeal membrane oxygenation** has been used with varying success. **Extracorporeal CO_2 removal** may be useful in life-threatening hypercapnia.
  - **prone ventilation** improves oxygenation and outcome in patients with severe hypoxaemia due to ARDS, especially in obese patients.
  - short-term use of **neuromuscular blocking drugs** may improve outcome.
  - diuresis and fluid restriction are often instituted to reduce lung water, although avoidance of initial fluid overload is thought to be more important.
  - **corticosteroid** therapy is controversial. There appears to be no benefit to its prophylactic administration, or in high-dose, short-term therapy at the onset of ALI/ARDS. However, corticosteroids may have a role in refractory ARDS.

- anti-inflammatory agents including nitric oxide, prostaglandins, prostacyclin, surfactant and N-acetylcysteine have not been shown to improve outcome.

MacSweeney R, McAuley DF (2016). Lancet; 388: 2416–30

Acute-phase response, A reaction of the haemopoietic and hepatic systems to inflammation or tissue injury, assumed to be of benefit to the host. There is a rise in the number/activity of certain cells (neutrophils, platelets) and plasma proteins (e.g. fibrinogen, **complement**, **C-reactive protein**, plasminogen, **haptoglobin**) involved in host defence, while there is a reduction in proteins with transport and binding functions (e.g. albumin, haemoglobin, transferrin). Initiated by actions of **cytokine** mediators such as interleukins (IL-1α, IL-1β, IL-6 and IL-11), tumour necrosis factors (α and β) and leukaemia inhibitory factor.

Serum levels of acute-phase proteins (e.g. C-reactive protein) can be helpful in diagnosis, monitoring and prognosis of certain diseases. The rise in fibrinogen levels causes an elevation in **ESR**. The fall in albumin is due to redistribution and decreased hepatic synthesis.

Acute physiology, age, chronic health evaluation, *see APACHE III scoring system*

Acute physiology and chronic health evaluation, *see APACHE scoring system; APACHE II scoring system*

Acute physiology score (APS). Physiological component of severity of illness scoring systems, such as **APACHE** II/III and Simplified APS. Weighted values (e.g. 0–4 in APACHE II) are assigned to each of a range of physiological variables (e.g. temperature, mean arterial blood pressure, serum creatinine) based on its derangement from an established 'normal' range, as measured either upon ICU admission or within 24 h of entry. The sum of all assigned weighted values for the physiological variables that comprise a given scoring system constitutes the acute physiological score. The higher the acute physiology score, the sicker the patient.

See also, Mortality/survival prediction on intensive care unit; Simplified acute physiology score

Acute respiratory distress syndrome (ARDS), *see Acute lung injury*

Acute tubular necrosis, *see Renal failure*

Acyclovir, *see Aciclovir*

Addiction, *see Alcoholism; Substance abuse*

Addison's disease, *see Adrenocortical insufficiency*

Adductor canal block. Distal approach to **femoral nerve block**, below the level at which the quadriceps motor innervation has left the **femoral nerve**. Thus provides analgesia to the anteromedial knee and lower leg while quadriceps strength is relatively preserved, aiding early postoperative mobilisation.

The adductor canal extends from the apex of the **femoral triangle** to the adductor hiatus. It contains the femoral vessels, saphenous nerve, obturator nerve (posterior division) and nerve to vastus medialis. With the patient supine and the leg to be blocked slightly flexed at the knee and externally rotated, 10–15 ml **local anaesthetic agent** is placed medial and 10–15 ml lateral to the **femoral artery** via a needle inserted midway down the medial aspect of the thigh, under **ultrasound** guidance.

Mariano ER, Perlas A (2014). Anesthesiology; 120: 530–2

ADEM, Acute demyelinating encephalomyelopathy, *see Demyelinating diseases*

Adenosine. Nucleoside, of importance in energy homeostasis at the cellular level. Reduces O_2 consumption, increases coronary blood flow, causes vasodilatation and slows atrioventricular conduction (possibly via increased potassium and reduced calcium **conductance**). Also an inhibitory CNS **neurotransmitter**.

The drug of choice for treatment of **SVT** (including that associated with **Wolff–Parkinson–White syndrome**), and diagnosis of other tachyarrhythmias by slowing atrioventricular conduction. Its short half-life (8–10 s) and lack of negative inotropism make it an attractive alternative to verapamil. Not included in the Vaughan Williams classification of **antiarrhythmic drugs**.

Has also been used as a directly acting **vasodilator drug** in **hypotensive anaesthesia**. Increases cardiac output, with stable heart rate. Its effects are rapidly reversible on stopping the infusion.

- Dosage:
  - SVT: 6 mg by rapid iv injection into a central or large peripheral vein; if unsuccessful after 1–2 min, may be followed by up to two further boluses of 12 mg.
  - hypotensive anaesthesia: 50–300 μg/kg/min. **ATP** has also been used.
- Side effects are usually mild and include flushing, dyspnoea and nausea. Bronchoconstriction may occur in asthmatics. Bradycardia is resistant to atropine. Adenosine's action is prolonged in **dipyridamole** therapy (because uptake of adenosine is inhibited) and reduced by **theophylline** and other **xanthines** (because of competitive antagonism). Transplanted hearts are particularly sensitive to adenosine's effects.

[EM Vaughan Williams (1918–2016), English pharmacologist]

Adenosine monophosphate, cyclic (cAMP). Cyclic adenosine 3′,5′-monophosphate, formed from **ATP** by the enzyme adenylate cyclase. Activation of surface receptors may cause a guanine nucleotide regulatory protein (**G protein**) to interact with adenylate cyclase with resultant changes in intracellular cAMP levels (Fig. 5). Many substances act on surface receptors in this way, including **catecholamines**, **vasopressin**, **ACTH**, **histamine**, **glucagon**, parathyroid hormone and **calcitonin**.

Some substances inhibit adenylate cyclase via an inhibitory regulatory protein, e.g. **noradrenaline** at **α_2-adrenergic receptors** (Fig. 5).

cAMP is termed a 'second messenger' as it causes phosphorylation of proteins, particularly enzymes, by activating protein kinases. Phosphorylation changes enzyme and thus cellular activity. cAMP is inactivated by phosphodiesterase to 5′-AMP. **Phosphodiesterase inhibitors**, e.g. **aminophylline** and **enoximone**, increase cAMP levels.

Adenosine triphosphate and diphosphate (ATP and ADP). ATP is the most important high-energy phosphate compound. When hydrolysed to form ADP, it releases **energy** that may be utilised in many cellular processes,

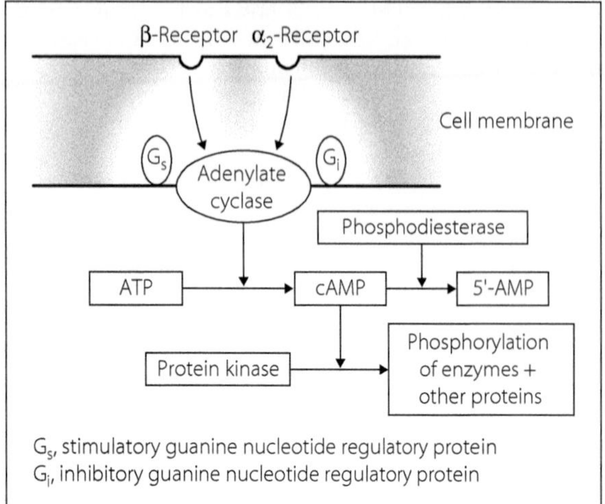

Fig. 5 cAMP involvement in transmembrane signalling

e.g. **active transport**, **muscle contraction**. Its phosphate bonds are formed using energy from catabolism; aerobic respiration generates 38 moles of ATP per mole of glucose, while anaerobic respiration (i.e., simple **glycolysis**) yields 2 moles of ATP.

Other high-energy phosphate compounds include phosphocreatine (in muscle), ADP itself, and other nucleotides.

See also, Cytochrome oxidase system; Metabolism; Tricarboxylic acid cycle

Adenylate cyclase, *see Adenosine monophosphate, cyclic*

ADH, Antidiuretic hormone, *see Vasopressin*

Adhesion molecules. Molecules normally sited on cell surfaces, involved in embryogenesis, cell growth and differentiation, and wound repair. Also mediate endothelial cell/leucocyte adhesion, transendothelial migration and cytotoxic T-cell-induced lysis. Four major families exist: integrins; cadherins; selectins (named after the tissues in which they were discovered: L-selectin [leucocytes], E-selectin [endothelial cells], P-selectin [platelets]); and members of the **immunoglobulin** superfamily.

In general, contact between an adhesion receptor and the extracellular milieu results in the transmission of information allowing the cell to interact with its environment. Defective interactions involving adhesion molecules are implicated in disease (e.g. certain skin diseases, metastasis of cancer cells). Many pathogens use adhesion receptors to penetrate tissue cells. Overexpression of intravascular adhesion molecules or receptors has been implicated in rheumatoid arthritis and rejection of transplanted organs. Control of vascular integrity and defence against invasive pathogens require regulation of adhesive interactions among blood cells and between blood cells and the vessel walls. Circulating leucocytes bind to the selectins of activated endothelial cells, become activated by chemoattractants and migrate through intracellular gaps to the site of inflammation. Thus adhesion molecules play a part in the inflammatory response in **sepsis**.

Adiabatic change. Volume change of a gas in which there is no transfer of heat to or from the system. Sudden compression of a gas without removal of resultant heat causes a rise in temperature. This may occur in the gas already present in the valves and pipes of an **anaesthetic machine** when a cylinder is turned on (hence the danger of explosion if oil or grease is present). Sudden adiabatic expansion of a gas results in cooling, as in the **cryoprobe**.

See also, Isothermal change

Adjustable pressure-limiting valves. Valves that open to allow passage of expired and surplus fresh gas from a breathing system, but close to prevent in-drawing of air. Ideally the opening pressure should be as low as possible to reduce resistance to expiration, but not so low as to allow the reservoir bag to empty through it. Most contain a thin disc held against its seating by a spring, as in the original Heidbrink valve. Adjusting the tension in the spring, usually by screwing the valve top, alters the pressure at which the valve opens. The valve must be vertical in order to function correctly.

Modern valves, even when screwed fully down, will open at high pressures (60 cmH_2O). Most are now encased in a hood for **scavenging** of waste gases.

[Jay A Heidbrink (1875–1957), US anaesthetist]

See also, Anaesthetic breathing systems; Non-rebreathing valves

ADP, *see Adenosine triphosphate and diphosphate*

Adrenal gland. Situated on the upper pole of the **kidney**, each gland is composed of an outer cortex and an inner medulla. The cortex consists of the outer zona glomerulosa (secreting **aldosterone**), the middle zona fasciculata (secreting **glucocorticoids**) and inner zona reticularis (secreting sex hormones). Hypersecretion may result in **hyperaldosteronism**, **Cushing's syndrome** and virilisation/feminisation, respectively. Hyposecretion causes **adrenocortical insufficiency**.

The adrenal medulla is thought to be derived from a sympathetic ganglion in which the postganglionic neurones have lost their axons, and secrete **catecholamines** into the bloodstream. Hypersecretion results in **phaeochromocytoma**.

See also, Sympathetic nervous system

Adrenaline (Epinephrine). **Catecholamine**, acting as a hormone and **neurotransmitter** in the **sympathetic nervous system** and brainstem pathways. Synthesised and released from the **adrenal gland** medulla and central adrenergic neurones (*for structure, synthesis and metabolism, see Catecholamines*). Called epinephrine in the USA because the name adrenaline, used in other countries, was too similar to the US-registered trade name Adrenalin that referred to a specific product (both adrenaline [Latin] and epinephrine [Greek] referring to the location of the adrenal gland 'on the kidney').

Stimulates both α- and β-**adrenergic receptors**; displays predominantly β-effects at low doses, α- at higher doses. Low-dose infusion may lower BP by causing vasodilatation in muscle via β_2-receptors, despite increased cardiac output via β_1-receptors. Higher doses cause α_1-mediated vasoconstriction and increased systolic BP, although diastolic pressure may still decrease.

- Clinical uses:
  - with **local anaesthetic agents**, as a vasoconstrictor.
  - in **anaphylaxis**, **cardiac arrest**, **bronchospasm**.
  - as an **inotropic drug**.
  - in **glaucoma** (reduces aqueous humour production).
  - in **croup**.

Adrenaline may cause cardiac **arrhythmias**, especially in the presence of hypercapnia, hypoxia and certain drugs, e.g. **halothane**, **cyclopropane** and **cocaine**. Adrenaline should not be used for ring blocks of digits or for penile nerve blocks, because of possible ischaemia to distal tissues.

- Dosage:
  - with local anaesthetic agents, 1:200 000 concentration is usual.
  - anaphylaxis: 50 µg iv (0.5 ml 1:10 000 solution), repeated as required, with ECG monitoring and only by practitioners familiar with its use. The recommended dosage in general medical guidelines is usually 0.5–1.0 ml of 1:1000 solution im into the middle third of the anterolateral thigh, repeated as required every 5 min, reflecting the risks of iv administration without appropriate monitoring. Dosage in children: <6 years, 0.15 ml of 1:1000 solution; 6–12 years, 0.3 ml; 12–18 years, 0.5 ml. For self-administration in adults, 0.3 ml of 1:000 solution im is recommended.
  - cardiac arrest: 1 mg (10 ml 1:10 000) iv.
  - by infusion: 0.01–0.15 µg/kg/min initially, increasing as required.
  - croup: 0.5 ml/kg (1:1000 solution) nebulised, up to 5 ml maximum, repeated after 30 min if required.

Subcutaneous injection in shocked patients results in unreliable absorption. Tracheal administration in the absence of iv access is no longer recommended; the intraosseous route is now the suggested alternative.

See also, Tracheal administration of drugs

α-Adrenergic receptor agonists. Naturally occurring **agonists** include **adrenaline** and **noradrenaline**, which stimulate both α_1- and α_2-**adrenergic receptors**.

Methoxamine and **phenylephrine** are synthetic α_1-receptor agonists, used to cause vasoconstriction, e.g. to correct hypotension in **spinal anaesthesia**.

Clonidine acts on central α_2-receptors. Clonidine and other α_2-receptor agonists (e.g. **dexmedetomidine**) have been shown to reduce pain and anaesthetic requirements, and have also been used for **sedation** in ICU. Other α_2-receptor agonists (e.g. xylazine, detomidine and medetomidine) have been used in veterinary practice as anaesthetic agents for many years.

β-Adrenergic receptor agonists. Include adrenaline, **dobutamine** and **isoprenaline**, which stimulate both β_1- and β_2-**adrenergic receptors** to varying degrees. **Dopamine** acts mainly at β_1-receptors.

Salbutamol and **terbutaline** predominantly affect β_2-receptors, and are used clinically to cause bronchodilatation in **asthma**, and as **tocolytic drugs** in labour. Formoterol and salmeterol are longer-acting agents given by inhalation for chronic asthma. Some β_1-receptor effects are seen at high doses, e.g. tachycardia. They have been used in the treatment of **cardiac failure** and **cardiogenic shock**; stimulation of vascular β_2-receptors causes vasodilatation and reduces afterload.

α-Adrenergic receptor antagonists (α-Blockers). Usually refer to **antagonists** that act exclusively at α-**adrenergic receptors**.

- Drugs may be:
  - selective:
    - α_1-receptors, e.g. **prazosin**, **doxazosin**, indoramin, **phenoxybenzamine**. Tamsulosin acts specifically at α_{1A}-receptors and is used in benign prostatic hypertrophy.
    - α_2-receptors: yohimbine, **atipamezole**.
  - non-selective, e.g. phentolamine.

Labetalol and carvedilol (a drug with similar effects) are antagonists at both α- and β-receptors. Other drugs may also act at α-receptors as part of a range of effects, e.g. **chlorpromazine**, **droperidol**.

Antagonism may be competitive, e.g. phentolamine, or non-competitive and therefore longer-lasting, e.g. phenoxybenzamine.

Used to lower BP and reduce **afterload** by causing vasodilatation. Compensatory tachycardia may occur.

- Side effects: postural hypotension, dizziness, tachycardia (less so with the selective α_1-antagonists, possibly because the negative feedback of noradrenaline at α_2-receptors is unaffected). **Tachyphylaxis** may occur.

β-Adrenergic receptor antagonists (β-Blockers). Competitive **antagonists** at β-**adrenergic receptors**.

- Actions:
  - reduce heart rate, **myocardial contractility** and O_2 consumption.
  - increase **coronary blood flow** by increasing diastolic filling time.
  - antiarrhythmic action results from β-receptor antagonism and possibly a membrane-stabilising effect at high doses.
  - antihypertensive action (not fully understood but may involve reductions in cardiac output, central sympathetic activity and renin levels).
  - some have partial agonist activity (**intrinsic sympathomimetic activity**), e.g. pindolol, acebutolol, celiprolol and oxprenolol.
  - practolol, **atenolol**, **metoprolol**, betaxolol, bisoprolol, nebivolol and acebutolol are relatively cardioselective, but all will block β_2-receptors at high doses. Celiprolol has β_1-receptor antagonist and β_2-receptor agonist properties, thus causing peripheral vasodilatation in addition to cardiac effects.
  - **labetalol** and carvedilol have α- and β-receptor blocking properties. The former is available for iv administration and is widely used for acute reduction in BP.
- **Half-lives:**
  - **esmolol**: a few minutes; hydrolysed by red cell esterases.
  - metoprolol, oxprenolol, pindolol, **propranolol**, timolol: 2–4 h.
  - atenolol, practolol, **sotalol**: 6–12 h.
  - nadolol: 24 h.

Most are readily absorbed enterally, and undergo extensive **first-pass metabolism**. Practolol, atenolol, celiprolol, nadolol and sotalol are water-soluble and largely excreted unchanged in the urine; propranolol and metoprolol are lipid-soluble and almost completely metabolised in the liver.

- Uses:
  - **hypertension**, **ischaemic heart disease**, **MI**, **arrhythmias**, **hyperthyroidism**, anxiety, **migraine** prophylaxis. Have been shown to improve outcome in **cardiac failure** when added to **ACE inhibitor** therapy. Acute perioperative withdrawal of β-blockers from patients already receiving them may worsen outcomes; they should therefore be continued.
  - perioperatively: to reduce the hypertensive response to laryngoscopy; to treat perioperative hypertension,

tachycardias and **myocardial ischaemia**; in **hypotensive anaesthesia.** The use of perioperative β-blockade to reduce perioperative cardiovascular morbidity and mortality in high-risk patients undergoing non-cardiac surgery is no longer advocated as the cardiovascular benefits are outweighed by the increased incidence of cerebrovascular accidents.

- Side effects:
  - cardiac failure, especially in combination with other negative inotropes.
  - **bronchospasm** and peripheral arterial insufficiency, via blockade of β_2-receptors.
  - increased risk of diabetes when used to treat hypertension and reduced cardiovascular (β_1) and metabolic (β_2) response to **hypoglycaemia** in diabetics.
  - depression and sleep disturbance: less likely with water-soluble drugs.
  - oral practolol was withdrawn because of the oculomucocutaneous syndrome following its use. The iv preparation has been withdrawn for commercial reasons.

β-Adrenergic receptor antagonist poisoning. Uncommon, but overdose is hazardous because of these drugs' low **therapeutic ratio.** General features include cardiac failure, bradycardia, cardiac conduction defects, hypotension, bronchospasm, coma and convulsions, the latter two especially with **propranolol. Sotalol** may cause ventricular tachyarrhythmias. **Hypoglycaemia** is rare.

- Treatment:
  - as for **poisoning and overdoses** generally.
  - CVS effects may require **CPR**, **glucagon** (2–20 mg [50–150 μg/kg in children up to 10 mg] iv followed by 50 μg/kg/h) or iv infusion of **isoprenaline. Atropine** is often ineffective but should be tried in vagal-blocking doses (3 mg iv [40 μg/kg in children]). **Cardiac pacing** may be required.

Adrenergic receptors. G protein-coupled receptors, activated by **adrenaline** and other **catecholamines**, and divided into α- and β-receptors. Further subdivided into $\beta_1/\beta_2/\beta_3$ and α_1/α_2 receptors (Table 3).

Their effects are mediated by '**second messengers**': α_1-receptor effects by increases in intracellular **calcium** ion concentration, α_2-receptor effects by reducing intracellular **cAMP**, and β_1- and β_2-receptor effects by increasing cAMP. There is evidence for mixed receptor populations at both pre- and postsynaptic membranes. α_2-Receptors have been further subdivided into α_{2A} (responsible for central regulation of BP, sympathetic activity, pain processing and alertness), α_{2B} (causes vasoconstriction) and α_{2C} (thought to be involved in behavioural responses).

See also, α-Adrenergic receptor agonists; β-Adrenergic receptor agonists; α-Adrenergic receptor antagonists; β-Adrenergic receptor antagonists; Sympathetic nervous system

Table 3 Classification and actions of adrenergic receptors

Receptor type	*Site*	*Effect of stimulation*
α_1	Vascular smooth muscle	Contraction
	Bladder smooth muscle (sphincter)	Contraction
	Radial muscle of iris	Contraction
	Intestinal smooth muscle	Relaxation, but contraction of sphincters
	Uterus	Variable
	Salivary glands	Viscous secretion
	Liver	Glycogenolysis
	Pancreas	Decreased secretion of enzymes, insulin and glucagon
α_2	Presynaptic membranes of adrenergic synapses	Reduced release of noradrenaline
	Postsynaptic membranes	Smooth muscle contraction
	Platelets	Aggregation
β_1	Heart	Increased rate and force of contraction
	Adipose tissue	Breakdown of stored triglycerides to fatty acids
	Juxtaglomerular apparatus	Increased renin secretion
β_2	Vascular smooth muscle (muscle beds)	Relaxation
	Bronchial smooth muscle	Relaxation
	Intestinal smooth muscle	Relaxation
	Bladder sphincter	Relaxation
	Uterus	Variable; relaxes the pregnant uterus
	Salivary glands	Watery secretion
	Liver	Glycogenolysis
	Pancreas	Increased insulin and glucagon secretion
β_3	Adipose tissue	Lipolysis

Adrenocortical insufficiency. May be due to:

- primary adrenal failure (Addison's disease, high **ACTH**) due to:
  - **autoimmune disease**: the most common cause; may be associated with other autoimmune disease, e.g. diabetes, thyroid disease, pernicious anaemia, vitiligo.
  - TB, amyloidosis, metastatic infiltration, haemorrhage, drugs or infarction, e.g. in **shock.** Waterhouse–Friderichsen syndrome comprises bilateral adrenal cortical haemorrhage associated with severe **meningococcal disease.**
- secondary adrenal failure (low ACTH) due to:
  - **corticosteroid** therapy withdrawal.
  - ACTH deficiency, e.g. due to surgery, **TBI**, disease of the **pituitary** or **hypothalamus.**

The term 'Addisonian' describes features of adrenal insufficiency irrespective of the cause.

- Features:
  - acute: hypotension and electrolyte abnormalities (**hyponatraemia**, **hyperkalaemia**, hypochloraemia, **hypercalcaemia** and **hypoglycaemia**), muscle weakness. In critically ill patients, treatment of occult adrenocortical insufficiency may be necessary for reversal of hypotension that is resistant to vasopressor drugs.
  - chronic: weight loss, vomiting, diarrhoea, malaise, postural hypotension, increased risk of infection, muscle weakness. Dark pigmentation in scars and skin creases occurs in primary disease. Acute insufficiency (crises) may develop following stress, e.g. infection, surgery, or any critical illness.

Diagnosed by measurement of plasma cortisol and ACTH levels, including demonstration of a 'failed' Synacthen test (an impaired cortisol response following administration of tetracosactide, a synthetic analogue of ACTH).

- Treatment:
  - acute: iv saline, **hydrocortisone** 100 mg iv 6–8-hourly (preferably as the sodium succinate).
  - chronic: hydrocortisone 20–30 mg/day, **fludrocortisone** 50–300 μg/day, both orally. Typically, both are required in primary insufficiency but only hydrocortisone in secondary insufficiency, although this may not always hold true.

[Thomas Addison (1793–1860) and Rupert Waterhouse (1873–1958), English physicians; Carl Friderichsen (1886–1979), Danish paediatrician]

Charmandari E, Nicolaides NC, Chrousos GP (2014). Lancet; 383: 2152–67

Adrenocorticotrophic hormone (ACTH). Polypeptide hormone (39 amino acids; mw 4500) secreted by corticotropic cells of the anterior **pituitary gland** in response to corticotropin releasing factor secreted by the **hypothalamus**. Release of ACTH is highest in the early morning and is increased by emotional and physical stress, including surgery. It increases corticosteroid synthesis in the **adrenal glands**, particularly **glucocorticoids** but also **aldosterone**. ACTH production is inhibited by glucocorticoids (i.e., negative feedback). ACTH or its synthetic analogue tetracosactide (Synacthen) has been used in place of **corticosteroid** therapy in an attempt to reduce adrenocortical suppression, and is used for diagnostic tests in endocrinology. They have also been given to treat or prevent **post-dural puncture headache** although the evidence is weak.

See also, Stress response to surgery

Adult respiratory distress syndrome, *see Acute lung injury*

Advance decision (Advance directive; 'Living will'). Statement, usually written, that provides for a mentally competent person to refuse certain future medical treatments, usually involving life-saving therapies, if he/she were subsequently to become mentally or physically incompetent. The directive may be triggered by certain background conditions such as dementia, **vegetative state** and terminal disease, or acute events including cardiorespiratory arrest, **pneumonia**, **acute kidney injury**, major **stroke** or **spinal cord injury**. Legal and ethical issues relate to the capacity (competence) of the individual, the possibility of changing one's mind, advances in medicine or techniques since the directive was written, the refusal of what might be considered basic care (e.g. feeding), difficulties anticipating the specific circumstances that may arise and therefore be covered/not covered, and the objections of doctors, other healthcare staff and relatives. Previously commonly referred to as advance directives, they were renamed 'advance decisions' in the **Mental Capacity Act 2005**, which enshrined them into statute for the first time. Healthcare guidance for advance decisions was issued in 2007 and revised in 2011. In order to be legally valid, an advance decision must:

- be made by a person ≥18 years old, with the capacity to make it.
- specify the treatment to be refused (can be in lay terms) and the circumstances in which this refusal would apply.
- be made freely without the influence of anyone else.
- be unaltered from when it was made.

Mullick A, Martin J, Sallnow L (2013). Br Med J; 347: 28–32

Advanced (Cardiac) Life Support (ACLS/ALS). System of advanced management of **cardiac arrest** and its training to paramedics, doctors, nurses and other healthcare professionals. Encompasses the recognition and management of periarrest arrhythmias and **post-resuscitation care**. In the UK, ALS courses are run by the **Resuscitation Council (UK)**. In the USA, the American Heart Association runs ACLS courses.

See also, Advanced life support, adult; Basic life support, adult; Cardiopulmonary resuscitation

Advanced life support, adult. Component of **CPR** involving specialised equipment, techniques (e.g. tracheal intubation), drugs, monitoring and 100% oxygen. Airway management may include use of tracheal intubation, **SADs**, **Combitube** or, rarely, tracheostomy.

- Recommendations of the **European Resuscitation Council** (2015):
  - attention to 'ABC' of **basic life support** ± advanced airway management, if there is a delay in getting a defibrillator. **Defibrillation** should take place without delay for a witnessed or in-hospital **cardiac arrest**. A precordial thump should be considered for witnessed, monitored collapse when a defibrillator is not immediately available.
  - actions then depend on the initial rhythm:
    - 'shockable', i.e., **VF**/pulseless **VT**:
      - defibrillation: a single shock of 150–200 J (biphasic) or 360 J (monophasic) followed by immediate resumption of CPR without reassessing the rhythm or feeling for a pulse. After 2 min of CPR, reassess and, if indicated, subsequent shocks of 150–360 J (biphasic) or 360 J (monophasic). If it is unclear whether the rhythm is asystole or fine VF, continue basic life support and do not attempt defibrillation.

        adrenaline 1 mg iv if VF/VT persists after the third shock, then 1 mg every 3–5 min if it still persists.
      - consider and correct potentially reversible causes (*see later*); if not already done, secure the airway, administer oxygen, get iv access. **Cardiac massage** and ventilation at 30:2; compressions should be uninterrupted once the airway has been secured.
      - in refractory VF despite three shocks, consider **amiodarone** 300 mg as an iv bolus; 150 mg as a second bolus followed by 900 mg/24 h. **Lidocaine** 1 mg/kg is an alternative if amiodarone is unavailable, but should not be used in addition (maximum 3 mg/kg in the first hour). Consider use of different pad positions/contacts, different defibrillator, buffers, if refractory. **Magnesium sulfate** 8 mmol may be indicated in **hypomagnesaemia**, **torsade de pointes** or **digoxin** toxicity.
    - 'non-shockable', i.e., asystole or pulseless electrical activity (PEA):
      - adrenaline 1 mg as soon as venous access obtained, repeated every 3–5 min. CPR for 2 min. Consider and correct potentially reversible causes; cardiac massage and ventilation as for VF (*see earlier*).
      - reassess after 2 min and repeat if necessary.
  - potentially reversible causes (4 'H's and 4 'T's): **hypoxaemia**; **hypovolaemia**; electrolyte and metabolic disorders (especially **hyper-/hypokalaemia**); **hypothermia**; tension **pneumothorax**; **cardiac tamponade**;

toxic/therapeutic disturbances (**poisoning and overdoses**); thromboembolic/mechanical obstruction (**PE**). A fifth 'H' (hydrogen ions, i.e., acidosis) and a fifth 'T' (coronary thrombosis) have also been suggested.
- drugs are usually given iv, preferably via a central vein. Peripheral lines should be flushed with 20 ml saline after each drug. Tracheal administration of drugs is no longer advocated; the intraosseous route is now recommended in the absence of iv access.
- consider buffers, e.g. **bicarbonate** 50 ml 8.4% solution in severe acidosis (pH <7.1 or **base excess** exceeding –10), or specific conditions, e.g. **tricyclic antidepressant drug poisoning**, hyperkalaemia.
- if unsuccessful, CPR is generally discontinued after 30–60 min depending on the circumstances (longer in treatable conditions and in children).
- successful resuscitation is characterised by return of spontaneous circulation (ROSC) and occurs in 50% of witnessed in-hospital arrests and 40% of witnessed out-of-hospital events. It is increasingly recognised that integrated **post-resuscitation care** can improve survival and neurological outcome by reducing **cerebral hypoxic ischaemic injury**.
- special situations:
  - **trauma**, **choking**, **near-drowning**, **electrocution**, **anaphylaxis**.
  - paediatric and neonatal CPR (see *Cardiopulmonary resuscitation, paediatric; Cardiopulmonary resuscitation, neonatal*).

- Changes made following 2015 review of 2010 recommendations:
  - increased emphasis on minimally interrupted high-quality chest compressions; interruptions for defibrillation or tracheal intubation should be <5 s.
  - waveform **capnography** must be used continuously to confirm correct tracheal tube placement, monitor the quality of CPR and provide early evidence of ROSC.
  - peri-arrest ultrasound may be used to identify reversible causes of cardiac arrest.

In addition:
- the decision to stop CPR may be difficult in certain circumstances, as may the decision not to start, e.g. terminally ill, elderly patients. Routine regular consideration of **do not attempt resuscitation orders** is becoming mandatory. **Advance decisions** may specify conditions under which patients do or do not wish to be resuscitated.
- controversy continues as to whether relatives of cardiac arrest victims should witness resuscitation attempts; discomfort of staff and possible hindrance of CPR may be offset by the beneficial effects of relatives' seeing that adequate efforts have been expended and being able to be present if the patient dies.
- manipulation of intrathoracic pressure has been suggested in order to improve cardiac output (*see Cardiac massage*).

Complications include trauma to abdominal organs and ribs and those associated with tracheal intubation/attempted intubation and vascular access.

European Resuscitation Council (2015). Resuscitation; 95: 1–312

See also, Acute Cardiac Life Support; Brainstem death; Cough-CPR; Resuscitation Council (UK)

Advanced Life Support Group. UK charity established in 1993, aiming to promote and provide both the public and healthcare professionals with training and education in life-saving techniques. Develops and administers several courses such as **APLS**, **MOET**, **STaR**.

Advanced Life Support in Obstetrics (ALSO). Training system developed in the USA and administered by the American Association of Family Physicians; introduced in the UK as part of the Maternal and Neonatal Emergency Training (MANET) project. Aimed at training medical and midwifery staff in the practical management of maternal and neonatal emergencies and provision of life support for the mother and child. Similar to other **CPR** training systems (e.g. **ACLS**, **ATLS**) in its approach and structure.

See also, Cardiopulmonary resuscitation, neonatal

Advanced Paediatric Life Support (APLS). System of management of the sick or injured child, devised by specialists in paediatrics, accident and emergency medicine, anaesthesia and paediatric surgery in the UK and administered by the **Advanced Life Support Group**. The system integrates basic and advanced resuscitation techniques, similar to those employed in ALS/**ACLS** and **ATLS**, to permit the assessment and treatment of paediatric emergencies (e.g. **airway obstruction**, **cardiac arrest**, **hypothermia**, **convulsions**, **poisoning** and **trauma**).

See also, Cardiopulmonary resuscitation, paediatric

Advanced Trauma Life Support (ATLS). System of **trauma** management devised by physicians in Nebraska, USA in 1978 and adopted by the American College of Surgeons in 1979. Based on the concept of reducing morbidity and mortality in the first ('golden') hour following trauma during which patients may die from potentially survivable injuries (**airway obstruction**, **hypovolaemia**, **pneumothorax**, **cardiac tamponade**), by teaching all members of the trauma team the same algorithms and procedures which are then carried out by rote on every patient. Has been criticised (mainly by senior doctors) because of its very didactic nature, although this is one of its strengths because those most likely to be in the 'front line' of trauma care are traditionally junior doctors who lack the expertise and judgement of their seniors.

Consists of the following phases:
- preparation.
- **triage**.
- primary survey: incorporates assessment of the integrity and function of the **airway**, **cervical spine**, breathing, circulation and neurological status. The patient is fully exposed to detect all life-threatening injuries, with resuscitation taking place in tandem with the primary survey. The need for radiographs of the chest, lateral cervical spine and pelvis should be considered during the primary survey but should not delay resuscitation (the cervical spine is assumed to require immobilisation for any injury above the clavicles until proven otherwise). This takes place simultaneously with the primary survey.
- resuscitation of life-threatening conditions.
- secondary survey: the patient is fully examined from 'head to toe' to exclude injuries to scalp, cranium, face, neck, shoulders, chest, abdomen, perineum, long bones, spine and spinal cord. Special procedures (e.g. abdominal ultrasound, diagnostic **peritoneal lavage**,

iv pyelogram, CT of brain) may be undertaken during this phase, before planning of definitive care.
- continued post-resuscitation monitoring and re-evaluation.
- definitive care: e.g. surgery, ICU admission or transfer to a specialist centre.

ATLS courses are administered in the USA by the American College of Surgeons and by the Royal College of Surgeons of England in the UK.
Carmont MR (2005). Postgrad Med J; 81: 87–91

Adverse drug reactions. Undesired drug effects, usually divided into:
- predictable (type A) dose-related side effects, e.g. hypotension following **thiopental**.
- unpredictable (type B; idiosyncratic) usually less common reactions. These are unrelated to known pharmacological properties of a drug (i.e., not due to common side effects or overdose), usually involving the immune system in some way (but not always, e.g. **MH**).

Suspected adverse reactions are voluntarily reported to the **Medicines and Healthcare products Regulatory Agency** on yellow cards, introduced in 1964 and updated in 2000. The yellow card system was extended to nurse reporters in 2002. Specific yellow cards for reporting anaesthetic drug reactions were introduced in 1988, to encourage reporting of serious reactions to established drugs and any reaction to new drugs. Anaesthetists give many different drugs iv to large numbers of patients, and therefore reactions are often seen. Reactions may be more likely if drugs are given quickly and in combination.
- Mechanisms:
  - on first exposure:
    - direct **histamine** release, e.g. **tubocurarine**, **atracurium**, thiopental, **Althesin**.
    - alternative pathway **complement** activation, e.g. Althesin.
  - apparently on first exposure: prior sensitisation by other (e.g. environmental) antigens may cause crossover sensitivity to subsequently administered drugs; e.g. reactions to **dextrans** may involve prior exposure to bacterial antigens.
  - requiring prior exposure:
    - **anaphylaxis**, e.g. to thiopental.
    - classical pathway complement activation, e.g. Althesin. Other drugs dissolved in **Cremophor EL** may crossreact.

Features range from mild skin rash to anaphylaxis. First exposure reactions tend to be milder and more frequent than those requiring prior exposure.

Reported incidence varies between countries and according to definitions but severe allergic reactions are thought to occur in about 1:10 000 to 1:20 000 cases.
- Management:
  - immediate medical management as for anaphylaxis.
  - testing:
    - a blood sample for **mast cell** tryptase levels should be taken as soon as possible and again at 1–2 h and 24 h after the reaction if anaphylaxis is suspected (99% of plasma tryptase arises from mast cells; normal plasma levels <1 ng/ml). A significant rise is suggestive of anaphylaxis, but its absence does not exclude it; conversely it can occur in non-allergic reactions, albeit to a lesser extent. Tryptase is stable in solution and its half-life is 2.5 h, so back-calculation to the time of the reaction should still be possible if the samples' actual times are accurately recorded. Histamine, complement and immunoglobulin levels may also be useful.
    - skin testing is the gold standard for the detection of IgE-mediated reactions and includes:
      - prick testing (placement of a drop of solution onto the skin of the forearm and gently lifting the underlying skin with a needle): has been suggested as the most useful investigation for specific agents. Because 'neat' solutions may cause flares in normal subjects, 1:10 dilutions or lower should also be used. Results are read after 15–20 min. A wide range of drugs should be tested. Waiting for ~6 months after the reaction has been suggested in order to allow recovery of the immune system.
      - intradermal testing (injection of 0.02–0.05 ml dilute solution into the skin of the forearm or back) has a higher **sensitivity** but lower **specificity** and is more likely to trigger a systemic reaction. Results are read after 20–30 min.
      - patch testing: not useful in suspected perioperative anaphylaxis, though useful for contact allergic reactions.
    - specific IgE antibodies may be assayed using fluorescence or (less commonly) radioactive detection systems and may be useful in reactions to **suxamethonium**, **antibacterial drugs** and latex; testing for other anaesthetic drugs is no longer considered specific enough. Less sensitive than skin testing.
    - the role of other tests, e.g. in vitro basophil studies, is controversial.

It is the anaesthetist's responsibility to arrange referral to an appropriate centre for further testing after a suspected severe reaction, and even after unexplained perioperative collapse/cardiac arrest.
Patton K, Borshoff DC (2018). Anaesthesia; 73: 76–84
See also, Latex allergy

AF, *see Atrial fibrillation*

Affinity. Extent to which a drug binds to a receptor. A drug with high affinity binds more avidly than one with lower affinity, whatever its **intrinsic activity**.

Afterload. Ventricular wall tension required to eject **stroke volume** during systole. For the left ventricle, afterload is increased by:
- an anatomical obstruction, e.g. **aortic stenosis**.
- raised **SVR**.
- decreased elasticity of the aorta and large blood vessels.
- increased ventricular wall thickness (greater tension is needed to produce the necessary pressure [**Laplace's law**]).

Increased afterload results in increased myocardial work/O_2 consumption, increased end-systolic ventricular volume and decreased stroke volume. Reduction of afterload may be achieved with **vasodilator drugs**.
See also, Preload

Agonist. Substance that binds to a receptor to cause a response within the cell. It has high **affinity** for the receptor and high **intrinsic activity**.

A partial agonist binds to the receptor, but causes less response; it may have high affinity, but it has less intrinsic

Table 4 Constituents of dry natural air by volume

Nitrogen	78.03%	Hydrogen	0.001%
O_2	20.99%	Helium	0.0005%
Argon	0.93%	Krypton	0.0001%
CO_2	0.03%	Xenon	0.000008%
Neon	0.0015%		

activity. It may therefore act as a competitive **antagonist** in the presence of a pure agonist.

An agonist–antagonist causes agonism at certain receptors and antagonism at others.
See also, Dose–response curves; Receptor theory

Agranulocytosis, *see Leucocytes*

AGSS, Anaesthetic gas scavenging system, *see Scavenging*

AIDS, Acquired immunodeficiency syndrome, *see Human immunodeficiency viral infection*

Air. Air contains mostly nitrogen and oxygen, with various other constituents (Table 4). **Density** is approximately 1.2 kg/m^3 (1.2 g/l).

'Medical' air may be supplied by a compressor or in **cylinders**. The latter (containing air at 137 bar) are grey with black and white shoulders. Piped air is normally at 4 bar.
See also, individual gases

Air embolism, *see Gas embolism*

Airway. The upper airway includes the mouth, **nose**, **pharynx** and **larynx**. Maintenance of the airway in the unconscious or anaesthetised patient is achieved by combined flexion of the neck and extension at the atlanto-occipital joint (the 'sniffing position'), and lifting the angles of the mandible forward. The **tongue** is lifted forward by the genioglossus muscle which is attached to the back of the point of the jaw; the hyoid bone and larynx are pulled forward by the hyoglossus, mylohyoid, geniohyoid and digastric muscles. Upward pressure on the soft tissues of the floor of the mouth may cause obstruction, particularly in children, and should be avoided. In the lateral (recovery) position, the tongue and jaw fall forward under gravity, improving the airway. **Airway obstruction** during anaesthesia has traditionally been attributed to the tongue falling back against the posterior pharyngeal wall. Radiological and electromyographic studies suggest that obstruction by the soft palate or epiglottis secondary to reduced local muscle activity may also be responsible.
See also, Airways; Tracheobronchial tree

Airway exchange catheter. Device placed into the trachea both to maintain oxygenation after tracheal **extubation** (i.e., inserted through the tracheal tube before the latter is removed), and to facilitate reintubation should it be required. Available devices share similar features: they are long, hollow catheters, able to be attached to an O_2 supply at their proximal end (e.g. using a detachable 15-mm connector) and stiff enough to act as a guide for a tracheal tube passed over them. The distal end may be angulated, allowing the catheter also to be used as an introducer, e.g. during direct laryngoscopy. A specific type of exchange catheter (the Aintree catheter) has been designed for exchanging a **LM** with a tracheal tube via a flexible fibrescope.

Airway obstruction. Obstruction may occur at the mouth, pharynx, larynx, trachea and large bronchi. It may be caused by the tongue, **laryngospasm**, strictures, tumours and soft tissue swellings, oedema, infection (e.g. **diphtheria**, **epiglottitis**) and **foreign objects**, including anaesthetic equipment. Hypotonia of the muscles involved in upper **airway** maintenance is common during anaesthesia. During IPPV, mechanical obstruction may occur at any point along the breathing system.

Airway obstruction results in **hypoventilation** and increased work of breathing. It may present as an acute medical emergency requiring immediate management.

- Features:
  - spontaneous ventilation:
    - dyspnoea, noisy respiration, **stridor**.
    - use of accessory muscles of respiration, with tracheal tug, supraclavicular and intercostal indrawing, and paradoxical 'see-saw' movement of abdomen and chest.
    - tachypnoea, tachycardia and other features of **hypoxaemia**, **hypercapnia** and **respiratory failure**.
    - **pulmonary oedema** may occur if negative intrathoracic pressures are excessive.
    - during anaesthesia, poor movement of the reservoir bag may occur.
  - IPPV:
    - increased **airway pressures** with reduced chest movement; noisy respiration or wheeze.
    - features of hypoxaemia and hypercapnia.
- Management:
  - **O_2 therapy** including **THRIVE**; increased F_IO_2 during anaesthesia.
  - spontaneous ventilation:
    - general measures in unconscious/anaesthetised patients:
      - turn to the lateral position if practical.
      - correct positioning of the head, elevation of the jaw, and use of oropharyngeal or nasopharyngeal **airways**. Tracheal intubation may be required as below.
    - specific treatment, e.g.:
      - **antibacterial drugs** for infection.
      - fresh frozen plasma or C1 esterase inhibitor for **hereditary angio-oedema**.
      - nebulised **adrenaline** for **croup**.
      - **Heimlich manoeuvre** for **choking**.
      - increasing **gas flow**: **helium–O_2** mixtures.
      - bypassing the obstruction: tracheal intubation, **tracheostomy** or **cricothyrotomy**. The last two may be difficult if the anatomy is distorted.
  - IPPV:
    - causes of increased airway pressure and hypoventilation other than obstruction due to equipment (e.g. **bronchospasm**, **pneumothorax**, inadequate neuromuscular blockade and coughing) should be considered.
    - while ventilating by hand, all tubing should be checked for kinks. A suction catheter will not pass down the **tracheal tube** if the latter is obstructed, e.g. by kinks, mucus, herniated cuff. If auscultation of the chest does not suggest bronchospasm or pneumothorax, the cuff should be deflated and

the tracheal tube pulled back slightly. If ventilation does not improve, the tube should be removed and ventilation attempted by facemask.

- Anaesthesia for patients with airway obstruction:
  - preoperatively:
    - **preoperative assessment** for the features and management as mentioned earlier.
    - useful pre-induction investigations include:
      - radiography, including tomograms, **thoracic inlet** views and **CT scanning**.
      - flexible nasendoscopy images.
      - arterial **blood gas interpretation**.
      - **flow–volume loops**.
    - **premedication** may aid smooth **induction of anaesthesia** but excessive sedation should be avoided.
  - perioperatively:
    - severe/critical obstruction may warrant securing of the airway using an awake technique (e.g. tracheostomy under local anaesthesia or awake fibreoptic intubation). The choice depends on patient compliance, operator experience and site/severity of the obstruction (e.g. large glottic tumours may be impassable with an endoscope).
    - if general anaesthesia is deemed preferable and/or necessary it should be induced with full **monitoring** and facilities for resuscitation and tracheostomy/cricothyrotomy immediately available.
    - patients with proximal airway obstruction usually adopt the optimal head and neck position for maximal air movement; muscle relaxation caused by iv induction may therefore lead to sudden complete obstruction. It may be impossible to ventilate the patient by facemask, and tracheal intubation may be difficult or impossible. **Intravenous anaesthetic agents** and **neuromuscular blocking drugs** should therefore be used with extreme caution. Inhalational induction (e.g. **sevoflurane** in O_2) is traditionally advocated, although induction may be slow and difficult. If obstruction worsens, anaesthesia is allowed to lighten. Tracheal intubation is performed without paralysis; **lidocaine** spray may be useful.
  - postoperatively: as for difficult intubation (*see Intubation, difficult*).

Classical management of patients with large airway compression, e.g. by mediastinal tumours, also employs inhalational induction and anaesthesia. This avoids acute exacerbation of airway obstruction caused by sudden muscle relaxation.

In the **recovery room** or casualty department, all unconscious patients should be positioned in the **recovery** position, to protect them from aspiration and airway obstruction.

See also, Intubation, awake; Extubation, tracheal

Airway pressure. Pressure within the breathing system and tracheobronchial tree. Useful as an indicator of mechanical obstruction to expiration during spontaneous ventilation. Factors affecting mean airway pressure during IPPV include **PEEP**, peak inflation pressure, inspiratory time and respiratory rate (because high rates decrease time for expiration). Changes in airway pressure during mechanical ventilation may indicate disconnection, **dynamic hyperinflation**, mechanical obstruction, decreased lung **compliance** or increased **airway resistance**, and the risk of **barotrauma**. The pressure measured at the mouth may considerably exceed alveolar pressure during positive pressure breaths, especially if airway resistance and gas flow rates are high. During expiration, mouth pressure falls to zero, but alveolar pressure may lag behind. In some ventilators airway pressure is measured in the expiratory limb of the breathing system.

Airway pressure release ventilation (APRV). **CPAP** with intermittent release to ambient pressure (or a lower level of CPAP) causing expiration. Spontaneous ventilation may continue between APRV breaths. Allows reduction of mean **airway pressure**, and has been used to support respiration in **ALI. Weaning** is achieved by reducing the frequency of CPAP release until the patient is breathing spontaneously with CPAP maintained.

Esan A, Hess DR, Raoof S, et al (2010). Chest; 137: 1203–16

Airway resistance.

$$\text{Resistance} = \frac{\text{driving pressure}}{\text{gas flow}}$$

Driving pressure is the difference between alveolar and mouth pressures, and may be measured using the **body plethysmograph**. Alternatively, gas flow may be halted repeatedly for a tenth of a second at a time with a shutter; during the brief period of no flow, alveolar pressure may be measured at the mouth. Gas flow can be measured with a **pneumotachograph**.

Most of the resistance resides in the large and medium-sized bronchi; severe damage to the small airways may occur before a measurable increase in resistance.

At low lung volumes, the radial traction produced by lung parenchyma surrounding the airways, and that holds them open, is reduced; thus airway calibre is reduced, and resistance increased. During forced expiration, some airways may close, causing air trapping. Bronchoconstriction and increased density or viscosity of the inspired gas also increase resistance (density because flow is partly turbulent in the airways). Resistance is increased in chronic bronchitis due to airway narrowing. In emphysema, the airways close because of lung parenchymal destruction.

Airway resistance increases during anaesthesia; this may be caused by bronchospasm, reduction in **FRC** and lung volume, or by the tubes and connections of the breathing system.

Kaminsky DA (2012). Respir Care; 57: 85–96

See also, Closing capacity; Compliance

Airways. Devices placed in the upper **airway** (but not into the larynx); used to:

- relieve **airway obstruction**.
- prevent biting and occlusion of the **tracheal tube**.
- support the tracheal tube.
- allow suction.
- act as a conduit for fibreoptic intubation.
- facilitate CPR.

Thus usually employed during anaesthesia and in unconscious patients.

- Types:
  - Oropharyngeal airways: **Guedel** airway is most commonly used. Modifications include a side port for attachment to a fresh gas source (**Waters** airway), 15-mm **connectors** for attachment to a breathing system, caps with side ports, and airways used for **fibreoptic intubation** (Fig. 6). A cuffed oropharyngeal airway (COPA) with a 15-mm connector was described in 1991 but was not widely used and is no

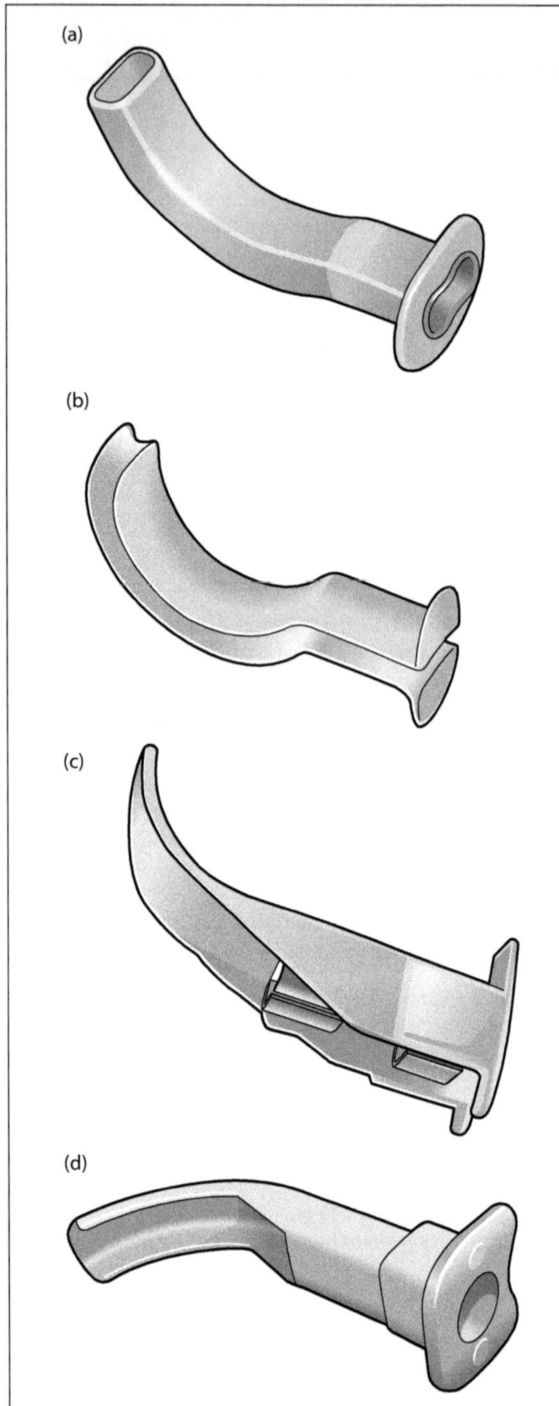

Fig. 6 Examples of oropharyngeal airways: (a) Guedel; (b) Berman intubating; (c) Ovassapian; (d) Williams. The latter three are used for fibreoptic intubation; the Berman and Ovassapian allow the airway to be removed without dislodging the tracheal tube once placed

longer available. Oropharyngeal airways are the commonest cause of damage to **teeth** in anaesthetised patients. They must be placed with care, particularly in children where soft tissue damage can easily occur.
- **SADs**: designed to be placed close to, but above, the larynx, resulting in a better seal and therefore the ability to control ventilation.
- nasopharyngeal: usually smooth non-cuffed tubes with a flange to prevent pushing them completely into the nose. Avoids risk to capped teeth, but may cause **epistaxis**. Cuffed nasal airways may be held in place by the inflated cuff, and allow attachment to a breathing system.

Insertion of an airway may cause gagging, coughing and laryngospasm unless the patient is comatose or adequately anaesthetised; these may also occur on waking.

[Robert Alvin Berman (1914–1999), US anaesthetist; Andranik Ovassapian (1936–2010), Iranian-born US anaesthetist; R Tudor Williams (1928–2017), Canadian anaesthetist]

Cook TM, Howes B (2011). Contin Educ Anaesth Crit Care Pain; 11: 56–61

AIS, *see Abbreviated injury scale*

AKI, *see Acute kidney injury*

Albendazole. Agent used (off-licence) in conjunction with surgery to treat **hydatid disease**. May be used alone in inoperable cases.
- Dose: up to 800 mg orally/day in divided doses for 28 days, followed by a 14-day treatment-free period. Up to three cycles may be given.
- Side effects: GIT upset, headache, dizziness, hepatic impairment, pancytopenia.

Albumin. The most abundant **plasma** protein (mw 69000): normal plasma levels: 35–50 g/l. Important in the maintenance of plasma **oncotic pressure**, as a **buffer**, and in the transport of various molecules such as bilirubin, hormones, fatty acids and drugs. It is synthesised by the liver and removed from the plasma into the interstitial fluid. It may then pass via lymphatics back to the plasma, or into cells to be metabolised. May have a role as a **free radical** scavenger. Depletion occurs in severe illness, infection and trauma. Available for transfusion as 4.5% and 20% solutions; currently the most expensive non-blood plasma substitute. Has been used as a **colloid** when providing iv fluid therapy for critically ill patients but hypoalbuminaemia in these patients usually results from increased metabolism of circulating albumin; administration does not generally result in maintained plasma albumin levels and no improvement in outcome has been found when compared with cheaper alternatives. The effect of albumin administration on mortality in critically ill patients remains controversial, although recent studies suggest mortality is not increased, except possibly in patients with **TBI**. The lack of any clear advantage of using albumin solutions for resuscitation, and its expense, have led to a decline in its use.

Vincent JL, Russell JA, Jacob M, et al (2014). Crit Care; 18: 231–41

See also, Blood products; Protein-binding

Albuterol, *see Salbutamol*

Alcohol, *see Alcohols*

Alcohol poisoning. Problems, features and management depend on the **alcohols** ingested:
- ethanol: commonly complicates or precipitates acute illness or injury, especially **trauma**. Results in depressed consciousness (hindering assessment of **head injury**), potentiation of depressant drugs and disinhibition. Patients are often uncooperative. Other effects of acute intoxication include vasodilatation, tachycardia, **arrhythmias**, **vomiting**, reduced **lower**

oesophageal sphincter pressure, gastric irritation, delayed **gastric emptying**, **hypoglycaemia** (typically 6–36 h after ingestion, especially in a starved or malnourished individual), metabolic **acidosis**, dehydration (due to diuretic effect), **coma** and **convulsions**. Intoxication occurs at blood levels ~100–150 mg/dl (22–33 mmol/l), loss of muscle coordination at ~150–200 mg/dl (33–43 mmol/l), decreased level of consciousness at ~200–300 mg/dl (43–65 mmol/l) and death at ~300–500 mg/dl (65–109 mmol/l). The fatal adult dose is about 300–500 ml absolute alcohol (500–1200 ml strong spirits) within 1 h.

Management is mainly supportive, as for **poisoning and overdoses. Haemodialysis** has been used in severe poisoning. Features of **alcoholism** require attention if present.

- methanol: toxicity results from hepatic metabolism of methanol to formaldehyde and thence formic acid, the latter being a potent inhibitor of mitochondrial cytochrome oxidase. Features occur after 8–36 h and include intoxication, vomiting, abdominal pain, coma, visual disturbances, severe metabolic acidosis with a large **anion gap** and **osmolar gap**, and **hyperglycaemia**. About 10 ml pure methanol may result in permanent blindness, with the fatal adult dose around 30 ml (methylated spirits contains 5% methanol and 95% ethanol, the latter causing the most toxicity). Blood levels greater than 500 mg/ml (15 mmol/l) indicate severe poisoning.

  Management includes **gastric lavage** if within 2 h of ingestion, administration of **bicarbonate**, inhibition of further methanol metabolism with ethanol (50 g orally/iv followed by 10–20 g/h iv to produce blood levels of 100–200 g/dl [20–30 mmol/l]). More recently, **fomepizole** has gained acceptance as an alternative to alcohol and may reduce the need for **haemodialysis**, which may still be required in severe cases. Folic acid or its metabolites have also been used (utilised in formate metabolism). Haemodialysis has been used in severe poisoning.
- isopropanol: effects are caused by the alcohol itself, not its metabolites. Effects are similar to those of ethanol but longer lasting. Gastritis, renal tubular acidosis, myopathy and haemolysis may occur.

  Management is with gastric lavage if within 2 h of ingestion and supportive thereafter.
- ethylene glycol: toxicity results from metabolism by alcohol dehydrogenase to glycoaldehyde and oxalic/formic acids. The former causes cerebral impairment, while the latter produce severe metabolic acidosis and acute tubular necrosis. The fatal adult dose is ~100 g, although patients have survived much larger doses. Features include intoxication, vomiting, haematemesis, coma, convulsions, depressed reflexes, myoclonus, nystagmus, papilloedema and ophthalmoplegia within the first 12 h; tachycardia, hypertension, **pulmonary oedema** and **cardiac failure** within the next 12 h; and **renal failure** over the subsequent 2–3 days. Investigations may reveal severe **lactic acidosis**, a large anion gap and osmolar gap, **hypocalcaemia** and **hyperkalaemia**. Blood levels exceeding ~200 mg/l (~35 mmol/l) indicate severe poisoning.

  Management includes haemodialysis, ethanol and fomepizole; thiamine and pyridoxine have also been used.

Kraut JA, Mullins ME (2018). New Engl J Med; 378: 270–80

Alcohol withdrawal syndromes. May be precipitated by acute illness or surgery, even if regular intake of alcohol (ethanol) is apparently not excessive and without the other features of **alcoholism**.

- Features:
  - most commonly, tremulousness, agitation, nausea, vomiting: usually within 6–8 h of abstinence.
  - hallucinations: usually visual; occur 10–30 h after abstinence and in under 10% of cases.
  - **convulsions**: occur up to 48 h after abstinence and in about 5% of cases.
  - **delirium tremens**: includes the above symptoms plus confusion, disorientation, sweating, tachycardia and hypertension. Occurs up to 3–10 days after abstinence and in about 5% of cases.

Management includes sedative drugs (e.g. **benzodiazepines**, **carbamazepine**, **clomethiazole**) and reassurance. More recently, **clonidine** has been used successfully to smooth withdrawal. **Vitamin B_6** supplements are usually administered, but if there is a risk of encephalopathy a mixture of vitamins is best prescribed.

Schuckit MA (2014). N Engl J Med; 371. 2109–13

Alcoholism. Form of **substance abuse** in which there is narrowing of the drinking repertoire (loss of day-to-day variation in drinking habits), increased **tolerance** to alcohol (ethanol), symptoms of **alcohol withdrawal syndromes** when intake is stopped, a craving for alcohol and drinking in the early part of the day/middle of the night. May precipitate admission to hospital as a consequence of acute **alcohol poisoning** or intoxication, or impaired organ function resulting from chronic abuse; may also complicate the management of incidental disease or surgery.

- Effects of chronic alcohol intake:
  - cerebral/cerebellar degeneration, **peripheral neuropathy**, psychiatric disturbances (Wernicke's encephalopathy, Korsakoff's psychosis).
  - withdrawal may lead to tremor, anxiety, hallucinations, **convulsions, delirium tremens**.
  - gastritis, **peptic ulcer disease, oesophageal varices**; may lead to **gastrointestinal haemorrhage**.
  - **pancreatitis**.
  - fatty liver, hepatic **enzyme induction**, cirrhosis causing **hepatic failure**, coagulopathy.
  - **malnutrition, immunodeficiency**.
  - increased risk of liver, bowel, breast, mouth and oesophageal malignancy.
  - although mild alcohol consumption may have cardioprotective effects, heavy consumption is associated with alcoholic **cardiomyopathy** and **cardiac failure**.

[Karl Wernicke (1848–1904), German neurologist; Sergei Korsakoff (1853–1900), Russian neurologist and psychologist]

Connor JP, Haber PS, Hall WD (2016). Lancet; 387: 988–98

Alcohols. Group of aliphatic (i.e., non-cyclic) organic chemicals that contain one or more hydroxyl (–OH) groups and that form esters (containing the –O–O– linkage) with acids. Used as solvents and cleaning agents. Those of particular medical/anaesthetic relevance include:

- ethanol (ethyl alcohol; C_2H_5OH): commonly referred to as 'alcohol'; widely drunk throughout the world and often abused, resulting in acute toxicity or **alcoholism**. Used in the past as an anaesthetic agent and as a **tocolytic drug**. May be added to irrigant solution to monitor the latter's uptake during **TURP**.

Also used for destructive injection, e.g. into neural tissue in chronic **pain management**. In the ICU, iv alcohol may be used to treat methanol poisoning; it may also be useful for sedating alcoholics (1–10 g/h of a 5%–10% solution).

Metabolised mostly to acetaldehyde, then acetate, acetyl coenzyme A and finally CO_2 and water via the **tricarboxylic acid cycle**. Five per cent is excreted unchanged, mostly in the urine but also in the breath. The rate of metabolism is 10 ml/h at concentrations above 100 mg/dl (22 mmol/l); below this level it is subject to first-order kinetics with a half-life of about 1 h (*see Michaelis–Menten kinetics*). Produces 30 kJ/g (7 Cal/g); it has been used as an iv energy source.

- methanol (methyl alcohol; CH_3OH): derived from distillation of wood or from coal or natural gas. Used in the petroleum and paint industries. Contained with ethanol in methylated spirits. Extremely toxic if ingested.
- isopropanol (isopropyl alcohol; $(CH_3)_2CHOH$): used as a solvent and to clean the skin before invasive procedures. Oxidised in the liver to acetone.
- ethylene glycol (glycol; $(CH_2OH)_2$): used as an antifreeze.
- **propylene glycol** ($CH_3.CHOH.CH_2OH$): used as a solvent in drugs, e.g. **etomidate**, **GTN**.

All are CNS depressants, rapidly absorbed from the upper GIT (also by inhalation and, to varying degrees, percutaneously) and metabolised by hepatic alcohol dehydrogenase to the aldehyde; all except isopropanol are metabolised further to the corresponding acid by aldehyde dehydrogenase.

See also, Alcohol poisoning; Alcohol withdrawal syndromes

Alcuronium chloride. Non-depolarising **neuromuscular blocking drug**, introduced in 1961 and withdrawn in the UK in 1994. Caused mild histamine release and hypotension, but anaphylaxis, when it occurred, was often severe.

Aldosterone. **Mineralocorticoid** hormone secreted by the outer layer (zona glomerulosa) of the cortex of the **adrenal gland**. Secreted in response to reduced renal blood flow (via **renin/angiotensin system**), trauma and anxiety (via **ACTH** release), and **hyperkalaemia** and **hyponatraemia** (direct effect on the adrenal cortex). Increases sodium and water reabsorption from renal tubular filtrate, sweat and saliva. Acts via mineralocorticoid receptors to up-regulate basolateral sodium/potassium pumps at the distal renal tubule and collecting duct. Sodium and water are retained while potassium and hydrogen ion excretion is increased.

Hyperaldosteronism results in **hypertension** and **hypokalaemia**. In cardiac failure and cirrhosis, aldosterone levels may be raised, although the mechanism is unclear.

Aldosterone antagonists, e.g. **spironolactone**, potassium canrenoate and eplerenone, cause sodium loss and potassium retention.

ALERT, *see Acute life-threatening events—recognition and treatment*

Alfentanil hydrochloride. **Opioid analgesic drug** derived from **fentanyl**. Developed in 1976. In comparison with fentanyl, alfentanil has a:

- faster onset of action (<1 min).
- lower p*K*a (6.5 vs. 8.4), rendering it mostly (90%) unionised at body pH.
- shorter elimination half-life due to its lower **volume of distribution** (despite a lower **clearance**).
- lower potency (approximately one-tenth).

Has minimal cardiovascular effects, although bradycardia and hypotension may occur. Other effects are like those of fentanyl. Metabolised in the liver to noralfentanil.

- Dosage:
    - for spontaneously breathing patients, up to 500 mg initially, followed by increments of 250 mg. Slow injection reduces the incidence of apnoea.
    - 30–50 μg/kg to obtund the hypertensive response to tracheal intubation. Up to 125 μg/kg is used in **cardiac surgery**.
    - for infusion, a loading dose of 50–100 μg/kg, followed by 0.5–1 μg/kg/min. Higher rates have been used in **TIVA**. The infusion is discontinued 10–30 min before surgery ends. Also used for **sedation** in ICU at 30–60 μg/kg/h initially.

Alimemazine tartrate (Trimeprazine). Phenothiazine-derived **antihistamine drug**, used for premedication in children. More sedative than other antihistamines. Has antiemetic properties.

- Dosage: up to 2 mg/kg orally 1–2 h preoperatively.
- Side effects include dry mouth, circumoral pallor and dizziness. May cause postoperative restlessness due to **antanalgesia**. Has been implicated in causing prolonged respiratory depression on rare occasions.

Aliskiren, *see Renin/angiotensin system*

Alkalaemia. Arterial **pH** >7.45 or H^+ concentration <35 nmol/l.

See also, Acid–base balance; Alkalosis

Alkalosis. A process in which arterial **pH** >7.45 (or H^+ concentration <35 nmol/l), or would be >7.45 if there were no compensatory mechanisms of **acid–base balance**.

See also, Alkalosis, metabolic; Alkalosis, respiratory

Alkalosis, metabolic. Inappropriately high **pH** for the measured arterial $P\text{CO}_2$.

- Caused by:
    - acid loss, e.g. vomiting, nasogastric aspiration.
    - base ingestion:
        - **bicarbonate** (usually iatrogenic).
        - citrate from **blood transfusion**.
        - milk–alkali syndrome.
        - forced alkaline diuresis.
    - potassium/chloride depletion leading to acid urine production.
- Primary change: increased bicarbonate/decreased hydrogen ion.
- Compensation:
    - **hypoventilation**: reaches its maximum within 24 h, usually with an upper limit for arterial $P\text{CO}_2$ of 7–8 kPa (50–60 mmHg). Initial increase in HCO_3^- is about 0.76 mmol/l per kPa change in arterial $P\text{CO}_2$ above 5.3 kPa (1 mmol/l per 10 mmHg above 40), although the level of compensatory change is less predictable than in metabolic acidosis.
    - decreased renal acid secretion.
- Effects:
    - confusion.
    - paraesthesia/**tetany** (reduced free ionised calcium concentration due to altered protein binding).

- Treatment:
  - correction of ECF and potassium depletion.
  - rarely, acid therapy, e.g. ammonium chloride or hydrochloric acid: deficit = **base excess** × body weight (kg) mmol.

Khanna A, Kurtzman NA (2006). J Nephrol; 19: S86–96
See also, Acid–base balance

Alkalosis, respiratory. **Alkalosis** due to decreased arterial $P\text{CO}_2$. Caused by alveolar **hyperventilation**, e.g. fear, pain, hypoxia, **pregnancy**, or during IPPV.
- Primary change: decreased arterial $P\text{CO}_2$.
- Compensation:
  - initial fall in plasma **bicarbonate** due to decreased carbonic acid formation and dissociation.
  - decreased acid secretion/increased bicarbonate excretion by the kidneys.

In acute **hypocapnia**, bicarbonate concentration falls by about 1.3 mmol/l per 1 kPa fall in arterial $P\text{CO}_2$. In chronic hypocapnia, the fall per 1 kPa is 4.0 mmol/l.
- Effects: those of hypocapnia.
- Treatment: of underlying cause.

See also, Acid–base balance

Alkylating drugs, *see Cytotoxic drugs*

Allen's test. Originally described for assessing arterial flow to the hand in thromboangiitis obliterans. Modified for assessment of ulnar artery flow before radial **arterial cannulation**. The ulnar and radial arteries are compressed at the wrist, and the patient is asked to clench tightly and open the hand, causing blanching. Pressure over the ulnar artery is released; the colour of the palm normally takes less than 5–10 s to return to normal, with over 15 s considered abnormal. A similar manoeuvre may be performed with the radial artery before ulnar artery cannulation. Although widely performed, it is inaccurate in predicting risk from ischaemic damage.
[Edgar Van Nuys Allen (1900–1961), US physician]
Brzezinski M, Luisetti T, London MJ (2009). Anesth Analg; 109: 1763–81

Allergic reactions, *see Adverse drug reactions*

Allodynia. **Pain** from a stimulus that is not normally painful. In mechanical allodynia, pain occurs in response to light touch or stroking, in thermal allodynia it results from mild temperature stimulus and in movement allodynia from joint movement. Seen in neuropathies, **complex regional pain syndrome**, **postherpetic neuralgia** and **migraine**, and paradoxically but rarely following chronic opioid use (**opioid-induced hyperalgesia**). Pathophysiology is unknown but reorganisation of nociceptors, mechanoreceptors, spinal interneurons and thalamic pathways has been suggested. Treatment includes analgesic agents and **anticonvulsant drugs** (e.g. **gabapentin**, **lamotrigine**).
Jensen TS, Finnerup NB (2014). Lancet Neurol; 13: 924–35
See also, Nociception; Pain; Pain pathways

Alpha-adrenergic..., *see α-Adrenergic ...*

Alprostadil. **Prostaglandin** E_1, used to maintain patency of a patent **ductus arteriosus** in neonates with congenital heart disease in whom the ductus is vital for survival, e.g. pulmonary atresia/stenosis, **Fallot's tetralogy**, coarctation, transposition of the great arteries.
- Dosage: 5–10 ng/kg/min initially via the umbilical artery or iv, titrated to a maximum of 100 ng/kg/min.
- Side effects include apnoea, brady- or tachycardia, hypotension, pyrexia, diarrhoea, convulsions, **DIC**, hypokalaemia. Undiluted preparation reacts with plastic containers, so care in preparation is required.

ALS, *see Advanced Cardiac Life Support; Advanced life support, adult; Advanced Life Support in Obstetrics; Advanced Paediatric Life Support; Advanced Trauma Life Support; Neonatal Resuscitation Programme*

ALSO, *see Advanced Life Support in Obstetrics*

Alteplase (rt-PA, tissue-type plasminogen activator). **Fibrinolytic drug**, used in acute management of **MI**, **PE** and acute ischaemic **stroke**. Becomes active when it binds to fibrin, converting plasminogen to plasmin, which dissolves the fibrin. Thought to be non-immunogenic.
- Dosage:
  - within 6 h of MI: 15 mg iv bolus followed by 50 mg/30 min, then 35 mg/60 min.
  - within 6–12 h of MI: 10 mg bolus, then 50 mg/60 min, then 40 mg/2 h.
  - PE: 10 mg followed by 90 mg/2 h.
  - acute stroke (within 4.5 h): 0.9 mg/kg (up to 90 mg); 10% by iv injection, the remainder by infusion/60 min.

Maximum dose: 1.5 mg/kg if under 65 kg body weight.
- Side effects: as for fibrinolytic drugs.

Althesin. **Intravenous anaesthetic agent** introduced in 1971, composed of two corticosteroids, alphaxalone and alphadolone. Withdrawn in 1984 because of a high incidence of **adverse drug reactions**, mostly minor but occasionally severe, thought to be due to **Cremophor EL**, the solubilising agent. Previously widely used because of its rapid onset and short duration of action; still used in veterinary practice.

Altitude, high. Problems include:
- lack of O_2: e.g. atmospheric pressure at 18 000 ft (5486 m) is half that at sea level. F_IO_2 is constant, but $P\text{O}_2$ is lowered. This effect is offset initially by the shape of the **oxyhaemoglobin dissociation curve**, which maintains haemoglobin saturation above 90% up to 10 000 ft (3048 m). Studies at 8400 m on Mount Everest have shown a mean P_aO_2 of 3.3 kPa. Compensatory changes due to hypoxia include hyperventilation and **respiratory alkalosis**, increased **erythropoietin** secretion resulting in **polycythaemia**, increased **2,3-DPG**, proliferation of peripheral capillaries and alterations in intracellular oxidative enzymes. **Alkalaemia** is reduced after a few days, via increased renal bicarbonate loss. CSF pH is returned towards normal. Pulmonary vasoconstriction may result in right heart strain.
- low temperatures, e.g. ambient temperature is –20°C at 18 000 ft (5486 m).
- expansion of gas-containing cavities, e.g. inner ear.
- acute high-altitude illness:
  - acute mountain sickness (AMS): occurs in 40% of people who have recently reached 3000 m. Symptoms include headache, GIT disturbance, insomnia, fatigue, dizziness.

- high-altitude cerebral oedema (HACE): symptoms of AMS plus ataxia or cognitive impairment (confusion, drowsiness, coma).
- high-altitude pulmonary oedema (HAPE): early symptoms including dry cough and dyspnoea are followed by orthopnoea and haemoptysis. Symptoms of AMS frequently coexist.

The incidence of AMS, HACE and HAPE may be reduced by controlling the rate of ascent e.g. 300 m/day above 3000 m, with rest days of 2–3 days. Symptoms should be treated with supplementary O_2 (so that S_aO_2 >90%) and descent by at least 500 m. **Acetazolamide** (250 mg tds) and **dexamethasone** (8 mg) may improve symptoms while awaiting descent.

- anaesthetic apparatus at high altitude:
  - **vaporisers**: **SVP** is unaffected by atmospheric pressure, thus the partial pressure of volatile agent in the vaporiser is the same as at sea level. Because atmospheric pressure is reduced, the delivered concentration is increased from that marked on the dial, but because anaesthetic action depends on alveolar partial pressure, not concentration, the same settings may be used as at sea level. However, reduced temperature may alter vaporisation.
  - **flowmeters**: because atmospheric pressure is reduced, a given amount of gas occupies a greater volume than at sea level; i.e., has reduced density. Thus a greater volume is required to pass through a Rotameter flowmeter to maintain the bobbin at a certain height, because it is the number of gas molecules hitting the bobbin that supports it. The flowmeters therefore under-read at high altitudes. However, because the clinical effects depend on the number of molecules, not volume of gas, the flowmeters may be used as normal.

Brown JPR, Grocott MPW (2013). Contin Educ Anaesth Crit Care Pain; 13: 17–22

Altitude, low. Problems are related to high pressure:
- **inert gas narcosis.**
- **oxygen toxicity.**
- pressure reversal of anaesthesia.
- effects on equipment:
  - implosion of glass ampoules.
  - deflation of air-filled tracheal tube cuffs.
  - functioning of **vaporisers** and **flowmeters** is normal, as above.

See also, Oxygen, hyperbaric

Alveolar air equation. In its simplified form:

$$\text{alveolar } P\text{O}_2 = F_\text{I}\text{O}_2(P_\text{B} - P_\text{A}\text{H}_2\text{O}) - \frac{P_\text{A}\text{CO}_2}{R}$$

$$\text{or } P_\text{I}\text{O}_2 - \frac{P_\text{A}\text{CO}_2}{R}$$

where P_B = ambient barometric pressure
P_AH_2O = alveolar partial pressure of water (normally 6.3 kPa [47 mmHg])
P_ACO_2 = alveolar PCO_2; approximately equals arterial PCO_2
R = respiratory exchange ratio, normally 0.8
P_IO_2 = inspired PO_2

Useful for estimating alveolar PO_2, e.g. when determining **alveolar–arterial O_2 difference** and **shunt** fractions. The equation also illustrates how **hypercapnia** may be associated with a lower P_AO_2. Another form of the equation allows for differences between inspired and expired gas volumes, and is unaffected by inert gas exchange:

$$\text{alveolar } P\text{O}_2 = P_\text{I}\text{O}_2 - P_A\text{CO}_2 - \left(\frac{P_\text{I}\text{O}_2 - P_\text{E}\text{O}_2}{P_\text{E}\text{CO}_2}\right)$$

where P_EO_2 = mixed expired PO_2
P_ECO_2 = mixed expired PCO_2

Table 5 Normal respiratory gas partial pressures and tensions in kPa (mmHg)

	Inspired	*Alveolar*	*Arterial*	*Venous*	*Expired*
O_2	21 (160)	14 (106)	13.3 (100)	5.3 (40)	15 (105)
CO_2	0.03 (0.2)	5.3 (40)	5.3 (40)	6.1 (46)	4 (30)
Nitrogen	80 (600)	74 (560)	74 (560)	74 (560)	75 (570)
H_2O	Variable	6.3 (47)	6.3 (47)	6.3 (47)	6.3 (47)

Alveolar–arterial oxygen difference (A–aDO_2). Alveolar PO_2 minus arterial PO_2. Useful as a measure of **$\dot{V}/\dot{Q}$ mismatch** and anatomical **shunt.** Alveolar PO_2 is estimated using the **alveolar air equation**; arterial PO_2 is measured directly. The small shunt and $\dot{V}/\dot{Q}$ mismatch in normal subjects result in a normal A–aDO_2 <2.0 kPa (15 mmHg) breathing air; this may reach 4.0 kPa (30 mmHg) in the elderly. It increases when breathing high O_2 concentrations because the shunt component is not corrected; i.e., normally up to 15 kPa (115 mmHg) breathing 100% O_2.

Alveolar gases. Normal alveolar gas partial pressures and intravascular gas tensions are shown in Table 5. End-tidal gas approximates to alveolar gas in normal subjects and may be monitored, e.g. during anaesthesia.
See also, End-tidal gas sampling

Alveolar gas transfer. Depends on:
- **alveolar ventilation.**
- **diffusion** across alveolar membrane, fluid interface and capillary endothelium (normally less than 0.5 µm).
- **solubility** of gases in blood.
- **cardiac output.**

For gases transferred from the bloodstream to the alveolus, e.g. CO_2, and anaesthetic vapours during recovery, the same factors apply.

With normal cardiac output, blood cells take about 0.75 s to pass through pulmonary capillaries. O_2 transfer is usually complete within 0.25 s; part of the time is taken for the reaction with **haemoglobin.** CO_2 diffuses 20 times more quickly through tissue layers; transfer is also complete within 0.25 s. Transfer of highly soluble gases, e.g. **carbon monoxide**, is limited by diffusion between alveolus and capillary, because large volumes can be taken up by the blood once they reach it. Transfer of insoluble gases, e.g. N_2O, is limited by blood flow from alveoli, because capillary blood is rapidly saturated.
See also, Carbon dioxide transport; Diffusing capacity; Oxygen transport

Alveolar hypoventilation syndrome, *see Obesity hypoventilation syndrome*

Alveolar recruitment manoeuvre. Technique used in patients receiving **IPPV**, aiming to recruit collapsed alveoli.

Typically, **CPAP** of 30–40 cmH_2O is applied for 20–40 s; alternatively, three 'sighing' breaths at a pressure of 45 cmH_2O may be given. May result in improved oxygenation, although evidence of outcome benefit in patients with **ALI** is inconsistent. May result in reduced cardiac output and hypotension due to reduced venous return.

Alveolar ventilation. Volume of gas entering the alveoli per minute; normally about 4–4.5 l/min. Equals (**tidal volume** minus **dead space**) × respiratory rate; thus rapid small breaths result in a much smaller alveolar ventilation than slow deep breaths, even though **minute ventilation** remains constant. In the upright position, apical alveoli receive less ventilation than basal ones, because the former are already expanded by gravity and are thus less able to expand further on inspiration. Because all the exhaled CO_2 comes from the alveoli, the amount exhaled in a minute equals alveolar ventilation × alveolar concentration of CO_2. Thus alveolar (and hence arterial) CO_2 concentration is inversely proportional to alveolar ventilation, at any fixed rate of CO_2 production.
See also, Ventilation/perfusion mismatch

Alveolitis. Generalised inflammation of lung parenchyma. Classified into:

- idiopathic fibrosing alveolitis: chronic fibroproliferative disease exclusively affecting the lungs, characterised by progressive irreversible fibrosis of the lung parenchyma. Prevalence is 30:100 000; it is most common at 50–60 years. Aetiology is thought to be partly genetic and partly environmental (risk factors include smoking and exposure to wood and metal dust). Recurrent microaspiration of gastric acid due to reflux may contribute. Definitive diagnosis is difficult but relies on **CT scanning** appearances with or without lung biopsy. Has an aggressive course with 50% mortality at 5 years, despite treatment.

  Symptoms include: progressive dyspnoea without wheeze; dry cough; weight loss; and lethargy. Clubbing occurs in 70%–80%. Most striking signs are the very distinctive, fine, end-expiratory crepitations heard at the lung bases and mid-axillary lines. Progresses to central cyanosis, **pulmonary hypertension**, **cor pulmonale** and a restrictive pattern of pulmonary impairment as for **pulmonary fibrosis**. **CXR** may reveal small lung fields with reticulonodular shadowing at lung peripheries and bases.

  Active treatment involves administration of the oral antifibrotic drug pirfenidone, which reduces the rate of fibrosis. **Lung transplantation** may be possible.
- extrinsic allergic alveolitis (hypersensitivity pneumonitis): causative agents include aspergillus (farmer's lung, malt-worker's lung), pituitary extracts (pituitary snuff taker's lung) and avian proteins (bird-fancier's lung). May be:
  - acute: requires initial sensitisation to an antigen. Subsequent exposure results in repeated episodes of dyspnoea, cough, malaise, fever, chills, aches and lethargy. Wheezing is uncommon. Severity depends on the dose of antigen; in very severe cases, life-threatening respiratory failure occurs. Recovery is accelerated by corticosteroids.
  - chronic: less dramatic onset, with a slow increase in dyspnoea with minimal other systemic upset and no acute episodes. May cause cor pulmonale.

  CXR may be normal, but widespread ground-glass appearance in mid and lower zones is common. Lung function is as mentioned earlier, although it may be normal between acute attacks. Other investigations and treatment as mentioned earlier.
- drug-induced alveolitis: patients may present with acute cough, fever and dyspnoea or with slowly progressive dyspnoea. Causal agents include: O_2, nitrofurantoin, **paraquat**, **amiodarone** and **cytotoxic drugs**.
- others: include physical agents (e.g. radiation), **connective tissue diseases**.

All forms may lead to pulmonary fibrosis, which may also occur without generalised alveolitis, e.g. following local disease or aspiration of irritant substances.

Alveolus. Terminal part of the respiratory tree; the site of gas exchange. About 3×10^8 exist in both **lungs**, with estimated total surface area 70–80 m^2. Their walls are composed of a capillary meshwork covered in cytoplasmic extensions of type I pneumocytes. Traditionally thought to conform to the bubble model; i.e., spherical in structure with a thin water lining, with **surfactant** molecules preventing collapse. Electron microscopy, and experimental and mathematical models, have led to alternative theories, e.g. pooling of water at septal corners with dry areas of surfactant in between, and surface tension helping return water to interstitial fluid.

Amantadine hydrochloride. Drug with both **antiparkinsonian** and **antiviral** effects. In **Parkinson's disease**, it improves tremor, rigidity and mild dyskinesia, but only in a small percentage of sufferers. Has been used for the treatment of herpes zoster infections, both during the acute phase and in the treatment of postherpetic pain. Has also been used for prophylaxis of influenza A in very selective groups, but is no longer recommended.

- Dosage:
  - parkinsonism: 100 mg orally od (doubled after 1 week).
  - herpes zoster: 100 mg bd for 14 days.
  - influenza A: 100 mg od for 4–5 days as treatment, 100 mg/day for 6 weeks as prophylaxis.
- Side effects: nausea, dizziness, convulsions, hallucinations, GIT disturbance.

Ambrisentan, *see Endothelin receptor antagonists*

Ambu-bag, *see Self-inflating bags*

Ambu-E valve, *see Non-rebreathing valves*

American Board of Anesthesiology (ABA). Recognised as an independent Board by the American Board of Medical Specialties in 1941, having been an affiliate of the American Board of Surgery since 1938. Issues the Diploma of the ABA.

American Society of Anesthesiologists (ASA). Formed from the American Society of Anesthetists in 1945, to distinguish medically qualified 'anesthesiologists' from 'anesthetists'. The American Society of Anesthetists had been formed in 1936 from the New York Society of Anesthetists, which until 1911 had been the Long Island Society of Anesthetists, founded in 1905. The ASA is concerned with improving the standards, education and audit of anaesthesia, and publishes the journal ***Anesthesiology***.

Amethocaine, *see Tetracaine*

Amfetamine poisoning. Increasingly seen with the rising popularity of crystalline methamphetamine (crystal meth; ice). Overdosage of **amfetamines** may cause anxiety, hyperactivity, tachycardia, hypertension, hallucinations and hyperthermia. Intracranial haemorrhage may accompany acute severe hypertension. The toxic dose is not well defined, as there is a wide variation in response related to tolerance in chronic abusers. Diagnosis is made on the history and clinical grounds, supported by qualitative laboratory analysis (plasma levels are unhelpful in guiding management). Patients should have continuous ECG and core temperature monitoring, and urine analysed for **myoglobin.** Treatment includes general supportive care as for **poisoning and overdoses**, and the use of **chlorpromazine** and **β-adrenergic receptor antagonists** (although β_2-receptor-mediated vasoconstriction in skeletal muscle vessels may increase BP). Forced acid diuresis increases excretion but this should not be undertaken if there is associated **rhabdomyolysis.**

Richards SJR, Albertson TE, Derlet RW, et al (2015). Drug Alcohol Depend; 150: 1–13

Amfetamines (Amphetamines). Group of drugs that promote the release and inhibit the uptake of noradrenaline, dopamine and serotonin at the synaptic cleft, thereby causing stimulation of the central and **sympathetic nervous systems.** Commonly abused, they cause addiction and are controlled drugs. Used in narcolepsy. Increase **MAC** of **inhalational anaesthetic agents.**

See also, Amfetamine poisoning

Amikacin. Antibacterial drug; an **aminoglycoside** with bactericidal activity against some gram-positive and many gram-negative organisms, including pseudomonas. Indicated for the treatment of serious infections caused by gram-negative bacilli resistant to **gentamicin.** Not absorbed from the GIT, it must be given parenterally. Excreted via the kidney.

- Dosage: 7.5 mg/kg im or slowly iv bd/tds up to 15 g over 10 days. One-hour (peak) concentration should not exceed 30 mg/l and predose (trough) level should be less than 10 mg/l.
- Side effects: as for gentamicin.

Amino acids. Organic acid components of **proteins**; they produce polypeptide chains by forming peptide bonds between the amino group of one and the carboxyl group of another, with the elimination of water.

Amino acids from the breakdown of ingested and endogenous proteins form an amino acid pool from which new proteins are synthesised. Amino acids are involved in **carbohydrate** and **fat** metabolism; amino groups may be removed or transferred to other molecules (deamination and transamination, respectively). Deamination results in the liberation of **ammonia,** which may be excreted as urea, or taken up by other amino acids to form amides.

Eight dietary amino acids are essential for life in humans: valine, leucine, isoleucine, threonine, methionine, phenylalanine, tryptophan and lysine. Arginine and histidine are required for normal growth. Other amino acids may be synthesised from carbohydrate and fat breakdown products.

Glutamine, the most abundant amino acid in the body, has a key role in muscle synthesis and immune function, as a **neurotransmitter** and as a major metabolic fuel for enterocytes. Inclusion of **glutamate** in enteral feeds appears to reduce gut permeability and prevents the mucosal atrophy that occurs when food is not given by the enteral route.

Synthetic crystalline amino acid solutions (containing the *l*-isomers) are used as a nitrogen source during **TPN.** The composition of solutions varies considerably by manufacturer, although all provide the essential, and most of the non-essential, amino acids. Enteral feed solutions also include a mixture of amino acids.

See also, Nitrogen balance; Nutrition

γ-Aminobutyric acid (GABA). Inhibitory **neurotransmitter** found in many parts of the CNS. Binds to specific **GABA receptors,** both pre- and postsynaptic, resulting in reduced neuronal excitability by increasing chloride conductance. Many **anticonvulsant drugs** facilitate the action of GABA, emphasising its role in **epilepsy** and the regulation of central activity. It is also an important regulator of muscle tone.

γ-Aminobutyric acid receptors (GABA receptors). Trans-membrane receptors activated by **GABA,** present throughout the CNS. Two classes have been identified:

- $GABA_A$: pentameric ligand-gated ion channel composed of numerous subunit isoforms (e.g. α, β, γ, δ, ε) arranged around a central chloride ion pore (Fig. 7). GABA binds at the interface between α and β subunits, allowing Cl^- to flow into the cell; this lowers the membrane potential and therefore neuronal excitability. Site of action for **benzodiazepines, barbiturates, propofol** and volatile anaesthetic agents, almost all of which potentiate the action of endogenous GABA at low concentrations, while directly activating the receptor at higher concentrations.
- $GABA_B$: G protein-coupled receptor, linked to K^+ and Ca^{2+} channels via phospholipase C and adenylate cyclase. Activation results in increased K^+ and decreased Ca^{2+} conductance, reducing neuronal excitability. Mediate long-acting, tonic inhibitory signalling. Site of action for **baclofen.**

Aminoglycosides. Group of bactericidal **antibacterial drugs.** Includes **amikacin, gentamicin, neomycin, netilmicin, streptomycin** and **tobramycin.**

Active against some gram-positive and many gram-negative organisms. Amikacin, gentamicin and tobramycin are also active against pseudomonas.

Not absorbed from the GIT; must be given parenterally. Excretion is via the kidney and delayed in renal impairment. Side effects include ototoxicity (especially with concurrent **furosemide** therapy) and nephrotoxicity. In pregnancy,

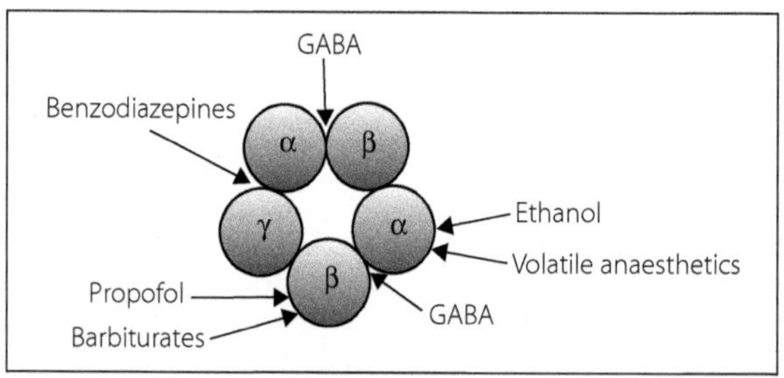

Fig. 7 $GABA_A$ receptor showing GABA and drug binding sites

they may cross the placenta and cause fetal ototoxicity. They may also impair neuromuscular function (by blocking presynaptic release of **acetylcholine**) and therefore avoidance has been suggested in **myasthenia gravis**. Monitoring of plasma levels should ideally be performed in all cases but is especially important in the elderly, children, those with renal impairment, the obese, and if high dosage or prolonged treatment is used. Monitored using 1 h (peak) and predose (trough) samples.

α-Amino-3-hydroxy-5-methyl-4-isoxazolepropionate receptors (AMPA receptors). Transmembrane tetrameric ligand-gated ion channel, activated by **glutamate**. Most abundant receptor in the CNS, it mediates fast synaptic transmission and has a major role in synaptic plasticity and memory formation. Activation by glutamate results in channel opening and influx of cations, mainly Na^+ and Ca^{2+} (depending on subunit composition). The AMPA receptor antagonist perampanel is used to treat **epilepsy**.

2-Amino 2 hydroxymethyl-1,3-propanediol (THAM/Tris). **Buffer** solution that acts both intra- and extracellularly, used extensively in molecular biology. Has been studied for the control of metabolic **acidosis** (e.g. post cardiac arrest) or increased **ICP**, but not currently recommended for clinical practice.

Aminophylline. Phosphodiesterase inhibitor, a mixture of **theophylline** and ethylenediamine, the latter conferring greater solubility than theophylline alone, hence its use iv. Used as a **bronchodilator drug** (but not as first-line therapy), and as an **inotropic drug**, especially in paediatrics.

Causes bronchodilatation, increased diaphragmatic contractility, vasodilatation, increased cardiac output (direct effect on the heart), diuresis (direct effect on the kidney), and CNS stimulation.

- Dosage:
  - 100–500 mg orally bd–qds (depending on the preparation), usually as slow-release preparations. Rectal preparations are no longer used, as they were associated with proctitis and unpredictable response.
  - for emergency iv use, injection of 5–7 mg/kg over 30 min (using ideal weight for height if obese) may be followed by an infusion of 0.5 mg/kg/h (up to 1 mg/kg/h in smokers), with ECG monitoring. Dosage should be reduced in cardiac and hepatic failure, and during therapy with **cimetidine**, **erythromycin** and **ciprofloxacin. Phenytoin**, **carbamazepine** and other enzyme inducers may decrease its **half-life**.
- Side effects: arrhythmias, agitation and convulsions, GIT disturbances.

Patients already on oral treatment should not be given an iv loading dose, because the drug has a low **therapeutic ratio**. Plasma levels should be measured; therapeutic range is 10–20 mg/l.

Amiodarone hydrochloride. Antiarrhythmic drug, used for treating **SVT**, **VT** and **Wolff–Parkinson–White syndrome**. Acts by blocking cardiac K^+ channels, thereby prolonging the cardiac **action potential** and **refractory period**. Hence traditionally designated a class III antiarrhythmic, although also demonstrates class I, II and IV activity. Causes minimal myocardial depression. **Half-life** is over 4 weeks. Acts rapidly following iv administration.

- Dosage:
  - 200 mg orally, tds for 1 week, then bd for a further week, then od for maintenance.
  - as an iv infusion: 5 mg/kg over 20–120 min followed by up to 1.2 g/24 h, with ECG monitoring. (Prefilled syringes of 300 mg are available for VT/**VF** at **cardiac arrest**, with a further 150 mg iv given if required + an infusion of 900 mg/24 h). Bradycardia and hypotension may occur. May cause inflammation of peripheral veins. The dose should be reduced after 1–2 days.
- Side effects: prolonged administration commonly results in corneal microdeposits (reversible, and rarely affecting vision), and may cause photosensitivity, peripheral neuropathy, hyper- or hypothyroidism, hepatitis and pulmonary fibrosis.

Amitriptyline hydrochloride. Tricyclic antidepressant drug. Competitively blocks neuronal uptake of noradrenaline and serotonin. Also has anticholinergic and antihistaminergic properties, thus has marked sedative effects and is well suited for patients with agitated depression. Also used in chronic neuropathic **pain management**, especially when pain prevents sleeping at night. Antidepressant and analgesic effects become apparent after 2–4 weeks' treatment.

- Dosage:
  - depression: 75 mg orally/day (less in the elderly), in divided doses or as a single dose at night, increased up to 150–200 mg/day.
  - pain: 10–75 mg at night.
- Side effects: muscarinic effects include arrhythmias, heart block, dry mouth, urinary retention, blurred vision, constipation; hypersensitivity, blood dyscrasias, hepatic impairment, confusion and convulsions may also occur. Should be avoided in cardiovascular disease.

See also, Tricyclic antidepressant drug poisoning

Ammonia (NH_3). Toxic, colourless, pungent-smelling gas, highly soluble in water. Produced in the GIT by the action of enteric organisms on dietary **proteins** and **amino acids**, and detoxified by transformation in the liver into **urea**. Normal blood level is 100–200 mg/l; levels rise in the presence of severe liver disease or a portal–systemic blood shunt. Ammonia intoxication causes tremor, slurred speech, blurred vision and coma. There is a weak association between blood ammonia level and the degree of hepatic encephalopathy in **hepatic failure**. Rare genetic disorders of the urea cycle (e.g. ornithine carbamoyltransferase deficiency) lead to hyperammonaemia; similarly, treatment with sodium **valproate** may result in raised ammonia levels due to interference with the urea cycle.

Ammonia is also produced in the proximal tubule of the kidney from the breakdown of glutamine. It combines intracellularly with H^+ to form the ammonium ion (NH_4^+), which is secreted by the proximal tubule cells into the tubular filtrate, thereby facilitating regulation of **acid–base balance** and cation conservation. Ammonia formed from the dissociation of NH_4^+ is reabsorbed, recycled and resecreted, primarily by the collecting tubule.

See also, Nitrogen balance

Amnesia. Impairment of **memory**. May occur with intracranial pathology, dementia, metabolic disturbances, **alcoholism** and psychological disturbances. May be caused by **head injury** and drugs. Patients who recover from critical illness may have poor recall of events afterwards.

Retrograde amnesia (between the causative agent/event and the last memory beforehand) is common after head injury. Anterograde amnesia (loss of memory for the period following the causative agent/event) may occur after head injury, and is common after administration of certain drugs, typically **benzodiazepines** and **hyoscine**. Amnesia for intraoperative events may be a factor reducing the incidence of reported **awareness** during anaesthesia.

Amniotic fluid embolism. Condition originally thought to be a mechanical embolic phenomenon caused by entry of amniotic fluid and fetal cells into the maternal circulation; now generally accepted to have a major immunologic component, involving an inflammatory response similar to **anaphylaxis**. The incidence has been quoted as 1:8000–1:80 000 deliveries, the wide range reflecting difficulty in diagnosis; more recent surveillance data, using stricter criteria, suggest an incidence ~1.7 per 100 000 (~1:59 000 deliveries). Traditionally quoted as having a high mortality (30%–60%), though a more recent figure of ~20% has been observed with modern management. May lead to permanent neurological morbidity in ~7% of survivors. Perinatal mortality rate is ~120 per 1000.

Associated with multiple pregnancy, older maternal age, placenta praevia, induction of labour and instrumental delivery. Usually occurs during labour or delivery, although it can present up to 48 h postpartum.

Typical features include fetal distress, **shock** (often profound), **cardiac arrest**, **pulmonary hypertension**, **pulmonary oedema**, **ALI**, cyanosis, **DIC**, vomiting, drowsiness, **convulsions**.

Management involves aggressive supportive treatment, including correction of DIC.

Fitzpatrick KE, Tuffnell D, Kurinczuk JJ, Knight M (2016). Br J Obstet Gynaecol; 123: 100–9

Amoebiasis, *see Tropical diseases*

Amoxicillin (Amoxycillin). Derivative of **ampicillin**, differing only by one hydroxyl group; has similar antibacterial activity but oral absorption is better and unaffected by food in the stomach. Enteral administration produces higher plasma and tissue levels than ampicillin. Combined with β-lactamase inhibitor **clavulanic acid** in **co-amoxiclav**.

- Dosage: 250–1000 mg orally, 500 mg im or 500 mg to 1 g iv tds.
- Side effects: as for ampicillin.

AMPA receptors, *see α-Amino-3-hydroxy-5-methyl-4-isoxazolepropionate (AMPA) receptors*

Ampere. SI **unit** of **current**, one of the seven base (fundamental) units. Defined as the current flowing in two straight parallel wires of infinite length, 1 m apart in a vacuum, that will produce a force of 2×10^{-7} N/m length on each of the wires. In practical terms, represents the amount of charge passing a given point per unit time; a flow of one **coulomb** of electrons per second equates to one ampere of current.

[Andre Ampère (1775–1836), French physicist]

Amphetamine poisoning, *see Amfetamine poisoning*

Amphetamines, *see Amfetamines*

Amphotericin (Amphotericin B). Polyene **antifungal drug**, active against most fungi and yeasts. Not absorbed enterally. Highly protein-bound, it penetrates tissues poorly. Administered orally as a treatment for intestinal candidiasis, or iv for systemic fungal infections. Amphotericin is available encapsulated in liposomes or as a complex with sodium cholesteryl sulfate, both of which reduce its toxicity.

- Dosage: 0.25–5 mg/kg/day iv, depending on the formulation.
- Side effects: renal and hepatic impairment, nausea and vomiting, electrolyte disturbance, especially hypokalaemia, arrhythmias, blood dyscrasias, convulsions, peripheral neuropathy, visual and hearing disturbances. A test dose is recommended before iv administration because of the risk of **anaphylaxis**.

Ampicillin. Broad-spectrum semisynthetic bactericidal **penicillin**. Active against many gram-positive and negative organisms; ineffective against β-lactamase producing bacteria, including *Staphylococcus aureus* and *Escherichia coli*. Only moderately well absorbed orally (~50% of dose) and this is further diminished by food in the gut. Excreted into bile and urine.

- Dosage: 250 mg–1 g orally qds; 500–2000 mg iv or im, 4–6-hourly, depending on indication.
- Side effects: nausea, rash, diarrhoea.

Amplifiers. Electrical devices used to increase the power of an input signal using an external energy source. Widely used in clinical measurement to amplify measured biological electrical potentials (e.g. **ECG**).

- May be described in terms of:
  - degree of **gain** (ratio of output to input signal amplitude).
  - bandwidth (range of frequencies over which the device provides reliable and constant amplification).
  - noise compensation (most clinical amplifiers employ common-mode rejection, whereby only the difference between two signal sources is amplified, and interference that is common to both signals is rejected).

Amrinone lactate. **Phosphodiesterase inhibitor**, used as an **inotropic drug**. Active iv and orally. Increases cardiac output and reduces SVR via inhibition of cardiac and vascular muscle phosphodiesterase. MAP and heart rate are unaltered. **Half-life** is 3–6 h. Not available in the UK. **Milrinone**, a more potent derivative, is less likely to cause side effects (e.g. GIT upset, **thrombocytopenia**).

Amylase. Group of **enzymes** secreted by salivary glands and the pancreas. Salivary amylase (an α-amylase, ptyalin) breaks down starch at an optimal pH of 6.7; consequently it is inactivated by gastric acid. In the small intestine, both salivary and pancreatic α-amylase act on ingested polysaccharides.

Plasma amylase measurements may be useful for the diagnosis of numerous conditions, particularly acute **pancreatitis**. Normal levels are <150 U/l. About 35%–40% of total plasma amylase activity is contributed by the pancreatic isoenzyme. Amylase levels >5000 U/l are suggestive of acute pancreatitis (peak reached within 24–48 h); other intra-abdominal emergencies (e.g. perforated peptic ulcer, mesenteric infarction) are usually associated with lower plasma levels.

See also, Carbohydrates

Anaemia. Reduced **haemoglobin** concentration; usually defined as less than 130 g/l for males, 120 g/l for females. In children, the figure varies: 180 g/l (1–2 weeks of age); 110 g/l (6 months–6 years); 120 g/l (6–12 years).

- Caused by:
  - reduced production:
    - deficiency of iron, **vitamin B_{12}**, folate.
    - chronic disease, e.g. **malignancy**, infection.
    - endocrine disease, e.g. **hypothyroidism, adrenocortical insufficiency**.
    - bone marrow infiltration, e.g. leukaemia, myelofibrosis.
    - aplastic anaemia, including drug-induced, e.g. **chloramphenicol**.
    - reduced **erythropoietin** secretion, e.g. **renal failure**.
    - abnormal red cells/haemoglobin, e.g. sideroblastic anaemia, **thalassaemia**.
  - increased **haemolysis**.
  - acute or chronic **haemorrhage**.
- Investigated by measuring the size and haemoglobin content of **erythrocytes**:
  - hypochromic, microcytic: e.g. thalassaemia, iron deficiency, including chronic haemorrhage, chronic disease.
  - normochromic, macrocytic: vitamin B_{12} or folate deficiency, alcoholism.
  - normochromic, normocytic: chronic disease, e.g. infection, malignancy, renal failure, endocrine disease; aplastic anaemia, bone marrow disease or infiltration.

  Other investigations include examination of blood film (e.g. for sickle cells, parasites, reticulocytes suggesting increased breakdown or haemorrhage), measurement of platelets and white cells, bone marrow aspiration and further blood tests, e.g. iron, vitamin B_{12}.
- Effects:
  - reduced O_2-carrying capacity of blood: fatigue, dyspnoea on exertion, angina.
  - increased cardiac output, to maintain **O_2 flux**: palpitations, tachycardia, systolic murmurs, cardiac failure. Reduced **viscosity** increases **flow** but turbulence is more likely.
  - increased **2,3-DPG**.
  - maintenance of blood volume by **haemodilution**.

Preoperative anaemia (Hb <100 g/l) is associated with a 30% increase in mortality and morbidity and therefore unexpected anaemia should be investigated before routine surgery. The traditional minimal 'safe' haemoglobin concentration for anaesthesia has been 100 g/l, unless surgery is urgent; below this level, reduced O_2 carriage was felt to outweigh the advantage of reduced blood viscosity and increased flow. More recently, 70–100 g/l has been suggested, reflecting the concerns over the complications of **blood transfusion** (except in **ischaemic heart disease**, in which postoperative mortality increases as preoperative haemoglobin concentration falls below around 100 g/l). Reduction of cardiac output during anaesthesia is particularly hazardous. F_IO_2 of 0.5 is often advocated to reduce risk of perioperative hypoxia by increasing the O_2 reserve within the lungs.

Anaemia is common in critical care patients, with 60% having Hb <90 g/l on admission and 80% below this level at 7 days. Multifactorial aetiology includes bone marrow suppression due to sepsis (with low serum iron and low total iron binding capacity) and iatrogenic blood loss due to blood sampling. Studies show that the default target for Hb in ICU patients should be 70–90 g/l unless specific comorbidities exist. Transfusing to above this level increases risk of **MODS** and possibly **ALI**.

Transfused stored blood takes up to 24 h to reach its full O_2-carrying capacity; ideally transfusion should occur at least 1 day preoperatively. Slow transfusion also minimises the risk of fluid overload in chronic anaemia.

Kotze A, Harris A, Baker C, et al (2015). Br J Haematol; 171: 322–31 and Retter A, Wyncoll D, Pearse R, et al (2013). Br J Haematol; 160: 445–64

Anaerobic infection. Caused by:
- obligate anaerobes: only grow in the absence of O_2.
- microaerophilic organisms: only grow under conditions of reduced O_2 tension.
- facultative anaerobes: capable of growing aerobically or anaerobically.

The most clinically important are species of clostridium, bacteroides and actinomyces. Predisposing factors include disruption of mucosal barriers, impaired blood supply, tissue injury and necrosis. Most infecting organisms are endogenous. Infections are accompanied by foul-smelling, putrid pus. Specimens for analysis of possible anaerobic infections may require special anaerobic transport systems as some anaerobic species die if exposed to O_2. **Metronidazole** is especially active against anaerobes.

See also, Clostridial infections

Anaerobic threshold. Conventionally defined as the work rate at which metabolic acidosis and associated changes in gas exchange occur. A theoretical measure of overall cardiopulmonary function, derived from **cardiopulmonary exercise testing**. Commonly estimated using the inflection point of the oxygen consumption/carbon dioxide production curve (Fig. 8). The sudden increase in $\dot{V}CO_2/\dot{V}O_2$ is traditionally ascribed to increased buffering of lactic acid by HCO_3^- (thereby generating 'excess' CO_2), although this is controversial. Has been used to predict outcome from major surgery, an anaerobic threshold of <10–11 ml/kg/min suggesting a greater risk of death, especially if associated with high risk surgery and/or **ischaemic heart disease**.

Hopker JG, Jobson SA, Pandit JJ (2011). Anaesthesia; 66: 111–23

***Anaesthesia*.** Official journal of the **Association of Anaesthetists of Great Britain and Ireland**, first published in 1946.

Anaesthesia (from Greek: an + aisthesis; without feeling). Term suggested by Oliver Wendell **Holmes** in 1846 to describe the state of sleep produced by ether; the word had been used previously to describe lack of feeling, e.g.

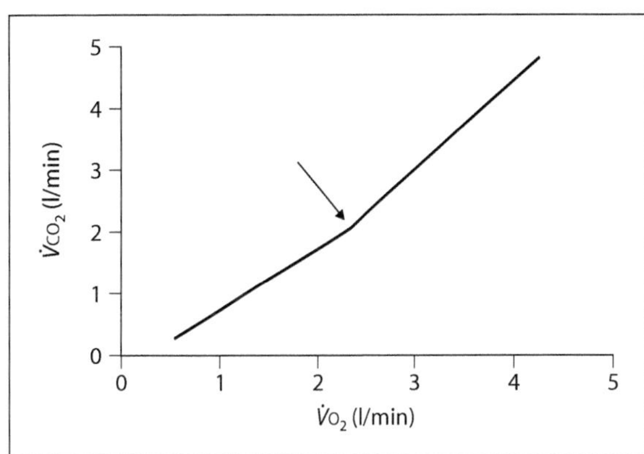

Fig. 8 Anaerobic threshold *(arrowed)*

due to peripheral neuropathy. He introduced derived terms, e.g. 'anaesthetic agent'.

Anaesthesia and Intensive Care. Official journal of the Australian Society of Anaesthetists (formed in 1935) since its launch in 1972. Also the official journal of the Australian and New Zealand Intensive Care Society and the New Zealand Society of Anaesthetists.

Anaesthesia, balanced, *see Balanced anaesthesia*

Anaesthesia crisis resource management, *see Crisis resource management*

Anaesthesia, depth of. Anaesthesia is generally accepted as being a continuum in which increasing depth of anaesthesia results in loss of consciousness, recall, and somatic and autonomic reflexes. It has also been argued that, while these are the effects of anaesthetic drugs in increasing dosage, 'anaesthesia' itself occurs at a particular undefined point, and is therefore either present or absent.

Assessment is important in order to avoid inadequate anaesthesia with **awareness** and troublesome reflexes, or overdose.

- Methods of assessment:
  - clinical:
    - stages of anaesthesia (see *Anaesthesia, stages of*).
    - signs of inadequate anaesthesia:
      - lacrimation.
      - tachycardia.
      - hypertension.
      - sweating.
      - reactive dilated pupils.
      - movement, laryngospasm.

      These signs may be altered by anaesthetic drugs themselves, and by others, e.g. opioids, **atropine**, neuromuscular blocking drugs.
    - **isolated forearm technique.**
  - **EEG**:
    - conventional EEG: bulky and difficult to interpret. Poor correlation between different anaesthetic agents.
    - **cerebral function monitor** and **analysing monitor**: easier to use and read, but less informative than conventional EEG. Rarely used now.
    - **power spectral analysis**: graphic display of complicated data; easier to interpret than conventional EEG. The **bispectral index monitor**, E-Entropy and Narcotrend-Compact M monitors are increasingly used. These monitors use proprietary algorithms to convert raw EEG data into a single number that is claimed to represent global activity; titration of anaesthesia in order to keep the value within defined limits may thus reduce both awareness and overdosage, although their efficacy remains controversial.
  - **evoked potentials**: similar effects are produced by different anaesthetic agents.
  - **oesophageal contractility**: affected by smooth muscle relaxants and ganglion blocking drugs, also by disease, e.g. **achalasia.**
  - **EMG**: particularly of the frontalis muscle. Requires separate monitoring of peripheral neuromuscular blockade in addition.

Stein EJ, Glick DB (2016). Curr Opin Anaesthesiol; 29: 711–6

Anaesthesia dolorosa. Pain in an anaesthetic area, typically following destructive treatment of **trigeminal neuralgia.** Unpleasant symptoms, ranging from paraesthesia to severe pain, develop in the area of the face rendered anaesthetic, and may be more distressing than the original symptoms. Anaesthesia dolorosa may develop many months after the lesion, and is often refractory to further treatment, including deep brain stimulation and **dorsal root entry zone procedures.** Limited success has been reported with **gabapentin.**

Anaesthesia, history of

- Early attempts at pain relief:
  - **opium** used for many centuries, especially in the Far East. First injected iv by Wren in 1665.
  - use of other plants and derivatives for many centuries, e.g. **cocaine (cocada), mandragora, alcohol.**
  - **acupuncture.**
  - unconsciousness produced by carotid compression.
  - analgesia produced by cold (**refrigeration anaesthesia**), compression and ischaemia: 1500–1600s.
  - **mesmerism**: 1700–1800s.
- General anaesthesia:
  - effects of **diethyl ether** on animals described by **Paracelsus**: 1540.
  - understanding of basic physiology, especially respiratory and cardiovascular, and isolation of many gases, e.g. O_2, CO_2, N_2O: 1600–1700s.
  - N_2O suggested for analgesia by **Davy** in 1799.
  - CO_2 inhalation to produce insensibility described by **Hickman** in 1824.
  - use of **diethyl ether** for anaesthesia by **Long, Clarke**: 1842.
  - use of N_2O for anaesthesia by **Wells, Colton**: 1844.
  - first public demonstration of ether anaesthesia in Boston by **Morton**: 16 October 1846 (*see Bigelow; Holmes; Warren*).
  - first UK use by Scott in Dumfries, Scotland, on 19 December 1846, news of Morton's demonstration in Boston having travelled to Dumfries with Fraser, ship's surgeon aboard the Royal Mail steamship *Acadia*. Used in London by Squire 2 days later (*see Liston*).
  - **chloroform** introduced by **Simpson**: 1847.
  - first deaths, e.g. **Greener**: 1848.
  - development in UK led by **Snow**, then **Clover.**
  - **rectal administration of anaesthetic agents** described.
  - iv anaesthesia produced with **chloral hydrate** by **Oré**: 1872.
  - ether versus chloroform: the former was favoured in England and northern USA, the latter in Scotland and southern USA. Other agents introduced (*see Inhalational anaesthetic agents*). **Boyle** machine described 1917.
  - iv anaesthesia popularised by Weese, **Lundy** and **Waters**: 1930s (*see Intravenous anaesthetic agents*). Neuromuscular blockade introduced by **Griffith**: 1942. **Halothane** introduced 1956.
  - UK pioneers: **Hewitt, Macewen, Magill, Rowbotham, Macintosh** (first UK professor), **Hewer, Organe.**
  - US pioneers: Waters (first university professor), **Guedel, McKesson, Crile, McMechan, Lundy.**
  - UK: **Association of Anaesthetists** founded 1932; **DA examination** 1935; **Faculty of Anaesthetists** 1948; **FFARCS** examination 1953; **College of Anaesthetists** 1988; **Royal College of Anaesthetists** 1992.
  - USA: **American Society of Anesthesiologists** founded 1945.

- **World Federation of Societies of Anaesthesiologists** founded 1955.
- Local anaesthesia:
  - cocaine isolated 1860.
  - topical anaesthesia produced by **Koller**: 1884.
  - **regional anaesthesia** performed by **Halsted** and **Hall**: 1884; **Cushing**: 1898.
  - **spinal anaesthesia** by **Corning**: 1885; **Bier**: 1898.
  - **epidural anaesthesia** 1901.
  - pioneers: **Braun, Lawen, Labat.**

[Sir Christopher Wren (1632–1723), English scientist and architect; William Scott (1820–1887) and William Fraser (1819–1863), Scottish surgeons; Helmut Weese (1897–1954), German pharmacologist]

See also, Cardiopulmonary resuscitation; Intermittent positive pressure ventilation; Intensive care, history of; Intubation, tracheal; Local anaesthetic agents

Anaesthesia, mechanism of. The precise mechanism is unknown, but theories are as follows:

- anatomical level:
  - midbrain **ascending reticular activating system**, thalamus, and cerebral cortex are considered the most likely anatomical sites of action as studies show preferentially depressed glucose uptake in these regions during anaesthesia.
  - **spinal cord** is also affected by anaesthetics, which decrease both afferent and efferent neuronal activity.
  - synaptic sites are thought to be more important than axonal sites, because the former are blocked more easily than the latter at clinically effective concentrations of anaesthetic agent. Inhalational agents inhibit excitatory presynaptic activity at nicotinic, glutaminergic and serotonergic receptors while also potentiating inhibitory glycine and **GABA receptors**.
- cellular level:
  - now accepted to act at specific neuronal protein targets, including:
    - $GABA_A$ receptors: known target for barbiturates, benzodiazepines, propofol and volatile agents, all of which potentiate GABA-mediated inhibition of neuronal activity.
    - **NMDA receptors**: known target for **ketamine**.
    - two-pore domain K^+ channels: activated by volatile agents, resulting in membrane hyperpolarisation and reduced excitability.

Previously suggested but now discarded theories:

- disruption of lipid bilayers/non-specific membrane expansion; initially suggested by the observation that the potency of volatile agents is related to their lipid solubility (**Meyer–Overton rule**). However, this does not explain the **cut-off effect** or the lack of potentiation of anaesthetics by heat.
- **clathrate** theory (water hydrates of anaesthetic agents).
- Ferguson's thermodynamic activity theory: related activity to the chemical composition of the agent concerned, by determining the energy contained within the chemical bonds of its molecules. Related to lipid solubility and other physical properties.
- **Bernard** suggested that anaesthetics caused intracellular protein coagulation.

[J Ferguson (described 1939), English scientist]

Brown EN, Lydic R, Schiff ND (2010). N Engl J Med; 363: 2638–50

Anaesthesia, one-lung, *see One-lung anaesthesia*

Anaesthesia Practitioners, *see Physician's Assistants (Anaesthesia)*

Anaesthesia, stages of. In 1847, **Snow** described five stages of narcotism, although a less detailed classification had already been described. The classic description of anaesthetic stages was by **Guedel** in 1937 in unpremedicated patients, breathing **diethyl ether** in air:

- stage 1 (analgesia):
  - normal reflexes.
  - ends with loss of the eyelash reflex and unconsciousness.
- stage 2 (excitement):
  - irregular breathing, struggling.
  - dilated pupils.
  - vomiting, coughing and laryngospasm may occur.
  - ends with the onset of automatic breathing and loss of the eyelid reflex.
- stage 3 (surgical anaesthesia):
  - plane I:
    - until eyes centrally placed with loss of conjunctival reflex.
    - swallowing and vomiting depressed.
    - pupils normal/small.
    - lacrimation increased.
  - plane II:
    - until onset of intercostal paralysis.
    - regular deep breathing.
    - loss of corneal reflex.
    - pupils becoming larger.
    - lacrimation increased.
  - plane III:
    - until complete intercostal paralysis.
    - shallow breathing.
    - light reflex depressed.
    - laryngeal reflexes depressed.
    - lacrimation depressed.
  - plane IV:
    - until diaphragmatic paralysis.
    - carinal reflexes depressed.
- stage 4 (overdose):
  - apnoea.
  - dilated pupils.

With modern agents and techniques, the stages often occur too rapidly to be easily distinguished.

The stages may be seen in reverse order on emergence from anaesthesia.

See also, Anaesthesia, depth of

Anaesthesia, total intravenous, *see Total intravenous anaesthesia*

Anaesthetic accidents, *see Anaesthetic morbidity and mortality*

Anaesthetic agents, *see Inhalational anaesthetic agents; Intravenous anaesthetic agents; Local anaesthetic agents*

Anaesthetic breathing systems

- Definitions:
  - open: unrestricted ambient air as the fresh gas supply.
  - semi-open: as above, but some restriction to air supply, e.g. enclosed mask.

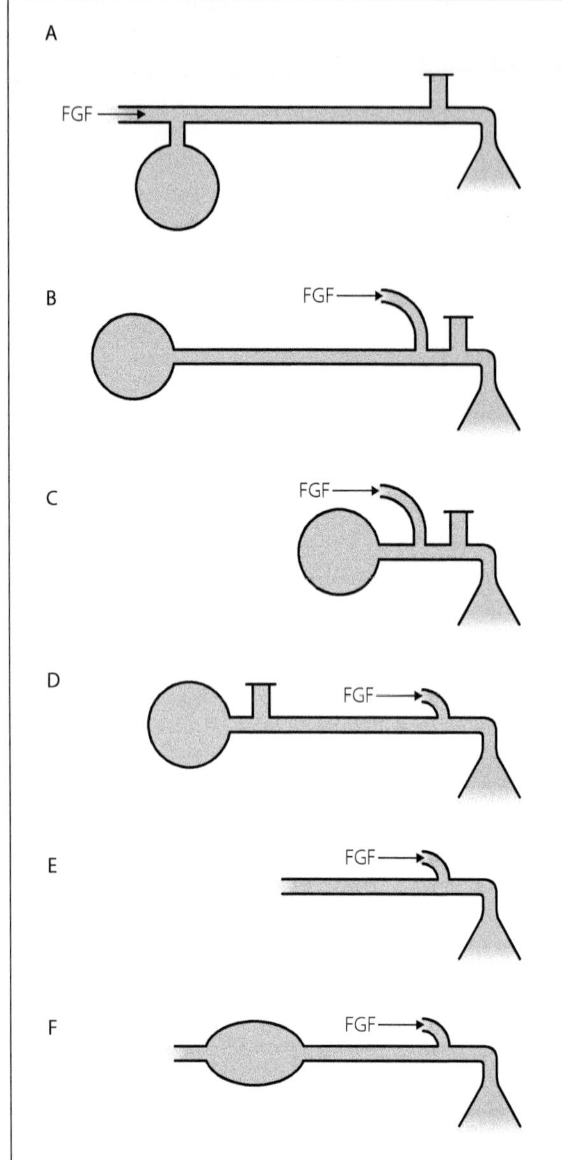

Fig. 9 Nomenclature of anaesthetic breathing systems (*see text*)

- closed: totally closed circle system.
- semi-closed: air intake prevented but venting of excess gases allowed. Divided by Mapleson into five groups, A to E, in 1954; a sixth (F) was added later (Fig. 9). Arranged in order of decreasing efficiency in eliminating carbon dioxide during spontaneous ventilation.

- Mapleson's nomenclature (excludes **open drop techniques**, **circle systems**, and use of **non-rebreathing valves**):
  - Mapleson A (**Magill** attachment):
    - most efficient for spontaneous ventilation, because exhaled dead-space gas is reused at the next inspiration, and exhaled alveolar gas passes out through the valve. Thus fresh gas flow (FGF) theoretically may equal alveolar minute volume (70 ml/kg/min).
    - inefficient for IPPV, because some fresh gas is lost through the valve when the bag is squeezed, and exhaled alveolar gas may be retained in the system and rebreathed. High gas flows are therefore needed (2–3 times minute volume).
  - Mapleson B and C: rarely used, other than for resuscitation. Inefficient; thus 2–3 times minute volume is required.
  - Mapleson D:
    - inefficient for spontaneous ventilation, because exhaled gas passes into the **reservoir bag** with fresh gas, and may be rebreathed unless FGF is high. Suggested values for FGF range from 150 to 300 ml/kg/min (i.e., 2–4 times minute ventilation); resistance to breathing may be a problem at high FGF.
    - efficient for IPPV; exhaled dead-space gas passes into the bag and is reused but when alveolar gas reaches the bag, the bag is full of fresh gas and dead-space gas; alveolar gas is thus voided through the valve. Theoretically, 70 ml/kg/min will maintain normocapnia.
  - Mapleson E (Ayre's T-piece): used for children, because of its low resistance to breathing. To prevent breathing of atmospheric air, the reservoir limb should exceed tidal volume. A FGF of 2–4 times minute volume is required to prevent rebreathing. May be used for IPPV by intermittent occlusion of the reservoir limb outlet.
  - Mapleson F (Jackson–Rees modification): adapted from Ayre's T-piece. The bag allows easier control of ventilation, and its movement demonstrates breathing during spontaneous ventilation. Suggested FGF: 2–4 times minute volume for spontaneous ventilation. For IPPV, 200 ml/kg/min has been suggested, although more complicated formulae exist.
- Modifications include:
  - coaxial versions of the A and D systems (Lack and Bain, respectively): the valve is accessible to the anaesthetist for adjustment and **scavenging**, and the tubing is longer and lighter.
  - Humphrey ADE system: valve and bag are at the machine end, with a lever incorporated within the valve block; may be converted into type A, D or E systems depending on requirements.
  - enclosed afferent reservoir system: resembles the Mapleson D with an additional reservoir placed on the FGF limb. This reservoir is enclosed within a chamber that connects to the main limb such that compressing the original reservoir bag (e.g. manually) causes the additional reservoir to be compressed too, increasing the tidal volume delivered. The system (in a more sophisticated form, including a bellows as the additional reservoir) has been incorporated within a ventilator system; although it has been shown to be efficient during both spontaneous and controlled ventilation, it is not widely used.

British and International Standard taper sizes of breathing system connections are 15 mm for tracheal tube **connectors** and paediatric components, and 22 mm for adult components. Some components have both external tapers of 22 mm, and internal tapers of 15 mm. Some paediatric equipment has 8.5 mm diameter fittings, although not standard. Upstream parts of connections are traditionally 'male', and fit into the 'female' downstream parts.

[William W Mapleson, Cardiff physicist; Philip Ayre (1902–1980), Newcastle anaesthetist; Gordon Jackson Rees

(1918–2000), Liverpool anaesthetist; David Humphrey, South African physiologist and anaesthetist]
Conway CM (1985). Br J Anaesth; 57: 649–57
See also, Adjustable pressure-limiting valve; Catheter mounts; Coaxial anaesthetic breathing systems; Facemasks; Tracheal tubes; Valveless anaesthetic breathing systems

Anaesthetic drug labels, *see Syringe labels*

Anaesthetic machines. Term commonly refers to machines providing continuous flow of anaesthetic gases (cf. **intermittent-flow anaesthetic machines**). The original **Boyle** machine was developed in 1917 at St Bartholomew's Hospital, although similar apparatus was already being used in America and France.

- Usual system:
  - **piped gas supply** or **cylinders**.
  - **pressure gauges** may indicate pipeline, cylinder or regulated (reduced) pressure (*see Pressure measurement*).
  - **pressure regulators** provide constant gas pressure, usually about 400 kPa (4 bar) in the UK. Pipelines are already at this pressure.
  - **flowmeters**, usually **Rotameters**. Some modern machines have electronically controlled gas flow, with visual displays that may resemble traditional 'tube' flowmeters or dials.
  - **vaporisers**.
  - pressure relief valve downstream from the vaporisers protects the flowmeters from excessive pressure; it opens at about 38–40 kPa. May be combined with a non-return valve.
  - O_2 flush; bypasses flowmeters and vaporisers, delivering at least 35 l/min.
  - **O_2 failure warning device.**
  - **ventilators**, **monitoring** equipment, **suction equipment** and various **anaesthetic breathing systems** may be incorporated.
- Modern safety features reduce the risk of:
  - delivering hypoxic gas mixtures:
    - to avoid incorrect gas delivery:
      - **pin index system** for cylinders and non-interchangeable connectors for piped gas outlet.
      - colour coding of pipelines and cylinders.
      - O_2 analyser.
      - O_2 flowmeter control is bigger and has a different profile from others; it is positioned in the same place on all machines (on the left in the UK; on the right in the USA).
      - linkage between N_2O and O_2 Rotameters, so that less than 25% O_2 cannot be 'dialled up', e.g. **Quantiflex apparatus** and newer machines.
    - to avoid O_2 leak: O_2 flowmeter feeds downstream from the others; thus a cracked CO_2 Rotameter leaks N_2O in preference to O_2.
    - to avoid risk of O_2 delivery failure:
      - O_2 pressure gauge.
      - O_2 failure warning device; preferably switching off other gas flows and allowing air to be breathed.
      - O_2 analyser.
  - delivering excessive CO_2 (e.g. caused by the CO_2 flowmeter opened fully, with the bobbin hidden at the top of the flowmeter tube):
    - maximal possible CO_2 flow is limited, e.g. to 500 ml/min.
    - bobbin is clearly visible throughout the length of the Rotameter tube.
    - CO_2 cylinder is connected to the machine only when specifically required.
  - delivering excessive pressures:
    - **adjustable pressure-limiting valve** on breathing systems: modern ones allow maximal pressures of ~70 cmH_2O when fully closed. Many ventilators also have cut-off maximal pressures.
    - distensible **reservoir bag**; maximal pressure attainable is about 60 cmH_2O. Pressure reaches a plateau as the bag distends, falling slightly (**Laplace's law**) before bursting.
- Other safety features:
  - switches to prevent **soda lime** being used with **trichloroethylene** (older machines).
  - **key filling system** for vaporisers. Interlocks between vaporisers prevent concurrent administration of more than one volatile agent.
  - negative and positive pressure relief valves within **scavenging** systems.
  - **antistatic precautions.**

Thompson PW, Wilkinson DJ (1985). Br J Anaesth; 57: 640–8
See also, Checking of anaesthetic equipment

Anaesthetic morbidity and mortality. Complications during and following anaesthesia are difficult to quantify, because many may be related to surgery or other factors. Many are avoidable, and may be more disturbing to the patient than the surgery itself.

- Examples:
  - tracheal intubation difficulties (*see Intubation, complications of*).
  - **sore throat.**
  - damage to **teeth**, mouth, **eyes**, etc.
  - respiratory complications: **hypoventilation**, **atelectasis**, **chest infection**, **PE**, **pneumothorax**, **aspiration pneumonitis**, **airway obstruction**, **bronchospasm.**
  - cardiovascular complications: **MI**, **hypertension/hypotension**, **gas embolism**, **arrhythmias.**
  - **blood transfusion** hazards.
  - thrombophlebitis/pain at injection or infusion sites.
  - extravasation of injectate/intra-arterial injection.
  - severe neurological complications: **stroke**, brain damage, spinal cord infarction; they often follow severe hypotension/cardiac arrest/hypoxia.
  - **awareness.**
  - drowsiness, confusion, psychological changes, **postoperative cognitive dysfunction.**
  - **PONV.**
  - headache: often related to perioperative dehydration and starvation. **Post-dural puncture headache.**
  - **nerve injury** and damage related to **positioning of the patient.**
  - muscle pains following **suxamethonium.**
  - backache: especially after lithotomy position. Reduced by lumbar pillows.
  - falls during transfer from/to trolleys.
  - burns, e.g. from **diathermy.**
  - **adverse drug reactions**, e.g. halothane hepatitis, **MH.**
  - drug overdose.
  - renal impairment, e.g. following uncorrected hypotension.
  - **death.**
- Mortality may be related to anaesthesia, surgery or the medical condition of the patient. Mortality studies in

the UK, USA, Canada, Scandinavia, Europe and Australia have tended to implicate similar factors:
- preoperatively:
  - inadequate assessment and/or involvement of senior staff.
  - hypovolaemia and inadequate resuscitation.
- perioperatively:
  - aspiration.
  - inadequate **monitoring**.
  - intubation difficulties.
  - delivery of hypoxic gas mixtures and equipment failure.
  - inexperience/inadequate supervision.
- postoperatively:
  - inadequate observation.
  - hypoventilation due to respiratory depression, residual neuromuscular blockade and respiratory obstruction.
- Morbidity and mortality are thus reduced by:
  - thorough **preoperative assessment** and adequate resuscitation.
  - **checking of anaesthetic equipment** and drugs.
  - adequate monitoring.
  - anticipation of likely problems.
  - attention to detail.
  - adequate **recovery** facilities.
  - adequate supervision/assistance.

Clear contemporaneous **record-keeping** promotes careful perioperative monitoring and assists retrospective analysis of complications and future anaesthetic management.
See also, Audit; Confidential Enquiries into Maternal Deaths, Report on; Confidential Enquiry into Perioperative Deaths

Anaesthetic rooms (Induction rooms). Usual in the UK but not used in many other countries.
- Advantages:
  - quiet area for induction of anaesthesia and teaching.
  - less frightening for the patient than lying on the operating table. Allows parents to be present during induction of anaesthesia in children.
  - anaesthetists' domain; i.e., without pressure from surgeons.
  - store for anaesthetic drugs and equipment.
  - increased throughput of the operating suite, if another anaesthetist is available to start while previous cases are being completed in theatre.
- Disadvantages:
  - expensive duplication of equipment is required, e.g. anaesthetic machine, monitoring, scavenging.
  - monitoring is disconnected during transfer of the patient.
  - transfer and positioning for surgery are more hazardous with the patient anaesthetised than when awake.
  - equipment, iv fluids and drugs may not be immediately available in the operating theatre.

The above disadvantages lead many anaesthetists to induce anaesthesia in the operating theatre for high-risk patients. Continued existence of anaesthetic rooms is controversial. Holding areas capable of processing many patients at once (allowing premedication and performance of regional blocks) have been suggested as an alternative.
Meyer-Witting M, Wilkinson DJ (1992). Anaesthesia; 47: 1021–2

Anaesthetic simulators, *see Simulators*

Anaesthetists' non-technical skills (ANTS). Defined as the cognitive, social and personal resource skills that complement technical skills, contributing to the safe and efficient delivery of anaesthesia. Long recognised to play a major role in crisis management and error prevention; recent interest in objectively assessing and developing these skills has led to the development of the ANTS taxonomy. This consists of an assessment system addressing skills relating to four categories: team working; decision-making; task management; and situation awareness. Each skill is assessed on a four-point scale.

Largely used in the **simulator** setting; elements of the system have recently been incorporated into formal workplace-based assessment tools.
Flin R, Patey R, Glavin R, Maran N (2010). Br J Anaesth; 105: 38–44
See also, Crisis resource management; Fixation error

Analeptic drugs. Drugs causing stimulation of the CNS as their most prominent action (many other drugs also have stimulant properties, e.g. **aminophylline**).
- Mechanism of action:
  - block inhibition, e.g. strychnine (via **glycine** antagonism), picrotoxin (via **GABA** antagonism).
  - increase excitation, e.g. **doxapram**, nikethamide.

Doxapram increases respiration via stimulation of peripheral chemoreceptors. All the analeptics may cause cardiovascular stimulation, and convulsions at sufficient doses.

Analgesia. Lack of sensation of **pain** from a normally painful stimulus.
See also, Analgesic drugs

Analgesic drugs. May be divided into:
- **opioid analgesic drugs.**
- inhibitors of **prostaglandin** synthesis:
  - **NSAIDs.**
  - **paracetamol.**
- others:
  - **inhalational anaesthetic agents**, e.g. N_2O, **trichloroethylene.**
  - **ketamine.**
  - **clonidine.**
  - **cannabis.**
  - **flupirtine.**
  - **nefopam.**
  - **local anaesthetic agents.**
- adjuncts: i.e., reduce pain or pain sensation by alternative means: e.g. **antidepressant drugs, corticosteroids, carbamazepine, gabapentin,** muscle relaxants, e.g. **diazepam.** Used widely in chronic **pain management. Caffeine** is often included in oral analgesic preparations.

Analgesic drugs are distinguished from anaesthetic agents by their ability to reduce pain sensation without inducing sleep; thus N_2O is a good analgesic but a poor anaesthetic, and sevoflurane has poor analgesic properties but is a potent anaesthetic. In practice the distinction is not precise, as analgesic drugs, e.g. opioids, will cause unconsciousness at high doses, and anaesthetic drugs, e.g. sevoflurane, will abolish pain sensation at deep planes of anaesthesia.

Anaphylaxis. Severe, life-threatening, generalised or systemic hypersensivity reaction. The term has traditionally been reserved for type I immune reactions in which cross-linking of two **immunoglobulin** type E (reagin) molecules by an antigen on the surface of **mast cells** results in the release of **histamine** and other vasoactive substances, e.g. **kinins, 5-HT** and **leukotrienes.** Type G immunoglobulin may also be involved. 'True' anaphylaxis requires previous exposure to the antigen responsible, sometimes many exposures; e.g. anaphylaxis to **thiopental** classically occurs after more than 10 exposures. However, in 80% of cases no prior exposure is evident.

Reactions not involving IgE cross-linking (and therefore not requiring prior exposure to the causative agent, unless the classical **complement** pathway is involved) have been termed 'anaphylactoid', but current European guidelines recommend avoidance of this term, because the clinical presentation and management of both types are identical. Such reactions may involve direct histamine release from mast cells (typically **radiological contrast media**, certain **neuromuscular blocking drugs**, e.g. **atracurium, tubocurarine**), or activation of complement via either classical or alternative pathways (e.g. **Althesin**).

More common when drugs are given iv. More common in women, which has led to the suggestion that exposure to cosmetics may 'prime' the reaction. Anaphylaxis to antibiotics is more common in smokers, possibly due to prior priming from multiple courses for chest infections. Patients with a history of atopy/asthma may have an increased risk of latex and radiological contrast media-associated anaphylaxis.

Incidence during anaesthesia is estimated at 1 in 10 000–20 000 anaesthetics, but with considerable variation between countries. Agents most commonly implicated are: neuromuscular blocking drugs (60%–70%), especially **suxamethonium; latex** (10%–20%); and **antibacterial drugs** (10%–15%; N.B. current opinion is that patients allergic to penicillin are not more likely to react to third- or fourth-generation **cephalosporins**). Mortality is approximately 5%.

Has been classified clinically into five grades:

- I: cutaneous: erythema, urticaria, angio-oedema.
- II: as above plus hypotension, tachycardia, bronchospasm.
- III: as above but severe; collapse, arrhythmias.
- IV: cardiac and/or respiratory arrest.
- V: death.

Clinical presentation is variable, although 70%–90% of patients have cutaneous features and 20%–40% have bronchospasm. Hypotension is the only feature in ~10%.

- Immediate management:
  - removal of potential triggers; call for help.
  - 'ABC' approach to assessment and treatment; intubation if necessary and administration of 100% O_2 and iv fluids. The patient's legs should be raised if there is hypotension. **CPR** if indicated.
  - **adrenaline** im (0.5–1.0 ml of 1:1000 every 10 min as required) or iv (0.5–1.0 ml of 1:10 000 slowly, repeated as required) (*see Adrenaline for more details of dosage*). IV infusion of adrenaline or **noradrenaline** may be required after initial treatment.

    Alternative vasoconstrictors in resistant cases include: **metaraminol**; **glucagon** (1–5 mg iv then 5–15 μg/min), e.g. if the patient is taking β-blockers; and **vasopressin** (5 IU, repeated as necessary). **Bronchodilator drugs**, e.g. **salbutamol**, may also be required.
- Secondary management includes **antihistamine drugs**, e.g. **chlorphenamine** 10–20 mg slowly iv (**H_2 receptor antagonists** have been suggested but current UK guidelines do not support their use), and **hydrocortisone** 100–200 mg iv. **Bicarbonate** therapy may be required according to **blood gas interpretation**.

Blood samples should be taken for subsequent testing (*see Adverse drug reactions*).

AAGBI (2009). Anaesthesia; 64: 199–211

Aneroid gauge, *see Pressure measurement*

***Anesthesia and Analgesia*.** Oldest current journal of anaesthesia, first published in 1922 as *Current Researches in Anesthesia and Analgesia* (the journal of the National Anesthesia Research Society, which became the International Anesthesia Research Society (IARS) in 1925). The official journal of the IARS; also affiliated with several other anaesthetic and related societies.

Craig DB, Martin JT (1997). Anesth Analg; 85: 237–47

***Anesthesiology*.** Journal of the **American Society of Anesthesiologists**, first published in 1940.

Anesthesiology. American term describing the practice of anaesthesia by trained physicians (anesthesiologists) as opposed to others who might administer anaesthetics (e.g. nurse anesthetists). Formally accepted as a specialty by the American Medical Association in 1940. In the UK, the term 'anaesthetist' implies medical qualification.

Angina, *see Ischaemic heart disease; Myocardial ischaemia*

Angio-oedema. Tissue swelling resulting from allergic reactions. Spread of oedema through subcutaneous tissue often involves the periorbital region, lips, tongue and oropharynx. Life-threatening **airway obstruction** may occur. Common precipitants include plants, foodstuffs (e.g. shellfish, nuts) and drugs (especially **angiotensin converting enzyme inhibitors**). Acute swelling often settles after about 6 h, although treatment of a severe life-threatening attack should follow the management of **anaphylaxis**.

Certain forms of angio-oedema result from a deficiency of C1-esterase inhibitor, either acquired or hereditary. Colicky abdominal pain or severe respiratory obstruction often occurs. Treatment of attacks resulting from these forms includes androgens (e.g. danazol), plasminogen inhibitors or replacement of C1-esterase inhibitor (as fresh frozen plasma or in a synthetic form).

See also, Complement; Hereditary angio-oedema

Angioplasty, *see Percutaneous coronary intervention*

Angiotensin converting enzyme inhibitors (ACE inhibitors). Originally isolated from snake venom. Used in the treatment of **hypertension** and **cardiac failure**, they have been shown to reduce mortality in cardiac failure associated with **MI**. They block the action of angiotensin converting enzyme; apart from converting angiotensin I to angiotensin II, this enzyme breaks down **kinins**, naturally occurring vasodilators. The ACE inhibitors cause vasodilatation and a drop in BP that may be profound after the first dose. Side effects include hypotension, rashes, leucopenia, renal and hepatic damage, loss of taste, **angio-oedema**, pancreatitis, GIT disturbance, myalgia, dizziness, headache and cough. Severe hypotension may follow induction of anaesthesia or perioperative haemorrhage, especially if the patient is fluid- and/or sodium-depleted (e.g. taking

diuretics). Should be used with caution in patients with renovascular disease.

Captopril and **enalapril** were the first and second ACE inhibitor introduced, respectively; others include benazepril, cilazapril, fosinopril, imidapril, lisinopril, moexipril, perindopril, quinapril, ramipril and trandolapril.
See also, Renin/angiotensin system

Angiotensin II receptor antagonists. **Antihypertensive drugs**, also shown to reduce mortality in **cardiac failure**; competitively inhibit angiotensin II at its AT_1 receptor subtype on arteriolar smooth muscle, thus less likely than **angiotensin converting enzyme inhibitors** to cause systemic side effects, including those related to interaction with other hormone systems (e.g. involving **kinins**), or **renin/angiotensin system** imbalance. However, may cause hypotension or **hyperkalaemia**, and should be used with caution in renal artery stenosis. Other side effects include rash, urticaria, **angio-oedema**, myalgia, GIT disturbance and dizziness. Losartan was the first to be developed; others include azilsartan, candesartan, eprosartan, irbesartan, olmesartan, telmisartan and valsartan.

Angiotensins, *see Renin/angiotensin system*

Anidulafungin. **Antifungal drug** used for treatment of invasive candida infection.
- Dosage: 200 mg by iv infusion on the first day, 100 mg daily thereafter.
- Side effects: GIT upset, headaches, seizures, coagulopathy, allergic reactions, electrolyte disturbances.

Animal bites, *see Bites and stings*

Anion gap. Difference between measured cation and anion concentrations in the plasma. Sodium concentrations exceed chloride plus bicarbonate concentrations by 4–11 mmol/l (the range has changed in recent years as modern methods of measuring electrolytes give rise to higher normal values for chloride concentrations). Anionic proteins, phosphate and sulfate make up the difference. Of use in the differential diagnosis of metabolic **acidosis**; anionic gap increases when organic anions accumulate, e.g. in **lactic acidosis**, **ketoacidosis**, uraemia. It does not increase in acidosis due to loss of bicarbonate or intake of hydrochloric acid. Not an infallible tool because other cations such as potassium, calcium and magnesium may influence the calculation. Anion gap has also been compared with alterations in plasma bicarbonate levels ($\delta AG/\delta HCO_3^-$ ratio). It has also been calculated for urine electrolytes.
Glasmacher SA, Stones W (2016). BMC Anesthesiol 30; 16: 68

Ankle–Brachial Pressure Index (ABPI). Measure of peripheral vascular disease, calculated by dividing the systolic pressure in the leg (best results are obtained if the dorsalis pedis and posterior tibial artery pressures are averaged) by the systolic pressure in the arms (average of left and right brachial artery pressures). Normally 0.91–1.3, with values >1.3 suggesting poor arterial compressibility due to medial arterial calcification while values of <0.9, <0.7 and <0.4 indicate mild, moderate and severe disease, respectively. Has been used to predict cardiovascular morbidity and mortality and distinguish **atherosclerosis** from other causes of leg pain.

Ankle, nerve blocks. Useful for surgery distal to the ankle.
- Nerves to be blocked are as follows (Fig. 10):
  - tibial nerve (L5–S3): lies posterior to the posterior tibial artery, between flexor digitorum longus and flexor hallucis longus tendons. Divides into lateral and medial plantar nerves behind the medial malleolus. Supplies the anterior and medial parts of the sole of the foot. A needle is inserted lateral to the posterior tibial artery at the level of the medial malleolus, or medial to the Achilles tendon if the artery cannot be felt. It is passed anteriorly and 5–10 ml **local anaesthetic agent** injected as it is withdrawn.
  - sural nerve (L5–S2): formed from branches of the tibial and common peroneal nerves. Accompanies the short saphenous vein behind the lateral malleolus and supplies the posterior part of the sole, the back of the lower leg, the heel and lateral side of the foot. Subcutaneous infiltration is performed from the Achilles tendon to the lateral malleolus, using 5–10 ml solution.
  - deep and superficial peroneal nerves (both L4–S2): the deep peroneal nerve supplies the area between the first and second toes. It lies between anterior tibial (medially) and extensor hallucis longus (laterally) tendons, lateral to the anterior tibial artery. A needle is inserted between these tendons; a click may be felt as it penetrates the extensor retinaculum.

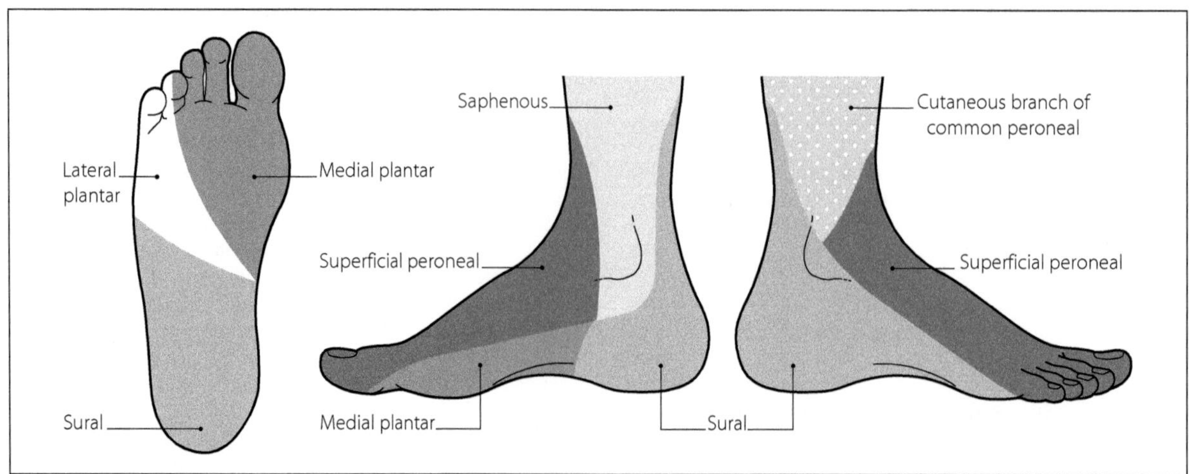

Fig. 10 Cutaneous innervation of the ankle and foot

5 ml solution is injected. The superficial peroneal nerve is blocked by subcutaneous infiltration from the lateral malleolus to the front of the tibia. It supplies the dorsum of the foot.
    - saphenous nerve (L3–4): the terminal branch of the femoral nerve; blocked by subcutaneous infiltration above and anterior to the medial malleolus. It supplies the medial side of the ankle joint.

Increasingly performed using **ultrasound** guidance, which allows more accurate placement and reduced volumes of local anaesthetic agent.

Purushothaman L, Allan AGL, Bedforth N (2013). Cont Educ Anaesth Crit Care Pain; 13: 174–8

Ankylosing spondylitis. Disease characterised by inflammation and fusion of the sacroiliac joints and lumbar vertebrae (resulting in 'bamboo spine'); may also involve the thoracic and cervical spine. Five times more common in males, with a high proportion carrying tissue type antigen HLA B27.

- Features:
    - backache and stiffness. Spinal cord compression may occur; atlantoaxial subluxation or cervical fracture may also occur. **Spinal/epidural anaesthesia** may be difficult.
    - restricted ventilation if thoracic spine or costovertebral joints are severely affected; increased diaphragmatic movement usually preserves good lung function. **Pulmonary fibrosis** is rare.
    - tracheal intubation may be difficult due to a stiff or rigid neck, or **temporomandibular joint** involvement. Cricoarytenoid involvement may result in stridor.
    - aortitis may occur (in less than 5% of chronic sufferers), causing **aortic regurgitation. Cardiomyopathy** and conduction defects are rare.
    - amyloidosis may occur.

Woodward JL, Kam PCA (2009). Anaesthesia; 64: 540–8

Anorexia nervosa. Psychiatric condition, most common in young women. Characterised by loss of weight, distortion of body image and amenorrhoea; the last results from weight loss, and psychological and endocrine factors. Quoted mortality is 4%–18%.

- Anaesthetic considerations:
    - electrolyte disturbances, especially **hypokalaemia**, are associated with laxative abuse or self-induced vomiting.
    - tendency towards hypothermia, hypotension and bradycardia.
    - ECG changes occur in 80% and include AV block, **prolonged Q–T syndrome**, ST wave depression and T wave inversion. **Mitral valve prolapse** more common.
    - **aspiration pneumonitis** and pneumomediastinum may result from self-induced vomiting.
    - increased risk of infection due to leucopenia.
    - reduced lean body mass, osteoporosis.
    - **anaemia**.
    - psychiatric co-morbidity, including depression.
    - rarer complications: myopathy, **cardiomyopathy**, peripheral neuritis, hepatic impairment, gastric dilatation. Treatment includes behavioural and psychotherapy; deep brain stimulation is under investigation. **Chlorpromazine** has also been used.

Hirose K, Hirose M, Tanaka K, et al (2014). Br J Anaesth; 112: 246–54

Anrep effect. Intrinsic regulatory mechanism of the heart; contractility increases in response to acute increases in **afterload**. Initial reduction in stroke volume and increase in left ventricular diastolic pressure are followed by restoration to near original values. May be related to changes in myocardial perfusion.

[Gleb V Anrep (1890–1955), Russian-born Egyptian physiologist]

Yentis SM (1998). J Roy Soc Med; 91: 209–12

Anrep, Vassily (1852–1927). Russian scientist and medico-politician. Described the pharmacology of **cocaine** in 1880 and was the first person to describe the numbing effect of sc injection; he went on to perform the first nerve blocks (intercostal), publishing his results in Russian in 1884 but failing to publicise his work more widely. His son Gleb described the **Anrep effect**.

Yentis SM (1999). Anesthesiology; 90: 890–5

Antacids. Used to relieve pain in **peptic ulcer disease**, **hiatus hernia** and **gastro-oesophageal reflux** by increasing gastric pH. Used preoperatively in patients at high risk of **aspiration of gastric contents** (e.g. in obstetrics) to reduce the risk/severity of ensuing pneumonitis, should aspiration occur. Also used on ICU as prophylaxis against **stress ulcers**. Many preparations are available; **sodium citrate** is most commonly used in anaesthetic practice. Chronic overuse of antacids may result in **alkalosis, hypercalcaemia** (calcium salts), constipation (aluminium salts) and diarrhoea (magnesium salts).

Antagonist. Substance that opposes the action of an agonist.

- Antagonism may be:
    - competitive: the substance reversibly binds to a receptor, and causes no direct response within the cell (i.e., has no **intrinsic activity**), but may cause a response by displacing an agonist, e.g. **naloxone**.
    - non-competitive: as above, but with irreversible binding, e.g. **phenoxybenzamine**.
    - physiological: opposing actions are produced by binding at different receptors, e.g. **histamine** and **adrenaline** causing bronchoconstriction and bronchodilatation, respectively.

See also, Dose–response curves; Receptor theory

Antanalgesia. Increased sensitivity to painful stimuli caused by small doses of depressant drugs, e.g. **thiopental.** Thought to result from suppression of the inhibitory action of the **ascending reticular activating system**, allowing increased cortical responsiveness (decreased pain threshold). Larger doses depress the activating system and induce sleep. Antanalgesia may also occur as blood drug levels fall, e.g. causing postoperative restlessness when barbiturates or **alimemazine** are used as premedication, especially in children. It may also be seen in opioid naïve subjects given **naloxone**.

Antecubital fossa (Cubital fossa). Triangular fossa, anterior to the elbow joint (Fig. 11).

- Borders:
    - proximal: a line between the humeral epicondyles.
    - lateral: brachioradialis muscle.
    - medial: pronator teres.
    - floor: supinator and brachialis muscles, with the joint capsule behind.
    - roof: deep fascia with the median cubital vein and medial cutaneous nerve on top.

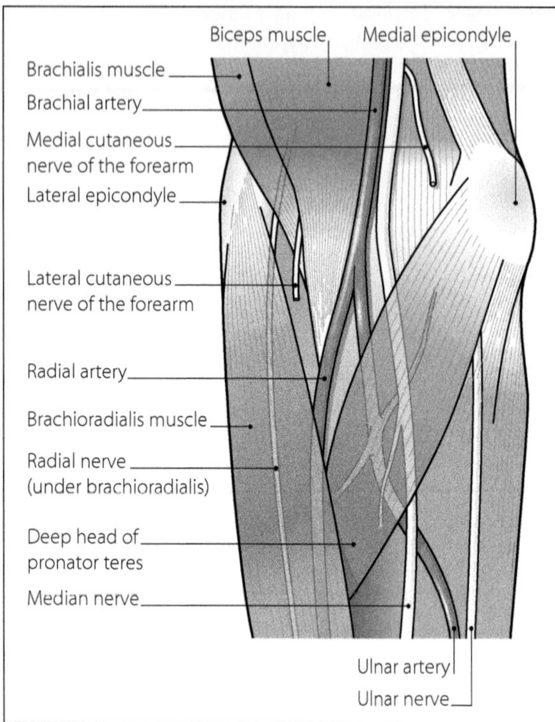

Fig. 11 Anatomy of the antecubital fossa

- Contents from medial to lateral (embedded in fat):
  - **median nerve**.
  - **brachial artery**, dividing into **radial** and **ulnar arteries**.
  - biceps tendon.
  - posterior interosseous and **radial nerves**.

The bicipital aponeurosis lies between the superficial veins and deeper structures, protecting the latter during venepuncture. Damage may still be caused to nerves and arteries during this procedure; anomalous branches are relatively common. Accidental intra-arterial injection of drugs is a particular hazard.
See also, Venous drainage of arm

Antepartum haemorrhage (APH). Defined as vaginal bleeding after 22 weeks' gestation. Occurs in up to 5% of all pregnancies. Most cases are not severe and are associated with various conditions, including infection. Two conditions affecting the **placenta** are of particular importance to the anaesthetist because they may cause sudden and severe collapse and rapid exsanguination, although this extreme is fortunately rare:
  - **placenta praevia**: the placenta encroaches upon or covers the cervical os. Presents with vaginal bleeding, usually in the third trimester; there may be fetal distress. Unless the mother is at risk of exsanguination, delivery of the fetus by **caesarean section** should wait until adequate blood has been obtained and appropriate staff are present, because the mother is not at risk of developing coagulopathy unless massive transfusion is required. Particularly high risk if associated with abnormal placentation; the placenta may invade (placenta accreta) or even penetrate (placenta percreta) the uterine wall. Haemorrhage may be torrential, requiring hysterectomy. Placenta accreta/percreta is more common if there has been prior uterine surgery, e.g. myomectomy or caesarean section, the risk increasing with each previous procedure.
  - **placental abruption**: haemorrhage behind the placenta. May present with abdominal pain and fetal distress, usually in the third trimester; vaginal bleeding is not always present. Caesarean section should not be delayed because there is a risk of developing **DIC** if the fetus is not delivered, this risk increasing the longer the wait. Has been associated with renal cortical necrosis.

Anaesthetic management includes standard resuscitation and techniques of **obstetric analgesia and anaesthesia**; the choice of regional versus general anaesthesia depends on the cardiovascular stability, estimated blood loss, presence of fetal distress, whether there is a coagulopathy and the preferences of the anaesthetist, obstetrician and patient. Postpartum observation is important because adequate fluid balance and urine output must be maintained; in addition placenta praevia in particular predisposes to **postpartum haemorrhage** because the uterine lower segment is not able to contract as effectively as the more muscular upper segment.

Anterior spinal artery syndrome. Infarction of the **spinal cord** due to anterior spinal artery insufficiency. May follow profound **hypotension**, e.g. in **spinal** or **epidural anaesthesia**. May also occur after aortic surgery. Results in lower **motor neurone** paralysis at the level of the lesion, and spastic paraplegia with reduced pain and temperature sensation below the level. Because the posterior spinal arteries supply the dorsal columns and posterior horns, joint position sense and vibration sensation are preserved.

Anthrax, *see Biological weapons*

Antiarrhythmic drugs. Classified by Vaughan Williams into four classes, depending on their effects on the **action potential** in vitro. A fifth class has been suggested that includes a number of miscellaneous drugs (e.g. **digoxin**, and other **cardiac glycosides**, **adenosine**, **magnesium**) that do not fit into the standard four classes (Table 6). More usefully classified for clinical purposes according to their site of action:
  - atrioventricular node: **calcium channel blocking drugs**, **digoxin**, **β-adrenergic receptor antagonists**, adenosine (used for supraventricular arrhythmias).
  - atria, ventricles and accessory pathways: **quinidine**, **procainamide**, **disopyramide**, **amiodarone** (used for supraventricular and ventricular arrhythmias) and dronedarone (used to maintain sinus rhythm after successful cardioversion for atrial fibrillation).
  - ventricles only: **lidocaine**, **mexiletine**, **phenytoin** (used for ventricular arrhythmias).

[EM Vaughan Williams (1918–2016), English pharmacologist]
See also, individual arrhythmias

Antibacterial drugs. Drugs used to kill **bacteria** (bactericidal) or inhibit bacterial replication (bacteriostatic).

Antibiotics are synthesised by micro-organisms and kill or inhibit other micro-organisms. Drugs synthesised in vitro, e.g. sulfonamides, are not antibiotics.
- Classified by mechanism of action into:
  - agents inhibiting cell wall synthesis (bactericidal):
    - **β-lactams**: include **penicillins**, **cephalosporins**, **aztreonam**, **carbapenems**.

Table 6 Classification of antiarrhythmic drugs

Class	Action	Examples
I	Slow depolarisation rate by inhibiting sodium influx	
a	Prolong action potential	Quinidine Procainamide Disopyramide
b	Shorten action potential	Lidocaine Mexiletine Phenytoin
c	No effect on action potential	Flecainide Propafenone Encainide
II	Diminish effect of catecholamines	β-Adrenergic receptor antagonists Bretylium
III	Prolong action potential, without affecting depolarisation rate	Amiodarone Sotalol Bretylium
IV	Inhibit calcium influx	Calcium channel blocking drugs
V	Miscellaneous	Digoxin Adenosine Magnesium

  - other cell wall inhibitors: **vancomycin**, β-lactamase inhibitors (**clavulanic acid**, tazobactam), **polymyxins**, **teicoplanin**, bacitracin.
- agents inhibiting protein synthesis:
  - anti-30S ribosomal unit: **aminoglycosides**, e.g. **gentamicin**, **netilmicin** (bactericidal), **tetracyclines** (bacteriostatic).
  - anti-50S ribosomal unit: **macrolides**, e.g. **erythromycin** (bacteriostatic), **chloramphenicol** (bacteriostatic), **clindamycin** (bacteriostatic), **linezolid** (variable), **quinupristin/dalfopristin** (combination bactericidal).
  - anti-70S ribosomal unit: **capreomycin**.
  - inhibition of amino acid transfer: **fusidic acid**.
- agents inhibiting nucleic acid synthesis (bacteriostatic):
  - DNA synthesis inhibitors: **4-quinolones** (e.g. **ciprofloxacin**, nalidixic acid), **metronidazole**.
  - RNA synthesis inhibitors: **rifampicin**.
- agents inhibiting mycolic acid synthesis (bacteriostatic): **isoniazid**, **ethambutol**.
- agents inhibiting folic acid synthesis: **sulfonamides**, **trimethoprim**: each alone is bacteriostatic; the combination (**co-trimoxazole**) is bactericidal.
- other mechanisms: **pyrazinamide**.

Choice of antibacterial drug depends on the organism involved (or suspected), the severity of the condition and the site of the infection. In many conditions, initial therapy is based on a 'best guess' principle with broad-spectrum drugs, narrower therapy being continued when the results of culture and sensitivity studies are known. The requirement for prompt treatment in severe illness may conflict with the need to obtain adequate samples for culture before therapy is started. Much concern exists about the increasing problem of **bacterial resistance**.

See also, Antifungal drugs; Antiviral drugs

Antibiotics, *see Antibacterial drugs*

Antibodies, *see Immunoglobulins*

Anticholinergic drugs. Strictly, should include all drugs impairing cholinergic transmission, although the term usually refers to **antagonists** at muscarinic **acetylcholine receptors** (antagonists at nicotinic receptors are classified as either **ganglion blocking drugs** or **neuromuscular blocking drugs**). In general, effects are 'antiparasympathetic', and include tachycardia, bronchodilatation, mydriasis, reduced gland secretion, smooth muscle relaxation, and sedation or restlessness. Anaesthetic uses include the treatment of **bradycardia**, as a component of **premedication** and antagonism of the cardiac effects of **acetylcholinesterase inhibitors**.

- In anaesthesia, the most commonly used agents are **atropine**, **hyoscine** and **glycopyrronium**. Comparison of actions:
  - atropine:
    - central excitation.
    - greater action than hyoscine on the heart, bronchial smooth muscle and GIT.
  - hyoscine:
    - central depression; amnesia (may cause excitement/confusion in the elderly).
    - greater action than atropine on the pupil and sweat, salivary and bronchial glands.
  - glycopyrronium:
    - minimal central effects (quaternary ammonium ion; crosses the **blood–brain barrier** less than atropine and hyoscine, both tertiary ions).
    - similar peripheral actions to atropine, but with greater antisialagogue effect and less effect on the heart. Less antiemetic action than hyoscine and atropine.
    - longer duration of action.
- Other uses of anticholinergic drugs include:
  - antispasmodic effect (on bowel and bladder), e.g. propantheline.
  - ulcer healing, e.g. pirenzepine.
  - bronchodilatation, e.g. **ipratropium**.
  - mydriasis and cycloplegia (dilatation of pupil and paralysis of accommodation), e.g. atropine.

Anticholinergic **antiparkinsonian drugs**, e.g. **benzatropine**, **procyclidine**, orphenadrine, are used for their central effects.

See also, Central anticholinergic syndrome

Anticholinesterases, *see Acetylcholinesterase inhibitors*

Anticoagulant drugs. Mechanisms of action:
- prevent synthesis of **coagulation** factors, e.g. **warfarin**.
- inhibit existing factors, e.g. **heparin**, **factor Xa inhibitors**, **thrombin inhibitors**.
- inhibit **platelet** aggregation, i.e., **antiplatelet drugs**.
- break down circulating fibrinogen, e.g. ancrod (snake venom derivative; not commonly used).

Fibrinolytic drugs break down thrombus once formed. Warfarin and heparin are more effective at preventing venous thrombus than arterial thrombus, as the former contains relatively more fibrin. Antiplatelet drugs are more effective in arterial blood, where thrombus contains many platelets and little fibrin.

Anticonvulsant drugs. Heterogeneous group of drugs used to treat **epilepsy**. Classified according to their main mechanism of action, although all act either to suppress excitatory neuronal activity or to facilitate inhibitory impulses:
- neuronal sodium channel blockade, e.g. **sodium valproate**, **phenytoin**, **carbamazepine**, oxcarbazepine, **lamotrigine**, zonisamide, **lacosamide**.

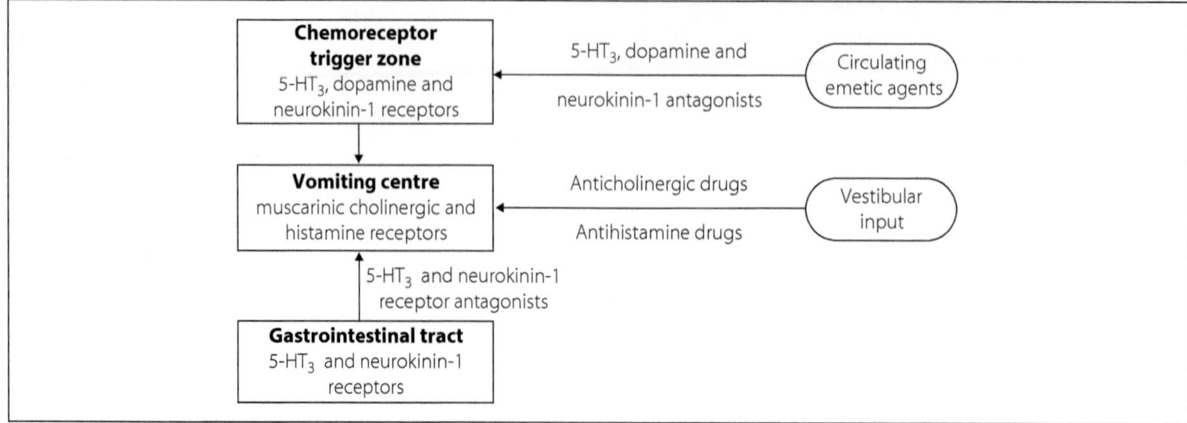

Fig. 12 Sites of action of different antiemetic drugs

- calcium channel blockade, e.g. carbamazepine, **ethosuximide**.
- increase in **GABA** levels:
  - $GABA_A$ receptor agonists, e.g. **benzodiazepines**, **barbiturates**.
  - GABA transaminase inhibitors, e.g. **vigabatrin**.
  - GABA uptake inhibitors, e.g. tiagabine.
  - glutamic acid decarboxylase inhibitors, e.g. **gabapentin**, sodium valproate.
- **glutamate** receptor blockers, e.g. felbamate, topiramate
- unknown action: **levetiracetam**.

Choice of drug depends on the type of seizures, absence of side effects and teratogenesis in women of child-bearing age. NICE guidelines (2012) suggest carbamazepine as the first-line drug for focal or generalised tonic–clonic seizures, sodium valproate for tonic or atonic seizures, levetiracetam for myoclonic seizures and ethosuximide for absence attacks. About 50% of epileptic patients can be managed with one anticonvulsant drug.

First-line management of **status epilepticus** involves use of iv **lorazepam. Diazepam**, phenytoin, **fosphenytoin** and **thiopental** are also used.

For patients undergoing surgery, anticonvulsant therapy should continue up to operation, and restart as soon as possible postoperatively. If oral therapy is delayed postoperatively, parenteral administration may be substituted. Phenobarbital and phenytoin cause hepatic **enzyme induction**, increasing the metabolism of certain drugs.

Bialer M, White HS (2010). Nat Rev Drug Discov; 9: 68–82

See also, γ-Aminobutyric acid (GABA) receptors

Antidepressant drugs. Most increase central amine concentrations (e.g. **dopamine**, **noradrenaline**, **5-HT**), supporting the theory that depression results from amine deficiency. Further evidence is that central depletion (e.g. by **reserpine**) may cause depression.

- May be classified into:
  - **tricyclic antidepressant drugs**: block noradrenaline and 5-HT uptake from synapses.
  - **selective serotonin reuptake inhibitors** (SSRIs): specifically block reuptake of 5-HT, e.g. citalopram, fluoxetine, sertraline.
  - serotonin and noradrenaline reuptake inhibitors e.g. venlafaxine, duloxetine.
  - noradrenaline and specific serotoninergic antidepressants e.g. mianserin, mirtazapine.
  - **monoamine oxidase inhibitors** (MAOIs): prevent catecholamine breakdown.
  - others, e.g. **lithium** (mechanism of action unknown), reboxetine (selective noradrenaline reuptake inhibitor).

Perioperative problems arising from concurrent antidepressant therapy may occur, particularly with MAOIs.

Antidiuretic hormone, *see Vasopressin*

Antiemetic drugs.

- Site of action (Fig. 12):
  - vomiting centre: **anticholinergic** and **antihistamine drugs**.
  - **chemoreceptor trigger zone** (CTZ): **dopamine receptor** antagonists (e.g. **phenothiazines**, **butyrophenones** and **metoclopramide**) and **5-HT$_3$ receptor antagonists**.
  - GIT: metoclopramide increases **lower oesophageal sphincter** tone and gastric emptying by a peripheral action.
  - **neurokinin-1 receptor antagonists** (e.g. **aprepitant**): originally developed for use in cancer chemotherapy.
  - others:
    - **dexamethasone**: mechanism of action is uncertain.
    - **cannabis** derivatives (e.g. **nabilone**) have been used in the treatment of chemotherapy-induced emesis.
    - **midazolam** on induction of anaesthesia has been shown to reduce **PONV**.

Dopamine antagonists are suitable for treatment of **vomiting** associated with **morphine**, which stimulates the CTZ. Increased vestibular stimulation of the vomiting centre, e.g. in motion sickness, is best treated with drugs acting on the vomiting centre, e.g. **hyoscine**. Sedation is a common side effect, particularly of antihistamines, anticholinergic drugs and phenothiazines. In addition, phenothiazines may cause hypotension, and all dopamine antagonists may cause **dystonic reactions**.

Anti-endotoxin antibodies. Antibodies directed against various parts of gram-negative **endotoxins**, investigated as possible treatment of severe **sepsis**. Theoretically, antibodies against the inner core of endotoxin (which is conserved among many different bacteria) should provide protecting against many organisms. One product (HA-1A; Centoxin) was introduced in 1991 for use in humans, but was withdrawn in 1993 following evidence that it might increase mortality in patients without gram-negative bacteraemia.

Antifibrinolytic drugs. Drugs that prevent dissolution of fibrin. Include **aprotinin**, ε-aminocaproic acid (no longer available in the UK) and **tranexamic acid**, which inhibit plasminogen activation and thus reduce fibrinolysis. Used perioperatively to reduce surgical blood loss (e.g. in cardiac surgery and obstetric haemorrhage), and in **trauma**.
Ortmann E, Besser MW, Klein AA (2013). Br J Anaesth; 111: 549–63
See also, Coagulation

Antifungal drugs. Heterogeneous group of drugs active against fungi. Includes:
- polyenes (**amphotericin**, **nystatin**).
- imidazoles (e.g. clotrimazole, **ketoconazole**, **miconazole**).
- triazoles (**fluconazole**, **itraconazole**, **voriconazole**).
- others (**anidulafungin**, **caspofungin**, **flucytosine**, griseofulvin).

Antigen. Substance that may provoke an immune response, then react with the cells or antibodies produced. Usually a protein or carbohydrate molecule. Some substances (called haptens), too small to provoke immune reactions alone, may combine with host molecules, e.g. proteins, to form a larger antigenic combination.

Antigravity suit. Garment used to apply pressure to the lower half of the body, in order to increase blood volume in the upper half and prevent hypotension, e.g. in the sitting position in **neurosurgery**. Systolic BP and CVP are increased; the latter may aid prevention of **gas embolism**. Modern suits are inflated pneumatically around the legs and abdomen, to a pressure of 2–8 kPa.

Military antishock trousers (MAST) have been used in **trauma** to produce similar effects. They also splint broken bones and apply pressure to bleeding points.

Antihistamine drugs. Usually refers to H_1 **histamine** receptor antagonists.
- Uses:
  - prevention or treatment of allergic disorders, e.g. hay-fever, urticaria, drug reactions, e.g. **chlorphenamine**.
  - for **sedation** or **premedication**, e.g. **promethazine** and **alimemazine**.
  - prevention/treatment of nausea and **vomiting**, e.g. cinnarizine, **cyclizine** (act on vomiting centre).

They have anticholinergic effects (e.g. dry mouth, blurring of vision, urinary retention). Newer drugs, e.g. terfenadine, cross the blood–brain barrier to a lesser extent, causing less sedation.
See also, H_2 receptor antagonists

Antihypertensive drugs. Drugs used to reduce BP may act at different sites (Fig. 13):
- **diuretics**: reduce **ECF** volume initially and cause vasodilatation (1).
- **vasodilator drugs**: act on the vascular smooth muscle (2), either directly, e.g. **hydralazine, sodium nitroprusside**, or indirectly, e.g. **α-adrenergic receptor antagonists, calcium channel blocking drugs, angiotensin II receptor antagonists, potassium channel activators.** A direct renin inhibitor, aliskiren, is now available. **Angiotensin converting enzyme inhibitors** also decrease water and sodium retention.

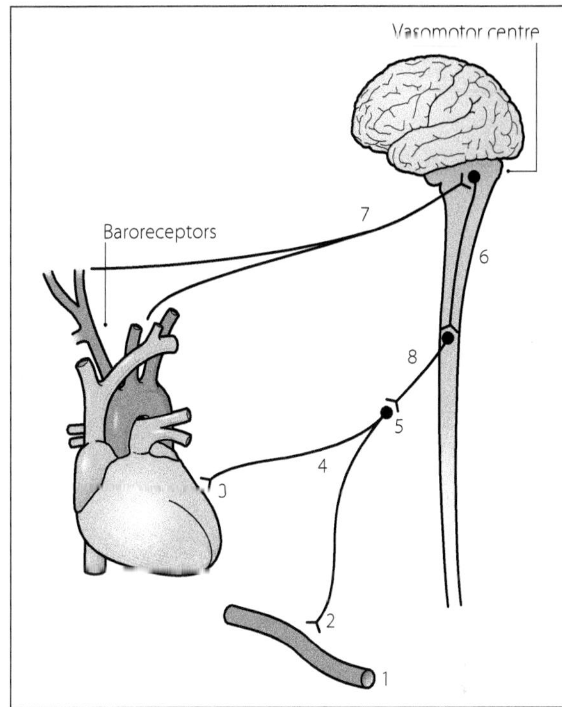

Fig. 13 Sites of action of antihypertensive drugs (*see text*)

- **β-adrenergic receptor antagonists**: lower cardiac output (3).
- adrenergic neurone blocking drugs (4): e.g. **guanethidine** depletes nerve endings of noradrenaline, preventing its release. **Reserpine** prevents storage and release of noradrenaline. **α-Methyl-p-tyrosine** inhibits dopa formation from tyrosine.
- **ganglion blocking drugs** (5).
- centrally acting drugs (6): reduce sympathetic activity, e.g. reserpine, **α-methyldopa, clonidine, moxonidine.**

In addition, anaesthetic agents and techniques may reduce BP; e.g. **halothane** depresses **baroreceptor** activity (7) and also reduces sympathetic activity and cardiac output; **spinal** and **epidural anaesthesia** block sympathetic outflow (8).

In the treatment of **hypertension**, oral vasodilators (except for α-adrenergic receptor antagonists) and thiazide diuretics are used most commonly. **NICE** (2011) suggests a stepwise introduction of various antihypertensive agents depending on age and ethnicity (*see* Fig. 86, **Hypertension**).

Ganglion blockers, adrenergic neurone blocking drugs and the centrally acting drugs are seldom used, because of their side effects.

In the treatment of a **hypertensive crisis**, vasodilator drugs are often given iv. For patients undergoing surgery, antihypertensive drugs should be continued up to operation, and recommenced as soon as possible postoperatively.
See also, Hypotensive anaesthesia

Anti-inflammatory drugs, *see Non-steroidal anti-inflammatory drugs; Corticosteroids*

Antimalarial drugs. Used for:
- prophylaxis: no drugs give absolute protection against **malaria**. Treatment should begin at least 1 week before travel to an endemic area (to ensure patient tolerance) and continued for at least 4 weeks after leaving. Drugs used depend upon

the area to be visited and include **chloroquine** + proguanil, atovaquone + proguanil, mefloquine and doxycycline.
- treatment:
  - falciparum malaria: for mild infection either oral **quinine** + doxycycline, co-artem (artemether + lumefantrine), or atovaquone + proguanil are equally effective. For severe infection: iv quinine followed by oral quinine + doxycycline when the patient is recovering.
  - benign (non-falciparum) malaria: chloroquine is the drug of choice ± primaquine.

White NJ, Pukrittayakamee S, Hien TT (2014). Lancet; 383: 723–35

Antimitotic drugs. *see Cytotoxic drugs*

Antiparkinsonian drugs, Drug treatment of **Parkinson's disease** is directed towards increasing central dopaminergic activity or decreasing cholinergic activity:
- increasing **dopamine**:
  - levodopa: crosses the **blood–brain barrier** and is converted to dopamine by dopa decarboxylase. Decarboxylase inhibitors (carbidopa, benserazide), which do not cross the blood–brain barrier, prevent peripheral dopamine formation, thus reducing the dose of levodopa required and the incidence of side effects. Entacapone prevents peripheral breakdown of levodopa by inhibiting **catechol-*O*-methyl transferase** and is used in combination with decarboxylase inhibitors in severe cases.

    Levodopa is most effective for bradykinesia. Its use may be limited by nausea and vomiting, dystonic movements, postural hypotension and psychiatric disturbances. Improvement is usually only temporary and may exhibit 'on–off' effectiveness.
  - bromocriptine, lisuride, pergolide and **apomorphine**: dopamine agonists. Ropinirole is a selective D_2 receptor agonist. Pramipexole is a D_2 and D_3 agonist.
  - **amantadine**: increases release of endogenous dopamine.
  - selegiline: monoamine oxidase inhibitor type B.
  - **amfetamines** have been used.
- anticholinergic drugs, e.g. **atropine**, **benzatropine**, **procyclidine**, trihexyphenidyl: most effective for rigidity, tremor and treatment of drug-induced parkinsonism. For acute drug-induced **dystonic reactions**, benzatropine 1–2 mg or procyclidine 5–10 mg may be given iv. There is a higher risk of intraoperative arrhythmias and labile BP in patients taking these drugs.

Connolly BS, Lang AE (2014). J Am Med Assoc; 311: 1670–83

Antiphospholipid syndrome, *see Coagulation disorders*

Antiplatelet drugs. Reduce **platelet** adhesion and aggregation, thereby inhibiting intraluminal thrombus formation. May act via different mechanisms:
- inhibition of platelet **cyclo-oxygenase** and **thromboxane** α_2 production; may be reversible (e.g. **prostacyclin**) or irreversible (e.g. low-dose **aspirin** and other **NSAIDs**).
- increased intraplatelet **cAMP** levels, e.g. **dipyridamole**.
- glycoprotein IIb/IIIa receptor antagonists (e.g. **abciximab**, **eptifibatide**, **tirofiban**); block the site at which fibrinogen, **von Willebrand** factor and adhesive proteins bind to platelets. Reversible and short-acting.
- platelet ADP receptor antagonists (e.g. **clopidogrel**, **prasugrel**, **ticagrelor**, ticlopidine). Inhibition blocks the glycoprotein IIb/IIIa pathway. Irreversible and long-acting.

Used to improve cerebral, peripheral and coronary blood supply in vascular disease, and to prevent thromboembolism. Glycoprotein IIb/IIIa inhibitors are recommended for high-risk patients with unstable angina or non-Q wave MI and for those undergoing **percutaneous coronary intervention**. **Dextran** also has an antiplatelet action and has been used to prevent postoperative **DVT** and **PE**.

Patients receiving these drugs who present for surgery may be at increased risk of bleeding. The place of regional anaesthesia in such patients is controversial because of the possibly increased risk of spinal haematoma. It has been suggested that two elimination half-lives should elapse between the last dose and performance of the block.

Hall R, Mazer CD (2011). Anesth Analg; 112: 292–318

See also, Anticoagulant drugs; Coagulation

Antipsychotic drugs (Neuroleptics). Drugs used for the management of psychosis (e.g. hallucinations, delusions, thought disorder) and acute agitation. Previously termed 'major tranquillisers'. All act via antagonism of D_2 **dopamine receptors**, with other effects (e.g. sedation, antimuscarinic effects) mediated via antagonism of other receptors (e.g. **histamine** receptors, 5-HT_2 receptors, muscarinic **acetylcholine receptors**). Other side effects include: **prolonged Q–T syndromes**; **dystonic reactions**; parkinsonian symptoms; **hyperglycaemia**; and **neuroleptic malignant syndrome**. Should be used with caution and at lower dosage in the elderly, in whom they have been shown to be associated with a slightly increased mortality and increased risk of **stroke**.
- Classification:
  - **phenothiazines** (e.g. **prochlorperazine**, **chlorpromazine**).
  - **butyrophenones** (e.g. **haloperidol**, **droperidol**).
  - atypical (e.g. clozapine, olanzapine, risperidone, quetiapine).

There is no evidence that any one agent is superior to any other; choice of drug is determined by individual response and tolerability of side effects.

Antispasmodic drugs. Used as adjunctive therapy in the management of non-ulcer dyspepsia, irritable bowel syndrome and diverticular disease. Also administered during GIT endoscopy and radiology, and when constructing bowel anastomoses.

Include:
- antimuscarinic agents (e.g. **atropine**, dicycloverine, **hyoscine**, propantheline). Produce dry mouth, blurred vision, urinary retention and constipation. Also relax the oesophageal sphincter, causing gastro-oesophageal reflux.
- others: e.g. alverine, mebeverine, peppermint oil: direct intestinal smooth muscle relaxants.

Antispasmodics should not be used in patients with **ileus**.

Antistatic precautions. Employed in operating suites, to prevent build-up of static electricity with possible sparks,

explosions and fires. Surfaces and materials should have relatively low electrical resistance, to allow leakage of charge to earth, but not so low as to allow **electrocution and electrical burns**.

- Precautions include:
  - avoidance of wool, nylon and silk, which may generate static charge. Cotton blankets and clothing are suitable (resistance is very low in moist atmospheres).
  - antistatic rubber (containing carbon) for tubing. Coloured black with yellow labels for identification. Resistance is 100 000–10 000 000 ohms/cm.
  - terrazzo floor (stone pieces embedded in cement and polished): resistance should be 20 000–5 000 000 ohms between two points 60 cm apart.
  - trolleys and other equipment have conducting wheels; staff wear antistatic footwear.

Sparks are more likely in cold, dry atmospheres, therefore relative **humidity** should exceed 50% and temperature exceed 20°C.

The requirement for expensive antistatic flooring and other precautions are rarely followed in modern UK operating suites, because flammable anaesthetic agents (e.g. **cyclopropane**) are no longer used, and although fires may still occur with other substances (e.g. alcohol skin cleansers), ignition is usually caused by a high-energy source such as **diathermy** or **laser** rather than static electricity.

Antithrombin III. Cofactor of **heparin** and natural inhibitor of **coagulation**. Often deficient in critical illness such as **sepsis**; hence its investigation as a possible treatment, though evidence suggests that therapy causes no improvement in outcome while increasing bleeding complications. A hereditary antithrombin III deficiency may result in recurrent thromboembolism; patients with the deficiency require higher doses of heparin.

Allingstrup M, Wetterslav J, Ravn FB (2016). Cochrane Database Sys Rev; 2: CD005370

Antituberculous drugs. Used for:

- prophylaxis: advised for susceptible close contacts or following treatment of **TB** in immunocompromised patients. Comprises **isoniazid** alone daily for 6 months, or combined with **rifampicin** daily for 3 months.
- treatment is carried out in two phases:
  - initial phase (2 months) using four drugs: intended to reduce the number of viable organisms as quickly as possible to avoid resistance. Usually includes isoniazid, rifampicin, **pyrazinamide** and **ethambutol. Streptomycin** is rarely used nowadays but is sometimes added if resistance to isoniazid is present.
  - continuation phase (further 4 months) using two drugs: intended to eradicate the bacteria from the body (longer treatment may be required in bone, joint, CNS and resistant infections). Usually comprises continuation of isoniazid and rifampicin therapy.

Other drugs used in resistant cases or when side effects are limiting include **capreomycin, cycloserine, azithromycin, clarithromycin, 4-quinolones** and **rifabutin**.

Treatment must be supervised if non-compliance is suspected, because partial completion of treatment courses is a major factor in producing resistance. During use of antituberculous drugs (especially pyrazinamide, isoniazid and rifampicin), monitoring of liver function is mandatory. Streptomycin and ethambutol should be avoided in patients with renal impairment. Multidrug resistant tuberculosis treatment requires close supervision by microbiologists and extended periods of treatment.

Zumla A, Raviglione M, Hafner R, et al (2013). N Engl J Med; 368: 745–55

Antiviral drugs. Heterogeneous group of drugs with generally non-specific actions. Parenteral use is usually reserved for severe life-threatening systemic infections, especially in immunocompromised patients. Available drugs can best be classified according to the infections in which they are used:

- herpes simplex/varicella zoster:
  - **aciclovir**: purine nucleoside analogue; after phosphorylation, it inhibits viral DNA polymerase. Phosphorylated by, and therefore active against, herpes simplex and varicella zoster viruses. Early initiation of treatment is important. May also be useful in **HIV infection**. May be given topically, orally or iv; side effects include GIT upset, rashes, and deteriorating renal and liver function.
  - famciclovir, valaciclovir, idoxuridine, inosine, **amantadine**: used for simplex and zoster infection of the skin and mucous membranes.
- HIV:
  - nucleoside reverse transcriptase inhibitors: e.g. **zidovudine**, abacavir, zalcitabine, didanosine, stavudine, lamivudine, tenofovir.
  - protease inhibitors: e.g. indinavir, ritonavir, lopinavir, nelfinavir, amprenavir, saquinavir. May cause metabolic derangement, including hyperlipidaemia and redistribution of body fat, insulin resistance and hyperglycaemia.
  - non-nucleoside reverse transcriptase inhibitors: e.g. efavirenz, nevirapine. May cause severe skin reactions and hepatic impairment.
- **cytomegalovirus: ganciclovir**, valganciclovir, **foscarnet**.
- respiratory syncytial virus: **tribavirin**.

In addition, **interferons** are used in **hepatitis** infections.

Antoine equation. Describes the theoretical variation of **SVP** with temperature. Empirically relates SVP to three constants, derived from experimental data for each substance.

[Louis Charles Antoine (1825–97), French scientist]

ANTS, *see Anaesthetists' Non-technical Skills*

Aortic aneurysm, abdominal. Manifestation of peripheral vascular disease, most often due to **atherosclerosis**. Usually occurs in males over 60 years old. Often presents with abdominal or back pain, or as an asymptomatic, pulsatile abdominal swelling, increasingly detected by ultrasound screening. May rupture or dissect acutely, leading to death; leakage is amenable to urgent surgical intervention. Elective surgery is indicated when the diameter of the aneurysm exceeds 5.5 cm (men) and 5.0 cm (women). The traditional open procedure is usually performed via an abdominal incision from xiphisternum to pubis. Alternatives include endoluminal repair (endovascular aneurysm repair, EVAR), in which a graft is placed via percutaneous arterial puncture, or a semi-laparoscopic method, in which much of the mobilisation is achieved laparoscopically via small incisions before grafting. Preparation should be as for the open technique, because the risk of proceeding or of severe, sudden haemorrhage is always present. Endoluminal repair in particular has been shown to reduce blood loss, organ dysfunction, hospital stay and early mortality, although mortality at 1 year is thought to be the same as after open repair.

- Anaesthetic considerations for elective repair:
  - **preoperative assessment** is particularly directed to the effects of widespread atherosclerosis, i.e., affecting coronary, renal, cerebral and peripheral arteries. **Hypertension** is also common.
  - perioperatively:
    - monitoring: ECG; direct arterial, central venous pressure measurement; temperature; **urine** output.
    - at least two large-bore iv cannulae.
    - warming blanket and warming of iv fluids. **Humidification** of inspired gases.
    - cardiovascular responses:
      - hypertension during tracheal intubation.
      - increased **afterload** caused by aortic cross-clamping. Hypertension and left ventricular failure may occur. Anticipatory use of **vasodilator drugs** may help to reduce hypertension and left ventricular strain.
      - reduction of afterload, return of vasodilator metabolites from lower part of the body, and possible haemorrhage following aortic unclamping (declamping syndrome). **Myocardial contractility** is reduced by the acidotic venous return. Anticipatory volume loading before unclamping, with termination of vasodilator therapy before slow controlled release of the clamp, may reduce hypotension. **Bicarbonate** therapy is guided by arterial acid–base analysis; it is often not required if clamping time is less than 1–1.5 h.
    - blood loss and effects of massive **blood transfusion.**
    - postoperative visceral dysfunction:
      - **renal failure** may follow aortic surgery; it is more likely to occur after suprarenal cross-clamping. **Mannitol**, **furosemide** or **dopamine** is often given before aortic clamping, to encourage diuresis.
      - GIT ischaemia and infarction may occur if the mesenteric arterial supply is interrupted. The **anterior spinal artery syndrome** may also occur.

    Attempts to reduce the effects of renal and GIT ischaemia have also included **hypothermia** and use of metabolic precursors, e.g. **inosine**.
  - postoperatively: ICU or HDU. Elective IPPV may be required. Epidural analgesia is often used.
- For **emergency surgery**, prognosis is generally poor; 50% die in the prehospital setting, and a further 50% die in hospital. The following are important:
  - wide-bore peripheral venous access (and ideally an arterial line) pre-induction; insertion of invasive monitoring should not delay surgery.
  - preparation and draping of the patient before induction.
  - availability of blood, O negative if necessary.
    - rapid sequence induction. **Etomidate** or **ketamine** is often used.

Abdominal muscular relaxation following induction of anaesthesia may result in decreased abdominal 'tamponade' of the leaking aneurysm, resulting in further haemorrhage and hypotension.

Recent evidence suggests that surgeons in England operate less often on aortic aneurysms than in the USA, possibly related to different aortic diameter thresholds in practice, and that the death rate in England is over twice that in the USA.

Vaughn SB, LeMaire SA, Collard CD (2011). Anesthesiology; 115: 1093–102

See also, Aortic aneurysm, thoracic; Blood transfusion, massive; Induction, rapid sequence

Aortic aneurysm, thoracic. Usually results from **aortic dissection.** Surgical approach is via left thoracotomy; **one-lung anaesthesia** facilitates surgery. Concurrent aortic valve replacement may be required. General anaesthetic management is as for abdominal aneurysm repair. Cardiovascular instability may be more dramatic because of the proximity of the aortic clamp to the heart, and the reduction of venous return and cardiac output during surgical manoeuvres. Complications include haemorrhage and infarction of spinal cord, liver, gut, kidneys and heart. Perioperative drainage of CSF is commonly performed to increase spinal cord **perfusion pressure** in an attempt to reduce spinal cord ischaemia. Operative techniques include atriofemoral **cardiopulmonary bypass**, or use of a shunt across the clamped aortic section. An endoluminal approach has also been described (thoracic endovascular aneurysm repair, TEVAR), similar to that for abdominal aneurysms.

See also, Aortic aneurysm, abdominal

Aortic bodies. Peripheral **chemoreceptors** near the aortic arch. Similar in structure and function to the **carotid bodies.** Afferents pass to the medulla via the vagus.

Aortic coarctation, *see Coarctation of the aorta*

Aortic counter-pulsation balloon pump, *see Intra-aortic counter-pulsation balloon pump*

Aortic dissection. Passage of arterial blood into the aortic wall, usually involving the media of the vessel. Degeneration of this layer is usually caused by **atherosclerosis** but is also seen in **Marfan's syndrome** and Ehlers–Danlos syndrome. Often associated with **hypertension.** Dissection may involve branches of the aorta, including the coronary arteries. Additionally, rupture into pericardium, pleural cavity, mediastinum or abdomen may occur. May also follow **chest trauma.** Classified originally by the DeBakey classification:

  - type I: starts in the ascending aorta, extending proximally to the aortic valve and distally around the aortic arch.
  - type II: limited to the ascending aorta.
  - type III: starts distal to the left subclavian artery, extending distally (commonly) or proximally (rarely).

The Stanford classification is more commonly used, as it relates more closely to surgical management:

  - type A: involves the ascending aorta.
  - type B: involves only the descending aorta.

About 65% start in the ascending aorta, ~20% in the descending thoracic aorta, ~10% in the aortic arch, and ~5% in the abdominal aorta.

- Features:
  - severe tearing central chest pain; may mimic **MI.** May radiate to the back or abdomen.
  - signs of **aortic regurgitation.**

- signs of **haemorrhage** or **cardiac tamponade**.
- progressive loss of radial pulses and **stroke** may indicate extension along the aortic arch. Coronary artery involvement may cause MI. Renal vessels may be involved.
- **CXR** may reveal a widened mediastinum or **pleural effusion. Echocardiography**, **CT/MRI scanning** and aortography may be used in diagnosis.

• Management:
- analgesia.
- control of BP, e.g. using **vasodilator drugs**.
- surgery is increasingly employed, especially if the aortic valve is involved, dissection progresses or rupture occurs. Management: as for thoracic aortic aneurysm.

[Edward Ehlers (1863–1937), Danish dermatologist; Henri Alexandre Danlos (1844–1912), French dermatologist; Michael E DeBakey (1908–2008), US cardiac surgeon]

Nienber CA, Clough RE (2015). Lancet; 385: 800–11

See also, Aortic aneurysm, thoracic

Aortic regurgitation. Retrograde flow of blood through the aortic valve during diastole. Causes left ventricular hypertrophy and dilatation, with greatly increased stroke volume. Later, compliance decreases and end-diastolic pressure increases, with ventricular failure.

• Caused by:
- **rheumatic fever**; usually also affects the mitral value.
- **aortic dissection.**
- **endocarditis** (especially acute regurgitation).
- **Marfan's syndrome.**
- congenital defect (associated with **aortic stenosis**).
- postsurgical (including after transcatheter aortic valve replacement).
- **chest trauma, ankylosing spondylitis, rheumatoid disease, syphilis, SLE.**

• Features:
- collapsing **pulse** with widened pulse pressure (water hammer). Bobbing of the head in synchrony with the pulse (Musset's sign) may occur.
- early diastolic murmur, high-pitched and blowing. Loudest in expiration and with the patient leaning forward, and heard at the left sternal edge, sometimes at the apex. The third **heart sound** may be present. A thrill is absent. An aortic ejection murmur is usually present, radiating to the neck; a mid diastolic mitral murmur may be present due to obstruction by aortic backflow (Austin Flint murmur).
- left ventricular failure.
- angina is usually late.
- investigations: **ECG** may show left ventricular hypertrophy; **CXR** may show ventricular enlargement/failure. **Echocardiography** and **cardiac catheterisation** are also useful.

• Anaesthetic management:
- antibiotic prophylaxis as for **congenital heart disease.**
- general principles: as for **cardiac surgery/ischaemic heart disease. Myocardial ischaemia** and left ventricular failure may occur.
- the following should be avoided:
  - bradycardia: increases time for regurgitation.
  - peripheral vasoconstriction and increased diastolic pressure: increase-afterload and therefore regurgitation. Peripheral vasodilatation reduces regurgitation and increases forward flow.
- **cardioplegia** solution is infused directly into the coronary arteries during cardiac surgery, because if injected into the aortic root it will enter the ventricle.
- **left ventricular end-diastolic pressure** may be much greater than measured **pulmonary capillary wedge pressure**, if the mitral valve is closed early by the regurgitant backflow.
- postoperative hypertension may occur.

[Alfred de Musset (1810–1857), French poet; Austin Flint (1812–1886), US physician]

Bobow RO, Leon MB, Doshi D, Moat N (2016). Lancet; 387: 1312–23

See also, Heart murmurs; Preoperative assessment; Valvular heart disease

Aortic stenosis. Narrowed aortic valve with obstruction to the left ventricular outflow, resulting in a pressure gradient between the left ventricle and aortic root. Initially, left ventricular hypertrophy and increased force of contraction maintain **stroke volume**. Compliance is decreased. **Coronary blood flow** is decreased due to increased **left ventricular end-diastolic pressure** and involvement of the coronary sinuses, while left ventricular work increases. Ultimately, contractility falls, with left ventricular dilatation and reduced cardiac output.

• Caused by:
- **rheumatic fever**: may present at any age (usually also involves the mitral valve).
- congenital bicuspid valve: usually presents in middle age.
- degenerative calcification: usually in the elderly.

• Features:
- angina (30%–40%), syncope, left ventricular failure.
- sudden death.
- low-volume, slow-rising pulse with reduced pulse pressure (plateau pulse). **AF** usually signifies coexistent mitral disease.
- ejection systolic murmur, radiating to the neck. Loudest in the aortic area, with the patient sitting forward in expiration. The second **heart sound** is quiet, with reversed splitting if stenosis is severe (due to delayed left ventricular emptying). A thrill, fourth sound and ejection click may be present.
- investigations: **ECG** may show left ventricular hypertrophy; **CXR** may show ventricular enlargement/failure, possibly with calcification and poststenotic dilatation. **Echocardiography** and **cardiac catheterisation** are especially useful, providing measurements of the gradient across the valve and valve area (normal is 2.6–3.5 cm^2; Table 7).

• Anaesthetic management:
- antibiotic prophylaxis as for **congenital heart disease.**
- general principles: as for **cardiac surgery/ischaemic heart disease.**

Table 7 American Heart Association/American College of Cardiology classification of aortic stenosis

	Mild	*Moderate*	*Severe*
Valve area (cm^2)	>1.5	1.0–1.5	<1.0
Valve area index (cm^2/m^2)	>0.85	0.6–0.85	<0.6
Jet velocity (m/s)	<3	3–4	>4
Peak gradient (mmHg)	36	36–64	>64
Mean gradient (mmHg)	<25	25–40	>40

- **Myocardial ischaemia**, ventricular arrhythmias and left ventricular failure may occur. Percutaneous transcatheter valve replacements are now being performed.
- the following should be avoided:
  - loss of sinus rhythm: atrial contraction is vital to maintain adequate ventricular filling.
  - peripheral vasodilatation: cardiac output is relatively fixed, therefore BP may fall dramatically, causing myocardial ischaemia.
  - excessive peripheral vasoconstriction: further reduces left ventricular outflow.
  - tachycardia: ventricular filling is impaired and coronary blood flow reduced.
  - myocardial depression.
- postoperative hypertension may occur.

Bobow RO, Leon MB, Doshi D, Moat N (2016). Lancet; 387: 1312–23

See also, Heart murmurs; Preoperative assessment; Valvular heart disease

Aortocaval compression (Supine hypotension syndrome). Compression of the great vessels against the vertebral bodies by the gravid uterus in the supine position in mid- to late **pregnancy**. Vena caval compression reduces venous return and cardiac output with a compensatory increase in SVR; this may be symptomless ('concealed'), or associated with hypotension, bradycardia or syncope ('revealed'). Reduced placental blood flow may result from the reduced cardiac output, vasoconstriction and compression of the aorta. During uterine contractions, the compression may worsen (**Poseiro effect**). Reduced cardiac output is more likely to occur if vasoconstrictor reflexes are impaired, e.g. during regional or general anaesthesia. May be reduced by manual displacement of the uterus or tilting the mother to one side (usually the left is preferred), e.g. with a wedge. Up to 45 degrees tilt may be required.

Lee A, Landau R (2017). Anesth Analg; 125: 1975–85

See also, Obstetric analgesia and anaesthesia

Aortovelography. Use of a **Doppler** ultrasound probe in the suprasternal notch to measure blood velocity and acceleration in the ascending aorta. Used for **cardiac output measurement**.

APACHE scoring system (Acute physiology and chronic health evaluation). Tool described in 1981 for assessing the severity of illness of individual patients and predicting the risk of hospital mortality for groups of patients treated in **ICUs**. Consists of two parts: an **acute physiology score** (APS) and an assessment of the patient's pre-illness health status. Rarely used now because of acknowledged superiority of other systems, e.g. **APACHE II**, **APACHE III**, **APACHE IV**, **SAPS**, **MPM**.

Vincent JL, Moreno R (2010). Crit Care; 14: 207–15

See also, Mortality/survival prediction on intensive care unit

APACHE II scoring system (Acute physiology and chronic health evaluation; version II). Revised version of the prototype **APACHE scoring system**, described in 1985. The number of physiological measurements used in the **acute physiology score** is reduced to 12, with weightings allocated for the degree of derangement of each physiological parameter in the first 24 h after ICU admission (range 0–4), age and chronic health (Table 8); selection of criteria and weightings is based upon the opinions of a panel of experts. Definitions of chronic health are more specific than in the original APACHE system. The assigned weights for all physiological measurements, age and chronic health are summated to give an APACHE II score (maximum 71), which is further integrated with the patient's diagnosis to calculate the predicted mortality.

APACHE II has been validated in many large centres and is thought to be a reliable method for estimating group outcome among ICU patients. Survival rates of 50% have been reported for an admission score of about 25 points, with 80% mortality for scores above 35 points. More recently, repeated assessments (i.e., change in APACHE II score over time) have been used to chart patients' progress.

Vincent JL, Moreno R (2010). Crit Care; 14: 207–15

See also, APACHE III scoring system; APACHE IV scoring system; Mortality/survival prediction on intensive care unit

APACHE III scoring system (Acute physiology, age and chronic health evaluation). Further development of the **APACHE II scoring system**, introduced in 1991. Consists of a numerical score (range 0–299) reflecting the weights assigned to the variables of three principal data categories: physiological measurements, chronological age (the emphasis on age reflected in the reassignment of the second 'A' in 'APACHE') and chronic health status. APACHE III uses data from 16 physiological measurements. Unlike earlier versions, weighting of physiological abnormalities is derived from multiple logistic regression. Physiological abnormalities have a greater relative importance in the APACHE III score and predictive equations. The chronic health component has been modified and is based on seven variables referring to the presence or absence of haematological malignancies, lymphoma, AIDS, metastatic cancer, immunosuppression, hepatic failure and liver cirrhosis.

APACHE III uses 78 mutually exclusive disease definitions to group patients according to the principal reason for ICU admission. Patients admitted directly from the operating or recovery room are classified as operative (surgical), and are further subdivided according to the urgency of the operation (elective versus emergency). All other patients are classified as non-operative (medical). The APACHE III score is integrated with the patient's diagnosis and source before ICU to calculate the estimate of hospital mortality and length of ICU stay. Although its performance is slightly better than that of APACHE II, APACHE III is less widely used because the predictive equations it employs are commercially protected.

Vincent JL, Moreno R (2010). Crit Care; 14: 207–15

See also, Mortality/survival prediction on intensive care unit

APACHE IV scoring system (Acute physiology, age and chronic health evaluation). Further development of the **APACHE III scoring system**, published in 2006. Derived from a more refined statistical analysis of data from 100 ICUs and >110 000 patients. Like the APACHE III, it utilises multiple logistic regression and generates an estimate of predicted mortality and length of ICU stay.

Vincent JL, Moreno R (2010). Crit Care; 14: 207–15

Table 0 APACHE II scoring system

Physiological variable	*High abnormal range* +4	+3	+2	+1	0	*Low abnormal range* +1	+2	+3	+4
Temperature, rectal (°C)	○ ≥41	○ 39–40.9		○ 38.5–38.9	○ 36–38.4	○ 34–35.9	○ 32.2–33.9	○ 30–31.9	○ ≤29.9
Mean arterial pressure (mmHg)	○ >160	○ 130–159	○ 110–129		○ 70–109		○ 50–69		○ ≤49
Heart rate (ventricular response)	○ ≥180	○ 140–179	○ 110–139		○ 70–109		○ 55–69	○ 40–54	○ ≤39
Respiratory rate (non-ventilated or ventilated)	○ ≥50	○ 35–49		○ 25–34	○ 12–24	○ 10–11	○ 6–9		○ ≤5
Oxygenation: A–adO_2 or P_aO_2 (kPa [mmHg])									
(a) F_IO_2 ≥0.5 record A–adO_2	○ >67 (>500)	○ 47–66.9 (350–499)	○ 27–46.9 (300–349)		○ <27 (<200)				
(b) F_IO_2 <0.5 record only P_aO_2					○ >9.3 (>70)	○ 8.1–9.3 (61–70)		○ 7.3–8.0 (55–60)	○ <7.3 (<55)
Arterial pH	○ ≥7.7	○ 7.6–7.69		○ 7.5–7.59	○ 7.33–7.49		○ 7.25–7.32	○ 7.15–7.24	○ <7.15
Serum sodium (mmol/l)	○ ≥180	○ 160–179	○ 155–159	○ 150–154	○ 130–149		○ 120–129	○ 111–119	○ ≤110
Serum potassium (mmol/l)	○ ≥7	○ 6–6.9		○ 5.5–5.9	○ 3.5–5.4	○ 3.5–5.4	○ 3.5–5.4		○ <2.5
Serum creatinine (μmol/l [mg/100 ml]) (double point score for *acute kidney injury*)	○ >301 (≥3.5)	○ 170–300 (2–3.4)	○ 130–169 (1.5–1.9)		○ 50–129 (0.6–1.4)		○ <50 (<0.6)		
Haematocrit (%)	○ ≥60		○ 50–59.9	○ 46–49.9	○ 30–45.9		○ 20–29.9		○ <20
Glasgow coma scale (GCS) Score = 15 minus actual GCS									
A Total acute physiology score (APS): a sum of the 12 individual variable points									
Serum HCO_3^- (venous mmol/l) (not preferred, use if no arterial blood gases)	○ ≥52	○ 41–51.9		○ 32–40.9	○ 22–31.9		○ 18–21.9	○ 15–17.9	○ <15

B Age points

Assign points to age as follows:

Age (years)	Points
≤44	0
45–54	2
55–64	5
65–74	5
≥75	6

C **Chronic health points**

If the patient has a history of severe organ system insufficiency or is immunocompromised, assign points as follows:

(a) for non-operative or emergency postoperative patients +5 points or

(b) for elective postoperative patients +2 points

Definitions

Organ insufficiency or immunocompromised state must have been evident before this hospital admission and conform to the following criteria:

Liver: Biopsy-proven cirrhosis and documented portal hypertension; episodes of past upper gastrointestinal bleeding attributed to portal hypertension, or prior episodes of hepatic failure/encephalopathy/coma

Cardiovascular: New York Heart Association Class IV (inability to perform physical activity)

Respiratory: Chronic restrictive, obstructive, or vascular disease resulting in severe exercise restriction, i.e., unable to climb stairs or perform household duties, or documented chronic hypoxia, hypercapnia, secondary polycythaemia, severe pulmonary hypertension (>40 mmHg), or respiratory dependency

Renal: Receiving chronic dialysis

Immunocompromised: The patient has received therapy that suppresses resistance to infection, e.g. immunosuppression, chemotherapy, radiation, long-term or recent high-dose corticosteroids, or has a disease that is sufficiently advanced to suppress resistance to infection, e.g. leukaemia, lymphoma, AIDS

APACHE II SCORE

Sum of:

A APS points

B Age points

C Chronic health points

Total APACHE II

Table 9 Apgar scoring system

Sign	Score 0	Score 1	Score 2
Heart rate (beats/min)	Absent	<100	>100
Respiratory effort	Absent	Weak cry	Strong cry
Muscle tone	Limp	Poor tone	Good tone
Reflex irritability	No response	Some movement	Strong withdrawal
Colour	Blue, pale	Pink body, blue extremities	Pink

Apgar scoring system. Widely used method of evaluating the condition of the neonate, described in 1953. Points are awarded up to a maximum total of 10 according to clinical findings (Table 9). Assessments are commonly performed at 1 and 5 min after birth, but may be repeated as necessary. Colour may be omitted from the observed signs to give a maximum score of 8 (Apgar minus colour score).
[Virginia Apgar (1909–1975), US anaesthetist]

Apixaban. Orally active direct factor Xa inhibitor, licensed in adults for **DVT** prophylaxis after elective hip or knee replacement surgery. More effective than **enoxaparin** at preventing DVT and **PE**, with comparable risks of haemorrhagic side effects. Also recommended by **NICE** (2013) for prophylaxis against stroke in certain patients with **AF**.

Rapidly absorbed via the oral route (peak plasma concentration within 3–4 h), with 50% oral **bioavailability**. **Half-life** is ~12 h; 70% undergoes hepatic metabolism (by the cytochrome P_{450} system) to inactive products, and 30% is excreted unchanged in urine. Thus caution is required in patients with severe hepatic or **renal failure**, or those taking drugs that cause hepatic **enzyme induction/inhibition**. Bleeding risk is increased with concomitant **antiplatelet drugs**.

- Dosage: 2.5 mg orally bd, starting 12–24 h after surgery, for 2 (knee) or 5 (hip) weeks after surgery, respectively.
- Side effects: nausea, haemorrhage.

APLS, *see Advanced Paediatric Life Support*

Apneustic centre, *see Breathing, control of*

Apnoea. Absence of breathing. In **sleep** studies, defined as cessation of breathing lasting >10 s (hypopnoea = reduction >30% for >10 s, together with a 3% drop in S_pO_2). Causes are as for **hypoventilation**. Results in **hypercapnia** and **hypoxaemia**. The rate of onset and severity of hypoxaemia are related to the F_IO_2, **FRC** and O_2 consumption. Thus **preoxygenation** delays the onset of hypoxaemia following apnoea. In **pregnancy**, hypoxaemia develops more quickly, due to reduced FRC and increased O_2 consumption.

Alveolar $P{CO_2}$ rises at about 0.5 kPa/min (3.8 mmHg/min) when CO_2 production is normal.

In paediatrics, prematurity is a major cause of recurrent apnoea. In newborn animals, induced hypoxaemia results in vigorous efforts to breathe, followed by primary apnoea and bradycardia, then secondary (terminal) apnoea after a few gasps. During primary apnoea, gasping and possibly spontaneous respiration may be induced by stimulation; the **gasp reflex** is also active. During secondary apnoea, active resuscitation and oxygenation are required to restore breathing.

See also, Cardiopulmonary resuscitation, neonatal; Obstructive sleep apnoea; Sleep-disordered breathing

Apnoea–hypopnoea index, *see Sleep-disordered breathing*

Apnoeic oxygenation. Method of delivering O_2 to the lungs by insufflation during apnoea. A catheter is passed into the trachea, its tip lying above the carina. O_2 passed through it at 4–6 l/min reaches the alveoli mainly by mass diffusion, with O_2 utilised faster than CO_2 is produced. The technique does not remove CO_2, which rises at a rate of approximately 0.5 kPa/min (3.8 mmHg/min) at normal rates of CO_2 production. **Hypercapnia** may therefore occur during prolonged procedures.

May be used to maintain oxygenation (e.g. during **bronchoscopy**) or during the diagnosis of **brainstem death**.
See also, Insufflation techniques; Transnasal humidified rapid-insufflation ventilatory exchange

Apomorphine hydrochloride. Alkaloid derived from **morphine**, with a powerful agonist action at both D_1 and D_2 **dopamine receptors**. Used to treat refractory motor fluctuations in **Parkinson's disease**. Causes intense stimulation of the **chemoreceptor trigger zone**, resulting in **vomiting**; thus previously used as an **emetic drug** to empty the stomach.

Aprepitant. Neurokinin-1 receptor antagonist, licensed as an **antiemetic drug** as part of combination therapy (with a **corticosteroid** and a **5-HT$_3$ receptor antagonist**) in cancer chemotherapy. Has been studied in **PONV**.

- Dosage: 125 mg, 80 mg and 80 mg orally on 3 successive days.
- Side effects: hiccups, fatigue, GIT upset.

Aprotinin. Proteolytic enzyme inhibitor. Inhibits:
- plasmin (at low dose, causing reduced **fibrinolysis**).
- **kallikrein** (at higher dose, causing reduced **coagulation**).
- trypsin.

Used (off license) to reduce perioperative blood loss in **cardiac surgery**; bolus loading followed by continuous infusion is usual, although dosing regimens vary. A test dose is usually given because of a relatively high risk of hypersensitivity reactions; **anaphylaxis** is particularly severe after repeat administration within 6 months. Other side effects include **hypotension** and renal impairment. Temporarily withdrawn in 2007 because of safety concerns, reintroduced in 2012 for selected patients undergoing cardiac surgery at high risk of bleeding.

APRV, *see Airway pressure release ventilation*

APS, *see Acute physiology score*

Apudomas. Tumours of amine precursor uptake and decarboxylation (APUD) cells, present in the anterior **pituitary gland, thyroid gland, adrenal gland** medulla, GIT, pancreatic islets, **carotid body** and **lung**. Originally thought to arise from neural crest tissue; now thought to be derived from endoderm. They have similar structural and biochemical properties, secreting polypeptides and amines. They may secrete hormones that cause systemic disturbances, e.g. **insulin, glucagon, catecholamines, 5-HT, somatostatin**, gastrin and **vasoactive intestinal peptide**.
See also, Carcinoid syndrome; Multiple endocrine adenomatosis; Phaeochromocytoma

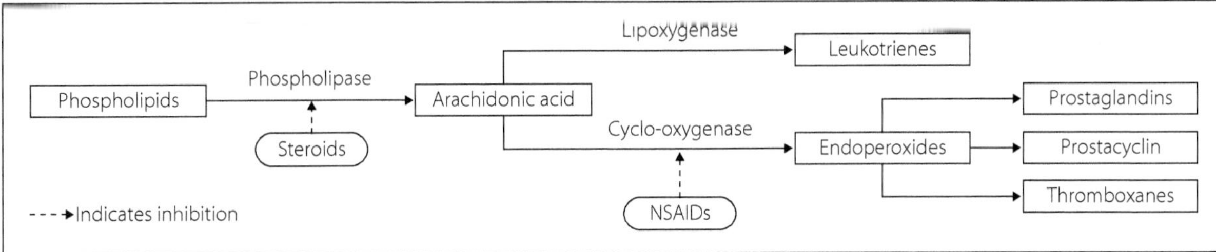

Fig. 14 Arachidonic acid pathways

Arachidonic acid. Essential fatty acid synthesised from phospholipids and metabolised by lipoxygenase and **cyclo-oxygenase** to **leukotrienes** and endoperoxides, respectively (Fig. 14). Endoperoxides form **prostaglandins**, **prostacyclin** and **thromboxanes** via separate pathways. The pathways are inhibited by **corticosteroids** and **NSAIDs** as shown.

Arachidonic acid may also undergo peroxidation during oxidative stress, under the action of **free radicals**, with the production of isoprostanes.

Arachnoiditis. Inflammation of the arachnoid and pial **meninges**. Diagnosed with high specificity and sensitivity with MRI. Has occurred after **spinal** and **epidural anaesthesia**; antiseptic solutions (especially alcoholic chlorhexidine) and preservatives in drug solutions (e.g. sodium bisulfite) have been implicated. Also occurs after radiotherapy, trauma and myelography with oil-based contrast media. May occur months or years after the insult. Progressive fibrosis may cause spinal canal narrowing, ischaemia and permanent nerve damage. The cauda equina is usually affected, with pain, muscle weakness and loss of sphincter control. May rarely spread cranially. Response to treatment is generally poor.

Killeen T, Kamat A, Walsh D, et al (2012). Anaesthesia; 67: 1386–94

See also, Cauda equina syndrome

ARAS, *see Ascending reticular activating system*

ARDS, Acute respiratory distress syndrome, *see Acute lung injury*

Argatroban monohydrate. Monovalent **thrombin inhibitor**, indicated as an alternative to **heparin** in heparin-induced thrombocytopenia. Similar to **lepirudin** but excreted via the liver as opposed to the kidneys. Half-life is 30–60 min, thus requiring administration by continuous infusion.

- Dosage: 2 μg/kg/min adjusted according to APTT up to 10 μg/kg/min.
- Side effects: nausea, haemorrhage, purpura, GIT upset, liver impairment.

Arginine vasopressin/argipressin, *see Vasopressin*

Arm–brain circulation time. Time taken for a substance injected into an arm vein (traditionally antecubital) to reach the brain. If a bile salt is injected, the time until arrival of the bitter taste at the tongue may be measured (normally 10–20 s; this may be greatly prolonged when cardiac output is reduced). Useful conceptually when comparing different **iv induction agents**; thus **thiopental** acts 'within one arm–brain circulation time', whereas **midazolam** takes longer.

Arrhythmias. Deviation from normal sinus rhythm.

- Classification:
  - disorders of impulse formation:
    - supraventricular:
      - **sinus arrhythmia**, **bradycardia** and **tachycardia**.
      - **SVT**.
      - **sick sinus syndrome**.
      - **AF**, **atrial flutter**, **atrial ectopic beats**.
    - **junctional arrhythmias**.
    - **VF**, **ventricular tachycardia**, **ventricular ectopic beats**.
  - disorders of impulse conduction:
    - slowed/blocked conduction (e.g. **heart block**).
    - abnormal pathway of conduction (e.g. **Wolff–Parkinson–White syndrome**).

Arrhythmias, especially tachycardias, are common in acute illness. During anaesthesia, ECG monitoring is mandatory. Bradycardia, junctional rhythm and ventricular ectopic beats (including bigeminy) are common, but usually not serious.

- Arrhythmias are more likely with:
  - pre-existing cardiac disease.
  - **hypoxaemia** and **hypercapnia**.
  - acid–base disturbances.
  - electrolyte abnormalities, especially of **potassium**, **calcium**, **magnesium**.
  - drugs, e.g. **inotropic drugs**, **antiarrhythmic drugs**, **theophylline**, **cocaine**.
  - mechanical stimulation of heart chambers (e.g. **central venous/pulmonary artery catheterisation**).
  - inherited rhythm disorders e.g. **prolonged Q–T syndromes**, Brugada syndrome (ventricular arrhythmias), catecholaminergic polymorphic ventricular tachycardia. All may result in sudden unexplained death syndrome, often in young people.
  - pacemaker malfunction.
  - certain diseases, e.g. **hyperthyroidism**, **subarachnoid haemorrhage**.
  - manoeuvres that activate powerful reflex pathways, e.g. during **dental surgery**, **oculocardiac reflex**, visceral manipulation, **tracheobronchial suctioning**.

[Pedro and Josep Brugada, Spanish cardiologists]

Arterial blood pressure. The pulsatile ejection of the **stroke volume** gives rise to the **arterial waveform**, from which systolic, diastolic and **mean arterial pressures** may be determined.

$$\text{MAP} = \textbf{cardiac output} \times \textbf{SVR}$$

Thus arterial pressure may vary with changes in cardiac output (stroke volume × **heart rate**) and vascular resistance.

- Control of BP:
  - short-term:
    - intrinsic regulatory properties of the heart: **Anrep effect**, **Bowditch effect**, **Starling's law**.

- autonomic pathways involving **baroreceptors**, **vasomotor centre** and **cardioinhibitory centre**.
- hormonal mechanisms:
  - **renin/–angiotensin system**.
  - **vasopressin**.
  - **adrenaline** and **noradrenaline** as part of the sympathetic response.
- intermediate/long-term: renin/–angiotensin system, **aldosterone**, vasopressin, **atrial natriuretic peptide**, endocannabinoids.

See also, Arterial blood pressure measurement; Diastolic blood pressure; Hypertension

Arterial blood pressure measurement. First attempted by Hales in 1733, who inserted pipes several feet long into the arteries of animals. The BP cuff was introduced by Riva-Rocci in 1896. Measurement and recording of BP were introduced into anaesthetic practice by **Cushing** in 1901.

- May be direct or indirect:
  - direct:
    - gives a continuous reading; i.e., changes may be noticed rapidly.
    - provides additional information from the shape of the **arterial waveform**.
    - requires **arterial cannulation**.
    - requires calibration and zeroing of the **monitoring** system.
    - **resonance** and **damping** may cause inaccuracy.
  - indirect:
    - palpation (unreliable).
    - mercury or aneroid manometer attached to a cuff: the brachial artery is palpated and the cuff inflated to 30–60 mmHg above the pressure at which the pulsation disappears. Cuff pressure is released at 2–3 mmHg/s, and pressure measured by detecting pulsation by using the **Korotkoff sounds**, a **pulse detector** or **Doppler** probe. The cuff width must be 20% greater than the arm's diameter or half its circumference; narrower cuffs will over-read. Error may arise between different observers. BP should be recorded to the nearest 2 mmHg.
    - **oscillotonometer**.
    - automatic oscillometry devices that use the same cuff for inflation and detection of movement of the arterial walls. Systolic pressure and diastolic pressures correspond to onset and offset of pulsations, respectively; MAP to the maximum oscillation amplitude. Some devices measure only systolic and mean pressures while calculating diastolic pressure. Tend to under-read when pressures are high and over-read when low. Inconsistencies occur if the cardiac cycle is irregular, e.g. in **atrial fibrillation**.
    - plethysmographic methods: a cuff is inflated around a finger, and its pressure varied continuously to keep its volume constant, using photometry/oximetry to measure volume. Cuff pressure is proportional to finger arterial pressure; a continuous display of the arterial pressure waveform is obtained. May be unreliable if peripheral vascular disease is present.
    - continuous arterial tonometry: a pressure transducer is positioned over the radial artery, compressing it against the radius. The transducer output voltage is proportional to the arterial BP, which is displayed as a continuous trace. Periodic calibration is performed using an automatic oscillometric cuff on the arm.

[Stephen Hales (1677–1761), English curate and naturalist; Scipione Riva-Rocci (1863–1937), Italian physician]
See also, Pressure measurement

Arterial cannulation. Used for direct **arterial BP measurement**, and to allow repeated arterial **blood gas interpretation**. Peripheral cannulation (e.g. of **radial** and **dorsalis pedis** arteries) produces higher peak systolic pressure than more central cannulation, but is usually preferred because of reduced complication rates. Other sites available include **brachial, ulnar, posterior tibial** and **femoral arteries. Allen's test** is sometimes performed before radial artery catheterisation, but is of doubtful value. Ultrasound-guided radial artery cannulation improves first attempt success rate but is not routinely used in adults. Continuous slow flushing with saline (3–4 ml/h) reduces blockage and is preferable to intermittent injection; recent systematic reviews suggest addition of heparin to the flush is unnecessary. Flushing with excessive volumes of solution may introduce air into the carotid circulation, especially in children. Dextrose solutions should not be used because of the risk of erroneous treatment of artefactual hyperglycaemia.

- System consists of:
  - cannula: ischaemia, emboli and tissue necrosis are uncommon if a 20–22 G parallel-sided Teflon cannula is used, and removed within 24–48 h.
  - connecting catheter: short and stiff to reduce **resonance**.
  - **transducer** placed level with the heart. Requires calibration and zeroing.
  - electrical monitor and connections. An adequate frequency response of less than 40 Hz is required.

Bubbles, clots and kinks may cause **damping**.

Intravascular transducers may be placed within large arteries, but are expensive and not routinely used.

Arterial gas tensions, *see Blood gas interpretation*

Arterial waveform. The shape of the pressure wave recorded directly from the aorta differs from that recorded from smaller arteries; the peak systolic pressure and **pulse pressure** increase, and the dicrotic notch becomes more apparent, peripherally (Fig. 15a). The aorta and large arteries are distended by the **stroke volume** during its ejection; during diastole, elastic recoil maintains diastolic blood flow (Windkessel effect). Smaller vessels are less compliant and therefore less distensible; thus the pressure peaks are higher and travel faster peripherally. In the elderly, decreased aortic compliance results in higher peak pressures.

- Abnormal waveforms (Fig. 15b):
  - anacrotic: **aortic stenosis**.
  - collapsing:
    - hyperdynamic circulation, e.g. **pregnancy**, fever, **anaemia**, **hyperthyroidism**, arteriovenous fistula.
    - **aortic regurgitation**.
  - bisferiens: aortic stenosis + aortic regurgitation.
  - alternans: left ventricular failure.
  - excessive **damping**: e.g. air bubble.
  - excessive **resonance**: e.g. catheter too long or flexible.
- Information that may be derived from the normal waveform:
  - arterial BP.
  - stroke volume and **cardiac output**, from the area under the systolic part of the waveform.

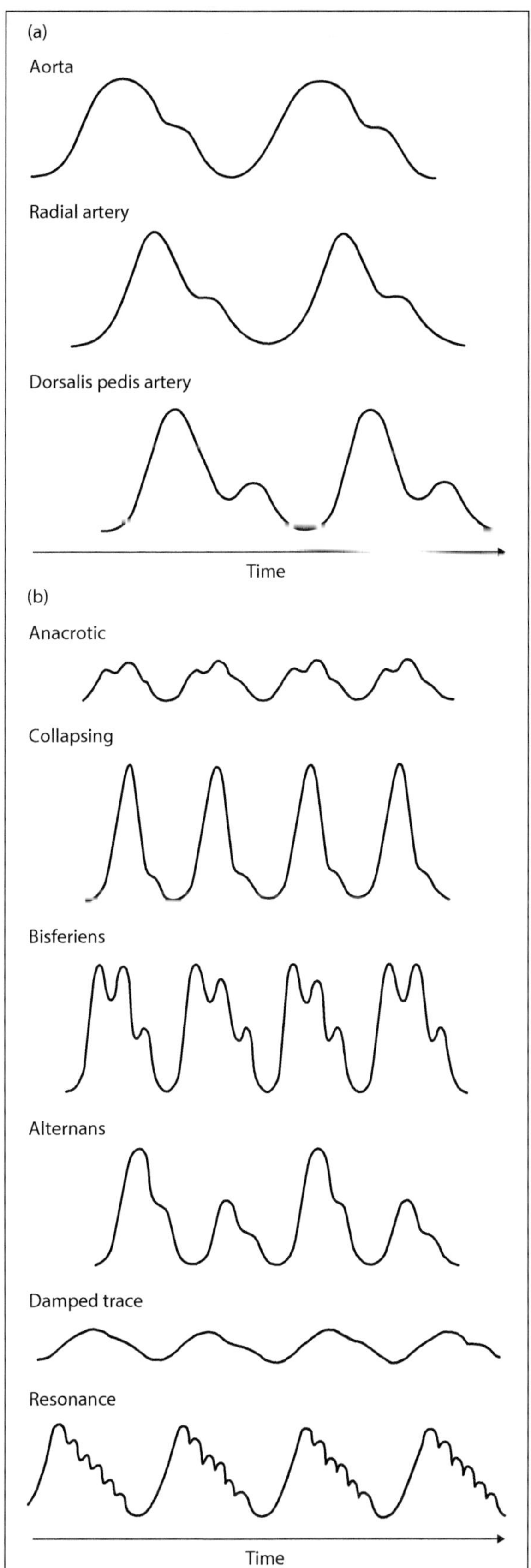

Fig. 15 (a) Arterial tracing from different sites. (b) Abnormal arterial waveforms

- **myocardial contractility**, as indicated by rate of pressure change per unit time (d*P*/d*t*).
- outflow resistance; estimated by the slope of the diastolic decay. A slow fall may occur in vasoconstriction, a rapid fall in vasodilatation.
- **hypovolaemia** is suggested by a low dicrotic notch, narrow width of the waveform and large falls in peak pressure with IPPV breaths.

[Windkessel, German, 'wind chamber']
See also, Arterial blood pressure; Cardiac cycle; Mean arterial pressure

Arteriovenous oxygen difference. Difference between arterial and mixed venous O_2 content, normally 5 ml O_2/100 ml blood. Increased with low cardiac output or exercise (high O_2 extraction). Decreased with peripheral arteriovenous shunting, or when tissue O_2 extraction is impaired, e.g. sepsis or **cyanide poisoning**.
See also, Oxygen transport

Arthritis, *see Connective tissue diseases; Rheumatoid arthritis*

Articaine hydrochloride (Carticaine). **Local anaesthetic agent** containing both ester and amide groups, first used clinically in 1974. Although used in Canada and continental Europe for several years, was only introduced in the UK (only in combination with **adrenaline**) in 2001. Chemically similar to **prilocaine** and of similar potency. Suggested as being particularly suitable for **dental anaesthesia** because of its low toxicity (maximal safe dose 7 mg/kg), an ability to diffuse readily through tissues and its metabolism by blood and tissue esterases. Elimination **half-life** is about 1.6 h, with 50% excreted in the urine. Duration of action is about 2–4 h.

Artificial heart, *see Heart, artificial*

Artificial hibernation, *see Lytic cocktail*

Artificial ventilation, *see Expired air ventilation; Intermittent positive pressure ventilation*

ASA physical status. Classification system adopted by the **American Society of Anesthesiologists** in 1941 for categorising preoperative physical status. Originally with six categories (the last two referring to emergency cases), a seventh (moribund patient) was later added and in 1962 the ASA adopted a modified five-category system with the postscript 'E' indicating emergency surgery. A sixth category was added in 1984–85 in the ASA's relative value guide for billing purposes:

- 1: normal healthy patient.
- 2: mild systemic disease.
- 3: severe systemic disease.
- 4: severe systemic disease that is a constant threat to life.
- 5: moribund patient; not expected to survive without the operation.
- 6: declared brain-dead organ donor.

Extremes of age, **smoking** and late **pregnancy** are sometimes taken as criteria for category 2.

Although not an indicator of anaesthetic or operative risk, there is reasonable correlation with overall outcome. Widely used in **clinical trials** to describe fitness of patients. However, use of the scoring system may be inconsistent between anaesthetists.
See also, Preoperative assessment

Ascending cholangitis, *see Cholangitis, acute*

Ascending reticular activating system (ARAS). Group of neuronal circuits extending from the upper cervical cord and medulla to midbrain, implicated in regulating sleep–wake transitions and level of cortical 'arousal' (and thus **consciousness**). Its main pathway is the central tegmental tract, conveying impulses to the hypothalamus and thalamus and thence to the cortex. Any lesion interrupting the ARAS tends to cause **coma**. Because of proximity to other brainstem nuclei, lesions often cause cardiovascular or respiratory disturbances. A possible site of action for general anaesthetic agents.

Ascites. Excessive free fluid within the abdominal cavity; may exceed 20–30 l in extreme cases. Initially asymptomatic but features include weight gain, abdominal discomfort, fullness in the patient's flanks, shifting dullness to percussion and a fluid thrill. May be sufficient to restrict ventilation, via increased intra-abdominal pressure or **pleural effusions**. There may be dependent **oedema** despite evidence of **hypovolaemia**.

Causes include: **hepatic failure**; **cardiac failure**; abdominal **malignancy**; hepatic vein or portal vein occlusion; constrictive **pericarditis**; **nephrotic syndrome**; **malnutrition**; **pancreatitis**; **trauma** (haemoperitoneum); **ovarian hyperstimulation syndrome**; and bacterial **peritonitis**. Analysis of the ascitic fluid may help in the differential diagnosis, as for pleural effusion.

- Management:
  - first-line: dietary sodium restriction (88 mmol/day), **spironolactone** ± **furosemide**.
  - fluid restriction: unnecessary unless serum sodium <125 mmol/l.
  - **paracentesis**: indicated at first presentation and for patients with tense ascites. However, repeated removal of ascitic fluid can result in refractory ascites. Large-volume paracentesis should be accompanied by blood volume replacement using albumin (6–8 g per litre of fluid removed).
  - transjugular intrahepatic portosystemic stent shunting: may be indicated in chronic refractory ascites.
  - antibacterial drug therapy: if coexisting bacterial **peritonitis** is suggested (e.g. high white cell counts in ascitic fluid).

ASCOT, *see A severity characterisation of trauma*

Aspiration of gastric contents. Potentially a risk in all unconscious, sedated or anaesthetised patients, as **lower oesophageal sphincter** tone decreases and laryngeal reflexes are depressed. Aspiration may follow passive regurgitation of **gastric contents** or **vomiting**, and is not necessarily prevented by the presence of a cuffed tracheal or tracheostomy tube.

- Factors predisposing to aspiration:
  - full stomach:
    - recent oral intake (see later). Certain foods e.g. those with high fat content, take longer to leave the stomach than others.
    - gastrointestinal obstruction.
    - gastrointestinal bleeding.
    - **ileus**.
    - trauma/shock/anxiety/pain. After **trauma**, **gastric emptying** may be delayed for several hours, especially in children.
    - **hiatus hernia**.
    - drugs, e.g. **opioid analgesic drugs**.
    - **pregnancy**.
  - inefficient lower oesophageal sphincter:
    - hiatus hernia.
    - drugs, e.g. opioids, **atropine**.
    - pregnancy with heartburn.
    - presence of a nasogastric tube.
  - raised intra-abdominal pressure:
    - pregnancy.
    - lithotomy position.
    - **obesity**.
  - **oesophagus** not empty:
    - **achalasia**.
    - strictures.
    - pharyngeal pouch.
  - ineffective laryngeal reflexes:
    - general anaesthesia/**sedation**.
    - **topical anaesthesia**.
    - neurological disease.
- May result in:
  - stimulation of the airway(s), causing breath-holding, cough, **bronchospasm**.
  - impaired laryngoscopy if it occurs during induction of anaesthesia.
  - complete or partial **airway obstruction**.
  - obstruction of smaller airways causing distal **atelectasis**.
  - **aspiration pneumonitis**. Silent and continuous aspiration of small amounts of material may cause repeated episodes of moderate respiratory impairment, especially in patients with chronically impaired protective reflexes. The diagnosis may be easy to confuse with other conditions, e.g. repeated small **PEs** or **chest infections**.
- Measures to reduce risk:
  - starvation: traditionally, 6 h of starvation has been recommended before anaesthesia in all but extreme emergencies, but actual periods have been considerably longer when audited. Current guidelines generally advise 4–6 h of no food intake, and 2 h for clear fluids. Milk in tea and coffee has been considered inadvisable although recent evidence suggests this may not be problematic.
  - empty stomach:
    - via nasogastric tube.
    - **metoclopramide**.
  - increase lower oesophageal sphincter tone, e.g. with metoclopramide, **prochlorperazine**.
  - rapid sequence induction of anaesthesia.
  - induction in the lateral or sitting position.
  - reduction of the severity of aspiration pneumonitis: e.g. **H_2 receptor antagonists**, **antacids**, **proton pump inhibitors**.
- If aspiration occurs:
  - the patient should be placed in the head-down lateral position.
  - material is aspirated from the pharynx and larynx, and O_2 administered.
  - tracheal intubation may be necessary to protect the airway, and to allow tracheobronchial suction.
  - further management is as for aspiration pneumonitis.

Smith I, Kranke P, Murat I, et al (2011). Eur J Anaesthesiol; 28: 556–69

See also, Induction, rapid sequence

Aspiration pneumonitis (Mendelson's syndrome). Inflammatory reaction of lung parenchyma following **aspiration**

of gastric contents, originally described in obstetric patients. A 'critical' volume of 25 ml of aspirate of pH 2.5, based on animal studies, is no longer considered relevant clinically; the more acidic the inhaled material, the less volume is required to produce pneumonitis. Should be distinguished from aspiration pneumonia, caused by aspiration of colonising bacteria from the oropharynx.

Particulate **antacids** (e.g. **magnesium trisilicate**) may themselves be associated with pneumonitis if aspirated.

The acid gastric contents cause chemical injury and loss of **surfactant**. Pneumonitis occurs within hours of aspiration, with decreased **FRC** and pulmonary **compliance**, **pulmonary hypertension, shunt** and increased **extravascular lung water**. Features include dyspnoea, tachypnoea, tachycardia, hypoxia and bronchospasm, with or without pyrexia. Crepitations and wheezes may be heard on chest auscultation. Irregular fluffy densities may appear on the **CXR** from 8 to 24 h. Movement of fluid into the lungs results in **hypovolaemia** and **hypotension**. The syndrome is often considered part of the **ALI** spectrum. Differential diagnosis includes **cardiac failure, sepsis, PE, amniotic fluid embolism** and **fat embolism**.

Treatment is mainly supportive, with **O_2 therapy**, **bronchodilator drugs**, and removal of aspirate and secretions by **physiotherapy** and suction. **Bronchoscopy** may be required to remove large particulate matter. Secondary infection may occur, and prophylactic **antibacterial drugs** are sometimes given, although this is controversial. Use of high-dose **corticosteroids** is declining but inhaled corticosteroids may be beneficial for treatment of bronchospasm. **CPAP** or **IPPV** with **PEEP** may be required in severe cases. Mortality remains high.

[Curtis L Mendelson (1913–2002), US obstetrician]

Raghavendran K, Nemzek J, Napolitano LM, et al (2011). Crit Care Med; 39: 818–26

Aspirin. Acetylsalicylic acid, synthesised in the early 1900s in Germany. Commonest **salicylate** in use. Uses, side effects and pharmacokinetics as for salicylates. Used widely as an **antiplatelet drug**. Due to the risk of **Reye's syndrome**, it is contraindicated in children under 16 years of age (except for the treatment of **Kawasaki disease** and as an antiplatelet agent after **cardiac surgery**).

- Dosage:
  - analgesia: 300–900 mg orally 4–6-hourly, up to a total of 4 g daily.
  - secondary prevention of thrombotic cerebrovascular or CVS disease: 75–100 mg orally od.
  - **acute coronary syndromes**: 150–300 mg orally od.
  - following **cardiac surgery**: 75–300 mg orally od.

Over-the-counter sale of 300-mg tablets/capsules in the UK is limited to packs of 32 (packs of 100 tablets/capsules may be purchased from pharmacists in special circumstances).

See also, Salicylate poisoning

Assisted ventilation. Positive pressure ventilation supplementing each spontaneous breath made by the patient. May be useful during transient **hypoventilation** caused by respiratory-depressant drugs in spontaneously breathing anaesthetised patients. Also used in ICU, e.g. in **weaning from ventilators**.

- Different modes:
  - assist mode ventilation: delivery of positive pressure breaths triggered by inspiratory effort.
  - assist-control mode ventilation: assist mode ventilation against a background of regular IPPV.
  - **inspiratory pressure support.**
  - **inspiratory volume support.**
  - **proportional assist ventilation.**

Association of Anaesthetists of Great Britain and Ireland. Founded in 1932 to represent anaesthetists' interests and to establish a diploma in anaesthetics (**DA examination**). Before this, the London Society of Anaesthetists (founded 1893) had formed the Anaesthetic Section of the Royal Society of Medicine in 1908, its purpose to advance the science and art of anaesthesia. Publishes the journal ***Anaesthesia*** and regular guidelines on various aspects of anaesthetic practice. Has over 11 000 members.

Helliwell PJ (1982). Anaesthesia; 37: 913–23

Asthma. Reversible airways obstruction, resulting from bronchoconstriction, bronchial mucosal oedema and mucus plugging. Causes high airways resistance, **hypoxaemia**, air trapping and increased work of breathing. Two main forms exist:

- extrinsic allergic: begins in childhood; may have an associated family history of atopy (e.g. hayfever, eczema), is episodic and tends to respond to therapy.
- intrinsic: adult onset; no allergic family history. Nasal polyps are common and exacerbations occur with infection and **aspirin**. Less responsive to treatment.

Patients' bronchi show increased sensitivity to triggering agents, constricting when normal bronchi may not. During anaesthesia, surgical stimulation or stimulation of the pharynx or larynx may cause **bronchospasm**.

- Chronic drug treatment:
  - **β_2-adrenergic receptor agonists**, e.g. **salbutamol**.
  - **aminophylline** and related drugs.
  - **corticosteroids**.
  - **sodium cromoglicate**.
  - **anticholinergic drugs**, e.g. **ipratropium**.
  - **leukotriene receptor antagonists**.
- Acute severe asthma:
  - signs of a severe attack:
    - inability to talk.
    - tachycardia >110 beats/min.
    - tachypnoea >25 breaths/min.
    - **pulsus paradoxus** >10 mmHg.
    - **peak expiratory flow rate** (PEFR) <50% of predicted normal.
  - signs of life-threatening attack:
    - silent chest on auscultation.
    - cyanosis.
    - bradycardia.
    - exhausted, confused or unconscious patient.
  - arterial blood gas measurement: hypoxaemia, largely from **$\dot{V}/\dot{Q}$ mismatch**, may be severe. It may worsen following bronchodilator treatment due to increased **dead space** and mismatch. Arterial $P\text{CO}_2$ is usually reduced because of hyperventilation, but may rise in severe cases, indicating requirement for IPPV. There is poor correlation between FEV_1 and arterial $P\text{CO}_2$.
  - other problems: **pneumothorax**, infection, **dehydration. Hypokalaemia** is common due to corticosteroids, **catecholamine** administration and respiratory **alkalosis**.
  - general medical and ICU management:
    - first-line therapies:
      - humidified O_2 with high $F_{I}O_2$.
      - nebulised salbutamol 2.5–5 mg or **terbutaline** 5–10 mg 4-hourly (may be given continuously

in severe asthma); iv salbutamol 250 μg may be given, followed by 5–20 μg/min, although in general, iv administration of β_2-agonists is thought to have no advantage over the inhaled route.
  - nebulised ipratropium 0.1–0.5 mg is traditionally alternated with β_2-agonists, although in modern practice they are often combined in the same nebuliser.
  - corticosteroids; e.g. **hydrocortisone** 100–200 mg 4-hourly iv, or by infusion.
- second-line therapies:
  - **magnesium sulfate** 1.2–2.0 g iv over 20 min as a single dose.
  - aminophylline 3–6 mg/kg iv, followed by 0.5 mg/kg/h (with caution if the patient is already taking **theophyllines**).
  - **inhalational anaesthetic agents**, **ketamine** and **adrenaline** have been used in resistant cases.
- supportive therapies:
  - **antibacterial drugs**, **physiotherapy**, iv rehydration.
  - **IPPV**:
    - intubation may provoke cardiac arrhythmias in severe hypoxia/hypercapnia.
    - **sedation** and neuromuscular blockade are required to aid IPPV.
    - high inflation pressures risk **barotrauma** and decreased cardiac output.
    - a flow generator **ventilator** is required, to ensure adequate **tidal volumes**.
    - because expiration may not be complete before the next breath, **FRC** increases with 'gas trapping', usually reaching equilibrium after 5–10 breaths. Despite the resultant auto-**PEEP** (intrinsic PEEP) and traditional teaching that PEEP should not be used in asthma because of the increased risk of barotrauma, PEEP has been applied to good effect and may actually reduce FRC by an unknown mechanism.
    - adequate ventilation may be difficult; **permissive hypercapnia** is often practised. Gas exchange may be improved by a slow inspiratory flow rate, low minute volume (6–8 l/min) and low ventilatory rate (12–14 breaths/min). Expiration should occupy at least 50% of the ventilatory cycle duration.
- **bronchoalveolar lavage** has been used.

- Anaesthetic management of patients with asthma:
  - preoperatively:
    - **preoperative assessment** is directed towards respiratory function, frequency and severity of attacks, and drug therapy (including corticosteroids).
    - investigations: **CXR**; PEFR/spirometry (especially pre- and post-bronchodilator); arterial **blood gas interpretation**.
    - **premedication**: nebulised bronchodilators may be given with premedication. Preoperative physiotherapy may also be useful. Steroid cover may be required.
  - perioperatively:
    - regional anaesthesia is often suitable.
    - **thiopental** has been implicated as causing bronchospasm, although this is controversial. **Propofol**, **etomidate** and ketamine are suitable alternatives. Volatile agents cause bronchodilatation. **Atracurium** may cause histamine release, while **vecuronium**, **pancuronium**, **rocuronium** and **fentanyl** do not.
    - although many **opioid analgesic drugs** may release **histamine**, they are commonly given. **Fentanyl** may be a good alternative if morphine has previously provoked bronchospasm.
    - tracheal intubation and the presence of a tracheal tube may cause bronchospasm. This may be reduced by spraying the larynx and trachea with **lidocaine**; iv lidocaine, 1–2 mg/kg, has been used to reduce the incidence of bronchospasm on intubation and extubation. Alternatively, techniques avoiding tracheal intubation may be employed.
    - **β-adrenergic receptor antagonists** should be avoided.
    - dehydration should be avoided.

Sellers WFS (2013). Br J Anaesth; 110: 183–90

See also, Bronchodilator drugs

Astrup method. Used for the analysis of blood acid–base status. The **pH** of a blood sample is measured, and the sample equilibrated with two gases of different CO_2 concentration, usually 4% and 8%. pH is measured after each equilibration, and the standard **bicarbonate** and **base excess** calculated. The original CO_2 tension is calculated from the pH of the original sample, using the **Siggaard-Andersen nomogram.**

[Poul Astrup (1915–2000), Danish chemist]

Asystole. Absent cardiac electrical activity. Common in **cardiac arrest** due to hypoxia or exsanguination, especially in children. Must be distinguished from accidental ECG disconnection. Management: as in **CPR**.

Atelectasis. Collapse of lung tissue affecting all or part of the **lung**. Caused by inadequate aeration of alveoli, with subsequent absorption of gas. The latter occurs because the total partial pressure of dissolved gases in venous blood is less than atmospheric pressure; gas trapped behind obstructed airways (e.g. by secretions) is therefore slowly absorbed. **Nitrogen**, being relatively insoluble in blood, tends to splint alveoli open when breathing air. Absorption atelectasis may follow high F_IO_2, because O_2 is readily absorbed into the blood and the nitrogen has been washed out of the alveoli.

Has been shown by CT scanning to occur in dependent parts of the lung during anaesthesia in normal patients, contributing to impaired gas exchange. May also follow accidental endobronchial placement of a tracheal tube. It may persist postoperatively, particularly in patients with poor lung function and sputum retention, and when chest movement is reduced, e.g. by pain after upper abdominal surgery or fractured ribs. **Hypoxaemia**, tachypnoea and tachycardia result, with reduced air entry to the affected area of lung that may then become infected. Treatment of atelectasis includes **physiotherapy**, **incentive spirometry**, **humidification**, intermittent lung inflations using a ventilator, **CPAP** and, occasionally, **bronchoscopy**.

Tusman G, Böhm SH, Warner DO, Sprung J (2012). Curr Opin Anaesthesiol; 25: 1–10

Atenolol. Water-soluble **β-adrenergic receptor antagonist**, available for oral and iv administration. Relatively selective for β_1-receptors. Uses and side effects are as for β-adrenergic receptor antagonists in general.

- Dosage:
  - hypertension: 25–50 mg/day orally; angina and arrhythmias: 50–100 mg/day.
  - acute arrhythmias: 2.5 mg iv over 3 min, repeated at 5-min intervals up to 10 mg, or 150 μg/kg iv over 20 min, repeated 12-hourly as required.
  - after acute MI: 5 mg iv over 5 min, then 50 mg orally after 15 min and 12 h, then 100 mg/day.
- Side effects: as for β-adrenergic receptor antagonists.

Atherosclerosis. Disease involving the intima of medium and large arteries, resulting in fat accumulation and fibrous plaques that narrow the vessel lumen. Further stenosis may follow thrombosis and haemorrhage. Thought to be at least partly inflammatory in aetiology, although the precise roles of proinflammatory and prothrombotic mediators are uncertain. Causes **ischaemic heart disease**, cerebrovascular disease and peripheral arterial insufficiency, especially in the legs. Thus patients with peripheral vascular disease frequently have occult atherosclerotic disease involving other organs.

A rigid arterial tree results in a high systolic arterial BP with normal diastolic pressure, a common finding in the elderly, because virtually all elderly patients have some atherosclerosis.

Atipamezole. Highly selective **α_2-adrenergic receptor antagonist** used to reverse the sedative, analgesic and cardiovascular effects of **dexmedetomidine** in dogs. Has been studied as a potential **antiparkinsonian drug**.

ATLS, *see Advanced Trauma Life Support*

Atmosphere. Unit of **pressure**. One atmosphere equals 760 mmHg (101.33 kPa), the average barometric pressure at sea level.
See also, Bar

ATN, **Acute tubular necrosis**, *see Acute kidney injury*

Atopy. Tendency to **asthma**, hayfever, eczema and other allergic conditions, including **adverse drug reactions**. Sufferers are sensitive to antigens that usually cause no reaction in normal subjects. May be familial. IgE levels may be raised. Drugs associated with **histamine** release should be avoided.

Atorvastatin, *see Statins*

ATP, *see Adenosine triphosphate and diphosphate*

ATPD and ATPS. Ambient temperature and pressure, dry; and ambient temperature and pressure, saturated with water vapour. Used for standardising gas volume measurements.

Atracurium besilate. Non-depolarising **neuromuscular blocking drug**, first used in 1980. A bisquaternary nitrogenous plant derivative. Initial dose: 0.3–0.6 mg/kg. Intubation is possible approximately 90 s after a dose of 0.5 mg/kg. Effects last 20–30 min. Supplementary dose: 0.1–0.2 mg/kg. Has been given by iv infusion at 0.3–0.6 mg/kg/h. May cause **histamine** release, usually mild, but severe reactions have been reported (an isomer of atracurium, **cisatracurium**, has similar neuromuscular properties but causes less histamine release). At body temperature and pH, undergoes spontaneous **Hofmann degradation** to **laudanosine**. Up to 50% ester hydrolysis also occurs. Often considered the drug of choice in renal or hepatic impairment. Its cardiostability, low risk of accumulation and spontaneous reversal are also advantages. Stored at 2°–8°C; at room temperature, activity decreases by only a few per cent per month.

Atrial ectopic beats. Impulses arising from abnormal pacemaker sites within the atria. The **P waves** are usually abnormal, and arise early in the **cardiac cycle**. They are usually conducted to the ventricles in the normal way, producing normal QRS complexes (Fig. 16). Very early ectopics may produce abnormal **QRS complexes**, because the ventricular conducting system may still be refractory when the ectopic impulse reaches it. The resultant QRS may then be mistaken for a **ventricular ectopic beat**. Several ectopic sites may give rise to the 'wandering pacemaker', producing differently shaped P waves with differing PR intervals. Rarely require treatment.
See also, Arrhythmias; Electrocardiography

Atrial fibrillation (AF). Lack of coordinated atrial contraction, resulting in impulses from many different parts of the atria reaching the atrioventricular (AV) node in quick succession, only some of which are transmitted. Ventricular response may be fast, resulting in inadequate ventricular filling, and reduced stroke volume and cardiac output. **Cardiac failure**, hypotension and systemic emboli from intra-atrial thrombus may occur.

- Features:
  - irregularly irregular pulse. Ventricular rate depends upon the conducting ability of the AV node; usually rapid, the ventricular activity is slow and regular if complete **heart block** exists.
  - no **P waves** on the **ECG** (Fig. 17).
- May be idiopathic or caused by:
  - **ischaemic heart disease** (most common cause), including acute **MI**.
  - mitral valve disease.
  - **hyperthyroidism**.
  - **PE**.
  - **cardiomyopathy**.
  - thoracic surgery/central venous cannulation.
  - acute **hypovolaemia**.
- Treatment:
  - drug therapy is aimed at rate rather than rhythm control although **sinus rhythm** may be restored. Initial

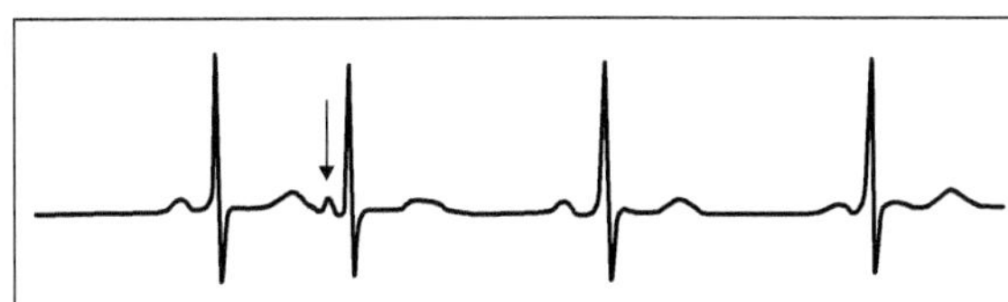

Fig. 16 Example of an atrial ectopic beat *(arrowed)*

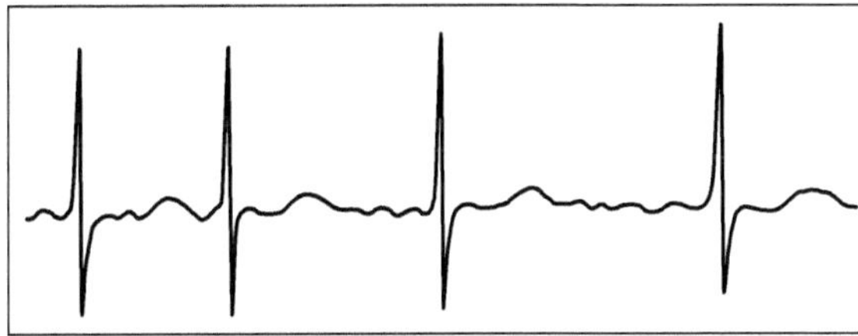

Fig. 17 Atrial fibrillation

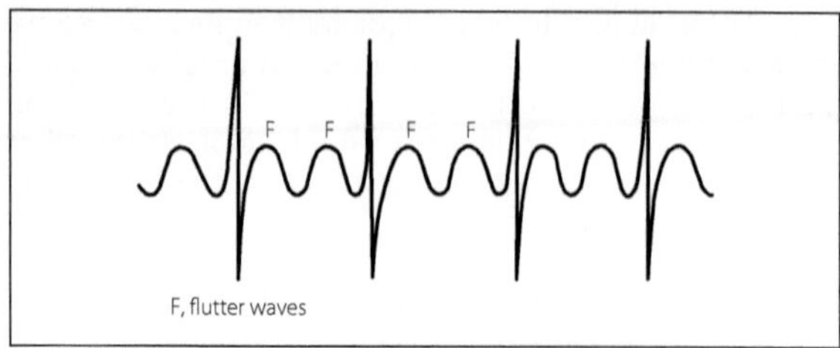

Fig. 18 Atrial flutter

monotherapy consists of **β-adrenergic receptor antagonists** or a rate-limiting **calcium channel blocking drug** (e.g. **verapamil**, **diltiazem**). Other agents used include **amiodarone** and **disopyramide**. **Digoxin** is used only in sedentary patients.
- **cardioversion** if haemodynamically unstable or recent onset (<3 days).
- catheter ablation of the AV node or atrial foci where AF originates; largely reserved for cases intolerant of or refractory to other treatment.
- anticoagulation should be considered if AF has persisted for more than 2–3 days, especially before cardioversion. In chronic AF, anticoagulation with **warfarin** (or newer agents e.g. **apixaban**, **dabigatran**, **rivaroxaban**) is used depending on the presence or absence of other risk factors, e.g. age >75, congestive cardiac failure, diabetes, hypertension, previous **stroke**, previous MI.

Jones C, Pollit V, Fitzmaurice D, et al (2014). Br Med J; 348: g3655
See also, Arrhythmias

Atrial flutter. **Arrhythmia** resulting from rapid atrial discharge (usually 300/min), caused by a re-entrant circuit within the atria and usually initiated by an **atrial ectopic beat**. May be paroxysmal or sustained. Commonly occurs with 4:1 or 2:1 atrioventricular block; i.e., with ventricular rates 75/min or 150/min, respectively.
- Features:
  - usually regular pulse.
  - saw-tooth flutter (F) waves on the **ECG** (Fig. 18); with 2:1 block the second flutter wave of each pair may be hidden in the QRS or T waves, leading to the incorrect diagnosis of **sinus tachycardia**. **Carotid sinus massage** may slow the ventricular rate enough to reveal rapid flutter waves.
- Causes: as for **AF**.
- Treatment:
  - aimed at restoring sinus rhythm: **cardioversion** using low-energy (25–50 J), rapid atrial pacing, and drug therapy as for AF.
  - **digoxin** may convert flutter to AF.

See also, Cardiac pacing

Atrial natriuretic peptide (ANP). Hormone isolated from myocytes of the right atrium; similar peptides are present in the cardiac ventricles and vascular endothelium. Released in response to atrial stretching, e.g. in fluid overload (i.e., not to increased atrial pressure per se), sympathetic stimulation and presence of angiotensin II.
- Actions:
  - increases **GFR** and urinary sodium and water excretion. Decreases reabsorption of sodium ions in the proximal convoluted tubule of the nephron.
  - relaxes vascular smooth muscle; renal vessels are more sensitive than others.
  - inhibits plasma renin activity and **aldosterone** release.
  - has immune and cytoprotective properties, increasing the rate of phagocytosis and decreasing production of oxygen **free radicals**.
  - releases free fatty acids from adipose tissue, possibly via specific receptors.

ANP and related peptides have been investigated as markers of **cardiac failure** and **myocardial ischaemia**. Inhibition of their breakdown has been investigated as possible therapy in **hypertension**, cardiac failure and myocardial ischaemia, while infusion of ANP has been investigated for its renal protective effect in oliguric acute tubular necrosis. A synthetic ANP is available for treatment of advanced heart failure.
DeVito P (2014). Peptides; 58: 108–16
See also, B-type natriuretic hormone

Atrial septal defect (ASD). Accounts for up to 10% of **congenital heart disease**.
- Normal septal development is as follows:
  - the septum primum grows down from the top of the heart, separating the right and left halves of the common atrium.
  - the ostium secundum appears in its upper part.
  - the septum secundum grows down to the right of the septum primum, usually just covering the ostium secundum.
  - the foramen ovale is formed from the ostium secundum and overlapping septum secundum.
- Features of ASD:
  - left-to-right shunting increases flow to the right heart, producing a pulmonary flow murmur with or without a tricuspid murmur, increasing on inspiration. Fixed splitting of the second **heart sound** may be heard.
  - right ventricular hypertrophy, right **bundle branch block** and right axis deviation may be present.
  - **pulmonary hypertension**.

Over 90% of defects are secundum ASDs; they may present in later life with pulmonary hypertension, right-sided cardiac failure, **Eisenmenger's syndrome** and **AF**. Suturing of the defect is usually quick if a patch is not required. Transcatheter surgery is being increasingly used.

Primum ASDs may involve the atrioventricular valves; they often present early. Repair is more complicated. Valve regurgitation and conduction defects may follow surgery.

Anaesthetic management: as for congenital heart disease and **cardiac surgery**.
Geva T, Martins JD, Wald RM (2014). Lancet; 383: 1921–32
See also, Heart murmurs; Preoperative assessment

Atrial stretch receptors, *see Baroreceptors*

Atrioventricular block, *see Heart block*

Atrioventricular dissociation. Unrelated ventricular and atrial activity. The term is usually reserved for when the ventricular rate exceeds the atrial rate, to distinguish it from complete **heart block** (in which the reverse occurs). Ventricular activity may arise from the atrioventricular node or an ectopic pacemaker. It may occur during bradycardia as an escape mechanism, and during anaesthesia. On the **ECG**, **P waves** and **QRS complexes** are unrelated, the former more widely spaced than the latter (Fig. 19). Rarely clinically significant.
See also, Arrhythmias

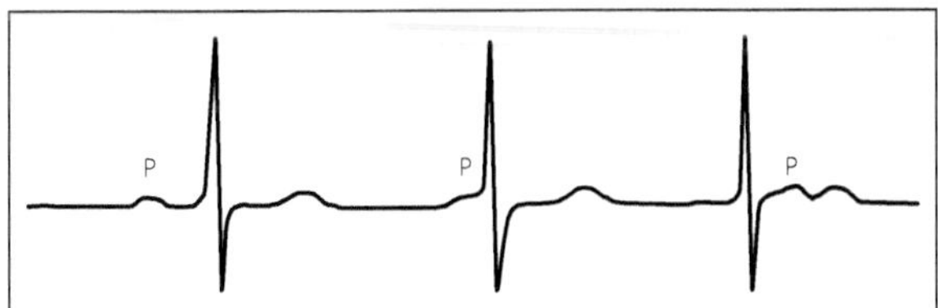

Fig. 19 Atrioventricular dissociation

Atrioventricular node, *see Heart, conducting system*

Atropine sulfate. **Anticholinergic drug** (competitive antagonist at muscarinic **acetylcholine receptors**), an ester of tropic acid and tropine. Found in deadly nightshade. Used to reduce muscarinic effects of **acetylcholinesterase inhibitors**, for **premedication** and in the treatment of bradycardia. Has also been used as an **antispasmodic drug** and as a mydriatic.

- Effects:
  - CVS:
    - tachycardia (may cause bradycardia initially; thought to be due to central vagal stimulation).
    - cutaneous vasodilatation (cause unknown).
  - CNS:
    - excitement, hallucinations and hyperthermia, especially in children.
    - antiparkinsonian effect.
  - RS:
    - bronchodilatation and increased dead space.
    - reduced secretions.
  - GIT:
    - reduced salivation.
    - reduced motility.
    - reduced secretion.
    - reduced **lower oesophageal sphincter** tone.
  - others:
    - reduced sweating.
    - mydriasis and cycloplegia.
    - reduced bladder and ureteric tone.
- Standard doses:
  - 0.1–0.6 mg increments iv for bradycardia. A larger maximum dose (3 mg) is no longer recommended for the management of **asystole/pulseless electrical activity**.
  - 0.3–0.6 mg im as premedication; 0.01–0.02 mg/kg for children.
  - 0.01–0.02 mg/kg when given with acetylcholinesterase inhibitors.
  - 0.6–1.2 mg orally at night in irritable bowel disease, diverticulitis.

Applied directly to the eye, it may provoke closed-angle glaucoma in susceptible patients, the iris obstructing drainage of aqueous humour when the pupil is dilated.

See also, Anticholinergic drugs, for comparison with hyoscine and glycopyrronium; Tracheal administration of drugs

Audit. Systematic process by which medical practice is assessed and improved. Involves the following steps:

- identification of a particular aspect of practice (e.g. reducing **PONV**).
- assessment of how that practice is carried out (e.g. measuring nausea scores, recording usage of antiemetics).
- judgement by peer review whether certain standards are being met (e.g. deciding in advance that more than 10% of patients suffering severe nausea is unacceptable. National standards exist for many areas of practice, e.g. issued by professional bodies).
- identification of areas for improvement where practice is substandard (e.g. prophylactic antiemetics not being given for high-risk surgery).
- addressing the deficiency (e.g. education, institution of protocols).
- reassessment after a period to check that practice has improved and standards are being met; i.e., 'closing the audit loop'. To be effective, specific audits require repeating regularly.

Audit (is the correct management being used?) should be distinguished from research (what is the correct management?), although both may involve similar methods of data collection and analysis, and distinction may be difficult. Because traditional 'audit' is intermittent and based only on reaching set standards, rather than continuing to improve beyond these, the continuous process of 'quality improvement' is now often seen as preferable in the clinical setting.

- Anaesthetic/ICU applications include monitoring:
  - organisation of services, e.g. appropriate allocation of trainees, cancellation of surgery because of insufficient staff, leave allocations and costs.
  - management of patients' drug usage and clinical policies.
  - complications, e.g. unplanned admission to ICU, specific events. Methods include analysis of currently held data (e.g. anaesthetic **record-keeping**) or specific studies into particular aspects of care (e.g. **National Confidential Enquiry into Patient Outcome and Death** and **Confidential Enquiries into Maternal Deaths**). Audit is now a mandatory part of medical practice in the UK, despite controversy over its value in relation to costs.

See also, National Audit Projects; Quality assurance/improvement; Risk management

Auriculotemporal nerve block, *see Mandibular nerve blocks*

Auscultatory gap, *see Korotkoff sounds*

Australia antigen, *see Hepatitis*

Autoimmune disease. Characterised by activation of the immune system, directed against host tissue. May involve antibody production, attacking intracellular, extracellular or cell membrane **antigens**. Pathogenesis is not fully understood, but involves imbalance of suppressor and helper T lymphocyte cell function. May affect specific organs, e.g. **adrenocortical insufficiency**, or many tissues, e.g. **connective tissue diseases**.

- May follow triggering agents, e.g.:
  - drugs: SLE-like syndrome after **procainamide** or **hydralazine** therapy, haemolytic anaemia after **α-methyldopa** therapy.
  - infection: **haemolysis** following mycoplasma pneumonia, **rheumatic fever** following streptococcal infection. Viral infections are often implicated.

Genetic factors are also important, hence the association between certain diseases and HLA types (e.g. **myasthenia gravis**) thyroid disease, pernicious anaemia and vitiligo. More than one of these diseases may occur in the same patient, suggesting common mechanisms. Testing for autoantibodies may be useful in the diagnosis and treatment of these conditions.

Autologous blood transfusion, *see Blood transfusion, autologous*

Autonomic hyperreflexia. Increased sensitivity of sympathetic reflexes in patients with **spinal cord injury** above T5/6. Cutaneous or visceral stimuli below the level of the lesion may result in mass discharge of sympathetic nerves, causing sweating, vasoconstriction and hypertension, with high levels of circulating **catecholamines. Baroreceptor** stimulation results in compensatory bradycardia. Distension of hollow viscera, especially of the bladder, is a potent stimulus. It may also occur during abdominal surgery and labour. Onset of susceptibility is usually within a few weeks of injury.

In anaesthesia, both general and regional techniques have been used; **spinal anaesthesia** has been suggested as the technique of choice, if appropriate. Control of hypertension has been successfully achieved with **vasodilator drugs**. Hypotension may also occur.

Autonomic nervous system. System that regulates non-voluntary bodily functions, by means of reflex pathways. Efferent nerves contain medullated fibres that leave the brain and spinal cord to synapse with non-medullated fibres in peripheral ganglia. Closely related to the CNS, anatomically and functionally; thus sensory input may affect autonomic activity and consciousness and voluntary behaviour, e.g. pain, temperature and sensation.

- Divided into the **parasympathetic** and **sympathetic nervous systems**, based on anatomical, pharmacological and functional differences (Fig. 20):
  - parasympathetic:
    - output in cranial and sacral nerves; ganglia near to target organs.
    - **acetylcholine** released as a transmitter at pre- and postganglionic nerve endings.
    - increases GIT activity, and reduces arousal and cardiovascular activity.
  - sympathetic:
    - output in thoracic and lumbar segments of the spinal cord; ganglia form the sympathetic trunk.
    - acetylcholine released at preganglionic nerve endings, **adrenaline** and **noradrenaline** (in general) at postganglionic nerve endings.
    - increases arousal and cardiovascular activity ('fight or flight' reaction), reduces visceral activity.

Some organs receive only sympathetic innervation (e.g. piloerector muscles, adipose tissue, **juxtaglomerular apparatus**), others only parasympathetic innervation (e.g. lacrimal glands); most are under dual control.

See also, Acetylcholine receptors

Autonomic neuropathy. May be:
- central:
  - primary, e.g. progressive autonomic failure (Shy–Drager syndrome).
  - secondary to **stroke**, infection or drugs.
- peripheral, e.g. due to **diabetes mellitus**, amyloidosis, **autoimmune diseases**, **porphyria**, **Guillain–Barré syndrome**, **myasthenic syndrome**.

Results in postural hypotension, cardiac conduction defects, bladder dysfunction and GIT disturbances, including delayed gastric emptying. Diabetics with autonomic neuropathy have increased risk of perioperative cardiac or respiratory arrest.

- Useful bedside tests of autonomic function include:
  - pulse and BP measurement lying and standing; a postural drop of over 30 mmHg indicates autonomic dysfunction.
  - **Valsalva manoeuvre.**
  - effect of breathing on pulse rate (normally slows on expiration).
  - sustained hand grip (normal response: tachycardia and over 15 mmHg increase in diastolic BP).

ECG is useful for the latter two tests. Other tests include observation of sweating and pupillary responses, and catecholamine studies.

Patients with autonomic neuropathy are at risk of developing severe hypotension during anaesthesia, particularly with **spinal** or **epidural anaesthesia**, and **IPPV**. They may also show reduced response to **hypoglycaemia**. There may be increased risk of **aspiration of gastric contents.**

[George Shy (1919–1967) and Glenn Drager (1917–1967), US neurologists]

Lankhorst S, Keet SW, Bulte CS, Boer C (2015). Anaesthesia; 70: 336–43

See also, Peripheral neuropathy

Autoregulation. Mechanism by which an organ maintains a constant **blood flow** despite variations in the mean arterial pressure perfusing the organ.

- Several theories exist:
  - myogenic theory: postulates that muscle in the vessel wall contracts as intraluminal pressure increases, thus maintaining wall tension by reducing radius, in accordance with **Laplace's law**.
  - metabolic theory: argues that vasodilator substances (**nitric oxide**, **hydrogen ions**, CO_2, **adenosine**) accumulate in the tissues at low blood flow; the resultant vasodilatation results in increased flow and the vasodilator metabolites are washed away.
  - tissue theory: states that, as blood flow increases, the vessels are compressed by the increased amount of interstitial fluid that has accumulated. Usually occurs at MAP of 60–160 mmHg in normotensive subjects; it may be impaired by volatile anaesthetic agents, **vasodilator drugs** or disease states (e.g. **cerebral blood flow in TBI**).

See also, Systemic vascular resistance

Autotransfusion, *see Blood transfusion, autologous*

Average, *see Mean*

Avogadro's hypothesis. At constant temperature and pressure, equal volumes of all ideal gases contain the same number of molecules. One **mole** of a substance at standard temperature and pressure contains 6.023×10^{23} particles (Avogadro's number), and one mole of a gas occupies 22.4 l.

[Count Amedeo Avogadro (1776–1856), Italian scientist]

AVP, Arginine vasopressin, *see Vasopressin*

AVPU scale. Simple scale of responsiveness, commonly used to assess the neurological status of patients, e.g. following **trauma**, **cardiac arrest**. Records whether the patient is alert (A), responsive only to vocal (V) or painful (P) stimuli, or unresponsive (U). Easier and faster to perform than other more complicated **trauma scales** and systems such as the **Glasgow coma scale.**

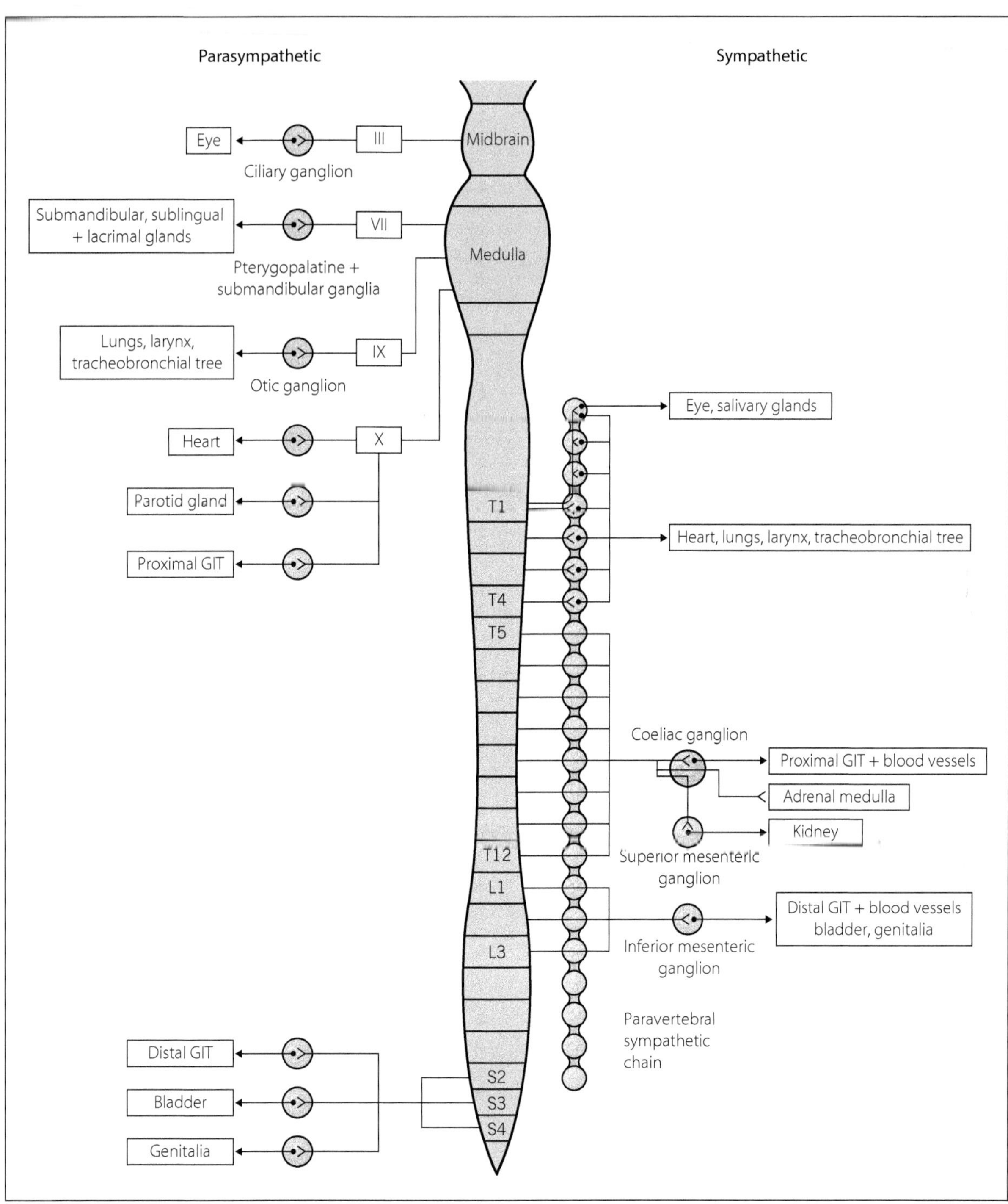

Fig. 20 Autonomic nervous system

Awareness. Accidental awareness during anaesthesia (AAGA) ranges from being fully conscious and in pain intraoperatively with explicit recall, to non-specific postoperative psychological symptoms with only vague recollections or dreams. Signs of inadequate anaesthesia (tachycardia, sweating, hypertension, dilated pupils, lacrimation) may not be present.

Quoted incidence is 0.01%–0.2%; its rarity and diagnostic variability contribute to the wide range, with the lower figures arising from studies in which only spontaneous reports are counted, and the higher figures arising from those in which patients are routinely questioned about recall postoperatively. The fifth **National Audit Project** (NAP 5) in 2014 found an overall incidence of reports of AAGA during a one-year period in the UK and Ireland of 1:19 000 (although this is not the incidence of AAGA because the denominator was extrapolated from brief 'snapshots' and the reported events were not limited to those actually occurring during that year). Other findings suggested that AAGA may be associated with:

- women, young adults, those with previous AAGA and **obesity**. Rare in paediatric practice.

- cardiothoracic anaesthesia and **caesarean section**.
- sedation, underlining the need for better explanation of the technique to patients.
- emergency surgery and junior anaesthetists.
- use of **neuromuscular blocking drugs**.
- use of **TIVA**, especially without target-controlled infusions.

About 50% of NAP5 reports were of awareness during induction, especially with contributory factors including the use of **thiopental**, rapid sequence induction, obesity, use of neuromuscular blocking drugs and difficulties with airway management. 20% occurred during emergence from anaesthesia and almost all were associated with residual neuromuscular block. Reports of awareness in ICU were almost all associated with neuromuscular blockade in conjunction with low-dose **propofol** infusions.

- AAGA may be reduced by:
  - ensuring adequate administration of anaesthetic agent, including use of end-expiratory gas monitoring (with alarms enabled).
  - thorough **checking of anaesthetic equipment**.
  - avoidance of neuromuscular blocking drugs when not necessary.
  - use of amnesic drugs, e.g. **benzodiazepines**.
  - use of cerebral function monitors (e.g. **bispectral index monitor**), especially if using TIVA.

In NAP5, 41% of patients experienced moderate to severe sequelae including **post-traumatic stress disorder**. Good outcomes are generally reported with early clinician acceptance of the patient's account and psychological support. The NAP5 authors recommended that **consent for anaesthesia** should include discussion of the incidence and risk factors of AAGA.

Tasbihgou SR, Vogels MF, Absalom AR (2018). Anaesthesia; 73: 112–22

See also, Anaesthesia, depth of; Isolated forearm technique; Traumatic neurotic syndrome

Axillary venous cannulation. Route of **central venous cannulation**, usually used when alternative sites are unsuitable. Advantages include venous puncture outside the ribcage, thus reducing the risk of **pneumothorax**, and the ability to compress the axillary artery directly if accidentally punctured. Several techniques have been described:

- proximal: with the arm abducted to 45 degrees, a needle is introduced three fingers' breadth (5 cm) below the coracoid process and directed at the junction of the medial one-quarter and lateral three-quarters of the clavicle.
- distal: with the arm abducted to 90 degrees, a needle is introduced 1 cm medial to the axillary arterial pulsation in the axilla. The medial cutaneous nerve may be at risk with this approach.

Fluoroscopy and increasingly, **ultrasound**, have been used to guide cannulation.

Ayre's T-piece, *see Anaesthetic breathing systems*

Azathioprine. Non-specific **cytotoxic drug**, used as an **immunosuppressive drug** in **organ transplantation**, **myasthenia gravis** and other **autoimmune diseases**. Metabolised to mercaptopurine.

- Dose: 3–5 mg/kg orally/iv initially; maintenance 1–4 mg/kg per day.
- Side effects: myelosuppression, fever, rigors, arthralgia, myalgia, interstitial nephritis, liver toxicity. Monitoring of therapy requires regular full blood counts. The iv preparation is alkaline and very irritant.

Azeotrope. Mixture of two or more liquids whose components cannot be separated by distillation. The boiling point of each is altered by the presence of the other substance; thus the components share the same boiling point, and the vapour contains the components in the same proportions as in the liquid mixture. Halothane and ether form an azeotrope when mixed in the ratio of 2:1 by volume.

Azidothymidine, *see Zidovudine*

Azithromycin. **Macrolide**, similar to **erythromycin** but less active against gram-positive bacteria and more active against certain gram-negative ones. Used in respiratory and other infections and as an **antituberculous drug** in resistant **TB**. Extensively tissue-bound.

- Dosage: 500 mg orally or by iv infusion od, for 2–3 days.
- Side effects: as for **clarithromycin**.

AZT, Azidothymidine, *see Zidovudine*

Aztreonam. Monocyclic **β-lactam** (monobactam) active against gram-negative aerobes (including pseudomonas) but not gram-positive or anaerobic organisms; thus reserved for specific (as opposed to 'blind') therapy. Resistant to some, but not all, β-lactamases. Synergistic with **aminoglycosides** against many bacteria.

- Dosage: 0.5–1.0 g iv over 3–5 min or by deep im injection tds/qds (or 2 g iv bd); in severe infections 2 g iv tds/qds.
- Side effects: as for **penicillin**. May cause phlebitis and pain on injection.

Azumolene sodium. Analogue of **dantrolene**; has been investigated as an alternative because of its greater water solubility and a smaller volume of administration.

B

BACCN, *see British Association of Critical Care Nurses*

Backward failure, *see Cardiac failure*

Baclofen. Synthetic **GABA$_B$** receptor agonist and skeletal muscle relaxant, used to treat muscle spasticity, e.g. following spinal injury and in multiple sclerosis. Acts at both spinal and supraspinal levels. Has also been used to treat **alcohol withdrawal syndromes**.

- Dosage: 5 mg orally tds, increased slowly up to 100 mg/day. Has also been given intrathecally: 25–50 μg over 1 min, increased by 25 μg/24 h up to 100 μg to determine an effective dose, then 12–2000 μg/day by infusion for maintenance.
- Side effects: sedation, nausea, confusion, convulsions, hypotension, GIT upset, visual disturbances, rarely hepatic impairment.

See also, γ-Aminobutyric acid receptors

Bacteraemia. Presence of **bacteria** in the blood. May be present in **sepsis**, but is not necessary for the diagnosis to be made.
See also, Blood cultures; Endotoxins

Bacteria. Micro-organisms with a bilayered cytoplasmic membrane, a double-stranded loop of DNA and, in most cases, an outer cell wall containing muramic acid. Responsible for many diseases; mechanisms include the initiation of inflammatory pathways by **endotoxins** or **exotoxins**; direct toxic effects on/destruction of tissues or organ systems; impairment of host defensive mechanisms; invasion of host cells; and provocation of autoimmune processes. For clinical purposes, classified phenotypically according to their ability to be stained by crystal violet after iodine fixation and alcohol decolourisation (Gram staining), their oxygen requirements for growth, and with serological testing in which selected antisera are used to identify carbohydrate or protein antigens in the bacterial cell wall:

- Gram-positive: cell wall consists of peptidoglycan (made up of glucosamine, muramic acid and amino acids), lipoteichoic acid and polysaccharides; include:
  - aerobes:
    - cocci (spherical-shaped), e.g. staphylococci, enterococci, streptococci species.
    - bacilli (rod-shaped), e.g. bacillus, corynebacterium, mycobacterium species.
  - anaerobes:
    - cocci, e.g. peptococcus species.
    - bacilli, e.g. actinomyces, propionibacterium, clostridium species.
- Gram-negative: have an additional outer cell wall layer containing lipopolysaccharide (endotoxin); include:
  - aerobes:
    - cocci, e.g. neisseria species.
    - bacilli, e.g. enterobacteria (enterobacter, escherichia, klebsiella, proteus, salmonella, serratia, shigella, yersinia), vibrio, acinetobacter, pseudomonas, brucella, bordetella, campylobacter, haemophilus, helicobacter, legionella, chlamydia, rickettsia, mycoplasma, leptospira, treponema species.
  - anaerobes:
    - cocci, e.g. veillonella species.
    - bacilli, e.g. bacteroides species.

Bacteria may also be classified genotypically using rRNA sequence analysis and molecular subtyping, and by their susceptibility to various viral phages and **antibacterial drugs**. **Bacterial resistance** is an increasing problem.
[Hans Gram (1853–1938), Danish physician]
See also, individual infections

Bacterial contamination of breathing equipment, *see Contamination of anaesthetic equipment*

Bacterial resistance. Ability of **bacteria** to survive in the presence of **antibacterial drugs**. An increasingly significant problem in terms of cost, pressure on development of new antibiotics and impaired ability to treat infections both in critically ill patients and the community as a whole.

- Mechanisms:
  - impermeability of the cell wall to the drug, e.g. pseudomonas and many antibiotics.
  - lack of intracellular binding site for the antibiotic, e.g. *Streptococcus pneumoniae* and **penicillin** resistance.
  - lack of target metabolic pathways, e.g. **vancomycin** is only effective against gram-positive organisms because it affects synthesis of the peptidoglycan cell wall components that gram-negative bacteria do not possess.
  - production of specific enzymes against the drug, e.g. penicillinase.
  - the presence of bacterial biofilms—communities of bacteria held within a polysaccharide and protein matrix that make them resistant to normal treatment regimens of antibacterial agents.

Resistance may be a natural or acquired property. Acquired resistance arises from chromosomal mutation leading to cross-resistance, gene transfer from one bacterium to another by conjugation or transduction via bacteriophages.

Factors that increase the likelihood of resistance include indiscriminate use of antibacterial drugs (possibly including prophylactic perioperative use), inappropriate choice of drug and use of suboptimal dosage regimens (including poor compliance by users, e.g. long-term anti-TB drug therapy). Regular consultation with microbiologists, use of antibiotic guidelines and **infection control** procedures, and microbiological surveillance may limit resistance. In the UK, the Department of Health has run several campaigns to increase awareness of the problem and encourages sensible prescribing of antibiotics. 'Antimicrobial stewardship' programmes (particularly in ICUs) strive to reduce

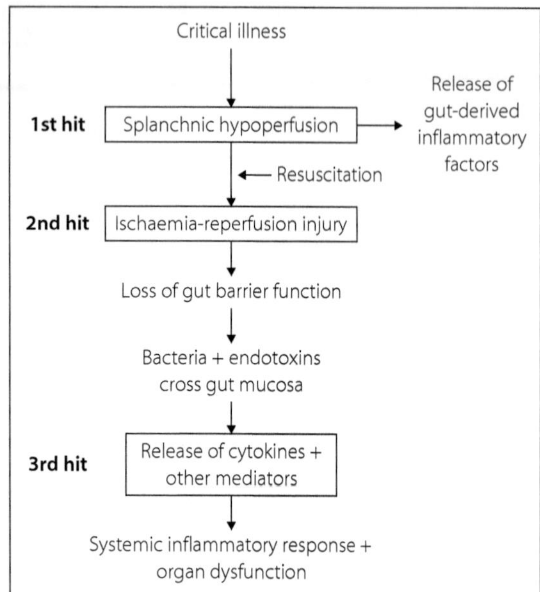

Fig. 21 Three-hit model of bacterial translocation

the emergence of bacterial resistance, improve clinical outcomes and control costs, through the logical prescribing of antibacterial drugs.

Resistance may also occur in other micro-organisms, although the problem is greatest in bacteria.
Holmes AH, Moore LSP, Sundsfjord A, et al (2016). Lancet; 387: 176–87

Bacterial translocation. Passage of **bacteria** across the normally relatively impermeable bowel mucosa into the bowel lymphatics, from where they gain access into the systemic circulation. Implicated in the pathophysiology of **intra-abdominal** or generalised **sepsis** and **MODS**. The '3 hit hypothesis' has been proposed as a possible mechanism (Fig. 21).

- Prevention and treatment:
  - early resuscitation to avoid splanchnic hypoperfusion.
  - early recognition and treatment of raised **intra-abdominal pressure** and **abdominal compartment syndrome.**
  - early enteral feeding.
  - administration of pro- and prebiotics.
  - immune-enhancing diets (e.g. with addition of glutamine, arginine, fish oils) have been studied.

Seraridou E, Papaioannou V, Kolios G, Pneumatikos I (2015). Ann Gastroenterol; 28: 309–22

Bactericidal/permeability-increasing protein. Protein normally released by activated polymorphonuclear leucocytes but also found in mucosal tissues. Binds to and neutralises **endotoxin** and is bactericidal against gram-negative organisms (by increasing permeability of bacterial cell walls). May have a role in the future treatment of severe gram-negative infections, e.g. meningococcal disease. Lipopolysaccharide-binding protein is closely related.
See also, Sepsis; Sepsis syndrome; Septic shock

Bailey manoeuvre, *see Extubation, tracheal*

Bain breathing system, *see Coaxial anaesthetic breathing systems*

Bainbridge reflex. Reflex tachycardia following an increase in central venous pressure, e.g. after rapid infusion of fluid. Activation of atrial stretch receptors results in reduced vagal tone and tachycardia. Absent or diminished if the initial heart rate is high. Of uncertain significance but has been proposed to be involved in respiratory **sinus arrhythmia** and to act as a counterbalance to the **baroreceptor reflex.**
[Francis Bainbridge (1874–1921), English physiologist]
Crystal GJ, Salem MR (2012). Anesth Analg; 114: 520–32

BAL, *see Bronchoalveolar lavage*

Balanced anaesthesia. Concept of using a combination of drugs and techniques (e.g. general and regional anaesthesia) to provide adequate analgesia, anaesthesia and muscle relaxation (triad of anaesthesia). Each drug reduces the requirement for the others, thereby reducing side effects due to any single agent, while also allowing faster recovery. Arose from **Crile**'s description of anociassociation in 1911, and **Lundy**'s refinement in 1926.

Ballistocardiography. Obsolete method for measurement of **cardiac output** and **stroke volume** via detection of body motion resulting from movement of blood within the body with each heartbeat.

Balloon pump, *see Intra-aortic counter-pulsation balloon pump*

Bar. Unit of **pressure.** Although not an SI unit, commonly used when referring to the pressures at which anaesthetic gases are delivered from **cylinders** and **piped gas supplies.**

$$1\ \text{bar} = 10^5\ \text{N/m}^2\ (\text{Pa}) = 100\ \text{kPa} = 10^6\ \text{dyn/cm}^2$$
$$= 14.5\ \text{lb/in}^2 \approx 1\ \text{atmosphere}$$

Baralyme. Calcium hydroxide 80% and barium octahydrate 20%. Used to absorb CO_2. Although less efficient than **soda lime**, it produces less heat and is more stable in dry atmospheres. Used in spacecraft. Carbon monoxide production may occur when volatile agents containing the CHF_2 moiety (**desflurane**, **enflurane** or **isoflurane**) are passed over dry warm baralyme (e.g. at the start of a Monday morning operating session) following prolonged passage of dry gas through the absorber.

Barbiturate poisoning. Causes CNS depression with **hypoventilation**, **hypotension**, **hypothermia** and **coma.**

Skin blisters and muscle necrosis may also occur.

- Treatment:
  - general measures as for **poisoning and overdoses.**
  - of the above complications.
  - forced alkaline diuresis, **dialysis** or **haemoperfusion** may be indicated.

Now rare, with the declining use of **barbiturates.**
See also, Forced diuresis

Barbiturates. Drugs derived from barbituric acid, itself derived from urea and malonic acid and first synthesised in 1864. The first sedative barbiturate, diethyl barbituric acid, was synthesised in 1903. Many others have been developed since, including **phenobarbital** in 1912, **hexobarbital** in 1932 (the first widely used iv barbiturate),

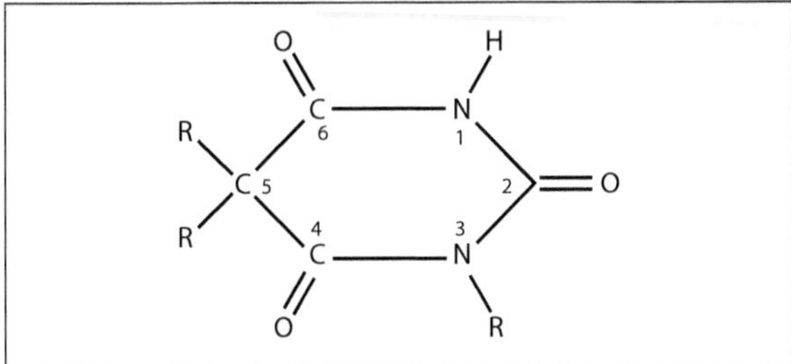

Fig. 22 Structure of the barbiturate ring

thiopental in 1934, and **methohexital** (methohexitone) in 1957.

- Substitutions at certain positions of the molecule confer hypnotic or other properties to the compound (Fig. 22). Chemical classification:
  - oxybarbiturates: as shown. Slow onset and prolonged action, e.g. phenobarbital.
  - thiobarbiturates: sulfur atom at position 2. Rapid onset, smooth action, and rapid recovery, e.g. thiopental.
  - methylbarbiturates: methyl group at position 1. Rapid onset and recovery, with excitatory phenomena, e.g. methohexital.
  - methylthiobarbiturates: both substitutions. Very rapid, but too high an incidence of excitatory phenomena to be useful clinically.

  Long side groups are associated with greater potency and convulsant properties. Phenyl groups confer anticonvulsant action.

Exist in two structural isomers, the enol and keto forms. The enol form is water-soluble at alkaline pH and undergoes dynamic structural **isomerism** to the lipid-soluble keto form upon exposure to physiologic pH (e.g. after injection).

- Divided clinically into:
  - long-acting, e.g. phenobarbital.
  - medium-acting, e.g. amobarbital.
  - very short-acting, e.g. thiopental.

  Speed of onset of action reflects lipid solubility, and thus brain penetration. The actions of long- and medium-acting drugs are terminated by metabolism; the shorter duration of action of thiopental and methohexital is due to redistribution within the body.

Bind avidly to the alpha subunit of the **GABA$_A$** receptor, potentiating the effects of endogenous GABA. Antagonism of AMPA-type glutamate receptors (**α-amino-3-hydroxy-5-methyl-4-isoxazolepropionic acid receptors**) and inhibition of **glutamate** release by blocking of high-voltage calcium channels also contribute to CNS depression.

- Actions:
  - general CNS depression, especially cerebral cortex and **ascending reticular activating system**.
  - central respiratory depression (dose-related).
  - **antanalgesia**.
  - reduction of rapid eye movement **sleep** (with rebound increase after cessation of chronic use).
  - anticonvulsant or convulsant properties according to structure.
  - cardiovascular depression. Central depression is usually mild; the hypotension seen after thiopental is largely due to direct myocardial depression and venodilatation.
  - hypothermia.

Oxidative and conjugative hepatic metabolism is followed by renal excretion. Cause hepatic **enzyme induction**.

Contraindicated in **porphyria**.

Used mainly for **induction of anaesthesia** and as **anticonvulsant drugs**. Have been replaced by **benzodiazepines** for use as sedatives and hypnotics, as the latter drugs are safer.

See also, γ-Aminobutyric acid receptors; Barbiturate poisoning

Bariatric surgery. Performed to induce significant and sustained weight loss in severe **obesity**, thereby preventing and indirectly treating the complications of obesity. Delivered as part of a multidisciplinary programme including diet/lifestyle modifications ± drug therapy.

- Indications (issued by **NICE** 2014):
  - **body mass index** (BMI) ≥40 kg/m^2 or 35–40 kg/m^2 in the presence of related significant disease (e.g. **diabetes, hypertension**), where non-surgical measures have failed.
  - BMI >50 kg/m^2 as first-line treatment.

  Patients must be fit for anaesthesia and surgery, able to receive intensive specialist management and be committed to long-term follow-up.
- Surgical techniques:
  - restrictive: laparoscopic adjustable gastric banding (AGB), sleeve gastrectomy, gastric balloon insertion.
  - malabsorptive: biliopancreatic diversion ± duodenal switch.
  - restrictive/malabsorptive: Roux-en-Y gastric bypass (laparoscopic or open).

  Of these, laparoscopic AGB and Roux-en-Y bypass constitute the vast majority of performed procedures. Some evidence suggests that the latter is more effective in severely obese patients, although there is increased potential for serious surgical complications. AGB is quicker and easier to perform and its adjustability and reversibility confer specific advantages. May achieve losses of 50% of excess weight and improvement of associated morbidity (e.g. hypertension, diabetes mellitus).

Anaesthetic considerations are as for all patients with morbid obesity.

[Jean Charles Roux (1857–1934), French surgeon]

Colquitt JL, Pickett K, Loveman E, Frampton GK (2013). Cochrane Database Syst Rev; 8: CD003641

Barker, Arthur E (1850–1916). English Professor of Surgery at University of London. Helped popularise **spinal anaesthesia** in the UK. In 1907 became the first to use hyperbaric solutions of **local anaesthetic agents**, combined with alterations in the patient's posture, to vary the height of block achieved. Studied the effects of baricity of various local anaesthetic preparations by developing a glass spine model. Used specially prepared solutions of **stovaine** (combined with 5% glucose) from Paris.

Lee JA (1979). Anaesthesia; 34: 885–91

Baroreceptor reflex (Pressoreceptor, Carotid sinus or Depressor reflex). Reflex involved in the short-term control of **arterial BP**. Increased BP stimulates **baroreceptors** in the **carotid sinus** and aortic arch, increasing afferent discharge in the glossopharyngeal and vagus nerves, respectively, that is inhibitory to the **vasomotor centre** and excitatory to the **cardioinhibitory centre** in the medulla. Vasomotor inhibition (reduced sympathetic activity) and increased cardioinhibitory activity (vagal stimulation) result in a lowering of BP and heart rate. The opposite changes occur following a fall in BP, with sympathetic stimulation and parasympathetic inhibition. Resultant peripheral vasoconstriction occurs mainly in non-vital vascular beds, e.g. skin, muscle, GIT.

The reflex is reset within 30 min if the change in BP is sustained. It may be depressed by certain drugs, e.g. **propofol.**

See also, Valsalva manoeuvre

Baroreceptors. Stretch mechanoreceptors in the walls of blood vessels and heart chambers. Respond to distension caused by increased pressure, and are involved in control of **arterial BP**.

- Exist at many sites:
  - **carotid sinus** and aortic arch:
    - at normal BP, discharge slowly. Rate of discharge is increased by a rise in BP, and by increased rate of rise.
    - send afferent impulses via the carotid sinus nerve (branch of glossopharyngeal nerve) and vagus (afferents from aortic arch) to the **vasomotor centre** and **cardioinhibitory centre** in the medulla. Raised BP invokes the **baroreceptor reflex**.
  - atrial stretch receptors:
    - found in both atria. Involved in both short-term neural control of **cardiac output** and long-term humoral control of **ECF** volume.
    - some discharge during atrial systole while others discharge during diastolic distension (more so when venous return is increased or during **IPPV**). The latter may be involved in the **Bainbridge reflex**. Discharge also results in increased urine production via stimulation of **ANP** secretion and inhibition of **vasopressin** release.
  - ventricular stretch receptors: stimulation causes reduced sympathetic activity in animals, but the clinical significance is doubtful. May also respond to chemical stimulation (**Bezold–Jarisch reflex**).
  - coronary baroreceptors: importance is uncertain. Other baroreceptors may be present in the mesentery, affecting local blood flow.

Barotrauma. Physical injury caused by an excessive pressure differential across the wall of a body cavity; in anaesthesia, the term usually refers to **pneumothorax**, pneumomediastinum, pneumoperitoneum or subcutaneous emphysema resulting from passage of air from the tracheobronchial tree and alveoli into adjacent tissues. Risk of barotrauma is increased by raised airway pressures, e.g. with **IPPV** and **PEEP** (especially if excessive tidal volume or air flow is delivered, or if the patient fails to synchronise with the ventilator). **High-frequency ventilation** may reduce the risk. Diseased lungs with reduced **compliance** are more at risk of developing barotrauma, e.g. in **asthma**, **ALI**; limiting inspiratory pressures at the expense of reduced minute volume and increased arterial $P\text{CO}_2$ is increasingly used to reduce the risk of barotrauma in these patients (**permissive hypercapnia**). Evidence of pulmonary interstitial emphysema may be seen on the **CXR** (perivascular air, hilar air streaks and subpleural air cysts) before development of severe pneumothorax. In all cases, N_2O will aggravate the problem.

Risk of barotrauma during anaesthesia is reduced by various pressure-limiting features of **anaesthetic machines** and breathing systems.

See also, Emphysema, subcutaneous; Ventilator-associated lung injury

Basal metabolic rate (BMR). Amount of **energy** liberated by **catabolism** of food per unit time, under standardised conditions (i.e., a relaxed subject at comfortable temperature, 12–14 h after a meal). May be expressed corrected for body surface area.

- Determined by measuring:
  - heat produced by the subject enclosed in an insulated room, the outside walls of which are maintained at constant temperature. The heat produced raises the temperature of water passing through coils in the ceiling, allowing calculation of BMR.
  - O_2 consumption: the subject breathes via a sealed circuit (containing a CO_2 absorber) from an O_2-filled **spirometer**. As O_2 is consumed, the volume inside the spirometer falls, and a graph of volume against time is obtained. O_2 consumption per unit time is corrected to standard temperature and pressure. Average energy liberated per litre of O_2 consumed = 20.1 kJ (4.82 Cal; some variation occurs with different food sources); thus BMR may be calculated. A similar derivation can be obtained electronically by the bedside 'metabolic cart', e.g. when calculating **energy balance** in critically ill patients.

Normal BMR (adult male) is 197 kJ/m^2/h (40 Cal/m^2/h). BMR values are often expressed as percentages above or below normal values obtained from charts or tables.

- Metabolic rate is increased by:
  - circulating catecholamines, e.g. due to stress.
  - muscle activity.
  - raised temperature.
  - **hyperthyroidism.**
  - pregnancy.
  - recent feeding (**specific dynamic action** of foods).
  - age and sex (higher in males and children).

Measurement of metabolic rate under basal conditions eliminates many of these variables.

See also, Metabolism

Basal narcosis, *see Rectal administration of anaesthetic agents*

Base. Substance that can accept **hydrogen ions**, thereby reducing hydrogen ion concentration.

Base excess/deficit. Amount of **acid** or **base** (in mmol) required to restore 1 l of blood to normal **pH** at $P\text{CO}_2$ of 5.3 kPa (40 mmHg) and at body temperature. Normally +2 to −2. By convention, its value is negative in **acidosis** and positive in **alkalosis**. May be read from the **Siggaard–Andersen nomogram**. Useful as an indication of severity of the metabolic component of acid–base disturbance, and in the calculation of the appropriate dose of acid or base in its treatment. For example, in acidosis:

Total **bicarbonate** deficit (mmol)
= base deficit (mmol/l) × 'treatable' fluid compartment (l); estimated to be 30% of body weight, comprised of **ECF** and exchangeable intracellular fluid

$$= \text{base deficit} \times \frac{\text{body weight}}{3}$$

Because of problems associated with bicarbonate administration, half the calculated deficit is given initially.

See also, Acid–base balance; Blood gas analyser; Blood gas interpretation

Basic life support, adult (BLS). Component of CPR without any drugs (i.e., suitable for anyone to administer), known as the 'ABC' of resuscitation. Use with simple equipment, e.g. **airways, facemasks, self-inflating bags, oesophageal obturators, SADs**, has been defined as 'basic life support with airway adjuncts'. May include the use of public automatic external defibrillators (AEDs). European Resuscitation Council recommendations (2015):

- ensure own and victim's safety.
- assess: e.g. shake the victim, ask if he/she is all right. If responsive, leave the patient in the same position (provided safe) and get help. If unresponsive, shout for help, turn the patient onto his/her back, open the airway and remove any obstruction.
- Airway: tilt the head back and lift the chin. Remove food and dentures from the airway. Use airway adjuncts if available.
- Breathing: check first—look, listen and feel for up to 10 s. If breathing, turn into the **recovery position**, unless **spinal cord injury** is suspected. Summon help, asking for an AED if one is available; a solo rescuer should 'phone first' because the chance of successful **defibrillation** falls with increasing delay (although children, trauma or drowning victims, and poisoned or choking patients may benefit from 1 min of CPR before calling for help). If patient is not breathing, summon help and, on returning, start **cardiac massage**; after 30 compressions give two slow effective breaths (700–1000 ml, each over 1 s) followed by another 30 compressions. Rapid breaths are more likely to inflate the stomach. **Cricoid pressure** should be applied if additional help is available. Risk of **HIV infection** and **hepatitis** is considered negligible. Inflating equipment and 100% O_2 should be used if available.
- Circulation: apply external cardiac massage (5–6 cm chest depressions) at 100–120/min, with the hands in the centre of the chest, stopping only if the patient starts breathing. It is important to deliver uninterrupted compressions because this improves chances of survival. Do not stop to check the victim or discontinue CPR unless the victim starts to show signs of regaining consciousness, e.g. coughing, eye opening, speaking or moving purposefully. External bleeding should be stopped and the feet raised.
- if there is a second rescuer, the two rescuers should swap every 1–2 min to minimise fatigue. The recommended ratio of compressions to breaths is 30:2 for both single- and two-operator CPR. Chest-compression-only CPR is acceptable if the rescuer is unable or unwilling to give rescue breaths.
- in cases of **choking**, encourage coughing in conscious patients; clear the airway manually and use ≤5 back slaps then ≤5 abdominal thrusts (**Heimlich manoeuvre**) if patient is not breathing or is unable to speak, repeated as necessary; use basic life support (as detailed earlier) if the patient becomes unconscious.

All medical and paramedical personnel should be able to administer basic life support (ideally every member of the public). Ability of hospital staff has been consistently shown to be poor. Regular training sessions are thought to be necessary, using training manikins.

Perkins GD, Travers AH, Considine J, et al (2015). Resuscitation; 95: e43–70

See also, Advanced life support, adult; Cardiac arrest; Cardiopulmonary resuscitation, neonatal; Cardiopulmonary resuscitation, paediatric; International Liaison Committee on Resuscitation; Resuscitation Council (UK)

BASICS, *see British Association for Immediate Care*

Batson's plexus. Valveless epidural venous plexus composed of anterior and posterior longitudinal veins, communicating at each vertebral level with venous rings that pass transversely around the dural sac. Also communicates with basivertebral veins passing from the middle of the posterior surface of each vertebral body, and with sacral, lumbar, thoracic and cervical veins. It thus connects pelvic veins with intracranial veins. Provides an alternative route for venous blood to reach the heart from the legs. Originally described to explain a route for metastatic spread of tumours. Distends when vena caval venous return is obstructed, e.g. in **pregnancy**, thus thought to reduce the space available for local anaesthetic solution in **epidural anaesthesia**.

[Oscar V Batson (1894–1979), US otolaryngologist]

See also, Epidural space

Beclometasone dipropionate (Beclomethasone). Inhaled **corticosteroid**, used to prevent **bronchospasm** in **asthma** by reducing airway inflammation.

- Dosage: 0.2–0.8 mg bd, depending on clinical severity and drug preparation. A nebuliser preparation is available but is relatively inefficient because the drug is poorly soluble.
- Side effects: as for corticosteroids, although systemic uptake is low. Hoarse voice and oral candidiasis may occur with high dosage.

Becquerel. SI **unit** of radioactivity. One becquerel = amount of radioactivity produced when one nucleus disintegrates per second.

[Antoine Becquerel (1852–1908), French physicist]

Bed sores, *see Decubitus ulcers*

Bee stings, *see Bites and stings*

Beer–Lambert law. Combination of two laws describing absorption of monochromatic light by a transparent substance through which it passes:

- Beer's law: intensity of transmitted light decreases exponentially as concentration of substance increases.
- Lambert's law: intensity of transmitted light decreases exponentially as distance travelled through the substance increases.

Forms the basis for spectrophotometric techniques, e.g. enzyme assays, **oximetry, near infrared spectroscopy**.

[August Beer (1825–1863) and Johann Lambert (1728–1777), German physicists]

Bell–Magendie law. The dorsal roots of the **spinal cord** are sensory, the ventral roots motor.

[Sir Charles Bell (1774–1842), Scottish surgeon; François Magendie (1783–1855), French physiologist]

Bellows. Expansible container used to deliver controlled volumes of pressurised gas. May describe bellows incorporated into **ventilators** or hand-operated devices. The latter have been used in **CPR** and animal experiments for several centuries. More modern devices allow manual-controlled ventilation, and are either applied directly to the patient's face or used in **draw-over techniques**.

- Examples:
  - Cardiff bellows: mainly used for resuscitation (rarely used now, **self-inflating bags** being preferred). Design:

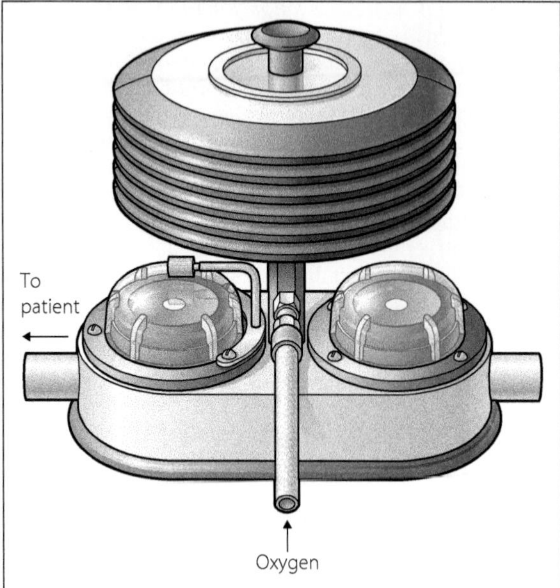

Fig. 23 Oxford bellows

- concertina bellows with a facemask at one end.
- **non-rebreathing valve** between the bellows and facemask.
- one-way valve at the other end of the bellows that prevents air or O_2 leaks during compression, while allowing fresh gas entry during expansion.

▸ Oxford bellows (Fig. 23): used for resuscitation or draw-over anaesthesia. Design:
- concertina bellows mounted on a block containing one-way valves.
- held open by an internal spring, but may be manually compressed. Expansion draws in air or O_2 through a side port.
- unidirectional gas flow is ensured by the one-way valves, one on either side of the bellows. A non-rebreathing valve is required between the bellows and patient.

In earlier models, an O_2 inlet opened directly into the closed bellows system. This could allow build-up of excessive pressure, with risk of **barotrauma**.

Bends, *see Decompression sickness*

Benzatropine mesylate (Benztropine). **Anticholinergic drug**, used to treat acute **dystonic reactions** and parkinsonism, especially drug-induced.
- Dosage:
  - 1–4 mg orally od.
  - 1–2 mg iv/im, repeated as required.
- Side effects: sedation, dry mouth, blurred vision, GIT upset, urinary retention, tachycardia. May worsen tardive dyskinesia.

Benzodiazepine poisoning. Commonest overdose involving prescription drugs. Generally considered to be less serious than overdose with other sedatives, although death may occur, usually due to respiratory depression and **aspiration of gastric contents**. Of the **benzodiazepines**, **temazepam** is most sedating, and oxazepam least sedating, when taken in overdose. Often accompanied by **alcohol poisoning**.

Features are mainly those of CNS depression; hypoventilation and hypotension may also be present. Treatment is largely supportive. **Flumazenil** may be used but large doses may be required and the effects may be temporary; acute withdrawal and **convulsions** may be provoked in patients on chronic benzodiazepine therapy, those with alcohol dependence, or in cases of mixed drug overdoses (**tricyclic antidepressants drug poisoning** in particular).

Benzodiazepines. Group of drugs with sedative, anxiolytic and anticonvulsant properties. Also cause **amnesia** and muscle relaxation. Bind to the α and γ subunits of the **$GABA_A$** receptor complex, potentiating the increase in chloride ion conductance caused by endogenous GABA. They thus enhance GABA-mediated inhibition in the brain and spinal cord, especially the **limbic system** and **ascending reticular activating system**.
- Anaesthetic uses:
  - **premedication**, e.g. **diazepam**, **temazepam**, **lorazepam**.
  - **sedation**, e.g. diazepam, **midazolam**.
  - as **anticonvulsant drugs**, e.g. diazepam, lorazepam, clobazam, **clonazepam**.
  - **induction of anaesthesia**, e.g. midazolam.
- **Half-life**:
  - midazolam: 1–3 h.
  - oxazepam: 3–8 h.
  - temazepam: 6–8 h.
  - lorazepam: 12 h.
  - diazepam, clonazepam: 24–48 h.
  - clobazam: 38–42 h.

Metabolism often produces active products with long half-lives that depend upon renal excretion, e.g. diazepam to temazepam and nordiazepam (the latter has a half-life of up to 900 h and is itself metabolised to oxazepam). In chronic use, benzodiazepines have largely replaced **barbiturates** as hypnotics and anxiolytics, because they cause fewer and less serious side effects. Overdosage is also less dangerous, usually requiring supportive treatment only. Hepatic **enzyme induction** is rare. A chronic dependence state may occur, with withdrawal featuring tremor, anxiety and confusion. **Flumazenil** is a specific benzodiazepine antagonist.
See also, γ-Aminobutyric acid receptors; Benzodiazepine poisoning

Benztropine, *see Benzatropine*

Benzylpenicillin (Penicillin G). **Antibacterial drug**, the first **penicillin**. Used mainly in infections caused by gram-positive and gram-negative cocci, although its use is hampered by increasing **bacterial resistance**. The drug of choice in **meningococcal disease**, **gas gangrene**, **tetanus**, anthrax and **diphtheria**. Inactivated by gastric acid, thus poorly absorbed orally.
- Dosage: 0.6–1.2 g im/iv qds; up to 2.4 g 4–6-hourly in meningococcal meningitis or anthrax.
- Side effects: allergic reactions, convulsions following high doses or in renal failure.

Bernard, Claude (1813–1878). French physiologist, whose many contributions to modern physiology include: demonstrating hepatic gluconeogenesis; proving that pancreatic secretions could digest food; discovering vasomotor nerves; and investigating the effects of **curare** at the **neuromuscular junction**. Also suggested the concept of the ‘internal environment’ (*milieu intérieur*) and **homeostasis**.
Lee JA (1978). Anaesthesia; 33: 741–7

Bernoulli effect. Reduction of pressure when a **fluid** accelerates through a constriction. As velocity increases during passage through the constriction, kinetic **energy** increases. Total energy must remain the same, therefore potential energy (hence pressure) falls. Beyond the constriction, the pressure rises again. A second fluid may be entrained through a side arm into the area of lower pressure, causing mixing of the two fluids (**Venturi principle**).
[Daniel Bernoulli (1700–1782), Swiss mathematician]

Bert effect. Convulsions caused by acute **O_2 toxicity**, seen with hyperbaric **O_2 therapy**. Although initially described at pressure >3 atm, it may occur at lower pressures on prolonged exposure.
[Paul Bert (1833–1896), French physiologist]
See also, Oxygen therapy, hyperbaric

Beta-adrenergic..., *see β-Adrenergic ...*

Beta-lactams, *see β-Lactams*

Bezold–Jarisch reflex. Bradycardia, vasodilatation and hypotension following stimulation of ventricular receptors by ischaemia or drugs, e.g. **nicotine** and veratridine. Thought to involve inhibition of the **baroreceptor reflex**. Although of disputed clinical significance, a role in regulation of BP and the response to hypovolaemia has been suggested. The reflex may be activated during **myocardial ischaemia** or **MI**, and in rare cases of unexplained cardiovascular collapse following spinal/epidural anaesthesia.
[Albert von Bezold (1836–1868), German physiologist; Adolf Jarisch (1850–1902), Austrian dermatologist]
Campagna JA, Carter C (2003). Anesthesiology; 98: 1250–60

Bicarbonate. Anion present in plasma at a concentration of 24–33 mmol/l, formed from dissociation of carbonic acid. Intimately involved with **acid–base balance**, as part of the major plasma **buffer** system. Filtered in the kidneys and reabsorbed to a variable extent, according to acid–base status. 80% of filtered bicarbonate is reabsorbed in the proximal tubule via formation of carbonic acid, which in turn forms CO_2 and water aided by **carbonic anhydrase**. The bicarbonate ion itself does not pass easily across cell membranes.

- Sodium bicarbonate may be administered iv to raise blood pH in severe acidosis, but with potentially undesirable effects:
  - increased formation of CO_2, which passes readily into cells (unlike bicarbonate), worsening intracellular acidosis.
  - increased blood pH shifts the **oxyhaemoglobin dissociation curve** to the left, with increased affinity of **haemoglobin** for O_2 and impaired O_2 delivery to the tissues.
  - solutions contain 1 mmol sodium ions per mmol bicarbonate ions, representing a significant sodium load.
  - 8.4% solution is hypertonic: increased plasma osmolality may cause arterial vasodilatation and hypotension.
  - severe tissue necrosis may follow extravasation.

For these reasons, treatment is usually reserved for pH below 7.1–7.2.

- Dose: $\dfrac{\text{base deficit} \times \text{body weight (kg)}}{3}$ mmol

  Half of this dose is given initially.

  Presented as 8.4%, 4.2% and 1.26% solutions (1000 mmol/l, 500 mmol/l and 150 mmol/l, respectively).

See also, Base excess/deficit

Bier, Karl August Gustav (1861–1949). German surgeon: Professor in Bonn and then Berlin. Introduced **spinal anaesthesia** using **cocaine**, describing its use on himself, his assistant and a series of patients, in 1899. Gave a classic description of the **post-dural puncture headache** he later suffered, and suggested CSF leakage during/after the injection as a possible cause. Also introduced **IVRA**, using **procaine**, in 1908. As consulting surgeon during World War I, he introduced the German steel helmet.
van Zundert A, Goerig M (2000). Reg Anesth Pain Med; 25: 26–33

Bier's block, *see Intravenous regional anaesthesia*

Bigelow, Henry Jacob (1818–1890). US surgeon at the Massachusetts General Hospital, Boston. Sponsored **Wells**' abortive attempt at anaesthesia in 1845 and promoted and published the first account of **Morton**'s use of **diethyl ether** anaesthesia for surgery in 1846. Described several operations and the intraoperative events that occurred during them. Later, as a professor, he became renowned for many contributions to surgery, including inventing a urological evacuator.
Malenfant J, Robitaille M, Schaefer J, et al (2011). Clin Anat; 24: 539–43

Biguanides. Hypoglycaemic drugs, used to treat non–insulin-dependent **diabetes mellitus**. Act by decreasing gluconeogenesis and by increasing **glucose** utilisation peripherally. Require some pancreatic islet cell function to be effective. May cause **lactic acidosis**, especially in renal or hepatic impairment. Lactic acidosis is particularly likely with phenformin, which is now unavailable in the UK. Metformin, the remaining biguanide, is used as first-line treatment in obese patients in whom diet alone is unsuccessful, or when a **sulfonylurea** alone is inadequate.

Biliary tract. Bile produced by the **liver** passes to the right and left hepatic ducts, which unite to form the common hepatic duct. This is joined by the cystic duct, which drains the gallbladder, to form the common bile duct; the latter drains into the duodenum (with the pancreatic duct) through the ampulla of Vater, the lumen of which is controlled by the sphincter of Oddi. Both infection of the biliary tree (**cholangitis**) and inflammation of the gallbladder (**cholecystitis**) may occur during critical illness.
[Ruggero Oddi (1845–1906), Italian physiologist and anatomist; Abraham Vater (1684–1751), German anatomist and botanist]
See also, Jaundice

Binding of drugs, *see Pharmacokinetics; Protein-binding*

Bioavailability. Fraction of an administered dose of a drug that reaches the systemic circulation unchanged; iv injection thus provides 100% bioavailability. For an orally administered dose, it equals the area under the resultant concentration-against-time curve divided by that for an iv dose (Fig. 24). Low values of bioavailability occur with poorly absorbed oral drugs, or those that undergo extensive

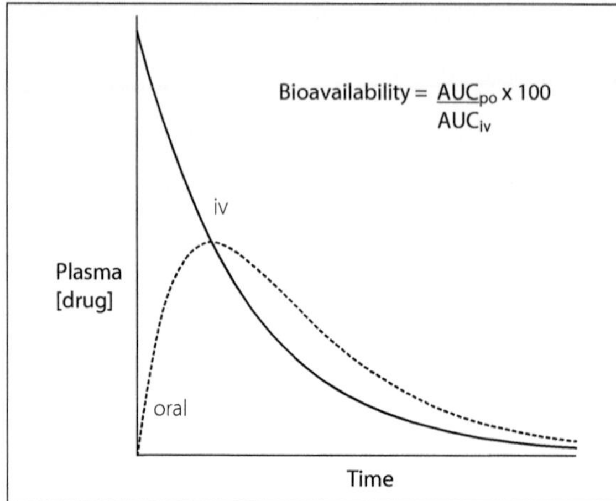

Fig. 24 Bioavailability

first-pass metabolism. Various formulations of the same drug may have different bioavailability. 'Bioinequivalence' is a statistically significant difference in bioavailability, whereas 'therapeutic inequivalence' is a clinically important difference, e.g. as may occur with different preparations of **digoxin**.
See also, Pharmacokinetics

Biofeedback. Technique whereby bodily processes normally under involuntary control (e.g. heart rate) are displayed to the subject, enabling voluntary control to be learnt. Has been used to aid relaxation, and in chronic **pain management** when increased muscle tension is present, using the **EMG** as the displayed signal.

Bioimpedance cardiac output measurement, *see Impedance plethysmography*

Biological weapons. Living organisms or infected material derived from them, used for hostile purposes, either by certain nations in 'legitimate' biological warfare or by (bio) terrorists. The agents depend for their effects on their ability to multiply in the person, animal or plant attacked. Although not pathognomonic of a bioterrorist attack, the following should raise suspicion:
- an unusual clustering of illness in time or space.
- an unusual age distribution of a common illness (e.g. apparent chickenpox in adults).
- a large epidemic.
- disease that is more severe than expected.
- an unusual route of exposure.
- disease outside its normal transmission season.
- multiple simultaneous epidemics of different diseases.
- unusual strains or variants of organisms or antimicrobial resistance patterns.

- Potential diseases include:
    - anthrax: gram-negative bacillus causing fever, skin eschars (dry scabs) and associated lymphadenopathy, chest pain, dry cough, nausea and abdominal pain, followed by sepsis, shock, widened mediastinum, haemorrhagic pleural effusions and respiratory failure. Mortality rates vary depending on exposure: approximately 20% for cutaneous anthrax without antibiotics, 25%–75% for gastrointestinal anthrax and over 80% for inhalation anthrax.
    - pneumonic plague: gram-negative bacillus causing mucopurulent sputum, chest pain and haemoptysis. If untreated, mortality approaches 100%.
    - tularaemia: gram-negative coccobacillus causing bronchopneumonia, pleuritis and hilar lymphadenopathy. Overall mortality for virulent strains is 5%–15%, but up to 30%–60% in pulmonic or septicaemic tularaemia without antibiotics.
    - viral haemorrhagic fevers: influenza-like illness with haemorrhage, petechiae and ecchymoses or multiple organ failure. Mortality approaches 100% for the most virulent forms.
    - **botulism**: paralytic illness characterised by symmetric, descending flaccid paralysis of motor and autonomic nerves, usually beginning with the cranial nerves. Mortality is approximately 6% if appropriately treated.
    - smallpox: febrile illness followed by a generalised macular or papular-vesicular-pustular eruption. Mortality is approximately 30%.

Management includes specific and general supportive measures; consideration should also be directed towards protection of staff, decontamination of clinical areas and equipment, disposal of bodies and other aspects of major incidents.
White SM (2002). Br J Anaesth; 89: 306–24
See also, Incident, major; Chemical weapons

Biotransformation, *see Pharmacokinetics*

BIPAP. Bi-level positive airway pressure, *see Non-invasive positive pressure ventilation*

Bispectral index monitor. Cerebral function monitor that uses a processed **EEG** obtained from a single frontal electrode to provide a measure of cerebral activity. Used to monitor anaesthetic depth to prevent **awareness**. Produces a dimensionless number (the BIS number) ranging from 100 (fully awake) to 0 (no cerebral activity). The algorithm used to calculate the BIS value is commercially protected but is based on **power spectral analysis** of the EEG, the synchrony of slow and fast wave activity and the burst suppression ratio. A BIS number of 40–60 suggests anaesthetic depth is appropriate. Recent guidance from the **Association of Anaesthetists of Great Britain and Ireland** advocates its use (or an alternative depth of anaesthesia monitor) in patients receiving **TIVA** with **neuromuscular blocking drugs**.
Chhabra A, Subamanian R, Srivastava A, et al (2016). Cochrane Database Syst Rev; 3: CD010135
See also, Anaesthesia, depth of

Bisphosphonates. Group of drugs that inhibit osteoclast activity; used in Paget's disease, osteoporosis, metastatic bone disease and **hypercalcaemia**. They are adsorbed on to hydroxyapatite crystals, interfering with bone turnover and thus slowing the rate of **calcium** mobilisation. May be given orally or by slow iv infusion, e.g. in severe hypercalcaemia of malignancy:
- pamidronate disodium: 15–60 mg, given once or divided over 2–4 days, up to a maximum of 90 mg in total.
- ibandronic acid: 2–4 mg by a single infusion.
- zoledronic acid: 4–5 mg (depending on the preparation) over 15 min by a single infusion.

Side effects include **hypocalcaemia**, **hypophosphataemia**, pyrexia, flu-like illness, vomiting and headache. Blood

dyscrasias, hyper- or hypotension, renal and hepatic dysfunction may rarely occur, especially with disodium pamidronate. Osteonecrosis of the jaw and atypical femoral fractures have also been reported, mainly associated with long-term administration and particularly in patients with cancer.
[Sir James Paget (1814–1899), English surgeon]

Bites and stings. May include animal bites, and animal or plant stings. Problems are related to:
- local tissue **trauma**: damage to vital organs, haemorrhage, oedema. Importance varies with the size, location and number of the wound(s).
- effect of venom or toxin delivered: may cause an intense immune and inflammatory reaction, usually with severe pain and swelling. Systemic features usually present within 1–4 h; they may vary but typically include:
  - respiratory: **bronchospasm**, **pulmonary oedema**, **respiratory failure** (type I or II), **airway obstruction** (from oedema).
  - cardiovascular: hypertension (from **neurotransmitter** release), hypotension (from cardiac depression, **hypovolaemia**, vasodilatation), **arrhythmias**.
  - neurological: confusion, **coma**, **convulsions**.
  - neuromuscular: **cranial nerve** palsies and peripheral **paralysis** (from pre- or postsynaptic neuromuscular junction blockade), muscle spasms (from neurotransmitter release), **rhabdomyolysis**.
  - gastrointestinal: nausea, vomiting.
  - haematological: **coagulation disorders**, **haemolysis**.
  - renal: impairment from **myoglobinuria**, hypotension and direct nephrotoxicity.
- wound infection, either introduced at the time of injury or acquired secondarily.
- systemic transmitted disease, e.g. **tetanus**, **rabies**, plague.

Venoms are typically mixtures of several compounds, including enzymes and other proteins, amino acids, peptides, carbohydrates and lipids. The age and health of the victim, and the site and route of envenomation, may affect the severity of the injury. Identification of the offending animal or plant is particularly important, because prognosis and management may vary considerably between species. Certain venoms may be identified by blood testing.
- Management:
  - initial resuscitation as for trauma, **anaphylaxis**. Rapid transfer of victims of envenomation to hospital is the most important prehospital measure. Jewellery should be removed from the affected limb as swelling may be marked.
  - specific management:
    - application of a pressure dressing and immobilisation of the affected body part to reduce systemic absorption.
    - neutralisation of venom already absorbed. Many antivenoms are derived from horses, and severe allergic reactions may occur.
    - previously employed measures, now agreed to be unhelpful or harmful, include suction to remove venom from the wound and application of limb tourniquets.
  - general supportive management according to the system affected. IV fluids are usually required. Blood should be taken early as certain venoms and antivenoms may interfere with grouping. Frequent assessment of all systems and degree of swelling are important. Antitetanus immunisation should be given. Broad-spectrum **antibacterial drugs** are often given.

Bivalirudin. Direct **thrombin inhibitor** and recombinant **hirudin**, used as an anticoagulant in **acute coronary syndromes**. Has few advantages over conventional **heparin** therapy following **percutaneous coronary intervention** (PCI), hence often reserved for patients with heparin-induced **thrombocytopaenia** or heparin resistance.
- Dosage:
  - in patients undergoing PCI, including those with S–T segment elevation **MI**: 750 µg/kg iv initially followed by 1.75 mg/kg/h for up to 4 h after procedure.
  - in patients with unstable angina or non-S–T segment elevation MI: 100 µg/kg iv initially followed by 250 µg/kg/h for up to 72 h. For those proceeding to PCI, an additional bolus dose of 500 µg is given followed by an infusion of 1.75 mg/kg/h.
- Side effects: bleeding, hypotension, angina, headache.

Bladder washouts. Main types used in ICU.
- to remove debris and exclude catheter blockage as a cause of **oliguria**: sterile saline. Various solutions are available to remove phosphate deposits.
- to dissolve blood clots: sterile saline or sodium citrate 3% irrigation. Streptokinase-streptodornase enzyme preparation may also be used (allergic reactions and burning may occur).
- for **urinary tract infection**: chlorhexidine 1:5000 (may cause burning and haemorrhage); ineffective in pseudomonal infections. Saline may also be used. **Amphotericin** may be used in fungal infection.

Also used to treat local malignancy.

Blast injury, *see Chest trauma*

Bleeding time, *see Coagulation studies*

Bleomycin. Antibacterial **cytotoxic drug**, given iv or im to treat lymphomas and certain other solid tumours. Side effects include **alveolitis**, dose-dependent progressive **pulmonary fibrosis**, skin and allergic reactions (common) and myelosuppression (rare). Pulmonary fibrosis is thought to be exacerbated if high concentrations of O_2 are administered, e.g. for anaesthesia. Suspicion of fibrosis (CXR changes or basal crepitations) is an indication to stop therapy.

Blood. Circulating body fluid composed of blood cells (red cells, white cells and platelets) suspended in plasma. Normal adult blood volume is 70–80 ml/kg, of which ~45% is cellular. Cell formation occurs in the liver, spleen and bone marrow before birth, after which it occurs in bone marrow only. In adults, active bone marrow is confined to vertebrae, ribs, sternum, ilia and humeral and femoral heads. Stem cells differentiate into mature cells over many divisions. Primary stem cells may give rise to the lymphocyte series of stem cells or to secondary stem cells. The secondary stem cells may give rise to the erythrocyte, granulocyte, monocyte or megakaryocyte series of stem cells (the latter forming platelets).
See also, Blood volume; Erythrocytes; Leucocytes; Plasma; Platelets

Blood, artificial. Synthetic solutions capable of O_2 transport and delivery to the tissues. Circumvent many of the complications of **blood transfusion** and avoid the need for **blood compatibility testing**. Two types have been investigated:

- **haemoglobin** solutions:
  - must be free of red cell debris (stroma-free) to avoid renal damage, which has also occurred with certain stroma-free solutions. Other effects may include impairment of macrophage activity, vasoconstriction and activation of various inflammatory pathways. Free haemoglobin solutions are also hyperosmotic and are quickly broken down in the blood.
  - the **oxyhaemoglobin dissociation curve** of free haemoglobin is markedly shifted to the left of that for intra-erythrocyte haemoglobin, reducing its usefulness.
  - must be stored in O_2-free atmosphere to avoid oxidisation to methaemoglobin.

  Various modifications of the haemoglobin molecule have been made to prolong its **half-life** from under 1 h to over 24 h, including polymerisation with glutaraldehyde, linking haemoglobin with **hydroxyethyl starch** or **dextran**, cross-linking the α or β chains, and fusing the chains end to end (the latter has been done with recombinant human haemoglobin). Bovine haemoglobin, and encapsulation of haemoglobin within liposomes, has also been used. Many of these preparations are currently undergoing clinical trials.
- **perfluorocarbon** solutions (e.g. Fluosol DA20) carry dissolved O_2 in an amount directly proportional to its partial pressure, and have been used to supplement O_2 delivery in organ ischaemia due to shock, arterial (including coronary) insufficiency and haemorrhage. Have been used for **liquid ventilation**. Even with high F_IO_2, O_2 content is less than that of haemoglobin (newer compounds may be more efficient at O_2 carriage). Accumulation in the reticuloendothelial system is of unknown significance. Clinical trials are continuing.

Blood–brain barrier. Physiological boundary between the cerebral vasculature and CNS, preventing transfer of hydrophilic substances from plasma to brain. The original concept was suggested by the lack of staining of brain tissue by aniline dyes given systemically. The barrier is formed by a cellular layer of pericytes that surround the parenchymal surface of the cerebral endothelium and is reinforced by a basement membrane composed of collagen and laminins. In addition, astrocytes extend processes that wrap around the blood vessels. **Active transport** occurs for specific molecules, e.g. **glucose**. Certain areas of the brain lie outside the barrier, e.g. the **hypothalamus** and areas lining the third and fourth ventricles (including the **chemoreceptor trigger zone**).

In the absence of active transport, the ability of chemicals to cross the barrier is proportional to their lipid solubility, and inversely proportional to molecular size and charge. Water, O_2 and CO_2 cross freely; charged ions and larger molecules take longer to cross, unless lipid-soluble. All substances eventually penetrate the brain; the rate of penetration is important clinically. Some drugs only cross the barrier in their unionised, non–protein-bound form, i.e., a small proportion of the injected dose, e.g. **thiopental**. Quaternary amines, such as **neuromuscular blocking drugs** and **glycopyrronium**, are permanently charged, and cross to a very limited extent (cf. **atropine**).

The effectiveness of the barrier is reduced in **neonates** compared with adults: hence the increased passage of drugs (e.g. **opioid analgesic drugs**) and other substances (e.g. bile salts, causing kernicterus). Localised pathology, e.g. trauma, malignancy and infection, may also reduce the integrity of the barrier.

Daneman R (2012). Ann Neurol; 72: 648–72

Blood compatibility testing. Procedures performed on donor and recipient blood before **blood transfusion**, to determine compatibility. Necessary to avoid reactions caused by transfusion of red cells into a recipient whose plasma contains antibodies against them. **ABO** and **Rhesus** are the most relevant **blood group** systems clinically, although others may be important.

Antibodies may be intrinsic (e.g. ABO system) or develop only after exposure to antigen (e.g. Rhesus).

- Methods:
  - group and screen: if red cells have serum added that contains antibody against them, agglutination of the cells occurs; serum of known identity is thus used to identify the recipient's ABO blood group and Rhesus status. The recipient's serum is also screened for atypical antibodies against other groups. Usually takes 30–40 min.
  - cross-match: in addition to group and screen, the recipient's serum is added to red cells from each donor unit to confirm compatibility. Usually takes 45–60 min.
  - computer cross-match (electronic issue): uncross-matched ABO and Rhesus-compatible blood may be issued within a few minutes with no further testing, provided the patient does not have irregular antibodies.

Uncross-matched O Rhesus-negative blood is reserved for life-threatening emergencies. Fresh frozen plasma is not cross-matched, but chosen as type-specific (ABO) so that antibodies are not infused into a recipient who might have the corresponding antigens on his or her cells. Platelets are suspended in plasma, so are also selected as type-specific, but also according to Rhesus type.

Green L, Allard S, Cardigan R (2014). Anaesthesia; 70 Suppl 1: 3–9

Blood cultures. Microbiological culture of blood, performed to detect circulating micro-organisms. Blood is taken under aseptic conditions and injected into (usually two) bottles containing culture medium, for aerobic and anaerobic incubation. Diluting the sample at least 4–5 times in the culture broth reduces the antimicrobial activity of serum and of any circulating drugs. Changing the hypodermic needle between taking blood and injection into the bottles is not now thought to be necessary, although contamination of the needle and bottles must be avoided. Sensitivity depends on the type of infection, the number of cultures and volume of blood taken. At least 2–3 cultures, each using at least 10–30 ml blood, are usually recommended. More samples may be required when there is concurrent **antibacterial drug** therapy (the sample may be diluted several times or the drug removed in the laboratory to increase the yield) or when **endocarditis** is suspected. False-positive results may be suggested by the organism recovered (e.g. bacillus species, coagulase-negative staphylococci, diphtheroids) and their presence in only a single culture out of many and after prolonged incubation.

Many different culture systems exist, some directed at particular organisms. Different systems may be used

together to increase their yield. Modern microbiological techniques may involve automatic alerting of staff when significant microbial growth interrupts passage of light through the bottles. The organisms may then be identified and sensitivity to antimicrobials determined.
See also, Sepsis

Blood filters. Devices for removing microaggregates during **blood transfusion.** Platelet microaggregates form early in stored blood, with leucocytes and fibrin aggregates occurring after 7 days' storage. Pulmonary microembolism has been suggested as a cause of **transfusion-related acute lung injury**.

- Types of filters:
  - screen filters: sieves with pores of a certain size.
  - depth filters: remove particles mainly by adsorption. Pore size varies, and effective filtration may be reduced by channel formation within the filter.
  - combination filters.

Most contain woven fibre meshes, e.g. of polyester or nylon. Filtration results from both a physical sieving effect and the presence of a positive or negative charge on the surface of the material that traps cellular components and large molecules.

Standard iv giving sets suitable for blood transfusion contain screen filters of 170–200 µm pore size. Filtration of microaggregates requires microfilters of 20–40 µm pore size. The general use of microfilters is controversial; by activating **complement** in transfused blood they may increase formation of microaggregates within the recipient's bloodstream. They add to expense, increase resistance to flow and may cause **haemolysis**. They have, however, been shown to be of use in **extracorporeal circulation.**

Leucodepletion filters are used in **cell salvage** (e.g. to remove cellular fragments) but their routine use has been questioned because of rare reports of severe hypotension in recipients, possibly related to release of bradykinin and/or other mediators when blood is passed over filters with a negative charge.

Filters capable of removing prion proteins that cause **Creutzfeldt–Jakob disease** have been developed and are under evaluation.

Blood flow. For any organ:

$$\text{flow} = \frac{\text{perfusion pressure}}{\text{resistance}}$$

thus representing the haemodynamic correlate of **Ohm's law**.

Perfusion pressure depends not only on arterial and venous pressures but also on local pressures within the **capillary circulation**.

- Resistance depends on:
  - vessel radius, controlled by humoral, neural and local mechanisms (**autoregulation**).
  - vessel length.
  - blood **viscosity**. Reduced peripherally due to plasma skimming, which results in blood with reduced **haematocrit** leaving vessels via side branches. Reduced in **anaemia.**

Flow is normally laminar (i.e., it roughly obeys the **Hagen–Poiseuille equation**), although blood vessels are not rigid, arterial flow is pulsatile and blood is not an ideal fluid. Turbulent flow may occur in constricted arteries and in the hyperdynamic circulation, particularly in anaemia, when viscosity is reduced (*see Reynolds' number*).

- Measurement.
  - direct measurement of blood from the arterial supply.
  - **electromagnetic flow measurement.**
  - **Doppler** measurement.
  - indirect methods:
    - **Fick principle.**
    - **dilution techniques.**
    - **plethysmography.**

Approximate blood flow to, and O_2 consumption of, various organs are shown in Table 10.

Table 10 Blood flow to and O_2 consumption of heart, brain, liver and kidneys

	Blood flow		O_2 consumption	
Organ	(ml/min)	(ml/100 g tissue/min)	(ml/min)	(ml/100 g tissue/min)
Heart	250	80	30	10
Brain	700	50	50	3
Liver	1400	50	50	2
Kidneys	1200	400	20	6

Blood/gas partition coefficients, *see Partition coefficients*

Blood gas analyser. Device used to measure blood gas tensions, **pH**, electrolytes, metabolites and haemoglobin derivatives. Incorporates a series of measuring electrodes ± a co-oximeter. Directly measured parameters include pH, PO_2, PCO_2. **Bicarbonate, standard bicarbonate** and **base excess/deficit** are derived. Inaccuracy may result from excess **heparin** (acidic), bubbles within the sample and metabolism by blood cells. The latter is reduced by rapid analysis after taking the sample, or storage of the sample on ice. O_2, CO_2 and pH electrodes require regular maintenance and two-point **calibration.**
See also Blood gas interpretation; Carbon dioxide measurement; Oxygen measurement; pH measurement

Blood gas interpretation. Normal ranges are shown in Table 11.

- Suggested plan for interpretation:
  - oxygenation:
    - knowledge of the F_IO_2 is required before interpretation is possible.
    - calculation of the alveolar PO_2 (from **alveolar gas equation**).
    - calculation of the **alveolar–arterial O_2 difference.**
  - **acid–base balance:**
    - identification of **acidaemia** or **alkalaemia**, representing **acidosis** or **alkalosis**, respectively.
    - identification of a respiratory component by referring to the CO_2 tension.
    - identification of a metabolic component by referring to the **base excess/deficit** or **standard bicarbonate** (both are corrected to a normal CO_2 tension, thus eliminating respiratory factors).
    - knowledge of the clinical situation helps to decide whether the respiratory or metabolic component represents the primary change.

Table 11 Normal values (ranges or mean ± 2 SD) for blood gas interpretation, for young adults breathing room air at sea level

Arterial	pH	7.35–7.45	
	Po_2	10.6–13.3 kPa	(80–100 mmHg)
	Pco_2	4.6–6.0 kPa	(35–45 mmHg)
	HCO_3^-	22–26 mmol/l	
	S_aO_2	95%–100%	
Mixed venous	pH	7.32–7.36	
	Po_2	4.7–5.3 kPa	(35–40 mmHg)
	Pco_2	5.6–6.1 kPa	(42–46 mmHg)
	HCO_3^-	24–28 mmol/l	
	$S_{\bar{v}}O_2$	60%–80%	

See also, Blood gas analyser; Carbon dioxide measurement; Carbon dioxide transport; Oxygen measurement; Oxygen transport; pH measurement

Blood groups. Red cells may bear antigens capable of producing an antibody response in another person. Some are only present on red cells, e.g. **Rhesus** antigens; others are also present on other tissue cells, e.g. **ABO** antigens. **Immunoglobulins** may be present intrinsically, e.g. ABO and Lewis, or following exposure to the antigen, e.g. Rhesus; they are usually IgG or IgM. Administration of blood cells to a recipient who has the corresponding antibody causes **haemolysis** and a severe reaction.

Minor blood groups may be important clinically following ABO-typed uncross-matched **blood transfusion**, or multiple transfusions; an atypical antibody in a recipient makes the finding of suitable donor blood difficult. Minor groups include the Kell, Duffy, Lewis and Kidd systems. Many more have been described; the significance of such diversity is unclear.

Daniels G, Reid ME (2010). Transfusion; 50: 281–9

See also, Blood compatibility testing

Blood loss, perioperative. Overall management consists of preoperative patient evaluation and preparation, pre-procedure preparation and intraoperative management of blood loss:

- preoperative patient evaluation:
  - history of previous **blood transfusion**, drug-induced coagulopathy (e.g. with **warfarin**, **clopidogrel**), congenital coagulopathy (e.g. **haemophilia**), thrombotic disease (**DVT**, **PE**).
  - presence or risk factors of **ischaemic heart disease** which may influence the transfusion trigger level.
  - review of blood results e.g. presence of **anaemia**, coagulopathy, etc.
- pre-procedure patient preparation:
  - consider iron therapy for iron deficient anaemia and **erythropoietin** and iron therapy for patients with anaemia of chronic illness.
  - stop anticoagulant drugs (e.g. warfarin, **factor Xa inhibitors**) and transfer patients to shorter-acting agents (e.g. **heparin**). If possible, stop non-aspirin antiplatelet drugs (e.g. clopidogrel) for an appropriate time before elective surgery except in patients who have undergone **percutaneous coronary intervention.** **Aspirin** may be continued if indicated by the patient's condition.
  - if indicated, the patient may donate blood for autologous transfusion (*see Blood transfusion, autologous*).
  - risks and benefits of transfusion should be explained and **consent** obtained.
  - a restrictive transfusion protocol (i.e., no allogeneic blood transfusion before haemoglobin level falls below 70 g/l) helps reduce transfusion but preoperative haemoglobin levels, the magnitude and rate of bleeding, the intravascular volume status and the patient's cardiorespiratory function must be considered.
  - appropriate number of units of blood should be ordered beforehand.
  - massive blood transfusion protocol must be in place (*see Blood transfusion, massive*).
  - **prothrombin complex concentrate** or fresh frozen plasma can be given for urgent reversal of warfarin.
  - consider **antifibrinolytic drugs** (e.g. **tranexamic acid**) in patients undergoing surgery with expected high blood loss (e.g. cardiopulmonary bypass, major joint replacement surgery, liver surgery).
  - consider **cell salvage** if large blood loss anticipated.
- intraoperative management:
  - measures to reduce blood loss:
    - **hypotensive anaesthesia.**
    - **tourniquets.**
    - local infiltration with **vasopressor drugs.**
    - appropriate positioning, e.g. head-up for **ENT surgery.**
    - **spinal** and **epidural anaesthesia.**
  - factors that may increase blood loss:
    - raised venous pressure:
      - raised intrathoracic pressure, e.g. due to respiratory obstruction, coughing, straining.
      - fluid overload and cardiac failure.
      - inappropriate positioning.
      - venous obstruction.
    - **hypercapnia.**
    - **hypertension.**
    - coagulopathy.
    - poor surgical technique.
  - monitoring required:
    - regular observation of surgical field for blood loss and 'oozing', which might suggest coagulopathy.
    - measurement of amount of **haemorrhage.**
    - standard physiological monitoring including urine output, ± arterial blood gas analysis, haemoglobin level, etc.
    - **coagulation studies** if coagulopathy suspected or blood loss is excessive.
    - for signs of reactions if transfusion is necessary.

American Society of Anesthesiologists Task Force on Perioperative Blood Management (2015). Anesthesiology; 122: 241–75

Blood patch, epidural. Procedure for the relief of **post-dural puncture headache.** The patient's blood is drawn from a peripheral vein under sterile conditions, and injected immediately into the **epidural space.** Blood is thought to seal the dura, thus preventing further **CSF** leak, although cranial displacement of CSF resulting from epidural injection may also be important, at least initially. Anecdotally, more effective with larger volumes; 15–25 ml is usually injected, with back or neck discomfort often limiting the volume used. Maintaining the supine position for at least 2–4 h after patching is recommended to reduce dislodgement of the clot from the dural puncture site. Should be avoided if the patient is febrile, in case of bacteraemia and subsequent epidural abscess.

Effective in 70%–100% of cases, although symptoms may recur in 30%–50%, sometimes necessitating a repeat blood patch. Relief of headache may occur immediately or within 24 h. Spectacular results have been claimed, even when performed up to several months after dural puncture. Prophylactic use has been less consistently successful. Complications are rare, and include transient bradycardia, back and neck ache, root pain, pyrexia, tinnitus and vertigo. Imaging studies have shown considerable blood in the paraspinal tissues. Subsequent epidural anaesthesia is thought to be unaffected.

Blood pressure, *see Arterial blood pressure; Diastolic blood pressure; Mean blood pressure; Systolic blood pressure*

Blood products Many products may be obtained from donated **blood** (Fig. 25), including:

- whole blood: stored at 2°–6°C for up to 35 days. 70 ml citrate preservative solution is added to 420 ml blood. The use of whole blood for **blood transfusion** is restricted in the UK. Heparinised whole blood (lasts for 2 days) has been used for paediatric cardiac surgery.
- packed red cells (plasma reduced): stored at 2°–6°C for up to 35 days. **Haematocrit** is approximately 0.55. Produced by removing all but 20 ml residual plasma from a unit of whole blood and suspending the cells in 100 ml SAG-M (saline–adenine–glucose–mannitol) solution to give a mean volume per unit of 280 ml. Since 1998, routinely depleted of leucocytes to decrease the risk of transmitting variant **Creutzfeldt–Jakob disease** (vCJD). One unit typically increases haemoglobin concentration in a 70-kg adult by 10 g/l.
- microaggregate-free blood: leucocytes, platelets and debris removed (i.e., the 'buffy coat'). Used to prevent reactions to leucocyte and platelet antigens.
- leucocytes: separated from blood donated by patients whose leucocyte count has been increased by pre-treatment with corticosteroids, or those with chronic granulocytic leukaemia.
- frozen blood: used by the armed forces but too expensive and time-consuming for routine use. Glycerol is added to prevent haemolysis. Requires thawing and washing. May be stored for many years.
- **platelets**: stored at 22°C for up to 5 days. Obtained either from a single donor by plateletpheresis (one donation yielding 1–3 therapeutic dose units) or from multiple units of donated whole blood (one unit of platelets derived from four male donors (to reduce the risk of **transfusion-related acute lung injury**). In the UK, a target of >80% of transfusions from single donors has been set. Transfusion thresholds vary according to the clinical situation, the level of platelet function and laboratory evidence of coagulopathy, but typically include a platelet count of 50 × 10^9/l or less for surgery, unless platelet function is abnormal. One therapeutic dose unit (approximate volume 210–310 ml) normally increases the platelet count by 20–40 × 10^9/l, although some patients may exhibit 'refractoriness' (e.g. those with circulating antiplatelet antibodies). Filtered by microfilters; ordinary iv giving sets are suitable. Preferably should be ABO-compatible. Contains added citrate.
- fresh frozen plasma (FFP): stored at −25°C for up to 3 years. Must be ABO-compatible. Once thawed, can be stored at 4°C and must be given within 24 h in the UK, or kept at room temperature and given within 4 h. Contains all clotting factors, including fibrinogen, and is also a source of plasma **cholinesterase**. Contains added citrate. Viral infection risk is as for whole blood. In the UK, one unit of FFP is derived from plasma from a single (male) donor, and FFP for patients born after 1995 is derived from donors from countries with a low risk of vCJD and treated (e.g. with methylene blue or detergent) to reduce the risk of viral transmission. Indicated for treatment of various coagulopathies, e.g. multifactor deficiencies associated with major haemorrhage

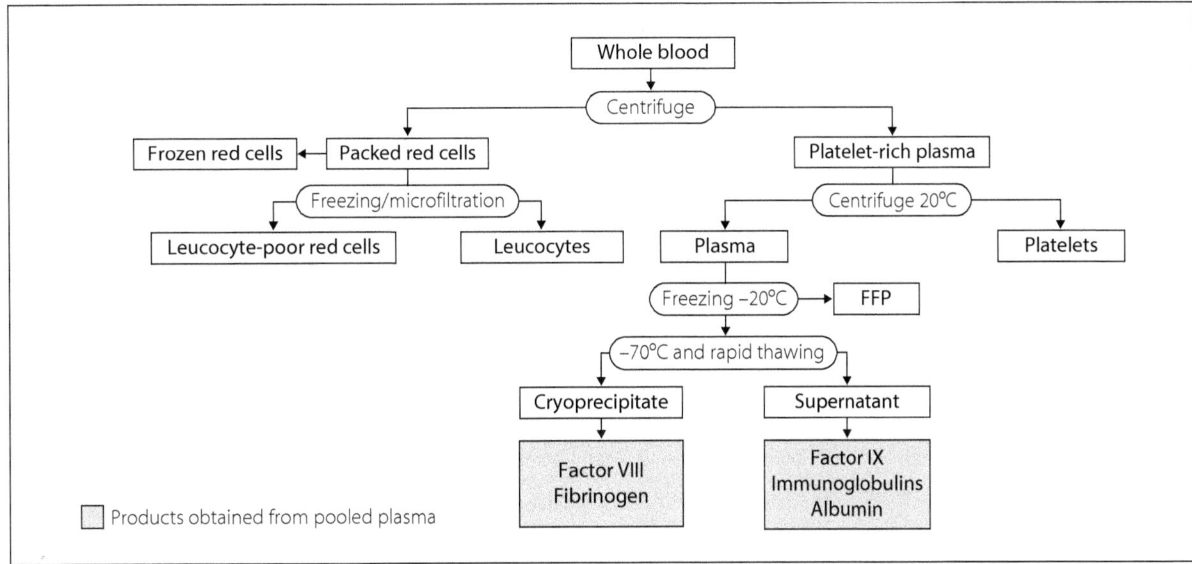

Fig. 25 Blood products available from whole blood

and/or **DIC**. One adult therapeutic dose is 12–15 ml/kg or 4 units for a 70-kg adult, and would typically increase the fibrinogen concentration by 1 g/l. Solvent detergent treated FFP is widely available as a licensed medicinal product (Octaplas LG); it is prepared from large donor pools (hence the need for pathogen inactivation) resulting in more standardised concentrations of clotting factors than standard FFP. Other plasma products include 'never frozen' or 'liquid' plasma (stored at 1°–6°C for up to 26 days), dried plasma and 'extended life plasma' (FFP that is thawed and stored for up to 5–7 days).

- cryoprecipitate: obtained by controlled thawing of FFP to precipitate high-molecular-weight proteins (e.g. factor VIII, fibrinogen and von Willebrand's factor). Frozen and stored at –25°C; thawed immediately before use. Indicated for the treatment of ongoing bleeding in the presence of low fibrinogen levels (<1 g/l). Concentration of fibrinogen is 5–6 times that of FFP. A typical adult dose is two 5-unit pools, in total containing ~3 g fibrinogen in ~500 ml; this would increase fibrinogen levels by ~1 g/l. Viral infection risk is as for whole blood.
- human **albumin** solution (HAS; previously called plasma protein fraction, PPF): stored at room temperature for 2–5 years depending on the preparation. Heat-treated to kill viruses. Contains virtually no clotting factors. Available as 4.5% and 20% (salt-poor albumin) solutions; both contain 140–150 mmol/l sodium but the latter contains less sodium per gram of albumin. Licensed for blood volume expansion with or without hypoalbuminaemia. Use is controversial owing to high cost and the absence of evidence demonstrating its superiority to other colloids. UK supplies are now sourced from the USA.
- factor concentrates, e.g. I (fibrinogen), VIII and IX: obtained by recombinant gene engineering, removing the risk of viral infection. **Recombinant factor VIIa** is licensed for the treatment of patients with acquired or congenital haemophilia, **von Willebrand's disease** and inhibitors to factors VIII or IX of the clotting cascade. It enhances thrombin generation on the surfaces of activated platelets, thus having a mainly local effect with little impact on systemic coagulation. Has been used off-licence for arresting major traumatic, surgical and obstetric haemorrhage, although use is restricted owing to high cost. Fibrinogen concentrate is licensed for treatment of congenital hypofibrinogenaemia but has also been used in trauma and obstetrics (particularly the latter, where a fall in plasma fibrinogen levels (which are normally raised in pregnancy) has been identified as a marker of and risk factor for severe haemorrhage).

Green L, Allard S, Cardigan R (2014). Anaesthesia; 70 Suppl 1: 3–9

See also, Blood, artificial; Blood storage

Blood storage. Viability of red cells is defined as at least 70% survival 24 h post-transfusion.

- The following occur in stored blood:
  - reduced pH, as low as 6.7–7.0, mainly due to high $P\text{CO}_2$.
  - increased lactic acid.
  - increased potassium ion concentration, up to 30 mmol/l.
  - reduced **ATP** and glucose consumption.
  - shift to the left of **oxyhaemoglobin dissociation curve** due to reduced **2,3-DPG** levels (**Valtis–Kennedy effect**).
  - reduced viability of other blood constituents (e.g. **platelets** and **leucocytes**) and formation of microaggregates. **Coagulation** factors V and VIII are almost completely destroyed, XI is reduced, and IX and X are reduced after 7 days.
- Storage solutions:
  - SAG-M (saline 140 mmol/l, adenine 1.5 mmol/l, glucose 50 mmol/l and mannitol 30 mmol/l). The standard solution used in the UK. Used to suspend concentrated red cells after removal of plasma from CPD anticoagulated blood (*see later*), allowing a greater amount of plasma to be removed for other blood products. Has similar preserving properties to CPD-A. Mannitol prevents haemolysis. BAGPM (bicarbonate-added glucose–phosphate–mannitol) is similar.
  - ACD (acid–citrate–dextrose): trisodium citrate, citric acid and dextrose. Introduced in the 1940s. Red cell survival is 21 days. 2,3-DPG is greatly reduced after 7 days.
  - CPD (citrate–phosphate–dextrose): citrate, sodium dihydrogen phosphate and dextrose. Described in the late 1950s. Red cell survival: 28 days. 2,3-DPG is greatly reduced after 14 days.
  - CPD-A. Addition of adenine increases red cell ATP levels. Red cell survival: 35 days. 2,3-DPG is low after 14 days. Used for whole blood.

Storage at 2°–6°C is optimum for red cells but reduces platelets and clotting factors. 22°C is optimum for platelets (survival time 3–5 days). Freezing of blood is expensive and time-consuming, but allows storage for many years. It requires 2 h of thawing, and removal of glycerol (used to prevent haemolysis).

After rewarming and transfusion, potassium is taken up by red cells. 2,3-DPG levels are restored within 24 h.

Plastic collection bags, permeable to CO_2, were introduced in the 1960s. In the closed triple-bag system, blood passes from the donor to the first collection bag, from which plasma and red cells are passed into separate bags if required. The closed system prevents exposure to air and infection.

Before transfusion, the correct identity of the unit of blood (including expiry date) and the patient must be confirmed (by checking against an identification band). The integrity of the bag should be checked. Blood left out of the fridge for more than 30 min should be transfused within 4 h or discarded. Details of each unit given and the total volume transfused should be recorded in the patient's notes and/or anaesthetic record.

Orlov D, Karkouti K (2014). Anaesthesia; 70: 29–e12

See also, Blood products; Blood transfusion

Blood substitutes, *see Blood, artificial*

Blood tests, preoperative, *see Investigations, preoperative*

Blood transfusion. Reports of transfusion between animals, and between animals and humans, date from the seventeenth century. Transfusions between humans were performed in the early nineteenth century. Adverse reactions in recipients and clotting of blood were major problems. **ABO blood groups** were discovered in 1900; improvements in **blood compatibility testing** and anticoagulation followed.

In the UK, NHS Blood and Transplant, a Special Health Authority, relies on voluntary donors, and is increasingly hard-pressed to meet demand for **blood products**. Perioperative use accounts for about 50% of total blood usage. Recent guidelines suggest that, under stable conditions, a perioperative haemoglobin concentration of 70–100 g/l should be maintained, depending on the circumstances.

- Complications of transfusion:
  - immunological (reactions are associated with 2% of all transfusions):
    - immediate **haemolysis** (e.g. ABO incompatibility). Incidence is 1 in 180 000. Features include rapid onset of fever, back pain, skin rash, hypotension and dyspnoea. **DIC** and **renal failure** may occur. Hypotension and increased oozing of blood from wounds may be the only indication of incompatible transfusion in an anaesthetised patient. Immediate treatment is as for **anaphylaxis**, although the underlying mechanisms are different. Samples of recipient and donor blood should be taken for analysis. Mortality is <20%. Most cases arise from clerical errors (e.g. incorrect labelling or administration to the wrong patient).
    - delayed haemolysis (e.g. minor groups). Usually occurs 7–10 days after transfusion, with fever, **anaemia** and jaundice. Renal failure may occur.
    - reactions to platelets and leucocytes (HLA antigens). Slow onset of fever, dyspnoea and tachycardia; shock is rare.
    - reactions to donor plasma proteins (often IgA). May cause anaphylaxis.
    - **transfusion-related acute lung injury** (TRALI): a major cause of mortality following transfusion. Incidence is 1 in 150 000.
    - **graft-versus-host disease** in immunosuppressed patients. Rare since universal leucocyte reduction of blood components was introduced in 1999. Irradiated products (by gamma or x-rays within 14 days of donation, after which it has a shelf life of 14 days) are indicated in: Hodgkin lymphoma (for life); certain congenital immunodeficiency states (e.g. DiGeorge syndrome); treatment with certain biological immunodepressants or purine analogues; intrauterine transfusion; and bone marrow transplant recipients.
    - febrile reactions of unknown aetiology, with or without urticaria.
    - infusion of Rhesus-positive blood into Rhesus-negative women of child-bearing age may cause haemolytic disease of the newborn in future pregnancies.
    - increased tumour recurrence has been reported in patients undergoing surgery for colonic, ovarian and prostatic cancer who receive perioperative transfusion, possibly via immunosuppression due to transfused leucocytes.
  - infective: transmission of infective agents is reduced/prevented by excluding certain groups from donating blood, and screening donated blood (Table 12). Bacterial contamination of donor units, typically with gram-negative organisms, e.g. pseudomonas or coliforms, may result in fever and cardiovascular collapse. Risk is 1 in 500 000 units transfused. Platelet concentrates harbouring staphylococcus, yersinia and salmonella have been reported. Risk is about 1 in 50 000.
  - metabolic:
    - **hyperkalaemia**: rarely a problem, unless with rapid transfusion in hyperkalaemic patients, as potassium is rapidly taken up by red cells after infusion and warming.
    - citrate toxicity: citrate is normally metabolised to bicarbonate within a few minutes. Rapid transfusion of citrated blood may cause **hypocalcaemia**, and **calcium** administration may be required. **Alkalosis** may follow citrate metabolism to bicarbonate. With the modern practice of using SAG-M (saline–adenine–glucose–mannitol) solution, citrate toxicity is rare unless large volumes of plasma or platelet preparations are given, because these do contain citrate.
    - **acidosis** due to transfused blood is rarely a problem (*see earlier*).
  - transfusion-associated circulatory overload (TACO): characterised by dyspnoea, tachycardia, pulmonary oedema and hypertension. Caused by hypervolaemia although may occur after transfusion of a single unit. Incidence 1 in 450 000. More common in infants and the elderly, especially those with cardiac and renal impairment. Often requires diuretic therapy.
  - **hypothermia**. Rapid infusion of cold blood may cause cardiac arrest. All transfused blood should be warmed, especially when infused rapidly. Excessive heat may cause haemolysis.
  - in the ICU, evidence suggests that lowering the threshold for transfusion from 100 g/l to 70 g/l decreases mortality, organ dysfunction and cardiac complications.
  - impaired O_2 delivery to tissues, due to the leftward shift of **oxyhaemoglobin dissociation curve** in stored blood that lasts up to 24 h. In addition, red cells in stored blood are thought to be more likely to cause blockage of capillaries owing to their reduced physical flexibility, further impairing O_2 delivery.
  - impaired **coagulation** caused by dilution and/or consumption of circulating clotting factors and platelets. DIC is rare.
  - microaggregates (*see Blood filters*).
  - thrombophlebitis and extravasation.
  - **gas embolism**.
  - iron overload (chronic transfusions).
  - interaction when stored blood is administered following iv fluids, e.g. clotting (**gelatin solutions, Hartmann's solution**), haemolysis (**dextrose solutions**).

Serious complications of blood transfusion are monitored in the UK by the Serious Hazards of Transfusion (SHOT) scheme.

Routine warning about the risk of blood transfusion—including the exclusion of recipients of blood products as future donors—has been recommended as part of the standard preoperative consent process.

[Angelo DiGeorge (1921–2009), American paediatric endocrinologist; Thomas Hodgkin (1798–1866), English pathologist]

Klein AA, Arnold P, Bingham RM, et al (2016). Anaesthesia; 71: 829–42

See also, Blood groups; Blood storage; Blood transfusion, massive; Intravenous fluid administration; Rhesus blood groups

Blood transfusion, autologous. Transfusion of a patient's own blood. For perioperative use, different methods may be used:

- 2–6 units are taken over a period of days or weeks before surgery. Concurrent oral iron therapy ensures

Table 12 Exclusions and screening applying to donation of blood (N.B. primarily applies to the UK, though similar procedures apply to other Western countries)

	Donors excluded	*Blood screening*	*Comments*
Brucellosis	Past history of infection		
Cytomegalovirus (CMV)		For intrauterine transfusion, neonates <28 days and during pregnancy if time permits (ordinary leucodepleted products acceptable otherwise)	About 55% of the population are CMV-positive
Glandular fever	Infection within last 2 years		
Hepatitis	Hepatitis or jaundice within last year Acupuncture (unless by registered practitioner), tattoo or other skin piercing within 6 months	Hepatitis B surface antigen/nucleic acid: routine Hepatitis C antibodies/RNA: routine Hepatitis E RNA: routine since 2017	No carrier state for hepatitis A, therefore not screened for If post-transfusion hepatitis occurs, the donor may be traced and further investigated Risk of transmission ~1:1.6 million units for hepatitis B and 1:26 million for hepatitis C. Risk for hepatitis E currently being assessed
HIV	Previous HIV-positive test; at-risk groups (iv drug users, sex workers, men with male sexual partners, men or women with sexual partners from a high-risk group or area where HIV is common): within 3 months of high-risk activity/ exposure	HIV-1 and HIV-2 antibodies/nucleic acid: routine	Risk of transmission ~1:6.25 million units
HTLV-I and II	Past history of infection	Antibodies: routine	Infection with HTLV-I may result in adult T-cell leukaemia
Malaria	Visit to endemic areas within last 6 months, with only plasma collected for next 5 years unless cleared by antibody testing		
vCJD	Recipients of: transfusion in the UK after 1980; iv immunoglobulins prepared from UK plasma; human pituitary extract Donors whose blood has been transfused to recipients who later develop vCJD without other explanation Family member with vCJD		Leucodepletion (removal of white cells) of all blood components Plasma for fractionation to make plasma derivatives imported from outside the UK FFP for patients <16 years old imported from outside the UK A filter that removes the prion protein responsible for vCJD is under investigation
Syphilis	Past history of infection	Antibodies: routine	
Others	Blood donation within last 12 weeks Chesty cough, sore throat, active cold sore or any infection within last 2 weeks Antibiotic medication within last week Currently pregnant or 9 months postpartum	*Trypanosoma cruzi* antibodies and West Nile virus RNA if recent travel to endemic areas	

HTLV-I, Human T-cell leukaemia and lymphoma virus type I; vCJD, variant Creutzfeldt–Jakob disease.

an adequate bone marrow response. **Erythropoietin** has been used. Pre-transfusion testing varies between centres, from ABO grouping to full cross-matching. Labelling of blood must be meticulous and this, together with wastage of unused blood (which may be up to 20%), results in higher administration costs than for allogeneic transfusion. Only suitable for elective surgery.

- perioperative **haemodilution**: simultaneous collection of blood and replacement of removed volume with colloid or crystalloid. The collected blood is available for transfusion when required, usually during or shortly after blood loss has stopped.
- peri- or postoperative transfusion of blood salvaged from the operation site during surgery. Washing and filtering remove debris and contaminants. Methods range from simple closed collecting/reperfusion systems to expensive centrifuging machines (the latter referred to as '**cell salvage**').

Attractive as it reduces: (i) the risks of transfusion related to compatibility and cross-infection; (ii) the shortfall between the demand and supply of donated blood; and (iii) the costs associated with donated blood products. However, the safety of blood products and their administration has improved markedly over the last 1–2 decades, while the additional demands and costs of running perioperative autologous transfusion schemes are also disincentives.

Ashworth A, Klein AA (2010). Br J Anaesth; 105: 401–16

See also, Blood transfusion

Blood transfusion, massive. Definitions vary but include:
- **blood transfusion** ≥10 units of packed red blood cells (PRBCs; i.e., the total blood volume of an average adult) within 24 h.
- transfusion of >4 units of PRBCs within 1 h, with anticipation of further need for **blood products**.
- replacement of >50% of total blood volume within 3 h.

May occur during surgery or because of the presenting condition e.g. **postpartum haemorrhage**, **GIT haemorrhage**, **trauma**. Approximately 40% of trauma-related mortality is due to massive haemorrhage and 5% of patients admitted to trauma centres require massive blood transfusion. Adverse effects are those of blood transfusion generally; in particular:
- impaired O_2 delivery to tissues.
- impaired **coagulation** due to a combination of:
  - coagulopathy related to the presenting condition, e.g. early trauma-induced coagulopathy (ETIC), **DIC** associated with **placental abruption**.
  - lack of coagulation factors and functioning **platelets** in transfused blood.
- **hypothermia**.
- **hypocalcaemia** (if rapid transfusion).
- **hyperkalaemia** may occur, although this is rarely a problem; **hypokalaemia** may follow potassium uptake by red cells.
- metabolic **acidosis** may occur initially; **alkalosis** may follow as citrate is metabolised to bicarbonate (rare with modern blood products).
- **hypovolaemia** or fluid overload.
- **transfusion-related acute lung injury**.

- Management of massive blood transfusion:
  - early resuscitation of circulating blood volume with blood products reduces mortality.
  - the use of institutional massive transfusion protocols to coordinate trauma, transfusion medicine, laboratory, transport and nursing teams has been shown to improve patient survival, reduce organ failure and decrease postoperative complications.
  - traditionally, early resuscitation is performed using **crystalloid** solutions. However, in trauma, survival is thought to be improved by transfusion with PRBCs/plasma/platelet solutions in a 1:1:1 combination. Whether this is the case for other causes of massive transfusion (e.g. obstetric) is less clear.
  - **antifibrinolytic agents** (e.g. **tranexamic acid**) may improve survival, especially when given early in the resuscitation process.

Pham HP, Shaz BH (2013). Br J Anaesth; 111(suppl 1): i71–82

See also, Blood storage

Blood urea nitrogen (BUN). Nitrogen component of blood urea. Gives an indication of renal function in a similar way to urea measurement. Normally 1.5–3.3 mmol/l (10–20 mg/dl).

Blood volume. Total blood volume is approximately 70 ml/kg in adults, 80 ml/kg in children and 90 ml/kg in neonates (although the latter may vary widely, depending on how much blood is returned from the placenta at birth. The formula: [% **haematocrit** + 50] ml/kg has been suggested for neonates).
- Distribution (approximate):
  - 60%–70% venous
  - 15% arterial
  - 10% within the heart
  - 5% capillary.

Measured by **dilution techniques**; plasma volume is found by injecting a known dose of marker (e.g. albumin labelled with dyes or radioactive iodine) into the blood and measuring plasma concentrations. Rapid exchange of albumin between plasma and interstitial fluid leads to slight overestimation using this method; larger molecules, e.g. immunoglobulin, may be used.

$$\text{Total blood volume} = \text{plasma volume} \times \frac{100}{100 - \%\text{haematocrit}}$$

Red cell volume may be found by labelling erythrocytes with radioactive markers, e.g. ^{51}Cr.

Bloody tap, *see Epidural anaesthesia*

Blow-off valve, *see Adjustable pressure-limiting valve*

BMI, *see Body mass index*

BMR, *see Basal metabolic rate*

Bodok seal. Metal-edged, rubber bonded disk, used to prevent gas leaks from the **cylinder**/yoke interface on **anaesthetic machines**.

Body mass index (BMI). Indication of body fat derived from a person's weight and height: BMI = weight (kg) ÷ height (m)^2. Widely used as a measure of **obesity**, although it does not account for body build and muscle mass. Varies with age and sex in children and adolescents, thus reference to growth reference charts is required. Also used to refer to degrees of underweight. Has been incorporated into most international and national classifications of obesity (Table 13), although some national variations in definitions exist.

Body plethysmograph. Airtight box, large enough to enclose a human, used to study **lung volumes** and pressures. Once a subject is inside, air pressure and volume may be measured before and during respiration.
- May be used to measure:
  - **FRC**: the subject makes inspiratory effort against a shutter. Box volume is decreased due to lung expansion, and box pressure increased because of the decrease in volume. Applying **Boyle's law**:

$$\text{original pressure} \times \text{volume} = \text{new pressure} \times \text{new volume}$$

where new volume = original volume − change in lung volume.

Table 13 World Health Organization classification of obesity according to body mass index (kg/m^2)

Underweight	<18.5
Normal	18.5–24.99
Overweight	25.0–29.9
Obese: class I	30.0–34.9
class II	35.0–39.9
class III	≥40.0

Thus, change in lung volume may be calculated. If airway pressures are also measured:

Original airway pressure × resting lung volume = new airway pressure × new lung volume

where resting lung volume = FRC, and new volume = FRC + change in lung volume
Thus, FRC may be calculated.

- **airway resistance**:

$$= \frac{\text{alveolar pressure} - \text{mouth pressure}}{\text{airflow}}$$

The subject breathes the air in the box. Box volume is reduced by the change in alveolar volume during inspiration, measured as above. Lung volume may be measured at the same time, as above:

lung volume × starting alveolar pressure = new lung volume × new alveolar pressure;

where starting alveolar pressure = box pressure, and new lung volume = lung volume + alveolar volume
Alveolar pressure may thus be calculated. Also, mouth pressure = box pressure, and flow may be measured using a **pneumotachograph**.

- pulmonary blood flow: the subject breathes from a bag containing N_2O and O_2 within the box. As the N_2O is taken up by the blood, the volume of the bag decreases. Because N_2O uptake is flow-limited (*see Alveolar gas transfer*), uptake occurs in steps with each heartbeat. The decrease in bag size therefore occurs in steps, and is calculated by measuring bag pressure, and box volume and pressure. If the N_2O-carrying capacity of blood is known, pulmonary blood flow may be calculated and displayed as a continuous trace showing pulsatile flow.

Body surface area, *see Surface area, body*

Body weight. Used as the basis for many anaesthetic and related drugs. In most cases, total (actual) body weight can be used, but difficulties may arise in **obesity**, in which the greater proportion of the body composed of fat, with its relatively low blood flow compared with other tissues, alters the **pharmacokinetics** of injected drug. Several different derived weights may be used for calculating appropriate dosage in obesity (Table 14), the lean or adjusted body weight (the latter accounting for the increased **volume of distribution** in obesity) being used most often. In practice, however, the most cautious approach is to titrate small doses against effect.
Nightingale CE, Margarson MP, Shearer E, et al (2015). Anaesthesia; 70: 859–76

Bohr effect. Shift to the right of the **oxyhaemoglobin dissociation curve** associated with a rise in blood $P\text{CO}_2$ and/or fall in pH. Results in lower affinity of **haemoglobin** for O_2, favouring O_2 delivery to the tissues, where CO_2 levels are high.

The double Bohr effect refers to pregnancy, when CO_2 passes from fetal to maternal blood at the placenta, causing the following changes:

- maternal blood: CO_2 rises, i.e., shift of curve to right and reduced O_2 affinity.
- fetal blood: CO_2 falls, i.e., shift of curve to left and increased O_2 affinity.

The net effect is to favour O_2 transfer from maternal to fetal blood.
[Christian Bohr (1855–1911), Danish physiologist]
See also, Oxygen transport

Bohr equation. Equation used to derive physiological **dead space**.

Expired CO_2 = inspired CO_2 + CO_2 given out by lungs,
or: $F_E \times V_T = (F_I \times V_T) + (F_A \times V_A)$

where F_E = fractional concentration of CO_2 in expired gas
F_I = fractional concentration of CO_2 in inspired gas
F_A = fractional concentration of CO_2 in alveolar gas
V_T = tidal volume
V_A = alveolar component of tidal volume.

Since inspired CO_2 is negligible, it may be ignored:
i.e., $F_E \times V_T = F_A \times V_A$

But $V_A = V_T - V_D$, where V_D = dead space

$$\text{Therefore: } F_E \times V_T = F_A \times (V_T - V_D) = (F_A \times V_T) - (F_A \times V_D)$$

$$\text{or: } F_A \times V_D = (F_A \times V_T) - (F_E \times V_T) = V_T(F_A - F_E)$$

$$\text{Therefore } \frac{V_D}{V_T} = \frac{F_A - F_E}{F_A}$$

Since partial pressure is proportional to concentration:

$$\frac{V_D}{V_T} = \frac{P_A\text{CO}_2 - P_E\text{CO}_2}{P_A\text{CO}_2}$$

where $P_A\text{CO}_2$ = alveolar partial pressure of CO_2
$P_E\text{CO}_2$ = mixed expired partial pressure of CO_2

Since alveolar $P\text{CO}_2$ approximately equals arterial $P\text{CO}_2$,

$$\frac{V_D}{V_T} = \frac{P_a\text{CO}_2 - P_E\text{CO}_2}{P_a\text{CO}_2}$$

where $P_a\text{CO}_2$ = arterial partial pressure of CO_2.

See also, Bohr effect

Boiling point (bp). Temperature of a substance at which its **SVP** equals external atmospheric pressure. Additional heat does not raise the temperature further, but provides

Table 14 Derived body weights used for calculating drug doses (all weights in kg)

Total body weight (TBW)	Actual measured weight
Ideal body weight (IBW)	Height (cm) − 100 (men) or 105 (women)
Lean body weight (LBW)	Men: (9270 × TBW) ÷ (6680 + (216 × BMI [kg/m²])
	Women: (9270 × TBW) ÷ (8780 + (244 × BMI [kg/m²])
Adjusted body weight (ABW)	IBW + (0.4 × TBW) − IBW

the **latent heat** of vaporisation necessary for the liquid to evaporate. If external pressure is raised, e.g. within a pressure cooker, bp is also raised; thus, the maximal temperature attainable is raised, and food cooks more quickly.

Bone cement implantation syndrome. Cardiovascular impairment associated with surgical instrumentation of the bony canal of the femur, e.g. during intramedullary nailing and fixation of fractured neck of femur. Originally thought to involve either direct cardiotoxicity of the monomer used in the cement (methylmethacrylate) or an allergic reaction to it, but now understood to be caused by embolism of cement, bone fragments, fat and/or bone marrow from the bone cavity into the vasculature. Ranges from mild desaturation ± hypotension (~20% of cases of cemented arthroplasty), through significant desaturation ± hypotension requiring treatment (~3%), to collapse requiring CPR (~1%). Reduced by washing and drying the interior femoral shaft before insertion of cement, which should be done retrogradely, and venting of air from the canal during cement insertion (e.g. using a suction catheter placed in the shaft) to avoid build-up of pressure. Requires good communication between surgeons and anaesthetists, with resuscitative drugs/fluids ready should they be required. Insertion of cement should be documented on the anaesthetic record.

Griffiths R, White SM, Moppett IK, et al (2015). Anaesthesia; 70: 623–6

Bone marrow harvest. Taking of bone marrow for **bone marrow transplantation**, from either a healthy donor (allograft) or the patient recipient before radio- or chemotherapy (autograft). Usually performed under general anaesthesia, especially in children, although regional anaesthetic techniques may be used.

- Anaesthetic considerations:
  - preoperatively:
    - allografts: donors are usually fit.
    - autografts: usually performed for blood malignancy; i.e., patients may be anaemic or thrombocytopenic and prone to infections. Cardiovascular, respiratory and renal function may be impaired. Drug treatment may include **cytotoxic drugs** and **corticosteroids**.
  - perioperatively:
    - marrow is usually taken from the posterior and anterior iliac crests and sternum, requiring **positioning** first supine, then prone, although the lateral position may suffice. Tracheal intubation and IPPV are usually employed. Avoidance of N_2O has been suggested, but this is controversial.
    - large-bore iv cannulation is required, because there may be large volume losses. Autologous **blood transfusion** is usually performed, especially for allografts. Non-autologous blood is irradiated before transfusion to kill any leucocytes present. The volume of marrow harvested is up to 20%–30% of estimated blood volume, to provide the required leucocyte count.
    - **heparin** may be given to stop the marrow clotting; it may also protect against **fat embolism**, which may occur during harvesting.
  - postoperatively: large volumes of iv fluids are often required.

Bone marrow transplantation. Performed for leukaemias, lymphomas, certain solid tumours, and various non-malignant disorders including aplastic anaemia, **haemoglobinopathies** and rare genetic diseases. Involves donation of bone marrow (usually under general anaesthesia), and its subsequent infusion via a central vein into the recipient, whose own bone marrow has been ablated with chemotherapy + radiotherapy.

- May be one of three types:
  - autologous: the recipient's own bone marrow is taken and treated to remove neoplastic cells before being frozen and stored while ablation is performed. Mortality is up to 10%.
  - syngeneic: the donor and recipient are identical twins. Treatment of the collected cells is not required.
  - allogeneic: the donor is HLA-matched as closely as possible to the recipient; they usually come from the same family or racial group. Mortality is up to 30%.
- Problems occur with all three types but to different extents, and may be related to:
  - the procedure itself:
    - ablative therapy includes **cyclophosphamide**, **busulfan** and other **cytotoxic and immunosuppressive drugs**. Toxic effects include **vomiting**, **cardiomyopathy**, **convulsions**, **pulmonary fibrosis**, GIT mucositis and hepatic veno-occlusive disease.
    - impaired bone marrow function: bacterial, viral, fungal and pneumocystis infections may be problems in the first 4–6 months after autologous and syngeneic transplantation; **immunodeficiency** may be especially prolonged after allogeneic transplantation, when prolonged immunosuppressive therapy is required. **Antibacterial** and **antiviral drugs** are often given prophylactically; **immunoglobulins** have also been used (*see Immunoglobulins, intravenous*). **Blood products** are often required to restore red cell, white cell and platelet numbers. Recently, macrophage and **granulocyte colony-stimulating factors** have been used.
  - rejection: may require repeat transplantation.
  - **graft-versus-host disease**.
  - interstitial **pneumonitis** may occur; it may be unclear whether this is related to **cytomegalovirus** or other atypical infection, or directly related to radiotherapy. Mortality is up to 80%.

Boott, Francis (1792–1863). US-born London physician; qualified in Edinburgh. Having read a letter from **Bigelow**'s father about **Morton**'s demonstration of **diethyl ether**, he arranged a dental extraction by Robinson (who also administered the ether) on 19 December 1846 at his house in Gower Street, London (now a nursing home and formerly the location of part of the **FCAnaes examination**). He then informed **Liston**, who operated using ether 2 days later.

[James Robinson (1813–1861), English dentist]

Ellis RH (1977). Anaesthesia; 32: 197–208

Bosentan, *see Endothelin receptor antagonists*

Bosun warning device, *see Oxygen failure warning devices*

Botulinum toxins. Group of **exotoxins** responsible for **botulism**. Act on presynaptic cholinergic nerve terminals blocking release of **acetylcholine**. Eight have been characterised (labelled A–H), each produced by a distinct strain of *Clostridium botulinum*. Types A, B and E (rarely, F and G) cause disease in humans. Types A and B have been used therapeutically in minute quantities to cause selective muscle weakness that may last for several months, e.g. in strabismus, blepharospasm, hemifacial spasm, torticollis, dystonias, spasmodic dysphonia and as a cosmetic procedure. Also used as a tool to investigate **neurotransmitter** function.

Botulism. Clinical syndrome caused by ingestion of **exotoxins** (**botulinum toxins**) produced by the anaerobic gram-positive bacillus *Clostridium botulinum*. Exotoxin binds irreversibly to cholinergic nerve endings, preventing **acetylcholine** release. Affects the **neuromuscular junction**, autonomic ganglia and parasympathetic postganglionic fibres. Classified according to the source of infection:
  - foodborne botulism: caused by ingestion of *Clostridium* spores or exotoxin produced under anaerobic conditions (e.g. home canning).
  - wound botulism: due to contamination of surgical or other wounds. Also seen in drug abusers injecting 'black-tar' heroin subcutaneously ('skin-popping').
  - infant botulism: due to absorption of exotoxin produced within the GIT, classically after eating contaminated honey.
  - adult infectious botulism: similar to the infant form but follows GIT surgery.
  - inadvertent botulism: follows accidental overdose of botulinum toxin given for treatment of movement disorders (e.g. dystonia).
- Features occur within 12–72 h:
  - nausea, vomiting and abdominal pain.
  - symmetrical descending paralysis initially affecting **cranial nerves**, with diplopia, fixed dilated pupils, facial weakness, dysphagia, dysarthria, limb weakness and respiratory difficulty.
  - autonomic disturbance: ileus, unresponsive pupils, dry mouth, urinary retention.
  - sensory deficit, mental disturbance and fever do not occur.

Diagnosed by inoculation of the patient's serum into mice that have been treated or untreated with antitoxin. Different strains of toxin may be identified. EMG studies may aid diagnosis while waiting for inoculation studies.
- Management:
  - supportive. Long periods of IPPV may be necessary, especially in cases of foodborne botulism.
  - wound debridement if indicated.
  - heptavalent botulinum antitoxin to neutralise circulating exotoxin. Hypersensitivity may occur. A human botulism immunoglobulin (BIG) is used for treatment of infant botulism and those allergic to the antitoxin.
  - **penicillin** to kill live bacilli.

Complete recovery may take months.
See also, Biological weapons, Paralysis, acute

Bougie, *see Intubation aids*

Bourdon gauge, *see Pressure measurement*

Bovie machine, *see Diathermy*

Bowditch effect. Intrinsic regulatory mechanism of cardiac muscle in response to increased rate of stimulation. As rate increases, contractility increases. Also called the treppe effect.
[Henry Bowditch (1840–1911), US physiologist; *Treppe*, German for steps]

Bowel ischaemia. May affect any part of the GIT (although rarely stomach) but usually affects the large bowel. May be caused by thrombus, embolism (e.g. from mural thrombus after **MI**), vascular spasm or low mesenteric perfusion with vasoconstriction (non-occlusive mesenteric ischaemia [NOMI]). May occur in patients with intra-abdominal pathology, especially following vascular surgery, or in any patient with low cardiac output. May also occur in severe **intestinal obstruction**. Vasoconstriction often persists after correction of the initial insult. Bowel infarction may follow secondary to reduced tissue oxygenation or **reperfusion injury**.

Associated with high mortality because diagnosis may be difficult, and bowel infarction may continue despite treatment. **Gastric tonometry** has been used to monitor GIT perfusion in critical illness.

Features include abdominal pain and distension, GIT bleeding, nausea and vomiting, tachycardia, pyrexia, leucocytosis and metabolic acidosis. Angiography may be useful to diagnose ischaemia and differentiate its causes.
- Treatment:
  - supportive measures, including **antibacterial drugs**, restoration of cardiac output ± **vasodilator drugs**.
  - intra-arterial infusion of vasodilators, e.g. **papaverine** 30–60 mg/h, has been used via the angiography catheter.
  - surgery to resect necrotic bowel ± remove embolus or thrombus.

Boyle, Henry Edmund Gaskin (1875–1941). English anaesthetist, best known for the **anaesthetic machine** named after him. Originally introduced in 1917, it consisted of N_2O and O_2 **cylinders**, pressure gauges, water-sight **flowmeters** and ether **vaporiser** ('Boyle's bottle') set in a wooden case. Being left-handed, he placed all controls on the left side of the machine, a practice that continues today. His name is also attached to the instrument used to maintain jaw opening during tonsillectomy (Boyle–Davis gag). Boyle practised at St Bartholomew's Hospital, London, was involved in the advancement and improvement of anaesthesia in the UK, and performed much work on the use of N_2O, including under battle conditions.
[John S Davis (1824–1885), US surgeon]
Hadfield CF (1950). Br J Anaesth; 22: 107–17

Boyle's law. At constant temperature, the volume of a fixed mass of a perfect gas varies inversely with pressure.
[Robert Boyle (1627–1691), Anglo-Irish chemist]
See also, Charles' law; Ideal gas law

Brachial artery. Continuation of the axillary artery, running from the lower border of teres minor to the **antecubital fossa**, where it divides into the **radial** and **ulnar arteries**. Lies at first medial, then anterior to the humerus. Around its midpoint, crossed from lateral to medial by the **median nerve**. Protected from the medial cubital vein in the antecubital fossa by the bicipital aponeurosis. Occasionally divides in the upper arm.

May be used for **arterial cannulation**, although seldom as the site of first choice because of possible distal ischaemia.

Brachial plexus. Nerve plexus supplying the arm. Arises from the ventral rami of the lower cervical and first thoracic **spinal nerves**, and emerges between the scalene

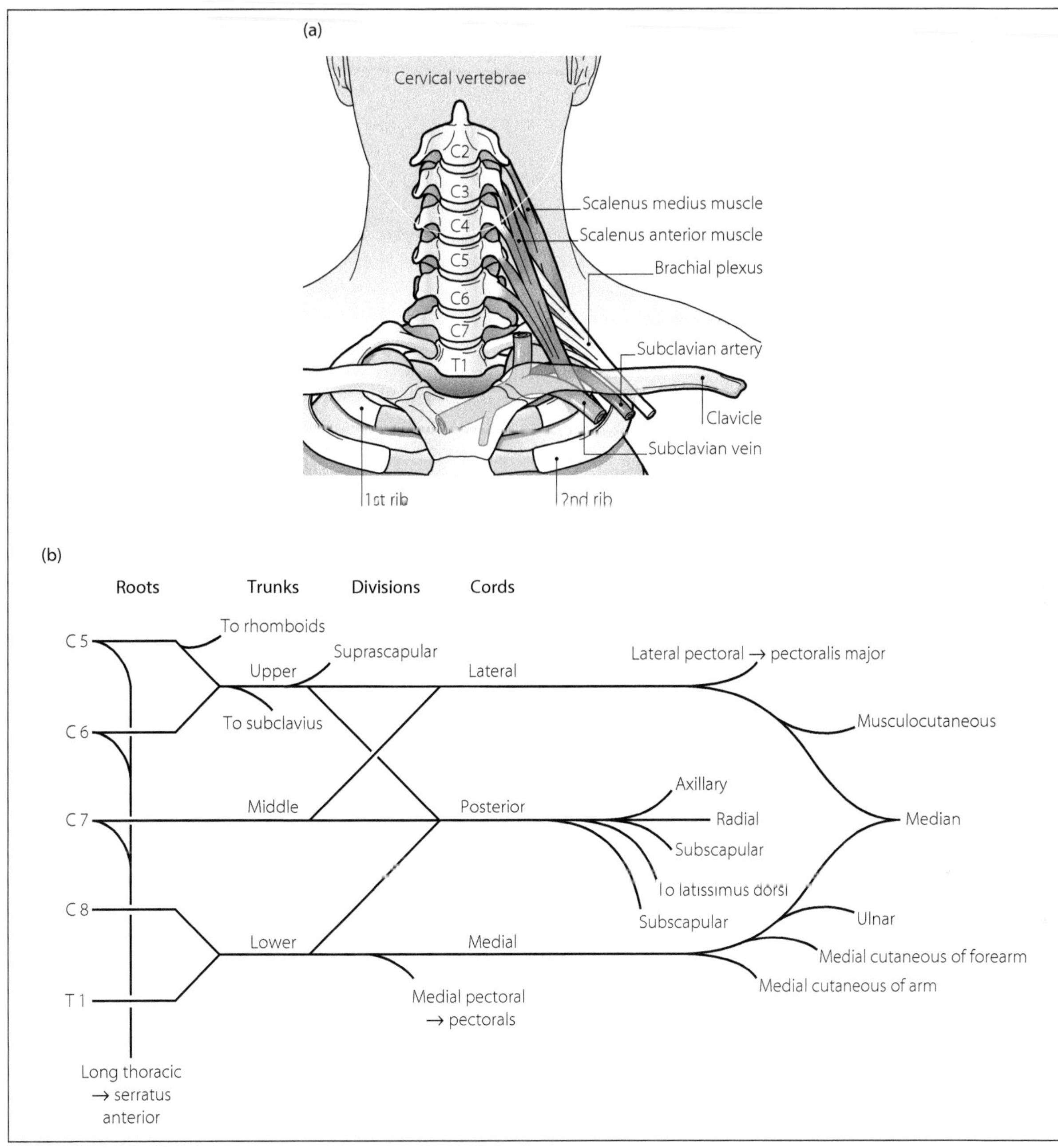

Fig. 26 (a) Relations of the upper brachial plexus. *Continued*

muscles in the neck. The plexus invaginates the scalene fascia and passes down over the first **rib** (Fig. 26a). It accompanies the subclavian artery (which becomes the axillary artery) within a perivascular sheath of connective tissue.

- Anatomy of the scalene muscles:
  - scalenus anterior arises from the anterior tubercles of the 3rd–6th cervical transverse processes, and inserts into the scalene tubercle on the first rib.
  - scalenus medius arises from the posterior tubercles of the 2nd–6th cervical transverse processes and inserts into the first rib behind the groove for the subclavian artery.
  - scalenus posterior is the portion of the previous muscle attached to the second rib.
- The roots lie in the interscalene groove; the trunks cross the posterior triangle of the neck; the divisions lie behind the clavicle; the cords lie in the axilla. Branches arise at different levels (Fig. 26b):
  - roots: nerves to the rhomboids, scalene muscles and serratus anterior (long thoracic nerve), and a contribution to the **phrenic nerve** (C5).
  - trunks: nerve to subclavius, and the suprascapular nerve (to supraspinatus and infraspinatus).
  - cords:
    - lateral:
      - lateral pectoral nerve to pectoralis major.
      - musculocutaneous nerve: passes through the belly of coracobrachialis in the upper arm, supplying coracobrachialis, biceps and brachialis

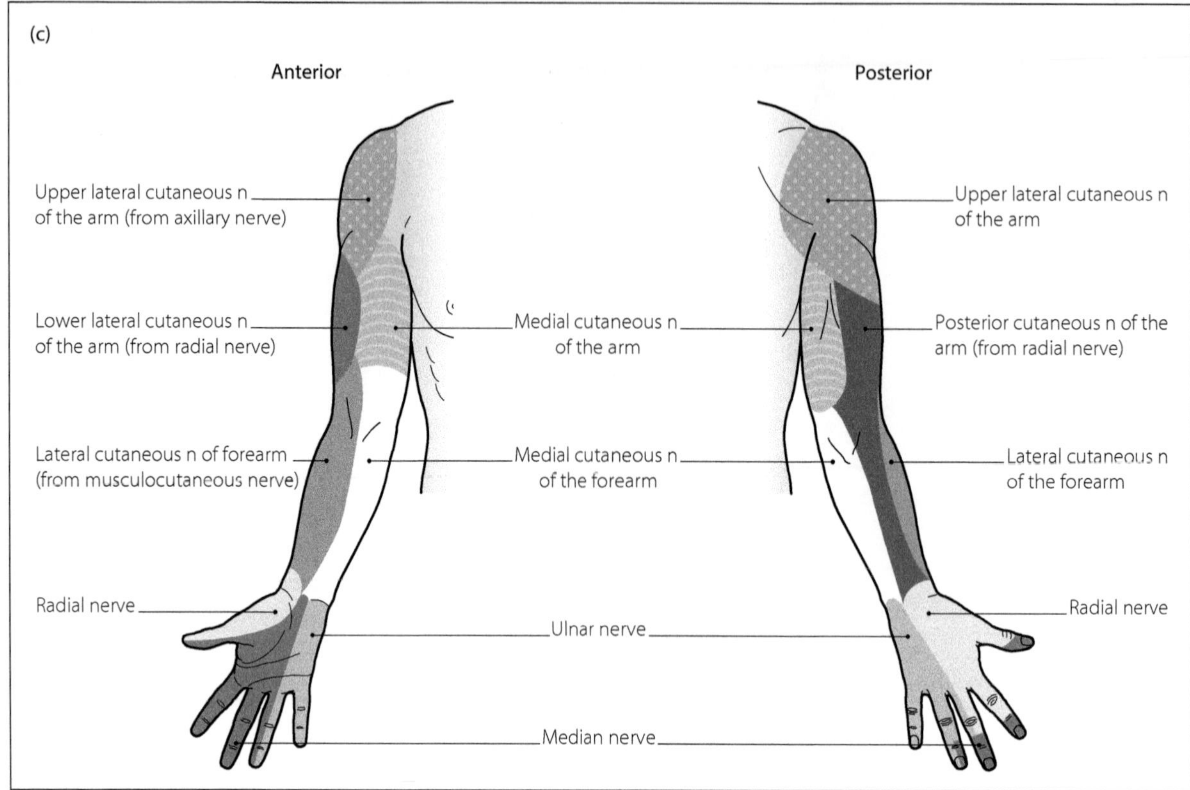

Fig. 26, cont'd (b) Plan of the brachial plexus. (c) Cutaneous nerve supply of the arm

muscles and the elbow joint. Continues as the lateral cutaneous nerve of the forearm, supplying the radial surface of the forearm.
  - lateral part of the **median nerve**.
- medial:
  - medial pectoral nerve to pectoralis major and minor.
  - medial cutaneous nerves of the arm and forearm: supply the medial aspect of the upper arm and forearm, respectively.
  - **ulnar nerve**.
  - medial part of median nerve.
- posterior:
  - subscapular nerves to subscapularis and teres major.
  - nerve to latissimus dorsi.
  - axillary nerve: passes posterior to the neck of the humerus. Supplies deltoid and teres minor and the shoulder joint, and continues as the upper lateral cutaneous nerve of the arm, supplying the skin of the outer shoulder.
  - **radial nerve**.

The plexus thus supplies the skin of the upper limb (Fig. 28c).

- Characteristic motor lesions of the plexus:
  - upper roots: 'waiter's tip' position; arm internally rotated and pronated, with wrist flexed (Erb's paralysis).
  - lower roots: claw hand (Klumpke's paralysis).

[Wilhelm Erb (1840–1921), German physician; Augusta Klumpke (1859–1927), French neurologist]

See also, Brachial plexus block; Dermatomes

Brachial plexus block. May be performed by injecting local anaesthetic solution into the fascial compartment surrounding the **brachial plexus** at several levels. Needle placement is routinely guided by use of a nerve stimulator (eliciting contractions in the appropriate muscle group), or increasingly by ultrasound imaging:
- interscalene:
  - with the patient's head turned away from the side to be blocked, a needle is inserted in the interscalene groove, lateral to the sternomastoid, and level with the cricoid cartilage. It is directed towards the transverse process of C6 (medially, caudally and posteriorly). Accidental epidural, intrathecal or intravascular injections are more likely if the needle is directed cranially.
  - 30–40 ml solution is injected when the needle position is confirmed. If a nerve stimulator is used, contractions should be sought in the shoulder, arm or forearm.
  - produces adequate block for shoulder manipulations.
  - **ulnar nerve** may be missed.
  - complications include phrenic nerve block, recurrent laryngeal nerve block, **Horner's syndrome**, inadvertent epidural or spinal block and injection into the vertebral artery. Bilateral blocks, or blocks in patients with contralateral phrenic nerve palsy, should be avoided.
- supraclavicular:
  - with the patient's head turned away from the side to be blocked, a needle is inserted immediately posterior and lateral to the subclavian pulsation behind the mid-clavicle. In the classic technique, it is directed caudally, medially and posteriorly to the upper surface of first rib, and 'walked' along the rib until the needle position is confirmed; 8–10 ml solution is injected per division.

- median nerve may be missed.
- complications: phrenic and recurrent laryngeal nerve blocks, Horner's syndrome, subclavian puncture, **pneumothorax**. Bilateral blocks should be avoided.

▸ subclavian perivascular:
- with the patient's head turned away from the side to be blocked, a needle is inserted in the interscalene groove, caudal to the level of the cricoid cartilage, and cranial and posterior to a finger palpating the subclavian artery. It is directed caudally only, until the needle position is confirmed (for nerve stimulation, contractions elicited in the arm/hand, not in the shoulder, which may be caused by stimulation of the suprascapular nerve).
- 20–30 ml solution is injected.
- complications: as for supraclavicular block, but pneumothorax is less likely.

▸ axillary:
- with the patient's head turned away, the arm abducted to 90 degrees and the hand under the head, a needle is inserted just above the axillary artery pulsation, as high in the axilla as possible. A click is felt as the perivascular sheath is entered.
- 25–50 ml solution is injected, with digital pressure or a tourniquet below the injection site to encourage upward spread of solution. Careful aspiration before application of digital pressure excludes placement of the needle in the axillary vein. The arm is returned to the patient's side after injection, to avoid compression of the proximal sheath by the humeral head, or before injection if a cannula technique is used.
- a cannula, e.g. iv type 18–20 G, may be inserted and used for repeated injection.
- may miss the musculocutaneous and axillary nerves. The former may be blocked thus:
  - upper arm: at the time of axillary block, 5–10 ml is injected above the perivascular sheath, into coracobrachialis muscle.
  - elbow: 10 ml is injected in the groove between biceps tendon and brachioradialis in the **antecubital fossa**, and infiltrated subcutaneously around the lateral elbow.
- the intercostobrachial nerve, supplying the inner upper arm, may be blocked by superficial infiltration as the needle is withdrawn from the axillary block.
- fascial sheets within the neurovascular sheath may cause a 'patchy' block. Puncture both above and below the artery has been suggested as a remedy. Alternatively, separate identification of the different nerves with a nerve stimulator has been advocated (median: causes contraction of flexor carpi radialis; ulnar: flexor carpi ulnaris; radial: extensor muscles of hand/wrist; musculocutaneous: biceps), with the total dose divided between them. Intentional transfixion of the artery has also been described: blood is aspirated as the needle is advanced through the artery; when aspiration ceases, solution is deposited posterior to the artery.

▸ infraclavicular:
- with the patient's arm abducted, a needle is inserted 2–3 cm caudal to the midpoint of a line drawn between the medial head of the clavicle and the coracoid process. The needle is advanced laterally parallel to this line and at 45 degrees to the skin until twitches are seen in the hand (pectoral contraction indicates superficial placement of the needle, and biceps contraction may be achieved by stimulating the musculocutaneous nerve outside the plexus sheath). Has also been described with the needle directed directly posteriorly at a point 1 cm medial and 2 cm caudal to the coracoid process.
- 30–45 ml solution is injected.

▸ posterior:
- with the patient sitting or lying, and the cervical spine flexed, a needle is inserted 3 cm from the midline level with the C6–7 interspace. A loss of resistance technique or nerve stimulation has been described, with injection of 20–40 ml solution at a depth of 5–7 cm. Horner's syndrome is common; difficulty breathing may also occur and epidural and spinal blockade have been reported.

- Suitable solutions:
  ▸ **prilocaine** or **lidocaine** 1%–1.5% with adrenaline: onset within 20–30 min and lasts for 1.5–2 h.
  ▸ **bupivacaine** 0.375%–0.5%: onset up to 1 h, lasts for up to 12 h. Combination with 1% lidocaine speeds onset.

The area blocked is increased by using larger volumes of solution. Motor block is increased by increasing concentration, and intensity of block by increasing total dose. Although maximal safe doses have been exceeded without serious effects or high blood levels of agent, this cannot be recommended routinely. Systemic uptake of agent is greatest following interscalene block, and least following axillary block. Incidence of neurological damage is thought to be reduced by using short bevelled needles, and using ultrasound guidance or a nerve stimulator rather than eliciting paraesthesia as the end-point for localisation.
See also, Regional anaesthesia

Bradycardia, *see Heart block; Junctional arrhythmias; Sinus bradycardia*

Bradykinin, *see Kinins*

Brain. Intracranial part of the CNS. Forms from tubular neural tissue, developing into hindbrain (rhombencephalon), midbrain (mesencephalon) and forebrain (prosencephalon):

▸ hindbrain:
- medulla: continuous with the **spinal cord**. Communicates with the cerebellum via the inferior cerebellar peduncle. Forms the posterior part of the fourth ventricle floor. Contains the decussation of pyramidal tracts, gracile and cuneate nuclei, nuclei of **cranial nerves** IX, X, XI and XII, and 'vital centres', e.g. for respiration and cardiovascular homeostasis.
- pons: communicates with the cerebellum via the middle cerebellar peduncle. Forms the anterior part of the fourth ventricle floor. Contains the nuclei of cranial nerves V, VI, VII and VIII, and pontine nuclei. Also houses the apneustic and pneumotaxic centres of breathing control.
- cerebellum: occupies the posterior cranial fossa. Consists of grey cortex covering white matter. Communicates via the medulla, pons and midbrain with the thalamus, cerebral cortex and spinal cord. Regulates posture, coordination and muscle tone. Lesions cause ipsilateral effects.

- midbrain: communicates with the cerebellum via the superior cerebellar peduncle. Contains the pineal body and cranial nerve nuclei III and IV.
- forebrain:
  - diencephalon: consists of the **hypothalamus** (forming the floor of the lateral wall of the third ventricle) with the **pituitary gland** below, and thalamus (lateral to the third ventricle). The thalamus integrates sensory pathways.
  - basal ganglia: grey matter within cerebral hemispheres. The internal capsule, containing the major ascending and descending pathways to and from the cerebral cortex, passes between the basal ganglia. They receive and relay information concerned with fine motor control.
  - cerebral cortex:
    - frontal lobes: contain motor cortices, including areas for speech and eye movement; areas for intellectual and emotional functions lie anteriorly.
    - parietal lobes: contain sensory cortices, and areas for association and integration of sensory input.
    - temporal lobes: contain auditory cortices, and areas for integration and association of auditory input and memory. Also constitutes part of the **limbic system**, which integrates endocrine, autonomic and motivational functions.
    - occipital lobes: contain the visual cortices, and areas for association and integration of visual sensory input.

See also, Ascending reticular activating system; Brainstem; Cerebral circulation; Cerebrospinal fluid; Motor pathways; Sensory pathways

Brainstem. Composed of midbrain, pons and medulla. Contains neurone groups involved in the control of breathing, cardiovascular homeostasis, GIT function, balance and equilibrium, and eye movement. Also integrates ascending and descending pathways between the **spinal cord**, **cranial nerves**, cerebellum and higher centres, partly via the **ascending reticular activating system**.

See also, Brain; Brainstem death; Breathing, control of

Brainstem death. Irreversible absence of **brainstem** function despite artificial maintenance of circulation and gas exchange. Clinical experience has shown that, once it is diagnosed, cardiac arrest is inevitable, usually within a few days. Diagnosis of brainstem death allows treatment to be legitimately withdrawn and enables the process of **organ donation** to be considered.

- UK guidelines include:
  - necessary preconditions before testing can be considered:
    - comatose patient dependent on mechanical ventilation.
    - irreversible brain damage of known aetiology (e.g. **subarachnoid haemorrhage**, **TBI**, **meningitis**).
  - exclusion of reversible causes of coma and apnoea:
    - absence of sedative drugs: can be difficult to determine whether levels of sedative drugs (e.g. **thiopental**) are appropriately low, especially with altered pharmacokinetics and renal function in critically ill patients. Serum levels may help.
    - absence of paralysis caused by neuromuscular blocking drugs (**neuromuscular blockade monitoring** is useful) or neuromuscular disorders (e.g. **Guillain–Barré syndrome**).
    - absence of primary **hypothermia**, i.e., core temperature >34°C (N.B. secondary hypothermia often follows brainstem death but temperatures of 32°–34°C are rarely associated with decreased levels of consciousness).
    - absence of severe electrolyte/glucose abnormalities: it is important to distinguish between primary electrolyte abnormalities and those secondary to brain injury (e.g. as a result of **diabetes insipidus**). UK guidelines recommend that plasma sodium is 115–160 mmol/l during testing. Blood glucose should be 3–20 mmol/l.
    - absence of primary endocrine disturbance (N.B. secondary endocrine abnormalities often follow brainstem death, e.g. **hypothyroidism**, hypoprolactinaemia).
  - necessary clinical findings:
    - absent **cranial nerve** reflexes:
      - pupillary light reflex (II and III).
      - corneal reflex (V and VII).
      - oculovestibular reflex (VIII), i.e., no eye movement following injection of 40–60 ml icy water into the ear canal (normal response is a tonic deviation of the eyes towards the side being irrigated followed by a faster phase back towards the midline). Each ear is tested in turn, having checked that the canal is not blocked. (In the UK, testing for **doll's eye movements** is not used as a component of brainstem testing.)
      - gag reflex (IX and X).
      - cough reflex (X).
    - absent motor responses following painful stimulus applied within the cranial nerve distribution (corticospinal tract runs through the brainstem). Painful stimuli applied to the periphery may cause limb movement due to spinal reflexes.
    - absent respiratory efforts despite arterial $P\text{CO}_2$ of 6.6 kPa (50 mmHg), and adequate oxygenation (e.g. with **apnoeic oxygenation**). Must be confirmed using blood gas analysis.

All of these requirements must be met for the diagnosis of brainstem death to be made. Two sets of tests should be performed by two doctors (registered for 5 years) who have skill in the field, one of whom is a consultant, neither of whom should be part of the organ donation team. There is no evidence that two tests are necessary, but this has been stipulated in all UK guidelines.

The tests may be carried out together or separately. No specific time interval has been recommended between testing. Although **EEG**, cerebral angiography and **oesophageal contractility** testing are performed in some countries, they are not required to make the diagnosis of brainstem death in the UK. The legal time of death is recorded as the time the first set of tests shows no activity.

Although the clinical criteria remain unchanged for paediatric patients, the interval between the two tests differs. No UK recommendations exist; therefore the US ones are usually followed for children of different ages:

- newborn to 2 months (usually performed for medicolegal reasons): interval 48 h.
- 2–12 months: 24 h.
- 1–18 years: 12 h.

Vegetative state associated with absent cortical function or cortical disconnection may occur with intact brainstem

reflexes. Such patients may have spontaneous respiration and may live for years without recovery, and do not satisfy the criteria for brainstem death.
Smith M (2015). Semin Neurol; 35: 145–51

Braun, Heinrich Friedrich Wilhelm (1862–1934). German surgeon who also practised and investigated anaesthesia. One of the pioneers of local anaesthesia, he described many local blocks, and published extensively on the subject. Introduced **adrenaline** to local anaesthetic solutions to prolong their action in 1902 and in 1903 suggested its possible use in resuscitation. Popularised **procaine** in 1905.

Breathing, control of. Control of breathing is under automatic and voluntary control. The exact origin of the signal for automatic breathing is unknown but three **brainstem** centres involved in the control of breathing have been identified:
- medullary centre:
  - dorsal respiratory group neurones arising from the nucleus tractus solitarius are involved in inspiration; when stimulated, they cause diaphragmatic contraction via contralateral phrenic nerves; they also project to ventral neurones.
  - ventral respiratory group neurones arising from the nucleus ambiguus are predominantly involved in expiration, causing contraction of ipsilateral accessory muscles (via vagus nerves) and intercostal muscles. They also inhibit the apneustic centre.
- apneustic centre in the lower pons: causes excitation of medullary dorsal respiratory group neurones causing inspiration while inhibiting ventral respiratory group neurones. Surgical section above it causes prolonged pauses at end-inspiration.
- pneumotaxic centre (nucleus parabrachialis) in the upper pons: curtails inspiration and thus regulates respiratory rate.

The 'respiratory centre' composed of these groups of neurones receives afferents from **chemoreceptors** and other structures:
- chemoreceptors:
  - peripheral (**aortic** and **carotid bodies**): afferents pass via the vagus and glossopharyngeal nerves, respectively. Stimulated by a rise in $P\text{CO}_2$, hydrogen ion concentration and a fall in $P\text{O}_2$. The rise in minute ventilation with increases in $P\text{CO}_2$ is roughly linear (Fig. 27, *solid line*). Volatile anaesthetic agents and opioid drugs decrease the ventilator response to **hypercapnia** in a dose-related manner (Fig. 27, *dotted line*). Minute ventilation remains at normal levels until $P\text{O}_2$ falls to <8 kPa, after which it increases markedly. If hypercapnia is accompanied by **hypoxaemia**, minute ventilation increases further (Fig. 28).
  - central: present on the ventral surface of the medulla, but separate from the respiratory centre. Stimulated by a rise in hydrogen ion concentration in CSF, due to increased $P\text{CO}_2$ or metabolic acidosis.

  Hypoxaemia causes direct depression of the respiratory centres, in addition to reflex stimulation. In chronic lung disease, the central chemoreceptors may not respond to increased CO_2 levels, either due to chemoreceptor 'resetting' or due to correction of CSF pH. Hypoxaemia then becomes the main drive to respiration (of importance in **O_2 therapy**).

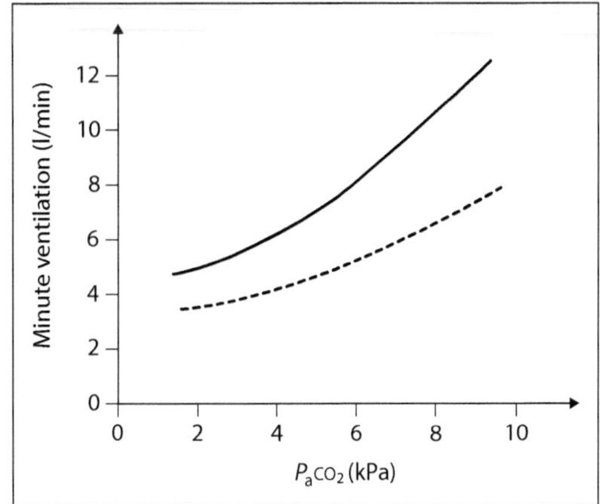

Fig. 27 CO_2 response curve (*see text*)

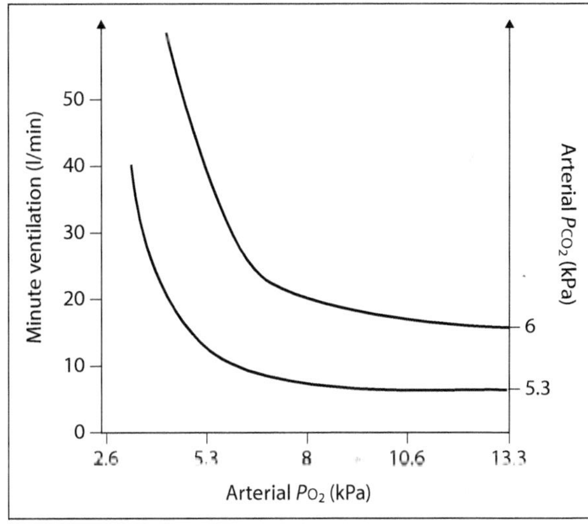

Fig. 28 Ventilatory response to hypoxaemia

- other structures:
  - lungs:
    - **pulmonary stretch receptors**, involved in the **Hering–Breuer** and **deflation reflexes**.
    - **juxtapulmonary capillary receptors**, involved in dyspnoea due to pulmonary disease and pulmonary oedema.
    - **pulmonary irritant receptors**, responding to noxious stimuli.
  - proprioceptors in joints and muscles, thought to be important during exercise.
  - **baroreceptors**; hypertension inhibits ventilation, but this is of little clinical significance.

Voluntary control of breathing comes from the cerebral cortex via the corticospinal tract to the respiratory muscles. In addition, the hyperventilation caused by emotion is generated by the **limbic system**.

During anaesthesia, the responses to hypercapnia and hypoxaemia are depressed, the latter severely.
See also, Hypoventilation

Breathing, muscles of, *see Respiratory muscles*

Breathing systems, *see Anaesthetic breathing systems*

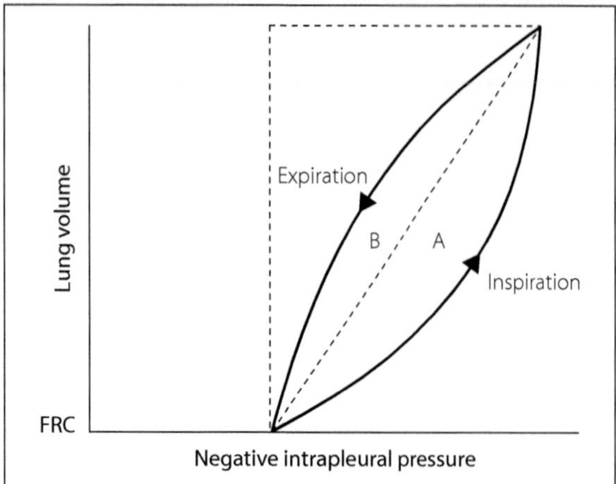

Fig. 29 Graph of intrapleural pressure against lung volume during breathing (see text)

Breathing, work of. Equals the product of pressure change across the lung and volume of gas moved. During inspiration, most of the work of breathing is done to overcome elastic recoil of the thorax and lungs, and the resistance of the airways and non-elastic tissues (Fig. 29):
- the area enclosed by the broken line represents work done to overcome elastic forces.
- area A represents work done to overcome resistance during inspiration.
- area B represents work done to overcome resistance during expiration.

The greater the tidal volume or lung volume, the more work is required to overcome elastic recoil. The faster the flow rates, the greater the amount of work required to overcome resistance. Normally, energy is provided for expiration by potential energy stored in the stretched elastic tissues (i.e., area B lies within the broken line), but extra energy may be required in **airway obstruction**.

Total work of breathing is difficult to measure in spontaneous respiration. Volume may be measured with a **pneumotachograph**; oesophageal pressure, indicating **intrapleural pressure**, may be measured with an oesophageal balloon. Normally, the work of breathing accounts for <3% of the total body O_2 consumption at rest, but may be much higher in disease states, e.g. **COPD**, **cardiac failure** and during exercise.

Expiratory valves in anaesthetic breathing systems increase work of expiration, particularly when not fully open. **Coaxial anaesthetic breathing systems** increase expiratory resistance, the Lack by virtue of its small-calibre expiratory tube, and the Bain because of the high flow rate of fresh gas directed at the patient's mouth.
Grinnan DC, Truwit C (2005). Crit Care; 9: 472–84
See also, Airway resistance; Compliance

Bretylium tosylate. Class II and III **antiarrhythmic drug**, originally introduced as an **antihypertensive drug**. Reduces sympathetic drive to the heart and prolongs the **action potential**; was reserved for treatment of resistant ventricular arrhythmias, but discontinued in 2011 because of supply problems.

Brewer–Luckhardt reflex. Laryngospasm in response to remote stimulation, e.g. anal or cervical dilatation.
[Nathan R Brewer (1904–2009) and Arno B Luckhardt (1885–1957), US physiologists]

Table 15 Bromage scale for motor block

1	Complete	Unable to move legs or feet
2	Almost complete	Able to move feet only
3	Partial	Just able to flex knees only
4	None	Full movement of legs and feet

British Association for Immediate Care (BASICS). Voluntary charitable organisation, formed in 1977, whose members provide medical assistance at the scene of an accident or medical emergency or during primary transport to hospital. Acts as the national coordinating body for schemes and individual doctors providing immediate care throughout the UK. Organises educational courses for doctors, nurses, paramedics, occupational health professionals, the emergency services and those involved in healthcare at sporting and other events.

British Association of Critical Care Nurses (BACCN). Formed in 1984 from the amalgamation of various groups of UK critical care nurses. Exists to support personal and professional development of members (who include nurses, managers, educationalists, researchers and others with an interest in critical care) and to promote the art and science of critical care nursing. Its official journal is *Nursing in Critical Care.*

***British Journal of Anaesthesia*.** Second oldest journal of anaesthesia (first published in 1923), and the first to be published monthly (in 1955). Previously unaffiliated with any association, institution or society, it became the official journal of the **College of Anaesthetists** in 1990.
Spence AA (1988). Br J Anaesth; 60: 605–7

Bromage scale. Scoring system used to assess the degree of motor block, originally described in the context of **epidural anaesthesia** for surgery. Consists of four grades (Table 15). Various modifications have been described, and the term 'Bromage scale/score' is often incorrectly applied to them, and to scales in which a decreasing score indicates decreasing block instead of decreasing motor power, as in the original description.
[Philip Bromage (1920–2013), English-born Canadian/US anaesthetist]

Bromethol (Tribromoethanol; Avertin). CBr_3CH_2OH. Obsolete rectal and iv sedative drug introduced in 1927 and used for deep sedation or anaesthesia.

Bronchial blockers, *see Endobronchial blockers*

Bronchial carcinoma. Commonest cause of death from cancer in Western men and women. Mostly associated with **smoking**, but also occurs following exposure to asbestos, and certain industrial chemical and radioactive substances. Air pollution may also be a causative factor. Five-year survival in the UK is 8%; in the USA and certain parts of Europe it is ~15%.
- Types:
  - small cell (~20%): may arise from APUD cells (*see Apudomas*), and secrete hormones. Extensive

spread is usual at presentation. Extremely poor prognosis.
- non–small cell:
  - adenocarcinoma (~40%).
  - squamous cell (~30%): most present with bronchial obstruction. Better prognosis than the other common forms.
  - large cell (~10%); particularly related to smoking.
  - others:
    - bronchiolar alveolar, carcinoid: least related to smoking.
    - carcinoma in situ.
- Features:
  - local:
    - haemoptysis, cough, dyspnoea.
    - wheeze, stridor, chest discomfort.
    - **chest infection**, **pleural effusion**.
  - invasion of:
    - mediastinum, chest wall. May cause **superior vena caval obstruction**, dysphagia, cardiac **arrhythmias**, pericardial effusion.
    - vertebrae.
    - recurrent laryngeal nerve, usually on the left.
    - sympathetic trunk at C8/T1, causing **Horner's syndrome**.
    - **brachial plexus** at lung apex, causing pain and wasting in the hand/arm (with Horner's syndrome, ± rib or vertebral erosion, ± superior vena caval obstruction, = Pancoast syndrome).
  - metastases: commonly lymph nodes, bone, liver, brain.
  - other features:
    - fatigue, anorexia, weight loss, anaemia.
    - hormone secretion, e.g. causing the **syndrome of inappropriate antidiuretic hormone secretion**, **Cushing's syndrome**, **hypercalcaemia** due to parathyroid hormone secretion, **carcinoid syndrome**. Most common with small cell tumours. Thyroid and sex hormone secretion may occur.
    - sensory or motor neuropathy; cerebellar atrophy.
    - **myasthenic syndrome**, muscle weakness, dermatomyositis.
    - finger clubbing and hypertrophic pulmonary osteoarthropathy.

May present for **bronchoscopy**, mediastinoscopy or **thoracic surgery**. Anaesthetic considerations are related to the earlier features, effects of smoking and **malignancy**; thus **preoperative assessment** of respiratory, cardiovascular and neurological systems, and hormonal and metabolic status, is particularly important.

Radiotherapy is used mainly for palliative treatment of pain and obstructive lesions (e.g. **superior vena caval obstruction**), especially due to small cell carcinoma. Chemotherapy is also used, particularly in small cell carcinoma. Immunotherapy is a promising avenue undergoing trials.

[Henry Pancoast (1875–1939), US radiologist]

Sculier JP, Berghmans T, Meert AP (2010). Am J Respir Crit Care Med; 181: 773–81

See also, Polymyositis

Bronchial tree, *see Tracheobronchial tree*

Bronchiectasis. Permanent abnormal bronchial dilatation, usually suppurative. May follow pneumonia, bronchial obstruction, chronic repeated chest infections, e.g. in **cystic fibrosis** and immunological impairment.
- Features:
  - haemoptysis.
  - chronic cough with purulent sputum.
  - chronic respiratory insufficiency, of restrictive and/or obstructive pattern.
  - empyema, abscesses, **cor pulmonale**, clubbing.
  - **CXR**: increased lung markings, patchy shadowing, thick-walled dilated bronchi.

Treatment includes antibiotic therapy, **physiotherapy** and postural drainage, and lung resection if disease is localised.
- Anaesthetic management:
  - preoperatively:
    - early admission for **preoperative assessment**, medical treatment and physiotherapy.
    - CXR, arterial **blood gas interpretation**, **lung function tests** as appropriate.
  - perioperatively: soiling of the unaffected lung is reduced by appropriate positioning. Double-lumen **endobronchial tubes** may assist surgery and allow isolation and suction of copious secretions.
  - postoperatively: adequate analgesia and physiotherapy to reduce risk of respiratory complications.

McShane PJ, Naureckas ET, Tino G, et al (2013). Am J Resp Crit Care Med; 188: 647–56

Bronchiolitis. Inflammation of the bronchioles; usually refers to acute infection in children but may also occur chronically in early **COPD** in adults. In children, respiratory syncytial virus (RSV) accounts for 70% of cases, but many other viruses may also be responsible. Usually affects children under 1 year old, causing non-specific upper respiratory tract symptoms that may progress over 1–2 days to respiratory distress with diffuse crackles ± persistent wheezing. **Hypoxaemia** results from **hypoventilation** and **$\dot{V}/\dot{Q}$ mismatch**. May be associated with apnoea, especially in premature babies. Treatment is supportive, including humidified **O_2 therapy**, fluid replacement and occasionally **IPPV**. **β-adrenergic receptor agonists** and **corticosteroids** are no longer advocated. Palivizumab, a monoclonal antibody directed against RSV, is licensed for use in susceptible infants.

Usually self-limiting, lasting under 10 days; mortality in infants admitted to hospital is about 1% if previously fit. Has been implicated in the development of subsequent **asthma**.

Meissner HC (2016). N Engl J Med; 374: 62–72

See also, Tracheobronchial tree

Bronchoalveolar lavage (BAL). Performed for pulmonary alveolar proteinosis, to remove accumulated lipoproteinaceous material. Has also been used in **asthma** and **cystic fibrosis**. Usually performed under general anaesthesia, and involves instillation and drainage under gravity of 20–40 litres warm buffered saline (**heparin** may be added) through one lumen of a double-lumen **endobronchial tube**, while ventilating via the other. The other lung is treated after a few days. Main problems are related to the pre-existing state of the patient, **one-lung anaesthesia** and avoidance of soiling of the ventilated lung. **Cardiopulmonary bypass** has also been used.

Lavage using small volumes is sometimes used to aid diagnosis of atypical chest infections, and may be carried out via flexible **bronchoscopy** under local anaesthesia.

Bronchodilator drugs. Drugs that increase bronchial diameter.

- Postulated mechanisms of action:
  - **β_2-adrenergic receptor agonists**, e.g. **salbutamol**:
    - inhibit degranulation of **mast cells.**
    - stimulate adenylate cyclase in smooth muscle cells, increasing **cAMP** levels and thus causing reduced intracellular **calcium** and relaxation.
  - **phosphodiesterase inhibitors**, e.g. **theophylline, aminophylline**:
    - inhibit the breakdown of cAMP in smooth muscle cells.
    - possible effect via release of **catecholamines** via **adenosine** inhibition.
    - possible effect on **myosin** light chains, reducing contraction.
  - **anticholinergic drugs**, e.g. **ipratropium**:
    - block muscarinic **acetylcholine receptors**, decreasing intracellular guanine monophosphate (cGMP; opposes the bronchodilating action of cAMP).
    - possible effect via reduction in intracellular calcium.
  - **corticosteroids**:
    - anti-inflammatory action.
    - reduced capillary permeability.
    - possibly increase the effects of β-adrenergic receptor agonists.

Sodium cromoglicate and **leukotriene receptor antagonists** are not bronchodilators, but help to prevent bronchoconstriction by reducing inflammation.

See also, Asthma; Bronchospasm

Bronchopleural fistula. Abnormal connection between the **tracheobronchial tree** and **pleura**. Most commonly occurs 2–10 days after pneumonectomy, although it may follow trauma, chronic infection and erosion by tumour.

- Features:
  - fever, productive cough, malaise.
  - x-ray evidence of infection in the remaining lung with fall in fluid level on the affected side.
- Problems caused:
  - source of (usually) infected material in one pleural cavity, with potential contamination of the normal lung through the fistula. Repeated spillage may cause pulmonary function impairment before corrective surgery.
  - IPPV may force fresh gas through the fistula, without inflating the remaining lung. Increased pressure in the affected pleura increases the likelihood of contamination, and may impair cardiac output.
- Management:
  - **chest drainage**.
  - sitting the patient up, with affected side lowermost.
  - classical method for induction of anaesthesia: inhalational induction and intubation with a double-lumen **endobronchial tube**, with spontaneous ventilation. IPPV may be started once the affected side has been isolated. However, deep anaesthesia with volatile agents may cause profound cardiovascular effects, and coughing may increase contamination risk. Alternatives include awake intubation under local anaesthesia, or preoxygenation, iv induction and intubation using **suxamethonium** or **rocuronium**.
  - postoperatively, IPPV may be necessary. **High-frequency ventilation** and **differential lung ventilation** have been used.

See also, Thoracic surgery

Bronchopulmonary lavage, *see Bronchoalveolar lavage*

Bronchoscopy. Inspection of the **tracheobronchial tree** by passing an instrument down its lumen. May be:

- rigid: usually performed in the operating theatre for diagnosis of bronchial disease, removal of foreign bodies and management of haemoptysis. Anaesthetic management:
  - preoperatively:
    - **preoperative assessment** is directed at the respiratory and cardiovascular systems. Many patients will have **bronchial carcinoma** or other **smoking**-related diseases. Secretions may be improved by preoperative **physiotherapy.** Neck mobility and the **teeth** should be assessed.
    - **premedication** reduces **awareness**. The antisialagogue effects of **anticholinergic drugs** may be useful.
  - perioperatively:
    - in the absence of a foreign body in the airway, iv **induction of anaesthesia** is usual. Inhalational induction may be indicated if **airway obstruction** is present, particularly in children. Neuromuscular blockade is usually achieved with a short-acting **neuromuscular blocking drug.**
    - spraying of the larynx with **lidocaine** may reduce perioperative and postoperative coughing and **laryngospasm.**
    - ventilation: several methods may be used:
      - **injector techniques**; air entrainment through the bronchoscope using intermittent jets of O_2. Automatic jet ventilators have been used for long procedures.
      - **IPPV** via a side arm on the bronchoscope, the proximal end of which is occluded by a window or the operator's thumb.
      - deep anaesthesia with spontaneous ventilation. Often used in children, classically using **diethyl ether**, then **halothane**, but now **sevoflurane.** Anaesthetic gases may be delivered via a side arm on the bronchoscope; before these 'ventilating bronchoscopes' became available, the patient breathed air and bronchoscopy was performed as anaesthesia lightened (a possible disadvantage of sevoflurane being that anaesthesia might lighten too quickly).
      - **insufflation techniques**, particularly **apnoeic oxygenation**. Suitable for short procedures only.
      - intermittent IPPV via a tracheal tube placed in the proximal end of the bronchoscope.
      - **high-frequency ventilation** has been used.
    - **monitoring** as standard.
    - **TIVA** is frequently used, typically **propofol** with **remifentanil.**
    - **recovery** should be in the lateral, head-down position, to encourage drainage of blood and secretions.
- fibreoptic: commonly performed for diagnostic purposes under local anaesthesia as for awake intubation, but also used by anaesthetists and intensivists during general anaesthesia and on the ICU. Uses:
  - airway management:
    - **tracheal intubation** in airway obstruction. Also useful for changing tracheal tubes.

    - confirmation of correct placement of tracheal/**tracheostomy/endobronchial tubes.** Also used in **percutaneous tracheostomy**.
    - assessment of the tracheobronchial tree before **extubation**. In cases of potential post-extubation airway obstruction (e.g. caused by oedema) the fibreoptic bronchoscope can be left in situ while the tracheal tube is removed and the airway assessed; the tube may be resited over the bronchoscope if required.
  - diagnostic:
    - **chest infection**, especially atypical. Washings, brushings or transbronchial/endobronchial biopsies or needle aspiration may be used. Repeated instillation of 20 ml sterile saline with subsequent aspiration (**bronchoalveolar lavage**) may be useful in both infective and non-infective processes.
    - other lesions, e.g. tumours, tears, thermal damage. May be used to investigate abnormalities on **CXR**.
  - therapeutic:
    - aspiration of sputum and aspirated material. **Mucolytic drugs** can be instilled onto mucus plugs. Bronchoalveolar lavage has been used in severe asthma.
    - removal of foreign body.
    - for haemoptysis; saline lavage may be useful for small areas of bleeding; the bronchoscope itself can be used to compress bleeding points; or it may facilitate passage of a balloon-tipped catheter into the affected segment.
- Management for bronchoscopy in the ICU:
  - coagulation studies should be performed if biopsies are planned. Electrolyte imbalance should be corrected.
  - secretions may be improved by physiotherapy. Anticholinergic drugs may reduce secretions but may also make them thick and difficult to aspirate.
  - awake patients may be managed under local anaesthesia as for awake intubation. In those with tracheal tubes, the bronchoscope may be passed through a rubber-sealed connector at the tube's proximal end and IPPV continued. Leaks may occur around the scope, especially if airway pressures are high; a swab coated in lubricant jelly wrapped around the leak may improve the seal. 5.0-mm diameter bronchoscopes require an 8.0-mm tracheal tube to ensure adequate gas flow around the bronchoscope. Passage of the bronchoscope alongside the tracheal tube has also been used, as has high-frequency ventilation.
  - increased **sedation** and neuromuscular blockade are usually required in ventilated patients.
  - **hypoxaemia** may worsen during bronchoscopy; 100% O_2 is usually administered. Severe hypoxaemia is usually considered a contraindication.
  - **arrhythmias, hypertension**, coughing, **bronchospasm** or laryngospasm may occur during and after stimulation of the tracheobronchial tree. Topical lidocaine may reduce airway irritation. Bleeding and **pneumothorax** may also occur.

Pawlowski J (2013). Curr Opin Anaesthesiol; 26: 6–12
See also, Foreign body, inhaled; Intubation, awake

Bronchospasm. May occur during anaesthesia due to:
  - surgical stimulation.
  - presence of airway adjunct or tracheal tube.
  - pharyngeal/laryngeal/bronchial secretions or blood.
  - **aspiration of gastric contents.**
  - **anaphylaxis.**
  - **pulmonary oedema.**
  - use of **β-adrenergic receptor antagonists.**

Particularly likely in smokers or in patients with **asthma** or **COPD**, and if anaesthesia is inadequate.
- Features:
  - polyphonic expiratory wheeze.
  - reduced movement of reservoir bag.
  - increased expiratory time.
  - increased airway pressures.
- Must be distinguished from:
  - **pneumothorax.**
  - mechanical obstruction.
  - **laryngospasm.**
  - pulmonary oedema.
- Treatment:
  - of primary cause.
  - increased F_IO_2.
  - increased inspired concentration of volatile **inhalational anaesthetic agent.**
  - **salbutamol** 250–500 µg sc/im or 250 µg iv slowly. Delivery by nebuliser or aerosol may also be used but may be technically difficult.
  - **aminophylline** 3–6 mg/kg iv slowly, followed by 0.5 mg/kg/h infusion.
  - further management as for asthma.

Brown fat. Specialised adipose tissue used for thermogenesis because of its chemical make-up and structural composition. Of particular importance in **temperature regulation in neonates.** Laid down from about 22 weeks of gestation around the base of the neck, axillae, mediastinum and between the scapulae; gradually replaced by adult 'white' adipose tissue after birth, the process taking several years. Fat breakdown and thermogenesis are increased by α-adrenergic neurone activity.
Enerbäck S (2009). N Engl J Med; 360: 2021–3

BTPS. Body temperature and pressure, saturated with water vapour.

Buccal nerve block, *see Mandibular nerve blocks*

Buffer base. Blood anions that can act as **bases** and accept **hydrogen ions.** Mainly composed of **bicarbonate, haemoglobin** and negatively charged proteins.
See also, Acid–base balance; Buffers

Buffers. Substances that resist a change in **pH** by absorbing or releasing **hydrogen ions** when **acid** or **base** is added to the solution. In aqueous solutions this comprises either a weak acid and its conjugate base (*see later*), or a weak base and its conjugate acid.

For the equation $HA \rightleftharpoons H^+ + A^-$, where HA = undissociated acid and A^- = anion, the equation shifts to the left if acid is added, and to the right if base is added; changes in H^+ concentration are thus minimised.

The **Henderson–Hasselbalch equation** describes these relationships:

$$pH = pK + \log\frac{[A^-]}{HA}$$

When pH equals pK of the buffer system, maximal buffering may occur, because HA and A^- exist in equal amounts.

- Body buffer systems:
  - blood:
    - carbonic acid/**bicarbonate**: $H_2CO_3 \rightleftharpoons H^+ + HCO_3^-$. The p*K* is 6.1; i.e., the system is not very efficient at buffering alkaline at body pH (although it is quite efficient at buffering acid, efficiency increasing as pH falls). However, because there is a large reservoir of plasma bicarbonate, and CO_2 may be readily eliminated via the lungs and bicarbonate excretion can be regulated via the kidneys, this system constitutes the main buffer system in the blood.
    - **haemoglobin**: dissociation of histidine residues gives haemoglobin six times the buffering capacity of plasma proteins. Deoxygenated haemoglobin is a better buffer than oxygenated haemoglobin (**Haldane effect**).
    - plasma proteins: carboxyl and amino groups dissociate to form anions; this accounts for a small amount of buffering capacity.
    - phosphate: $H_2PO_4 \rightleftharpoons H^+ + HPO_4^{2-}$. Plays a small part in buffering in the ECF.
  - intracellular:
    - proteins.
    - phosphate.

See also, Acid–base balance

Bumetanide. Loop **diuretic**, like **furosemide** in its actions. 1 mg is approximately equivalent to 40 mg furosemide. Diuresis begins within minutes of an iv dose and lasts for 2 h.
- Dosage:
  - 1–5 mg orally od–tds.
  - 1–2 mg iv, repeated after 20 min if required. May also be given by infusion at 1–5 mg/h.
- Side effects: as for furosemide; myalgia may also occur, especially with high doses.

BUN, *see Blood urea nitrogen*

Bundle branch block (BBB). Interruption of impulse propagation in the **heart conducting system** distal to the atrioventricular node. Causes are as for **heart block.**
- May involve right or left bundles:
  - right BBB:
    - common; usually clinically insignificant.
    - **ECG** findings (Fig. 30a):
      - QRS duration >0.12 s.
      - large S wave, lead I.
      - RSR pattern, lead V_1.
    - incomplete BBB may be due to an enlarged right ventricle, e.g. due to **cor pulmonale** or **ASD.**
  - left BBB:
    - represents more widespread disease, as the left bundle is a bigger and less discrete structure, consisting of anterior and posterior fascicles. If present preoperatively, it serves as an indicator of existing heart disease.
    - ECG findings (Fig. 30b):
      - QRS duration >0.12 s.
      - wide R waves, leads I and V_{4-6}.
      - may be due to left ventricular hypertrophy, e.g. due to hypertension or valvular heart disease.
  - hemiblock (involving individual fascicles of the left bundle):
    - left anterior hemiblock:
      - QRS may be normal or slightly widened.
      - left axis deviation >60 degrees.

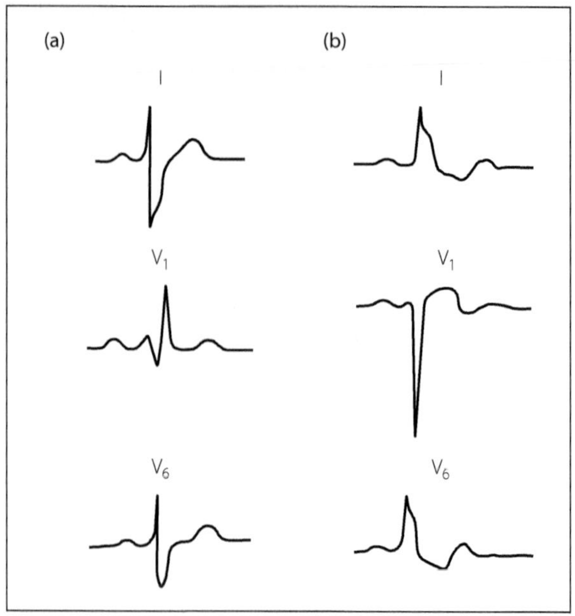

Fig. 30 ECG findings in bundle branch block: (a) right BBB; (b) left BBB

    - left posterior hemiblock:
      - less common, because the posterior fascicle is better perfused than the anterior.
      - QRS normal or slightly widened.
      - right axis deviation >120 degrees.
  - bifascicular block:
    - composed of right BBB and one hemiblock:
      - anterior:
        - right BBB ECG pattern and left axis deviation.
        - may lead to complete heart block later in life, but this is rare during anaesthesia.
      - posterior:
        - right BBB ECG pattern and right axis deviation.
        - rare.
        - at risk of developing complete heart block.
    - bifascicular block plus prolonged P–R interval (i.e., partial trifascicular block) is particularly likely to progress to complete heart block.

BBB itself is not a contraindication to anaesthesia, but progression to complete heart block during anaesthesia remains the main risk. Temporary perioperative **cardiac pacing** should be considered if BBB is associated with either a history of syncope or a prolonged P–R interval. Anaesthetic management is as for heart block.

Bungarotoxins. Snake venom neurotoxins. α-Bungarotoxin binds irreversibly to postsynaptic **acetylcholine receptors** at the **neuromuscular junction**; β-bungarotoxin acts presynaptically to block acetylcholine release. They have been used to study **neuromuscular transmission.**

Bupivacaine hydrochloride. Amide **local anaesthetic agent**, introduced in 1963. Widely used for peripheral nerve/plexus blocks, **spinal** and **epidural anaesthesia.** In comparison with lidocaine, bupivacaine:
  - has a slower onset of action (pK_a 8.1).
  - is more potent (~6× more lipid-soluble); 0.5% bupivacaine is equivalent to 2% lidocaine.

- causes less vasodilatation; addition of **adrenaline** neither prolongs the effect nor restricts systemic absorption of bupivacaine.
- is extensively bound to tissue and plasma proteins (95%); thus has a longer duration of action (3–4 h for epidural block and up to 12 h for some nerve blocks, e.g. **brachial plexus**).
- is more cardiotoxic.

Mainly metabolised by the liver; a small amount is excreted unchanged in the urine. 0.25%–0.5% solutions are used for most purposes. 0.75% produces more prolonged motor block when given epidurally; this concentration is contraindicated in obstetric practice because of toxicity. Contraindicated for use in **IVRA** because of its cardiotoxicity. A hyperbaric 0.5% solution (with glucose 8%) spinal administration was introduced in 1982. Maximal safe dose: 2 mg/kg; toxic plasma levels: >2–4 μg/ml.

The original preparation of bupivacaine is a racemic mixture of *l*- and *d*-isomers. A preparation of the pure enantiomer *l*-bupivacaine (levobupivacaine) was developed in 1997 and is equivalent to the racemic mixture in terms of action and potency, while having reduced propensity to CVS and CNS toxicity. It is available in the same concentrations as the racemic preparation.

See also, Isomerism; individual blocks

Buprenorphine hydrochloride. **Opioid analgesic drug** derived from thebaine, with partial **agonist** properties. Synthesised in 1968. 0.4 mg is equivalent to 10 mg **morphine**; it has slower onset and its effects last longer (about 8 h). May be given iv or im (0.3–0.6 mg), or sublingually (0.2–0.4 mg) 6–8-hourly. Slow-release patches (5–70 μg/h) have been produced for severe chronic pain. Respiratory depression does occur, but reaches a plateau that cannot be exceeded by increasing the dose. Respiratory depression is not readily reversed by **naloxone** and may persist for up to 24 h after removal of patches. Carries a low risk of dependence and has been used in the treatment of drug addiction.

See also, Opioid receptors

Burns. Burned patients may suffer from:

- direct thermal injury to body and airway. Heat and steam injury may result in facial, tongue, epiglottis and laryngeal swelling that develops over a few hours and usually subsides over 3–6 days.
- **smoke inhalation**, with e.g. **carbon monoxide** (CO) or **cyanide** (CN) **poisoning**, the latter suggested by a large **anion gap** metabolic **acidosis**. Inhalation injury significantly increases morbidity and mortality.
- extensive loss of intravascular fluid (mainly plasma) into the dermis and blisters, and from skin surfaces. Burn areas >25% of total body surface area result in generalised oedema even in non-injured tissue. Fluid loss causes 'burn **shock**' that is worsened by the myocardial depression seen in severe burns. This phase lasts 24–72 h and is followed by a hypermetabolic phase characterised by increased cardiac output, tachycardia, decreased SVR and increased protein catabolism. These changes are exacerbated by coexisting **sepsis**.

Patients suffering from **electrocution and electrical burns** may have suffered widespread internal tissue injury, while those suffering from chemical burns may also have features of systemic toxicity/metabolic disturbance. General management of electrical and chemical burns is similar to that for thermal burns.

- Management:
  - high F_IO_2 O_2 therapy. Early tracheal intubation and IPPV are required in:
    - severe CO or CN poisoning. It has been suggested that CN poisoning should be assumed if there is unexplained severe metabolic acidosis, and treated accordingly.
    - apparent or impending upper **airway obstruction** due to inhalational injury. Obstruction due to oedema may develop over a few hours; tracheal intubation with an uncut tube should be performed early if burns to the airway are present. The latter may be indicated by burns or soot around the face and in the mouth, and are confirmed by fibreoptic bronchoscopy. Although obstruction usually resolves within 4–6 days, **tracheostomy** may be indicated if extensive laryngeal injury is present.
    - an unconscious patient.
    - **respiratory failure**.

    Measurement of blood gas tensions, carboxyhaemoglobin and possibly CN levels, should be performed. A CXR is mandatory.
  - assessment of the extent of burns (**rule of nines** is appropriate for adults; a paediatric burn chart is used for children). Burns are designated first, second or third degree depending on whether there is superficial, partial or full-thickness damage of the skin; fourth degree burns damage deeper structures e.g. muscle, bone.
  - fluid replacement: many different regimens exist, but most advocate isotonic **crystalloid** solutions initially followed by **colloid** solutions after 12–24 h. **Hartmann's solution** is favoured over 0.9% saline solution because of the risk of hyperchloraemic metabolic acidosis with the large volumes of fluid needed. Although prominent loss of plasma following burns tends to cause haemoconcentration, blood transfusion may be necessary at some stage. Average total requirements = water 2–4 ml/kg/% burn + sodium 0.5 mmol/kg/% burn. The most common UK regimen calculates the replacement volume (V) in ml:

    $$V = \frac{\text{body weight (kg)} \times \text{\%surface area burnt}}{2}$$

    $3 \times V$ is infused in the first 12 h from the time of burn;

    $2 \times V$ in the next 12 h;

    $1 \times V$ in the next 12 h.

    Frequent reassessment is crucial. Urine output should be maintained at 0.5–1 ml/kg/h with osmolality 600–1000 mosmol/kg (high due to high circulating levels of **vasopressin**). Low urine flow with high osmolality indicates under-replacement; high flow with low osmolality indicates overreplacement, in the absence of **renal failure**. The fluid regimen is altered as necessary.

    Oral rehydration is acceptable in burns of up to 10% (children) to 15% (adults). Oral rehydration fluid mixtures are suitable for children. For adults, water containing 75 mmol/l sodium chloride and 15 mmol/l sodium bicarbonate has been suggested, at 2–3 times normal water intake.
  - escharotomy (incision of contracted full-thickness burn that prevents ventilation or limb perfusion) may be necessary.

- monitoring of:
  - urine output (via catheter if >25% burn).
  - haematocrit and plasma electrolytes.
  - respiratory function.
  - **CVP**.
- analgesia: opioid infusions are often required.
- adequate **nutrition** (enteral if possible via a nasogastric or nasojejunal tube) to combat the hypercatabolic state. A high carbohydrate, high protein, low fat feed is advocated.
- prevention of **Curling ulcers**, e.g. with **H_2 receptor antagonists**.
- **tetanus** toxoid as necessary.
- consider transfer to a specialist burns unit if:
  - burn >10% total body surface area (adult) or >5% (child), or any full-thickness burn >5%.
  - burn to face, hands, genitalia, major joints.
  - significant inhalational injury.
  - <5 and >60 years of age (poorer prognosis).
  - circumferential burn to limbs or chest.
  - high-voltage electrical or chemical burn >5% total body surface area.

• Complications:
  - infection and sepsis.
  - respiratory failure and **ALI**.
  - renal failure, with **myoglobinuria** or haemoglobinuria. Suggested by low urine osmolarity and urine/blood urea ratio <10.

Mortality is related to the extent and site of burn, and age. Recent evidence suggests that area of burn >40%, age >60 years and the presence of inhalational injury are the three risk factors most strongly associated with death; absence of these risk factors is associated with 0.3% mortality; a single risk factor with 3% mortality, two risk factors with 33% mortality, and all three risk factors with 90% mortality.

• Anaesthetic considerations:
  - patients often require repeat anaesthetics, e.g. for change of dressings, plastic surgery.
  - difficult airway and/or intubation if burns exist around the head and neck, especially if contractures develop.
  - a life-threatening enhanced increase in plasma potassium may follow use of **suxamethonium**; cardiac arrest has been reported. Current recommendation is that suxamethonium should be avoided in patients >48 h after a burn injury.
  - increased requirement for non-depolarising **neuromuscular blocking drugs** occurring 3–7 days after the burn injury. The mechanism is unclear but may involve altered **pharmacokinetics**, e.g. changes in **protein-binding**, hepatic and renal **clearance**, **volume of distribution** and an upregulation of **acetylcholine receptors**.
  - limited venous access.
  - hypermetabolism/catabolism.
  - **heat loss** during prolonged surgery.
  - extensive blood loss is possible; e.g. during grafting procedures approximately 2% blood volume lost per 1% surface burn.
  - suggested techniques:
    - iv **opioid analgesic drugs**, traditionally combined with **butyrophenones** (**neuroleptanaesthesia**), though this is less common now.
    - inhalational analgesia with **Entonox** or volatile agents.
    - **ketamine** ± other iv agents, e.g. **midazolam**, **propofol**.
    - standard general anaesthesia.

Bittner EA, Shank E, Woodson L, Martyn JAJ (2015). Anesthesiology; 122: 448–64

Burns, during anaesthesia, *see Diathermy; Electrocution and electrical burns; Explosions and fires; Laser surgery*

BURP, Backward, upward and rightward pressure, *see Intubation, difficult*

Burst suppression, *see Electroencephalography*

Busulfan (Busulphan). Alkylating agent **cytotoxic drug**, given orally to treat chronic myeloid leukaemia. Causes myelosuppression that may be irreversible, and, rarely, **pulmonary fibrosis**. Thus, important in patients presenting for **bone marrow transplantation**.

Butorphanol tartrate. Obsolete **opioid analgesic drug** with partial agonist properties, withdrawn in the UK in 1983, similar in actions to **pentazocine**.
See also, Opioid receptors

Butyrophenones. Group of centrally acting drugs, originally described with **phenothiazines** as 'major tranquillisers' (a term no longer used). They produce a state of detachment from the environment and inhibit purposeful movement via **$GABA_A$ receptor** antagonism. They may cause distressing inner restlessness that may be masked by outward calmness. They are powerful **antiemetic drugs**, acting as dopamine antagonists at the **chemoreceptor trigger zone**. Although some α-adrenergic blocking effect has been shown, cardiovascular effects are minimal. May cause extrapyramidal side effects, and the **neuroleptic malignant syndrome**, especially after chronic usage. Used to treat psychoses (especially schizophrenia and mania), in **neuroleptanaesthesia** and as antiemetics. **Droperidol** has a faster onset of action and shorter **half-life** than **haloperidol**.

Bypass, cardiopulmonary, *see Cardiopulmonary bypass*

C

C1-esterase deficiency, *see Hereditary angio-oedema*

CABG, *see Coronary artery bypass graft*

Cachectin, *see Cytokines*

Cachexia, *see Malnutrition*

Caesarean section (CS). Operative delivery of a fetus by surgical incision through the abdominal wall and uterus. Usually done via a transverse lower segment incision as this is associated with lower rates of ileus, infection and bleeding than the classic midline upper uterine segment approach. The CS rate in the UK has steadily increased from ~8%–10% in the 1980s to ~26%. Rates vary widely across Europe (~20%–50%); in the USA and Australia the rate is ~30%–33%.

Indications include: previous CS; maternal morbidity (e.g. severe cardiac disease); complications of pregnancy (e.g. **pre-eclampsia**); obstetric disorders (e.g. **placenta praevia**); fetal compromise; failure to progress.

- Specific anaesthetic considerations:
  - physiological changes of **pregnancy**.
  - difficult tracheal intubation and **aspiration of gastric contents** associated with general anaesthesia (GA) have been major anaesthetic causes of maternal mortality, especially in emergency CS.
  - **aortocaval compression** must be minimised by avoiding the supine position at all times.
  - uterine tone is decreased by volatile anaesthetic agents; however, consideration of this should not result in the administration of inadequate anaesthesia.
  - placental perfusion may be reduced by severe and/or prolonged hypotension and/or reduction in cardiac output.
  - contraction of the uterus upon delivery results in autotransfusion of about 500 ml blood, helping to offset the average blood loss of 500–1000 ml (GA) or 300–700 ml (regional anaesthesia).
  - neonatal depression should be avoided, but maternal **awareness** may occur if depth of anaesthesia is inadequate.
- The usual **preoperative assessment** should be made, with particular attention to:
  - the indication for CS (e.g. pre-eclampsia) and other obstetric or medical conditions.
  - whether CS is elective or emergency, and whether the fetus is compromised. A widely used classification of urgency is:
    - 1: immediate threat to life to mother or fetus.
    - 2: fetal or maternal compromise that is not immediately life threatening
    - 3: needs early delivery but no compromise.
    - 4: at a time to suit the team/mother.
  - assessment of the airway.
  - maternal preference for general or regional anaesthesia.
  - the quality of existing **epidural analgesia**.
  - assessment of the lumbar spine and any contraindications to regional anaesthesia.

These points inform the decision to employ general or regional anaesthesia.

- Regimens used to reduce the risk of **aspiration pneumonitis**:
  - fasting during labour: most centres no longer have a general fasting policy because the use of GA is infrequent so few women will benefit. Instead, women should be stratified according to risk and informed of the reasons for/against fasting, with those at higher risk of surgical intervention advised to fast. Women who wish to eat or drink should be encouraged to take clear fluids or foods with low fat and sugar content.
  - **antacid** therapy: 0.3 M **sodium citrate** (30 ml) directly neutralises gastric acidity; it has a short duration of action and should be given immediately before induction of general anaesthesia.
  - **H_2 receptor antagonists**: most units reserve these for prophylaxis (e.g. with **ranitidine**) in women at risk of operative intervention or receiving **pethidine** (causing reduced gastric emptying). For elective CS, ranitidine 150 mg orally the night before and 2 h before surgery is usual. For emergency CS, ranitidine 50 mg iv or **cimetidine** 200 mg im may be given.
  - **omeprazole** and **metoclopramide** have also been used, to reduce gastric acidity and increase gastric emptying, respectively.

Sedative **premedication** is usually avoided because of the risk of neonatal respiratory depression and difficulties over timing.

- Anaesthetic techniques:
  - for all types of anaesthesia:
    - wide-bore iv access (16 G or larger).
    - cross-matched blood available within 30 min.
    - routine **monitoring** and skilled anaesthetic assistance, with all necessary equipment and resuscitative drugs available and checked.
    - aortocaval compression is reduced by positioning the patient laterally during transport to theatre and surgery.
    - **oxytocin** has superseded **ergometrine** as the first-line uterotonic following delivery because of the latter's side effects (e.g. hypertension and vomiting).
  - general anaesthesia:
    - **rapid sequence induction** with an adequate dose of anaesthetic agent is required to prevent awareness; a 'maximal allowed dose' based on weight may be insufficient. **Thiopental** has been traditionally used but unfamiliarity with its use and the risk of syringe-swap with antibiotic (and in the USA, the unavailability of thiopental) has led to increasing use of **propofol**. Neonatal depression due to iv induction agents is minimal. **Suxamethonium** has

been considered the **neuromuscular blocking drug** of choice for many years, although **rocuronium** (especially with the advent of **sugammadex**) is an increasingly used alternative.

- difficult and failed intubation (the latter ~1:300–500) is more likely in obstetric patients than in the general population. Contributory factors include a full set of **teeth**, increased fat deposition, enlarged breasts and the hand applying cricoid pressure hindering insertion of the laryngoscope blade into the mouth. Laryngeal oedema may be present in pre-eclampsia. **Apnoea** rapidly results in **hypoxaemia** because of reduced **FRC** and increased O_2 demand, especially for CS during labour.
- IPPV with 50% O_2 in $\mathbf{N_2O}$ is commonly recommended until delivery; however, in the absence of fetal distress, 33% O_2 is associated with similar neonatal outcomes.
- 0.5–0.6 MAC of volatile agents (with 50% N_2O) reduces the incidence of awareness to 1% without increasing uterine atony and bleeding, or neonatal depression; however, at 0.8–1.0 MAC, awareness falls to 0.2% and the uterus remains responsive to uterotonics. Placental blood flow is thought to be maintained by vasodilatation caused by the volatile agents, and high levels of vasoconstricting **catecholamines** associated with awareness are avoided. Delivery of higher concentrations of volatile agents ('overpressure') in 66% N_2O has been suggested for the first 3–5 min while alveolar concentrations are low, to reduce awareness. Factors increasing the likelihood of awareness include lack of premedication, reduced concentrations of N_2O and volatile agents, and withholding opioid analgesic drugs until delivery. Up to 26% awareness was reported in early studies using 50% N_2O and no volatile anaesthetic agent. Obstetric cases were overrepresented in cases of awareness in the 5th **National Audit Project**.
- normocapnia (4 kPa/30 mmHg in pregnancy) is considered ideal; excessive **hyperventilation** may be associated with fetal hypoxaemia and acidosis due to placental vasoconstriction, impairment of O_2 transfer associated with low $P\text{CO}_2$, and reduced venous return caused by excessive IPPV.
- all **neuromuscular blocking drugs** cross the **placenta** to a very small extent. Shorter-acting drugs (e.g. **vecuronium** and **atracurium**) are usually employed (unless rocuronium is used for intubation), because postoperative residual paralysis associated with longer-lasting drugs has been a significant factor in some maternal deaths.
- **opioid analgesic drugs** are withheld until delivery of the infant, to avoid neonatal respiratory depression (unless indicated during induction of anaesthesia).
- aspiration may also occur during recovery from anaesthesia (when the effect of sodium citrate may have worn off). Routine gastric aspiration during anaesthesia has been suggested in emergency cases. Before tracheal extubation, the patient should be awake and on her side.
- advantages: usually quicker to perform in emergencies. May be used when regional techniques are inadequate or contraindicated, e.g. in **coagulation disorders**. Safer in hypovolaemia.
- disadvantages: risk of aspiration, difficult intubation, awareness and neonatal depression. Hypotension and reduced cardiac output may result from anaesthetic drugs and IPPV. Postoperative pain, drowsiness, **PONV**, blood loss and **DVT** risk all tend to be greater.

- epidural anaesthesia (EA):
  - facilities for GA should be available.
  - **bupivacaine**/levobupivacaine 0.5% or **lidocaine** 2% (the latter with adrenaline 1:200 000) is most commonly used in the UK, often in combination. Addition of opioids (e.g. **fentanyl**) is common (though may not be necessary if many epidural doses have been given during labour). **Bicarbonate** has also been added to shorten the onset time (e.g. 2 ml 8.4% added to 20 ml lidocaine or lidocaine/bupivacaine mixture), but risks errors from mixing drugs, especially in an emergency. Commercial premixed solutions of lidocaine/bupivacaine and adrenaline may be unsuitable as they have a low pH (3.5–5.5) and contain preservatives. **Ropivacaine** 0.5%–0.75% is also used. 0.75% bupivacaine is associated with a high incidence of toxicity, and has been withdrawn from obstetric use. **Chloroprocaine** is available in the USA and a small number of European countries (but not the UK); it has a rapid onset and offset. **Etidocaine** has also been used in the USA.
  - L3–4 interspace is usually chosen.
  - on average, 15–20 ml solution is required for adequate blockade (from S5 to T4–6). Loss of normal light touch sensation is a better predictor of intraoperative comfort than loss of cold sensation, although either may be used to assess the block. Smaller volumes are required for a specified level of block than in non-pregnant patients, as dilated epidural veins reduce the available volume in the **epidural space**.
  - injection of solution in 5-ml increments at 5-min intervals reduces the risk of hypotension and extensive blockade (e.g. due to accidental spinal injection), but increases anaesthetic time and total dose. A single injection of 15–20 ml over 2 min (after a 2–4 ml test dose) is advocated by some as producing a more rapid block. A catheter technique is used most frequently, although injection through the epidural needle may be performed.
  - opioids (e.g. **diamorphine** 2–4 mg or fentanyl 50–100 µg) may be given epidurally for peri- and **postoperative analgesia**.
  - hypotension associated with blockade of sympathetic tone may be reduced by preloading with **iv fluid**; however, the use of vasopressors to prevent and treat hypotension in the euvolaemic patient is thought to be a more effective and rational approach. **Ephedrine** 3–6 mg or **phenylephrine** 50–100 µg is commonly given by intermittent bolus, the latter drug increasingly given by infusion. Phenylephrine is associated with a better neonatal acid–base profile than large doses of ephedrine (thought to be due to ephedrine crossing the placenta and causing increased anaerobic **glycolysis** in the fetus via β-adrenergic stimulation).
  - nausea and vomiting may be caused by hypotension and/or bradycardia.
  - routine administration of O_2 by facemask has been questioned on the grounds of being ineffective

and even possibly harmful to the fetus, due to generation of free radicals.
- during surgery many women feel pressure and movement, which may be unpleasant; all women should be warned of this possibility and of the potential requirement for general anaesthesia. Inhaled N_2O, further epidural top-ups, small doses of iv opioid drugs (e.g. fentanyl or **alfentanil**), iv **paracetamol** and **ketamine** may be useful. Shoulder-tip pain may result from blood tracking up to the **diaphragm** and may be reduced by head-up tilt. Good communication between mother, anaesthetist and obstetrician is especially important when performing CS under regional anaesthesia, and the obstetrician should warn the anaesthetist before exteriorising the uterus or swabbing the paracolic gutters.
- advantages: the risks of GA are avoided. Onset of hypotension is usually slow, the mother may be able to warn of it early and it may be corrected before becoming severe. Minimal neonatal depression occurs compared with GA. The mother is not drowsy and is able to hold the baby soon after delivery. Her partner is able to be present during the procedure. Epidural analgesia provided in labour can be extended for operative delivery. The catheter can be used for further 'top-up' during surgery if required, and for postoperative analgesia.
- disadvantages: risk of **dural tap**, total spinal blockade, local anaesthetic toxicity, severe hypotension. It may be slow to achieve adequate blockade with a risk of patchy block. Inability to move the legs may be disturbing.

▸ **spinal anaesthesia** (SA):
- general considerations as for EA.
- 0.5% bupivacaine is used in the UK; plain bupivacaine (e.g. 3 ml) produces a more variable block than hyperbaric bupivacaine (e.g. 1.8–2.8 ml), which is the only form licensed for spinal anaesthesia. Plain levobupivacaine is also licensed in the UK. Hyperbaric bupivacaine 0.75% (1.4–1.8 ml) is commonly used in the USA.
- injection is usually at the L3–4/L4–5 interspace.
- advantages: as for EA, but of quicker onset, and blockade is more intense and less likely to be patchy. Smaller doses of local anaesthetic drug are used.
- disadvantages: single shot; i.e., may not last long enough if surgery is prolonged. Spinal catheter techniques allow more control over spread and duration but are technically more difficult. Risk of **post-dural puncture headache** (reduced to under 1% if 25–27 G pencil-point **needles** are used). Hypotension is of faster onset and thus may be more difficult to control; has been associated with poorer neonatal acid–base status compared with EA/GA. Remains the most popular anaesthetic technique for CS in the UK.

▸ **combined spinal–epidural anaesthesia** (CSE):
- general considerations: as for EA and SA.
- allows the fast onset and dense block of SA but with the flexibility of EA. Also allows a small subarachnoid injection to be extended by epidural injection of either saline (thought to act via a volume effect) or local anaesthetic, with greater cardiovascular stability.
- usually performed at a single vertebral interspace (needle-through-needle method).
- increased flexibility must be weighed against increased cost and the suggestion that the spinal component may be less effective than a single-shot spinal (possibly related to less rapid return to the horizontal position after injection).

(*For contraindications and methods, see individual techniques*)

CS is possible using local anaesthetic infiltration of the abdominal wall (e.g. with 0.5% lidocaine or prilocaine). Large volumes are required, with risk of toxicity. Infiltration of each layer is performed in stages. The procedure is lengthy and uncomfortable, but may be used as a last resort if other techniques are unavailable or unsuccessful. It may also be used to supplement inhalational anaesthesia following failed intubation. **Transversus abdominis plane block** has been used, e.g. for postoperative analgesia.

[Julius Caesar (100–44 BC), Roman Emperor; said to have been born by the abdominal route; his name allegedly derived from *caedare* (Latin, to cut). An alternative suggestion is related to a law enforced under the Caesars concerning abdominal section following death in late pregnancy]

See also, Confidential Enquiries into Maternal Deaths; Fetus, effects of anaesthetic agents on; I–D interval; Induction, rapid sequence; Intubation, difficult; Intubation, failed; Obstetric analgesia and anaesthesia; U–D interval

Caffeine. **Xanthine** present in tea, coffee and certain soft drinks; the world's most widely used psychoactive substance. Also used as an adjunct to many oral **analgesic drug** preparations, although not analgesic itself. Causes CNS stimulation; traditionally thought to improve performance and mood, while reducing fatigue. Increases cerebral vascular resistance and decreases cerebral blood flow. **Half-life** is about 6 h. Has been used iv and orally for treatment of **post-dural puncture headache**. Acts via inhibition of phosphodiesterase, increasing levels of cAMP and as an antagonist at adenosine receptors.
- Dosage: up to 30 mg in compound oral preparations. 150–300 mg orally tds/qds for post-dural puncture headache; 250 mg iv (with 250 mg sodium benzoate).
- Side effects: as for **aminophylline**, especially CNS and cardiac stimulation.

Caisson disease, *see Decompression sickness*

Calcitonin. Hormone (mw 3500) secreted from the parafollicular (C) cells of the **thyroid gland**. Involved in **calcium** homeostasis; secretion is stimulated by **hypercalcaemia**, **catecholamines** and gastrin. Decreases serum calcium by inhibiting mobilisation of bone calcium, decreasing intestinal absorption and increasing renal calcium and phosphate excretion. Acts via a **G protein-coupled receptor** on osteoclasts. Calcitonin derived from salmon is used in the treatment of severe hypercalcaemia, postmenopausal osteoporosis, Paget's disease and intractable pain from bony metastases. Has also been used in chronic pain states e.g. **phantom limb** pain and **complex regional pain syndrome**.

[Sir James Paget (1814–1899), English surgeon]

See also, Procalcitonin

Calcium. 99% of body calcium is contained in bone; plasma calcium consists of free ionised calcium (50%) and calcium bound to proteins (mainly **albumin**) and other ions. The free ionised form is a **second messenger** in many cellular processes, including **neuromuscular transmission**, **muscle contraction**, **coagulation**, cell division/movement and certain oxidative pathways. Binds to intracellular proteins (e.g. calmodulin), causing configurational changes and enzyme activation. Intracellular calcium levels are much higher than extracellular, due to relative membrane impermeability and **active transport** mechanisms. Calcium entry via specific channels leads to direct effects (e.g. **neurotransmitter** release in neurones), or further calcium release from intracellular organelles (e.g. in cardiac and skeletal **muscle**). Extracellular hypocalcaemia has a net excitatory effect on nerve and muscle; hypocalcaemic **tetany** can result in life-threatening **laryngospasm**.

Ionised calcium increases with **acidosis**, and decreases with **alkalosis**. Thus for accurate measurement, blood should be taken without a tourniquet (which causes local acidosis), and without hyper-/hypoventilation. Ionised calcium is measured in some centres, but total plasma calcium is easier to measure; normal value is 2.12–2.65 mmol/l. Varies with the plasma protein level; corrected by adding 0.02 mmol/l calcium for each g/l albumin below 40 g/l, or subtracting for each g/l above 40 g/l.

- Regulation:
  - **vitamin D**: group of related sterols. Cholecalciferol is formed in the skin by the action of ultraviolet light, and is converted in the liver to 25-hydroxycholecalciferol (in turn converted to 1,25-dihydroxycholecalciferol in the proximal renal tubules). Formation is increased by parathyroid hormone and decreased by **hyperphosphataemia**. Actions:
    - increases intestinal calcium absorption.
    - increases renal calcium reabsorption.
    - increases bone mineralisation.
  - parathyroid hormone: secretion is increased by **hypocalcaemia** and **hypomagnesaemia**, and decreased by **hypercalcaemia** and **hypermagnesaemia**. Actions:
    - mobilises bone calcium.
    - increases renal calcium reabsorption.
    - increases renal phosphate excretion.
    - increases formation of 1,25-dihydroxycholecalciferol.
  - **calcitonin**: secreted by the parafollicular cells of the **thyroid gland**. Secretion is increased by hypercalcaemia, **catecholamines** and gastrin. Actions:
    - decreases intestinal absorption of dietary calcium.
    - inhibits mobilisation of bone calcium.
    - increases renal calcium and phosphate excretion.

Calcium is used clinically to treat hypocalcaemia, e.g. during massive **blood transfusion**. It is also used as an **inotropic drug**. Although ionised calcium concentration may be low after **cardiac arrest**, its use during **CPR** is no longer recommended unless persistent hypocalcaemia, **hyperkalaemia** or overdose of **calcium channel blocking drugs** is involved. This is because of its adverse effects on ischaemic myocardium and on coronary and cerebral circulations.

Calcium chloride 10% contains 6.8 mmol/10 ml and 14.7% contains 10 mmol/10 ml; calcium gluconate 10% contains 2.2–2.3 mmol/10 ml, depending on the formulation. 5–10 ml calcium chloride or 10–20 ml calcium gluconate is usually recommended by slow iv bolus. The chloride preparation is usually recommended for CPR, although equal rises in plasma calcium are produced by gluconate, if equal amounts of calcium are given. Arrhythmias and prolonged hypercalcaemia may follow their use.

Aguilera IM, Vaughan RS (2000). Anaesthesia; 55: 779–90

Calcium channel blocking drugs. Structurally diverse group of drugs that block Ca^{2+} flux via specific Ca^{2+} channels (largely L-type, slow inward current). Effects vary according to relative affinity for cardiac or vascular smooth muscle Ca^{2+} channels.

- Classified according to pharmacological effects in vitro and in vivo:
  - class I: potent negative inotropic and chronotropic effects, e.g. **verapamil**. Acts mainly on the myocardium and conduction system; reduces **myocardial contractility** and O_2 consumption and slows conduction of the **action potential** at the SA/AV nodes. Thus mainly used to treat angina and SVT (less useful in hypertension). Severe myocardial depression may occur, especially in combination with **β-adrenergic receptor antagonists**.
  - class II: acts on vascular smooth muscle, reducing vascular tone; minimal direct myocardial activity (although may cause reflex tachycardia):
    - **nifedipine**: acts mainly on coronary and peripheral arteries, with little myocardial depression. Used in angina, hypertension and Reynaud's syndrome. Systemic vasodilatation may cause flushing and headache, especially for the first few days of treatment.
    - **nicardipine**: as nifedipine, but with even less myocardial depression.
    - amlodipine and felodipine: similar to nifedipine and nicardipine, but with longer duration of action and therefore taken once daily.
    - **nimodipine**: crosses the **blood–brain barrier** and is particularly active on cerebral vascular smooth muscle; it is used to prevent cerebral vasospasm following **subarachnoid haemorrhage**.
  - class III: slight negative inotropic effects, without reflex tachycardia: **diltiazem** is used in angina and hypertension.

These drugs act mainly on the L-type calcium (long-lasting) channels; these are more widely distributed than the T-type (transient) channels, which are confined to the sinoatrial node, vascular smooth muscle and renal neuroendocrine cells. N-type calcium channels are concentrated in neural tissue and are the binding site of omega toxins produced by certain venomous spiders and cone snails. A derivative of the latter, **ziconotide**, is available for the treatment of chronic pain.

Additive effects might be expected between these drugs and the volatile anaesthetic agents, all of which decrease calcium entry into cells. Reduction in cardiac output, decreased atrioventricular conduction and vasodilatation may occur to different degrees, but severe interactions are rarely a problem in practice. Non-depolarising neuromuscular blockade may be potentiated.

Overdose causes hypotension, bradycardia and **heart block**. Treatment includes iv calcium chloride, glucagon and **catecholamines**. Heart block is usually resistant to **atropine** and hypotension may not respond to inotropes or vasopressors. High-dose **insulin** has been successful in reversing refractory hypotension as has **levosimendan**, a **calcium sensitiser**.

[Maurice Reynaud (1834-1881), French physician]

Calcium resonium, *see Polystyrene sulfonate resins*

Calcium sensitisers. Class of **inotropic drugs**, now established as effective treatment of acute **cardiac failure**; examples include **levosimendan** and pimobendan. Act directly on cardiac myofilaments without increasing intracellular **calcium**, thus improving **myocardial contractility** without impairing ventricular relaxation. Levosimendan also has vasodilatory effects through opening of K^+ channels.

Calibration. Process of standardising the output of a measuring device against another measurement of known and constant magnitude. Reduces measurement error due to drift. One-point calibration is sufficient to address offset drift; two-point calibration is required for the mitigation of gradient drift. Essential for the accurate functioning of many measurement devices (e.g. **arterial blood pressure** monitor, **blood gas analyser**, expired gas analyser).

Calorie. **Unit** of **energy**. Although not an SI unit, widely used, especially when describing energy content of food.

1 cal = energy required to heat 1 g water by 1°C.

1 kcal (1 Cal) = energy required to heat 1 kg water by 1°C = 1000 cal.

1 cal = 4.18 **joules**.

Calorimetry, indirect, *see Energy balance*

CAM-ICU, *see Confusion in the intensive care unit*

cAMP, *see Adenosine monophosphate, cyclic*

Campbell–Howell method, *see Carbon dioxide measurement*

Canadian Journal of Anesthesia. Official journal of the Canadian Anesthetists' Society. Launched in 1954 as the *Canadian Anaesthetists' Society Journal*. Became the *Canadian Journal of Anaesthesia* in 1987 and the *Canadian Journal of Anesthesia* in 1999.

Candela. SI **unit** of luminous intensity, one of the base (fundamental) units. Definition relates to the luminous intensity of a radiating black body at the freezing point of platinum.

Candida infection, *see Fungal infection in the ICU*

Cannabis. Hallucinogenic drug obtained from the *Cannabis sativa* plant. A mixture of at least 60 chemicals (cannabinoids), including the main psychoactive δ-9-tetrahydrocannibinol. Cannabinoid receptors have been identified in central and peripheral neurones (CB_1 receptors) and lymphoid tissue (e.g. spleen) and macrophages (CB_2); both types are **G protein-coupled receptors**.

Therapeutic uses include treatment of glaucoma and as an antiemetic agent during chemotherapy. Also has analgesic, anticonvulsant and possibly antispasmodic properties, hence its use in chronic pain and multiple sclerosis. Mild psychological dependence is common, although physiological withdrawal states do not occur. Cognitive impairment, including psychosis with chronic usage, has been reported. Usually combined with tobacco and smoked; anaesthetic concerns are as for **smoking** generally.

Present law prohibits prescription of cannabis without a Home Office Licence and has hampered clinical trials; there has been pressure to allow freer administration in certain chronic conditions and even to decriminalise it altogether. Reclassified as a Class C drug under the **Misuse of Drugs Act 1971** in 2004. **Nabilone** is a synthetic cannabinoid used as an antiemetic in chemotherapy-induced nausea and vomiting.

Schrot RJ, Hubbard JR (2016). Ann Med; 48: 128–41

Capacitance. Ability to retain electrical charge; defined as the charge stored by an object per voltage difference across it. The unit of capacitance is the farad (F), 1 farad being the capacity to store 1 coulomb of charge for an applied potential difference of 1 volt.

A capacitor composed of conductors separated by an insulator may be charged by a potential difference across it, but will not allow direct current to flow. Its stored charge may subsequently be discharged, e.g. in **defibrillation.** Repeated charging and discharging induced by an alternating current results in current flow across a capacitor.

[Michael Faraday (1791–1867), English chemist]

Capacitance vessels. Composed of venae cavae and large veins; normally only partially distended, they may expand to accommodate a large volume of blood before venous pressure is increased. Innervated by the **sympathetic nervous system** in the same way as the arterial system (**resistance vessels**), they act as a blood reservoir. 60%–70% of **blood volume** is within the veins normally.

Capacitor, *see Capacitance*

Capillary circulation. Contains 5% of circulating **blood volume**, which passes from arterioles to venules via capillaries, usually within 2 s. Controlled by local autoregulatory mechanisms, and possibly by autonomic neural reflexes. Substances that readily cross the capillary walls (mainly by **diffusion**) include water, O_2, CO_2, glucose and urea. Hydrostatic pressure falls from about 30 mmHg (arteriolar end) to 15 mmHg (venous end) within the capillary. Direction of fluid flow across capillary walls is determined by hydrostatic and osmotic pressure gradients (**Starling forces**).

Capillary refill time. Time taken for capillaries to refill after blanching pressure is applied for 5 s. Normally <2 s; prolonged in hypoperfusion and hypothermia. May be measured centrally, over the sternum, or peripherally, on the soft pad of a digit.

Capnography. Continuous measurement and pictorial display of CO_2 concentration (capnometry refers to measurement only). During anaesthesia, used to display end-tidal CO_2; this may be achieved using:

- **spectroscopy** (most commonly infrared).
- **mass spectrometer.**

The equipment used must have a very short response time in order to produce a continuous display (for uses and capnography traces, *see Carbon dioxide, end-tidal*).

Whitaker DK (2011). Anaesthesia; 66: 544–9

See also, Carbon dioxide measurement

Capreomycin. Cyclic polypeptide **antibacterial drug** used to treat **TB** resistant to other therapy (especially in immunocompromised patients). Also used in other mycobacterial infections. Poorly absorbed orally, peak levels occur within 2 h of im injection. Excreted unchanged in the urine.

- Dosage: 1 g/day by deep im injection for 2–4 months, then 1 g 2–3 times weekly, reduced in renal failure.

- Side effects: renal and hepatic impairment, ocular disturbances, ototoxicity, blood dyscrasias, electrolyte disturbances, neuromuscular blockade.

Capsaicin. Component of hot chilli peppers used in the treatment of neuropathic **pain.** Topical application causes initial sensitisation followed by prolonged desensitisation of local pain nerves. Acts via the transient receptor potential ion channel vanilloid 1 (TRPV1). Applied topically for the treatment of neuralgias (e.g. **postherpetic neuralgia**) and arthritis. Should be applied 6–8-hourly. Takes 1–4 weeks to produce its effect. Application of a single high-concentration (8%) capsaicin patch can produce 3 months' relief from neuropathic pain.
Smith H, Brooks JR (2014). Prog Drug Res; 68: 129–46

Captopril. Angiotensin converting enzyme inhibitor, used to treat **hypertension** and **cardiac failure** (including following **MI**), and diabetic nephropathy. Shorter acting than **enalapril**; onset is within 15 min, with peak effect at 30–60 min. **Half-life** is 2 h. Interferes with renal **autoregulation**; therefore contraindicated in renal artery stenosis or pre-existing renal impairment.
- Dosage: 6.25–75 mg orally bd/tds.
- Side effects: severe hypotension after the first dose, cough, taste disturbances, rash, abdominal pain, agranulocytosis, hyperkalaemia, renal impairment. Severe hypotension may occur after induction of anaesthesia and in hypovolaemia.

Contraindicated in pregnancy and **porphyria.**

Carbamazepine. Anticonvulsant drug, used as first-line treatment of focal and generalised tonic clonic **epilepsy.** Acts by stabilising the inactivated state of voltage-gated sodium channels. Has fewer side effects than **phenytoin**, and has a greater **therapeutic index**. Also used for **pain management** (e.g. in **trigeminal neuralgia**) and in bipolar disorders.
- Dosage: initially 100–200 mg orally od/bd, increasing to up to 1.6 g/day in divided doses. Monitoring plasma levels may help determination of optimal dosage (target levels 20–50 µmol/l).
- Side effects: dizziness, visual disturbances, GIT upset, rash, **hyponatraemia**, cholestatic jaundice, hepatitis, **syndrome of inappropriate ADH secretion.** Blood dyscrasias may occur rarely. **Enzyme induction** may cause reduced effects of other drugs, e.g. **warfarin.**

Contraindicated in atrioventricular conduction defects and **porphyria.**

Carbapenems. Group of bactericidal **antibacterial drugs**; contain the **β-lactam** ring and thus, like the **penicillins**, impair bacterial cell wall synthesis. Include imipenem, **meropenem** and **ertapenem.**

Carbetocin. Analogue of human **oxytocin**, with a longer half-life (~90–100 min compared with 3–4 min), licensed for prevention of uterine atony after delivery by **caesarean section.** Acts within 2 min of injection, its effects lasting over an hour.
- Dosage: 100 µg iv.
- Side effects: as for oxytocin.

Carbicarb. Experimental **buffer** composed of 0.3 M sodium carbonate and 0.3 M sodium **bicarbonate**; unlike bicarbonate, there is no net generation of CO_2 when treating acidosis.

Carbocisteine, *see Mucolytic drugs*

Carbohydrates (Saccharides). Class of compounds with the general formula $C_a(H_2O)_b$, hence their name, although they are not true hydrates. a usually exceeds 3, and may or may not equal b. Notable examples of monosaccharides are ribose and glucose, where a = 5 and 6, respectively (pentoses and hexoses). Disaccharides are formed from condensation reactions between two monosaccharides (e.g. sucrose = glucose + fructose). Large polysaccharides include starch, cellulose and **glycogen.** Metabolites often contain phosphorus. Some polysaccharides are combined with proteins, e.g. mucopolysaccharides. Act as a source of **energy** in food, e.g.:

$$C_6H_{12}O_6 + 6O_2 \rightarrow 6CO_2 + 6H_2O + \text{energy}$$

1 g carbohydrate yields about 17 kJ energy (4 Cal).
- Ingested carbohydrates are broken down thus:
  - mouth: salivary **amylase**: starch → smaller units
  - small intestine:
    - pancreatic amylase: starch as above.
    - maltase: maltose → glucose.
    - lactase: lactose → glucose + galactose.
    - sucrase: sucrose → glucose + fructose.

Hexoses and pentoses absorbed from the GIT pass to the liver for storage molecule synthesis or use in alternative metabolic pathways.
See also, Metabolism

Carbon dioxide (CO_2). Gas produced by oxidation of carbon-containing substances. Average rate of production under basal conditions in adults is about 200 ml/min, although it varies with the energy source (*see Respiratory quotient*).
- Partial pressures of CO_2:
  - inspired: 0.03 kPa (0.2 mmHg).
  - alveolar: 5.3 kPa (40 mmHg).
  - arterial: 5.3 kPa (40 mmHg).
  - venous: 6.1 kPa (46 mmHg).
  - expired: 4 kPa (30 mmHg).

Isolated in 1757 by Black. **CO_2 narcosis** was used for anaesthesia in animals by **Hickman** in 1824. Used to stimulate respiration during anaesthesia in the early 1900s, to maintain ventilation and speed uptake of volatile agents during induction; also used to assist blind nasal tracheal intubation. Administration is now generally considered hazardous because of the adverse effects of **hypercapnia**; CO_2 **cylinders** have now been removed from anaesthetic machines. Manufactured by heating calcium or magnesium carbonate, producing CO_2 and calcium/magnesium oxide.
- Properties:
  - colourless gas, 1.5 times denser than air.
  - **mw** 44.
  - **boiling point** –79°C.
  - **critical temperature** 31°C.
  - non-flammable and non-explosive.
  - supplied in grey cylinders; pressure is 50 **bar** at 15°C, about 57 bar at room temperature.
- Effects: as for hypercapnia.

[Joseph Black (1728–1799), Scottish chemist]
See also, Acid–base balance; Alveolar gas transfer; Breathing, control of; Carbon dioxide absorption, in anaesthetic breathing systems; Carbon dioxide dissociation curve;

Carbon dioxide, end-tidal; Carbon dioxide measurement; Carbon dioxide transport

Carbon dioxide absorption, in anaesthetic breathing systems. Investigated and described by **Waters** in the early 1920s, although used earlier. Exhaled gases are passed over **soda lime** or a similar material (e.g. **baralyme**) and reused. In closed systems, only basal O_2 requirements need be supplied; absorption may also be used with low fresh gas flows and a leak through an expiratory valve.

- Advantages:
  - less wastage of inhalational agent.
  - less pollution.
  - warms and humidifies inhaled gases.
- Disadvantages:
  - if N_2O is also used, risk of hypoxic gas mixtures makes an O_2 analyser mandatory.
  - failure of CO_2 absorption may be due to exhaustion of soda lime or inefficient equipment; thus **capnography** is required.
  - resistance and **dead space** may be high with some systems, and inhalation of dust is possible.
  - **trichloroethylene** is incompatible with soda lime.
  - chemical reactions between the volatile agent and soda lime if the latter dries out excessively (*see Soda lime*).
- Methods:
  - **circle systems.**
  - Waters canister: cylindrical drum containing 0.45 kg soda lime. Reservoir bag at one end, facemask with fresh gas supply and expiratory valve at the other; exhaled gases pass to and fro through it. Most efficient when tidal volume equals the contained air space (400–450 ml). Smaller canisters are used for children. Dead space equals the volume between the patient and soda lime; it increases during use as the soda lime nearest the patient is exhausted. Efficiency is also reduced by channelling of exhaled gases through gaps in the soda lime if loosely packed and allowed to settle. Also heavy and bulky to use.

Carbon dioxide dissociation curve. Graph of blood CO_2 content against its $P\text{CO}_2$ (Fig. 31). The curve is much steeper than the **oxyhaemoglobin dissociation curve**, and more linear. Different curves are obtained for oxygenated and deoxygenated blood, the latter able to carry more CO_2 (**Haldane effect**). The difference between the dissolved CO_2 and the oxygenated haemoglobin curves represents the CO_2 carried as bicarbonate ion and carbamino compounds.

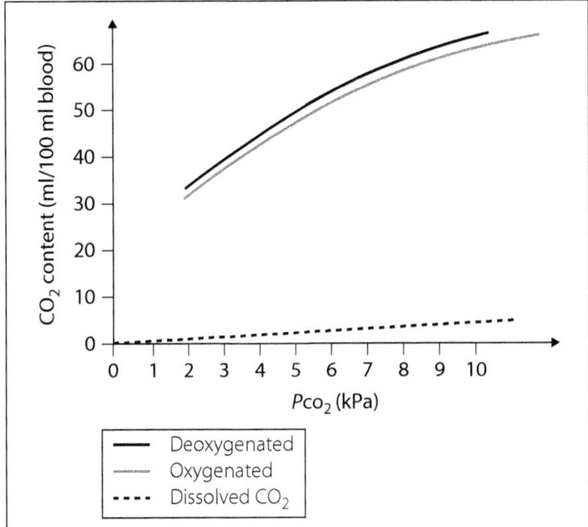

Fig. 31 Carbon dioxide dissociation curve

Carbon dioxide, end-tidal. Partial pressure of CO_2 measured in the final portion of exhaled gas. Approximates to alveolar $P\text{CO}_2$ in normal anaesthetised subjects; the difference is normally 0.4–0.7 kPa (3–5 mmHg), increasing with **$\dot{V}/\dot{Q}$ mismatch** and increased CO_2 production. Continuous monitoring (e.g. using infrared **capnography** or **mass spectrometry**) is considered mandatory during general anaesthesia.

- Measurement is useful for assessing adequacy of ventilation, whether controlled or spontaneous, and allows normo- or hypocapnia to be produced as required during IPPV. Measurement also aids detection of:
  - efficient **cardiac massage** or return of spontaneous cardiac output in **CPR**.
  - oesophageal intubation, because CO_2 is only present in the oesophagus and stomach in small amounts, if at all.
  - **PE** (including **fat** and **gas embolism**): $P_E\text{CO}_2$ falls due to increased alveolar **dead space** and reduced cardiac output.
  - rebreathing.
  - disconnection.
  - **MH**: $P_E\text{CO}_2$ rises as muscle metabolism increases.
- Display of a continuous trace is more useful than values alone (Fig. 32a):
  - phase 1: zero baseline during inspiration; a raised baseline indicates rebreathing (Fig. 32b).
  - phase 2: dead-space gas (containing no CO_2) is followed by alveolar gas, represented by a sudden rise to a plateau. Excessive sloping of the upstroke may indicate obstruction to expiration (Fig. 32c).
  - phase 3: near-horizontal plateau indicates mixing of alveolar gas. A steep upwards slope indicates obstruction to expiration or unequal mixing, e.g. **COPD** (Fig. 32c).
  - phase 4: rapid fall to zero at the onset of inspiration.
  - additional features may be present:
    - superimposed regular oscillations corresponding to cardiac contractions (Fig. 32d).
    - small waves representing spontaneous breaths between ventilator breaths, e.g. if neuromuscular blockade is insufficient (Fig. 32e).

See also, Carbon dioxide measurement

Carbon dioxide measurement. Estimation of arterial $P\text{CO}_2$:

- direct: Severinghaus CO_2 electrode consisting of a glass pH electrode separated from arterial blood sample by a thin membrane. CO_2 diffuses into bicarbonate solution surrounding the glass electrode, lowering pH. pH is measured and displayed in terms of $P\text{CO}_2$. Requires maintenance at 37°C, and **calibration** with known mixtures of CO_2/O_2 before use. Samples are stored on ice or analysed immediately, to reduce inaccuracy due to blood cell metabolism.

  Indwelling intravascular CO_2 electrodes are available for continuous monitoring of $P\text{CO}_2$.

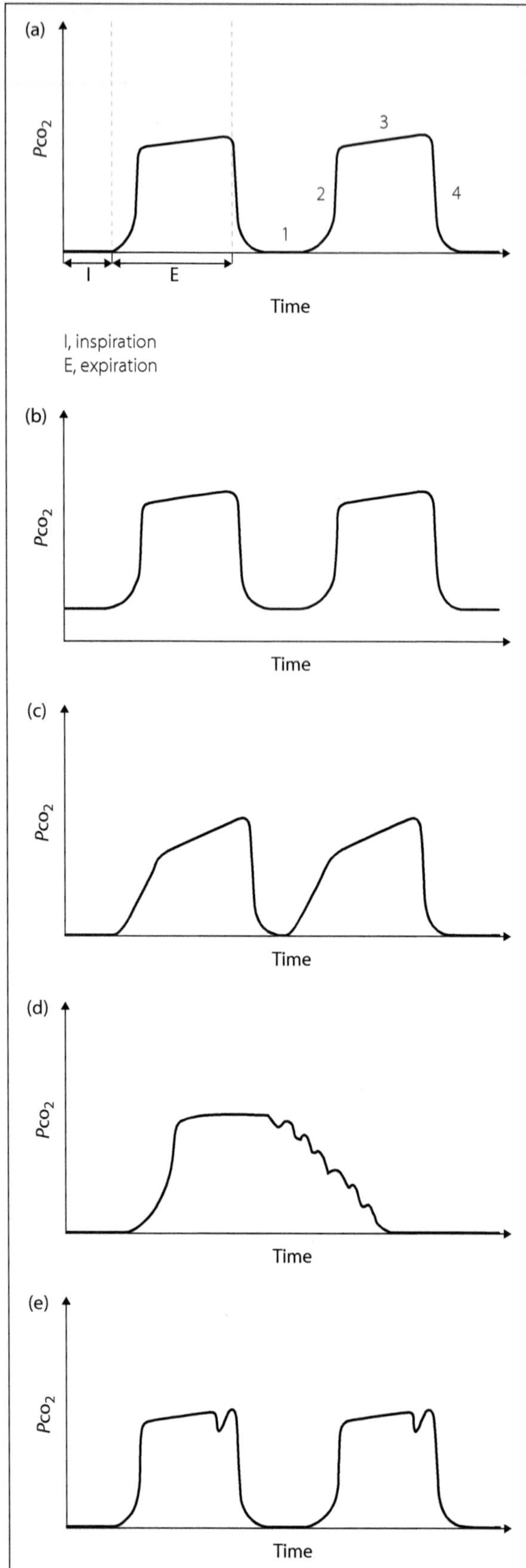

Fig. 32 End-tidal P_{CO_2} traces: (a) normal; (b) rebreathing; (c) expiratory obstruction; (d) superimposed heartbeats; (e) spontaneous breaths

- indirect:
  - from gas:
    - to obtain gas for analysis:
      - **end-tidal gas sampling** (end-tidal P_{CO_2} approximates to alveolar P_{CO_2}, which approximates to arterial P_{CO_2}).
      - rebreathing technique of Campbell and Howell: rebreathing from a 2 l bag containing 50% O_2 for 90 s, then a further 30 s after 3 min rest. Bag P_{CO_2} then approximates to mixed venous P_{CO_2}. Arterial P_{CO_2} is normally 0.8 kPa (6 mmHg) less than mixed venous P_{CO_2}.
    - subsequent **gas analysis**:
      - chemical: formation of non-gaseous compounds, with reduction of overall volume of the gas mixture (**Haldane apparatus**).
      - physical: **capnography** and **mass spectrometry** are most widely used. An **interferometer** or **gas chromatography** may also be used.
  - from blood/tissues:
    - transcutaneous electrode: requires heating of the skin; relatively inaccurate and slowly responsive.
    - measurement of venous P_{CO_2} and capillary P_{CO_2}: inaccurate and unreliable.
    - **Siggaard–Andersen nomogram**: equilibration of the blood sample with gases of known P_{CO_2}.
    - **van Slyke apparatus**: liberation of gas from blood sample with subsequent chemical analysis.
    - fibreoptic sensors: under development.

[John W Severinghaus, San Francisco anaesthetist; EJ Moran Campbell (1925–2004), English-born Canadian physiologist; John BL Howell (1926–2015), Southampton physician]

Carbon dioxide narcosis. Loss of consciousness caused by severe **hypercapnia**, i.e., arterial P_{CO_2} exceeding approximately 25 kPa (200 mmHg). Thought to be due to a profound fall in pH of **CSF** (under 6.9). Increasing central depression is seen at arterial P_{CO_2} greater than 13 kPa (100 mmHg), and CSF pH under 7.1. Other features of hypercapnia may be present.

Used by **Hickman** in 1824 to enable painless surgery on animals.

Carbon dioxide response curve, *Breathing, control of*

Carbon dioxide transport. In arterial blood, approximately 50 ml CO_2 is carried per 100 ml blood, as:
- **bicarbonate**: 45 ml.
- carbonic acid: 2.5 ml.
- carbamino compounds with proteins, mainly **haemoglobin**: 2.5 ml.

In venous blood, 54 ml is carried per 100 ml blood, as:
- bicarbonate: 47.5 ml.
- carbonic acid: 3.0 ml.
- carbamino compounds: 3.5 ml.

CO_2 is rapidly converted by **carbonic anhydrase** in red cells to carbonic acid, which dissociates to bicarbonate and **hydrogen ions**. Bicarbonate passes into plasma in exchange for chloride ions (**chloride shift**); hydrogen ions are buffered mainly by haemoglobin. Haemoglobin's buffering ability increases as it becomes deoxygenated, as does its ability to form carbamino groups (**Haldane effect**).

See also, Acid–base balance; Buffers; Carbon dioxide dissociation curve

Carbon monoxide (CO). Colourless, odourless and tasteless gas produced by the partial oxidation of carbon-containing substances. Produced endogenously from the breakdown of **haemoglobin**, it acts as a **neurotransmitter** and may have a role in modulating inflammation and mitochondrial activity. **Carbon monoxide poisoning** may result from exposure to high levels of exogenous CO (e.g. in **smoke inhalation**).

Carbon monoxide diffusing capacity, *see Diffusing capacity*

Carbon monoxide poisoning. May result from inhalation of fumes from car exhausts, fires, heating systems or coal gas supplies. Often coexists with **cyanide poisoning** during **burns**. Although not directly toxic to the lungs, carbon monoxide (CO) binds to **haemoglobin** with 200–250 times the affinity of O_2, forming carboxyhaemoglobin, which dissociates very slowly. The amount of carboxyhaemoglobin formed depends on inspired CO concentration and duration of exposure.

Production of CO in **circle systems** has been reported under certain circumstances.

- Effects:
  - reduced capacity for O_2 transport.
  - **oxyhaemoglobin dissociation curve** shifted to the left.
  - inhibition of the cellular **cytochrome oxidase system**; tissue toxicity is proportional to the length of exposure.
  - **aortic** and **carotid bodies** do not detect hypoxia, because the arterial $P\text{O}_2$ is unaffected.
- Features:
  - non-specific if chronic, e.g. angina, headache, weakness, dizziness, GIT disturbances.
  - if acute: as described earlier, with hypoxia, convulsions and coma if severe.
  - the 'cherry red' colour of carboxyhaemoglobin may be apparent.
  - **O_2 saturation** measured by **pulse oximetry** may be misleading because carboxyhaemoglobin (which has a unique spectrophotometric profile) is interpreted as oxygenated haemoglobin by some devices. Newer co-oximeters (e.g. Masimo Rainbow) are specifically able to determine blood carboxyhaemoglobin levels by measuring the absorbance of light across a range of wavelengths, thus distinguishing between different species of haemoglobin.
  - neurological symptoms (e.g. dystonia, ataxia, parkinsonism), personality changes and impaired memory may follow recovery from CO coma.
- Treatment:
  - **O_2 therapy**: speeds carboxyhaemoglobin dissociation. Tracheal intubation and **IPPV** may be necessary. Elimination **half-life** of carbon monoxide is reduced from 4 h to under 1 h with 100% O_2; it is reduced further to under 30 min with hyperbaric O_2 at 2.5–3 atm. At this pressure, dissolved O_2 alone satisfies tissue O_2 requirements. Hyperbaric O_2 has been recommended if the patient is unconscious, has arrhythmias, is pregnant or has carboxyhaemoglobin levels above 40%.
  - carboxyhaemoglobin levels correlate poorly with severity of symptoms, because of variable effects of tissue toxicity. Values often quoted:
    - 0.3%–2%: normal non-smokers (some CO from pollution, some formed endogenously).
    - 5%–6%: normal smokers.
    - 10%–30%: mild symptoms common.
    - above 60%: severe symptoms common.

Hampson NB, Piantadosi CA, Thom SR, Weaver LK (2012). Am J Respir Crit Care Med; 186: 1095–101

Carbon monoxide transfer factor, *see Diffusing capacity*

Carbonic anhydrase. Zinc-containing **enzyme** catalysing the reaction of CO_2 and water to form carbonic acid, which rapidly dissociates to **bicarbonate** and **hydrogen ions**. Absent from plasma, but present in high concentrations in:
- red blood cells: important in buffering, **CO_2 transport** and **O_2 transport**.
- renal tubular cells: important for maintaining **acid–base balance**.
- gastric mucosa: important in hydrochloric acid production.
- ciliary body: involved in aqueous humour formation.

Inhibited by **acetazolamide** and sulfonamides.

Carboprost. **Prostaglandin** $F_2\alpha$ analogue, used for the induction of second-trimester abortion; also used to treat **postpartum haemorrhage** unresponsive to first-line therapy. Given as the trometamol salt.
- Dosage: 250 µg by deep im injection, repeated as required at intervals of at least 15 min, up to 2 mg. Injection directly into the myometrium is no longer recommended as this risks accidental iv administration.
- Side effects: vomiting, diarrhoea, leucocytosis, fever, bronchospasm, uterine rupture.

Carboxyhaemoglobin, *see Carbon monoxide poisoning*

Carcinogenicity of anaesthetic agents, *see Environmental safety of anaesthetists; Fetus, effects of anaesthetic agents on*

Carcinoid syndrome. Results from secretion of vasoactive and other substances from certain tumours, found in the GIT (70%) or the bronchopulmonary system. Secreted compounds are metabolised by the liver so that symptoms are absent until hepatic metastases are present. May be associated with **neurofibromatosis**.
- Features:
  - flushing, mainly of the head and neck. May be associated with vasodilatation, hypotension, wheezing, skin wheals and sweating.
  - diarrhoea, sometimes with nausea and vomiting. Typically episodic, along with flushing. Weight loss is common.
  - endocardial fibrosis involving the tricuspid and pulmonary valves may cause right-sided **cardiac failure**.

Symptoms are traditionally ascribed to secretion of **5-HT** (diarrhoea) and **kinins** (flushing), but many more substances have been implicated, e.g. **dopamine**, **substance P**, **prostaglandins**, **histamine** and **vasoactive intestinal peptide**. Diagnosis includes measurement of urinary 5-hydroxyindole acetic acid, a breakdown product of 5-HT.
- Anaesthetic management:
  - perioperative treatment with various drugs has been used to reduce hyper-/hypotensive episodes and bronchospasm:

- **somatostatin** analogues, e.g. **octreotide**: inhibits release of inflammatory mediators and has become the first-line treatment of many authorities.
- 5-HT antagonists: **ketanserin**, cyproheptadine, methysergide.
- **antihistamine drugs**.

▸ invasive cardiovascular monitoring and careful fluid balance.
▸ use of cardiostable drugs where possible; avoidance of drugs causing histamine release.
▸ **suxamethonium** has been claimed to increase mediator release via fasciculations but this is uncertain.
▸ drugs should be prepared for treatment of bronchospasm and hyper-/hypotension.
▸ admission to HDU/ICU postoperatively.

Powell B, Al Mukhtar A, Mills GH (2011). Contin Educ Anaesth Crit Care Pain; 11: 9–13

Cardiac arrest. Sudden circulatory standstill. Common cause of death in cardiovascular disease, especially **ischaemic heart disease**. May also be caused by **PE**, electrolyte disturbances (e.g. of **potassium** or **calcium**), **hypoxaemia**, **hypercapnia**, **hypotension**, vagal reflexes, **hypothermia**, **anaphylaxis**, **electrocution**, drugs (e.g. **adrenaline**) and instrumentation of the heart.

- Features: unconsciousness within 15–30 s, apnoea or gasping respiration, pallor, cyanosis, absent pulses. Pupillary dilatation is usual.
- May be due to:
  ▸ **VF**: usually associated with **myocardial ischaemia**. The most common ECG finding (about 60%), with the best prognosis.
  ▸ **asystole**: occurs in about 30%. More likely in hypovolaemia and hypoxia, especially in children. May also follow vagally mediated bradycardia.
  ▸ **electromechanical dissociation** (EMD)/**pulseless electrical activity** (PEA). May occur in widespread myocardial damage. The least common ECG finding, with the worst prognosis, unless due to mechanical causes of circulatory collapse, e.g. PE, **cardiac tamponade**, **pneumothorax**.

  Asystole and EMD/PEA may convert to VF, which eventually converts to asystole if untreated.

Only 15%–20% of patients leave hospital after cardiac arrest. Up to 30%–40% survival is thought to be possible if prompt **CPR** is instituted. Permanent **cerebral hypoxic ischaemic injury** usually occurs within 4–5 min unless CPR is instituted. Factors suggesting poor outcome following cardiac arrest include:

▸ duration of arrest >6 min.
▸ increased age and presence of co-morbidity (e.g. cardiovascular disease, diabetes, renal disease, obesity).
▸ out of hospital arrest.
▸ delayed defibrillation and number of defibrillations.
▸ VT/VF have a better prognosis than PEA/asystole.

See also, Advanced life support, adult; Basic life support, adult; Postresuscitation care

Cardiac asthma. Acute **pulmonary oedema** resembling asthma. Both may feature dyspnoea, decreased lung compliance and widespread rhonchi, although pink frothy sputum is suggestive of pulmonary oedema. Increased airway resistance may result from true bronchospasm or from bronchial oedema.

Cardiac catheterisation. Passage of a catheter into the heart chambers for measurement of intracardiac pressures and O_2 saturations, or for injection of **radiological contrast media** for radiological imaging (angiocardiography). Used to investigate **ischaemic heart disease**, **valvular heart disease** and **congenital heart disease**; also used therapeutically (e.g. balloon valvotomy, atrial septostomy for **transposition of the great arteries** and **percutaneous coronary intervention**).

- Technique:
  ▸ commonly performed under local anaesthesia except in small children, in whom general anaesthesia is required.
  ▸ access is via a peripheral vein or artery (e.g. femoral or brachial vessels) using either a cut-down technique or percutaneous guide-wire (**Seldinger technique**).
  ▸ the right side of the heart is approached as for **pulmonary artery catheterisation**.
  ▸ the left side of the heart is approached retrogradely under x-ray control, via a peripheral artery or from the right side through the atrial septum or a defect thereof.
- Information gained:
  ▸ pressure values, waveforms and gradients between chambers.
  ▸ saturation values; greater than expected values on the right side indicate a left-to-right **shunt**.
  ▸ **cardiac output** may be measured using the **Fick principle**.
  ▸ **pulmonary vascular resistance** may be calculated.
  ▸ angiocardiography: cardiac function may be assessed on cine film, or the coronary vessels filled with dye to assess patency.

Approximate normal pressures and measurements are shown in Table 16.

Cardiac compressions, *see Cardiac massage*

Cardiac contractility, *see Myocardial contractility*

Cardiac cycle. Sequence of events occurring during cardiac activity; often represented by the Wiggers' diagram, which details changes in vascular pressures (especially **arterial BP**), **heart** chamber pressures, **ECG** and **phonocardiography** tracings during normal **sinus rhythm** (Fig. 33).

- Divided into five phases:
  ▸ phase 1: atrial contraction: responsible for about 30% of ventricular filling. Some blood regurgitates into the venae cavae and pulmonary veins.
  ▸ phase 2: isometric ventricular contraction: lasts from the closing of the tricuspid and mitral valves until ventricular pressures exceed aortic and pulmonary artery pressures, and the aortic and pulmonary valves open.

Table 16 Normal pressures and O_2 saturations obtained during cardiac catheterisation

Site	*Pressure (mmHg)*	*Saturation (%)*
Right atrium	1–4	75
Right ventricle	25/4	75
Pulmonary artery	25/12	75
Left atrium	2–10	97
Left ventricle	120/10	97
Aorta	120/70	97

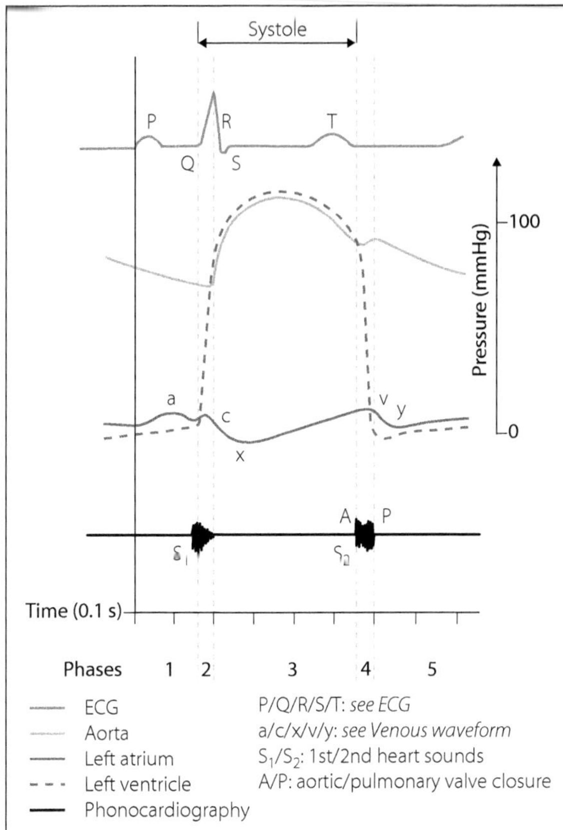

Fig. 33 Cardiac cycle (*see text*)

- phase 3: ventricular ejection: most rapid at the start of systole. Lasts until the aortic and pulmonary valves close.
- phase 4: isometric ventricular relaxation: lasts until the tricuspid and mitral valves open.
- phase 5: passive ventricular filling: most rapid at the start of diastole.

- May also be described in terms of the changes in pressure and volume within the left ventricle during the cardiac cycle—the left ventricular pressure–volume 'loop' (Fig. 34):
  - consists of four phases corresponding to phases 2–5 of the Wigger's diagram, as described earlier—the transition between phases is marked by opening/closure of mitral/aortic valves (MV/AV) (Fig. 34a).
  - **stroke volume** (SV) is the difference between end-diastolic volume (EDV) and end-systolic volume (ESV).
  - **stroke work** corresponds to the area within the loop.
  - changes in **preload**, **afterload** and **myocardial contractility** result in predictable changes in the shape of the loop, with corresponding changes in SV and work (Fig. 34b–d):
    - increased **preload** or EDV results in increased force of contraction (*see Starling's law*); SV and work increase.
    - increased **afterload** results in increased ESV; SV decreases.
    - increased contractility results in decreased ESV; stroke volume and work are increased.

[Carl J Wiggers (1883–1963), US physiologist]

See also, Arterial waveform; Pulse; Venous waveform

Cardiac enzymes. Enzymes normally within cardiac cells; released into the blood after injury (e.g. after **MI** or cardiac contusion), thus aiding diagnosis:

- creatine kinase (CK or CPK):
  - normally <190 IU/l.
  - rises 4–6 h after MI, peaks at 12 h, falls at 2–3 days.
  - three specific isoenzymes exist for skeletal muscle (CKMM), brain (CKBB) and myocardium (CKMB). Presence of CKMB in the plasma indicates myocardial necrosis.
- aspartate aminotransferase (AST):
  - normally <35 IU/l.
  - rises after 12 h, peaks at 1–2 days.
- lactate dehydrogenase (LDH):
  - normally <300 IU/l (depends on the assay).
  - rises after 12 h, peaks at 2–3 days, falls after 5–7 days.
  - five isoenzymes exist; an increase in the level of LDH1 or the ratio of LDH1:LDH2 indicates myocardial necrosis.

Have been largely replaced by troponins as indicators of myocardial damage (*see Acute coronary syndromes*).

Cardiac failure. Syndrome in which patients have typical symptoms (e.g. breathlessness, ankle swelling, fatigue) and signs (e.g. raised **JVP**, fluid retention, pulmonary congestion) resulting from an abnormality of cardiac structure or function leading to an inability to deliver enough oxygen to meet the requirements of metabolising tissues. This may be due to left ventricular systolic dysfunction (LVSD) or diastolic dysfunction (called heart failure with preserved **ejection fraction**; HF-PEF). Other terms such as forward or backward failure, congestive failure and high output failure have largely been superseded by this simpler classification. Diagnosis is largely clinical, ranging from mild symptoms on exertion only to **cardiogenic shock**. Estimated European prevalence is 2%–4% but this is increasing due to an ageing population and increasing prevalence of **diabetes** and **hypertension**.

Acute heart failure can present as new-onset cardiac failure or as a decompensation of chronic heart failure.

- Caused by:
  - increased workload:
    - **preload:**
      - **aortic/mitral regurgitation.**
      - **ASD/VSD.**
      - severe **anaemia**, fluid overload, **hyperthyroidism.**
    - **afterload:**
      - **hypertension.**
      - pulmonary/**aortic stenosis**, hypertrophic obstructive **cardiomyopathy.**
      - **pulmonary hypertension, PE.**
  - reduced force of contraction:
    - **MI, ischaemic heart disease.**
    - cardiomyopathy.
    - **arrhythmias.**
    - **myocarditis.**
  - reduced filling:
    - tricuspid/**mitral stenosis.**
    - **cardiac tamponade**, constrictive **pericarditis** (right side).
    - reduced ventricular compliance, e.g. amyloid infiltration.

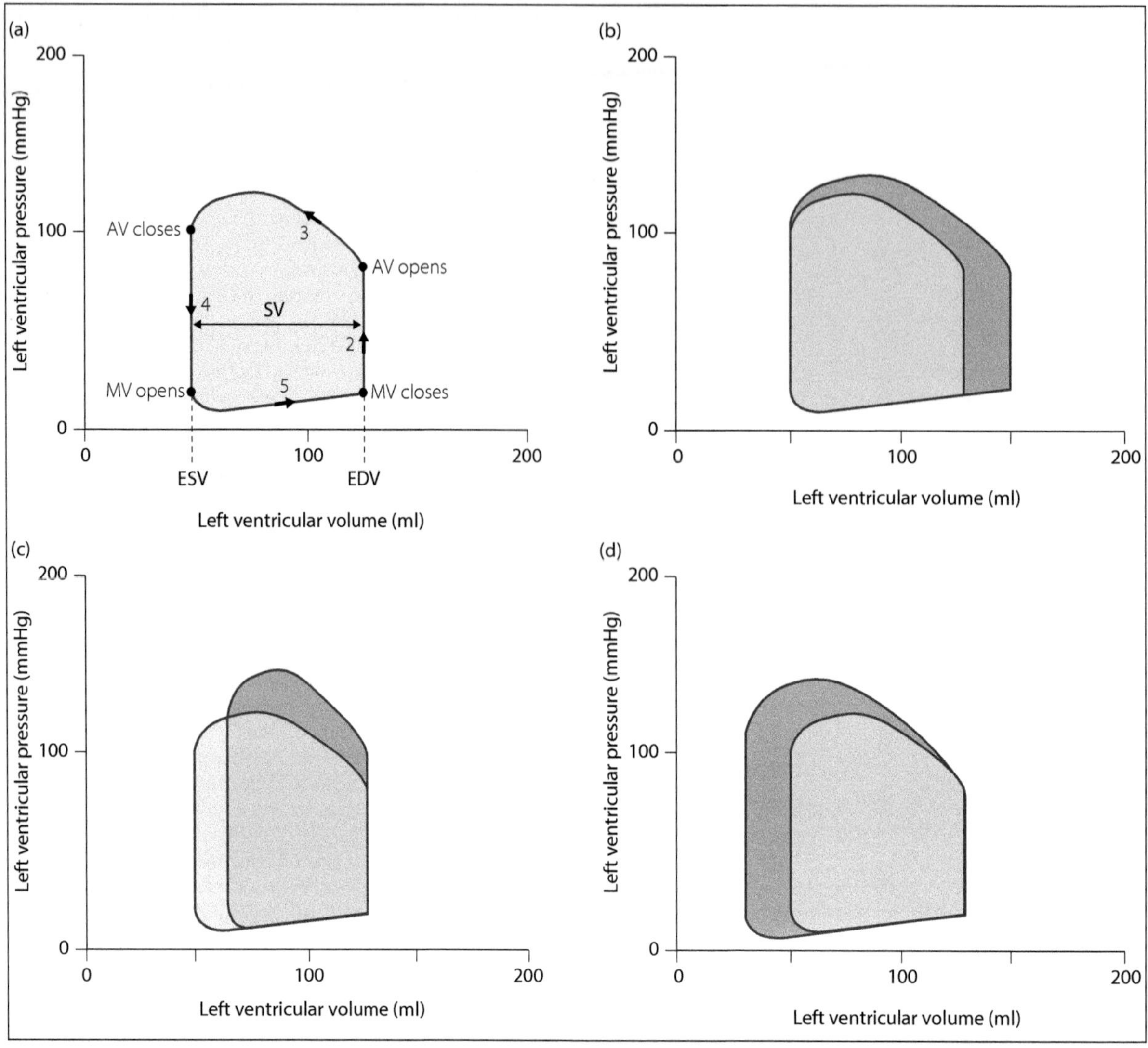

Fig. 34 Left ventricular pressure–volume 'loops' (*see text*): (a) baseline; (b) increased preload; (c) increased afterload; (d) increased contractility (darker shaded loops show the effect of changes)

- Effects:
  - ventricular end-diastolic pressure increases, leading to compensatory mechanisms:
    - ventricular hypertrophy.
    - increased force of contraction (**Starling's law**).
    - neuroendocrine response: mainly increased sympathetic activity, with tachycardia, vasoconstriction and increased contractility. **Aldosterone, renin/angiotensin** and **vasopressin** activity are increased, especially in chronic failure, but mechanisms are unclear. Salt and water retention result.
  - ventricular **compliance** is reduced, leading to increased atrial pressure and atrial hypertrophy. Eventually, ventricular dilatation occurs, with higher wall tension required to produce a given pressure (**Laplace's law**).
  - **coronary blood flow** is reduced by tachycardia, raised ventricular end-diastolic pressure and increased muscle mass.
  - left-sided failure may lead to **pulmonary oedema**, pulmonary hypertension, **$\dot{V}/\dot{Q}$ mismatch**, decreased lung compliance and right-sided failure.
  - right ventricular failure: **CVP** and **JVP** increase, with peripheral oedema and hepatic engorgement.
  - reduced peripheral blood flow leads to increased O_2 uptake and reduction of mixed venous Po_2.
  - sodium and water retention exacerbate oedema.
- Features:
  - reduced cardiac output may result in hypotension, confusion and coma.
  - left-sided failure:
    - dyspnoea, typically worse on lying flat (orthopnoea) and sometimes waking the patient at night (paroxysmal nocturnal dyspnoea).
    - peripheral vasoconstriction, basal crepitations, left ventricular hypertrophy. Extra **heart sounds**, e.g. gallop rhythm and **heart murmurs**, may be present. **Cheyne–Stokes respiration** may accompany low output.
    - acute pulmonary oedema.
  - right-sided failure:
    - raised JVP.
    - dependent oedema, e.g. ankles if ambulant, sacrum if bed-bound.

- hepatomegaly/ascites; the liver may be tender.
- right ventricular hypertrophy.
  - **CXR** may reveal cardiomegaly, upper-lobe blood diversion, fluid in the pulmonary fissures, **Kerley lines**, **pleural effusion** and pulmonary oedema. **ECG** may reveal ventricular hypertrophy and strain and arrhythmias.
- Management of acute heart failure:
  - confirm diagnosis using natriuretic peptide levels. Brain natriuretic peptide >100 ng/l or N-terminal pro-B-type natriuretic peptide >300 ng/l have high sensitivity and specificity.
  - in persistent hypoxaemia despite oxygen therapy or if acidosis present, consider **non-invasive positive pressure ventilation**.
  - give iv diuretic if peripheral or pulmonary oedema present, ± **ultrafiltration** if unsuccessful.
  - give iv nitrates (e.g. **glyceryl trinitrate**) if hypertension or myocardial ischaemia present.
  - perform transthoracic ultrasound:
    - if severe mitral regurgitation or critical aortic stenosis present, consider valve replacement.
    - if left ventricular systolic dysfunction present, start **ACE inhibitors** and **angiotensin II receptor antagonists** and titrate against effect. **Spironolactone** can be added in non-responsive failure. Start (or restart) **β-adrenergic receptor antagonists** once stable (i.e., when iv diuretics are no longer needed).
  - treat cardiogenic shock with iv inotropes and vasopressors and consider mechanical circulatory support (including **intra-aortic counter-pulsation balloon pump**).
- Response to treatment (Fig. 35):
  - 1: inotropic drugs/arterial vasodilators.
  - 2: diuretics/venous vasodilators.
  - 3:
    - drug combinations, e.g. inotropes + vasodilators; often produce the greatest improvement
    - intra-aortic counter-pulsation balloon pump.
- Management of chronic heart failure:
  - sympathetic nervous system blockade: β-adrenergic receptor antagonists (e.g. metoprolol, carvedilol, bisoprolol) have been shown to reduce mortality.

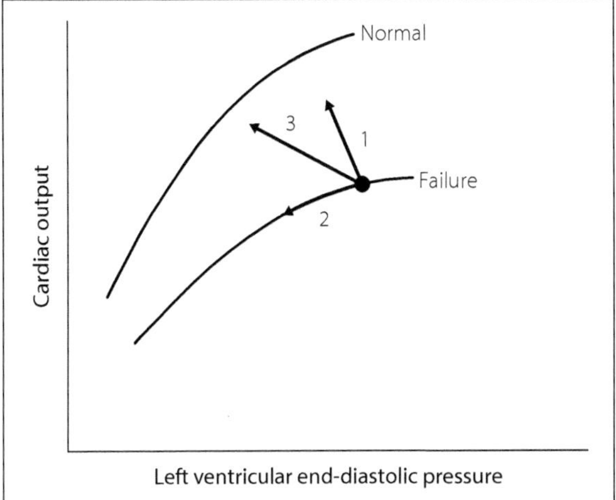

Fig. 35 Response to treatment of cardiac failure by Starling's curve (*see text*)

  - renin-angiotensin system blockade (e.g. with ACE inhibitors or angiotensin II receptor antagonists) improves survival. Direct renin inhibitors (e.g. aliskiren) and spironolactone also reduce mortality and morbidity.
  - **digoxin** can be of use in patients with severe functional limitation or ejection fractions <25%.
  - biventricular **cardiac pacing** improves exercise tolerance and quality of life in patients with unresponsive cardiac failure, even those in sinus rhythm.
- Anaesthetic considerations:
  - cardiac failure is associated with increased perioperative morbidity and mortality; it should therefore be treated preoperatively whenever possible.
  - treatment as above. Electrolyte disturbances and digoxin toxicity may occur.
  - anaesthetic drugs should be given in small doses and slowly, because:
    - **arm–brain circulation time** is increased.
    - increased proportion of cardiac output goes to vital organs, e.g. brain and heart; greater effects are seen on these organs than in normal cardiac output states.
  - danger of myocardial depression, hypoxia, arrhythmias.
  - use of epidural/spinal anaesthesia is controversial; the benefit of reduction of SVR may be offset by the risk of hypotension. Perioperative risk is not diminished.

Metra M, Teerlink JR (2017). Lancet; 390: 1981–95

Cardiac glycosides. Drugs derived from plant extracts; used to control ventricular rate in **atrial fibrillation** and **atrial flutter** and for symptomatic relief in **cardiac failure**. Actions are due to inhibition of the **sodium/potassium pump** and increased **calcium** mobilisation. The drugs have long **half-lives** (e.g. **ouabain** 20 h; **digoxin** 36 h; digitoxin 4 days), large **volumes of distribution** (e.g. digoxin 700 l) and low **therapeutic index**.

- Actions:
  - increase **myocardial contractility** and **stroke volume**.
  - decrease heart rate via direct effects on atrioventricular conduction and sinus node discharge; also act indirectly by increasing vagal tone.
- Side effects: as for **digoxin**. They are increased by **hypokalaemia**, **hypercalcaemia** and **hypomagnesaemia**. Toxicity is also more likely in **renal failure** and pulmonary disease.

Cardiac index (CI). **Cardiac output** corrected for body size, expressed in terms of body **surface area**:

$$CI = \frac{\text{cardiac output (l/min)}}{\text{surface area (m}^2\text{)}}$$

Normal value is 2.5–4.2 l/min/m^2.

Cardiac massage. Periodic compression of the heart or chest in order to maintain **cardiac output**, e.g. during **CPR**. Both open (internal) and closed (external) cardiac massage were developed in the late 1800s. The latter became more popular in the 1960s following clear demonstration of its value in dogs and humans, and was subsequently adopted by the American Heart Association and the **Resuscitation Council (UK)** as method of choice.

- Closed cardiac massage:
  - with the patient supine on a rigid surface, the heel of one hand is placed on the lower half of

the sternum. The other hand is placed on the first, with fingers clear of the chest. With elbows straight and shoulders vertically above the hands, regular compressions are applied, with a compression:relaxation ratio of 1:1. The sternum should be depressed 5–6 cm at each compression, at a rate of 100–120/min.

- efficacy is assessed by feeling the femoral or carotid pulse, although palpable peak pressures may not reflect blood flow. End-tidal CO_2 measurement should be used to assess adequacy of massage; an increase reflects improved cardiac output.
- may produce up to 30% of normal cardiac output with corresponding carotid and cerebral blood flow. Coronary flow is low during cardiac massage, and falls rapidly when massage is stopped.
- Technique in children up to 8 years:
  - under 1 year: tips of two fingers placed on the sternum, one finger's breadth below a line joining the nipples. The sternum is depressed by one-third of the depth of the child's chest at a rate of 100–120/min.
  - up to 8 years: heel of one hand placed over the lower half of the sternum, the fingers lifted to avoid applying pressure on the ribs. The sternum is depressed by one-third of the depth of the child's chest at a rate of 100–120/min.
- theories of mechanism (both may occur):
  - cardiac pump (as originally suggested): the heart is squeezed between sternum and vertebrae during compressions, expelling blood from the ventricles. During relaxation, blood is drawn into the chest by negative intrathoracic pressure, and the ventricles fill from the atria ('thoracic diastole'). Thought to be more important in children and when the heart is large.
  - thoracic pump: the theory arose from arterial and cardiac chamber pressure measurements during CPR, and from the phenomenon of **cough-CPR**. Positive intrathoracic pressure pushes blood out of heart and chest during compressions; reverse flow is prevented by cardiac and venous valves, and collapse of the thin-walled veins. During relaxation, blood is drawn into the chest by negative intrathoracic pressure.

  Intrathoracic pressures may be maximised by synchronising compressions with IPPV breaths, with or without abdominal binding or compression ('new' CPR). Devices used to augment the thoracic pump mechanism include:
  - automatic chest compressor ('chest thumper').
  - 'active compression/decompression' device: applies suction to the chest wall between compressions to increase venous return.
  - impedance valve inserted in the ventilating system: impedes passive inspiration during the 'release' phase, thus increasing intrathoracic negative pressure and increasing venous return. During compression the extra venous return results in greater cardiac output.

  Improved blood flows and outcome have been claimed but further studies are awaited.
- Open cardiac massage:
  - increasingly used, because blood flows and cardiac output are greater than with closed massage. Also, direct vision and palpation are useful in assessing cardiac rhythm and filling, and **defibrillation** and intra-cardiac injection are easier.
  - skin and muscle are incised in an arc under the left nipple in the fourth or fifth intercostal space, stopping 2–3 cm from the sternum to avoid the internal thoracic artery. Pericardium is exposed using blunt dissection and pulling the ribs apart. The heart is squeezed from the patient's left side using the left hand, with fingers anteriorly over the right ventricle and thumb posteriorly over the left ventricle. The rate of compressions is determined by cardiac filling. The descending aorta may be compressed with the other hand. The pericardium is opened for defibrillation or intracardiac injection. Because of the emergency nature of the procedure and the low risk of infection, sterile precautions are usually waived.
  - may also be performed per abdomen through the intact diaphragm; the heart is compressed against the sternum. **Minimally invasive direct cardiac massage** via a small thoracostomy has been described.
  - usually reserved for trauma, perioperative use, intra-abdominal or thoracic haemorrhage, massive PE, hypothermia, chest deformity and ineffective closed massage.

European Resuscitation Council (2015). Resuscitation; 95: 1–312

See also, Cardiac output measurement

Cardiac output (CO). Volume of blood ejected by the left ventricle into the aortic root per minute. Equals **stroke volume** (l) × **heart rate** (beats/min). Normally about 5 l/min (0.07 l × 70 beats/min) in a fit 70-kg man at rest; may increase up to 30 l/min, e.g. on vigorous **exercise**. Often corrected for body **surface area** (**cardiac index**).

Of central importance in maintaining **arterial BP** (equals cardiac output × **SVR**) and **O_2 delivery** to the tissues (**O_2 flux**).

Affected by metabolic rate (e.g. increased in **pregnancy**, **sepsis**, **hyperthyroidism** and exercise), drugs, and many other physiological and pathological processes that affect heart rate, **preload**, **myocardial contractility** and **afterload**.

- Distribution of normal CO (approximate values):
  - heart: 5%.
  - brain: 15%.
  - muscle: 20%.
  - kidneys: 20%.
  - liver: 25%.
  - rest: 15%.

  (for comparisons of blood flow and oxygen consumption, see Blood flow)
- Effects of **iv anaesthetic agents** on CO:
  - reduced by **propofol** > **thiopental** > **etomidate**, mostly via decreased contractility, though propofol may also cause vasodilatation and bradycardia.
  - increased by **ketamine**.
- Effects of **inhalational anaesthetic agents** on CO:
  - reduced by **enflurane** > **halothane** > **isoflurane**/**desflurane** > **sevoflurane** > **N_2O**. Proposed mechanisms include direct myocardial depression (via reduced concentration or modified activity of intracellular **calcium** ions during systole), inhibition of central or peripheral **sympathetic nervous system** outflow, and altered baroreceptor activity.
  - maintained by **diethyl ether** via sympathetic stimulation despite a direct myocardial depressant effect.

See also, Cardiac output measurement; Cardiac cycle

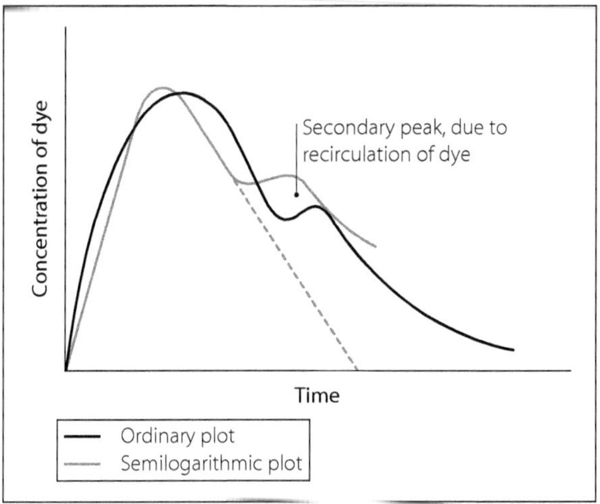

Fig. 36 Dilution technique for measuring cardiac output

Cardiac output measurement. Increasingly used in critically ill patients and as an important component of goal-directed therapy e.g. in the assessment of **fluid responsiveness**. The ideal monitor should be minimally or non-invasive, give a continuous reading, be accurate and reliable, cost effective and have a fast response time.

- Methods that have been used include:
  - **Fick principle**: most commonly O_2 consumption is measured using samples of mixed venous and arterial blood. Alternatively, CO_2 production may be measured, deriving arterial $P\text{CO}_2$ from end-tidal expired partial pressure. Mixed venous $P\text{CO}_2$ may be derived from analysis of expired gas collected in a closed rebreathing bag, using a **mass spectrometer**. Both methods are lengthy, complicated and unsuitable for routine use. A newer technique, **NiCO**, employs partial $P\text{CO}_2$ rebreathing and end-expiratory **CO_2 measurement**.
  - **dilution techniques**:
    - dye dilution: a known amount of dye is injected into the pulmonary artery, and its concentration measured peripherally using a photoelectric spectrometer. **Indocyanine green** is used because of its low toxicity, short half-life and absorption characteristics (i.e., unaffected by changes in O_2 saturation). Semilogarithmic plotting of the data curve is required, with extrapolation of the straight line obtained to correct for recirculation of the dye (Fig. 36). **Cardiac output** is calculated from the injected dose, the area under the curve within the extrapolated line and its duration. Curves of short duration are produced by high cardiac output; curves of long duration are produced by low cardiac output. Recirculation of dye may cause data from repeated injections to be affected by previous ones.

      The LiDCO system uses lithium as an alternative to indocyanine green; it is injected via a central venous catheter and measured by a lithium-sensitive electrode incorporated into an arterial cannula, e.g. placed in the radial artery. It combines pulse contour analysis with lithium indicator dilution to give continuous reading of **stroke volume**. The system requires recalibration every 8 hours and its calibration is affected by non-depolarising neuromuscular blocking agents.
    - thermodilution: suitable for use in the ICU or operating theatre:
      - intermittent: 5–10 ml cold dextrose or saline is injected through the proximal port of a pulmonary artery catheter, with temperature changes measured by a thermistor at the catheter tip. Injection is usually performed at end-expiration. A plot of temperature drop against time is produced as for dye dilution but without the secondary peak. Cardiac output is calculated by a bedside computer using the **Stewart–Hamilton equation** and an average of at least three measurements. Sources of inaccuracy include: the presence of intracardiac shunts or tricuspid regurgitation; inaccurate measurement of injectate volume or temperature; variation in the speed of injection; or if the thermistor is against a vessel wall. Repeated measurements are not affected by previous ones.

        In transpulmonary thermodilution cardiac output measurement (e.g. **PiCCO**), cold saline is injected via a central venous catheter and is dispersed into both intra- and extravascular spaces during passage through the lungs. Pulse contour cardiac output derived from rapid beat-to-beat analysis of the arterial (aortic) pressure wave is calibrated with an arterial thermodilution measurement to give a continuous indication of cardiac output. Use of an intra-arterial fibreoptic catheter and injection of cold dye allows measurement of intrathoracic blood volume and **extravascular lung water**.
      - continuous: employs a specially modified pulmonary artery catheter, containing a thermal filament extending 14–25 cm from its distal tip (thus lying within both the right atrium and the right ventricle during use), which adds an average of 7.5 W heat to the blood in a repetitive on–off sequence every 30–60 s. Changes in blood temperature are measured by a thermistor 4 cm from the catheter tip. A typical thermodilution 'washout' curve is constructed by applying a formula to correlate the thermistor temperature with the thermal energy input sequence. Cardiac output is computed from the curve as above.
  - FloTrac system: a pulse contour device that only requires an arterial line and is based on the principle that there is a linear relationship between pulse pressure and stroke volume. No external calibration is needed.
  - pressure recording analytic method (PRAM): measures the area under the curve of the arterial waveform.
  - **echocardiography**: two-dimensional echocardiography can be used to measure left ventricular **ejection fraction** and subsequent derivation of stroke volume. This relies on the shape of the ventricular cavity being ellipsoid, which may not always be the case. Three-dimensional and **transoesophageal echocardiography** may produce better results.
  - Doppler probe (oesophageal or suprasternal) may be used; the velocity of blood in the ascending aorta is measured using the **Doppler effect**, allowing estimation of the length of a column of blood passing through the aorta per unit time. This is multiplied by the cross-sectional area of the aorta to give cardiac output.

- **cardiac catheterisation** and angiography allow estimation of left ventricular volume and ejection fraction, as does **radioisotope** scanning.
- **impedance plethysmography** and **inductance cardiography**: thought to be useful in estimating changes in individual subjects, but not useful for absolute measurements.
- **aortovelography** and **ballistocardiography**: inaccurate.
- **electromagnetic flow measurement** may be achieved during surgery by placing a probe around the root of the aorta, but its use is limited.

Thermodilution and Doppler-based techniques have similar accuracy; devices based on bioimpedance, contour analysis, partial rebreathing and pulse wave analysis appear to be less reliable.

Thiele RH, Bartels K, Gan TJ (2015). Crit Care Med; 43: 177–85

Cardiac pacing. Repetitive electrical stimulation of myocardium, usually used to treat brady- or tachyarrhythmias.

- May be:
  - temporary:
    - transvenous: pacing wire passed via a central vein to the right ventricle under x-ray control. Usually bipolar, with two electrodes at the end of the wire; current passes from the distal to the proximal electrode, stimulating adjacent myocardium. Wires may be rigid, or flexible and balloon-tipped. Complications and technique of insertion are as for **central venous cannulation**; the procedure may be technically difficult. In biventricular pacing (for **cardiac failure**) a lead is also placed in the left ventricle via the coronary sinus.

      Indications include acute **MI** (inferior MI often requires temporary pacing; anterior often requires permanent pacing). Preoperative use should be considered in:
      - **heart block**: third-degree, sometimes second-degree (e.g. if Mobitz type II, associated with symptoms or intended surgery is extensive).
      - **bundle branch block**, e.g. symptomatic bifascicular block or P–R prolongation.
      - bradyarrhythmias.

      Technique of pacing:
      - bradyarrhythmias: once the wire is in place, the pacemaker box is set to V00 (*see later*) and the minimal current is determined (usually about 1–2 mA). The pacing output is set 2–3 times higher and the system changed to VVI. Failure to pace may result from disconnections, oversensing or failure to capture. The pacing box should be converted to V00 and the wire repositioned if necessary. Dual-chamber pacing may be achieved using a special atrial wire in addition to the ventricular one.
      - tachyarrhythmias, e.g. **SVT**, **atrial flutter**: A00 pacing is used, stimulating via a right atrial lead. The rate is slowly increased from 60/min to the spontaneous rate, held for 30 s, and pacing stopped. If unsuccessful, pacing at 400–800/min may be used to provoke **AF**, which usually reverts spontaneously to sinus rhythm. **VT** may be treated by slow ventricular V00 pacing, atrial pacing or ventricular pacing at 10%–30% faster rate than spontaneous for 5–10 beats only (burst pacing), with **defibrillation** available. Advantages over **cardioversion** include avoidance of anaesthesia and the adverse effects of electrical shock, easier repetition if unsuccessful and availability of pacing if bradycardia or asystole occurs.

      The pacing wire may conduct extraneous currents directly to the heart (e.g. from diathermy) with risk of **electrocution** (microshock).
    - transthoracic pacing may also be used, with large surface area skin electrodes (e.g. one over the cardiac apex, one over the right scapula or clavicle) and pulse duration of up to 50 ms to reduce cutaneous nerve and muscle stimulation. Avoids complications of transvenous pacing, and is quicker to perform.
    - transoesophageal pacing has also been used but is less reliable.
  - permanent: a pulse generator (**pacemaker**) is implanted subcutaneously. Electrodes are usually unipolar, i.e., one intracardiac electrode, with current returning to the pacemaker via the body. The heart electrode is usually endocardial, passed via a central vein; epicardial electrodes have been used.

Cardiac risk indices. Scoring systems for preoperative identification of patients at risk from major perioperative cardiovascular complications. The first, described by Goldman in 1977, was derived retrospectively from data from 1001 patients undergoing non-cardiac surgery; analysis identified nine differentially weighted variables correlating with increased risk:

- third **heart sound**/elevated **JVP**: 11 points.
- **MI** within 6 months: 10 points.
- **ventricular ectopic beats** >5/min: 7 points.
- rhythm other than sinus: 7 points.
- age >70 years: 5 points.
- emergency operation: 4 points.
- severe **aortic stenosis**: 3 points.
- poor medical condition of patient: 3 points.
- abdominal or thoracic operation: 3 points.

Patients with scores above 25 points had 56% incidence of death, with 22% incidence of severe cardiovascular complications. Corresponding figures for scores below 26 points were 4% and 17%, respectively, with 0.2% and 0.7% for scores less than 6.

The more recent Revised Cardiac Risk Index identifies six independent predictors of major cardiac complications following non-cardiac surgery:

- high-risk surgery (intraperitoneal, intrathoracic or suprainguinal vascular surgery).
- history of ischaemic heart disease.
- history of heart failure.
- cerebrovascular disease.
- insulin-dependent **diabetes mellitus**.
- preoperative serum creatinine >177 μmol/l.

Relative risk of major cardiac events for no factors is ~0.4%; for one factor it is ~1%, for two factors ~2% and for three or more factors ~6%.

Confirmed by other studies as having high specificity but low sensitivity; i.e., high-scoring patients are high risk, but not all high-risk patients are identified.

Other scoring systems are used for patients undergoing cardiac surgery (e.g. Parsonnet risk stratification scheme).

[Lee B Goldman, New York physician; Victor Parsonnet, New Jersey cardiac surgeon]

Fleisher LA, Fleischmann KE, Auerbach AD, et al (2014). Circulation; 130: 2215–45

See also, Ischaemic heart disease; Preoperative assessment

Cardiac surgery. First performed in the late 1800s but limited by the effects of circulatory interruption. Use of **hypothermia** increased the range of surgery possible, but 'open' heart surgery, i.e., employing **cardiopulmonary bypass** (CPB), was not developed until the 1950s.

- Indications:
  - requiring CPB:
    - **ischaemic heart disease**, i.e., **coronary artery bypass graft** (CABG; *but see later*).
    - **congenital heart disease**, e.g. **VSD, ASD, Fallot's tetralogy**.
    - others, e.g. **heart transplantation**, pulmonary embolectomy for **PE, chest trauma**.
  - not requiring CPB: patent **ductus arteriosus, coarctation of the aorta, pericarditis, cardiac tamponade**. CABG is increasingly performed 'off-pump'.
  - percutaneous procedures, e.g. **percutaneous coronary intervention** and stent insertion and pacemaker insertion, are usually performed under local anaesthesia. General anaesthesia is usually required for electrophysiological studies and insertion of implantable defibrillators.
- **Preoperative assessment** and management:
  - as for ischaemic and congenital heart disease. **Cardiac risk index** may be used for assessing risk. **Cardiac failure** is particularly important. Respiratory and cerebrovascular disease is common. Investigations include assessment of respiratory, renal, and liver function and coagulation studies. **CXR, ECG, cardiac catheterisation** studies and **echocardiography** are routine. Carotid **Doppler** studies may be indicated.
  - most cardiovascular drugs are continued. Oral **anticoagulant drugs** are usually stopped or changed to **heparin**.
  - traditional 'heavy' **premedication** regimens have largely been replaced with single-agent anxiolysis (e.g. temazepam) if required. Premedication is often omitted in emergency surgery. Antibiotic prophylaxis is usual.
- Induction and maintenance of anaesthesia:
  - **preoxygenation** is usually employed.
  - venous and **arterial cannulation** is usually performed under local anaesthesia. **Central venous cannulation** is often reserved until the patient is anaesthetised.
  - **opioid analgesic drugs** are used to provide a smooth induction and avoid the hypertensive response to intubation, e.g. **fentanyl** 5–10 μg/kg, **alfentanil** 30–50 μg/kg or **remifentanil** 1 μg/kg followed by 0.05–2 μg/kg/min. High-dose techniques (e.g. fentanyl or alfentanil up to 100–125 μg/kg) have been used but may necessitate prolonged postoperative IPPV.
  - iv induction with standard agents in small doses, as for ischaemic heart disease. Benzodiazepines and **etomidate** are commonly used.
  - standard **neuromuscular blocking drugs** are suitable; **pancuronium** has often been used as it is long-acting and maintains BP, although it may cause tachycardia.
  - N_2O is often avoided because of myocardial depression, especially in combination with high-dose opioids. It may also increase SVR and the size of air bubbles. Volatile **inhalational anaesthetic agents** are commonly used. **Isoflurane** was found to cause **coronary steal** in early animal models, but this concern has been refuted; there is now good evidence that volatile agents (including isoflurane) protect against subsequent ischaemic injury (**ischaemic preconditioning**). **TIVA** with propofol is also commonly used. No primary anaesthetic agent has been found to be superior to any other.
  - maintenance of myocardial oxygen balance and minimisation of ischaemia are of overriding importance; aims include avoidance of tachycardia, maintenance of oxygenation and adequate diastolic coronary perfusion pressure.
- **Monitoring**:
  - 5-lead ECG.
  - direct arterial BP measurement.
  - **CVP** measurement.
  - **pulmonary artery catheterisation** may be used in complex cases. Left-sided pressures may be measured directly via a needle during surgery.
  - **transoesophageal echocardiography** is routinely used. An oesophageal Doppler probe may be used to assess perioperative myocardial workload and **myocardial ischaemia**.
  - **temperature measurement** (core and peripheral).
  - electrolyte and **blood gas interpretation** should be readily available. Activated clotting time (ACT) may be determined in the operating theatre (*see Coagulation studies*).
  - a urinary catheter is usual.
- Pre-CPB management:
  - stimulation during sternotomy may require further analgesia to prevent tachycardia and hypertension.
  - after baseline ACT measurement, **heparin** 300–400 units/kg is injected via a tested central line. **Prostacyclin** has been used but is expensive and its role is uncertain. ACT measured after 1 min should be >480 s or three times baseline; aortic and right atrial cannulation may then be performed for CPB.
- Management during CPB:
  - circulation is gradually taken over by the pump.
  - drugs are diluted by the crystalloid prime, thus further iv boluses are often required, e.g. opioid, benzodiazepine, induction agent, neuromuscular blocking drug. Fentanyl may be taken up by the oxygenator membrane. Drugs, including inhalational agents, may be added to the CPB circuit.
  - **haemodilution** occurs.
  - hypothermia is used to reduce myocardial O_2 requirements and provide neuroprotection; the aorta is cross-clamped and **cardioplegia** used, lowering heart temperature to 10°–15°C. Intentional fibrillation is sometimes used, avoiding cardioplegia. Mild hypothermia (32°–35°C) is often used to provide some neuroprotection while avoiding problems of moderate (28°–32°C) and profound (22°–27°C) hypothermia, especially disturbed coagulation. Lower temperatures (15°–20°C) are used during circulatory arrest.
  - IPPV is stopped; continuous positive pressure is sometimes applied to maintain some lung expansion. Air is thought to be better than 100% O_2 because of increased **atelectasis** with the latter; N_2O is avoided because of the risk of **gas embolism**.
  - optimal perfusion pressure is controversial; 50 mmHg is generally thought to be the minimum. CPB details are also controversial, e.g. type of oxygenator, pulsatile/non-pulsatile flow.
  - SVR decreases as haemodilution occurs; vasopressor drugs (e.g. **phenylephrine** or **metaraminol**) may be needed to maintain perfusion pressure. SVR then slowly increases due to absorption of the crystalloid

and vasodilatation with GTN or **phentolamine** may be needed. Some cardiovascular drugs such as **nicorandil** and **angiotensin converting enzyme inhibitors** may exacerbate hypotension.
- solubility of CO_2 increases as temperature falls, causing a reduction in arterial $P\text{CO}_2$ (and therefore a respiratory **alkalosis**). Hypocapnia causes cerebral vasoconstriction and reduces **cerebral blood flow**. Thus acid–base management during hypothermic CPB may involve addition of CO_2 to the circuit in order to maintain a constant pH ~7.4 ('pH stat'), thereby preserving cerebral blood flow. As blood samples are heated to 37°C in most analysers, this approach requires the analysis results to be temperature-corrected. The alternative is to manage pH uncorrected for the patient's temperature ('alpha stat'). The superiority of one approach over the other is controversial.
- ACT is checked every 30 min, with further heparin given if necessary, e.g. one-quarter to one-half initial dose. **Potassium** is added as required. **Bicarbonate** is usually not administered unless **base deficit** exceeds 7–8 mmol/l. Blood is transfused to keep the **haematocrit** above 0.2–0.3.
- after repair of the lesion, the cross-clamp is removed and rewarming undertaken. Cardiac activity (usually **VF** but sometimes sinus rhythm) usually returns spontaneously. Internal **defibrillation** is performed if required; 5–10 J (biphasic) or 10–20 J (monophasic) is usually adequate. **Cardiac pacing** is sometimes required; epicardial wires may be inserted prophylactically for postoperative use. Adequate haematocrit and normal $P\text{O}_2$, pH and electrolyte concentrations are ensured.
- CPB blood flow is gradually decreased as **cardiac output** increases. Drug boluses are given iv as before; inotropic support is often required. Manual IPPV helps expel air from the pulmonary vessels.
- transoesophageal echocardiography is routinely used to exclude residual defects, assess myocardial function and ensure adequate de-airing of the left heart.

- Post-CPB and postoperative care:
  - left atrial pressure is optimised to 8–12 mmHg; vasodilators are used to accommodate CPB fluid volume.
  - a low-output state may occur, especially if ventricular function was poor preoperatively and ischaemia time prolonged. It may be improved by:
    - **inotropic drugs**: **calcium** is often used as a temporary measure but may worsen **reperfusion injury**. Others include **dopamine**, **dobutamine**, **adrenaline** and **isoprenaline**; more recently **enoximone**, **milrinone** and **dopexamine**. The choice is according to individual patient and drug characteristics, and clinician preference.
    - vasodilators (often combined with inotropes).
    - correction of potassium/acid–base imbalance.
    - **intra-aortic counter-pulsation balloon pump** may be required.
  - heparin is reversed with **protamine**, injected slowly to reduce side effects, especially **pulmonary hypertension**. 1 mg/mg heparin is usually used.
  - hypertension is common if left ventricular function is good, especially in aortic valve disease; vasodilators may be required.
  - temperature may fall as core heat is transferred to the periphery.
  - **arrhythmias** and **heart block** may occur.
  - pericardial and pleural drains are inserted before sternal closure.
  - transfer to ICU must be carefully managed because of the potential dangers from interrupted monitoring and infusions, and movement.
  - specific postoperative concerns include:
    - bleeding: may be surgical, or caused by consumption or dilution of **platelet** and **coagulation** factors during CPB, the effects of massive **blood transfusion**, or inadequate reversal of heparin. Perioperative **antifibrinolytic drugs** and **desmopressin** are routinely used to reduce bleeding.
    - treatment of hyper-/hypotension and arrhythmias.
    - low-output state, as earlier. Cardiac tamponade may necessitate thoracotomy on ICU.
    - maintenance of fluid balance and urine output. The crystalloid load from CPB usually causes diuresis but **pulmonary oedema** may occur, especially if cardiac output is low.
    - rewarming; central/peripheral temperature difference is a useful indication.
    - maintenance of electrolyte, acid–base and blood gas balance. Hypokalaemia is common.
    - IPPV is usually continued for a few hours, sometimes overnight. Opioid/benzodiazepine boluses are commonly used for **sedation**. Immediate extubation after surgery is increasingly performed in appropriately selected cases. Usual criteria for **weaning** include cardiovascular and respiratory stability, adequate warming and perfusion, good urine output, minimal blood loss and good conscious level. Impaired gas exchange may be associated with pre-existing lung disease, atelectasis, and CPB-related factors (e.g. embolisation with bubbles and platelet aggregates, complement activation), especially if CPB was prolonged.
    - CNS changes: **stroke** occurs in less than 2% of patients undergoing open-heart surgery, but subtle changes are found in up to 60%, thought to be related to embolisation (e.g. bubbles, aggregates during CPB) and/or inadequate perfusion. Effects are possibly reduced by filtering the arterial inflow line.

See also, Targeted temperature management

Cardiac tamponade. Compression of the heart by fluid (e.g. blood) within the pericardium, restricting ventricular filling and reducing **stroke volume** and **cardiac output**.

Myocardial O_2 supply is reduced by hypotension, increased end-diastolic pressure, tachycardia and compression of epicardial vessels. Tamponade should be differentiated from **pneumothorax** and **cardiac failure**.
- Features:
  - dyspnoea, restlessness, oliguria, hypotension, peripheral vasoconstriction. **JVP**, **CVP** and **left atrial pressure** are raised, and **pulsus paradoxus** is present. Jugular venous distension may occur during inspiration or when pressure is applied over the liver (Kussmaul's sign). Cardiovascular collapse and death may occur, especially if acute (e.g. following **chest trauma**).
  - **ECG** complexes may be small, and the heart shadow globular and enlarged on the **CXR**. Confirmed by **echocardiography**.

Immediate management is **pericardiocentesis**; surgery may be required subsequently.

- Anaesthetic considerations: drugs or manoeuvres that reduce **venous return**, **heart rate** or **myocardial contractility** should be avoided, especially with coexistent **hypovolaemia**. **IPPV** should be performed cautiously, if at all; techniques allowing spontaneous ventilation (e.g. with **ketamine**) may be safer.

[Adolf Kussmaul (1822–1909), German physician]
See also, Cardiac surgery

Cardiogenic shock. **Shock** due to primary cardiac pump failure. Most severe form of acute **cardiac failure**, accounting for <5% of cases. Diagnosis is suggested by signs of organ hypoperfusion and acute haemodynamic changes, including:
- systolic BP 30 mmHg below basal levels for more than 30 min.
- **cardiac index** <2.2 l/min/m^2.
- **arteriovenous oxygen difference** >5.5 ml/100 ml.
- **pulmonary capillary wedge pressure** (PCWP) >15 mmHg.

In 80% of adults, caused by **acute coronary syndromes** (including **MI**) affecting either right or left ventricle; other causes include decompensation of chronic cardiac failure and valvular disease but it may also follow **cardiac surgery**, **chest trauma** and acute **myocarditis**. **Heart rate** and **SVR** are usually increased to compensate for hypotension, exacerbating myocardial O_2 supply/demand imbalance. Lactic acidosis resulting from poor perfusion further impairs **myocardial contractility**.

- Features:
    - as for shock.
    - increased left ventricular end-diastolic pressure and **pulmonary oedema** are usual. However, relative **hypovolaemia** may be present due to redistribution of fluid to lungs, pathological vasodilatation, previous fluid restriction, diuretic therapy and sweating. Right-sided failure may occur, e.g. in right ventricular infarction.
- Management:
    - treatment of underlying cause; if caused by coronary artery occlusion, early **percutaneous coronary intervention** or **coronary artery bypass graft** improves prognosis.
    - direct arterial BP measurement and assessment of organ perfusion using lactate levels.
    - optimising left ventricular end-diastolic pressure; PCWP is a more useful guide than **CVP**, unless failure is predominantly right-sided. A PCWP of 18–22 mmHg is thought to be optimal for the failing heart, even though this is higher than normal. Fluids are given if PCWP is low. **Inotropic drugs** (e.g. **dobutamine**, **levosimendan** or **milrinone**) and **vasodilator drugs** are given if PCWP is high but evidence of their efficacy is lacking.
    - **intra-aortic counter-pulsation balloon pump** has been used in the past but does not improve mortality. **Extracorporeal membrane oxygenation** and/or ventricular assist devices may be considered as a 'bridge' to recovery (e.g. in acute myocarditis) or **heart transplantation**. Newer ventricular assist devices (e.g. Heartware) are now being trialled as 'destination therapies'.

Prognosis has improved over the last decade but mortality remains about 40%; early death is associated with the development of **SIRS** and **MODS**, older age, lower left ventricular ejection fraction, increased lactate levels and **renal failure**.

Mebazaa A, Tolppanen H, Mueller C, et al (2016). Int Care Med; 42: 147–63
See also, Cardiac failure

Cardioinhibitory centre (Cardioinhibitory area). Consists of the nucleus ambiguus and adjacent neurones in the ventral medulla, with some input from the dorsal motor nucleus and nucleus of the tractus solitarius. Produces vagal 'tone', increased by **baroreceptor** discharge. Also receives afferents from higher centres. Efferents pass to the vasomotor centre, inhibiting it, and thence to the heart via the **vagus nerve**. Thus involved centrally in controlling **arterial BP**.

Cardiomyopathy. Defined by the American Heart Association (AHA) as a myocardial disorder in which the heart muscle is structurally and functionally abnormal (not caused by **ischaemic heart disease**, **hypertension**, valvular disease or congenital heart disease).

- Classified by the AHA into:
    - primary:
        - genetic (N.B. a proportion of cases are not associated with an identified familial/genetic transmission):
            - hypertrophic (obstructive; HOCM):
                - characterised by left ventricular hypertrophy especially affecting the upper interventricular septum, causing left ventricular outflow obstruction. Epidemiological screening studies suggest a prevalence of 1 in 500 in the general population, with the majority undiagnosed. Usually familial.
                - causes **arrhythmias**, syncope, angina, **cardiac failure** and sudden **cardiac arrest**, especially in otherwise fit young adults. Infective **endocarditis** may occur.
                - treatment includes **diuretics**, **antiarrhythmic drugs** and **β-adrenergic receptor antagonists**; the latter reduce force and rate of contraction, reducing outflow obstruction. Conversely, **digoxin** should be avoided. **Anticoagulant drugs** are often used in sustained arrhythmias. Surgical myectomy or alcohol ablation is used to relieve obstruction and severe refractory symptoms; **heart transplantation** may be required.
                - anaesthetic management includes avoidance of tachycardia and increased myocardial work, arrhythmias, hypovolaemia and reduced SVR.
            - arrhythmogenic right ventricular cardiomyopathy (ARVC):
                - characterised by progressive replacement of right ± left ventricular myocardium with adipose and fibrous tissue. Usually familial.
                - may result in sudden death from arrhythmias, usually arising from the right ventricle.
                - treated mainly with antiarrhythmic drugs, catheter ablation or implantable cardioverter defibrillators; heart transplantation has been used.
            - dilated (congestive)
                - most common in men aged 20–60. About a third of cases are thought to be familial. The most common form of non-ischaemic cardiomyopathy.

- causes reduced contractility and **ejection fraction**, with ventricular dilatation, cardiac failure, arrhythmias, angina and systemic embolism from mural thrombus.
- prognosis is poor; death is usually within a few years of presenting with cardiac failure.
- treatment includes digoxin, diuretics, antiarrhythmic drugs, implantable defibrillators, **vasodilator drugs** and anticoagulant drugs.
- anaesthetic management: as for ischaemic heart disease and cardiac failure.
- myocardial depression, **hypovolaemia** and increased SVR are particularly hazardous.

- restrictive:
  - due to fibrosis or infiltration causing stiffness of the cardiac chambers. Thought to be the least common type of cardiomyopathy.
  - effects and management are as for constrictive **pericarditis.** Ion channelopathies and conduction disorders have been suggested as suitable for inclusion in the classification, and there is evidence of overlap (e.g. between cardiomyopathy and Brugada syndrome) but the precise relationship is not clear.
- acquired: **myocarditis**; peripartum (cardiac failure occurring in the last month of **pregnancy** or 5 months after delivery, in the absence of other causes); stress (Takotsubo) cardiomyopathy.

- secondary:
  - infiltrative e.g. **amyloidosis**, Gaucher's disease.
  - storage diseases e.g. haemochromatosis, Fabry's disease.
  - toxicity: drugs, **alcoholism, heavy metal poisoning**, chemotherapy (e.g. anthracyclines).
  - inflammatory: **sarcoidosis**; endocrine disease (**diabetes mellitus**, thyroid disease); neuromuscular disease (e.g. **muscular dystrophies**); nutritional deficiencies; autoimmune disease.

Definitive diagnosis requires exclusion of other causes of heart failure and careful history-taking to identify hereditary causes. Genetic testing is increasingly used. **ECG** is usually non-specific, showing arrhythmias, **bundle branch block**, ventricular hypertrophy and ischaemia. **CXR** may show cardiac enlargement and pulmonary oedema. **Echocardiography**, **cardiac catheterisation** and **nuclear cardiology** may be useful.

[Pedro and Josep Brugada, Spanish cardiologists; 'takotsubo', Japanese word for round-bottomed pot used to catch octopuses (because the left ventricle takes on a similar shape on imaging); Phillipe Gaucher (1854–1918), French physician; Johannes Fabry (1860–1930), German dermatologist]

See also, Defibrillators, implantable cardioverter

Special issue (2017). Circ Res; 121: 711–891

Cardioplegia. Intentional **cardiac arrest** caused by coronary perfusion with cold electrolyte solution, to allow **cardiac surgery**. After establishment of **cardiopulmonary bypass**, a cannula is inserted into the ascending aorta and connected to a bag of solution (traditionally at 4°C), having excluded air bubbles. After aortic cross-clamping distal to the cannula, the solution is passed under 200–300 mmHg pressure into the aortic root, closing the aortic valve and perfusing the coronary arteries. In aortic valve incompetence, individual coronary artery cannulation may be required. Severe coronary stenosis may require further injection of solution through a bypass graft or retrograde perfusion via the coronary sinus. **Asystole** usually occurs after 100–200 ml, but 1 l is used (15–20 ml/kg in children) in order to cool the heart to 10°–12°C.

Further infusion may be required in prolonged surgery. Cold saline is placed around the heart to maintain **hypothermia.**

- Solutions used may contain:
  - NaCl 110–140 mmol/l: prevents excess water accumulation. May increase calcium entry if sodium concentration is too high.
  - KCl 10–20 mmol/l: causes depolarisation and cardiac arrest in diastole, reducing myocardial O_2 demand. Higher concentrations may cause arterial spasm.
  - $MgCl_2$ 16 mmol/l and $CaCl_2$ 1.2–2.2 mmol/l: reduce automatic rhythmogenicity and protect against potassium-induced damage post-bypass. Excessive calcium may cause persistent myocardial contraction (stone heart). Magnesium reduces calcium entry.
  - $NaHCO_3$ 0–10 mmol/l.
  - procaine 0–1 mmol/l: membrane stabiliser, reducing arrhythmias postbypass.
  - other additives are more controversial, and include:
    - buffers, e.g. histidine and tromethamine: help maintain normal intracellular pH and encourage ATP generation.
    - metabolic substrates, e.g. glucose and amino acids: increase ATP generation.
    - **mannitol**: reduces water accumulation and may improve cardiac function.
    - **free radical** scavengers.
    - **corticosteroids.**
    - **calcium channel blocking drugs.**
- Other controversies:
  - use of blood instead of crystalloid: improved oxygenation with optimal osmotic, buffer and metabolic make-up, but increased viscosity limits the use of hypothermia.
  - oxygenation of the solution.
  - use of warm solution: may cause better myocardial relaxation, with reduced membrane and protein damage associated with low temperatures.
  - continuous versus intermittent injection.

Usual solution pH is 5.5–7.8 and osmolality 285–300 mosmol/kg.

Cardiopulmonary bypass (CPB). Developed largely by Gibbon in the 1950s from animal experiments performed in 1937. Haemolysis was caused by initial disc/bubble oxygenators; improved membrane oxygenators were developed in the late 1950s. Used in **cardiac surgery**; similar techniques are used for **extracorporeal membrane oxygenation** and **extracorporeal CO_2 removal in respiratory failure.**

- Principles:
  - venous drainage: under gravity via a right atrial cannula or separate superior/inferior vena caval cannulae if the right atrium is opened. Blood also drains via right atrial and left heart suckers/vents to avoid pooling of blood in the operative field. Blood passes through a filter and defoaming chamber, which may be combined with a reservoir and/or oxygenator.
  - oxygenator: older bubble oxygenators have been replaced by membrane oxygenators since the 1980s, the latter being associated with greater haemodynamic stability, reduced coagulopathy and fewer embolic phenomena.

Consist of hollow capillary fibres through which blood passes, with gas exchange across their walls. Flat membrane oxygenators are also available. Can also be used for concurrent **ultrafiltration**. Most incorporate temperature exchangers, and may therefore be used in the treatment of severe, refractory **hypothermia**. CO_2 and O_2 are supplied independently to the oxygenator as required, e.g. 2.5% CO_2 in O_2.
    - pumps: usually rotating roller pumps using wide tubing. Rotating chambers (centrifugal pumps) are also used, reducing damage to blood components. Flow is traditionally non-puslatile but pulsatile flow may provide better organ perfusion, with lower **vasopressin** and angiotensin levels; however, the equipment required is more complex and expensive. Pulsations may be synchronised with the ECG if the heart is pumping. Flows used vary between centres but are usually 1.0–2.4 l/min/m^2 surface area (up to 80 ml/min/kg).
    - arterial return: via ascending aorta (rarely, femoral artery) using a short, wide cannula to reduce resistance and avoid accidental cannulation of aortic branches. The return is filtered to remove platelet aggregates, fibrin and debris. 5–40 μm filters are standard; the smaller filters reduce microemboli but increase platelet consumption and risk of **complement** activation.
    - ultrafilter/haemoconcentrator: after separation from CPB, modified **ultrafiltration** may be performed to remove inflammatory mediators, reduce extravascular lung water (improving pulmonary compliance) and raise haematocrit.
- Use:
    - disposable systems are usually employed.
    - the system is primed with **crystalloid** usually, although **colloid** or blood (in neonatal circuits) may be used. The resulting haemodilution improves perfusion at low temperatures, and is usually corrected postoperatively by an appropriate diuresis.
    - anticoagulation, introduction and termination of CPB: as for cardiac surgery.
- Complications:
    - technical, e.g. leaks, bubbles, disconnections, obstruction, coagulation, power failure. Vascular damage may occur during cannulation.
    - embolisation with clot, debris, bubbles and defoaming agent. Bubbles may enter via the heart cavity during surgery, especially at end of bypass. Subtle neurological changes are thought to be related to microembolisation.
    - related to surgery or anticoagulation.

[John H Gibbon (1903–1974), US surgeon]

Cardiopulmonary exercise testing (CPX/CPEX testing; CPET). Integrated assessment of cardiopulmonary function at rest and during incrementally increasing levels of exercise. BP, ECG, ventilatory parameters and respiratory gases are measured throughout, and used to derive two major indicators of cardiopulmonary function: maximum oxygen uptake ($\dot{V}O_2$max) and **anaerobic threshold**. Several protocols exist, most utilising a treadmill or exercise bicycle for approximately 10 min. A bicycle is most commonly used for perioperative assessment as it is more stable and measurements are less prone to movement artefact; arm pedals have been used for those unable to use a standard bicycle.

- Indications include:
    - preoperative evaluation and risk stratification to help guide decisions regarding **prehabilitation**, choice of surgical and anaesthetic techniques, optimising medication preoperatively etc., i.e., as a valuable tool in enhanced **recovery** after surgery (ERAS) programmes
    - evaluation for heart/lung transplantation.
    - investigation of undiagnosed exercise intolerance.
    - evaluation of exercise tolerance, functional capacity, disability or response to treatment.

Thought to predict the patient's capacity to respond to the physiological stress of major surgery. Is now considered an established predictor of perioperative morbidity and mortality in patients undergoing pulmonary resection, aortic aneurysm surgery and major colonic and urological surgery.

Levett DZ, Grocott MP (2015). Can J Anaesth; 62: 131–42

Cardiopulmonary resuscitation (CPR). Over many centuries, numerous techniques have been tried in order to restore life; early attempts included use of heat, smoke, cold water, beating and suspension from ropes.

- Historical aspects:
    - Artificial ventilation was developed within the last ~500 years:
        - use of **bellows** via the mouth or nose is attributed to **Paracelsus** in the early 1500s. Used via tracheal tubes in the 1700s, e.g. by **Kite**.
        - postural techniques, e.g. compressing the chest and abdomen from behind with the victim prone, moving the arms, or using tilting boards: used from the 1850s.
        - **expired air ventilation**: developed in the 1700s, although reported earlier.
    - **cardiac massage**, external and internal, was first attempted in the late 1800s; external massage was popularised in the early 1960s.
    - **defibrillation** was investigated in animals in the 1700s/1800s; internal defibrillation was performed in humans in the 1940s and external defibrillation in the 1950s.
- CPR is divided into:
    - **basic life support** (BLS): traditionally without any equipment, and therefore suitable for 'lay-person resuscitation'. Increasingly includes the use of simple equipment (defined as 'basic life support with airway adjuncts'), e.g. **airways, facemasks, self-inflating bags, oesophageal obturators, SADs.**
    - **advanced life support**: as described previously, plus use of specialised equipment, techniques (e.g. tracheal intubation), drugs and monitoring.

Regular updates on guidelines are provided by the **Resuscitation Council (UK), European Resuscitation Council, International Liaison Committee on Resuscitation** and the American Heart Association (*see Basic life support, adult; Advanced life support, adult*).

See also, Brainstem death; Cardiopulmonary resuscitation, neonatal; Cardiopulmonary resuscitation, paediatric; Cough-CPR

Cardiopulmonary resuscitation, neonatal. Prompt resuscitation is important in order to prevent permanent mental or physical disability. Neonatal **cardiac arrest** is almost always caused by **hypoxaemia** and thus prompt management of **apnoea** and airway obstruction is vital.

- Equipment required includes:
  - a tilting resuscitation surface, with radiant heater, clock and pulse **oximetry**.
  - **suction equipment**.
  - O_2 with funnel and **facemasks**.
  - **self-inflating bag** (volume 250 ml, with pressure relief valve set at 30–35 cmH_2O).
  - pharyngeal **airways** (sizes 000, 00 and 0).
  - **tracheal tubes** (uncuffed). Suitable sizes:
    - 2.0–2.5 mm for babies under 750 g weight or 26 weeks' gestation.
    - 2.5–3.0 mm for 750–2000 g or 26–34 weeks.
    - 3.0–3.5 mm for over 2000 g or 34 weeks.
  - **laryngoscope**, usually with straight blade (size 0–1).
  - iv cannulae, including umbilical venous and arterial catheters.

Requirement for resuscitation may be anticipated from the course of pregnancy and labour and **fetal monitoring**. Elements of the **Apgar score** may also be useful.

Greater emphasis is placed on maintaining a patent airway and providing adequate ventilation than for adult **CPR**; **cardiac massage** is only started once adequate ventilation has been achieved.

- 2015 recommendations of the **Resuscitation Council (UK)**:
  - resuscitation is the immediate priority in all babies unless they are uncompromised, when a delay in cord clamping of >1 min from delivery is recommended.
  - dry, stimulate and wrap the baby. Body temperature should be kept at 36.5°–37.5°C unless therapeutic hypothermia is intended. All neonates should be placed under a radiant heater in the first instance; other measures include using warmed humidified gases, thermal mattresses, increased room temperature and wrapping in food-grade plastic, especially in babies <32 weeks' gestation.
  - airway management: early aggressive suctioning of pharynx and trachea is no longer recommended, and emphasis is on initiating lung inflation within the first minute of life. Suction is only indicated if there is copious thick meconium visible in the mouth and the baby is non-vigorous. To open the airway the head should be placed in the neutral position (with the aid of a towel placed under the shoulders) and a jaw thrust manoeuvre applied if required.
  - initial assessment of respiratory effort, heart rate (ideally using ECG or oximetry), colour and tone:
    - adequate respiration, heart rate >100 beats/min, the baby is centrally pink with good tone: no further treatment required.
    - heart rate <100 beats/min or absent/inadequate respiration: 5 inflation breaths lasting for 2–3 s, to aid lung expansion. Airway pressures should not exceed 30-35 cmH_2O (20 cmH_2O in the preterm neonate). Air should be used in the first instance (up to 30% O_2 if preterm), switching to oxygen if there is poor initial response (ideally guided by oximetry. Acceptable pre-ductal O_2 saturations: 60% at 2 min; 70% at 3 min; 80% at 4 min; 85% at 5 min; and 90% at 10 min). If there is no response, adequacy of ventilation (i.e., good chest wall movement) should be checked and a further 5 inflations attempted, with airway adjuncts if appropriate. If still no response, tracheal intubation should be considered.
  - subsequent management:
    - if heart rate <60 beats/min despite good ventilation, **cardiac massage** should be instituted, with both hands encircling the chest or using two fingers (*see Cardiopulmonary resuscitation, paediatric*). Compressions should occur at 120 beats/min, depressing the sternum one-third of the depth of the chest, and with a compression:ventilation ratio of 3:1. Standard ventilation breaths are 1 s in duration. Cardiac massage is futile unless adequate ventilation is provided.
    - if heart rate remains <60 beats/min after 30 s of cardiac massage, drugs should be given:
      - umbilical venous catheterisation is usually the most accessible route for iv administration of drugs (N.B. the umbilical cord contains a single vein and two arteries).
      - initial iv drugs: adrenaline 1:10 000:0.1 ml/kg initially, then 0.3 ml/kg, then 1 ml/kg after 4.2% **bicarbonate** 1–2 ml/kg (higher concentrations have been associated with intraventricular haemorrhages). The cannula should be flushed with saline after each drug.
      - administration of adrenaline via the tracheal tube is not recommended, but if it is given would require doses of 0.5–1 ml/kg. Bicarbonate must not be given via the tracheal route.
      - others:
        - crystalloid (e.g. NaCl 0.9%) 10 ml/kg if hypovolaemia or sepsis is suspected.
        - 10% **dextrose** 2–2.5 ml/kg if **hypoglycaemia** is present.
        - **naloxone** 10 mg/kg im, iv or sc, repeated every 2–3 min or 60 µg/kg im as a single injection, if the mother has received opioids during labour.
    - in babies breathing spontaneously who have or are at risk from respiratory distress, nasal **CPAP** is preferred to tracheal intubation.

Congenital abnormalities (e.g. **diaphragmatic hernia**, **tracheo-oesophageal fistula**) should be considered in babies who do not respond to resuscitation.

Wyllie J, Bruinenberg J, Roehr CC, et al (2015). Resuscitation; 95: 242–62

See also, Pugh, Benjamin

Cardiopulmonary resuscitation, paediatric. The same principles apply as for adult **CPR**, but primary cardiac disease is uncommon. **Sinus bradycardia** progressing to **asystole** is more common, especially if due to **hypoxaemia** or **haemorrhage**. Thus **cardiac arrest** is often secondary to respiratory arrest or exsanguination, and usually represents a severe insult.

- 2015 Recommendations of the **Resuscitation Council (UK)**:
  - basic life support (BLS):
    - assess as for adults. A lone rescuer should continue for about a minute before seeking help.
    - 'ABC' of resuscitation:
      - Airway: as for adults.
      - Breathing: 5 initial rescue breaths by **expired air ventilation**, each over 1 s; mouth to mouth and nose if <1 year, mouth to mouth otherwise. Only 5 breaths should be attempted; if unsuccessful, move on to circulation.
      - Circulation: up to 10 s to check for pulse or signs of life, then external **cardiac massage** at 100/min. In infants this may be delivered using two fingers; in older children the heel of the palm or both hands may be used. Whatever the technique, compressions should be applied to the lower half

of the sternum, compressing the chest by one-third of the anterior–posterior diameter of the chest (4 cm for an infant, 5 cm for a child).
  - ratio for cardiac massage:breaths of 15:2.
- advanced life support:
  - iv access/monitoring/airway management as for adults. An intraosseous needle should be used if venous access is difficult (*see Intraosseous fluid administration*). For monitoring small children via the defibrillator, it may be easier to apply the paddles to the front and back of the chest.
  - asystole/**pulseless electrical activity**:
    - **adrenaline** 10 μg/kg iv/im, repeated every 3–5 min. Tracheal administration is no longer recommended, but was previously given at 10 times the iv dose.
    - BLS for a further 2 min.
  - **VF/VT**:
    - **defibrillation** using 4 J/kg (one paddle below the right clavicle, the other at the left anterior axillary line).
    ventilation and chest compressions for further 2 min, then repeat the above.
    - repeat as necessary; after the third shock give amiodarone 5 mg/kg and an immediate fourth shock. Consider reversible causes of cardiac arrest.
- Special situations: **choking**, **electrocution**, **near-drowning**, **trauma**, neonatal CPR (*see Cardiopulmonary resuscitation, neonatal*).
- Other drugs:
  - **atropine** is no longer recommended for non-shockable rhythms.
  - bicarbonate: 1 mmol/kg iv (1 ml/kg 8.4% solution).
  - **calcium** chloride: 0.2 mmol/kg iv (0.3 ml/kg 10% solution).
  - glucose 10%: 1 g/kg iv (10 ml/kg).

Fluid bolus in hypovolaemia: 10 ml/kg colloid (traditionally 4.5% albumin initially).

Maconochie I, Bingham R, Eich C, et al (2015). Resuscitation; 95: 222–47

See also, Paediatric anaesthesia

Cardioversion, electrical. Restoration of sinus rhythm by application of synchronised DC current across the heart. Current delivery is synchronised to occur with the **R wave** of the **ECG**, because delivery during ventricular repolarisation may produce VF (**R on T phenomenon**).
- Used for:
  - **AF**, particularly of recent onset.
  - **atrial flutter**; usually successful with low energy.
  - **VT**, usually successful with low energy.
  - **SVT**.

Energy levels of 20–200 J are usually used.

Digoxin-induced arrhythmias may convert to serious ventricular arrhythmias; therefore digoxin is usually withheld for at least 24 h.

In chronic atrial arrhythmias, anticoagulation is often administered to reduce risk of systemic embolisation. Preparation of the patient, drugs and equipment, and monitoring should be as for any anaesthetic. The procedure is painful, therefore requiring brief sedation/anaesthesia. A single iv agent is commonly used, e.g. **propofol**. Further injections may be required if repeated shocks are delivered.

See also, Defibrillation

Care bundles. Group of evidence-based clinical interventions used in the management of specific conditions or procedures. Originally conceived in the critical care setting, they aim to improve outcomes by standardising care. Although broadly similar between institutions, each care bundle is adapted for local use. Commonly used as criteria for clinical **audit**; implementation of a care bundle element is a dichotomous state, and compliance requires completion of all elements. Examples include: the ventilator care bundle for the prevention of **ventilator-associated pneumonia**; the **central venous cannulation** care bundle for the prevention of **catheter-related sepsis**; and the severe **sepsis** care bundle.

Care of the critically ill surgical patient (CCrISP). Course run by the Royal College of Surgeons of England, primarily aimed at basic surgical trainees. Using a systematic means of patient assessment (similar to other **ALS**, **ATLS**, **APLS** courses), candidates are taught to manage immediate life-threatening events (e.g. airway obstruction, haemorrhage, sepsis, injury) and to organise subsequent care (monitoring, pain relief, nutrition) in the general ward, operating theatre, **HDU** or **ICU**. Consists of lectures, workshops and simulated patient assessments.

Care Quality Commission (CQC). Body responsible for regulating health and adult social care in England. In 2009, it replaced the Commission for Social Care Inspection, the Mental Health Act Commission, and the Healthcare Commission (which itself replaced the Commission for Health Improvement, the National Care Standards Commission and the Audit Commission in 2004). The CQC registers, monitors, inspects and rates care providers and services, with the aim of ensuring safe, effective and high-quality care, and encouragement of improvement. Other bodies have similar roles in the devolved nations e.g. Healthcare Improvement Scotland, Healthcare Inspectorate Wales, and the Regulation and Quality Improvement Authority in Northern Ireland.

Carfentanil. **Opioid analgesic drug**, developed in 1974. About 10 000 times as potent as **morphine**, and used to immobilise large animals. Reportedly used (with **remifentanil**) by aerosol to end a hostage crisis in a Moscow theatre in 2002, with ~130 deaths.

Carotid arteries. Anatomy is as follows (*see Fig. 116;* **Neck, cross-sectional anatomy**):
- common carotids:
  - right: arises from the brachiocephalic artery behind the sternoclavicular joint.
  - left: arises from the aortic arch medial to the left lung, **vagus** and **phrenic nerves**, then passes behind the sternoclavicular joint.
  - ascends in the neck within the carotid sheath.
  - divides level with C4 into internal and external carotids.
- internal carotid:
  - bears the **carotid sinus** at its origin.
  - runs firstly lateral, then behind and medial to the external carotid, with the internal **jugular vein** laterally and vagus and sympathetic chain posteriorly.
  - passes medial to the parotid gland, styloid process, glossopharyngeal nerve and pharyngeal branches of the vagus (with the external carotid lateral to these structures).
  - passes through the carotid canal at the base of the **skull**, with the internal jugular now lying posteriorly. After a tortuous path through the canal, it divides into the middle and anterior cerebral arteries.

- external carotid:
  - lies first deep, then lateral to the internal carotid, with the internal jugular posteriorly.
  - enters the parotid gland, ending behind the neck of the mandible.
  - branches, from below upwards:
    - ascending pharyngeal.
    - superior thyroid.
    - lingual.
    - facial.
    - occipital.
    - posterior auricular.
    - superficial temporal.
    - maxillary.

See also, Carotid body; Carotid endarterectomy; Cerebral circulation

Carotid body. Small (2–3 mm) structure situated above the carotid bifurcation on each side; involved in the chemical control of breathing. Contains:

- glomus cells (type I cells): depolarise in response to hypoxia and **cyanide**, releasing **dopamine** that stimulates the nerve endings via D_2 receptors.
- glial cells (type II cells): provide structural support to glomus cells.
- nerve endings: glossopharyngeal nerve afferents.

Afferents pass via the glossopharyngeal nerve to the **brainstem** regulatory centres.

Below arterial $P\text{O}_2$ of 13.3 kPa (100 mmHg), rate of discharge rises greatly for any further decrease. Response time is rapid enough to cause fluctuations in discharge rate with breathing. Discharge rate is also increased by a rise in arterial $P\text{CO}_2$, or fall in arterial pH.

Each carotid body receives 0.04 ml blood/min, equivalent to 2 l/100 g tissue/min (the highest blood flow per 100 g tissue in the body). Because of such high blood flow, dissolved O_2 alone is enough to provide the requirement for O_2; thus discharge is not increased by **anaemia** or **carbon monoxide poisoning**, where O_2 carriage by haemoglobin is reduced but arterial $P\text{O}_2$ is not.

Fitzgerald RS, Eyzaquirre C, Zapata A (2009). Adv Exp Med Biol; 648: 19–28

See also, Breathing, control of

Carotid endarterectomy. Performed in patients with carotid stenosis, with the aim of reducing the risk of **stroke**. Endarterectomy significantly reduces the risk of stroke in symptomatic patients with severe stenosis (>70% occlusion); surgery is less beneficial in moderate (50%–70%) stenosis and harmful in minor (<30%) stenosis and near-occlusion. Benefit in asymptomatic stenosis is less well established. Perioperative stroke occurs in up to 7% of cases; risks are greatest in the elderly (though the benefits of surgery have also been shown to be greatest in this group). Nerve injury in the neck (usually transient) may occur in up to 20% of cases. Perioperative mortality is about 5% for symptomatic and 3%–4% for asymptomatic stenosis, mostly from **MI** or stroke. Mortality is greatest in older women and those with symptomatic cardiovascular co-morbidity. The role and indications for percutaneous carotid artery stenting continue to be evaluated; the incidence of minor stroke following the procedure is higher than for endarterectomy (*see Neuroradiology*).

- Anaesthetic considerations:
  - preoperatively: often elderly patients with generalised arteriopathy. **Smoking, diabetes mellitus** and **hypertension** are common. Drug therapy may include **aspirin, dipyridamole** and other **antiplatelet drugs**.
  - intraoperatively:
    - direct arterial BP monitoring is mandatory, with meticulous avoidance of hypotension.
    - performed under general or regional anaesthesia (**cervical plexus block**); choice of technique does not affect outcomes. Regional anaesthesia in the awake patient allows early recognition of ischaemic symptoms, but may not be tolerated by all patients. General anaesthesia with **inhalational anaesthetic agents** may provide a degree of neuroprotection; methods of neurological monitoring include **transcranial Doppler ultrasound, EEG** and measurement of **evoked potentials** and internal carotid artery stump pressure.
    - evidence of cerebral ischaemia (e.g. after carotid clamping) should prompt consideration of shunt insertion or administration of **vasopressor drugs** to increase perfusion pressure.
    - **positioning of the patient** and restricted access, with risks of tracheal tube kinking/displacement and injury to the eyes. Vertebrobasilar insufficiency (often occurring with cervical spondylosis) is common and necessitates careful positioning of the neck during intubation and surgery.
    - **capnography** allows adjustment of IPPV to normocapnia and aids detection of **gas embolism.**
    - manipulation of the **carotid sinus** may lead to bradycardia and hypotension. Infiltration of **lidocaine** around the sinus prevents this, but may be followed by hypertension postoperatively.
  - postoperatively:
    - patients may require HDU/ICU admission for monitoring and further care.
    - assessment of neurological function: deficit occurs in <7% of patients. The hyperperfusion syndrome is caused by increased blood flow (in vessels with poor **autoregulation**) following relief of stenosis. It may result in headache, convulsions and intracranial haemorrhage.
    - control of BP: hypertension is common and may be related to pain, agitation, dysfunction of **carotid sinus** baroreceptors or impending neurological damage. Commonly used agents include **labetalol** and **hydralazine**. Hypotension is less common and may be associated with bradycardia.
    - **airway obstruction** may occur if bleeding occurs. Even after uncomplicated cases, some degree of airway oedema is common.

Erickson KM, Cole DJ (2013). Curr Opin Anaesthesiol; 26: 523–8

Carotid sinus. Dilatation of the internal **carotid artery**, just above the carotid bifurcation. **Baroreceptors** present in the walls respond to increased distension caused by raised **arterial BP** by increasing the rate of discharge via the carotid sinus nerve, a branch of the glossopharyngeal nerve. Resultant inhibition of the **vasomotor centre** and stimulation of the **cardioinhibitory centre** cause reduction in sympathetic tone and increase in vagal tone, respectively. BP and heart rate therefore fall (the **baroreceptor reflex**). The baroreceptors also respond to the rate of increase of BP. Similar baroreceptors exist in the walls of the aortic arch.

See also, Carotid sinus massage

Carotid sinus massage. Manual stimulation of the **carotid sinus** baroreceptors, causing reflex inhibition of the **vasomotor centre** and activation of the **cardioinhibitory centre.**

Depression of sinoatrial (SA) and atrioventricular (AV) nodes results in bradycardia and may reduce myocardial contractility.

The sinus is gently massaged below the angle of the jaw, where the carotid pulse is palpable. Concurrent ECG recording should be available. Only one side (the right is usually more effective) should be massaged at one time and for not longer than 5 s, or excessive reduction in **cerebral blood flow** may occur. It should be performed with care in patients with evidence of cerebrovascular disease. May restore sinus rhythm in **SVT**, and may aid diagnosis of other arrhythmias by slowing the ventricular rate, e.g. **AF** and **atrial flutter**. In sinus tachycardia, it causes gradual slowing of rate with speeding up when massage is stopped. May also demonstrate SA and AV node disease by causing severe bradycardia or sinus arrest.

Syncope, transient ischaemic attacks and **stroke**, **asystole** and **VT** are rare complications.

Carticaine, *see Articaine*

Caspofungin. Echinocandin **antifungal drug** used for treatment of invasive candidiasis and aspergillosis.
- Dosage: 70 mg by iv infusion on the first day, 50 mg daily thereafter.
- Side effects: GIT upset, tachycardia, flushing, dyspnoea, electrolyte disturbances, allergic reactions.

Catabolism. Metabolic breakdown of complex molecules into simple, smaller ones, often associated with the liberation of **energy**.
- Includes:
  - digestion of foodstuffs as in **metabolism** of **carbohydrate**, **fat** and **protein**.
  - mobilisation of body stores, e.g. in **malnutrition**, severe illness and the **stress response to surgery**. These may occur in combination in ICU because of:
    - inadequate **nutrition**, e.g. nil by mouth, ileus, fluid restriction.
    - increased energy and O_2 consumption associated with injury, especially multiple **trauma**, **burns** and **sepsis**.

  Includes breakdown of:
    - protein: causes increased urinary urea excretion and may contribute to reduced plasma **albumin**. Nitrogen loss may exceed 20–30 g/day, i.e., up to 5-kg body weight/week (mainly lost from muscle). **Amino acids** produced are used for synthesis of **glucose**, acute-phase reactants and cell components.
    - fat: triglycerides from adipose tissue are broken down to fatty acids (used as an energy source) and glycerol (used to synthesise glucose).
    - carbohydrates: **glycogen** is broken down to glucose.

See also, Nutrition, total parenteral

Catecholamines. Group of substances containing catechol (benzene ring with OH groups at positions 1 and 2) and amine portions; includes naturally occurring (e.g. **dopamine**, **adrenaline**, **noradrenaline**) and synthetic (e.g. **dobutamine**, **isoprenaline**) compounds. Catecholamines act at dopaminergic and **adrenergic receptors** in the CNS and **sympathetic nervous system**; although many other substances may produce similar effects (i.e., are **sympathomimetic drugs**), they may not be true catecholamines.

Synthesis of naturally occurring catecholamines proceeds in many steps from the amino acid phenylalanine (Fig. 37a). The rate-limiting step is the hydroxylation of

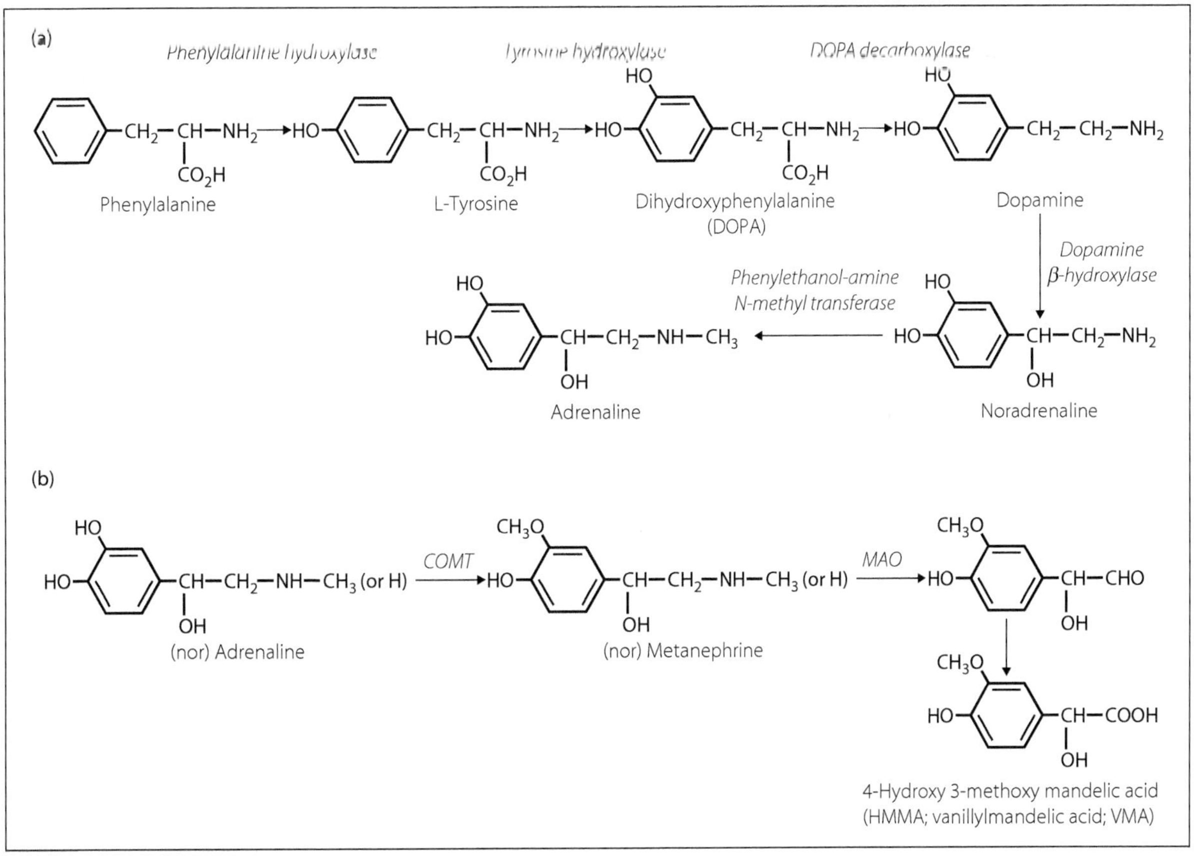

(a)
Phenylalanine hydroxylase · *Tyrosine hydroxylase* · *DOPA decarboxylase*
Phenylalanine → L-Tyrosine → Dihydroxyphenylalanine (DOPA) → Dopamine
Dopamine β-hydroxylase: Dopamine → Noradrenaline
Phenylethanol-amine N-methyl transferase: Noradrenaline → Adrenaline

(b)
(nor) Adrenaline → *COMT* → (nor) Metanephrine → *MAO* → 4-Hydroxy 3-methoxy mandelic acid (HMMA; vanillylmandelic acid; VMA)

Fig. 37 (a) Catecholamine synthesis. (b) Catecholamine metabolism

tyrosine to DOPA (dihydroxyphenylalanine). Formation of dopamine occurs in the cytoplasm; it is then taken up by an active process into vesicles and converted to noradrenaline.

Catecholamines are metabolised via **catechol-*O*-methyl transferase** (COMT) and **monoamine oxidase** (MAO) (Fig. 37b).

See also, Inotropic drugs

Catechol-O-methyl transferase (COMT). **Enzyme** present in most tissues (especially liver and kidneys) except nerve endings; catalyses the transfer of a methyl group from adenosylmethionine (a **methionine** derivative) to the 3-hydroxy group of the catechol part of **catecholamines**. Involved in the metabolism of circulating catecholamines and their derivatives, while catecholamines at nerve endings are metabolised by **monoamine oxidase**.

Inhibitors of COMT (e.g. entacapone) are used as adjuncts to levodopa in **Parkinson's disease**; they block metabolism of levodopa in the tissues, thus increasing its activity.

Catheter mounts (Tracheal tube adaptors). Original term refers to adaptors connecting the fresh gas supply to a catheter passed through the larynx into the trachea (**insufflation technique**), before tracheal intubation became popular. Now refers to adaptors connecting the **tracheal tube** to the end of the **anaesthetic breathing system**. Various **connectors** fit between the distal end and the tracheal tube; the proximal end should be of standard 22-mm taper. Some contain **heat–moisture exchangers**.

Catheter-related sepsis. Strictly, **nosocomial infection** involving a catheter at any site, but the term usually refers to intravascular devices (peripheral, central venous or arterial). Defined in clinical practice as isolation of the same organism from both a percutaneous blood culture and a catheter segment from a patient with symptoms and signs of bloodstream infection, in the absence of any other septic focus. Occurs in about 5% of cases in ICU. Should be differentiated from colonisation (growth of >15 colony-forming units from a catheter segment in the absence of local or systemic infection), which occurs in about 25% of cases, and local infection (erythema, tenderness, induration and purulence within 2 cm of the skin insertion site). In all cases, organisms are thought to grow in 'biofilms' on the surface of the catheter.

- Risk factors include:
  - site of catheter: affects central lines > arterial lines > peripheral lines. Subclavian lines are the least likely to become infected. Femoral lines are usually considered more susceptible to infection but this may not be so if proper care is taken during and after placement.
  - age <1 year or >60 years.
  - **immunodeficiency** or use of **immunosuppressive drugs**.
  - severity of underlying illness.
  - presence of other focus of infection.
  - emergency insertion or use of cut-down to insert line.
  - use of the line for parenteral feeding.
  - length of time the line is in situ is usually cited as a risk factor, but evidence is weak if adequate attention is paid to aseptic insertion and line handling/maintenance.

Organisms involved usually come from the patient's own skin flora or from medical or nursing staff. *Staphylococcus aureus* or *S. epidermidis* are most commonly responsible, although gram-negative organisms may be involved. Candida may also be responsible.

- Management:
  - taking of **blood cultures** peripherally and via the line. Use of an endoluminal brush has been described.
  - exclusion of other sources of infection.
  - **antibacterial drugs**.
  - removal, and sending for culture, of the distal part of the line involved.
  - if possible, insertion of a new line at the same site should be avoided, as should changing a suspected line over a guide-wire.
  - the following has been used for lines whose removal is considered especially undesirable (e.g. being used for long-term parenteral nutrition and poor venous access elsewhere): concomitant antibiotic (in high concentration) and fibrinolytic agent into the catheter as a 'lock', with parenteral antibacterial therapy. The line should be removed if the patient's condition has not improved after 36 h; use of the catheter may be restarted after 48 h if improvement occurs.
- Prevention:
  - use of **care bundles** to support best practice.
  - use of intravascular catheters only when definitely indicated, and removal when no longer needed.
  - scrupulous aseptic technique during insertion and aftercare. Chlorhexidine 2% is more effective than 10% povidone–iodine and 70% alcohol for cleansing the skin.
  - regular replacement of catheters (e.g. every 3–7 days) is often advocated, but there is little evidence supporting this.
  - daily inspection of insertion sites and regular changing of sterile dressings (24–48 h). Clear plastic dressings have been associated with increased rates of infection in some studies, but evidence is conflicting. Use of antimicrobial ointment or chlorhexidine-impregnated sponges at the skin entry sites may be beneficial.
  - use of a separate dedicated lumen for parenteral nutrition.
  - measures of unproven benefit include tunnelling of catheters, routine flushing and the use of in-line filters. Catheters incorporating antibacterial or heparin-treated coatings have been claimed to reduce colonisation with organisms, especially when tunnelling is also performed.

Chittick P, Sherertz RJ (2010). Crit Care Med; 38(Suppl): S363–72

See also, Central venous cannulation; Central venous cannulation, long-term; Infection control; Intravenous fluid administration; Sepsis

Cauda equina syndrome. Syndrome characterised by so-called 'red flag' symptoms of severe lower back pain, sciatica (usually bilateral), saddle and/or genital sensory disturbance and bladder, bowel and sexual dysfunction. Caused by radiculopathy affecting the nerve roots of the cauda equina (L2–S5). Has been associated with central intervertebral disc prolapse, spinal stenosis, vertebral fracture and malignancy, and requires rapid spinal decompression.

May also follow **spinal anaesthesia**, especially if a continuous microcatheter infusion technique is used. Possible mechanisms of injury include:
- direct trauma from lumbar puncture, intraneural injection, trauma from the catheter or epidural haematoma.
- poor mixing of local anaesthetic, especially hyperbaric, in the CSF. This results in pooling of anaesthetic in the terminal dural sac, with associated neurotoxicity (especially with **lidocaine**).
- passage of the catheter into the subdural space with high local concentrations of local anaesthetic around the cauda equina.

It has been suggested that the cauda equina nerve fibres are more vulnerable to damage because they lack protective sheaths. Symptoms may appear soon after surgery and may be permanent.

Todd NV (2017). Br J Neurosurg; 31: 336–9

See also, Transient radicular irritation syndrome

Caudal analgesia Produced by injection of **local anaesthetic agent** into the **sacral canal**, a continuation of the **epidural space**. First described independently by Cathelin and Sicard in 1901, predating lumbar **epidural anaesthesia**. Easily performed, but with a high failure rate in adults due to variations in sacral anatomy. Produces block of the sacral and lumbar nerve roots; thus ideal for perineal surgery. Higher blocks require greater volumes of anaesthetic solution, and are more unpredictable. Useful as a supplement to general anaesthesia, and for provision of postoperative analgesia. Also used for treatment of chronic back pain. Catheter insertion has been performed for continuous caudal block.

- Technique:
  - usually performed with the patient in the lateral position, with the knees drawn up to the chest. The prone and knee–elbow positions may also be used.
  - the sacral hiatus lies at the third point of an equilateral triangle formed with the two posterior superior iliac spines (each overlain by a skin dimple). The sacral cornua are palpable on either side of the hiatus.
  - using an aseptic technique, a needle is introduced in a slightly cranial direction through the hiatus. Ordinary iv needles and cannulae are commonly used, although specific caudal needles are available.
  - when the canal is entered (a click may be felt as the sacrococcygeal membrane is pierced), the needle is directed cranially, and advanced not more than 2 cm into the canal (in adults). The dura normally ends at S2, level with the posterior superior iliac spines, but may extend further.
  - after aspirating to confirm absence of blood or CSF, local anaesthetic is injected, feeling for accidental subcutaneous injection with the other hand. There should be little resistance to injection with a 19–21 G needle. If the patient is awake, pain is felt if the needle tip is under the periosteum of the anterior wall of the canal. Caudal needles may bear a side hole to prevent this complication.
- Doses:
  - 20–30 ml 0.25%–0.5% **bupivacaine**, or 1%–2% **lidocaine** with adrenaline, in young adults, reduced in the elderly. The average volume of the sacral canal is 30–35 ml.
  - 0.5 ml/kg 0.25% bupivacaine is used for sacrolumbar block in children; 1 ml/kg for upper abdominal blockade and 1.25 ml/kg for midthoracic blockade (using saline to increase the volume of injectate without exceeding the maximum safe dose of bupivacaine). 0.125% bupivacaine provides analgesia with less motor block.

Complications are as for epidural anaesthesia, but much less common. Insertion of the needle into the rectum, or presenting part of the fetus in obstetrics, has been reported.

[Fernand Cathelin (1873–1945), French surgeon; Jean-Athanase Sicard (1872–1929), French neurologist and radiologist]

See also, Vertebral ligaments

Causalgia, *see Complex regional pain syndrome*

Caval compression, *see Aortocaval compression*

Cave of Retzius block, *see Retzius cave block*

CAVH, Continuous arteriovenous haemofiltration, *see Haemofiltration*

CAVHD, Continuous arteriovenous haemodiafiltration, *see Haemodiafiltration*

CCF, Congestive cardiac failure, *see Cardiac failure*

CCrISP, *see Care of the critically ill surgical patient*

CCT, Central conduction time, *see Evoked potentials*

CCU, *see Coronary care unit*

Cefazolin (Cephazolin). **Antibacterial drug**; first-generation **cephalosporin** used to treat respiratory, urinary tract and soft tissue infections. Not recommended in meningitis as it crosses the blood–brain barrier poorly. 80% protein-bound and excreted largely unchanged in the urine.
- Dosage: 0.5–1.0 g iv/im bd/qds.
- Side effects: blood dyscrasias, hepatic impairment.

Cefotaxime. Antibacterial drug; third-generation **cephalosporin** active against gram-positive and gram-negative organisms including haemophilus, klebsiella, streptococcus, staphylococcus (but less so than **cefuroxime**), proteus, serratia, enterobacter and escherichia species. Also used for empirical treatment of bacterial **meningitis** in adults and children. **Half-life** is about 1 h; extensively protein-bound, it undergoes hepatic metabolism to an active metabolite, with 50%–80% excreted unchanged in the urine.
- Dosage: 1–2 g bd iv/im, up to 12 g/day in divided doses in severe infections.
- Side effects: phlebitis, rash, GIT upset, colitis.

Cefpirome. Fourth-generation **cephalosporin** with good activity against gram-positive organisms, including staphylococcus. Excreted largely unchanged by the kidney; thus reduced dosage is required in renal impairment.
- Dosage: 1–2 g iv bd.
- Side effects: headache, nausea, hepatic impairment, skin rashes, taste disorders.

Cefradine (Cephradine). First-generation **cephalosporin** similar to **cefazolin**. 10% protein-bound and excreted unchanged in the urine.

- Dosage: 0.5–1.0 g iv/im bd/tds/qds.
- Side effects: as for cefazolin.

Ceftazidime. Third-generation **cephalosporin** especially active against multiresistant gram-negative bacteria and pseudomonas. Largely unmetabolised and 90% excreted in the urine. Also available in combination with avibactam, a non-**β-lactam** β-lactamase inhibitor (2 g ceftazidime + 0.5 g avibactam).
- Dosage: 1–2 g iv/im bd/tds.
- Side effects: painful im injections, diarrhoea, hepatic impairment.

Ceftriaxone. Third-generation **cephalosporin** structurally related to **cefotaxime**, with similar spectrum of activity, although more active against enterobacter. Increasingly used as the first choice for empirical treatment of bacterial **meningitis**. Has the longest **half-life** of all the cephalosporins (5–9 h). Undergoes biliary and renal excretion.
- Dosage: 1–4 g iv/im od.
- Side effects: pain on injection, leucopenia, hepatic and renal impairment, precipitation (as calcium salt) in urine or gallstones.

Cefuroxime. Second-generation **cephalosporin**, most closely related to cefamandole. Has a wide spectrum of activity against both gram-positive and gram-negative organisms, including β-lactamase-producing staphylococcus, haemophilus and some enterobacter species. Penetrates well into **CSF**. The only second-generation agent that achieves therapeutic CSF levels. Excreted unchanged in the urine.
- Dosage: 0.75–1.5 g iv/im tds/qds. Surgical prophylaxis: 1.5 g iv (two further doses of 750 mg may be given for high-risk procedures).
- Side effects: GIT upset, rashes, rarely blood dyscrasias.

Cell salvage. Intraoperative collection and processing of blood from the surgical field for subsequent reinfusion of autologous red cells. Used during procedures known to involve significant blood loss (e.g. cardiac, complex orthopaedic) and for patients who refuse allogeneic **blood products** (e.g. **Jehovah's Witnesses**).
- Consists of three phases:
  - collection; via a dedicated double-lumen suction tube. One lumen is used for collection of blood, while the other is used to add heparinised saline to it.
  - processing; the anticoagulated salvaged blood is then filtered, centrifuged (to separate out the red cell component), washed (to remove free haemoglobin, plasma and heparin) and suspended in normal saline. The final **haematocrit** is 50%–80%.
  - storage/transfusion; recommended maximum storage time of salvaged blood is 6 h.

The main benefit of cell salvage is the reduction of the need for allogeneic **blood transfusion** and its associated risks/costs. Autologous blood may also provide superior oxygen delivery compared with allogeneic blood owing to higher levels of **2,3-DPG** and greater mean red cell viability. There is evidence of improved outcomes (e.g. cardiac events, infection rates) in specific types of surgery (e.g. major orthopaedic, oesophagectomy).

General risks include **gas embolism**, haemolysis, contamination with infective agents and **coagulation disorders**. Complications are rare and are no greater than with allogeneic transfusion.
- Areas of controversy:
  - obstetrics: despite theoretical risk of **amniotic fluid embolism** during **caesarean section**, now considered safe because levels of amniotic fluid in washed, salvaged blood are very low.
  - malignancy: previously an absolute contraindication due to risk of disseminating tumour cells; now increasing evidence supports its use (with leucocyte depletion filters, LDFs) in specific procedures (e.g. radical prostatectomy/cystectomy for urological malignancies).
  - microbiological contamination: although contraindicated by manufacturers, use in the presence of contamination with enteric contents and systemic sepsis is not associated with increased adverse outcomes; use of LDFs, prophylactic antibiotics and increased saline wash volumes significantly reduces infection risk.
  - **sickle cell anaemia**: generally avoided in these patients, but has been safely used in those with sickle cell trait.
  - Jehovah's Witnesses: potentially life-saving in these patients, cell salvage is usually acceptable to them, although consent must be sought on an individual basis. May require a special set-up, e.g. continuous flow of blood rather than intermittent.

Ashworth A, Klein AA (2010). Br J Anaesth; 105; 401–16

Cellulitis. Skin infection resulting in local inflammation (warmth, erythema and pain), usually with fever and leucocytosis. Lymphangitis and lymphadenitis may be present. Modes of pathogen entry include local trauma (including insertion of iv catheters) and abrasions. More common in those with impaired lymphatic drainage and in iv drug abusers. Organisms commonly responsible include β-haemolytic streptococci and *Staphylococcus aureus*, thus guiding initial **antibacterial drug** therapy if microbiological identification is uncertain (e.g. **phenoxymethylpenicillin** with **flucloxacillin**, or **erythromycin** or **co-amoxiclav** alone).

Burnham JP, Kirby JP, Kollef MH (2016). Int Care Med; 42: 1899–911

See also, Staphylococcal infections; Streptococcal infections

CEMACH, Confidential Enquiries into Maternal and Child Health, *see Confidential Enquiries into Maternal Deaths*

CENSA, *see Confederation of European National Societies of Anaesthesiologists*

Central anticholinergic syndrome. Syndrome caused by the use of **anticholinergic drugs** (especially **hyoscine**), thought to be due to a decrease in inhibitory **acetylcholine** activity in the brain. Other drugs with anticholinergic activity may cause it, including **antihistamine drugs**, **phenothiazines**, **antidepressant drugs**, **antiparkinsonian drugs** and **pethidine**. Has also been reported after volatile anaesthetic agents, **ketamine** and **benzodiazepines**. Reported incidence varies but has been up to 5%–10% after general anaesthesia.
- Features:
  - **confusion**, agitation, restlessness, anxiety, amnesia, hallucinations.
  - speech disturbance, ataxia.
  - nausea, vomiting.

- muscle incoordination.
- **convulsions, coma.**
- peripheral anticholinergic effects, e.g. tachycardia, dry mouth and skin, blurred vision, urinary retention.

- Treatment: **physostigmine** 0.5–1 mg slowly iv; 0.02 mg/kg in children. It usually acts within 5 min; features may recur after 1–2 h.

Central conduction time, *see Evoked potentials*

Central pain, *see Pain, central*

Central pontine myelinolysis. Demyelination occurring within the pons. Most commonly associated with **hyponatraemia** with resultant osmotic shifts. Risk factors include a serum sodium <120 mmol/l for >48 h and rapid (>12 mmol/l) correction or over-correction of sodium levels. May also occur in **alcoholism, malnutrition, HIV infection, burns**, following **diuretic** therapy. It may also follow **liver transplantation** (30% of patients showing pontine demyelination at postmortem examination). Accompanied by extrapontine demyelination in 10% of cases. Diagnosis is confirmed by MRI scanning.

May be asymptomatic, but usually presents with confusion, **coma**, horizontal gaze paresis, bulbar palsy and spastic quadriplegia. Large pontine lesions may result in the **locked-in syndrome**.

Treatment is largely supportive although high-dose **corticosteroids** have been used.

Singh TD, Fugate JE, Rabinstein AA (2014). Eur J Neurol; 12: 1443–50

Central venous cannulation.

- Performed for:
  - vascular access, e.g. for **dialysis**, TPN, infusion of irritant or potent drugs
  - measurement of **CVP**.
  - **cardiac catheterisation, pulmonary artery catheterisation** and transvenous **cardiac pacing**.

For intrathoracic lines, the catheter tip should ideally lie in the superior vena cava above the pericardial reflection, to reduce risk of **arrhythmias** and **cardiac tamponade** should erosion and bleeding occur. However, a tip placed too high may be associated with thrombosis.

- May be performed at different sites:
  - internal jugular vein:
    - easy to perform and reliable.
    - may cause **pneumothorax** or damage the common **carotid artery, vertebral artery, brachial plexus, phrenic nerve**, thoracic duct (on left) or sympathetic chain.
    - uncomfortable for the patient.
  - subclavian vein:
    - more convenient and comfortable for long-term use.
    - less chance of correct placement.
    - greater chance of pneumothorax or haemothorax.
    - may damage the subclavian artery; direct pressure cannot be applied to stop bleeding.
  - external jugular vein:
    - easy to perform because the vein is more superficial than the internal jugular or subclavian veins.
    - it may be difficult to thread the catheter through the junction with the subclavian vein. A J-shaped guide-wire may help.
  - femoral vein:
    - often easier than other routes, especially in obese patients.
    - avoids the pleura and lungs completely.
    - useful in **superior vena caval obstruction**.
    - thromboembolism and femoral arterial puncture may also occur.
  - axillary vein:
    - because venepuncture is extrathoracic, risk of pneumothorax is reduced.
    - the axillary artery may be compressed directly if accidentally punctured.
    - may damage the medial cutaneous nerve.
  - arm vein:
    - minimal risk of serious complications.
    - threading of a 'long line' is often difficult, especially via the cephalic vein because of valves at the junction with the axillary vein. Abduction of the arm may help.

Gas embolism, subcutaneous emphysema, retained guide-wire within the patient and sepsis are risks of all techniques. Patients should be in the head-down position for jugular and subclavian cannulation to prevent ingress of air. An aseptic technique is used to avoid **catheter-related sepsis**. Introduction of a catheter into the heart may cause arrhythmias (therefore **ECG** monitoring is required) or cardiac perforation. Reintroduction of the needle into the cannula while the tip is in the patient risks shearing off pieces of cannula. Endocardial damage and central vein thrombosis may also occur, especially with pulmonary artery catheters and with prolonged placement.

Successful placement is suggested by easy aspiration of non-pulsatile blood and obtaining the **venous waveform**. Placement of the catheter in the right ventricle results in excessive swinging of central venous pressure with each heartbeat. Catheter position must be checked by x-ray, and pneumothorax excluded. Guidelines issued by **NICE** support the routine use of ultrasound guidance for internal **jugular venous cannulation**, while AAGBI guidance is to consider ultrasound for other routes as well.

Smith RN, Nolan JP (2013). Br Med J; 347: f6570

See also, Axillary venous cannulation; Central venous cannulation, long-term; Femoral venous cannulation; Subclavian venous cannulation

Central venous cannulation, long-term. Usually employed for long-term **TPN**, administration of drugs (e.g. chemotherapy and antibiotics) and blood sampling. First developed in the 1970s. Silastic catheters (Hickman–Broviac) are usually inserted via the subclavian vein and tunnelled subcutaneously (emerging from the skin between the sternum and nipple). A Dacron cuff on the subcutaneous part incites an inflammatory reaction, providing fixation and a possible barrier to infection within 1–2 weeks. Single- and double-lumen catheters are available. These subcutaneous central venous access devices (or 'ports') are increasingly introduced using radiological control. Alternatively, a peripherally inserted central catheter (PICC) can be introduced via the basilic, cephalic or brachial vein and advanced into the superior vena cava; successful placement can be confirmed with CXR or by using fluoroscopy.

Catheters are inserted under sterile conditions via a surgical cut-down procedure, or percutaneously using the **Seldinger technique**. In the latter, the catheter is passed into the vein through a sheath that is split and peeled away as the catheter is advanced.

Catheters may remain in place for years if required, with regular heparinised flushing and aseptic handling.

[John W Broviac, US physician; Robert O Hickman, US paediatrician]

Walser EM (2012). Cardiovasc Intervent Radiol; 35: 751–64

See also, Central venous

Central venous pressure (CVP). Pressure within the right atrium and great veins of the thorax. Measured via **central venous cannulation**, using a manometer or **transducer**. An estimate may be made by observing the distension of neck veins (JVP). CVP is measured relative to a point 5 cm below the sternal angle, or the mid-axillary line (if the patient is supine). Normally 0–8 cmH_2O in the spontaneously breathing patient. By convention, it is measured at the end of expiration. The **venous waveform** may be seen on a pressure tracing, with the effects of ventilation superimposed (*see later*).

- Increased by:
  - raised intrathoracic pressure, e.g. **IPPV**, coughing. CVP normally rises in expiration during spontaneous ventilation.
  - impaired cardiac function, e.g. outlet obstruction, **cardiac failure**, **cardiac tamponade**. Primarily reflects right-sided function; thus CVP may be normal in the presence of left ventricular failure and **pulmonary oedema**, or raised in right-sided failure with normal left-sided function. With normal cardiac function, pressures on both sides move together. Left-sided function may be assessed by pulmonary artery catheterisation.
  - circulatory overload.
  - venoconstriction.
  - **superior vena caval obstruction** (the normal venous waveform may be lost).
- Decreased by:
  - reduced **venous return**, e.g. due to **hypovolaemia**, venodilatation.
  - reduced intrathoracic pressure, e.g. in inspiration during spontaneous ventilation.

Although useful in indicating right ventricular **preload**, its correlation with right ventricular stroke volume and cardiac output is poor because the latter variables are also dependent on myocardial contractility, diastolic function and pulmonary vascular resistance.

Extensively used in the past, routine measurement of CVP to guide volume resuscitation in anaesthetic and critical care settings is no longer recommended and has been superseded by measuring the effect of passive leg raising on stroke volume and other methods of **cardiac output measurement**.

Magder S (2015). Curr Opin Crit Care; 21: 369–75

Centre for Maternal and Child Enquiries (CMACE), *see Confidential Enquiries into Maternal Deaths*

Cephalosporins. Semisynthetic **antibacterial drugs**, derived from the natural substance cephalosporin C. Bactericidal, they act by inhibiting the synthesis of bacterial cell walls. Similar in pharmacology to **penicillins**; cross-sensitivity in penicillin-allergic individuals is rare with second- to fourth-generation cephalosporins. The 'generation' classification is based partly on their antibacterial activity and when they were introduced (generally, successive generations have greater activity against gram-negative organisms):

- first-generation, e.g. cefalotin (largely replaced by **cefazolin** and **cefradine**): good activity against gram-positive organisms, including penicillinase-producing staphylococci; poor activity against enterococci and gram-negative organisms.
- second-generation, e.g. **cefamandole**, **cefuroxime**: slightly less active than cephalothin against gram-positive organisms but greater stability against enterobacteria and *Haemophilus influenzae*. The cephamycin antibacterial drugs (e.g. cefoxitin) are classified as second-generation, although they have greater activity against anaerobes, especially *Bacteroides fragilis*.
- third-generation, e.g. **cefotaxime**, **ceftriaxone**: yet more stable against gram-negative bacteria, although less active against gram-positive organisms than first-generation drugs (but still very active against streptococci). **Ceftazidime** has enhanced activity against pseudomonas.
- fourth-generation, e.g. **cefpirome**.

CEPOD, *see National Confidential Enquiry into Patient Outcome and Death*

Cerebral abscess. Collection of infected material, often encapsulated, within the brain parenchyma. More common in the young (when it is associated with **congenital heart disease**) and those >60 years. Infection often arises from local spread (e.g. following paranasal sinusitis, otitis or cerebral trauma) or metastatic spread (e.g. following bacterial endocarditis or lung abscess) when cerebral abscesses are often multiple. May also occur in cyanotic heart disease when cardiac output is no longer 'filtered' by the lungs.

- Causative organisms (often multiple):
  - most commonly: gram-positive *Streptococcus milleri* (accounts for 70% of cases); gram-negative anaerobic bacteroides species; and aerobic gram-negative organisms (e.g. proteus, *Escherichia coli* and pseudomonas).
  - in immunocompromised patients: toxoplasma, **TB**, cryptococcus.
- Features:
  - Pyrexia (in 50%), headache (in 75%), nausea, vomiting, seizures, **coma**. Rupture of abscesses into the subarachnoid space causes meningism. Large abscesses may result in raised **ICP**. Focal neurological signs depend on the location of the abscess.
  - CT scan with contrast reveals typical ring enhancement of the abscess. MRI scan will show the extent of surrounding oedema.
  - **lumbar puncture** is rarely performed as it may cause cerebral herniation and has a poor diagnostic yield.
- Treatment:
  - urgent neurosurgical image-guided aspiration of the abscess for therapeutic and diagnostic purposes.
  - **antibacterial drugs** directed against the most likely organism (must be able to penetrate the abscess wall), e.g. **benzylpenicillin**, **metronidazole** and **cefotaxime** if otitis/sinusitis is suspected; may be required for up to 2 years.
  - **dexamethasone** is controversial but may be indicated if extensive cerebral oedema is present.

Overall mortality is 15% but rises to 80% if rupture of the abscess has occurred. 30% of patients have significant residual neurological morbidity.
Brouwer MC, Tunkel AR, McKhann GM, et al (2014). N Engl J Med; 371: 447–56

Cerebral blood flow (CBF). Normally 14% of **cardiac output**, approximately 700 ml/min (50 ml/100 g/min). Grey matter receives about 70 ml/100 g/min whereas white matter receives about 20 ml/100 g/min. Maintenance of CBF is critical: EEG slows if it falls to 20 ml/100 g/min; at 15 ml/100 g/min EEG is flat, and at 10 ml/100 g/min irreversible cerebral damage occurs.

- Measurement of CBF:
  - applying the **Fick principle**, using N_2O (**Kety–Schmidt technique**). Values are obtained for the whole brain; regional variations in flow are not demonstrated.
  - detection of radioactive decay over different parts of the head, following inhalation of radioactive xenon or injection of dissolved radioactive xenon into a carotid artery. Regional differences are detected.
  - regional flow may also be measured by **positron emission tomography**, specific **MRI** sequences and **transcranial Doppler ultrasound.**
- Control of CBF:
  - flow–metabolism coupling: local neuronal activity results in increased regional blood flow to match glucose and oxygen requirement and delivery. Mechanism involves changes of calcium and potassium flux within astrocytes that occurs with increased neuronal activity. These ion changes result in signalling to vascular smooth muscle producing dilatation and increased CBF to match metabolic needs.
  - chemical factors:
    - arterial $P\text{CO}_2$ (Fig. 38a): **hypercapnia** (with resultant acidosis) increases CBF via cerebral vasodilatation. **Hypocapnia** decreases CBF; a reduction from 5.3 to 4 kPa (40 to 30 mmHg) reduces CBF by 30%. Reduction may not be sustained for more than 24–48 h of hypocapnia.
    - arterial $P\text{O}_2$ (Fig. 38a): minimal effect until $P\text{O}_2$ falls below 6.7 kPa (50 mmHg).
  - **autoregulation** (Fig. 38b): CBF remains constant between a MAP of 60 and 160 mmHg (limits are raised in the hypertensive patient). Autoregulation is impaired by cerebral trauma, hypoxaemia, hypercapnia and **inhalational anaesthetic agents**.
  - temperature: **hypothermia** decreases cerebral metabolism, which results in a decrease in CBF (a ~5% drop per °C drop in temperature).
  - neural control (minor effect): sympathetic stimulation causes cerebral vasoconstriction, parasympathetic stimulation causes cerebral vasodilatation.
  - drugs: all volatile anaesthetic agents cause dose-dependent increase in CBF due to vasodilatation and loss of autoregulation. **Ketamine** also increases CBF; **thiopental, etomidate, benzodiazepines** and **propofol** reduce it. Opioid drugs cause little change if $P_a\text{CO}_2$ is kept within normal levels.

See also, Cerebral circulation; Cerebral ischaemia; Cerebral steal

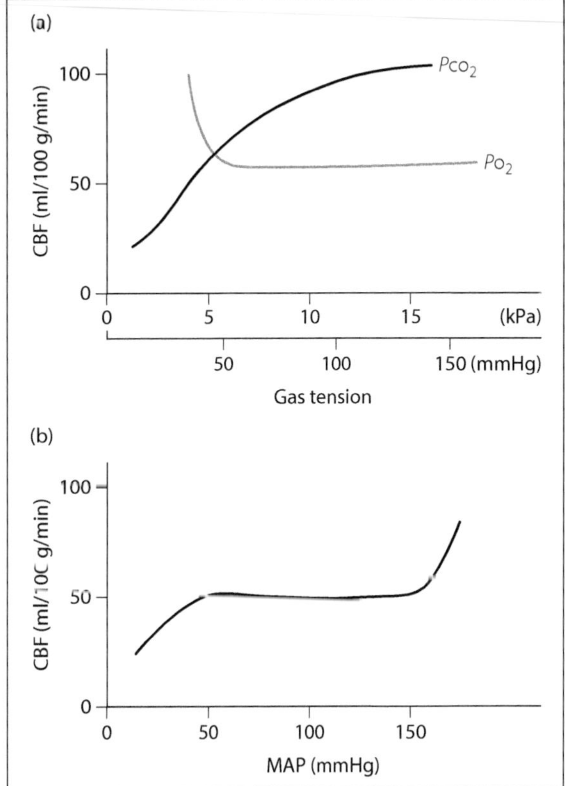

Fig. 38 Variation of cerebral blood flow with: (a) arterial $P\text{O}_2$ and $P\text{CO}_2$; (b) blood pressure

Cerebral circulation.

- Arterial supply: two-thirds via the two internal **carotid arteries** and one-third via the two vertebral arteries. These two systems are connected via the anterior and posterior communicating arteries, thus forming the anastomosis (patent in 50% of individuals) known as the circle of Willis (Fig. 39a):
  - anterior cerebral artery: supplies superior and medial parts of the cerebral hemisphere.
  - middle cerebral artery: supplies most of the lateral side of the hemisphere. Internal branches supply the internal capsule, through which most ascending and descending pathways pass. Commonly affected by **stroke.**
  - posterior cerebral artery: supplies the occipital lobe and the medial side of the temporal lobe.
- Venous drainage (Fig. 39b):
  - deep structures drain via the internal cerebral vein on each side; these form the midline great cerebral vein, which passes back to join the inferior sagittal sinus.
  - cerebral and cerebellar cortices drain via dural sinuses:
    - superior and inferior sagittal sinuses in the midline, between the layers of dura of the falx cerebri. The superior usually drains into the right transverse sinus; the inferior via the straight sinus into the left transverse sinus.
    - transverse sinuses within the tentorium cerebelli: pass via the sigmoid sinuses through the jugular foramina to become the internal **jugular veins.**
    - cavernous sinuses on either side of the pituitary fossa: receive blood from the eyes and nearby parts of the **brain**, draining into the transverse sinuses and internal jugular veins.

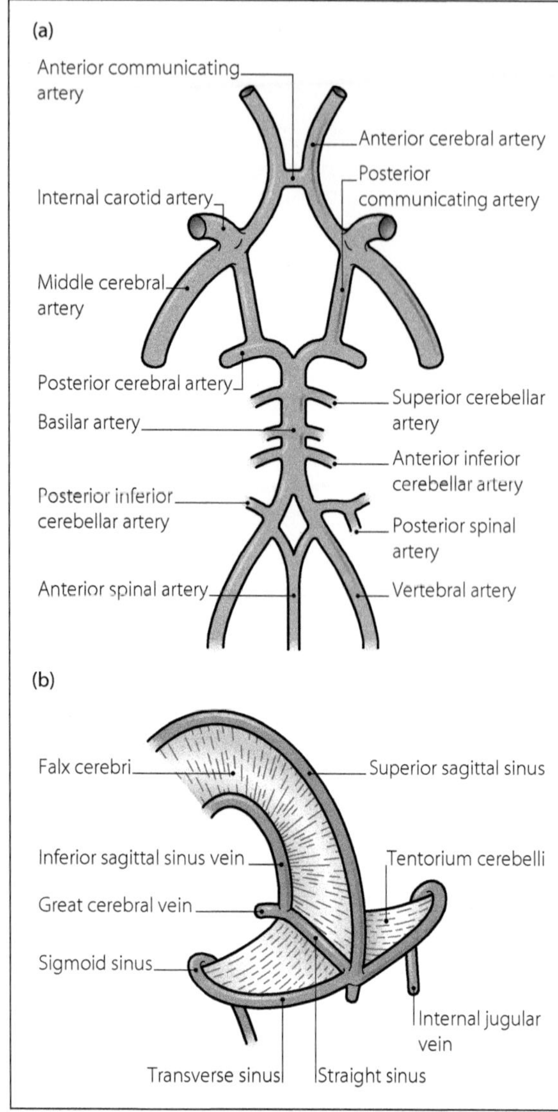

Fig. 39 Cerebral circulation: (a) arterial; (b) venous

Both arterial and venous circulations may be imaged using conventional or CT or MRI angiography.
[Thomas Willis (1621–1675), English physician]

Cerebral function analysing monitor. Development of the **cerebral function monitor** that provides information about the frequency distribution of the **EEG** signal as well as overall activity. Thus the relative proportions of the four standard EEG waveforms are presented. Said to be more useful than the cerebral function monitor, but suffers from similar drawbacks.

Cerebral function monitor. Device adapted from the conventional **EEG**. The signal from two parietal electrodes is filtered and amplified to produce a display of average peak voltage, charted on slow-moving paper. Thus monitors overall cerebral activity. Main use is in neonatology units to monitor seizure activity in hypoxic ischaemic encephalopathy. Has been used to monitor depth of anaesthesia, but has been superseded by the **bispectral index monitor**, which has more appropriate response times.
See also, Anaesthesia, depth of

Cerebral hypoxic ischaemic injury. Cerebral ischaemic injury refers to brain damage resulting from an acute reduction of cerebral oxygen delivery due to reduced **cerebral blood flow**; in addition, there is a limited or absent removal of toxic metabolites (e.g. **lactate**, H^+ ions, **glutamate**, **free radicals**) that contributes to the injury (*for mechanism, see Cerebral ischaemia*). Most common causes are **cardiac arrest** or severe hypotension (e.g. following **PE**, **sepsis**, drug overdose, severe haemorrhage).

Cerebral hypoxic injury is caused by a reduction in cerebral oxygen supply but with preserved cerebral blood flow. Causes include suffocation, airway obstruction, strangulation, **near-drowning**, chemical exposure (e.g. **carbon monoxide poisoning**, **cyanide poisoning**). Potential recovery is better than that of ischaemic injury.

- Management of hypoxic ischaemic injury following cardiac arrest:
  - following resuscitation, use fluids and vasopressor drugs to maintain a mean arterial pressure of 80–100 mmHg to ensure adequate CBF; the latter is compromised by loss of **autoregulation** following arrest.
  - monitor and treat raised **ICP** if present.
  - maintain adequate oxygenation while avoiding excessively high P_aO_2. Sedation is often necessary to allow effective mechanical ventilation.
  - blood glucose should be kept within the normal range.
  - treat pyrexia and seizures aggressively.
  - **targeted temperature management** (i.e., to 32°–34°C) has not been shown to reduce mortality.

  Other **cerebral protection** measures have proved disappointing.

The outcome of hypoxic ischaemic injury varies from mild neurocognitive deficits to **vegetative states**. In the absence of sedation, a poor prognosis is suggested by:
  - clinical features: unresponsive coma >6 h, no spontaneous limb movements or localisation to pain, prolonged loss of pupillary reflexes, sustained conjugate eye deviation and abnormal eye movements, myoclonic seizures, absent bulbar reflexes.
  - investigations: **EEG** showing electrical silence or generalised low voltage, burst suppression, generalised **status epilepticus**, predominance of alpha rhythm ('alpha coma') are all reliable indicators of poor recovery. Imaging (especially diffusion-weighted **MRI**) can show the extent of cerebral damage.
  - somatosensory **evoked potentials** are not influenced by the presence of sedation but have a poorer predictive value.
  - raised biomarkers e.g. neuron-specific enolase, predict poor outcome.

Howard RS, Holmes PA, Koutroumanidis MA (2011). Pract Neurol; 11: 4–11
See also, Brainstem death; Cerebral circulation; Cerebral metabolism; Cerebral steal

Cerebral ischaemia. Inadequate blood supply to brain. May be:
  - global:
    - complete, e.g. **cardiac arrest** or severely raised **ICP** with **hypotension** resulting in **cerebral hypoxic ischaemic injury**.
    - incomplete, e.g. hypotension and cerebrovascular disease.
  - focal or regional, e.g. cerebrovascular disease, emboli, local lesions, e.g. tumours; may also be complete or incomplete. The periphery of a focal infarct is termed

the penumbra; recovery of this area is the focus of therapeutic interventions.

- Effects of ischaemia:
  - anaerobic metabolism increases, with greater **acidosis** if a **glucose** source is available (e.g. with incomplete ischaemia).
  - impaired cell membrane pump activity results in depolarisation due to leak of **potassium** out of cells, and **calcium** into cells.
  - excitatory **neurotransmitters** (e.g. **glutamate**) are released and accumulate, contributing to 'excitotoxic' cell death.
  - **free radicals** are liberated.
  - permanent histological damage and associated neurological deficits occur after about 4–5 min.
  - reduction in **cerebral blood flow** from the normal 50 ml/100 g/min causes the following changes:
    - 30–40 ml/100 g/min: EEG slows.
    - 20 ml/100 g/min: no spontaneous electrical activity. **Lactate** rises.
    - 15 ml/100 g/min: **evoked potentials** disappear. Anaerobic metabolism occurs and pH decreases. Ionic changes begin.
    - 10 ml/100 g/min: oedema and irreversible damage occur if flow is not rapidly restored.

Hypoxaemia with uninterrupted blood supply is better tolerated because of continued removal of waste products despite O_2 lack.

Damage is thought to result from increased intracellular calcium levels, free radicals, **arachidonic acid** metabolites or lactic acid production; these have been the targets of investigated lines of treatment (**cerebral protection/resuscitation**). Severity depends on duration, site and cause of ischaemia, and patient factors, e.g. age, co-morbidity. Watershed areas between the main cerebral arteries are most at risk from ischaemia, particularly in the elderly, if vessels are diseased, or if **blood viscosity** is high. Chronic ischaemia may predispose to transient ischaemic attack, **stroke** or dementia. During anaesthesia, excessive **hyperventilation** combined with hypotension may cause ischaemia.

Sekhon MS, Ainslie PN, Griesdale DE (2017). Crit Care; 21: 90

See also, Brainstem death; Cerebral circulation; Cerebral metabolism; Cerebral steal

Cerebral metabolic rate for oxygen ($CMRO_2$). Volume of O_2 consumed by the brain per unit time. Equals **cerebral blood flow** × arteriovenous O_2 content difference (*see Fick principle*). Normally about 50 ml/min (20% of total basal requirement), or 3.5 ml/100 g/min. Indicative of global **cerebral metabolism**, over 90% of which is aerobic; the relationship may not hold if O_2 or glucose supplies are reduced and alternate metabolic pathways employed.

Reduced by **hypothermia** (about 5% reduction per °C drop). Also reduced in old age and by certain drugs, e.g. **barbiturates, benzodiazepines**, volatile anaesthetic agents; increased by seizures, **ketamine** and possibly N_2O.

Cerebral metabolism. **Glucose** is the main substrate, although **ketone bodies, amino acids** and **fats** may be utilised, e.g. in starvation. 90%–95% of **glycolysis** is aerobic, hence the requirement for a continuous supply of O_2. O_2 consumption is about 3.5 ml/100 g/min; CO_2 output is the same.

Cerebral metabolic rate for O_2 ($CMRO_2$) is used as a measure of global cerebral metabolism, and does not reflect regional variations; neuronal cells consume more O_2 than glial cells, grey matter more than white. Similar measurements may be made using glucose consumption (cerebral metabolic rate for glucose; normally about 4.5 mg/100 g/min) and lactate production (cerebral metabolic rate for lactate; normally about 2.3 mg/100 g/min).

Under normal conditions **cerebral blood flow** is closely related to cerebral metabolism.

See also, Cerebral ischaemia

Cerebral microdialysis. Method of measuring levels of **neurotransmitters** or metabolites present in the ECF of the brain, e.g. glucose, pyruvate, lactate, glycerol and glutamate. First used in humans in 1990, with bedside analysers becoming available in the 2000s. Has been used to detect and measure physiological and pathophysiological chemical changes, e.g. in **Parkinson's disease, cerebral ischaemia**, cerebral neoplasia, **subarachnoid haemorrhage** and **TBI**. A small microdialysis catheter is placed in the brain tissue and a 'perfusion' fluid passed through it. Substances within the ECF pass into the perfusion fluid by diffusion, forming a dialysate, chemical analysis of which allows assessment of the local, as opposed to global, cerebral metabolism.

Hutchinson PJ, Jalloh I, Helmy A, et al (2015). Int Care Med; 41: 1517–28

Cerebral oedema. Increased brain water content with associated tissue swelling. May be diagnosed by **CT scanning**.

- Different types:
  - vasogenic oedema: increased vascular permeability and defective **blood–brain barrier**, e.g. associated with inflammatory conditions, tumours, trauma. Plasma protein and fluid penetrate the brain, tracking along fibre tracts. Exacerbated by raised hydrostatic pressures.
  - cytotoxic oedema: astrocyte damage due to **cerebral ischaemia, hypoxia, encephalitis**, toxins, metabolic disturbances; cells become depleted of **ATP** and accumulate water and sodium. Involves aquaporin-4 glial water channel malfunction.
  - osmotic oedema: occurs when brain **osmolality** exceeds plasma osmolality, e.g. severe **hyponatraemia**, during **haemodialysis**, rapid reduction of plasma glucose in diabetic ketoacidosis.
  - hydrostatic oedema: seen in severe hypertension when fluid is forced out of cerebral capillaries.
  - interstitial oedema: in **hydrocephalus** the **CSF** may be forced from the ventricular system into white matter.
  - high-**altitude** cerebral oedema (HACE): may have similar mechanism to vasogenic cerebral oedema.
- Effects:
  - raised **ICP**: reduced **cerebral perfusion pressure**, compression of blood vessels and vital structures, papilloedema and **coning**.
  - increased distance for O_2 diffusion from capillaries to cells.
  - impaired consciousness, **convulsions** and **coma**.
- Management:
  - of primary cause.
  - **IPPV**, with **hypocapnia** to arterial P_{CO_2} 3.8–4.2 kPa (28–32 mmHg). The beneficial effects of **hyperventilation** may be reduced after 24 h. Fluid restriction to 1.5–2 l/day is usually instituted. Venous drainage is encouraged by head-up posture, good sedation/

neuromuscular blockade and unobstructed jugular veins, as for ICP reduction. Measures are usually carried out for 24–48 h after the insult.
- **corticosteroids** (e.g. **dexamethasone**) are effective in vasogenic oedema but have limited or no effect in other types.
- **diuretics**:
  - **mannitol** 0.25–1 g/kg iv; relies on an intact blood–brain barrier. Effective in vasogenic and cytotoxic oedema. **Urea** is rarely used now.
  - **furosemide** 10–40 mg. Effective in cytotoxic but not vasogenic oedema.
- **hypertonic intravenous solutions** (e.g. 3% saline) are also used.

Cerebral perfusion pressure (CPP). Difference between **MAP** and **ICP**; represents the pressure head available for **cerebral blood flow**. Normally 70–75 mmHg; critical level for **cerebral ischaemia** is thought to be 30–40 mmHg. In the presence of raised ICP, MAP increases in order to maintain CPP (**Cushing's reflex**).
Smith M (2015). Br J Anaesth; 115: 488–90

Cerebral protection/resuscitation.
- Possible techniques:
  - general measures:
    - maintaining normotension and oxygenation.
    - maintaining metabolic stability and other organ function.
  - increasing or maintaining **cerebral perfusion pressure**:
    - **nimodipine** in **subarachnoid haemorrhage**: thought to reduce vasospasm and maintain blood flow. Of uncertain benefit in other intracranial pathology.
    - reduction of **ICP**, e.g. **hypocapnia** or **mannitol**.
    - **haemodilution**.
    - cerebral angioplasty/endovascular thrombolysis in focal ischaemia.
  - reducing **cerebral metabolic rate for O_2**:
    - **targeted temperature management**: used in cardiac surgery and following **cardiac arrest** or **TBI**. Although it reduces **ICP**, no improvement in outcome has been demonstrated.
    - **barbiturates**: efficacy in animal studies has not been repeated in human trials; routine use is thus controversial, unless for sedation or treatment of convulsions. Profound hypotension is a major side effect.
    - **isoflurane**: possibly beneficial in incomplete global ischaemia; **cerebral steal** is possible in focal ischaemia. Efficacy has not been established in humans.
  - reducing cell damage:
    - avoidance of **hyperglycaemia**. Shown to have sustained benefits pre- and post-ischaemic injury.
    - **xenon** has a neuroprotective effect via NMDA receptor antagonism.
    - experimental agents include **free radical** scavengers (e.g. lazaroids) and **glutamate** antagonists.

Stocchetti N, Taccone FS, Citerio G, et al (2015). Crit Care; 19: 186–97

Cerebral salt-wasting syndrome. Loss of sodium (and water) via the kidneys associated with intracranial disease (e.g. **subarachnoid haemorrhage, TBI**). May be mediated by excessive secretion of **atrial natriuretic peptide**. Results in **hyponatraemia** and decreased plasma volume (unlike the **syndrome of inappropriate antidiuretic hormone secretion**, in which plasma volume is increased). Treatment is with fluid and sodium replacement.
Buffington MA, Abreo K (2016). J Int Care Med; 31: 223–36

Cerebral steal. Diversion of blood flow away from abnormal areas of brain (e.g. tumours and infarcts), secondary to vasodilatation of normal cerebral blood vessels, e.g. due to **hypercapnia**. The reverse may occur in **hypocapnia**; thus general vasoconstriction may increase blood flow to abnormal areas (inverse steal).

Cerebral venous thrombosis. Most commonly affects the superior sagittal, lateral, cavernous or straight sinuses, although cerebral veins may be involved (*see Cerebral circulation*).
- Aetiology:
  - infective:
    - local, e.g. **cerebral abscess, meningitis, sinusitis**, otitis.
    - systemic, e.g. **endocarditis, TB, HIV infection, bacteraemia**, viraemia.
  - non-infective:
    - local, e.g. **TBI, neurosurgery**, cerebral tumour, hyperosmolar infusion via jugular veins.
    - general, e.g. hypercoagulable **coagulation disorders**, including pregnancy.

Clinical features include headache, nausea, vomiting and seizures. Other features depend on the site but include those of raised **ICP, cranial nerve** palsies and **stroke**. Cavernous sinus thrombosis results in facial oedema and swelling of the eye.

Diagnosed clinically and by **CT scanning** or **MRI**, and cerebral angiography. Magnetic resonance venography is now the investigation of choice.

Heparin (either unfractionated or low molecular weight) is the mainstay of treatment and is given even if there is evidence of haemorrhagic transformation of a venous cerebral infarct. Direct infusion of **fibrinolytic drugs** into the venous sinuses has also been used.
Saposnik G, Barinagarrementeria F, Brown RD Jr, et al (2011). Stroke; 42: 1158–92

Cerebrospinal fluid (CSF). Clear fluid bathing the CNS, providing hydromechanical support for the brain and helping to maintain cerebral interstitial fluid homeostasis by regulating electrolytes. Adult CSF volume is 150 ml with 30 ml in the ventricles, 45 ml in the cranial subarachnoid space and 75 ml in the spinal subarachnoid space.
- Production:
  - 75% by the choroid plexuses of the lateral ventricle, but also in the third and fourth ventricles, at about 500 ml/day.
  - remainder is secreted by cerebral vessels across the **blood–brain barrier**. Formation is largely independent of **ICP**.
- Circulation (Fig. 40):
  - from the lateral ventricles to the third ventricle via the foramina of Monro, thence to the fourth ventricle via the aqueduct.
  - leaves the fourth ventricle via the foramina of Magendie (midline posteriorly) and Luschka (laterally) to pass down to the spinal cord or up over the cerebral hemispheres.

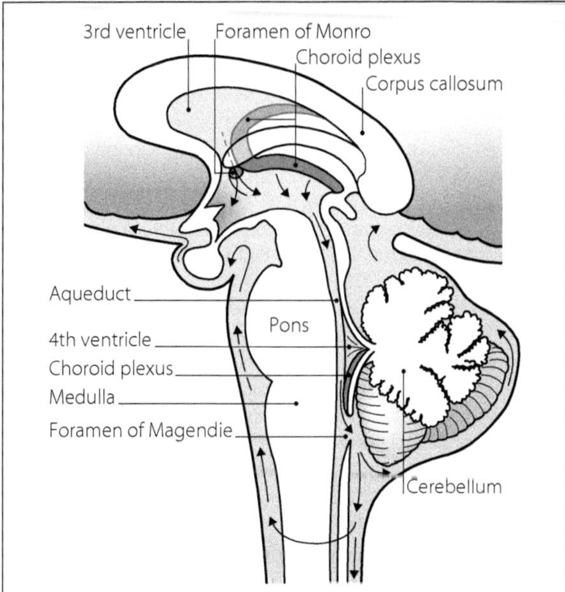

Fig. 40 Circulation of CSF

- Reabsorption:
  - reabsorbed into the venous system via the arachnoid granulations, finger-like invaginations projecting into the cerebral venous sinuses. Most absorption is into the superior sagittal sinus. In health, rate of production equals rate of absorption.
  - increases as CSF pressure increases and decreases if cerebral venous sinus pressure increases.

Imbalance of CSF production/reabsorption or defects in circulation may result in **hydrocephalus** and raised ICP.

- Normal constituents:
  - sodium: 135–145 mmol/l.
  - chloride: 115–125 mmol/l.
  - calcium: 1–1.5 mmol/l.
  - potassium: 2.5–3.5 mmol/l.
  - glucose: 2.7–4.2 mmol/l (if blood glucose normal).
  - pH: 7.3–7.5.
  - protein: 0.2–0.4 g/l.
  - urea: 1.5–6.0 mmol/l.
  - lymphocytes: 0–5 × 10^6/l.

[Alexander Monro (1733–1817), Scottish anatomist; Francois Magendie (1783–1855), French physiologist; Hubert von Luschka (1820–1875), German anatomist]
See also, Lumbar puncture

Cerebrovascular accident, *see Stroke*

Certoparin, *see Heparin*

Cervical plexus block. Provides analgesia of the upper cervical **dermatomes**; used for head and neck surgery and treatment of chronic **pain.**

The plexus is formed from the anterior branches of the upper four cervical nerves, lying between the anterior and posterior tubercles of the cervical vertebral transverse processes.

- Technique:
  - the patient is placed supine, looking away from the side to be blocked, with the neck partially extended. The transverse processes of C2–4 are palpated posterior to a line between the mastoid process and transverse process of C6.
  - a fine needle is introduced perpendicular to the skin, 1–3 cm towards each transverse process in turn until contact is made or paraesthesia elicited (or the needle tip position is confirmed on ultrasound).
  - after careful aspiration, 3–5 ml solution (e.g. 0.5% **lidocaine** with adrenaline) is injected at each level to block the deep branches. A further 3–5 ml is injected as the needle is withdrawn. The superficial branches are blocked by injecting 15–20 ml along the posterior border of the middle third of the sternomastoid muscle.

Complications include intravascular injection or puncture (e.g. vertebral artery), subarachnoid injection, sympathetic block, phrenic nerve block and recurrent laryngeal nerve block.

Cervical spine. Composed of seven cervical **vertebrae.** Important in the positioning of the neck in **airway** management, including tracheal intubation. Injury may often accompany **head injury.**
See also, Intubation, difficult; Spinal cord injury; Vertebral ligaments

CFAM, *see Cerebral function analysing monitor*

CFM, *see Cerebral function monitor*

cgs system of units. System based on the centimetre, gram and second; replaced in 1960 by the SI system based on the metre, kilogram and second.
See also, Units, SI

Charcoal, activated. Charcoal that has been processed to meet high-adsorbance standards via having multiple small pores, thus increasing the available surface area (1 g having a surface area of 500–3000 m^2 depending on its preparation/use).

- Has multiple uses in industry, agriculture and in medical practice:
  - administered orally or via a nasogastric tube to reduce gastrointestinal absorption of certain toxic compounds (e.g. **barbiturates, tricyclic antidepressant drugs**) in the treatment of **poisoning and overdoses.** In addition to adsorbing toxins present in the stomach, it reduces blood levels by preventing enterohepatic recirculation. Most effective when substances toxic in small amounts have been ingested, and within 1 h of ingestion (prehospital administration has been suggested). Dosage: 50 g (1 g/kg in children up to 50 g). May be repeated 4-hourly for overdosage with carbamazepine, dapsone, phenobarbital, quinine or theophylline, because it enhances these drugs' elimination. Tolerance may be improved by reducing the dose and increasing the frequency, e.g. 25 g 2-hourly, but efficacy may be reduced.

    May cause severe pneumonitis if aspirated, and contraindicated after ingestion of acidic, alkaline, corrosive or petroleum products, and metal salts.
  - during anaesthesia, containers of activated charcoal (the Aldasorber) have been used in breathing systems to adsorb volatile agents, thereby reducing pollution. **N_2O** is not adsorbed. Remaining adsorption capacity is monitored by weighing the container.
  - coated activated charcoal is used during **haemoperfusion.**

Juurlink DN (2016). Br J Clin Pharmacol; 81: 482–7

Charge, electric. Physical property of matter causing it to experience a force when in proximity to other charged matter. May be positive or negative, indicating a relative deficit or excess of electrons, respectively. Flow of charge constitutes a **current**. SI **unit** is the **coulomb**.

Charles' law. At constant pressure, the volume of a fixed mass of gas is proportional to its temperature.
[Jacques Charles (1746–1823), French chemist]
See also, Boyle's law; Ideal gas law

Chassaignac's tubercle. Transverse process of C6, against which the common **carotid artery** may be felt and compressed. Useful landmark for **stellate ganglion block**.
[Charles Chassaignac (1804–1879), French surgeon]

Checking of anaesthetic equipment. Should be performed before anaesthetising any patient. The requirement for following a checklist is mandatory in many countries, including the UK.

- The following should be checked before every operating theatre session (Association of Anaesthetists' guidelines):
  - **anaesthetic machine**:
    - check electricity supply/back-up as appropriate.
    - note any information/service labels present.
    - check the identity and attachments of all pipelines.
    - CO_2 cylinders should only be present if specifically requested. Blanking plugs should be fitted to unused yokes.
    - check the O_2 supply and reserve **cylinders**.
    - check the other gases are connected (confirm with a 'tug test') and that all pipeline pressure gauges read 400 kPa (4 bar).
    - check each flow valve and flowmeter throughout its whole range.
    - check the antihypoxic device linking the O_2 and N_2O flowmeters, and the O_2 flush.
    - check the vaporisers are seated properly, filled and able to be turned on. Test the vaporiser fittings for leaks by setting a gas flow of 5 l/min and obstructing the common gas outlet with the vaporiser turned on and off (unless the manufacturer suggests alternative testing).
    - obstruct the gas outlet with a set gas flow of 5 l/min, ensuring that the flowmeter bobbin 'dips' (indicating pressurisation of the machine back bar) and that the pressure relief valve opens (unless the manufacturer suggests alternative testing, e.g. using a negative-pressure leak-testing device consisting of a rubber bulb to be fitted to the gas outlet).
  - **scavenging**: check correct connection.
  - **anaesthetic breathing system**:
    - ensure correct configuration and firm attachment of connections.
    - ensure there is no obstruction by foreign material.
    - close the expiratory valve. Obstruct the distal end of the tubing to fill the reservoir bag; ensure no leaks. Use a 'two-bag' test to confirm.
    - open the valve, checking the bag empties.
    - **coaxial breathing systems**: as earlier, plus testing for correct attachment of the inner tubing of Bain system:
    - obstruct the distal end of the inner tube; the flowmeters should sink as pressure builds up behind the obstruction.
    - close the expiratory valve and fill the bag by occluding the distal end of the outer tube. Use the O_2 flush with the tube now unobstructed: the reservoir bag should empty due to gas entrainment, unless the inner tube is detached (Pethick's test; N.B. has been shown to be less efficient at detecting leaks from the inner tube than the obstruction test).
    - **circle systems**: check one-way valves and bag. Ensure the **soda lime** is properly packed and not expired.
    - **ventilator**: check on manual settings as earlier, and on automatic settings with the outlet obstructed, for adequate ventilating pressures and pressure relief. Check the disconnect alarm and that alternative means of IPPV are available, e.g. self-inflating bag.
  - ancillary equipment (before each case):
    - drugs, iv fluids.
    - **tracheal tubes**, **cuffs**, introducers, **laryngoscopes** (including spare), **suction equipment**, tipping trolley. Check the entire breathing system, including catheter mount, angle piece, filter and connections are patent (i.e., no obstructions) before each case. Single-use equipment should be kept packaged until the point of use to avoid obstruction with solid objects.
    - check all monitoring devices, including O_2 analyser, are functioning and have appropriate alarm limits (and for BP, an appropriate measuring frequency) set.

It is also recommended that the check is documented on each patient's anaesthetic chart, and a logbook kept with each anaesthetic machine.
[Simon L Pethick, Canadian anaesthetist]
Hartle A, Anderson E, Bythell V, et al (2012). Anaesthesia; 67: 660–8

Chelating agents. Chemicals that bind to certain metal ions forming soluble complex molecules; the bound ions are usually rendered inactive as a result.

- Examples (with the metals chelated):
  - **dimercaprol** (antimony, arsenic, bismuth, mercury, gold).
  - **sodium calcium edetate** (lead, copper, radioactive metals).
  - **penicillamine** (copper, lead, gold, mercury, zinc).
  - **desferrioxamine** (iron, aluminium).
  - **trisodium edetate** (calcium).

Chemical weapons. Substances used for hostile purposes, either by certain nations in 'legitimate' chemical warfare or by terrorists. The agents may be targeted at people, animals and/or plants. Usually classified according to their physiological effects:
  - toxins derived from living organisms, e.g. **botulinum toxins**, ricin (derived from castor bean), saxitoxin (derived from marine organisms).
  - nerve agents, e.g. **acetylcholinesterase inhibitors** (e.g. sarin, soman, VX gas and tabun).
  - blood agents, e.g. cyanide.
  - blistering or choking agents, e.g. mustard gas, chlorine, phosgene.
  - vomiting agents, e.g. adamsite.

- tear gas.
- radioactive compounds e.g. polonium.

Management includes specific and general supportive measures; consideration should also be directed towards protection of staff, decontamination of clinical areas and equipment, disposal of bodies and other aspects of major incidents.

White SM (2002). Br J Anaesth; 89: 306–24

See also, Biological weapons; Cyanide poisoning; Incident, major

Chemoreceptor trigger zone (CTZ). Area situated in the area postrema of the medulla, on the lateral walls of the fourth ventricle. Lies outside the **blood–brain barrier**; chemoreceptor cells within it are thus directly exposed to blood-borne chemicals. Stimulated by **noradrenaline**, **dopamine**, **acetylcholine**, **5-HT** and **opioid receptor** agonists. Circulating emetics (e.g. **opioid analgesic drugs**) may cause **vomiting** by stimulating the CTZ, which sends efferents to the vomiting centre of the medulla. Some **antiemetic drugs** (e.g. **phenothiazines**) act by inhibiting receptors within the CTZ.

Chemoreceptors. Receptors responding to chemical stimulation, producing **action potentials** when triggered by certain (often specific) molecules.

- Examples:
  - taste and smell receptors.
  - O_2, CO_2 and hydrogen ion receptors.
  - **chemoreceptor trigger zone** cells.

See also, Aortic bodies; Breathing, control of; Carotid bodies

Chest drainage. Removal of air or liquid from the pleural space via pleural aspiration (thoracocentesis) or chest drain insertion. Used in the management of **pneumothorax**, haemothorax and **pleural effusions**.

- Pleural aspiration:
  - indications include: spontaneous pneumothorax; diagnosis or symptomatic relief of malignant effusion; and diagnosis of parapneumonic effusion.
  - technique:
    - choice of patient position is dependent on the site of the pathology and operator preference. Options include: seated and leaning forward (with elbows resting on a table); lying semi-supine on a bed; and lateral decubitus.
    - use of ultrasound guidance reduces failure and complication rates, and is now strongly recommended where available.
    - insertion point is almost always either in the second intercostal space in the mid-clavicular line, or within a triangle bound by the lateral border of pectoralis major, the lateral edge of latissimus dorsi and the line of the fifth intercostal space (the 'triangle of safety').
    - after infiltration with **local anaesthetic agent** down to the periosteum of the upper surface of the chosen **rib**, the needle or cannula (with syringe attached) is advanced above the upper edge of the rib to avoid the nerve and vessels in the **intercostal space**. Air entry is prevented by continuous aspiration during advancement, until the pleura is penetrated and fluid/air is withdrawn.
    - a three-way tap may then be connected to the cannula and used to aspirate and expel fluid/air. Aspiration should be stopped if the patient develops chest discomfort or 1.5 l fluid is withdrawn (larger volumes are associated with post-expansion **pulmonary oedema**).
  - complications: pneumothorax, failure, visceral injury and bleeding.
- Chest drain insertion:
  - indications include: pneumothorax in a ventilated patient; tension pneumothorax (after initial needle decompression); empyema; traumatic haemopneumothorax.
  - technique:
    - positioning is as for pleural aspiration; insertion site is within the 'triangle of safety' described above.
    - when draining effusions, use of ultrasound guidance is recommended where available.
    - small-bore drains (e.g. 10–16 FG [French **gauge**]) are associated with lower complication rates and greater comfort (while having similar efficacy in most situations) and are recommended as first choice for drainage of pneumothorax, simple pleural effusion and empyema. They are inserted using a **Seldinger** technique, employing the same approach as for pleural aspiration, described earlier. Minimal force should be used and the dilator inserted no more than 1 cm beyond the depth of the pleura.
    - large-bore drains (>20 FG) are usually chosen in haemopneumothorax and if blockage of smaller drains is problematic. After local anaesthetic infiltration as described earlier, the chest wall is incised about 2 cm below the proposed site of pleural incision, cutting down onto the rib below. Blunt dissection with artery forceps is performed through to the pleural cavity, and the tip of a finger inserted to sweep adherent lung away from the insertion site. If possible, IPPV should be paused at end-expiration when the pleura is actually punctured, to reduce damage to the lung. The drain is inserted into the pleural cavity and slid into position (aimed apically for pneumothorax or basally for fluid). Use of a rigid trocar has been abandoned due to high risk of trauma to the lung. Analgesia (e.g. iv **morphine**) should be given to cover the procedure and prescribed regularly when the chest drain is in place.
  - complications: pain; visceral injury; bleeding; infection; blockage. Rates for all complications (except drain blockage) are higher with large-bore drains.
  - the drain is connected to an underwater seal device (*see later*), observing the water level for swinging/bubbling with respiration. One-way flutter valves may also be used, e.g. **Heimlich valve** (flattened rubber tube within a clear plastic tubing).
  - a suture is inserted around the puncture site to aid sealing after removal, and dressings are applied.
  - plastic tubes are most commonly employed. Most tubes have side holes to aid drainage, and a radio-opaque longitudinal line.
  - CXR demonstrates the position and effect of the drain.
  - the drain is usually removed 12–24 h after cessation of air or fluid loss, often after a trial period of clamping. CXR is mandatory following removal.
- Features of the underwater seal (Fig. 41a):
  - tube A must be wide to minimise resistance. Its volumetric capacity should exceed half of the patient's maximal inspiratory volume or water may be aspirated into the chest during inspiration.

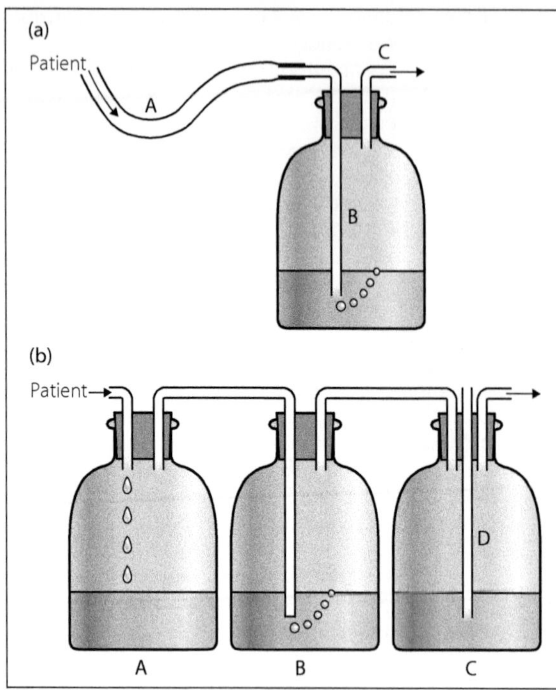

Fig. 41 Chest drainage systems: (a) one-bottle; (b) three-bottle

- the volume of water above the end of tube B should exceed half of the patient's maximal inspiratory volume to prevent indrawing of air during inspiration.
- the end of tube B should not be more than 5 cm below the surface of the water, or its resistance may prevent air being blown off.
- the drain should always be at least 45 cm below the patient.
- tube A should be temporarily clamped when the underwater seal's integrity may be disrupted, e.g. during transfer from bed to trolley.
- suction may be applied to tube C, although this is controversial. 10–20 cmH_2O suction is usually employed.
- a three-bottle system is often used, especially after cardiac or thoracic surgery (Fig. 41b). Bottle A acts as a fluid trap, e.g. for accurate measurement of blood. Bottle B provides the underwater seal. Bottle C allows suction; the height of the water level determines the amount of suction applied before air is drawn in through tube D as a safety suction-limiting device. Modern systems incorporate all three bottles in one plastic unit.

Havelock T, Teoh R, Laws D, Gleeson F (2010). Thorax; 65 (Suppl 2): ii61–76

Chest infection (Lower respiratory tract infection). Includes tracheitis, laryngotracheobronchitis (**croup**), acute bronchitis, **bronchiolitis**, acute exacerbations of **COPD/ bronchiectasis** and pneumonia.

- Commonly used classification for pneumonia:
  - community-acquired: often due to one of a limited number of pathogens, which may be deduced from epidemiological factors (e.g. exposure to animals, **alcoholism**, iv drug abuse):
    - bacteria, e.g. *Streptococcus pneumoniae* (the commonest causative agent, often resulting in classical lobar pneumonia), *Haemophilus influenzae*, *Klebsiella pneumoniae*.
    - viruses, e.g. influenza, parainfluenza, measles.
    - others, e.g. legionella, mycoplasma, rickettsia, chlamydia, *Mycobacterium tuberculosis*.
  - opportunistic: occurs in **immunodeficiency**, e.g. haematological malignancies and **AIDS**. Bacterial pneumonia with the usual organisms is common; other pathogens more likely to cause disease in the immunocompromised include *Pneumocystis jirovecii*, **cytomegalovirus**, herpes, **tuberculosis** and fungi (e.g. aspergillus and candida).
  - **nosocomial pneumonia**: up to 5% of hospital inpatients develop pneumonia, e.g. following anaesthesia, ICU admission, **atelectasis**, **aspiration of gastric contents** and **hypoventilation**. Thought to result from microaspiration of bacteria from the GIT and **bacterial translocation**; gram-negative (e.g. *Pseudomonas aeruginosa* and *Escherichia coli*) and anaerobic bacteria are commonly responsible.
- Features:
  - malaise, pyrexia, tachycardia. **Legionnaires' disease** may cause back pain and renal impairment.
  - cough, sputum, haemoptysis, dyspnoea, tachypnoea.
  - increased **$\dot{V}/\dot{Q}$ mismatch** and shunting causing **hypoxaemia** and **respiratory failure**.
  - clinical and radiological features of consolidation and collapse, possibly leading to **pleural effusion** and empyema. Severe pulmonary destruction and abscess formation may follow, especially in **staphylococcal infection**.
  - may lead to severe **sepsis** and **MODS**.
  - may also produce no systemic signs of infection (particularly in the elderly).
- Assessment and investigations include:
  - clinical assessment combined with **CXR**, arterial **blood gas interpretation**, full blood count, **C-reactive protein**, renal and liver function tests.
  - **blood cultures**, sputum culture, urinary legionella and pneumococcal antigen. HIV serological testing should be considered if indicated.
  - severity scoring systems e.g. **CURB-65 score**.

Microbiological diagnosis should not delay prompt empirical treatment according to the most likely organism. Serology or bronchial biopsy/washings may be useful in atypical cases.

- Treatment:
  - antimicrobial drugs.
  - supportive therapy; i.e., **O_2 therapy**, **iv fluids**, **physiotherapy**.
- Anaesthetic/ICU relevance:
  - **preoperative assessment** and optimisation of chest disease.
  - prevention of aspiration and atelectasis.
  - postoperatively: physiotherapy, adequate analgesia and avoidance of hypoventilation are important, especially in pre-existing chest disease.
  - treatment of respiratory failure on **ICU**, or development of **nosocomial pneumonia** in patients receiving IPPV. **Selective decontamination of the digestive tract** may help to reduce the incidence of nosocomial pneumonia on ICU, although its use is not routine.

See also, Mycoplasma infections; Nosocomial infection; Pseudomonas infections; Streptococcal infections

Chest trauma. Causes include road traffic accidents (RTAs), falls, assault including stabbings and shootings, and explosions. **Trauma** may be:
- penetrating: in stabbing injuries, trauma tends to be localised to the track of the implement. In gunshot wounds, a small entry point may disguise major internal disruption (because of rapid dissipation of kinetic injury).
- non-penetrating:
  - blunt trauma, e.g. deceleration injury in RTAs. Damage is caused by direct impact (e.g. **rib fractures**, myocardial contusion) and shearing forces (e.g. aortic rupture, tracheobronchial tears).
  - blast injuries: sudden external chest and abdominal compression may cause alveolar and pulmonary vessel rupture, with oedema and haemorrhage.

- Immediately life-threatening conditions:
  - severe **hypoventilation** caused by:
    - **airway obstruction** (especially likely with associated **head injury**).
    - **pneumothorax**/haemothorax.
    - **flail chest**.
  - reduced **cardiac output** caused by:
    - **hypovolaemia** caused by **haemorrhage**. Major vessel damage often accompanies fracture of the first two ribs. Aortic rupture usually occurs just beyond the left subclavian artery.
    - **cardiac tamponade**.
    - tension pneumothorax.
- Other conditions less immediately dangerous:
  - respiratory:
    - sternal/rib fractures.
    - tracheobronchial tears.
    - diaphragmatic rupture.
    - lung contusion.
    - **aspiration of gastric contents** (especially with head injury).
    - blast injury: symptoms may occur 2–3 days later. There may be associated **smoke inhalation**.
    - **$\dot{V}/\dot{Q}$ mismatch** and **shunt** result in **hypoxaemia**. Ventilatory failure may also occur. Infection and **ALI** may ensue.
  - cardiovascular:
    - myocardial contusion: may present as **arrhythmias**, **cardiac failure** or valve rupture.
    - damage to the coronary vessels and great vessels.
  - other injuries: head injury, vertebral and limb injuries. Oesophageal rupture may occur, with risk of mediastinitis.
- Management:
  - immediate assessment and management of the above life-threatening conditions, i.e., sealing of any penetrating wound with dressings, **O_2 therapy**, **iv fluid administration**. Airway patency and adequate respiratory movement should be checked. Chest percussion and auscultation may suggest pneumothorax or haemothorax. Heart sounds may be muffled in tamponade. **Pulsus paradoxus** may indicate tamponade or tension pneumothorax, while unequal pulses may suggest **aortic dissection** or rupture. Hypotension may occur in hypovolaemia, tamponade, tension pneumothorax and myocardial contusion.
  - subsequent assessment:
    - **CXR**: may reveal pneumothorax, surgical emphysema, fractures, evidence of aspiration and widened mediastinum (may represent aortic rupture, especially if associated with left haemothorax, depressed left main bronchus and oesophageal displacement to the right). Lung contusion may appear as fluffy, patchy shadowing within a few hours of injury.
    - arterial **blood gas interpretation**/pulse **oximetry** are especially useful.
    - **ECG** as a baseline. Serial ECG and **cardiac enzyme** changes may occur in myocardial contusion.
    - for other injuries.
  - **chest drainage**/**pericardiocentesis** as appropriate.
  - methods of analgesia include iv **opioid analgesic drugs** in small doses (but with risk of respiratory and cerebral depression), **intercostal nerve block**, **interpleural analgesia** and **epidural anaesthesia** with **local anaesthetic agent** or opioids.
  - nasogastric tube to prevent gastric dilatation.
  - surgery may be required for severe haemorrhage or trauma to the aorta, diaphragm, tracheobronchial tree or oesophagus.
  - **physiotherapy**/antibiotics. Lung contusion is exacerbated by overhydration, but hypovolaemia must be avoided.

Bernardin B, Troquet JM (2012). Emerg Med Clin North Am; 30: 377–400

Chest x-ray (CXR). Commonly performed diagnostic and screening test. Usually taken on deep inspiration; an expiratory film may be used to aid identification of a pneumothorax.
- Plan for the interpretation of CXRs (Fig. 42):
  - describe the film:
    - the date, patient's name and clinical history should be noted.
    - orientation (i.e., right/left marker) and projection. In posteroanterior (PA) films the scapulae shadows are projected laterally. Anteroposterior (AP) films are usually portable films. Lateral films allow three-dimensional localisation of pathology.
    - penetration/exposure: appropriate penetration should allow the thoracic spine to be just visible behind the heart.
    - rotation: clavicular heads should be equidistant from vertebral processes; particularly important for assessment of the mediastinum.
    - position (upright/supine): important when commenting on pneumothoraces and pleural effusions.
    - inspiratory effort: 9–10 posterior rib portions or 5–6 anterior ribs should be visible; inadequate inspiration may give the appearance of basal lung consolidation.
  - describe any obvious abnormality first; otherwise continue with the plan.
  - heart shadow:
    - normal width is <50% of thoracic diameter (PA film).
    - abnormal border may indicate aneurysm, chamber dilatation or overlying lesion; indistinct border may represent lung collapse/consolidation.
    - calcified/prosthetic valves: the aortic valve lies above a line drawn from the anterior costophrenic angle to the hilum on the lateral x-ray; the mitral valve lies below.
  - upper **mediastinum** (i.e., width, aortic shadow, hila):
    - hilar enlargement may be due to pulmonary vascular or lymph node enlargement, or overlying

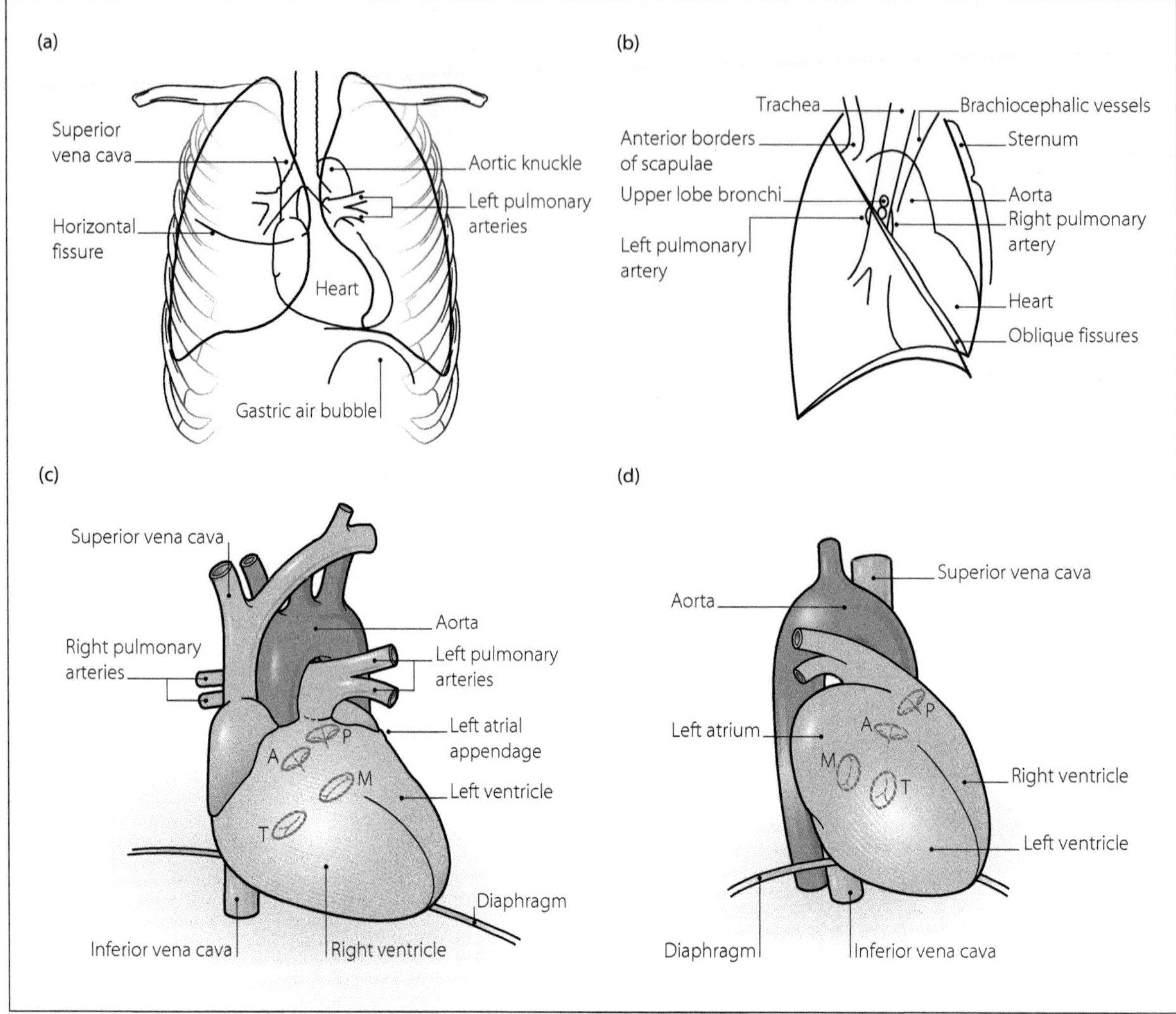

Fig. 42 Normal-appearance chest x-ray: (a) PA; (b) lateral; (c) mediastinal structures, PA; (d) mediastinal structures, lateral. Position of valves: *P*, pulmonary; *A*, aortic; *M*, mitral; *T*, tricuspid

lesion. The left hilum is usually higher than the right by 1–2 cm.
- the carina usually overlies T4–5 on inspiration.
- lung fields:
  - upper zone (above anterior part of second rib).
  - midzone (between second and fourth rib).
  - lower zone (below fourth rib).
  - compare each with the other side for translucency. Look for **pneumothorax** or hyperexpansion.
  - the left hemidiaphragm is usually lower than the right by 2 cm.
  - lung consolidation: a distinct border with neighbouring structures is lost, aiding identification of the affected lung portion; e.g. an indistinct heart border represents consolidation anteriorly, because the heart lies anteriorly in the chest.
  - lung collapse: as for consolidation, with volume loss on the affected side, mediastinal shift or tracheal deviation. The collapsed portion of lung may be visible against neighbouring structures.
  - **pleural effusion**: seen as an opacity sloping upwards and outwards at the lung base; if horizontal, it represents a gas/fluid interface.
  - **Kerley's lines** may be present.
  - prominent upper lobe pulmonary veins (upper lobe blood diversion), caused by raised pulmonary venous pressure; may be visible in left ventricular failure and left-to-right cardiac **shunts**. Proximal dilatation with peripheral narrowing (pruning) may represent **pulmonary hypertension**.
- bones: **ribs** (metastases, fractures, notching); scapulae; **vertebrae**; humerus.
- soft tissues: below **diaphragm**; above clavicles; neck; axillae; breasts.
- foreign bodies, including central lines, tracheal tubes.
- 'review' areas: apices; behind the heart; costophrenic angles.

See also, Thoracic inlet

Cheyne–Stokes respiration. Abnormal pattern of breathing characterised by alternating periods of **hyperventilation** and apnoea. Ventilation increases in depth and frequency to a peak, then decreases to apnoea. The cycle then repeats.
- Caused by:
  - central disturbance of control of breathing. **Hypoventilation** causes **hypercapnia**, which causes hyperventilation. Resultant **hypocapnia** causes apnoea until the arterial $P\text{CO}_2$ rises again. May occur in cerebral

disease, **head injury** and **opioid poisoning**. Also a major component of **sleep-disordered breathing**.
- prolonged circulation time between the lungs and brain, e.g. in **cardiac failure**. Hyperventilation continues until hypocapnia is registered by central **chemoreceptors**, although the CO_2 tension at the lungs is much lower. When the CO_2 content of blood arriving centrally is high enough to restart breathing, the CO_2 content of blood at the lungs is much higher, causing hyperventilation as it arrives at the chemoreceptors.

[John Cheyne (1777–1836), Scottish-born Irish physician; William Stokes (1804–1878), Irish physician]

Cherniack NS, Longobardo G, Evangelista CJ (2005). Neurocrit Care; 3: 271–9

See also, Breathing, control of

CHI, Commission for Health Improvement, *see Care Quality Commission*

Chi square analysis, *see Statistical tests*

Chloral hydrate. Sedative **prodrug**, introduced in 1869. Metabolised to trichloroethanol, which has a **half-life** of 8–10 h. Causes minimal cardiovascular or respiratory depression. Gastric irritation may occur; it is less frequent with **triclofos** or dichloralphenazone, both of which are also metabolised to trichloroethanol.
- Dosage: 25–50 mg/kg (children) orally/rectally; 0.5–2 g (adults).

Chloramphenicol. Bacteriostatic **antibacterial drug**; inhibits bacterial 50S ribosomal activity and thus protein synthesis. Has a broad spectrum of activity but, because of its potential toxicity, systemic use is usually reserved for life-threatening infections, e.g. due to *Haemophilus influenzae* and typhoid. Penetrates into CSF extremely well, thus used in **meningitis**. 70% protein-bound, it undergoes extensive hepatic metabolism. **Half-life** is 4 h.
- Dosage: 12.5–25 mg/kg orally/iv, qds.
- Side effects:
  - aplastic anaemia (often irreversible and may be fatal), peripheral or optic neuritis, nausea, vomiting, diarrhoea, erythema multiforme, nocturnal haemoglobinuria.
  - the 'grey-baby syndrome' (cardiovascular collapse) may occur in neonates unable to metabolise the drug. Plasma concentrations should be monitored in children under 4 years old; recommended peak (2 h after administration) and trough levels are 10–25 µg/ml and <15 µg/ml, respectively.
  - may enhance the effect of **warfarin**.

Chlordiazepoxide hydrochloride. Benzodiazepine, used for anxiolysis and treatment of **alcohol withdrawal syndromes. Half-life** is 6–30 h, with formation of active metabolites (that are renally excreted) including demoxepam (half-life up to 78 h), desmethyldiazepam and oxazepam. As with other benzodiazepines, drowsiness, respiratory depression, anterograde **amnesia**, **tolerance** and dependence may occur.
- Dosage:
  - for severe anxiety: 10 mg orally tds (increased to 100 mg daily if necessary).
  - for alcohol withdrawal: 10–50 mg orally qds, reduced over 7–10 days.

Chloride shift (Hamburger shift). Movement of chloride ions into red blood cells as O_2 is given up and exchanged for CO_2 in the tissues. CO_2 enters the cells, is converted to carbonic acid by **carbonic anhydrase** and dissociates into **hydrogen ions** and **bicarbonate**. H^+ ions are buffered by the reduced **haemoglobin**; HCO_3^- ions pass into the plasma. Chloride ions enter the cells to maintain electrical equilibrium. The reverse occurs in the lungs.

[Hartog J Hamburger (1859–1924), Dutch physiologist]

See also, Carbon dioxide transport

Chlormethiazole, *see Clomethiazole*

Chloroform. $CHCl_3$. **Inhalational anaesthetic agent**; used in 1847 by **Simpson**, although it had been used earlier. Rapidly became more popular than **diethyl ether**, and was administered to Queen **Victoria** during childbirth. Sweet-smelling and pleasant to inhale, with similar properties to **halothane**, including non flammability. Given by pouring onto a towel or by inhalers. Risk of sudden death, usually during induction, was attributed to respiratory depression in Scotland and cardiac standstill in England. The First and Second Hyderabad Commissions in 1888 and 1889, respectively, financed by the Nizam of Hyderabad (1866–1911), concluded that sudden death by respiratory depression preceded cardiac arrest. The reverse was generally accepted over 20 years later. **VF** occurred most commonly. Also caused severe **hepatic failure**. Gradually replaced by diethyl ether by the early/mid-1900s.

Payne JP (1981). Br J Anaesth; 53: 11S–15S

For physical properties, see Inhalational anaesthetic agents

See also, Greener, Hannah

Chloroprocaine hydrochloride. Ester **local anaesthetic agent**, introduced in 1952. Of rapid onset and short duration of action (approximately 45 min), with low systemic toxicity. Hydrolysed by plasma **cholinesterase**. Used for **epidural anaesthesia**, particularly for **caesarean section** in the USA and a few European countries, but not available in the UK. Used in 2%–3% solutions. Neurological deficits (after accidental intrathecal injection) and backache have followed use of preparations containing preservative. Maximal safe dose is about 15 mg/kg.

Chloroquine. Antimalarial drug, also used to treat **rheumatoid arthritis**. Should be used with caution in patients with hepatic or renal impairment, pregnancy and epilepsy. Used in combination with proguanil for prophylaxis and for treatment of non-falciparum **malaria**.
- Dosage:
  - treatment: 600 mg orally, then 300 mg after 6 h and 300 mg daily for 2 days.
  - prophylaxis: 300 mg once weekly 1 week before travel and for 6 weeks after returning.
- Side effects: GIT upset, headache, visual disturbance, skin and hair reactions, blood dyscrasias, psychosis, ECG changes, neuromuscular and myopathic weakness. Has a low therapeutic index and overdosage may cause rapidly developing arrhythmias and convulsions.

Chlorphenamine maleate (Chlorpheniramine). **Antihistamine drug**; competitive antagonist at **histamine** H_1 receptors. Used to treat allergic reactions, both mild (e.g. hayfever) and severe (e.g. **anaphylaxis**). Also used to treat

generalised itching, e.g. in obstructive jaundice or after **spinal opioids**. Duration of action is up to 6 h.
- Dosage:
  - 4 mg orally 4–6-hourly.
  - 10–20 mg im, sc or iv by slow injection, up to 40 mg/day.
- Side effects:
  - drowsiness, anticholinergic effects.
  - hypotension and CNS excitability may follow iv injection.

Chlorpromazine hydrochloride. **Phenothiazine**, used primarily as an **antipsychotic drug**. First used in the early 1950s, and called Largactil because of its large number of actions. Has been used before and during anaesthesia (e.g. **lytic cocktail**). Has powerful sedative and antiemetic properties, with anticholinergic, antidopaminergic and **α-adrenergic receptor antagonist** effects.
- Dosage: 25–50 mg orally or im tds (larger doses may be required). May also be given iv ('off-licence'), diluted to avoid thrombophlebitis. Hypotension may follow iv injection. May be given rectally as chlorpromazine base 100 mg.
- Side effects are as for phenothiazines.

Choanal atresia. Congenital blockage of one or both nasal passages. Incidence is 1:8000 births. If bilateral, it causes severe **airway obstruction** from birth, because **neonates** are obligate nose breathers. Respiratory distress and **cyanosis** are characteristically reduced during crying, when mouth breathing occurs. May be demonstrated by attempting to pass a soft catheter through the nostrils. Other congenital defects and syndromes may be associated, e.g. **VSD**.
- Management:
  - oropharyngeal airway insertion, with secure taping to the face.
  - puncture of membrane/bone is usually performed within a few days, and plastic tubes inserted.
- Anaesthetic management: classically, awake tracheal intubation is performed following **preoxygenation**, using an oral tube and throat pack; modern management and general considerations are as for any neonate. Extubation is performed awake.

Choking. Acute **airway obstruction** in a conscious person. May be due to foreign body, upper airway pathology or strangulation. There may be wheezing, coughing and obvious distress; if obstruction is complete the victim is silent.
- Management of choking by foreign body:
  - blind finger sweeps inside the mouth may push objects further down the **airway** and should be avoided.
  - adults:
    - assess severity; if able to cough or speak, encourage coughing while continuing to observe for deterioration.
    - if unable to cough or cough is inadequate, support chest with one hand, lean victim forward and, with the heel of the other hand, deliver a series of up to five sharp slaps between the shoulder blades.
    - if this is unsuccessful, perform the **Heimlich manoeuvre** (or upper abdominal thrusts aiming towards the diaphragm if the victim is supine) up to five times, then five back slaps, etc.
    - if the victim becomes unconscious or has a respiratory arrest, start **CPR**.
  - children: as for adult management but chest thrusts are performed in children <1 year; abdominal thrusts may cause visceral rupture in infants.

Perkins GD, Travers AH, Considine J, et al (2015). Resuscitation; 95: e43–70

Cholangitis, acute. Acute bacterial infection of the **biliary tract**. Varies from mild illness to acute fulminant cholangitis, with 40% mortality. Almost always associated with complete or partial biliary obstruction, e.g. caused by gallstones, pancreatic or ampullary cancer or surgery. May occur in critically ill patients due to 'biliary sludging' and be responsible for unexplained **sepsis**.
- Features:
  - Charcot's triad: fever (in 90%); right upper quadrant abdominal pain; and jaundice. Reynolds pentad adds altered mental state (in 20%) and hypotension (in 30%).
  - increased bilirubin, alkaline phosphatase and transaminases in 90% of cases.
  - positive blood culture (most commonly *Escherichia coli*, enterococci, klebsiella) in 20%–30% of cases.
  - increased **procalcitonin** levels indicate the need for emergency biliary drainage.

Ultrasound and/or hepatobiliary scanning confirms the diagnosis.
- Management:
  - supportive: iv fluids, O_2 therapy, analgesia, **antibacterial drugs**. Full ICU support may be required in fulminant cases.
  - endoscopic retrograde cholangiopancreatography (ERCP) to re-establish biliary drainage is the mainstay of treatment.

[Jean M Charcot (1825–1893), Paris neurologist; Benedict M Reynolds, US surgeon]

Cholecystitis, acute. Inflammation of the wall of the gallbladder. A recognised complication of critical illness, it may occur in the absence of gallstones (acalculous cholecystitis). Aetiology includes gallbladder ischaemia, biliary 'sludging' and cystic duct obstruction; contributory factors include fever, **sepsis**, **dehydration**, **opioid analgesic drugs** and **TPN**. Diagnosis should be considered in all ICU patients with unexplained sepsis. Untreated, it leads to gallbladder necrosis, gangrene and perforation; mortality is >50%.
- Features:
  - fever, leucocytosis, abdominal pain/tenderness and loss of bowel sounds.
  - increased alkaline phosphatase and bilirubin in 50% of cases.
  - diagnosis is confirmed by ultrasonography and/or hepatobiliary CT scanning.
- Management:
  - broad-spectrum **antibacterial drugs** to cover aerobic and anaerobic organisms.
  - Definitive treatment is cholecystectomy but percutaneous cholecystostomy is performed if the patient is unstable.

Morse BC, Smith JB, Lawdahl RB, Roettger RH (2010). Am Surg; 76: 708–12

See also, Biliary tract

Cholinergic crisis. Syndrome caused by relative overdose of **acetylcholinesterase inhibitors** causing excess nicotinic (muscle weakness, fasciculation) and muscarinic (sweating, miosis, lacrimation, abdominal colic) stimulation by **acetylcholine**. May occur in **myasthenia gravis** but rarely seen with good management. Also seen in **organophosphorus poisoning**.

Cholinergic receptors, *see Acetylcholine receptors*

Cholinesterase, plasma (Pseudocholinesterase). Circulating **enzyme** produced by the liver, of unknown primary function but which hydrolyses **suxamethonium**. Removes choline groups to produce first succinylmonocholine and then succinic acid. Also present in other tissues, e.g. brain and kidneys.

- Reduced enzyme activity causes prolonged paralysis after suxamethonium, and may be due to:
  - inherited atypical cholinesterase. Several autosomal recessive genes have been identified, using the degree of enzyme inhibition by various substances (e.g. dibucaine or fluoride) to describe the enzyme characteristics:
    - normal enzyme (designated E1u): 94% of the population are homozygotes. **Dibucaine number** (DN) is 75–85, and fluoride number (FN) is 60.
    - atypical enzyme (E1a): 0.03% of the population are homozygotes, with DN 15–25 and FN 20.
    - silent gene (E1s): 0.001% of the population are homozygotes, with no plasma cholinesterase activity.
    - fluoride-resistant enzyme (E1f): 0.0001% of the population are homozygotes; DN is 65–75 but FN is 30.

    Paralysis may last 2–4 h in homozygotes for silent and atypical genes, and 1–2 h in homozygotes for the fluoride-resistant gene. In addition, heterozygotes with one normal and one abnormal gene (e.g. E1u/E1a; 5% of the population) with DN 40–60 may show prolonged paralysis of about 10–20 min. Most of these have the atypical gene. Combinations of abnormal genes comprise less than 0.01% of the population and also show slight or marked prolongation of paralysis.
  - acquired deficiency of normal cholinesterase, e.g. in **hepatic failure**, **hypoproteinaemia**, **pregnancy**, **malnutrition**, **burns** and following **plasmapheresis**.
  - inhibition of cholinesterase by drugs, e.g. **echothiophate**, **cyclophosphamide**, **tetrahydroaminacrine**, **hexafluorenium** or phenelzine.

Plasma cholinesterase also hydrolyses other drugs, e.g. **mivacurium**, ester **local anaesthetic drugs**, **diamorphine**, **aspirin** and **propanidid**. Although **esmolol** and **remifentanil** are readily hydrolysed by non-specific cholinesterases, plasma cholinesterase itself is not important in their breakdown.

Chronic bronchitis, *see Chronic obstructive pulmonary disease*

Chronic obstructive airways disease (COAD), *see Chronic obstructive pulmonary disease.*

Chronic obstructive pulmonary disease (COPD; Chronic obstructive airways disease; COAD). Term encompassing chronic bronchitis and emphysema, which, although different histologically, often coexist. Aetiology is increasingly recognised as multifactorial, including genetic influences, respiratory illness during childhood, as well as environmental factors (e.g. **smoking**, air pollution). The main features are lower airway obstruction, hyperinflated lungs and impaired gas exchange.

- Chronic bronchitis:
  - defined clinically by productive cough each morning for at least 3 months per year, for at least 2 successive years.
  - results from chronic bronchial irritation (e.g. by smoke, dust or fumes), causing mucosal hypersecretion, mucosal oedema and bronchoconstriction.
  - features: cough, dyspnoea, wheeze. Sufferers are typically described as 'blue bloaters' because of cyanosis and oedema.
  - **FEV_1**, expiratory flow rate and FEV/**FVC** are decreased, with increased **residual volume** and **FRC**, and **$\dot{V}/\dot{Q}$ mismatch**.
  - **hypoxaemia** and **hypercapnia** result, with possible loss of the central response to CO_2 (the mechanism is unclear). **Hypoxic pulmonary vasoconstriction** may lead to **pulmonary hypertension** with **cor pulmonale** and right ventricular failure.
- Emphysema:
  - defined histologically by dilated alveoli and/or respiratory bronchioles, often in upper areas of the lungs. Different patterns of dilatation are identified. Elastic recoil is reduced.
  - causes: as above, plus α_1-antitrypsin deficiency; the latter typically affects the lung bases.
  - features: dyspnoea. Air trapping and increased airflow resistance result from airway collapse during forceful expiration. Breath sounds are usually quiet. Sufferers are typically described as 'pink puffers' because of absent cyanosis and marked dyspnoea.
  - work of breathing is markedly increased, with hypocapnia (i.e., hyperventilation as opposed to hypoventilation as in chronic bronchitis), but only mild hypoxaemia.
  - FEV_1 is reduced and FRC increased, as described earlier.

Diffusing capacity is decreased in both conditions. **Respiratory muscle fatigue** may be a factor. Acute exacerbations are often associated with **chest infection**; patients may present with **respiratory failure**.

- Management:
  - long-term treatment includes avoidance of precipitating factors if possible, pulmonary rehabilitation/exercise programmes, inhaled bronchodilators/steroids, and if severe, O_2 therapy. Mucolytics and antibiotics may also be used to reduce exacerbations. Lung volume reduction surgery and even transplantation have been used in very severe cases and in younger patients.
  - management of acute exacerbations is as for respiratory failure. Supplemental oxygen is titrated to achieve an arterial oxygen saturation of 88%–92% and medical therapy optimised. Frequent arterial **blood gas interpretation** monitors the success of medical management. If acidotic ventilatory failure persists, the treatment of choice is **non-invasive positive pressure ventilation**.
  - the decision to intubate/ventilate is sometimes difficult, because **weaning from ventilators** may be impossible. Useful information in making the decision concerning IPPV includes: the patient's level of normal activity and lifestyle; the nature and course of previous admissions; and whether the current crisis represents gradual decline or an acute treatable event, e.g. superimposed acute infection.

- Anaesthetic management:
  - preoperatively:
    - **preoperative assessment** for exercise tolerance, bronchospasm, cor pulmonale and history of previous admissions. Patients are likely to be smokers; thus cardiovascular assessment including **ECG** is important. **CXR** may reveal a hyperexpanded chest, flattened diaphragm, narrow mediastinum, emphysematous bullae or infection. Arterial blood gas interpretation and **lung function tests** may be useful.
    - improvement by **physiotherapy** and antibiotics if infection is present, and **bronchodilator drugs** if there is a reversible element to airway obstruction. Preoperative smoking cessation for >4 weeks decreases postoperative pulmonary complications. Nutritional supplementation is useful if serum albumin is low.
    - premedication: increased sensitivity to respiratory depressants, especially in chronic bronchitis, is rarely a problem. **Pethidine**, **promethazine** and **atropine** are often used; the latter may help prevent perioperative **bronchospasm** and reduce secretions, but may increase their tenacity.
  - perioperatively:
    - regional techniques are often suitable; problems may include inability to lie flat, possibility of coughing and sensitivity to sedative drugs if used.
    - general anaesthesia:
      - inhalational techniques with a facemask are suitable for short procedures, with minimal airway manipulation.
      - if tracheal intubation is undertaken, topical or iv **lidocaine** may be used to reduce irritation by the tracheal tube. Tracheal suction is often required. Bronchospasm and coughing may occur. **Capnography** allows maintenance of expired PCO_2 at the patient's normal (i.e., preoperative) level.
      - IPPV techniques should avoid excessive inflation pressures to reduce the risk of **barotrauma** and also to reduce air trapping. These include allowing greater time for expiration by decreasing the **inspiratory:expiratory ratio**, decreasing respiratory rate (and allowing **permissive hypercapnia**), judicious use of **PEEP** and using pressure-controlled ventilation.
      - drugs causing **histamine** release are usually avoided.
  - postoperative problems include:
    - sputum retention, bronchospasm, **atelectasis** and infection. Physiotherapy and bronchodilator therapy are important. Respiratory failure may occur. **Doxapram** may be useful. Ventilation is often improved in the sitting position.
    - hypoventilation may be exacerbated by pain, depressant drugs and high F_IO_2. Adequate **postoperative analgesia** is vital; regional techniques are particularly useful, as excessive use of systemic opioids must be avoided. Parenteral opioids should be given cautiously.
    - patients with severe disease or those receiving **spinal opioids** may require management on ICU/HDU.
    - elective IPPV may allow adequate gas exchange while depressant anaesthetic drugs are cleared. It also 'covers' the period of worst postoperative pain and allows stabilisation before weaning.

Spieth PM, Guldner A, de Abreu MG (2012). Curr Opin Anaesthesiol; 25: 24–9

Churchill, Frederick, *see Liston, Robert*

Ciclosporin (Cyclosporin). Isomerase-binding **immunosuppressive drug** that interferes with proliferation of activated T lymphocytes. Main use is to prevent and treat rejection following organ **transplantation**. Has also been used in **myasthenia gravis** and other **autoimmune diseases**. Oral administration has 30% **bioavailability**.

Eliminated via hepatic metabolism, its **half-life** (assuming normal liver function) is 19 h.

- Dosage: 2–5 mg/kg/day iv, followed by 12–15 mg/kg/day orally. After 1–2 weeks, the dose is reduced by 5%–10% per week. Therapeutic blood levels vary between centres and should be monitored.
- Side effects:
  - reduces GFR by at least 20% in almost all patients; renal function returns to normal within 2 weeks of stopping the drug, even following prolonged use. Irreversible nephrotoxicity occurs in a minority of cardiac and renal transplant patients.
  - GIT upset, gum hyperplasia, hirsutism, hyperkalaemia, mild hepatic impairment, hypertension, tremor, occasionally convulsions and encephalopathy.
  - interacts with other drugs that cause hyperkalaemia or nephrotoxicity, and increases plasma concentrations of several drugs, including **diclofenac** and **digoxin**.

Cigarette smoking, *see Smoking*

Ciliary activity. Continuous beating of the cilia of respiratory epithelial cells results in flow of thick mucus from the nose to the pharynx, and from the bronchi to the larynx. The mucus is then swallowed or expectorated. A more watery mucus layer lies between the thick layer and the epithelium, lubricating the cilia. Important in aiding removal of foreign particles and microbes and clearing of the airways. Reduced by **smoking**, extremes of temperature, volatile **inhalational anaesthetic agents**, **opioid analgesic drugs** and prolonged exposure to high O_2 levels. Prolonged inhalation of dry gases, anticholinergic drug administration and volatile agents may impair mucus production or flow.

Patients with inborn deficiency of cilia protein are predisposed to **bronchiectasis**; if associated with decreased spermatic activity, situs inversus and chronic sinusitis, this constitutes Kartagener's syndrome.
[Manes Kartagener (1897–1975), Swiss physician]

Cimetidine. **H_2 receptor antagonist**, of faster onset and shorter-acting than **ranitidine**, lasting about 4 h. **Half-life** is 2 h; up to 5 h in **renal failure**.

- Dosage:
  - 400 mg orally od/bd. Effective if given 90 min preoperatively.
  - 200 mg im/iv by infusion (may cause bradycardia and hypotension after rapid iv injection).
- Side effects:
  - gynaecomastia, rarely impotence (binds to androgen receptors).
  - hepatic **enzyme inhibition** (binds to microsomal cytochrome P_{450}). The actions of drugs such as **warfarin**, **phenytoin** and **theophylline** may be prolonged, and toxic effects seen.

- confusion, especially in the elderly and very ill.
- rarely, liver impairment and blood dyscrasias.

Cinchocaine hydrochloride. Amide **local anaesthetic agent**, synthesised in 1925. Formerly widely used in the UK for **spinal anaesthesia** and also for **epidural anaesthesia**, infiltration, nerve blocks and surface analgesia. Of slower onset and duration of action than lidocaine, and more toxic.

Used to estimate plasma **cholinesterase** activity (**dibucaine number**).

Ciprofloxacin. **4-Quinolone** type **antibacterial drug**; acts by inhibiting bacterial DNA replication. Has a broad spectrum of activity, but especially against gram-negative bacteria, including klebsiella, escherichia, salmonella, shigella, campylobacter, neisseria, pseudomonas, haemophilus and enterobacter species. Less active against gram-positive bacteria (e.g. streptococcus) and anaerobes. Also active against chlamydia and certain mycobacteria.

- Dosage:
  - 250–750 mg orally bd.
  - 400 mg iv bd (given over 60 min).
- Side effects:
  - GIT upset, skin reactions, renal/hepatic impairment, tendon inflammation/damage; less commonly, blood dyscrasias, haemolytic anaemia, convulsions.
  - may enhance the effects of **theophyllines** and **warfarin**.

Circle of Willis, *see Cerebral circulation*

Circle systems. **Anaesthetic breathing systems** incorporating unidirectional valves and **CO_2 absorption** with **soda lime**. First used by Sword in 1926.

- Features:
  - consist of CO_2 absorber, two one-way valves, **adjustable pressure-limiting** (APL) **valve**, **reservoir bag**, tubing to and from the patient and for fresh gas flow (FGF). Efficiency is increased by placing:
    - FGF downstream to APL valve (avoids venting of fresh gas).
    - bag and patient on opposite sides of the one-way valves (maintains circulatory gas flow).

    Examples of arrangements (Fig. 43): system A is efficient for spontaneous ventilation and IPPV; **dead space** gas is conserved beyond the APL valve during expiration while alveolar gas is flushed by FGF via the APL valve. System B is less efficient because the APL valve is further away from the patient; dead space and alveolar gases mix more before reaching it. System B is more convenient practically, however, because all components are away from the patient.
  - ready-assembled circle systems are usual now, arranged as in system B within one housing. Older systems had a switch that could bypass the soda lime; to prevent this happening accidentally these are not present on newer systems.
  - resistance is reduced by using wide-bore tubing.
- Advantages:
  - low gas flows may be used, allowing conservation of volatile agent with reduced cost and pollution.
  - reduced risk of **explosions and fires** with inflammable agents.
  - warmth and humidity of expired gases are retained, with further warming and humidification in the CO_2 absorber, although efficiency is reduced by passage through lengths of tubing.
  - spontaneous/controlled ventilation is easily performed without changing the system.
  - allows easy monitoring of O_2 uptake/CO_2 output.
- Disadvantages:
  - production of **carbon monoxide** may occur when volatile agents containing the CHF_2 moiety (**desflurane**, **enflurane** or **isoflurane**) are passed over dry warm absorbent (especially **baralyme**), e.g. at the start of a Monday morning operating session following prolonged passage of dry gas through the absorber.
  - accumulation of other substances in the system (especially if very low fresh gas flows are used over a long time): alcohol derived from the patient; compound A and bromochlorodifluoroethylene following use of **sevoflurane** and halothane, respectively; acetone in some starved patients. None of these has been associated with adverse clinical effects.
  - higher resistance and thus work of breathing.
  - bulky equipment.
  - slow changes in anaesthetic concentrations at low gas flows.
  - risk of hypoxic gas mixtures if N_2O is used.
  - more connections to come apart and valves to stick.
- Use:
  - if N_2O is used, nitrogen contained in the lungs and dissolved in the body will be washed out; build-up of nitrogen in the system may lead to a low F_IO_2. A high initial FGF (5–7 l/min) for 7–10 min is sufficient to remove most body nitrogen. N_2O concentration within the system as its uptake decreases may also contribute to low F_IO_2.
  - if only O_2 is used, hypoxic mixtures do not occur, but absorption **atelectasis** and **O_2 toxicity** are more likely.
  - with high flow, the APL valve is open.
  - low flow is defined as <1–1.5 l/min FGF:
    - APL valve totally closed: FGF supplies basal requirements only, i.e., 220–250 ml/min O_2 ('closed system').
    - APL valve slightly open, i.e., allowing a small leak: 1–3 l/min is often used as a compromise between the closed and high-flow systems ('semiclosed').
  - IPPV is achieved by hand or by switching the reservoir bag to a **bellows** that may be compressed intermittently by an integral **ventilator** (if present in the **anaesthetic machine**). If there is no integral ventilator, a suitable ventilator (e.g. Penlon Nuffield)

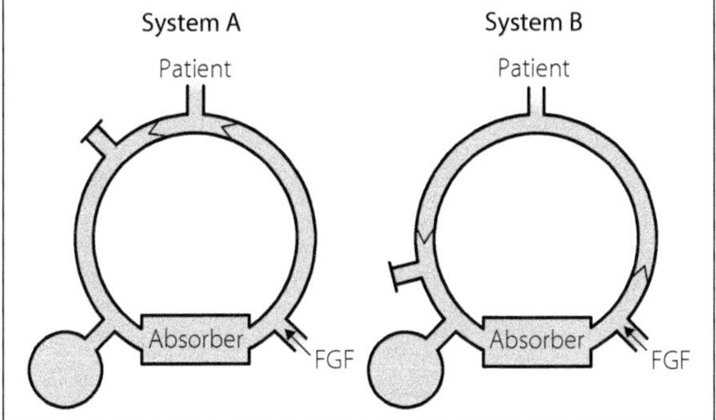

Fig. 43 Examples of circle systems (*see text*)

may be attached to the reservoir bag attachment by tubing of adequate length to prevent mixing of the driving gas (O_2) and the FGF.
- continuous **gas analysis** is particularly important.
- **vaporisers:**
  - out of circle (VOC):
    - usual plenum vaporisers are used on the back bar of the anaesthetic machine.
    - the concentration of volatile agent within the circle is less than that delivered by the vaporiser, because of dilution by exhaled gas. The difference is highest initially, when uptake of agent is greatest, unless high FGFs are used. The time to reach equilibrium is least for less soluble agents.
  - in circle (VIC):
    - low-resistance vaporisers are required, e.g. Goldman's (*see Vaporisers*). Delivered concentration is related to gas flow through the vaporiser.
    - as volatile agent is present in exhaled gas entering the vaporiser, high concentrations are possible. During spontaneous ventilation, respiratory depression increases as the concentration increases, reducing gas flow through the vaporiser. Thus dangerous levels of agent are not reached. During IPPV, this feedback mechanism is absent; i.e., dangerous levels are attainable.
    - liquid anaesthetic may be injected directly into the tubing.

[Brian Sword (1889–1956), US anaesthetist]

Circulation, respiration, abdomen, motor and speech scale (CRAMS scale). **Trauma scale** for use in adult prehospital **triage** when categorising severity of injury. Scores of 2 (normal), 1 or 0 are assigned to each of the five systems assessed. Rarely used in isolation now.

Cisapride. **Prokinetic drug** chemically related to **metoclopramide** but without antidopaminergic activity or CNS-depressant effects. Withdrawn from use in 2000 in the UK because of reports of **prolonged Q–T syndromes**, often resulting from concomitant use of other drugs such as antifungal and antibacterial drugs.

Cisatracurium besilate. Non-depolarising **neuromuscular blocking drug**, one of the 10 stereoisomers of **atracurium** (the 1R *cis*-1′R *cis* isomer; makes up 15% of atracurium, contributing about 60% of its activity). Introduced in 1995, it causes minimal **histamine** release with cardiovascular stability. Also, although up to 70% metabolized by **Hofmann degradation** (cf. atracurium, 50%–60%), produces about 10 times less **laudanosine** than atracurium after prolonged infusion, because of its greater potency and thus smaller total dosage. Initial dose: 150 μg/kg, with intubation possible ~120 s later. Effects last 30–40 min. Supplementary dose: 30 μg/kg. Has been given by iv infusion at 60–120 μg/kg/h. Storage requirements are as for atracurium. Faster degradation occurs when diluted in Hartmann's solution and 5% dextrose than in other iv fluids.
See also, Isomerism

Citrate and citrate solutions, *see Blood storage; Sodium citrate*

CJD, *see Creutzfeldt–Jakob disease*

Clapeyron–Clausius equation. Equation characterising the discontinuous phase change between two states of matter. Describes the relationship between **SVP**, temperature and **latent heat** (LH). Used practically to predict changes in state in response to alterations in pressure/temperature. Assumes LH is independent of temperature, and that the volume of liquid is negligible compared with that of the vapour.
[Benoit-Paul Clapeyron (1799–1864), French engineer; Rudolf Clausius (1822–1888), German physicist]

Clarithromycin. **Macrolide**, **antibacterial drug** derived from **erythromycin** and with similar mechanism of action and spectrum of activity, although more active against *Streptococcus pneumoniae* and *Staphylococcus aureus*, and with greater penetration of tissues. GIT side effects are less common than with erythromycin.
- Dosage: 250–500 mg orally or 500 mg iv bd.
- Side effects: nausea, vomiting, hepatic impairment, phlebitis, **Stevens–Johnson syndrome**.

Clark electrode, *see Oxygen measurement*

Clarke, William E (1818–1878). US physician; used **diethyl ether** to allow dental extraction in January 1842 in New York, but only reported this after **Morton**'s demonstration in 1846.

Clathrates. Compounds comprising a crystal lattice of one type of molecule trapping and containing another. Formation of clathrates consisting of volatile agent and water (gas hydrates) in neuronal cell membranes (thereby disrupting their function) was suggested by Pauling and Miller in 1961 as a basis for the mechanism of action of **inhalational anaesthetic agents.**

Now considered incorrect because:
- for some fluorocarbons, potency is not related to clathrate formation.
- some inhalational agents do not form clathrates at body temperature and pressure.
- effects of combining different agents are not accounted for.

[Linus Pauling (1901–1994) and Stanley L Miller (1930–2007), US chemists]
See also, Anaesthesia, mechanism of

Clavulanic acid. β-Lactamase inhibitor, used in combination with **amoxicillin** (as **co-amoxiclav**) and **ticarcillin** in order to prevent their breakdown by penicillinase produced by *Staphylococcus aureus* and other **bacteria.** Has been associated with cholestatic jaundice.

Clearance. Theoretical value representing removal of a substance from plasma or blood by passage through an organ. Defined as the volume of plasma completely cleared of a given substance per unit time. Thus for the kidney it equals (in ml/min):

$$\frac{\text{amount of substance excreted in urine per unit time}}{\text{plasma concentration of substance}}$$

$$= \frac{\text{urinary concentration (mmol/l)} \times \text{urine volume (ml/min)}}{\text{plasma concentration (mmol/l)}}$$

The concept is useful in comparing excretion rates of different drugs; it is also used to determine **renal blood flow** and **GFR.**

If there is incomplete removal by the kidney, clearance for a substance is less than GFR. If the substance is secreted into the urine by tubular cells, clearance exceeds GFR.
See also, Pharmacokinetics

Clearance, creatinine, *see Creatinine clearance*

Clearance, free water. Volume of plasma cleared of solute-free water per minute. Equals urine volume (ml/min) minus osmotic **clearance** (ml/min). Normally negative, i.e., water is being conserved, and hypertonic urine produced. Positive in **water diuresis**.
See also, Clearance, osmotic

Clearance, osmotic. Volume of plasma cleared of solute per unit time. Equals:

$$\frac{\text{urine osmolality (mosmol/l)} \times \text{urine volume (ml/min)}}{\text{plasma osmolality (mosmol/l)}}$$

If urine is hypotonic, urine volume exceeds osmotic **clearance**; if hypertonic, osmotic clearance is greater. The difference between them is free water clearance. Normally under 3 ml/min; increased by osmotic diuretics.
See also, Clearance, free water

Cleft lip and palate, *see Facial deformities, congenital*

Clindamycin. Bacteriostatic **antibacterial drug**, a semi-synthetic derivative of lincomycin. Although active against aerobic and anaerobic gram-positive organisms, its use is limited to the treatment of staphylococcal bone and joint infection, peritonitis and endocarditis because of its side effects, especially infection with *Clostridium difficile*. 95% protein-bound, it undergoes hepatic metabolism to inactive metabolites, with 20% excreted unchanged in the urine. Poor levels are attained in CSF.

- Dosage:
  - 150–450 mg orally qds.
  - 0.6–2.7 g/day in 2–4 divided doses by deep im injection (maximal single dose 600 mg) or by iv infusion (maximal single dose 1.2 g).
- Side effects: GIT upset, pseudomembranous colitis, hepatic impairment, rashes, blood dyscrasias, pain on injection, thrombophlebitis.

See also, Clostridial infections

Clinical governance. Term denoting a particular aspect of **risk management** and **quality assurance/improvement** in which responsibility for maintaining standards of care is defined and placed with specified individuals and departments. In the NHS, the chief executive of each Trust is responsible for the care provided, although each department is expected to take steps to ensure high standards and both detect and act upon deficiencies at individual and departmental levels. Requires that evidence-based medicine is in routine use, that good practice and innovations are systematically disseminated and applied, and that high-quality data are collected to monitor clinical care. Two bodies were set up in 1999 to monitor these processes: the National Institute for Clinical (now Health and Care) Excellence (**NICE**) and the Commission for Health Improvement (subsequently the **Care Quality Commission**). The concept arose formally from political and medical reactions to well-publicised examples of inadequate care, its introduction achieving particular impetus following the high death rate after paediatric cardiac surgery in Bristol in the 1980s/early 1990s. As a result of disciplinary rulings following this case, all clinicians are now expected to monitor their own performance and undergo regular appraisal and revalidation.
Halligan A, Donaldson L (2001). Br Med J; 322: 1413–7

Clinical trials. Performed to determine whether an intervention is useful, how it compares with others, whether it affects different groups of patients differently and how it is best delivered (e.g. drug dosage regimen, route, timing).

- Setting up a trial:
  - aims of the trial are defined.
  - the number of patients is defined; ideally, the number is calculated by first defining the size of difference considered clinically important, and then the sample size required to enable such a difference to be revealed if present (i.e., **power** analysis). Groups should usually be of equal size if possible.
  - subjects:
    - patients with other diseases and those taking other drugs are excluded where possible.
    - controls:
      - pairs may be matched for age, sex, race, degree and duration of illness and one of each pair assigned to each treatment.
      - cross-over studies: patients act as their own controls by receiving first one treatment then another. The effect of the first treatment on the second must be excluded.
      - **randomisation** into groups.
      - historical controls are avoided where possible.
      - treatment is compared with no treatment, placebo or existing treatment.
  - bias is further reduced by blinding:
    - single-blind (patient is unaware of group allocation).
    - double-blind (care-provider and patient are unaware).
    - triple-blind (as double-blind, plus those assessing outcome data are unaware)
  - variability is reduced by using the same location, time of day, medical/nursing staff and technique for all patients.
  - approval by a Research Ethics Committee (in the USA, Institutional Review Board): includes qualified and lay persons. Considers whether exposure of patients to the new treatment or denial of the old treatment to controls, or vice versa, is justified, whether adequate information is given to potential participants, and whether proper **consent** is obtained.
  - approval is also required from the organisation (e.g. Trust Research and Development Department) and regulatory authorities if drugs or devices are involved (in the UK, the **Medicines and Healthcare products Regulatory Agency**; in the USA, the **Food and Drug Administration**).
  - **data**:
    - what to measure, according to defined aims.
    - objective measurements are less prone to observer bias than subjective assessment.
    - how many measurements; measurement of too many variables increases the likelihood of at least one being significantly different due to chance alone (false positive).

  - which **statistical test** to use, and how to express results, e.g. use of the **null hypothesis** or **confidence intervals**.
- end-point of the trial:
  - according to the numbers studied.
  - sequential analysis: the trial stops when results attain significance.
  - if any predetermined stopping criteria are met, e.g. the treatment is found to have drastically superior or inferior outcomes compared with control.

See also, Drug development; Meta-analysis; Statistics

Clomethiazole edisylate (Chlormethiazole). Sedative drug, structurally related to vitamin B_1. Has been used for sedation and as an **anticonvulsant drug**. Traditionally used to treat acute **alcohol withdrawal syndromes**. No longer available for iv use because of the risk of severe CVS/RS depression.

- Dosage: 1–4 capsules (equivalent to 5–20 ml elixir that contains 50 mg/ml) orally, 3–4-hourly.
- Side effects: nasal irritation, GIT upset, headache, agitation.

Clonazepam. **Benzodiazepine**, used mainly to treat **epilepsy**. Has also been used in disorders of movement (e.g. dystonias) and as an adjunct to **pain management**. Has similar effects to **diazepam**. 50% protein-bound after iv injection. Metabolised in the liver and excreted in the urine. Elimination **half-life** is 24–48 h.

- Dosage:
  - 1–8 mg/day orally in adults, titrated to response.
  - 0.25–1 mg/day in infants.
  - 0.5–1 mg diluted in water for iv injection.
- Side effects include sedation (occasionally excitation), bronchial and salivary hypersecretion, and, rarely, hepatic impairment and blood dyscrasias.

Clonidine hydrochloride. **α-Adrenergic receptor agonist**, used as an analgesic, sedative and **antihypertensive drug**. Previously used in the prophylaxis of **migraine**. Licensed in the USA for use via the epidural route for pain therapy. Also used as an adjuvant drug in **spinal anaesthesia**, **caudal analgesia** and peripheral nerve blockade.

Stimulates central presynaptic **α_2-adrenergic receptors**, causing suppression of **catecholamine** release (i.e., activates a negative-feedback control system). Its main effect is on **vasomotor centre** output, but also has analgesic and sedative actions. It reduces **MAC** of **inhalational anaesthetic agents** and postoperative analgesic requirements. May have some α_1-agonist action peripherally, causing initial transient hypertension.

Its **half-life** is about 23 h. Metabolised in the liver, with about 65% excreted unchanged in the urine and 20% in the faeces.

- Dosage:
  - 50–100 µg/day tds, up to 1.2 mg.
  - 150–300 µg by slow iv injection. Effects occur within 10 min, and last 3–7 h. Transient hypertension and bradycardia may occur.
  - 30 µg/h via epidural route, adjusted according to response (boluses of 100–300 mg have been used for acute pain, although not licensed for this use). Hypotension may occur.
- Side effects: sedation, dry mouth, depression, urinary retention, reduced gastric motility. 'Rebound' hypertension can occur if it is suddenly withdrawn.

Clopidogrel besilate/hydrochloride/hydrogen sulfate. Thienopyridine **antiplatelet drug**; acts by inhibiting the P2Y12 class of ADP receptors on the platelet surface. Used for the treatment of **acute coronary syndromes**, secondary prevention of ischaemic events or primary prevention in patients with **atrial fibrillation** for whom **warfarin** is unsuitable. Usually combined with aspirin. Recently shown to be less effective than newer ADP receptor antagonist antiplatelet drugs, e.g. **prasugrel**, **ticagrelor**.

Oral **bioavailability** is approximately 50% but is highly variable. Clopidogrel itself is an inactive prodrug; it is converted to an active metabolite by the P_{450} cytochrome system (mostly CYP3A4/5). Has reduced activity when given with other CYP3A substrates (e.g. atorvastatin) and increased activity with P_{450} enzyme inducers (e.g. **rifampicin**). The active metabolite is rapidly excreted in bile and urine but irreversibly antagonises platelet $P2Y_{12}$ ADP receptors, thereby inhibiting ADP-mediated platelet aggregation by blocking the glycoprotein IIb/IIIb pathway. Restoration of platelet function requires synthesis (or transfusion) of new platelets. Withdrawal for a week before surgery has been recommended (unless the patient has coronary artery stents in situ; *see Percutaneous coronary intervention for details*).

- Dosage:
  - acute coronary syndromes: 300 mg orally initially followed by 75 mg od.
  - prevention of ischaemic events: 75 mg orally od.
- Side effects: bleeding, GI upset, rash, rarely **thrombotic thrombocytopenic purpura**.

Closing capacity. **Lung volume** at which airway closure occurs, mainly in the dependent parts of the lung. Equals closing volume plus **residual volume**. In fit young adults, closing capacity (CC) is considerably less than **FRC**; thus airway closure does not occur during normal quiet breathing. Airway closure occurring within FRC results in increased **shunt**.

- Measurement: inspiration of a bolus of marker gas (e.g. helium; He) at the end of maximal expiration (i.e., residual volume), followed by inspiration of air to total lung capacity (Fig. 44). Expired He concentration is measured during slow expiration: the same phases are seen as in **Fowler's method** (which may also be used to measure CC). Initially, **dead space** gas is exhaled, containing no He. Then, a mixture of dead space and alveolar gas, followed by alveolar gas. As CC is reached there is a sharp rise in expired He; this is because the alveoli that are still open at CC contain

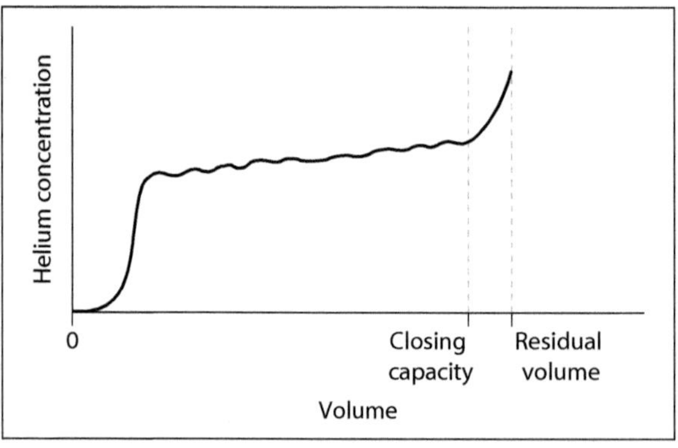

Fig. 44 Measurement of closing capacity

a higher concentration of He than the mean (because they received a larger amount of the initial inspired bolus).

- Increased by:
  - age: CC = FRC in neonates and infants.
    CC = FRC in the supine position at 40 years.
    CC = FRC in the upright position at 65 years.
  - increased intrathoracic pressures, e.g. **asthma**.
  - **smoking**.

CC may encroach upon a FRC reduced by **obesity**, the supine position and anaesthesia. **PEEP** and **CPAP** may reduce airway closure.

Drummond GB, Milic-Emili J (2007). Br J Anaesth; 99: 772–4

Closing volume, *see Closing capacity*

Clostridial infections. Caused by **bacteria** of the genus *Clostridium*. They are gram-positive, anaerobic, spore-forming and toxin-producing. Species include:

- *C. difficile*: increasingly common nosocomial pathogen that colonises the colon and releases **exotoxins** (Tcd A & B). Carriers may be asymptomatic but usually results in **diarrhoea**. Less commonly an acute and severe inflammation of the large bowel (pseudomembranous colitis) occurs. Transmission between humans is via the faecal–oral route. The dramatic increase in incidence in hospital patients since 2000 reflects the emergence of virulent strains. 30% of cases are community acquired.
  - risk factors:
    - **antibacterial drug** use: common drugs implicated include **clindamycin**, **amoxicillin**, **ampicillin**, **cephalosporins** (especially **ceftriaxone**) and **4-quinolones** (especially **ciprofloxacin**).
    - severity of illness, hence commonly seen in ICU.
    - advanced age: ten times more common in age >65 years.
    - possibly use of gastric acid lowering drugs e.g. **proton pump inhibitors, H_2 receptor antagonists.**
    - concurrent chemotherapy.
  - diagnosed using enzyme immunoassay of toxin or DNA-based tests to identify the microbial toxin genes in unformed stool.
  - prevention:
    - minimise antibacterial drug use through antibiotic stewardship programmes.
    - prohibit certain antibacterial agents unless absolutely necessary.
    - ensure strict handwashing with soap and water (alcohol-based preparations do not eradicate clostridium spores).
    - isolate known and suspected infected cases.
    - use of probiotics may decrease incidence.
  - treatment: involves stopping antibacterial drugs if possible and administration of **vancomycin** (which is superior to **metronidazole**). **Teicoplanin** may also be used. Faecal transplantation (given via a nasoduodenal tube or, more recently, a capsule) is effective for patients with severe and recurrent infection. Colectomy may be necessary for severe pseudomembranous colitis.
- *C. perfringens*: causes **gas gangrene**.
- *C. tetani*: causes **tetanus**.
- *C. botulinum*: causes **botulism**.

Leffler DA, Lamont JT (2015). N Engl J Med; 372: 1539–48

Clover, Joseph Thomas (1825–1882). Pioneering English anaesthetist. A medical student at University College Hospital, London, said to have been present at **Liston**'s historic operation in 1846. Devised inhalers for **chloroform** and later **diethyl ether** that delivered accurate concentrations of agent. Also described the use of **N_2O**, alone or in combination with volatile agents.

Buxton DW (1923). Br J Anaesth; 1: 55–61

C_m, *see Minimal blocking concentration*

CMACE, Centre for Maternal and Child Enquiries, *see Confidential Enquiries into Maternal Deaths*

$CMRO_2$, *see Cerebral metabolic rate for oxygen*

CMV, *see Cytomegalovirus*

COAD, Chronic obstructive airways disease, *see Chronic obstructive pulmonary disease*

Coagulation. Clot formation; follows vasospasm and platelet plug formation, which cause temporary haemostasis.

- Normal sequence of events:
  - vasospasm, thought to be mediated by vasoconstrictor substances released from **platelets**, e.g. **5-HT** and **thromboxane**.
  - platelet plug: platelets are attracted by collagen exposed by damaged vascular endothelium. Adherence is followed by release of 5-HT and **ADP**, the latter causing further aggregation.
  - clot formation: the platelet plug is bound by resultant fibrin to form the definitive clot. Clot retraction is caused by platelet contractile microfilaments. The classical explanation of the coagulation pathway involves many circulating factors in a cascade mechanism; each factor, when activated, activates the next in turn (Fig. 45). Most are produced by the liver. Nomenclature of factors is largely historical, according to the chronological order of discovery. The intrinsic pathway is initiated by exposure of blood to collagen, or in vitro by contact with glass, e.g. test tubes. The extrinsic pathway is initiated by substances released from damaged tissues. Each may activate the common pathway, which culminates in formation of a tight fibrin clot.

A single pathway has been proposed, in which tissue factor (TF; a membrane glycoprotein not normally exposed on the surface of intact blood vessels) binds to circulating factor VII, resulting in a complex (VII/TF), which then activates the coagulation cascade mainly via factors IX and X (and thence the common pathway). The central role of **recombinant factor VIIa** is reflected in its use in haemophilia and intractable haemorrhage.

Normally, the clotting mechanism is balanced by opposing reactions preventing coagulation, e.g. antithrombin III (formed from activated factor X), which inhibits active factors II, IX, X, XI and XII. **Prostacyclin** secreted by the vascular endothelium inhibits platelet aggregation.

Other pathways may be involved in the coagulation cascade, e.g. active factor XII leads to activation of **fibrinolysis** and **kinin** formation.

Versteeg HH, Heemskerk JWM, Levi M, Reitsma PH (2013). Physiol Rev; 93: 327–58

See also, Anticoagulant drugs; Coagulation disorders; Coagulation studies

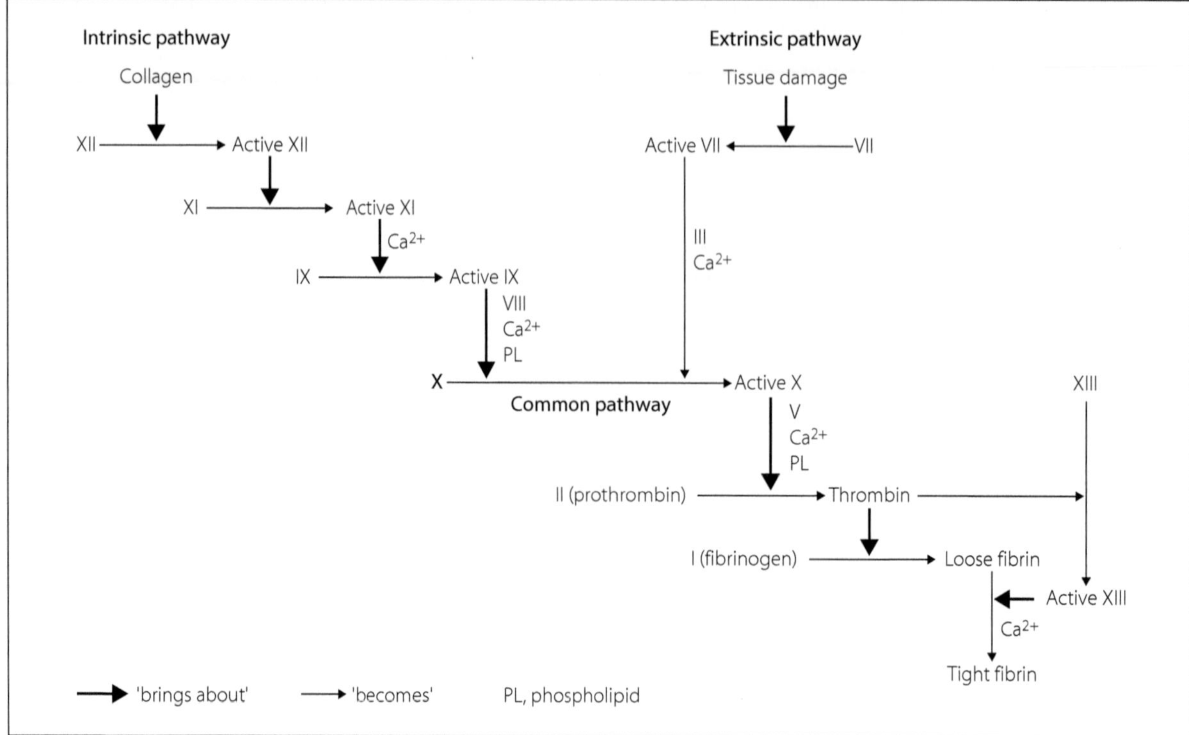

Fig. 45 Classical coagulation cascade

Coagulation disorders. May result in impaired coagulation or hypercoagulability. The former is more common and may arise from defects in:
- blood vessels:
  - infection, e.g. **meningococcal disease**, **sepsis**.
  - metabolic disease, e.g. **hepatic failure**, **renal failure**, scurvy.
  - congenital, e.g. hereditary telangiectasia.
- **platelets**:
  - **thrombocytopenia**.
  - **DIC**.
  - impaired function, e.g. **antiplatelet drugs**.
- **coagulation**:
  - congenital, e.g. **haemophilia**, **von Willebrand's disease** (also associated with blood vessel and platelet defects).
  - **heparin**, **warfarin**, hepatic failure, **vitamin K** deficiency, DIC.
  - increased **fibrinolysis**.

Blood transfusion may be associated with dilution of platelets and coagulation factors by fluid and blood components deficient in them. Impaired organ function and DIC may contribute.

Diagnosed by the underlying problem, aided by **coagulation studies** (Table 17).

- Treatment:
  - of underlying disease.
  - administration of appropriate blood products.

Table 17 Change in prothrombin time (PT), activated partial thromboplastin (APPT), thrombin time (TT), fibrin degradation products (FDPs), platelet count and fibrinogen levels in various coagulation disorders

Disorder	*PT*	*APPT*	*TT*	*FDPs*	*Platelets*	*Fibrinogen*
Thrombocytopenia	→	→	→	→	↓	→
DIC	↑	↑	↑	↑	↓	↓
Heparin therapy	↑	↑	↑	→	→[a]	→
Warfarin therapy	↑	↑	→	→	→	→
Hepatic failure	↑	↑	↑	→	→	↓
Massive blood transfusion	↑	↑	↑	→	↓	→
Primary fibrinolysis	↑	↑	↑	↑	→	↓

Note: DIC may complicate hepatic failure and massive blood transfusion.
[a]But thrombocytopenia may follow several days of heparin therapy.
↑, Increase; ↓, decrease; →, no change.

Abnormal hypercoagulability may lead to recurrent **DVT** and **PE**. It may result from:
- primary disorders:
  - **protein C** deficiency: protein C is a circulating anticoagulant protein; when activated by thrombin it inactivates factors V and VIII. Deficiency (the extent of which is variable) thus results in increased tendency to thrombosis.
  - protein S deficiency: protein S is a cofactor for protein C; deficiency also results in thrombophilia.
  - activated protein C resistance: inherited abnormality of factor V, resulting in resistance to cleavage by protein C. A particular form of factor V, factor V Leiden, is present in about 2% of Northern European individuals; the risk of thrombosis in homozygotes is estimated at up to 50%.
  - antithrombin III deficiency: may result in thrombophlebitis, thrombosis and PE.
  - others, e.g. prothrombin gene variants, deficiency of fibrinolytic components or factor XII.
- secondary to **malignancy**, **pregnancy**, **diabetes mellitus**, platelet and vessel wall abnormalities,

hyperviscosity and venous stasis. Circulating inhibitors (lupus anticoagulant and anticardiolipin antibodies) may develop spontaneously or in patients with **SLE**, resulting in the antiphospholipid syndrome. In this condition, activated partial thromboplastin time may be prolonged, although patients are at increased risk of thrombosis, possibly related to inhibition of factor XII activation or **prostacyclin** production from vascular endothelium.

Coagulopathy is commonly seen in ICU patients, with 40% developing thrombocytopenia and 60% having an INR >1.5. Such patients are more likely to develop **acute kidney injury** and **MODS**. Trauma patients who present with abnormal coagulation have an increased risk of **ALI** and a fourfold increase in mortality.

- Causes of abnormal coagulation in ICU:
  - acquired platelet dysfunction, e.g. liver failure, renal failure, extracorporeal circuits.
  - thrombocytopenia, e.g. haemorrhage, massive blood transfusion, increased consumption (e.g. in DIC), myelosuppression associated with sepsis.
  - deranged coagulation, e.g. dilution of coagulation factors in massive blood transfusion, vitamin K deficiency, or secondary to **anticoagulant drugs**.

[Leiden; city in the Netherlands where the factor was first identified in 1993]

Mensah PK, Gooding R (2015). Anaesthesia; 70 (suppl 1): 112–20 and Retter A, Barrett NA (2015). Anaesthesia; 70 (suppl 1): 121–7

Coagulation studies. May test different parts of the **coagulation** pathways:

- whole blood coagulation:
  - whole blood clotting time: bedside test of intrinsic and common pathways (i.e., spontaneous coagulation occurring in a glass tube without external reactive substances, e.g. tissue fluid). 1 ml blood is added to each of three glass tubes, kept at body temperature. The first is tilted every 15 s until clotted, then the second, third, etc. The time until the third is clotted is normally about 9–12 min.
  - activated clotting time (ACT): bedside test; commonly used to monitor **heparin** anticoagulation during **cardiopulmonary bypass** and **extracorporeal membrane oxygenation**. Similar to whole blood clotting time, but Celite is added to the blood for quicker results. Automated devices are usually used to detect fibrin formation, with a small bar magnet within the test tube. The tube is placed within the device and rotated slowly; when fibrin forms in the tube, the magnet starts to rotate, thereby activating the detector. Normal value is 100–140 s. Values of 3–4 times the baseline value are considered adequate during **extracorporeal circulation**.
- clotting factors: performed on fresh citrated plasma, with cells and platelets removed; physical activation of coagulation is avoided by using non-wettable plastic tubes. Normal plasma is used as a control:
  - prothrombin time (PT): tests the extrinsic and common pathways. Plasma, then calcium, is added to brain extract and phospholipid. Normal value is 11–15 s. International Normalised Ratio (INR; formerly British Ratio) is the ratio of sample time to a standard. A target ratio of 2–2.5 is used for prophylaxis of **DVT** with **warfarin**; 2–3 for treatment of DVT, **PE** and transient ischaemic attacks; 3–4.5 for prophylaxis of recurrent DVT or PE, and for patients with prosthetic heart valves and other arterial prostheses. A ratio of 1.5 is considered safe for surgery.
  - activated partial thromboplastin time (APTT; also partial thromboplastin time with kaolin, PTTK): tests the intrinsic and common pathways. Plasma, phospholipid and calcium are added to kaolin. Normal value is 35–40 s. A target ratio of 2–4 compared with normal plasma is used for treatment of DVT or PE with heparin. A ratio of 1.5 is considered safe for surgery.
  - mixture tests: if PT or APTT is prolonged, the patient's plasma may be mixed with normal plasma and the test repeated. If the test is normal, factor deficiency is present; if still prolonged, the sample plasma contains an inhibitor, e.g. antibody.
  - specific factor assays, e.g. factor VIII assay.
  - reptilase time (RT): snake venom is added to plasma, converting fibrinogen to fibrin. Unaffected by heparin; thus if normal but the thrombin time is prolonged, presence of heparin is suggested. A prolonged RT suggests fibrinogen deficiency.
- **platelets**:
  - platelet count: normally 150–400 × 10^9/l.
  - bleeding time: a standard incision is made on the forearm using a pricking device or template; a BP cuff is inflated around the upper arm to 40 mmHg. The incision is dabbed with filter paper every 30 s until the bleeding stops. Normal value is 2–9 min. Susceptible to considerable variation; therefore infrequently used.
  - commercially available devices: used as a rapid indicator of coagulation status, e.g. during **liver transplantation**:
    - **thromboelastography** (TEG).
    - Sonoclot: a tubular probe oscillates up and down within the sample and the resistance to motion encountered is plotted on a graph. As the blood clots, resistance increases; it then peaks and falls as a result of clot retraction and disruption of the clot, giving a characteristic tracing ('clot signature').
    - PFA-100: blood is aspirated through a microscopic hole in a membrane coated with collagen and adrenaline or ADP; the time for a platelet plug to occlude the hole completely is the 'closure time' and is related to platelet function.
- **fibrinolysis**:
  - fibrinogen assay: normally 1.5–4.0 g/l.
  - thrombin time (TT): tests conversion of fibrinogen to fibrin. Exogenous thrombin is added to plasma. Normal value is 10–15 s. Inhibited by heparin and **fibrin degradation products**.
  - fibrinogen degradation products: normally <10 mg/l. D-dimer concentration is normally <500 ng/ml.
  - plasminogen assay.
  - clot lysis times: euglobulin is precipitated from plasma by adding acid. Contains fibrinogen, plasminogen and plasminogen activator. Addition of thrombin causes clot formation; subsequent lysis depends on the amount of plasminogen-activating capacity present. Whole blood clot lysis and other variants are also used.

Co-amoxiclav. Broad-spectrum **antibacterial drug**; a mixture of **amoxicillin** and **clavulanic acid** in varying proportion. Active against gram-negative and gram-positive organisms; uses include respiratory, middle ear and urinary infections.

- Dosage: (expressed as amoxicillin):
  - 250–500 mg orally tds.
  - 1 g iv tds/qds.
- Side effects: as for amoxicillin; also cholestatic jaundice, erythema multiforme and interstitial nephritis.

Coanda effect. Development of reduced pressure between a fluid jet from a nozzle and an adjacent surface, resulting in adherence of the jet to the surface. Reduced pressure results from entrainment of surrounding molecules into the turbulent jet, with those next to the surface quickly 'used up'. If the jet has two surfaces to which it might adhere, it will attach to one only, without splitting. A small signal jet across the nozzle may switch the main jet from one surface to the other; this has formed the basis of control mechanisms in **fluidics**, e.g. control of ventilators.

Similar behaviour of fluids has been suggested to occur beyond constrictions in blood vessels, e.g. coronary arteries, contributing to ischaemia and infarction.

The effect was originally applied to the development of jet engines.

[Henri Coanda (1885–1972), Romanian engineer]

Coarctation of the aorta. Accounts for 6%–8% of **congenital heart disease**, with an incidence of 1:2500. More common in males. May be associated with **Turner's** and **Marfan's syndromes**. Acquired coarctation is rare and usually follows **chest trauma** or **vasculitides**.

Over 95% are post-ductal, often presenting in later life. May be associated with cerebral aneurysms and a bicuspid aortic valve.

- Features:
  - **hypertension**, left ventricular hypertrophy and **cardiac failure**. BP is high in the arms, normal or low in the legs. **Stroke** and **endocarditis** may occur.
  - weak femoral pulses, delayed compared with the radials.
  - systolic **heart murmur**, loudest posteriorly.
  - **ECG** findings include left ventricular hypertrophy.
  - characteristic **CXR** findings:
    - double aortic knuckle ('3' sign).
    - small descending aorta.
    - rib notching; seen at the middle of the lower border of the ribs posteriorly; caused by enlarged collateral vessels.
    - left ventricular enlargement/failure.

The pre-ductal (proximal to the **ductus arteriosus**) form is more severe, usually presenting in infancy with cardiac failure. Often associated with cerebral aneurysms, bicuspid aortic valve, patent ductus arteriosus, **VSD** and mitral and aortic abnormalities.

Repaired surgically via left thoracotomy; more recently, balloon angioplasty and stenting of the constricted segment have been performed.

- Anaesthetic management is similar to that for thoracic **aortic aneurysm**, in particular:
  - preoperative treatment of hypertension and cardiac failure.
  - antibiotic prophylaxis as for congenital heart disease.
  - arterial BP should be monitored in the right arm as the left subclavian artery is usually clamped during resection. Simultaneous BP measurement in the arms and legs is often performed.
  - complications include:
    - haemorrhage.
    - hypertension following aortic clamping, ischaemia to the spinal cord, bowel and kidneys, and acidosis and hypotension following unclamping.
  - hypertension may persist postoperatively and require treatment, especially in older patients.

See also, Cardiac surgery

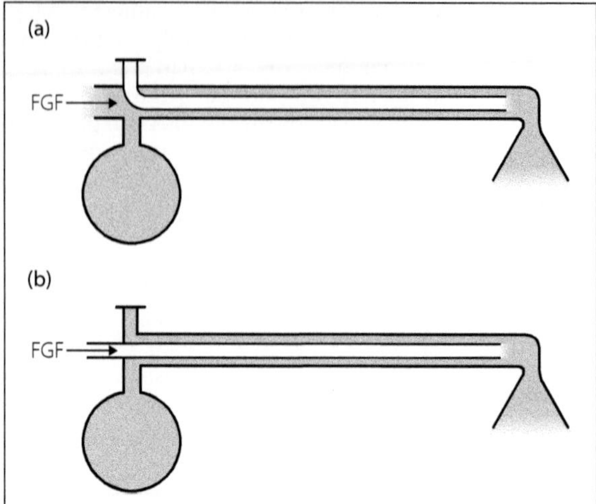

Fig. 46 Coaxial breathing systems: (a) Lack; (b) Bain

Coaxial anaesthetic breathing systems. Functionally, they are versions of Mapleson A (Lack) and D (Bain) **anaesthetic breathing systems**, but more convenient to use:

- Lack (Fig. 46a): the expiratory valve is at the anaesthetic machine end (cf. **Magill** system). Thus easier to adjust and scavenge waste gases, especially when the patient's head is covered. The patient end is also lighter. The outer tube is wider than usual to accommodate the inner tube, itself as wide as possible to reduce resistance to expiration. The system is therefore bulky and relatively inflexible. It has greater resistance to expiration than the Magill system. Required fresh gas flows are as for the Magill system. Parallel versions are also available, in which the inner tube is replaced by a second external tube running alongside the main tube. Both tubes are wide bore and thus of low resistance.
- Bain (Fig. 46b): lighter and longer than the standard systems, with the expiratory valve at the machine end, allowing easy adjustment and scavenging. Some resistance to expiration results from the flow of fresh gas directed at the patient's mouth from the inner tube. Ideal fresh gas flow rates for spontaneous ventilation are controversial, as high flows cause greater resistance. Suggested values range from 100 to 250 ml/kg. May be used for IPPV using a ventilator, e.g. Penlon Nuffield attached to the reservoir bag fitting (bag removed) by a length of tubing whose volume exceeds tidal volume. Disconnection of the inner tube from the fresh gas source (resulting in the whole length of tubing becoming dead space) must be excluded before use (*see Checking of anaesthetic equipment*).

A coaxial version of the **circle system** is available, which connects to the inspiration and expiration ports of a standard CO_2 absorber. It is claimed that the countercurrent heat exchange mechanism, in which the expiratory gases warm the inspiratory gases as they pass in opposite directions along the coaxial tube's length, results in greater transfer of heat to the inspiratory gas than in the conventional non-coaxial circle.
[J Alastair Lack, Salisbury anaesthetist; JA Bain, Canadian anaesthetist]

Cocada. Ball of coca leaves, mixed with guano and cornstarch, thought to be chewed by South American Incas to release free **cocaine** base. Dribbling of saliva onto wounds then allowed relatively painless surgery.

Cocaine/cocaine hydrochloride. Ester **local anaesthetic agent**, the first one discovered. An alkaloid originally extracted from the leaves and bark of South American coca plants. Used in 1884 for topical analgesia of the eye (by **Koller**), intercostal nerve block (by **Anrep**), mandibular nerve block (by **Halsted** and Hall) and other uses, including local infiltration. Now restricted to topical anaesthesia because of its toxicity. Used as a 10% spray or as component of **Moffet's solution** to reduce bleeding caused by nasal intubation. Causes vasoconstriction by preventing uptake of **noradrenaline** by presynaptic nerve endings; also inhibits **monoamine oxidase**.

- Toxicity:
  - CNS stimulation: **convulsions** at high doses, followed by central depression and **apnoea**.
  - sympathetic stimulation: **arrhythmias**, tachycardia, hypertension and **myocardial ischaemia** may occur.
  - addiction occurs with chronic use. Cerebral aneurysms, **cardiomyopathy** and sudden death are associated with chronic abuse.
- Maximum safe dose: 3 mg/kg.

Excreted mainly via the liver; a small amount is excreted unchanged in the urine.
[Richard J Hall (1856–1897), Irish-born US surgeon]
See also, Cocaine poisoning

Cocaine poisoning. Increasing problem in the developed world, especially with the production of the more addictive freebase cocaine (crack) by dissolution of the salt in alkaline solution and extraction with organic solvents (e.g. ether). Illegally obtained cocaine may contain **caffeine**, phencyclidine, **ephedrine**, **amfetamines**, strychnine and other contaminants.

The toxic dose depends on the individual's tolerance and route of administration but doses above 1 g are likely to be fatal. Effects are enhanced and prolonged by **alcohol**. Detectable in urine but serum levels are unhelpful because of a large **volume of distribution** and rapid metabolism.

- Clinical features:
  - CNS: euphoria, anxiety, agitation, psychosis, hallucinations, **convulsions**, **hyperthermia**, intracranial haemorrhage, coma. **Status epilepticus** suggests continued drug absorption (e.g. following rupture of cocaine-filled packets swallowed for smuggling purposes), intracranial haemorrhage or hyperthermia.
  - CVS: ventricular tachyarrhythmias, severe hypertension (may result in **stroke** or **aortic dissection**), **MI** caused by coronary thrombosis or spasm, dilated **cardiomyopathy**. The actions of **sympathomimetic drugs** may be greatly enhanced.
  - RS: non-cardiogenic **pulmonary oedema**, **bronchospasm**, pulmonary infiltrates ('crack lung'), pulmonary haemorrhage, pneumothorax/pneumomediastinum.
  - renal: **renal failure** caused by renal artery spasm, hypotension or rhabdomyolysis.
- Management:
  - supportive: resuscitation, sedation, **antiarrhythmic drugs**, **antihypertensive drugs** (avoiding β-blockade alone because it may result in cardiovascular collapse due to unopposed α_1-agonism), general management as for **poisoning and overdoses**.
  - laparotomy may occasionally be required to remove ingested bags of the drug.
  - general anaesthesia may be hazardous because of the risk of severe hypertension and arrhythmias following laryngoscopy and tracheal intubation.

Shanti CM, Lucas CE (2003). Crit Care Med; 31: 1851–9

'Cockpit drill', *see Checking of anaesthetic equipment*

Codeine phosphate. Naturally occurring **opioid analgesic drug**, isolated in 1832. Used to relieve mild to moderate **pain**. Also used in **diarrhoea**, and to suppress the cough reflex, e.g. in palliative care. Has similar effects to **morphine**, but with lower potency and efficacy.

About 5%–10% is metabolised to morphine via the CYP2D6 enzyme in the cytochrome P_{450} system, with alternative routes of metabolism to norcodeine (via CYP3A4) and codeine-6-glucuronide (via glucuronide transferase)—both of which have mild analgesic properties. A minority of the population (from 1%–2% in northern Europe to 7%–12% in Mediterranean and 29% in North African/Saudi Arabian populations) carry more than two functional copies of the CYP2D6 gene; metabolism via CYP2D6 is thus 'ultra-rapid', with increased risk of sedation and other effects. About 5%–10% of the population carry two non-functioning alleles and metabolism is reduced to <3%, resulting in reduced analgesia. The specific enzyme involved is also inhibited by a number of drugs, including antidepressants.

Partly excreted unchanged via the kidneys, and partly metabolised in the liver.

- Dosage: 30–60 mg orally or im, 4-hourly as required, <240 mg/day; in children 12–18 years old, 30–60 mg 6-hourly <240 mg, for up to 3 days. Available in combination with **paracetamol** (8 mg, 15 mg and 30 mg with 500 mg paracetamol). Codeine should not be given iv (severe hypotension may follow).

Since 2013, contraindicated in: all children <12 years; children <18 years undergoing tonsillectomy/adenoidectomy for sleep apnoea; adults/children known to be CYP2D6 ultra-rapid metabolisers; and breast-feeding mothers.

Co-dydramol, *see Dihydrocodeine*

COELCB, *see Current-operated earth-leakage circuit breaker*

Coeliac plexus block. **Sympathetic nerve block** involving blockade of the coeliac ganglions, one lying on each side of L1 (aorta lying posteriorly, pancreas anteriorly and inferior vena cava laterally) and closely related to the coeliac plexus. Through them pass afferent fibres from abdominal (but not pelvic) viscera.

Performed for relief of **pain** from non-pelvic intra-abdominal organs, especially due to pancreatic and gastric malignancies. Has also been used in acute/chronic pancreatitis (relaxes the sphincter of Oddi) and to provide intra-abdominal analgesia during surgery. Usually performed percutaneously with the patient prone, under x-ray guidance. CT scanning and ultrasound have also been used.

- Technique: point of needle insertion is 5–10 cm from the midline, level with the spinous process of L1, below the 12th rib. A long (>10 cm) needle is inserted at 45 degrees to the skin, directed medially and slightly cranially. It is passed until the needle tip lies anterior to the upper part of the body of L1. 15–25 ml **local anaesthetic agent** is injected on each side (e.g. **prilocaine** or **lidocaine** 0.5% with adrenaline) followed by 25 ml 50% alcohol if required, e.g. on the following day if the block is successful. Flushing with saline prevents alcohol deposition during needle withdrawal. Severe hypotension may result, even after unilateral block.

[Ruggero Oddi (1845–1906), Italian surgeon]
See also, Sympathetic nervous system

Co-fluampicil. Broad-spectrum **antibacterial drug**; a mixture of **ampicillin** and **flucloxacillin** in equal parts.

Cognitive behavioural therapy (CBT). Psychological therapy focused on examining how individuals' thoughts, beliefs and attitudes affect their feelings and behaviours. Focuses on identifying current patterns and problems, and developing coping strategies and skills. Particularly useful in disorders associated with anxiety and depression; frequently used in chronic **pain management** and **post-traumatic stress disorder** following, e.g. **awareness** under anaesthesia, ICU experiences, etc. Can be delivered by a trained therapist in individual or group sessions, through a computer system (CCBT) or as a self-help tool.
See also, Operant conditioning

COLD, Chronic obstructive lung disease, *see Chronic obstructive pulmonary disease*

Colistin (Colistimethate). **Antibacterial drug**, also known as **polymyxin** E. Acts on the **lipopolysaccharide** and phospholipid components of gram-negative bacterial cell walls, including pseudomonas. Not absorbed when given orally; therefore has been used in **selective decontamination of the digestive tract**. Rarely given iv because of its side effects.

- Dosage:
  - 1.5–3 million units orally tds.
  - 1 million units by nebulised solution bd (dose halved if under 40 kg).
  - 1–2 million units iv/im tds.
- Side effects: paraesthesia, vertigo, neuromuscular blockade, renal impairment, dysarthria, visual disturbance, confusion.

Colitis, *see Bowel ischaemia; Clostridial infections; Inflammatory bowel disease*

College of Anaesthetists. Founded in 1988, replacing the **Faculty of Anaesthetists, Royal College of Surgeons of England**; became the **Royal College of Anaesthetists** in 1992. Similarly, the Faculty of Anaesthetists at the Royal College of Surgeons in Ireland (founded in 1959) became the College of Anaesthetists of Ireland in 1998.
Mushin W (1989). Anaesthesia; 44: 291–2

Colligative properties of solutions. Those properties varying with the number, and not character, of solute particles present. Thus as concentration increases:
  - freezing point decreases.
  - **osmotic pressure** increases.
  - **boiling point** increases.
  - **vapour pressure** of solvent decreases (**Raoult's law**).

Measurement of **osmolality and osmolarity** may utilise any of the above properties, because the changes produced by addition of solute are proportional to the amount added.

Colloid. Substance unable to pass through a semipermeable membrane, being a suspension of particles rather than a true solution (cf. **crystalloid**). When given as **iv fluids**, have a greater tendency to remain in the intravascular compartment, at least initially. For many years, considered more useful than crystalloids when replacing a vascular volume deficit (e.g. in **haemorrhage**), but of less use correcting specific water and electrolyte deficiencies, e.g. in **dehydration**. Also more expensive. Sometimes called plasma substitutes or **plasma expanders**, because the increase in plasma volume may be greater than the volume of colloid infused, due to their higher **osmolality** than plasma.

- Available products:
  - **blood products**, e.g. blood, **albumin**, plasma: due to cost and risks of **blood transfusion** they should only be used for specific blood component deficiency. Approximate cost per unit (in 2015): red cells £120; platelets £200; fresh frozen plasma £30.
  - **hydroxyethyl starch**: solutions with differing degrees of substitution (40%–74%) have been produced, with varying duration of action and effects on circulating volume. Incidence of severe reactions is about 1/10 000–16 000; cost is £10–20/500 ml.
  - **gelatin solutions.** Effects last a few hours only. Severe reactions: 1/13 000 (succinylated), 1/2000 (urea-linked; lower incidence with the newer formulation since 1981). Cost: £3–5/500 ml.
  - **dextrans.** May affect renal function and coagulation. Severe reactions: 1/4500, reduced to 1/84 000 with hapten pretreatment. Cost: £4–5/500 ml.

See also, Colloid/crystalloid controversy

Colloid/crystalloid controversy. Arises from conflicting theoretical, experimental and clinical evidence concerning the use of iv **colloid** or **crystalloid** in **shock**, mostly in the context of **haemorrhage**.

- Arguments in favour of:
  - colloid:
    - more logical choice for intravascular volume replacement, because a greater proportion remains in the intravascular space for longer after infusion.
    - less volume is required to restore cardiovascular parameters, e.g. BP, **CVP**, **pulmonary artery capillary wedge pressure**. Thus initial resuscitation is more rapid.
    - less peripheral/**pulmonary oedema** follows its use for the above reasons, and also because there is less reduction of plasma **oncotic pressure**.
  - crystalloid:
    - expands the intravascular compartment adequately if enough is used (traditionally said to be 2–4 times the colloid requirements, although more recent evidence suggests a ratio nearer 1.5:1 for the same degree of intravascular expansion).

- in haemorrhage, fluid moves from the interstitial space into the vascular compartment and **third space**; this **ECF** depletion is better replenished by crystalloid.
- if vascular permeability is increased, colloids will enter the interstitial space and increase interstitial oncotic pressure, thus exacerbating **oedema**. Crystalloids do not increase interstitial oncotic pressure to the same extent.
- peripheral oedema is usually not a problem.
- risk of allergic reactions to colloids.
- crystalloid is much cheaper than colloid.

- Current opinion tends to favour crystalloids for routine fluid replacement:
  - a large US retrospective study of 1 million patients undergoing joint surgery in 2009–2013 showed that the use of hydroxyethyl starch was associated with an increased risk of renal, cardiac and pulmonary complications and ICU admission. Results are similar for albumin, which also showed an increased incidence of thromboembolic events.
  - large randomised controlled trials have shown that the use of hydroxyethyl starch in critically ill patients impairs kidney function and coagulation and probably increases mortality. This has resulted in restricted usage in ICU.
  - some industry-sponsored research supporting colloids has been found to be unreliable/fraudulent, due to one particular researcher (no aspersions made on the manufacturers).

It has been suggested that until large-scale randomised controlled trials comparing colloids and crystalloids in the perioperative setting have been undertaken, the perioperative use of colloids should be suspended.

Haase N, Perner A (2015). Br Med J; 350: h1656

Colloid oncotic pressure, *see Oncotic pressure*

Colton, Gardner Quincy (1814–1898). US lecturer and showman; studied medicine but never qualified. Demonstrated the exhilarating effects of N_2O inhalation for entertainment in 1844, inspiring **Wells** to suggest its use for dental analgesia. Said to have administered N_2O to Wells while the latter's tooth was painlessly removed. Stopped lecturing to prospect for gold, returning to N_2O and popularising its reintroduction by founding the Colton Dental Association in 1863.

Smith GB, Hirsch NP (1991). Anesth Analg; 72: 382–91

Coma. Disorder of **consciousness** in which the patient is totally unaware of both self and external surroundings, and unable to respond meaningfully to external stimuli. Results from gross impairment of both cerebral hemispheres, and/or the **ascending reticular activating system**.

- Caused by:
  - focal brain dysfunction, e.g. tumour, vascular events, demyelination, infection, **head injury**.
  - diffuse brain dysfunction:
    - infection, e.g. **meningitis, encephalitis**.
    - **epilepsy**.
    - **hypoxia** and **hypercapnia**.
    - drugs, **poisoning and overdoses**.
    - metabolic/endocrine causes (e.g. **diabetic coma**; **hepatic** or **renal failure**; **hypothyroidism**), electrolyte disturbance (e.g. **hyponatraemia, hypercalcaemia**).
    - **hypotension, hypertensive crisis**.
    - head injury.
    - **subarachnoid haemorrhage**.
    - **hypothermia, hyperthermia**.

Assessment of the **pupils, doll's eye movements**, posture and motor responses (e.g. **decerebrate** and **decorticate postures**) and respiratory pattern is especially useful. Investigations are directed towards the above causes.

Initial management includes respiratory and cardiovascular support as for **CPR**, and treatment of the underlying cause. In addition, longer-term management includes attention to pressure areas, mouth, eyes, physiotherapy, prophylaxis against **DVT**, **nutrition** and **fluid balance**.

Coma may be followed by complete recovery, **vegetative state** or **brainstem death**.

McClenathan BM, Thakor NV, Hoesch RE (2013). Semin Neurol; 33: 91–109

See also, Coma scales

Coma scales. Scoring systems for assessing the degree of **coma** in unconscious patients and charting their progress; may also give an indication of outcome.

- Include general scales, e.g. **AVPU** scale or a simple 1–5 scoring system:
  - 1 = fully awake.
  - 2 = conscious but drowsy.
  - 3 = unconscious but responsive to pain with purposeful movement, e.g. flexion.
  - 4 = unconscious; responds to pain with extension.
  - 5 = unconscious with no response to pain.
- Other data (e.g. from eye reflexes) are ignored; hence more complex or specific scoring systems are used:
  - **Glasgow coma scale** (GCS).
  - **FOUR score**.
  - for specific conditions, e.g. **hepatic failure, subarachnoid haemorrhage**.

Kornbluth J, Bhardwaj A (2011). Neurocrit Care; 14: 134–43

Combined spinal–epidural anaesthesia (CSE). Technique in which **spinal anaesthesia** is accompanied by the placement of a catheter into the **epidural space**. May be achieved by two completely separate punctures or, more commonly, combined into a single one, in which the epidural space is located in the usual way as for **epidural anaesthesia**, and spinal anaesthesia is performed either alongside or, more commonly, by inserting a long spinal needle through, the epidural needle to puncture the dura. The epidural catheter is then sited in the normal way.

- Advantages: speed of onset/density of block associated with spinal anaesthesia, combined with the flexibility of epidural anaesthesia. Also facilitates use of low-dose spinal anaesthesia with 'epidural volume expansion' (*see later*).
- Disadvantages (compared with 'single-shot' spinal injections): risk of dural puncture with epidural needle; longer time to perform; the possibility that the epidural catheter is inserted through the dural hole; inadequate block if the catheter cannot be threaded easily (with the patient in the same position for a long time); and a theoretical increased risk of infection. If saline is used to identify the epidural space, the appearance of clear fluid at the hub of the spinal needle may cause confusion if free flow is not obtained.

Used commonly in **obstetric analgesia and anaesthesia** and other types of surgery. Different needle systems exist to ease CSE, including epidural needles with a 'back hole' at the distal end to allow the spinal needle to pass through the epidural needle without being bent by the latter's curved tip, and double-lumen epidural needles to enable the catheter to be threaded before intrathecal injection. Various locking devices, to prevent the spinal needle from moving relative to the epidural needle once the intrathecal space has been located, are also available. Many practitioners prefer to use a long spinal needle placed through an ordinary epidural needle.

In epidural volume expansion (EVE), a bolus of epidural saline, injected via either the needle or catheter, is used to increase the cranial spread of a (usually small) spinal dose of local anaesthetic. The mechanism is thought to be compression of the dural sac by the epidural fluid, and has been implicated in the occasionally very high block when a spinal is performed after (inadequate) epidural anaesthesia. EVE has been claimed to produce a reliably extensive block from a smaller than usual dose of drug, while reducing side effects such as hypotension and motor block. However, it is not universally employed because the extra spread is usually relatively modest (a few segments only) and use of a smaller dose increases the risk of discomfort/inadequate block.

Cook TM (2000). Anaesthesia; 55: 42–64

Combitube, *see Oesophageal obturators and airways*

Commission for Health Improvement (CHI), *see Care Quality Commission*

Committee on Safety of Medicines (CSM). Advisory body, originally set up as the Committee on Safety of Drugs in 1963 after the thalidomide disaster. Became the CSM in 1971 when the Medicines Act became law. Was the body responsible for granting certificates to new drugs before **clinical trials** and product licences, and for monitoring post-marketing safety. Joined with the Medicines Commission in 2005 to form the Commission on Human Medicines (CHM), a committee of the **Medicines and Healthcare products Regulatory Agency**, charged with advising ministers on licensing policy, taking responsibility for drug safety issues, advising on appointments related to human medicines and hearing evidence from drug companies if licence applications are rejected.

See also, Adverse drug reactions; Drug development

Compartment syndromes. Impaired circulation and function of tissues within a fascial compartment, associated with increased pressure within the compartment. May be caused by external compression (e.g. **tourniquets**, limb plasters) or increased volume of compartment contents (e.g. following **trauma**, severe exercise, prolonged immobility, bleeding or ischaemia of the underlying tissues). May lead to disruption of capillaries, leakage of intravascular fluid into the tissues, impaired perfusion, **myoglobinuria** (**crush syndrome**) and **gangrene**. Total ischaemia leads to irreversible muscle changes after 4 h. The forearm or lower leg is most commonly affected. Pressure within the lower leg compartments is normally under 15 mmHg when supine, and may be monitored using a simple manometer.

- Features:
  - increasing pain despite immobilisation of the limb.
  - altered sensation in **dermatomes** corresponding to nerves running through the compartment.
  - increased pressure within the compartment on palpation and also when measured.
  - peripheral pulses may be present.

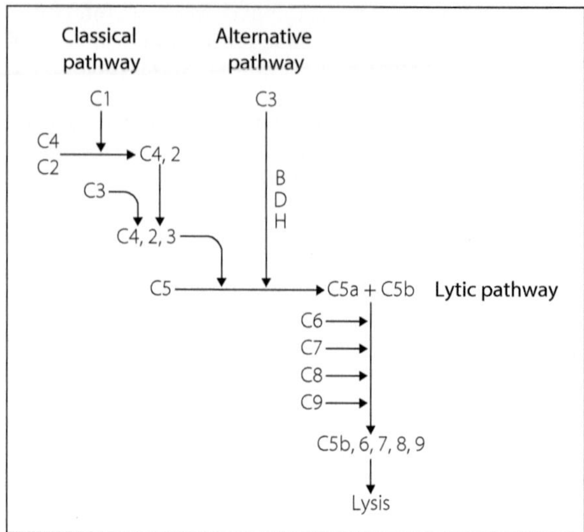

Fig. 47 Complement system

Treatment includes release of tourniquets, dressings and plaster casts; surgical fasciotomy may be required. The **abdominal compartment syndrome** may occur, e.g. in **abdominal trauma**.

Harvey EJ, Sanders DW, Shuller MS, et al (2012). J Orthop Trauma; 26: 699–702

Competition, drug, *see Antagonist; Dose–response curves*

Complement. Part of the innate immune system; describes a series of plasma proteins (labelled C1–C9) synthesised in the liver and involved in immunological and inflammatory reactions. Activation of the system causes a cascade of protein cleavage and further activation events, amplifying the initial stimulus.

- Pathways (Fig. 47):
  - classical (discovered first):
    - activated by antigen–antibody complexes (i.e., requires prior exposure to antigen), although it may follow prior exposure to a cross-reacting antigen.
    - antibody–antigen complex binds to C1.
    - via C4, C2 and C3, forming a complex that activates C5.
    - C1 activity is regulated by circulating C1 inhibitor; deficiency results in **hereditary angio-oedema**.
  - alternative:
    - activated by aggregated IgA, infections or spontaneous reaction.
    - via other factors: B, D and H forming a complex activating C5.
    - may amplify itself or the classical pathway via C3b formation.
  - lytic:
    - activated by products of the above pathways, causing C5 to form C5a and C5b. The latter binds to the target membrane.
    - C5b binding in turn by C6, C7, C8 and C9.
    - the resultant complex causes membrane lysis.
- In addition, activated factors produced during all pathways may:
  - bind to **mast cells** and basophils, causing degranulation and release of **histamine**.
  - be chemotactic for neutrophils and macrophages.

- cause vasodilatation and increase capillary permeability. Complement activation may be involved in many disease processes. IgM and IgG both bind complement, and are involved in hypersensitivity reactions, e.g. **adverse drug reactions**. Assays for individual components may assist determination of the pathways involved; e.g. low levels of C4 indicate classical pathway activation.

Complex regional pain syndrome (CRPS). Chronic **pain** disorder involving vasomotor, sudomotor (stimulation of sweat glands), trophic, sensory and, less frequently, motor abnormalities, in one or more extremity. CRPS type 1 (previously known as reflex sympathetic dystrophy or Sudeck's atrophy) describes the condition in the absence of an identifiable injury. In CRPS type 2 (causalgia), symptoms can be attributed to an injury; it usually develops weeks to months after the injury and is often out of proportion to severity of trauma.

- Clinical presentation is variable but includes:
  - pain (in 90%), usually burning and shooting initially, changing to aching or boring over time. Often associated with **allodynia** or **hyperalgesia** and worsened by movement.
  - sensory loss to thermal and mechanical stimuli.
  - excessive sweating and local changes in hair growth.
  - erythematous or cyanotic-looking limb with or without oedema.
  - atrophy of the limb, sometimes with radiological evidence of osteoporosis.
  - joint immobility and stiffness. Dystonia, tremors and weakness may also occur.
- Proposed pathophysiological mechanisms include:
  - peripheral nerve injury: small fibre damage (can be identified in skin biopsies even in CRPS 1), leading to peripheral sensitisation and sensory abnormalities.
  - central sensitisation: constant pain input 'resets' part of the central pain pathway, which now mis-recognises non-noxious inputs as painful, resulting in allodynia. **NMDA receptors** are thought to be involved.
  - neurogenic inflammation: nociceptor activation is thought to cause local release of proinflammatory neuropeptides and cytokines (e.g. **calcitonin**-related gene peptide, **substance P** and tumour necrosis factor alpha) causing vasomotor change and oedema.
  - sympathetic-mediated upregulation of adrenoreceptors, leading to vasoconstriction.
  - other proposed mechanisms include a regional autoimmune process and motor cortex adaptation.

Treatment may be extremely challenging and includes physiotherapy, rehabilitation and **cognitive behavioural therapy**. Drugs found to be helpful include **gabapentin**, **amitriptyline**, **bisphosphonates**, **ketamine** and **corticosteroids** for acute exacerbations. **Sympathetic nerve blocks** may allow physiotherapy and spinal cord stimulation may have a role, although evidence is currently lacking.

[Paul HM Sudeck (1866–1945), German surgeon]

Bruehl S (2015). Br Med J; 351: h2730

Compliance. Volume change per unit pressure change; thus a measure of distensibility, e.g. of lungs, chest wall, heart. For measurement of lung compliance, transmural pressure is required, i.e., the difference between alveolar and **intrapleural pressures**. The former is measured at the mouth during periods of no gas flow (e.g. with the lungs held partially inflated and a few seconds allowed for stabilisation) or using a shutter at the mouth to interrupt flow momentarily. Intrapleural pressure is measured using a balloon positioned in the lower third of the oesophagus. The resulting pressure/volume curve is approximately linear at normal tidal volumes (Fig. 48). Different curves are measured during lung inflation and deflation (hysteresis); this is thought to represent the effects of **surface tension**.

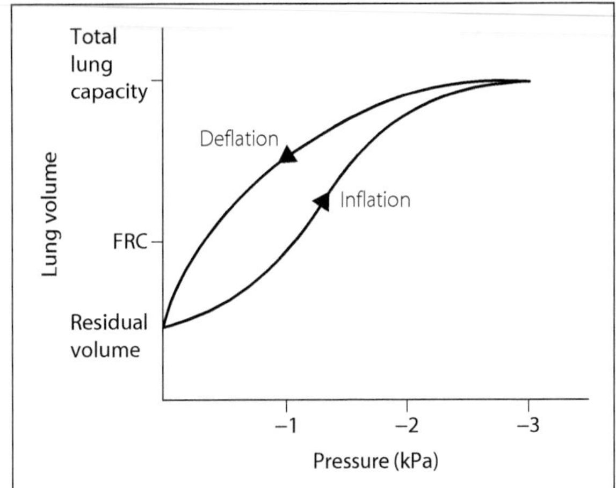

Fig. 48 Pressure/volume curve of lung

Human lung compliance is about 1.5–2 l/kPa (150–200 ml/cmH_2O); reduced when supine because of decreased **FRC**. Chest wall compliance is thought to be similar, but measurement is difficult because of the effects of respiratory muscles. Total thoracic compliance requires measurement of alveolar and ambient pressure difference, and equals about 0.85 l/kPa (85 ml/cmH_2O).

- Compliance measurements are related thus:

$$\frac{1}{\text{total thoracic}} = \frac{1}{\text{chest wall}} + \frac{1}{\text{lung}}$$

- Lung compliance is divided into two components:
  - static; i.e., alveolar 'stretchability'; measured at steady state, as earlier.
  - dynamic; related to **airway resistance** during equilibration of gases throughout the lung at end-inspiration or expiration.

Time constant (resistance × compliance) is a reflection of combined static and dynamic compliance.

Compliance is related to body size; thus specific compliance is often referred to (compliance divided by FRC). It increases in old age and emphysema, due to destruction of elastic lung tissue. It is reduced in pulmonary fibrosis, vascular engorgement and oedema; dynamic compliance is decreased in chronic bronchitis. It is also reduced at the extremes of lung volume, as well as at the lung apices and bases in upright subjects.

See also, Breathing, work of

Complications of anaesthesia, *see Anaesthetic morbidity and mortality*

Compound A, Pentafluoroisopropenyl fluoromethyl ether, *see Sevoflurane*

Compressed spectral array, *see Power spectral analysis*

Computed (axial) tomography (CAT scanning; CT scanning). Imaging technique in which an x-ray source and detector are held opposite each other, with the patient midway between. The source and detector are rotated stepwise about the midpoint, thus scanning the patient from different angles. At each step, the amount of x-rays reaching the detector is measured, and the spatial arrangement of structures within the patient 'slice' computed and displayed on a screen. In spiral CT scanning, the x-ray tube and detector are able to rotate around the patient as the latter moves through the scanner, resulting in a helical scan from which axial slices may be reconstructed. Spiral scanning is quicker than conventional scanning and allows greater detail, especially during contrast studies. Used initially for brain scanning, now for all parts of the body. Spiral CT scanning is increasingly used to diagnose **PE**.

Patients must remain still during scanning, and may require sedation or general anaesthesia, e.g. children and patients with **head injury**. Choice of techniques and drugs is dictated by the patient's condition; monitoring and maintenance of the airway are particular concerns. Management is similar to that for **radiotherapy**.

Whiting P, Singatullina N, Rosser JH (2015). Br J Anaesth Education; 15: 299–304 and Rosser JH, Singatullina N, Whiting P (2016). Br J Anaesth Education; 16: 15–20

See also, Radiology, anaesthesia for

COMT, *see Catechol-O-methyl transferase*

Concentration effect. Phenomenon whereby increased inspired concentration of **inhalation anaesthetic agent** results in earlier equilibrium of pulmonary uptake. As concentration increases, the effect of alveolar absorption of agent between breaths is reduced.

Conductance. Reciprocal of **resistance**. For electrical circuits, the SI **unit** is the siemens. The term is often used to describe the permeability of cell **membranes** to various ions.

[Sir William Siemens (1823–1883), German-born English engineer]

Confederation of European National Societies of Anaesthesiologists (CENSA). Organisation founded in 1998, originally created as the European Regional Section of the **World Federation of Societies of Anaesthesiologists**. Organised European congresses and was involved in various educational projects throughout Europe. Amalgamated with the European Society of Anaesthesiologists and the **European Academy of Anaesthesiology** to form the **European Society of Anaesthesiology** in 2005.

Confidence intervals. Range of values derived from sample data, relating the data to the actual population. 95% confidence intervals (95% CI) contain the true (population) value with a **probability** (*P* value) of 0.05.

When used to express the results of **statistical tests**, confidence intervals differ from **null hypothesis** testing thus:

- null hypothesis testing indicates whether a difference in data is statistically significant (i.e., unlikely to be due to chance alone); the significance is expressed as a *P* value.
- confidence intervals indicate the likely magnitude of such a difference, by giving a range within which the true value is likely to lie. By using the same units as the data, they allow estimations of clinical relevance to be made; for example, a statistically very significant result may be clinically irrelevant if the actual differences involved are very small.

Confidence intervals are wide if the sample size is small or **standard deviation** is large. If the 95% CI of a difference between groups does not include zero, this is equivalent to the difference having a *P* value <0.05; if it includes zero then $P > 0.05$.

Asai T (2002). Br J Anaesth; 89: 807–9

See also, Statistical significance

Confidential Enquiries into Maternal Deaths. Report into all maternal deaths in the UK (Scotland and Northern Ireland were excluded until 1985), originally conducted by the Royal College of Obstetricians and Gynaecologists in the 1930s. Published initially by the Department of Health, its first report covered 1952–1954. In 2003, combined with the Confidential Enquiries into Stillbirths and Deaths in Infancy (CESDI) to form the Confidential Enquiries into Maternal and Child Health (CEMACH). This became an independent charity, the Centre for Maternal and Child Enquiries (CMACE), in 2009, with its enquiries commissioned by the **National Patient Safety Agency**. After a series of reviews in 2010–2011, the enquiries are now commissioned by the **Healthcare Quality Improvement Partnership** (HQIP) and run by a consortium, MBRRACE-UK (Mothers and Babies: Reducing Risk through Audits and Confidential Enquiries in the UK), involving a number of centres, groups and individuals around the UK and led by the National Perinatal Epidemiology Unit in Oxford. Since 2013 the reports have included data from the Irish Maternal Death Enquiry programme.

Details of cases are collected from all involved clinical staff, observing strict confidentiality, and assessors (in anaesthetics, obstetric medicine, emergency medicine, psychiatry, general practice, pathology and midwifery) review and categorise the deaths according to cause. Causes of deaths may be:

- direct: arising directly from pregnancy or an intervention relating to it.
- indirect: resulting from disease that pre-exists or develops during pregnancy, and is aggravated by pregnancy, or from an intervention not related to the pregnancy but influenced by it.
- late: occur between 42 days and 1 year after the end of pregnancy.
- coincidental (previously fortuitous): unrelated to pregnancy.

For many years, reports were published every 3 years; the new MBRRACE-UK system reports annually, presenting data from the previous 3 years in a rolling surveillance programme together with chapters on selected topics. Numbers of direct deaths in the UK have fallen from ~100–130 to ~70–80 per triennium in the last 20 years, while indirect deaths have increased from ~80–90 to ~150–160 per triennium. In the last 5–6 years, mortality rates per 100 000 maternities have been 3–4 for direct deaths, 5–6 for indirect deaths, and 8–10 for total deaths.

In the last decade, the main causes of death have been cardiac disease, thrombosis/thromboembolism, suicide/psychiatric disease/substance abuse, **pre-eclampsia/eclampsia**, haemorrhage, **sepsis** (particularly genital tract and **chest infection** including **influenza**), **amniotic fluid embolism** and ectopic pregnancy. Obesity and increasing maternal age are particularly highlighted as recent contributing factors.

Anaesthesia was a consistent direct cause of death for many years, ranking third after hypertensive disease and thromboembolism up to the ~mid-1980s. In recent reports, ~4–8 deaths per triennium have been ascribed to anaesthesia, although the allocation of deaths to specific causes is difficult in complex cases and less useful than concentrating on the generic lessons to be learned. Improvements in anaesthetic mortality are thought to reflect better training and facilities, and are likely to be greater than suggested by numbers of deaths alone, because the number of anaesthetic procedures performed has markedly increased. Most direct and indirect anaesthetic deaths in previous reports have involved **caesarean section**; common factors have been lack of senior involvement, difficulty with tracheal intubation, aspiration of gastric contents, haemorrhage and lack of ICU or HDU facilities. The need for proper training, facilities and help is repeatedly stressed. In the more recent reports, communication failures, lack of senior availability, underestimation of severity of illness by trainees, delayed resuscitation and administration of blood products, inadequate ICU/HDU facilities, drug error and the risks of rapid iv injection of large doses of oxytocin have been highlighted.

See also, Audit; Obstetric analgesia and anaesthesia

https://www.npeu.ox.ac.uk/mbrrace-uk/reports

Confidential enquiry into perioperative deaths, *see National Confidential Enquiry into Patient Outcome and Death*

Confusion in the Intensive Care Unit. Increasingly recognised as an acute form of organ dysfunction. The term is often used interchangeably with 'delirium'. Occurs in 60%–80% of patients receiving mechanical ventilation. Characterised by disturbances of consciousness (e.g. decreased awareness of environment, reduced attention) and cognition (e.g. memory impairment, language difficulties) that arise over hours/days and fluctuate during the day. Associated with increased risk of prolonged IPPV, self-extubation and unintended removal of intravascular and urinary catheters. Also correlates with long-term cognitive impairment and physical disability.

- Risk factors:
  - premorbid factors: increased age, **hypertension**, hearing/visual impairment, alcohol use, smoking, history of depression.
  - illness-related factors:
    - severe illness, respiratory disease (especially **chest infection**), requirement for IPPV.
    - **hypoxaemia**, **hypercapnia**, **hypotension**, metabolic disorders (e.g. **hypo/hyperglycaemia**, **hypo/hypernatraemia**, **hypercalcaemia**).
    - CNS disease, e.g. **encephalitis**, **meningitis**, **head injury**, space-occupying lesions, post-ictal states.
    - pain.
    - use of sedative drugs.
  - environment-related factors: sleep deprivation, lack of daylight, lack of visitors, isolation in single rooms.

The CAM-ICU (confusion assessment method for ICU) is a tool for determining whether a patient is suffering from delirium by assessing if there is (1) an acute mental status change, (2) inattention to visual and auditory prompts, (3) an altered level of consciousness and (4) any disorganised thinking as assessed by set questions.

- Prevention:
  - intermittent waking of patients by stopping sedation combined with trials of spontaneous breathing significantly decreases duration of acute brain dysfunction.
  - avoidance of **benzodiazepine** sedation if possible. The incidence of delirium is decreased if **dexmedetomidine** is used for sedation.
  - effective treatment of pain. Opioids decrease the incidence of delirium if given for treatment of pain but increase it if given for sedation alone.
  - provision of hearing aids/spectacles to reduce sensory deprivation.
  - encouragement of visitors and prompts from home (photographs, etc.).
  - early mobilisation.
  - improved sleep hygiene e.g. establishing day/night cycles, darkening rooms and minimising noise at night. **Melatonin** may be useful.

Once it has occurred, treatment with **antipsychotic drugs** (e.g. **haloperidol**, olanzapine, risperidone) may be necessary.

Trogrlić Z, van der Jagt M, Bakker J, et al (2015). Crit Care; 19: 157

Confusion, postoperative. Occurs in 10%–60% of patients undergoing surgery, especially in the elderly. May be subdivided into: emergence delirium (related to drugs, pain and acute physiological derangements); delirium associated with postoperative complications; and longer-term impairment (**postoperative cognitive dysfunction**; POCD).

- Possible causes/contributing factors include:
  - type of surgery: more common with major surgery, especially cardiac.
  - drugs: e.g. opioids, **ketamine**, and those associated with the **central anticholinergic syndrome**.
  - **hypoxaemia**, **hypercapnia**.
  - **hypotension**.
  - restlessness due to pain or full bladder.
  - metabolic disturbances, e.g. **hypoglycaemia**, **hypernatraemia**, **hyponatraemia**, **acidosis**.
  - **alcohol** and **benzodiazepine** withdrawal.
  - **sepsis**.
  - intracranial pathology, e.g. raised **ICP**, **stroke**, post-ictal state.
  - pre-existing confusion e.g. due to dementia.
  - reduced **cerebral blood flow** resulting from perioperative **hyperventilation** (especially in the elderly) has been suggested as a contributory cause.

Confusion within a few days of surgery may be caused by any illness (e.g. sepsis, pulmonary disease). Appropriate investigation and treatment are required, rather than simply administering sedation, which may exacerbate the confusion. POCD may occur (often after an initial lucid period), particularly in the elderly and those with pre-existing cognitive deficit. The mechanism for this is unclear, but may involve an inflammatory process within the CNS as well as cerebrovascular impairment.

Sanders RD, Pandharipande PP, Davidson AJ, et al (2011). Br Med J; 343: d4331

Congenital heart disease. Incidence: up to 1% of live births; 15% survive to adulthood without treatment. May be associated with other congenital defects or syndromes.

- Simple classification:
  - acyanotic (no **shunt**):
    - **coarctation of the aorta** (6%–8%).
    - pulmonary and **aortic stenosis** (10%–15% together).
  - potentially cyanotic (i.e., left-to-right shunt); may reverse and become cyanotic if **pulmonary hypertension** develops (**Eisenmenger's syndrome**):
    - **ASD** (10%–15%).
    - **VSD** (20%–30%).
    - patent **ductus arteriosus** (10%–15%).
  - cyanotic, due to:
    - right-to-left shunt:
      - **Fallot's tetralogy** (5%–10%).
      - pulmonary atresia with septal defect.
      - **tricuspid valve lesions**, including **Ebstein's anomaly**, with septal defect.
      - abnormal connections (e.g. **transposition of the great arteries**, 5%).
      - mixing of systemic and pulmonary blood, e.g. single atrium or ventricle.
- Has also been classified functionally as:
  - obstructive: e.g. coarctation, valve stenosis.
  - shunt; defects may be:
    - restrictive: small defects entail shunt flow that is relatively unaffected by changes in downstream resistance e.g. small VSD.
    - non-restrictive: with large defects, amount of shunt depends largely on the relationship between pulmonary and systemic vascular resistance, because flow through the connection is variable, e.g. large VSD.
  - complex, i.e., involving both obstruction and shunt, e.g. Fallot's tetralogy.

Patients may present soon after birth. Common features include feeding difficulty, failure to thrive, **cyanosis**, **dyspnoea**, **heart murmurs** and **cardiac failure**. Investigation includes **echocardiography** and **cardiac catheterisation**. Increased risk of surgery within first year of life may be offset by a high mortality without surgery, depending on the lesion. Palliative procedures are sometimes performed early, with later corrective surgery, e.g.:
  - pulmonary balloon valvuloplasty in pulmonary stenosis.
  - shunt procedures to increase pulmonary blood flow in severe right-to-left shunt, e.g. Fallot's tetralogy. A prosthetic graft is inserted between the subclavian and pulmonary arteries (formerly involved direct anastomosis of the subclavian artery itself [Blalock–Taussig procedure]). Balloon atrial septostomy is sometimes performed in transposition of the great arteries, to allow oxygenated blood to pass from left to right sides of heart.
  - pulmonary artery banding to reduce pulmonary blood flow and prevent pulmonary hypertension in large left-to-right shunts.

Principles of anaesthesia are as for **cardiac surgery** and **paediatric anaesthesia**. Inhalational or iv techniques are suitable. Uptake of inhalational agents is slower when right-to-left shunts exist. **Ketamine** is preferred by some anaesthetists. Air bubbles in iv lines are particularly hazardous in right-to-left shunts, due to risk of systemic embolism. Nasal tracheal tubes are preferred when postoperative IPPV is required.

Antibiotic prophylaxis for **endocarditis** in patients with congenital heart disease was previously routinely administered for dental, genitourinary and gastrointestinal surgery. Current **NICE** guidance no longer recommends this practice, unless the procedure involves operating on an area of suspected infection in which prophylaxis for surgical site infection would normally be given; in these cases antibiotics should also be given that cover organisms known to cause endocarditis.

[Alfred Blalock (1899–1964), US surgeon; Helen Taussig (1898–1986), US physician]

Cannesson M, Collange V, Lehot JJ (2009). Curr Opin Anesth; 22: 88–94

See also, Preoperative assessment; Pulmonary valve lesions; Valvular heart disease

Congestive cardiac failure, *see Cardiac failure*

Coning. Herniation of **brain** structures caused by increased **ICP**. May be:
  - supratentorial, e.g. caused by **stroke**, **subarachnoid haemorrhage**, **cerebral abscess**, **encephalitis**, neoplasm, **trauma**. Supratentorial pressure may result in:
    - central herniation: the diencephalon is forced through the tentorial opening. Early signs include altered alertness, sighing and yawning, small pupils and conjugate roving eye movements. Appropriate motor responses give way to **decorticate posture**. As midbrain compression occurs, **Cheyne–Stokes respiration** appears, pupils become moderately dilated and **decerebrate posture** is seen. Medullary compression results in hypertension, bradycardia and respiratory arrhythmias (**Cushing's reflex**) and is a terminal event.
    - uncal herniation: usually caused by a rapidly expanding mass (e.g. traumatic haematoma) in the middle fossa or temporal lobe, which pushes the medial uncus over the edge of the tentorium. Decreased consciousness occurs later and the earliest consistent sign is a unilateral dilating pupil caused by compression of the ipsilateral oculomotor nerve (**cranial nerve** III) against the tentorial edge. Delay in decompression at this stage results in irreversible brainstem damage.
  - infratentorial: caused by posterior fossa masses. May result in:
    - upward cerebellar herniation causing midbrain compression, cerebellar infarction and **hydrocephalus**.
    - tonsillar herniation: the cerebellar tonsils are forced through the foramen magnum resulting in medullary compression. May follow lumbar puncture in the presence of increased ICP.

Conjoined twins. Incidence is about 1 in 200 000 births. Radiological assessment may require repeat anaesthesia. Each twin requires a separate anaesthetic team. Tracheal intubation and access may be difficult, depending on the site of union. If circulation is shared, induction of the first twin may be delayed, as anaesthetic drugs are taken up by the second twin. Induction of the second twin may thus be rapid. Blood loss at separation may be massive. Adrenal insufficiency may be present in one twin.

Kobylarz K (2014). Anaesthesiol Intensive Ther; 46: 124–9

Connective tissue diseases. Group of diseases sharing certain features, particularly inflammation of connective tissue and features of **autoimmune disease**. **Rheumatoid**

arthritis, SLE and **systemic sclerosis** (SS) are more common in women; **polyarteritis nodosa** (PN) is more common in men. In mixed connective tissue disease, features of SLE, SS and myositis coexist.

- Features may include the following:
  - autoimmune involvement: immunoglobulins may be directed against IgG (rheumatoid factors) and cell components, e.g. nuclear proteins, phospholipids. Organ-specific antibodies are also common, e.g. against thyroid and gastric parietal cells, smooth muscle and mitochondria. T- and B-cell dysfunction, immune complex deposition and **complement** activation may also occur. Diagnosis of specific disease is aided by the pattern of immune disturbance.
  - systemic involvement:
    - musculoskeletal: arthropathy, myopathy.
    - skin: rash, mouth ulcers. Thickening in SS, with characteristic 'pinched' mouth.
    - renal: **glomerulonephritis**, vasculitis, **nephrotic syndrome**.
    - fever, malaise
    - cardiovascular: **pericarditis**, **myocarditis**, conduction defects, vasculitis (affecting any organ). Raynaud's phenomenon (fingers turn white, then blue, then red on exposure to cold, stress or vibration) is common.
    - haematological: **anaemia**, leucopenia, **thrombocytopenia**. Lupus anticoagulant may be present in SLE.
    - hepatosplenomegaly.
    - central and peripheral nervous involvement, e.g. central lesions, neuropathies and psychiatric disturbances (especially with SLE).
    - pulmonary: fibrosis, pleurisy, pleural effusions and pulmonary infiltrates. **Pulmonary hypertension** may occur. Haemorrhage with PN.
    - Sjögren's syndrome (reduced tear and saliva formation and secretion) may occur.
    - GIT: reduced oesophageal motility, oesophagitis and risk of regurgitation, especially in SS.

Treatment includes **corticosteroids** and other **immunosuppressive drugs**. **Antimalarial drugs** are used in SLE.

- Anaesthetic considerations:
  - systematic **preoperative assessment** to identify the above features, complications and drugs, with appropriate management.
  - mouth opening may be difficult in SS.
  - general management: as for rheumatoid arthritis.

Other conditions without circulating rheumatoid factors may have systemic manifestations, e.g. **ankylosing spondylitis** and associated conditions. Arthritis may accompany **inflammatory bowel disease** and intestinal infection.

[Maurice Raynaud (1834–1881), French physician; Henrik Sjögren (1899–1986), Swedish ophthalmologist]

See also, Vasculitides

Connectors, tracheal tube. Adaptors for connecting **tracheal tubes** to **anaesthetic breathing systems**. Modern connectors are plastic, and 15 mm in size distally. They fit to any standardised 15/22-mm equipment, e.g. directly to breathing tubing or to **catheter mounts**. They may connect directly or via angle pieces, which may swivel. Some incorporate a capped port for tracheobronchial suction or insertion of fibreoptic instruments.

Conn's syndrome, *see Hyperaldosteronism*

Consciousness. State of awareness of self and surroundings that gives significance to stimuli from the internal and external environment.

- Consists of:
  - cognitive content: the sum of cortical functions (e.g. the expression of psychological functions of sensations, emotions and thought). Damaged by disorders affecting both cerebral hemispheres and, depending on aetiology, may result in akinetic syndrome or **vegetative states**.
  - arousal: arises from the **ascending reticular activating system** in the **brainstem**. Disorders of arousal due to temporary or permanent damage of the system result in obtundation, **confusion** or **coma**.

Consent for anaesthesia. Required before general and local anaesthetic techniques may be performed. Failure to obtain consent before touching (or making to touch) another person may result in a charge of assault or battery, although clinically a claim of **negligence** arising from inadequacy of the consent process is much more likely.

- Consent requires:
  - capacity of the patient to understand: the patient should be over 16 years (in England and Wales) and 'of sound mind', i.e., unaffected by drugs or extreme pain (this decision should be made by the treating doctor, although it may be aided by consulting with colleagues). Consent on behalf of children is given by their parents or legal guardians, although this may be overruled by the courts. The 'emancipated minor' is a child under the age of majority who is able to understand and therefore make decisions about his/her treatment (though in English law he/she may consent to treatment but not refuse it ['Gillick competent']).

    If the patient lacks capacity (e.g. is unconscious) then life-saving treatment may proceed if it is felt to be in his/her 'best interests' (N.B. these may not be the same as 'medical best interests') and every attempt should be made to find out the patient's views and wishes. In England and Wales, the **Mental Capacity Act 2005** laid down formal procedures for the appointment of advocates for persons lacking capacity, and also strengthens the status of **advance decisions** (in Scotland, advocates for incapacitated patients already had legal status).
  - disclosure of relevant information: traditionally, in the UK, doctors have used their discretion to explain risks and benefits as they feel appropriate, as long as their decision was judged reasonable according to current medical opinion. This has gradually moved towards divulging the information that a 'reasonable patient' would want to know, and then to what each particular patient would want to know. Following a landmark 2015 UK Supreme Court judgement (Montgomery), a doctor now needs to take 'reasonable care to ensure that the patient is aware of any material risks', defined as those to which the particular patient or a reasonable patient would attach significance. The options for treatment should also be discussed. The discussion about anaesthetic risks should therefore include general risks (e.g. **sore throat**, **postoperative nausea and vomiting**, **postoperative pain**, **shivering**, **teeth**, gum, lip and eye damage, serious allergy, **awareness**, brain damage and death) and specific risks relating to the proposed

technique and alternatives (e.g. **post-dural puncture headache**, nerve damage following regional anaesthesia) or surgery (e.g. transfer to **ICU**)—guided at each stage by what the patient wants to know. There should be some written evidence of the discussion (usually recorded on the anaesthetic chart).
    - patient's understanding of the options and their implications.
    - voluntary decision and the time in which to make it. Presentation of detailed information immediately before induction of anaesthesia (e.g. in the anaesthetic room) is not considered acceptable for elective surgery.
- Consent may be:
    - verbal or written. The latter serves as proof of consent afterwards, but is no 'stronger' than verbal consent, which should be witnessed if possible.
    - express or implied (i.e., by allowing treatment or insertion of a cannula, the patient is demonstrating consent, without having specifically expressed it).

Consent forms are standard for surgery, although there is disagreement about the requirement for consent forms for other procedures (e.g. epidural analgesia in labour requires written consent only in some UK units). Separate anaesthetic consent forms have been suggested but are not routine in the UK. **Association of Anaesthetists** guidance (2017) does not recommend a separate anaesthetic consent form, although the importance of recording the discussion around consent is stressed.

In the ICU/emergency setting, consent for invasive interventions (e.g. tracheal intubation, venous cannulation, surgery) often cannot be obtained from the patient and similar procedures apply as discussed earlier. Until the Mental Capacity Act, no person could legally give consent for another, although it has been customary to obtain 'informed assent' from the next of kin, though it had no legal status.

[Victoria Gillick, British campaigner against the policy that contraception could be prescribed to children below the age of 16 without parental consent; Sam Montgomery, born 1999 in Scotland; suffered cerebral hypoxia at delivery through shoulder dystocia]

Yentis SM, Hartle AJ, Barker IR, et al (2017). Anaesthesia; 72: 93–105

See also, Medicolegal aspects of anaesthesia

Constipation. Common postoperatively as a result of **opioid analgesic drug** administration and immobility. In addition, ICU factors include sedative drugs, dehydration and lack of fibre in some enteral diets, altered GIT flora and impaired neurological function, e.g. **spinal cord injury**. Resulting abdominal distension may impair **weaning from ventilators** and increase the risk of **bacterial translocation**. Patients should undergo rectal examination to exclude faecal impaction. Treatment is with oral or rectal **laxatives** and attention to any underlying cause. Manual evacuation may be required in unconscious patients.

Contamination of anaesthetic equipment. The role of cross-infection involving anaesthetic equipment is uncertain, although a common breathing system has been implicated in the cross-infection of patients with **hepatitis** C. Treatment of anaesthetic apparatus varies between hospitals, although disposable equipment is now routinely used for convenience and cheapness. Breathing system filters are routinely placed between the patient and breathing system.

Particularly important in **ICU**, **immunodeficiency** states and in high-risk infectious cases, e.g. **HIV infection**, hepatitis, **chest infection**, **TB** (equipment is changed after use and other precautions taken, e.g. bacterial filters).
- Methods of killing contaminating organisms:
    - disinfection: kills most organisms but not spores. Achieved by:
        - pasteurisation: 30 min at 77°C. Rubber/plastic items may be distorted.
        - chemical agents:
            - formaldehyde, formalin (no longer used).
            - alcohol 70%.
            - chlorhexidine 0.1%–0.5%.
            - glutaraldehyde 2%: expensive and may irritate skin.
            - hypochlorite 10%: may corrode metal.
            - hydrogen peroxide, phenol 0.6%–2%.

      Must be followed by rinsing and thorough drying.
    - sterilisation: kills all organisms and spores. The term sterility assurance level (SAL) is a measure of the probability of complete sterility of the item. A SAL of 10^{-6} (i.e., probability of an organism surviving on the item following sterilisation is one in a million) is considered acceptable. Methods include:
        - dry heat, e.g. 150°C for 30 min.
        - moist heat:
            - autoclave (most common method), e.g.:
                - 30 min at 1 atm at 122°C;
                - 10 min at 1.5 atm at 126°C;
                - 3 min at 2 atm at 134°C.

              Steam is used to increase temperature. Indicator tape or tubes are used to confirm that the correct conditions are achieved.
            - low-temperature steam + formaldehyde.
    - ethylene oxide: expensive and flammable (the latter risk is reduced by adding 80%–90% fluorohydrocarbons or CO_2). Toxic and taken up by plastics; up to 2 weeks' elution time is suggested before use.
    - γ-irradiation: used commercially but expensive and inconvenient for most hospital use.
    - gas plasma sterilisation: exposure of equipment to a mixture of highly ionised gas and free radicals. Provides low-temperature, dry sterilisation with short cycle times.

The above methods do not destroy the prion protein responsible for variant **Creutzfeldt–Jakob disease**; this has led to increasing interest in disposable instruments. New enzyme-based agents that disrupt prion structure are under investigation.

[Louis Pasteur (1822–1895), French bacteriologist]

See also, COSHH regulations

Continuous positive airway pressure (CPAP). Application of positive airway pressure throughout all phases of spontaneous ventilation. May be achieved with various systems, applied via a tightly fitting mask or tracheal tube. In order to apply positive pressure throughout ventilation, a reservoir bag, or a fresh gas flow exceeding maximal inspiratory gas flow, must be provided. The latter may be achieved using a **Venturi** mixing device. Increases **FRC**, thereby reducing airway collapse and increasing arterial oxygenation. F_IO_2 may thus be reduced.
- Uses:
    - to aid **weaning from ventilators**.
    - to improve oxygenation during **one-lung anaesthesia**.
    - in the treatment of some **sleep-related breathing disorders**, e.g. **obstructive sleep apnoea**.

- in acute exacerbations of **COPD** to avoid tracheal intubation.
- in neonates (e.g. in **respiratory distress syndrome**, bronchomalacia and tracheomalacia), especially if associated with apnoeic episodes. May be applied via nasal cannulae.

- Complications: as for PEEP, but less severe. **Barotrauma** and reduction in cardiac output are more likely in neonates. Some patients cannot tolerate the sensation of CPAP.

See also, BiPAP

Contraceptives, oral. Main anaesthetic considerations are related to the risk of venous thromboembolism, which is 2–6 times more common in patients taking the combined contraceptive pill. Patients taking the combined pill containing third-generation progesterones (desogestrel or gestodene) are at greatest risk. Other risk factors (e.g. inherited hypercoagulable states, smoking, obesity) compound this risk. Although 4 weeks' discontinuation of therapy before major or leg surgery has traditionally been advocated, it has been claimed that this is based on insufficient evidence. If other risk factors exist, discontinuation of therapy (or sc **heparin** in view of the risk of pregnancy) has been suggested. The pill is restarted after the first period beyond a fortnight postoperatively. No extra precautions are generally thought to be necessary for minor surgery, e.g. dilatation and curettage, or with oestrogen-free therapy.

Stone J (2002). Anaesthesia; 57: 606–25

See also, Hormone replacement therapy

Contractility, myocardial, *see Myocardial contractility*

Contrast media, *see Radiological contrast media*

Controlled drugs (CDs). Refers to drugs covered by the **Misuse of Drugs Act 1971** (the term is often reserved for drugs described in Schedule 2 of the Misuse of Drugs Regulations, 1985). **Association of Anaesthetists** guidelines (2006) on the handling of CDs in the operating theatre suite recommend:

- preference for prefilled syringes or similar devices to be licensed medicinal products rather than special items produced in a licensed facility for individual patients, with medicines prepared in an unlicensed site (e.g. pharmacy) being least preferable.
- local guidelines for ordering, storage, handling and administration of CDs, including doctors' signatures in the CD register; recording in the notes the amount given; return of unopened ampoules; and disposal of unused drug (e.g. by discarding onto absorbent material before disposal).
- ability for **ODPs** to issue and handle CDs (along with registration of ODPs, etc.).
- an end to the sharing of ampoules between patients.

See also, Abuse of anaesthetic agents

Convulsions. Usually refer to tonic–clonic epileptic seizures. They increase cerebral and whole-body O_2 demand and CO_2 production, while **airway obstruction** and chest wall rigidity may result in **hypoventilation.** Thus **hypoxaemia, acidosis, hypercapnia** and increased sympathetic activity may occur. Patients may also injure themselves. Fits may be generalised or focal. Anaesthetic involvement is usually necessary when they occur perioperatively, or in **status epilepticus**.

- Caused by:
  - pre-existing **epilepsy** (i.e., a continuing susceptibility to fits; may include other causes listed later).
  - hypoxaemia.
  - metabolic, e.g. **hypoglycaemia**, **hyponatraemia**, **hypocalcaemia**, **uraemia**.
  - anaesthetic drugs:
    - **diethyl ether**; convulsions classically occurred postoperatively in pyrexial children.
    - **enflurane**, especially following perioperative **hyperventilation** and **hypocapnia**.
    - **ketamine**, **methohexital** and **doxapram** in susceptible patients. Although **propofol** may cause myoclonic jerking, initial reports of epileptic seizures following its use are now thought to be unfounded. Similarly, **etomidate** may cause non-epileptic twitching.
    - **local anaesthetic drugs** in overdose.
    - **pethidine** in very high or prolonged dosage. Convulsions may also follow its interaction with **monoamine oxidase inhibitors**.
  - other drugs, e.g. **alcohol**, **phenothiazines**, **tricyclic antidepressant drugs**, **cocaine**.
  - **fat embolism**, also clot or **gas embolism**.
  - **TBI**, **stroke**, cerebral infections, **meningitis**, **neurosurgery**, brain tumours and other cerebral disease.
  - **eclampsia**.
  - pyrexia in children.
  - acute O_2 **toxicity** (**Bert effect**).
- Management:
  - protection of the airway and maintenance of oxygenation, with positioning on the side if possible. Tracheal intubation and IPPV may be required, e.g. if large doses of depressant drugs are needed.
  - **anticonvulsant drugs**:
    - **diazepam** 5-mg increments iv up to 20 mg; may be given rectally. **Midazolam** 5–10 mg im has been used as an alternative when iv cannulation is impossible. **Lorazepam** iv 75 µg/kg is the first-line treatment for status epilepticus.
    - **phenytoin** iv, 15 mg/kg slowly, with ECG monitoring.
  - other drugs used in the control of seizures include **paraldehyde** and **magnesium sulfate** (in eclampsia). If seizures persist following phenytoin the patient should be treated as for status epilepticus.

Cooley, Samuel, *see Wells, Horace*

COPD, *see Chronic obstructive pulmonary disease*

Copper kettle, *see Vaporisers*

Co-proxamol, *see Dextropropoxyphene*

Cordotomy, anterolateral. Destruction of lateral spinothalamic tracts, classically in the cervical region (C1–2) providing contralateral pain control below C4; used in chronic **pain management**. Usually performed percutaneously with x-ray guidance, under sedation. Electrical stimulation is used to confirm correct positioning of the needle before thermocoagulation.

Indicated for unilateral cancer pain (e.g. in malignant pleural mesothelioma, bronchial carcinoma, brachial plexus pain due to a Pancoast tumour) in patients with a life expectancy <12 months. Descending respiratory fibres lie close to the sectioned fibres and therefore cordotomy is usually not performed in patients with respiratory disease.

May damage pyramidal pathways or cause **Horner's syndrome**, bladder disturbances and paraesthesiae. Headache in a C2 distribution is common. Complications are more likely if cordotomy is bilateral.
[Henry Pancoast (1875–1939), US radiologist]
Feizerfan A, Antrobus JHL (2014). Cont Educ Anaesth Crit Care Pain; 14: 23–26
See also, Sensory pathways

Corning, James Leonard (1855–1923). New York neurologist; first described (and coined the term) **spinal anaesthesia** in 1885. He had intended to observe the effects of **cocaine** on the spinal cord by injecting it into the interspinal space of a dog, believing erroneously that the interspinal blood vessels communicated with those of the cord. Hindquarter paralysis and anaesthesia followed. Repeated the experiment on a human, and subsequently suggested its use in the treatment of neurological disease. **Epidural anaesthesia** may have been produced in some of his studies. Published the first textbook on local anaesthesia in 1886.
Gorelick PB, Zych D (1987). Neurology; 37: 672–4

Coronary angioplasty, *see Percutaneous coronary intervention*

Coronary artery bypass graft (CABG). Performed for **ischaemic heart disease** unresponsive to medical treatment and unsuitable for **percutaneous coronary intervention** (*see later*). A vascular conduit (most frequently long saphenous vein, internal thoracic [internal mammary] artery or radial artery) is grafted between the aorta and coronary artery distal to its obstruction.

'Minimal access' coronary surgery involves internal thoracic artery grafting through tiny incisions in the left side of the chest, offering the advantages of arterial grafts to the left anterior descending coronary artery without the need for **cardiopulmonary bypass**, although **one-lung ventilation** is still required. A technique of 'off-pump' CABG is increasingly used, in which median sternotomy is carried out enabling multiple grafts on the beating heart. Surgery requires good access (cardiac displacement), stabilisation of the heart's wall at the site of anastomoses using special devices, and the use of intracoronary shunts or strategies to limit periods of arterial occlusion. Anaesthesia is complicated by the need for cardiovascular stability, normothermia and bradycardia during anastomoses to reduce movement (bradycardia is less important with stabilising devices). Complications and costs are felt to be less than with traditional CABG but long-term randomised trials are relatively lacking.

- Life expectancy is improved following CABG (vs. **percutaneous coronary intervention** [PCI]) in:
    - moderate/severe angina, triple-vessel disease and impaired ventricular function.
    - double-vessel disease including severe stenosis of the proximal left anterior descending artery.
    - severe stenosis of the left main stem coronary artery.

  Life expectancy is not improved in single-vessel disease or if angina is not present.

PCI is an alternative but emergency CABG may be required if unsuccessful.

Anaesthesia is as for ischaemic heart disease and **cardiac surgery**. Combinations of **aspirin**, **dipyridamole** and **clopidogrel** are used postoperatively to maintain graft patency.

Mortality is under 1% for 1–2 grafts, but increases if more grafts are anastomosed. Mortality is greater in women.

Coronary artery disease, *see Ischaemic heart disease*

Coronary blood flow. Normally approximately 5% of **cardiac output**, i.e., 250 ml/min or 80 ml/100 g/min. May increase up to five times in exercise. The inner 1 mm of the left ventricle obtains O_2 via diffusion from blood in the ventricular cavity; the remainder of the ventricle is supplied via epicardial vessels. The left coronary vessels are compressed by the contracting myocardium during systole; thus **flow** to the subendocardium occurs during diastole only. Superficial areas receive more constant flow. Atrial and right ventricular flow occurs throughout the **cardiac cycle**. The left ventricle is therefore most at risk from **myocardial ischaemia**.

- Left ventricular blood flow is related to:
    - difference between aortic end-diastolic pressure and **left ventricular end-diastolic pressure**.
    - duration of diastole (inversely related to **heart rate**).
    - patency/radius of the coronary arteries; related to:
        - **autoregulation**: normally maintains blood flow above MAP of 60 mmHg, possibly via the action of adenine nucleotides, **potassium**, **hydrogen ions**, **prostaglandins**, lactic acid or CO_2 released from myocardial cells.
        - autonomic neural input: has little direct influence, being overridden by the effect on **SVR** and **myocardial contractility**.
        - coronary stenosis/spasm and the state of collateral vessels (e.g. **coronary steal**).
        - drugs causing vasoconstriction/dilatation.
    - blood **viscosity**.

The oxygen extraction of the myocardium is almost 75% and therefore increased O_2 demand can only be met by increased flow and is important if ischaemia is to be prevented. Reductions in flow may be minimised by controlling the above factors. Coronary perfusion pressure and duration of diastole may be assessed by the **diastolic pressure–time index**.

- Measurement:
    - **Fick principle** using N_2O or argon. Requires **coronary sinus catheterisation**.
    - thermodilution techniques to estimate coronary sinus flow, thus providing an indication of left ventricular drainage.
    - **nuclear cardiology** may be used to indicate regional flow.

See also, Coronary circulation; Ischaemic heart disease; Myocardial metabolism

Coronary care unit (CCU). Specialised hospital ward, originally proposed in 1961 for the management of patients with acute **MI**; introduction halved in-hospital mortality. Features include continuous ECG monitoring and availability of defibrillators, drugs and specially trained staff. Renamed 'acute cardiac care unit', reflecting its increasing role in treating patients with **cardiac failure**, **cardiogenic shock**, adult **congenital heart disease** and prolonged **arrhythmias**. Allows surveillance and prompt treatment of arrhythmias and cardiac failure, and limitation of infarct size and restoration of coronary blood flow using **fibrinolytic drugs**.

Coronary circulation

- Arterial supply (Fig. 49a):
    - right coronary artery: arises from the anterior aortic sinus. Passes between the pulmonary trunk and right atrium, and runs in the right atrioventricular groove

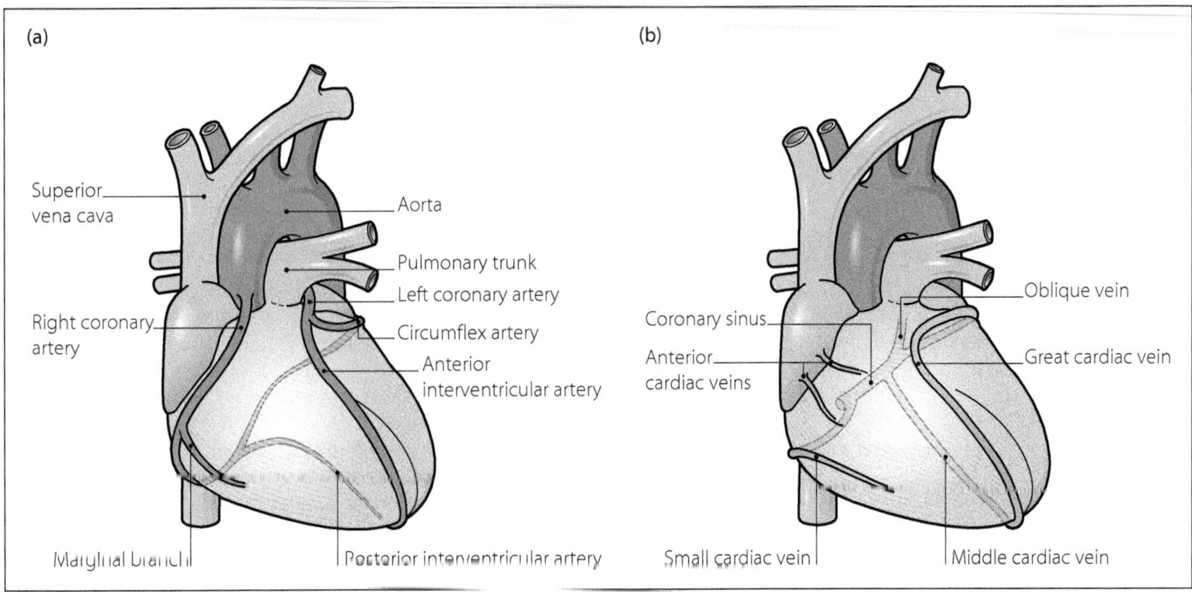

Fig. 49 Coronary circulation: (a) arterial; (b) venous

between the right atrium and ventricle. Descends the anterior surface of the heart, continuing inferiorly to anastomose with the left coronary artery. Supplies the right ventricle and sinoatrial node and, in 90% of the population, the atrioventricular node and posterior and inferior parts of the left ventricle.
- left coronary artery: arises from the left posterior aortic sinus. Passes lateral to the pulmonary trunk and runs in the left atrioventricular groove. Supplies the anterior wall of the left ventricle and the interventricular septum via its left anterior descending branch, and the lateral wall of the left ventricle via its circumflex branch.

The artery that supplies the posterior descending and the posterolateral arteries determines the dominant coronary artery; in 60% of the population, the right coronary artery is dominant.

- Venous drainage (Fig. 49b):
  - one-third via venae cordis minimae (thebesian veins) and anterior cardiac veins—small veins draining directly into the heart chambers (right atrium receiving most; left ventricle least). Those draining into the left heart are a source of anatomical **shunt**.
  - two-thirds via the coronary sinus, draining into the right atrium near the opening of the inferior vena cava.

[Adam Thebesius (1686–1732), German physician]
See also, Coronary blood flow

Coronary sinus catheterisation. Performed using fluoroscopy. May be used to determine:
- coronary sinus blood flow, using a thermodilution technique.
- **coronary blood flow**, using the **Fick principle**.
- blood O_2 and **lactate** levels. The latter are raised in **myocardial ischaemia**, due to decreased uptake by myocardial tissue and increased production.

Coronary steal. Diversion of blood from poorly perfused areas of myocardium to those already adequately perfused. May be caused by vasodilator substances acting on small coronary arteries but not on larger epicardial vessels. Poorly perfused areas supplied by stenosed vessels may be dependent on collateral vessels for blood flow. Dilatation of normal small arteries increases flow to normal areas, but the stenosed vessels are unable to dilate sufficiently, resulting in steal. Anti-anginal drugs (e.g. nitrates) are thought to increase collateral flow by acting predominantly on the large epicardial vessels. **Adenosine**, **dipyridamole**, **papaverine** and **isoflurane** have all been shown to cause steal in animal models, but the significance of this in humans is disputed. Recent work has demonstrated that isoflurane in fact has a protective effect against myocardial ischaemia (**ischaemic preconditioning**).

Coronary stents, *see Percutaneous coronary intervention*

Coroner. Independent judicial officer of the Crown who has a duty to investigate the circumstances of some deaths. Coroners are barristers, solicitors or legally qualified medical practitioners, and are assisted by Coroner's Officers. Cases are referred mostly from doctors, but also from registrars of births and deaths and from other sources, e.g. police. A death should be reported if:
- its cause is unknown.
- the deceased was not seen by the certifying doctor after death or within the fortnight preceding it.
- it was violent, unnatural or suspicious.
- it may have been caused by an accident (whenever it occurred).
- it may have been caused by neglect (by self or others).
- it may have been caused by industrial disease or related to employment.
- it may have been caused by abortion.
- it occurred during an operation or before recovery from an anaesthetic.
- it may have been suicide.
- it occurred during or shortly after detention in police or prison custody.

In England and Wales, about 45% of deaths are referred to the coroner, of which 14% proceed to an inquest; a conclusion (previously termed 'verdict') may then be issued as to the manner and cause of death. Potential conclusions that can be issued are: natural causes; suicide; accidental death; unlawful or lawful killing; death due to an industrial disease; open (not enough evidence available to determine cause of death); and narrative (a description of how an individual met his death).

The coroner may send a Prevention of Future Deaths Report (formerly 'Rule 43 Report') to an individual(s) or organisation(s)—e.g. hospital or Trust—if he/she considers that action is required; the recipient is required to respond within 56 days to say what action is planned.

Fundamental reform of the coroners' service came into effect in 2013, designed to increase the interaction between coroner and the bereaved by disclosing and recording information and keeping all informed about inquest arrangements.

Bass S, Cowman S (2016). BJA Education; 16: 130–3

Cor pulmonale. Right ventricular hypertrophy, dilatation or failure secondary to increased **pulmonary vascular resistance** due to respiratory disease. **COPD** is the commonest cause, but any disease that causes chronic **hypoxaemia** (e.g. **pulmonary fibrosis**) may result in **hypoxic pulmonary vasoconstriction**, eventually with pulmonary vascular muscle hypertrophy and **pulmonary hypertension**. **PE** is included in some definitions.

- Features:
  - those of the underlying disease, including cyanosis and hypoxaemia.
  - those of right-sided **cardiac failure**: peripheral oedema, raised **JVP**, hepatomegaly, third **heart sound**.
  - of pulmonary hypertension and underlying disease on **CXR**. The **ECG** may show right ventricular hypertrophy and axis deviation, peaked **P waves** (P pulmonale), and **T wave** and **S–T segment** changes in the right chest leads.
- Anaesthetic management:
  - as for COPD/underlying disease.
  - as for **cardiac failure**.
  - as for pulmonary hypertension.

Correlation, *see Statistical tests*

Corticosteroids. Steroid hormones released from the cortex of the **adrenal gland**. Classified according to activity:
  - **mineralocorticoids**: mainly **aldosterone**. Synthetic mineralocorticoids include **fludrocortisone**, used for replacement therapy and in congenital adrenal hyperplasia and postural hypotension.
  - **glucocorticoids**: mainly cortisone (**hydrocortisone**). The term '(cortico)steroid therapy' usually refers to use of drugs with predominantly glucocorticoid activity, although most have mineralocorticoid activity also. Corticosteroids are used in **adrenocortical insufficiency**, and to suppress inflammatory and immunological responses, including: **connective tissue diseases**; raised **ICP** due to tumours; skin diseases; blood dyscrasias; allergic reactions; **asthma**; **myasthenia gravis**; and following organ **transplantation**. Have been used in **ALI** but their efficacy is disputed. Use in severe **sepsis** remains controversial and is usually reserved for patients with confirmed adrenocortical insufficiency and/or high vasopressor requirements.

    Prednisolone 5 mg has equivalent anti-inflammatory activity to 20 mg hydrocortisone, 4 mg **methylprednisolone** and 0.75 mg **dexamethasone**. All except hydrocortisone have little mineralocorticoid activity and are thus suitable for long-term disease suppression.
- The drugs have many side effects:
  - related to mineralocorticoid activity: water and sodium retention, **hypokalaemia**, hypertension.
  - **hyperglycaemia** and **diabetes mellitus**, osteoporosis and pathological fractures, skeletal muscle wasting with proximal myopathy.
  - GIT effects: dyspepsia, **peptic ulcer disease**.
  - mental changes: euphoria, depression.
  - spread of infection. Severe chickenpox is a particular risk.
  - impaired wound healing.
  - cataract formation.
  - growth suppression in children.
  - **Cushing's syndrome** may occur with high dosage.
  - adrenal suppression, due to inhibition of **ACTH** release. Pituitary–adrenal axis function may take 6 months to recover following withdrawal of therapy; during this time patients are unable to mount a normal cortisone response to stress (secretion increases from 25 mg/day to 300 mg/day), and may develop circulatory collapse. Patients at risk are those who have:
    - received corticosteroid therapy for longer than 2 weeks within the previous 2 months (up to 1 year has been suggested).
    - adrenocortical insufficiency or adrenalectomy.

Based on studies of normal cortisone responses following surgery, estimated amounts required are 25 mg hydrocortisone equivalent for minor surgery; 50–75 mg/day for 1–2 days for moderate surgery; and 100–150 mg/day for 2–3 days for major surgery. These estimates include current medication; thus patients already taking the required amount do not need supplementation.

See also, Stress response to surgery

Corticotropin (Corticotrophin), *see Adrenocorticotrophic hormone*

COSHH regulations (Control of Substances Hazardous to Health). Came into force in 1989 in Scotland, England and Wales, and in 1991 in Northern Ireland. The latest regulations were published in 2011. Stipulate that employers must identify and control any substances that may be hazardous to health, e.g. chemicals and micro-organisms. Important guidance is given to allow employers to assess the risk to employees, eliminate or control the risk (e.g. with protective clothing, adequate ventilation), monitor the exposure and health of employees, and provide information and training. Employees must make full use of any control measure provided. Anaesthetic implications include concerns about the **environmental safety of anaesthetists**, **scavenging** and **contamination of anaesthetic equipment**.

Costs of anaesthesia. Intraoperative anaesthetic cost constitutes about 5%–6% of total hospital costs, whereas the total cost for intraoperative patient care is approximately 30%. Anaesthetic costs may be divided into:
  - overhead costs:
    - capital equipment, e.g. ventilators, anaesthetic machines. Often difficult to quantify because the life of equipment may be uncertain.
    - maintenance.

- staff salaries, e.g. anaesthetists, anaesthetic assistants, recovery nurses.
- running costs:
  - drugs, e.g. iv and inhalational anaesthetic agents, neuromuscular blocking drugs, opioids, antiemetics, iv fluids.
  - piped gases (and those in cylinders).
  - consumable items, e.g. iv cannulae, tracheal tubes, airways.

Estimates of the total costs of individual procedures have been made but vary widely according to the country and hospital, and the methods used for the calculations. In addition, techniques or drugs that appear more expensive may have cost savings elsewhere, e.g. by reducing postoperative complications and hospital stay. With increasing scrutiny of healthcare costs, calculations of anaesthetic costs and 'value-based anaesthetic care' may become more common and pressure applied to anaesthetic departments to reduce their costs, despite the relatively small amounts compared with those incurred by the surgeons. However, it has been estimated that about half the intraoperative anaesthetic costs could be influenced by the choice of drugs and anaesthetic techniques.

Rinehardt EK, Sivarajan M (2012). Curr Opin Anaesthesiol; 25: 221–5

Costs of intensive care. Actual costs of ICU treatment are difficult to quantify because no standardised model of costing has been validated as being applicable to all types of unit. Methods used have included dividing the total annual expenditure by the number of patients treated and the use of severity of illness and workload scoring systems. Costs have been divided into six 'cost blocks':

- capital equipment: includes depreciation, maintenance and lease charges (~6%).
- estates: includes building depreciation, water, sewage, energy and maintenance charges (~3%).
- non-clinical support: includes administration and cleaning (~8%).
- clinical support: includes physiotherapy, radiology, laboratory services, pharmacy, dietetics (~8%).
- consumables: includes drugs, fluids, nutrition, disposables (~25%).
- staff: medical, nursing, technical (~50%).

ICU costs are significantly higher in the first 24 h after admission and for patients with greater severity of illness as defined by the various scoring systems.

Co-trimoxazole. Synthetic **antibacterial drug** containing one part **trimethoprim** to five of the **sulfonamide** sulfamethoxazole. The drugs inhibit bacterial DNA replication and protein synthesis, respectively. Previously widely used to treat exacerbations of **COPD** and **urinary tract infections**; due to its toxicity and unfavourable side-effect profile, routine use is now restricted to prophylaxis and treatment of **pneumocystis pneumonia** and toxoplasmosis.

- Dosage: 960 mg–1.44 g orally/iv bd.
- Side effects: nausea, diarrhoea, erythema multiforme, pancreatitis, hepatic impairment, blood dyscrasias.

Cough. Reflex partially under voluntary control. A deep inspiration is followed by forceful expiration against a closed glottis which is suddenly opened to allow explosive exhalation. An intrathoracic pressure of up to 40 kPa may be produced, and the peak expiratory flow may exceed 900 l/min. Solid objects, liquids and mucus are thus expelled from the airways. Afferent pathways for coughing are from the mucosa of the **larynx**, trachea and large bronchi via the **vagus nerve** and medulla, and are stimulated by physical or chemical irritants.

- Factors associated with coughing during anaesthesia include:
  - insertion of a pharyngeal **airway** or **tracheal tube** if depth of anaesthesia is inadequate.
  - introduction of **inhalational anaesthetic agents** (e.g. **isoflurane**) at too high a concentration.
  - use of certain **iv anaesthetic agents**, e.g. **methohexital**.
  - presence/aspiration of blood, saliva or gastric contents.
  - increased airway reactivity, e.g. **asthma**, **COPD**, upper respiratory tract infection, **smoking**.

In ICU, cough may be produced by airway manoeuvres such as tracheobronchial suctioning, especially if the carina is stimulated. Persistent coughing may cause inadequate ventilation, and excessive intrathoracic pressures may reduce cardiac output (causing 'cough syncope' in non-anaesthetised patients). Deepening of anaesthesia, increased F_IO_2 and neuromuscular blockade may be required.

The reflex is protective, helping to prevent sputum retention and atelectasis. Postoperatively, it may be reduced by:

- impaired mechanical movement, e.g. due to pain, muscle weakness, neuromuscular blockade or disease, central and peripheral nervous disorders.
- depressed cough reflex, e.g. depressant drugs, central lesions.

Opioid analgesic drugs, e.g. **codeine**, are sometimes used to suppress cough, e.g. in malignant disease.

Cough-CPR. Maintenance of cerebral perfusion and consciousness during severe **arrhythmias** (e.g. **VF**) by repeated coughing. Each **cough** increases intrathoracic pressure and expels arterial blood from the thorax; each gasp draws in venous blood. Has been successful for up to 1–2 min pending availability of a defibrillator.

See also, Cardiopulmonary resuscitation

Coulomb. **Unit** of **charge**. One coulomb is the amount of charge passing any point in a circuit in 1 s when a **current** of 1 **ampere** is flowing. Equivalent to the charge carried by 6.242×10^{18} electrons.

[Charles Coulomb (1738–1806), French physicist]

COX, *see Cyclo-oxygenase*

CPAP, *see Continuous positive airway pressure*

CPD/CPD-A, Citrate–phosphate–dextrose/Citrate–phosphate–dextrose–adenine, *see Blood storage*

CPET/CPEX, *see Cardiopulmonary exercise testing*

CPR, *see Cardiopulmonary resuscitation*

CPX, *see Cardiopulmonary exercise testing*

CQC, *see Care Quality Commission*

Crack, *see Cocaine*

CRAMS scale, *see Circulation, respiration, abdomen, motor and speech scale*

Cranial nerves. Composed of 12 pairs, passing from the **brain** via openings in the **skull**. Convey motor and sensory fibres involved in somatic, parasympathetic (visceral) and special visceral (e.g. taste sensation) pathways:

- I: olfactory nerves (convey smell sensation from the nasal mucosa); pass through the cribriform plate of the ethmoid bone to the olfactory bulb.
- II: optic nerve (conveys visual sensation from the retina); passes through the optic canal and via the optic chiasma, tract and radiation to the visual cortex in the occipital lobe of the brain (*see Pupillary reflex*).
- III: oculomotor nerve (somatic motor fibres supply the extraocular muscles except superior oblique and lateral rectus; parasympathetic fibres supply the pupillary sphincter and ciliary muscles after synapsing in the ciliary ganglion). In the posterior fossa, the nerve passes from the upper midbrain between the cerebral peduncles and lies near the edge of the tentorium cerebelli (hence the early ipsilateral pupillary dilatation that occurs in acute rises of **ICP**, when the nerve is compressed against the edge of the tentorium [Hutchinson's pupil]). In the middle cranial fossa, it passes forwards on the lateral wall of the cavernous sinus as far as the supraorbital fissure. Before entering the fissure it divides into superior and inferior branches.
- IV: trochlear nerve (motor supply to the superior oblique muscle). Passes from the dorsum of the lower midbrain, then forwards in the lateral wall of the cavernous sinus to enter the supraorbital fissure.
- V: trigeminal nerve (sensory fibres supply the anterior dura, scalp and face, nasopharynx, nasal and oral cavities and air sinuses; motor fibres supply the muscles of mastication). The sensory nuclei are in the medulla, midbrain and pons. The nerve passes from the pons to the trigeminal ganglion lateral to the cavernous sinus, where it divides into ophthalmic, maxillary and mandibular divisions. The motor nucleus is in the pons; the root bypasses the ganglion to join the mandibular division. Branches:
  - ophthalmic division (V_1): branches (lacrimal, frontal and nasociliary nerves) pass via the superior orbital fissure. Associated with the ciliary ganglion.
  - maxillary division (V_2): passes via the foramen rotundum. Associated with the pterygopalatine ganglion. Branches (nasal, nasopalatine, palatine, pharyngeal, zygomatic, posterior superior alveolar and infraorbital nerves) are involved with lacrimation and sensory and sympathetic supply to the nose, nasopharynx, palate and orbit.
  - mandibular division (V_3): passes via the foramen ovale. Associated with the otic (parotid gland) and submandibular (submandibular and sublingual glands) ganglia. Sensory branches are the meningeal, buccal, auriculotemporal, inferior alveolar and lingual nerves. Somatic motor fibres supply the muscles of mastication (masseter, pterygoids, temporalis).

  (See Gasserian ganglion block; Mandibular nerve blocks; Maxillary nerve blocks; Ophthalmic nerve blocks.)
- VI: abducens nerve (motor supply to the lateral rectus). Passes from the lower pons through the cavernous sinus and supraorbital fissure. Often involved in injury to the skull.
- VII: facial nerve (mixed sensory and motor nerve): passes laterally from the lower pons through the internal acoustic meatus to the geniculate ganglion. Passes through the temporal bone to emerge through the stylomastoid foramen. Runs forward to the parotid gland. Branches:
  - motor supply to the muscles of facial expression: divides within the parotid gland into temporal, zygomatic, buccal, mandibular and cervical branches from above down. Branches also pass to the digastric, stylohyoid, auricular and occipital muscles.
  - greater petrosal nerve: passes from the geniculate ganglion to the pterygopalatine ganglion and fossa, to supply the lacrimal gland.
  - chorda tympani: leaves the facial nerve before it enters the stylomastoid foramen; conveys taste sensation from the anterior two-thirds of the **tongue** and parasympathetic fibres to the submandibular gland.
- VIII: vestibulocochlear nerve (special somatic sensory nerve): cochlear and vestibular components are involved in hearing and balance, respectively. The nerve is formed in the internal acoustic meatus and passes to nuclei in the floor of the fourth ventricle. Connects centrally with cranial nerves III, IV, VI, XI and descending pathways to the upper cervical cord.
- IX: glossopharyngeal nerve (conveys sensation from the pharynx, back of the tongue and tonsil, middle ear, **carotid sinus** and **carotid body**, taste from the posterior one-third of the tongue, and parasympathetic fibres to the parotid gland; provides motor supply to stylopharyngeus). Passes from the medulla through the jugular foramen, and then passes between the internal and external **carotid arteries** to the pharynx.
- X: **vagus nerve** (provides parasympathetic afferent and efferent supply to the heart, lungs and GIT as far as the splenic flexure, motor supply to the larynx, pharynx and palate, and conveys taste sensation from the valleculae and epiglottis, and sensation from the external ear canal and eardrum). Passes from the medulla via the jugular foramen.
- XI: accessory nerve (motor supply to the sternomastoid and trapezius muscles). Arises from the upper five cervical segments of the spinal cord, passing upwards through the foramen magnum to join the smaller cranial root. Leaves the skull through the jugular foramen; the cranial root joins the vagus (to the pharynx and larynx) and the spinal root passes to the sternomastoid.
- XII: hypoglossal nerve (motor supply to all muscles of the tongue except palatoglossus). Passes from the medulla, then through the hypoglossal canal behind the carotid sheath to the tongue.

- Cranial nerves may be assessed by testing:
  - I: ability to smell substances, e.g. peppermint, cloves. Irritant substances are avoided, because they may act via the Vth nerve.
  - II:
    - visual acuity using distant objects/charts.
    - visual fields, e.g. ability to discern peripheral movement while looking straight ahead. Size of blind spot.
    - appearance of optic discs.
    - pupillary reflex to light and accommodation.
  - III, IV, VI: full eye movements without diplopia. Results of specific lower **motor neurone** lesions:
    - III: eye displaced downwards and outwards, pupil dilated, ptosis.

- IV: downward gaze impaired; eyeball rotated inwards by inferior rectus when attempted.
- VI: lateral gaze impaired. Upper motor neurone lesions may cause impaired conjugate movements.

- V:
  - skin sensation in each division (*see Fig. 79;* **Gasserian ganglion block**), e.g.:
    - ophthalmic: forehead, corneal reflex (afferent arc V, efferent pathway VII).
    - maxillary: cheek next to nose.
    - mandibular: side of jaw.
  - ability to open/close jaw against resistance.
- VII:
  - facial expression: ability to show teeth, raise eyebrows, screw up eyes against resistance, blow out cheeks. Movement in the upper part of the face is preserved in upper motor neurone lesions, and lost in lower motor neurone lesions.
  - taste sensation of the anterior tongue, e.g. to salt, sugar, citric acid.
- VIII.
  - ability to hear, e.g. fingers rubbing next to the ear.
  - using a tuning fork: air conduction is lost in middle ear disease, with preservation of bone conduction (Rinne's test). Both are impaired in nerve damage. If the tuning fork is placed on the forehead, the sound is heard best on the affected side in middle ear disease, on the unaffected side in nerve disease (Weber's test).
- IX, X:
  - taste sensation of the posterior tongue.
  - soft palate elevation is equal on both sides.
  - **gag reflex**.
  - voice and phonation.
- XI: ability to raise shoulders, and rotate head to the side, against resistance.
- XII: protrusion of tongue in the midline (to the affected side if abnormal). Absence of wasting and ability to move from side to side.

[Sir Jonathan Hutchinson (1828–1913), English surgeon; Friedrich Rinne (1819–1868) and Friedrich Weber (1832–1891), German otologists]

'Crash induction', *see Induction, rapid sequence*

C-reactive protein (CRP). Plasma protein, so called because it reacts with the C polysaccharide of pneumococci. Complexes formed when CRP binds to saccharides of micro-organisms activate the classical **complement** pathway and stimulate cell-mediated cytotoxicity. Part of the **acute-phase response**, it is synthesised in the liver in response to the **cytokine** interleukin-6. Plasma levels are normally under 10 mg/l but increase within 6–10 h of tissue damage. Has therefore been used to aid diagnosis of acute inflammation (e.g. infection) and to monitor the response to treatment. Although in the ICU, because of underlying critical illness, 'resting' plasma levels may not lie within the 'normal' <10 mg/l range (e.g. may exceed 200 mg/l), a 25% change from the previous day's value may still be used to indicate acute changes in inflammatory status.

Póvoa P (2002). Intensive Care Med; 28: 235–43

Creatinine. Basic compound formed mainly in skeletal **muscle** from phosphorylcreatine. The latter is formed from **ATP** and creatine, and is a source of ATP during exercise. Creatinine production remains fairly constant, hence the value of plasma creatinine measurement as a reflection of renal function (cf. urea, whose production varies with the amount of protein breakdown occurring). Normal value: 60–130 μmol/l; serial values are more useful indicators of renal function than single measurements. As **GFR** decreases, creatinine levels rise slowly up to about 200 μmol/l (GFR below 40 ml/min), rising greatly thereafter for small decreases of GFR. Thus measurement is less useful at high values, and values above 200 μmol/l represent severe renal impairment.

See also, Creatinine clearance

Creatinine clearance. Clearance of **creatinine**, used as an approximation for **GFR**. Although some creatinine is secreted by renal tubules, this source of error tends to be cancelled out by the over-measurement of plasma creatinine at low levels. Commonly estimated, because creatinine is easily measured. Usually averaged over 24 h to reduce error from inaccurate urine volume measurement. Normal value: 90–130 ml/min.

Cremophor EL. Polyoxyethylated castor oil, formed from ethylene oxide and castor oil. Used as an emulsifying agent in preparations of certain drugs. Implicated in causing **adverse drug reactions**, sometimes severe, after iv injection. Has led to the withdrawal of iv induction agents (e.g. **Althesin**, **propanidid** and the original formulation of **propofol**), although injectable preparations of other drugs may still contain it (e.g. ciclosporin, vitamin K).

CREST syndrome, *see Systemic sclerosis*

Creutzfeldt–Jakob disease (CJD). Group of transmissible human encephalopathies caused by infectious proteins known as prions. Infection results in the formation of an abnormal form of a cellular membrane protein (prion-related protein) that causes destruction of neuronal tissue and overgrowth of glial cells.

- Classified thus:
  - sporadic (sCJD): cause is unknown, accounts for 85% of cases. Occurs in the elderly; incidence is 1 per million population/year. Dementia is prominent and death occurs within 6 months. Definitive diagnosis requires brain biopsy.
  - familial: caused by prion protein gene mutations, accounts for ≤10% of cases
  - acquired:
    - iatrogenic: identical to sCJD but occurs following implantation of prion protein-infected tissue (e.g. dura mater and corneal grafts) or from administration of human growth hormone taken from affected cadavers. Kuru, a prion disease caused by ingestion of infected neural tissue during cannibalism, continues to be seen in the Fore tribe of Papua New Guinea despite the practice being outlawed in 1947.
    - variant (vCJD): first described in 1996 in young people. Due to ingestion of beef from cattle affected by bovine spongiform encephalopathy (BSE); the prion causing vCJD is identical to that present in BSE. sCJD is caused by a different prion. 228 cases were reported in the UK between 1990 and 2011, with the peak incidence in 2000. Clinical features of vCJD include early psychiatric changes, sensory disturbances, ataxia, stimulus-sensitive myoclonus, dystonia and dementia. Diagnosis is supported by MRI findings and confirmed by tonsillar biopsy.

The incubation period of prion diseases is variable and may be >40 years with Kuru, but is considerably shorter with other forms (e.g. vCJD).

- Anaesthetic implications:
  - high exposure rate of the population to BSE-infected beef may result in an epidemic of vCJD, although this is now considered unlikely given the decline in the number of cases since 2003.
  - conventional decontamination of instruments does not destroy the prion protein; thus transmission may occur via contaminated surgical and anaesthetic instruments. Tissues with high prion concentrations (e.g. brain, spinal cord, tonsils, lymph nodes and lower GIT) present greater risk. Disposable instruments are available for high-risk cases and care must be taken to use disposable or sheathed laryngoscope blades in these cases.
  - vCJD has been transmitted by **blood transfusion** and, since 1998, all donated blood has been leukodepleted, which reduces prion infectivity by 60%–70%. Since 1999, all non-cellular blood products except fresh frozen plasma and cryoprecipitate are sourced from the USA and Germany. UK donors are banned from giving blood if they have received a transfusion since 1980. A filter that removes prion protein is undergoing trials.

[Hans G Creutzfeldt (1885–1964), German psychiatrist; Alfons M Jakob (1884–1931), German neurologist. Kuru, derived from Fore word *kuria*—to shake]
Farling P, Smith G (2003). Anaesthesia; 58: 627–9

Cricoid pressure (Sellick's manoeuvre). Digital pressure against the cricoid cartilage of the **larynx**, pushing it backwards. The **oesophagus** is thus compressed between the posterior aspect of the cricoid and the **vertebrae** behind. The cricoid cartilage is used because it forms the only complete ring of the larynx and trachea. Used to prevent passive regurgitation of gastric and oesophageal contents (e.g. during **induction of anaesthesia**) although no randomised controlled trials concerning its necessity, safety or effectiveness have been conducted.

The cricoid cartilage is identified level with C6, and the index finger is placed against the cartilage in the midline, with the thumb and middle finger on either side. Moderate pressure may be applied before loss of consciousness, and firmer pressure maintained until the **cuff** of the tracheal tube is inflated.

Estimates of the force required vary from 20 N to over 40 N (approximately corresponding to a mass of 2 kg to over 4 kg), most recent guidance suggesting 20–30 N as optimal. It must be released during active vomiting, to reduce risk of oesophageal rupture. Incorrectly performed cricoid pressure may hinder laryngoscopy either by distorting the laryngeal anatomy or flexing the neck; the latter may be prevented by the assistant's second hand being placed behind the patient's neck. Cricoid pressure may also hinder placement of a **SAD**.

[Brian A Sellick (1918–1996), London anaesthetist]
Salem MR, Khorasani A, Zeidan A, Crystal GJ (2017). Anesthesiol; 126: 738–52
See also, Induction, rapid sequence

Cricothyroidotomy (Cricothyrotomy). Puncture or incision of the cricothyroid membrane (passes between the thyroid cartilage above and the cricoid cartilage below) of the **larynx**. Performed to allow ventilation in **airway obstruction**, e.g. in a 'can't intubate can't oxygenate' (CICO) situation.

Scalpel cricothyroidotomy is recommended by the Difficult Airway Society as the technique of choice in the emergency setting. The technique depends on whether the cricothyroid membrane is palpable or not:

- palpable cricothyroid membrane:
  - stabilise the larynx using the left hand and with the left index finger identify the cricothyroid membrane.
  - using a scalpel in the right hand, make a transverse incision through the skin and cricothyroid membrane.
  - rotate the scalpel through 90 degrees so that the sharp edge points caudally. Swap hands and with the right hand, slide the tip of a bougie down the side of the scalpel into the trachea.
  - remove the scalpel and 'railroad' a 6-mm cuffed tracheal tube into the trachea. Remove the bougie and confirm correct tube placement using **capnography**.
- impalpable cricothyroid membrane (e.g. in the obese):
  - attempt to identify laryngeal anatomy with the right hand. Ultrasound may be useful if immediately available.
  - make a 8–10 cm vertical midline incision.
  - use blunt dissection with both hands to separate the tissues and identify the cricothyroid membrane.
  - proceed with the scalpel method as described earlier.

Although cannula techniques (narrow- or wide-bore introduced using the **Seldinger technique**) have been used, they are associated with higher rates of misplacement and complications including **barotrauma**.

Cricothyroid puncture is also performed for transtracheal injection of **lidocaine**, during awake intubation. The **minitracheotomy** device may also be useful for sputum aspiration.
Frerk C, Mitchell VS, McNarry AF, et al (2015). Br J Anaesth; 6: 827–48

Crile, George Washington (1864–1943). Eminent US surgeon, a major contributor to regional anaesthesia. Described the combination of opioids, regional block and general anaesthesia, calling the concept anociassociation (led to the concept of **balanced anaesthesia**). Also investigated the pathogenesis and treatment of **shock**, and described a pneumatic garment for its treatment in 1903.
Tetzlaff JE, Lautsenheiser F, Estafanous FG (2005). Reg Anesth Pain Med; 29: 600–5

Crisis resource management. Strategy for coping with **critical incidents**, developed initially in the airline industry (as Cockpit and then Crew resource management) as a means of dealing effectively with crises and preventing them from evolving into disasters. Has since been adapted to other high-risk industries and also to anaesthesia. Consists of a number of components:

- being aware of the immediate and wider environment, e.g. knowing what equipment and staff are available; manipulating the environment as required (e.g. turning on the light in a dark operating theatre).
- use of all available resources and allocating them appropriately, e.g. using cognitive aids (e.g. printed algorithms); delegating personnel according to their skills.
- planning and anticipation, e.g. rehearsing drills; mobilising resources when likely to be needed rather

than when they are actually needed; calling for help early.
- effective leadership.
- effective communication, including specific and directed requests/orders (and receiving confirmation that they have been understood correctly).

Commonly forms part of training programmes involving **simulators** but can be incorporated into many **risk management** programmes.

Gaba DM (2010). Br J Anaesth; 105: 3–6

Critical care. System designed to look after seriously ill patients, with levels of care allocated according to clinical need (and not to staffing levels or location). Four levels are recognised in the UK:
- level 0: patients whose needs can be met by normal ward care in an acute hospital, e.g. those requiring oral or iv bolus medication or patient-controlled analgesia. Observations required less frequently than 4 h.
- level 1: patients recently discharged from a higher level of care, in need of additional and more frequent monitoring and clinical advice, or requiring critical care **outreach** services.
- level 2: patients requiring single organ monitoring or support (e.g. nasal **CPAP**), preoperative optimisation or extended postoperative care, or those with major uncorrected physiological abnormalities (e.g. increased respiratory rate, tachycardia, hypotension, decreased **Glasgow coma scale** score) and at risk of deterioration.
- level 3: patients requiring advanced respiratory monitoring and support, e.g. **IPPV** (but excluding electively IPPV for <24 h postoperatively), those requiring monitoring and support of two or more organ systems, or those with chronic impairment of one or more organ systems who require support for an acute reversible failure of another organ system (e.g. severe ischaemic heart disease and major perioperative haemorrhage).

Thus the term encompasses care provided on both **ICUs** and **HDUs**.

***Critical Care Medicine*.** Monthly journal of the **Society of Critical Care Medicine**. First published in 1972.

Critical damping, *see Damping*

Critical flicker-fusion test, *see Recovery testing*

Critical illness polyneuropathy/myopathy. Major cause of ICU acquired weakness (ICUAW). Occurs in up to 65% of patients receiving mechanical ventilation >5 days. Associated with prolonged ventilation and ICU/hospital stays, and increased hospital mortality.
- Comprises:
    - critical illness polyneuropathy: main finding is axonal degeneration. Mechanisms include microvascular changes in endoneurium caused by **sepsis**, neural oedema reducing energy delivery to nerves, mitochondrial dysfunction and sodium channelopathy.
    - critical illness myopathy: occurs early and is due to muscle atrophy resulting from increased breakdown and decreased synthesis of muscle proteins. Mechanisms include inflammation, immobilisation, nutritional deficit and denervation.

Often the above coexist (critical illness neuromyopathy).
- Risk factors:
    - increased age and severity of illness.
    - presence of sepsis, bacteraemia and **MODS**.
    - **hyperglycaemia**.
    - use of **corticosteroids** and non-depolarising **neuromuscular blocking drugs** have been implicated but may not be independent risk factors.
    - long duration of bed rest and prolonged mechanical ventilation.
- Clinical signs:
    - symmetrical limb weakness, especially affecting proximal muscles.
    - sensory symptoms may be present.
    - reflexes are usually reduced.
    - respiratory muscle weakness and failure to wean from ventilation.

Diagnosis is largely clinical but supported by nerve conduction studies and electromyography. Treatment of ICUAW is largely supportive. Preventive measures include aggressive treatment of sepsis, avoiding hyperglycaemia, reducing duration of immobilisation (e.g. by stopping sedation as soon as possible), early **physiotherapy** and providing early and sufficient nutrition.

The majority of patients recover within months, reaching a plateau at 1 year; patients with severe **ALI** may have significantly impaired function at 5 years.

Hermans G, Van den Berghe G (2015). Crit Care; 19: 274–83

Critical incidents. Term derived from the airline industry; usually defined as any event that results in actual harm, or would do so if not actively managed.

In the NHS, the term now preferred is 'serious incidents', defined as 'events in healthcare where the potential for learning is so great, or the consequences to patients, families and carers, staff or organisations are so significant, that they warrant using additional resources to mount a comprehensive response'—thus moving away from actual or potential harm alone, to include the (in)ability to provide safe healthcare at an organisational or health system level. Although not specifying a finite list of events that might trigger the declaration of a 'serious incident', they include:
- unexpected/avoidable death(s) or injury resulting in serious harm (or treatment to avoid it).
- actual or alleged abuse.
- **Never Events.**
- any major disruption to an organisation/healthcare system (including loss of public confidence).

Critical/serious incident reporting schemes are a central part of **risk management** and a ready topic for **audit**, and have become a useful tool in **quality assurance/improvement**. A problem common to reporting schemes is the underreporting of incidents, although this may be improved by education and guarantees of anonymity and lack of blame. In addition, they may not always suggest a means of improving care.

Critical/serious incidents require appropriate investigation and analysis, with/without formation of a multidisciplinary panel (which may be external to the 'host' organisation) depending on the healthcare system and severity of the incident. The aim of the investigation is to identify contributory factors and the root causes that need addressing to prevent repeat/similar incidents.
- Terms used in incident reporting schemes include:
    - latent errors: within the 'system', e.g. having two drugs presented in very similar ampoules stored next to each other.

- active errors: produce immediate effects.
- human errors: those involving direct human contribution, e.g. the giving of the incorrect drug; may be caused by:
  - slips: the action is unintended, e.g. picking up the wrong syringe.
  - lapses: the action is intended but the error is related to memory, e.g. forgetting the patient is allergic to penicillin.
  - violations: e.g. not checking the drug with another person when that is the policy of the department.

  In addition, human errors may be classified as knowledge-based, rule-based or skill-based.

In the UK, the **National Patient Safety Agency** was established in 2001 to coordinate national reporting of critical incidents and dissemination of lessons learned from them. The new NHS Serious Incident Framework was introduced in 2010 (revised 2015) and sets out the procedure for the identification, reporting and management of serious incidents.
See also, Anaesthetists' non-technical skills; Crisis resource management

Critical pressure. Pressure required to liquefy a **vapour** at its **critical temperature**. Examples:
- O_2: 50 bar.
- N_2O: 72 bar.
- CO_2: 73 bar.

Critical temperature. Temperature above which a **vapour** cannot be liquefied by any amount of pressure. Above this temperature, the substance is a gas; below it, the substance is a vapour. Examples:
- O_2: −118°C.
- N_2O: 36.5°C.
- CO_2: 31°C.

See also, Isotherms; Pseudocritical temperature

Critical velocity. Velocity above which laminar **flow** in a tube becomes turbulent.

Proportional to

$$\frac{\textbf{viscosity}\text{ of fluid}}{\textbf{density}\text{ of fluid} \times \text{radius of tube}}$$

thus refers to a specific fluid within a tube of specific radius.

At critical velocity, **Reynolds' number** is greater than 2000.

Crohn's disease, *see Inflammatory bowel disease*

Cromoglicate (Cromoglycate), *see Sodium cromoglicate*

Cross-matching, *see Blood compatibility testing*

Croup (Laryngotracheobronchitis). Upper respiratory obstruction and **stridor** in children due to viral infection affecting the larynx, trachea and bronchi; most commonly due to parainfluenza (especially type I), respiratory syncytial and influenza viruses. The typical barking 'croupy' cough, the child's age (usually 6 months–2 years) and the gradual onset help distinguish it from **epiglottitis,** which is usually of more acute onset, affects children of 2–5 years and is associated with greater systemic illness.

Treatment is with **corticosteroids**; a single dose of **dexamethasone** (0.15 mg/kg to a maximum of 10 mg) iv, im or orally within 24 hours of onset reduces the severity. Nebulised **adrenaline** may be helpful: racemic solution (equal amounts of *d*- and *l*-isomers) is widely used in the USA: 0.5 ml of 2.25% solution is diluted to 4 ml in saline. In the UK (0.4 ml) 400 μg/kg of the generally available non-racemic preparation (comprising mostly the more active *l*-isomer) has been used, up to a maximum of 5 ml (5 mg). It may be repeated after 30 min if required. ECG monitoring should be instituted and therapy stopped if the heart rate exceeds 180 beats/min. Mucosal swelling may recur after treatment so careful monitoring is required. **Helium**/oxygen mixtures may provide short-term improvement. Tracheal intubation and mechanical ventilation may be required.

Bjornson CL, Johnson DW (2008). Lancet; 371: 329–39

CRP, *see C-reactive protein*

CRPS, *see Complex regional pain syndromes*

Crush syndrome. Acute oliguric **renal failure** following **trauma**, usually involving impaired perfusion of a limb. May occur in direct trauma and in comatose patients who lie on a limb for a prolonged period. Muscle swelling and necrosis lead to release of myoglobin with resultant **myoglobinuria**. Renal impairment is compounded by any associated **hypotension** and **dehydration.** Potassium is also released from the damaged muscle; severe **hyperkalaemia** may be fatal unless **dialysis** is instituted. **Hyperphosphataemia** and **hypocalcaemia** also occur.

Gonzalez D (2005). Crit Care Med; 33: S34–41

Cryoanalgesia. Use of extreme cold to damage peripheral nerves and provide pain relief lasting up to several months. Causes axonal degeneration without epineurial or perineurial damage, allowing slow regeneration of the axon without neuritis or neuroma formation. Has been used in chronic **pain management**, and perioperatively to provide prolonged **postoperative analgesia**, e.g. applied to intercostal nerves in **thoracic surgery**.
See also, Cryoprobe; Refrigeration anaesthesia

Cryoprecipitate, *see Blood products*

Cryoprobe. Instrument used to freeze tissues. Compressed gas (e.g. CO_2 or N_2O) is passed through a narrow tube and allowed to expand suddenly at its tip. Work done by the gas as it expands results in a temperature drop (**Joule–Thomson effect**; an example of an **adiabatic change**) to as low as −70°C in the metal sheath of the probe. Used to destroy superficial lesions, e.g. in gynaecology and dermatology; also used in ophthalmology and to provide **cryoanalgesia**.

Crystalloid. Substance that, in solution, may pass through a semipermeable membrane (cf. **colloid**). **Saline solutions, dextrose solutions** and **Hartmann's solution** are commonly used clinically as **iv fluids.**
See also, Colloid/crystalloid controversy

CSE, *see Combined spinal–epidural anaesthesia*

CSF, *see Cerebrospinal fluid*

CSF filtration. Therapeutic removal of cellular and soluble components known to be involved in the pathophysiology of certain diseases. First used in 1991 in severe

Guillain–Barré syndrome unresponsive to other therapies. CSF is removed through an intrathecal catheter into a closed system via a syringe and pump and then reinjected through a filter with a pore size of 0.2 µm. Is now used in some cases of acute and chronic inflammatory demyelinating polyneuropathies, multiple sclerosis, amyotrophic lateral sclerosis and bacterial meningitis.

CSM, *see Committee on Safety of Medicines*

CT scanning, *see Computed (axial) tomography*

CTZ, *see Chemoreceptor trigger zone*

Cuffs, of tracheal tubes. Seal the trachea to avoid gas leakage and contamination from above, e.g. blood, gastric contents. Popularised by **Waters** and **Guedel** in the 1920s. Usually inflated with air following tracheal intubation, until the audible gas leak is just eliminated. The degree of distension of a pilot balloon, or measurement of cuff pressure, indicates the extent of cuff inflation.

- Main problems are related to pressure exerted by the cuff on the tracheal walls causing mucosal ischaemia:
  - may occur if capillary pressure is exceeded (i.e., greater than about 25 mmHg). Cuff pressures of up to 60 mmHg have been measured with high-volume low-pressure cuffs, and up to 200 mmHg with low-volume high-pressure cuffs (*see Laplace's law*). The former are therefore preferable, especially for prolonged intubation, e.g. in ICU. Handheld cuff inflators may incorporate pressure gauges to indicate cuff pressure during inflation.
  - cuff pressure may increase during anaesthesia due to increased temperature or diffusion of **N_2O** into the cuff. Saline/N_2O mixtures have been used for cuff inflation, to avoid the latter. Monitoring of cuff pressure, or intermittent deflation and inflation, has been suggested during long operations and in ICU.
  - mucosal inflammation may lead to ulcer formation over cartilaginous rings; infection, tracheal dilatation and erosion of tracheal walls may follow. Tracheal stenosis may occur after extubation.
  - damage is worst after prolonged use, although some degree of ciliary damage may occur within a few hours of inflation.
  - damage is worse if wrinkles are formed by the cuff.

Similar problems may occur with **tracheostomy** tubes. Recurrent **laryngeal nerve** injury may be caused by a cuff inflated just below the vocal cords. Cuff placement should be 1.5–2 cm below the cords. Trauma may be caused if tracheal extubation is performed without prior deflation of the cuff. Uncuffed tracheal tubes are traditionally used for **paediatric anaesthesia**, although cuffed tubes are increasingly being used.

Similar considerations apply to bronchial cuffs of **endobronchial tubes**; bronchial rupture may follow excessive inflation.

Longitudinal wrinkles in the cuff may allow passage of secretions from the pharynx into the tracheobronchial tree; new cuffs have thus been designed in which wrinkles do not form, thereby reducing the risk of aspiration pneumonia in patients requiring chronic ventilatory support.

Filling the cuff with **lidocaine** (4%–10%) has been reported to reduce coughing on extubation.

See also, Tracheal tubes

Cuirass ventilator, *see Intermittent negative pressure ventilation*

Curare. Dried plant extract used by South American Indians as arrow poison, containing **tubocurarine** and other alkaloids. Described in Raleigh's writings in 1596. Used experimentally by **Waterton** and **Bernard**, among others, from the early/mid-1800s onwards. Used to treat **tetanus** and in psychiatric convulsive therapy. First used in anaesthesia by **Lawen** in 1912, but remained in short supply for many years. Its use became more widespread after **Griffith**'s famous description in 1942; his supply was brought back from Ecuador by Gill.

[Sir Walter Raleigh (1552–1618), English explorer; Richard Cochran Gill (1901–1958), US explorer]

CURB-65 score. Scoring system for stratification of patients with community-acquired **chest infection**. Consists of five criteria, scoring one point for each if present.

- confusion.
- urea >7 mmol/l.
- respiratory rate >30 breaths/min
- BP <90 mmHg systolic or 60 mmHg diastolic
- age >65 years.

A score of 0 predicts a 30-day mortality rate of 0.6%; this rises to 17% with a score of 3, and 57% with a score of 5.

Has also been applied to infection of any type, a score of 0–1 associated with <5% mortality; 2–3 with <10% mortality; and 4–5 with 15%–30% mortality.

Loke YK, Kwok CS, Niruban A, Myint PK (2010). Thorax; 65: 884–90

Curling ulcers. Peptic ulcers occurring after severe **burns**. Most common in children.

[Thomas Curling (1811–1888), English surgeon]

Current. Flow of electrical **charge**. Direct current describes flow of charge continuously in one direction, e.g. from a battery. Direction of flow alternates in an alternating current, e.g. mains power supply. SI **unit** is the **ampere**.

Current density. Current per unit area. Important in **electrocution and electrical burns** as heat production is directly proportional to current density. Thus there is no tissue damage at the site of a **diathermy** plate, but intense heat at the site of the probe or forceps, where area of contact is very small. Similarly, a small current delivered directly to the heart over a very small area may produce the same current density as a much larger current delivered to the whole body, and may therefore be as dangerous (microshock).

Current-operated earth-leakage circuit breaker (COELCB). Device containing equally sized coils of live and neutral wires, used in electrical circuits to prevent **electrocution**. The current in each wire induces magnetic flux equal and opposite to that induced by the other, as long as each wire carries the same current. Imbalance between the two currents, e.g. due to leakage of current to earth, results in unequal magnetic fluxes that do not cancel each other out. Resultant magnetic flux induces current in a third coil, causing rapid (within 5 ms) breakage of the circuit via a solenoid.

Cushing, Harvey Williams (1869–1939). US neurosurgeon, professor of surgery at Harvard University. A pioneer in

neurosurgery, he developed many techniques, including the use of **diathermy**, and clips for cerebral vessels. Advocated **record-keeping** and **monitoring** during anaesthesia, and investigated many aspects of neurophysiology and neuropathology, several of which bear his name. Won the Pulitzer Prize for his biography of Osler, and published many books and articles.
[Joseph Pulitzer (1847–1911), Hungarian-born US journalist; Sir William Osler (1849–1919), Canadian-born US and English physician]

Cushing's disease. **Cushing's syndrome** caused by ACTH-secreting adenoma of the pituitary gland. Incidence is 2–4 per million population; 80% occur in women.
- Treatment:
    - pituitary surgery (effective in up to 80% of cases).
    - radiotherapy to the pituitary gland.
    - bilateral adrenalectomy in resistant cases (carries the risk of Nelson's syndrome: hyperpigmentation owing to secretion of melanocyte-stimulating hormone).
    - medical treatment: metyrapone inhibits 11β-hydroxylase and reduces cortisol production. May be used before surgery, to improve the patient's condition, or after irradiation.

[Don H Nelson (1925–2009), US endocrinologist]
Smith M, Hirsch NP (2000). Br J Anaesth; 85: 3–14

Cushing's reflex. Hypertension with compensatory bradycardia occurring with acutely raised **ICP**. Due to the effect of local **hypoxia** and **hypercapnia** on the **vasomotor centre** as **cerebral perfusion pressure** falls.
Fodstad H, Kelly PJ, Buchfelder M (2006). Neurosurgery; 59: 1132–7/8
See also, Cushing, Harvey Williams

Cushing's syndrome. Clinical syndrome resulting from excessive endogenous or exogenous corticosteroid levels.
- Features:
    - central obesity, i.e., limbs are spared. 'Buffalo hump' of fat behind the neck.
    - 'moon face', greasy skin, acne, hirsutism.
    - skin atrophy and poor wound healing, with increased susceptibility to infection.
    - abdominal striae.
    - osteoporosis.
    - proximal muscle weakness.
    - psychiatric disturbances.
    - **hypertension**.
    - **hypernatraemia** and **hypokalaemia**.
    - **diabetes mellitus**.
- Caused by:
    - **Cushing's disease** (the most common non-iatrogenic cause).
    - adrenal tumours.
    - other hormone-secreting tumours, e.g. **bronchial carcinoma** secreting **ACTH**.
    - **corticosteroid** therapy.
- Investigation:
    - raised urinary cortisol and 17-oxogenic corticosteroids (cortisol precursors).
    - raised plasma cortisol levels; normally low at midnight, and low the morning after dexamethasone administration.
    - ACTH levels are raised in Cushing's disease and ACTH-secreting tumours. Metyrapone decreases adrenal cortisol production, causing ACTH to increase: this does not occur with adrenal tumours or ACTH-secreting tumours, but does occur in Cushing's disease. The ACTH increase is measured directly, or cortisol precursors (17-oxogenic corticosteroids) are measured in the urine.

Hypertension and **cardiac failure**, hypernatraemia, hypokalaemia and diabetes, although not always present, may cause problems during anaesthesia. Steroid cover is required, as in corticosteroid therapy. Fragile skin and veins may be easily damaged. Postoperative fluid and electrolyte balance is particularly important.
Loriaux DL (2017). New Engl J Med; 376: 1451–9
See also, Cushing, Harvey Williams

Cushing's ulcers. Peptic ulcers occurring after **head injury**, associated with increased gastric acid secretion.
See also, Cushing, Harvey Williams

Cut-off effect. Reduced anaesthetic potency of larger molecules in a homologous series, despite increasing lipid solubility.
See also, Anaesthesia, mechanism of

CVA, Cerebrovascular accident, *see Stroke*

CVVH, Continuous venovenous haemofiltration, *see Haemofiltration*

CVVHD, Continuous venovenous haemodiafiltration, *see Haemodiafiltration*

Cyanide poisoning. May result from industrial accidents, self-administration, **smoke inhalation**, prolonged use of **sodium nitroprusside** or use as a **chemical weapon**. Absorption may occur via stomach, skin and lungs (the latter may be rapidly fatal). Causes inhibition of the **cytochrome oxidase system** and other **enzymes**, interrupting cellular respiration. Tissues are thus unable to utilise delivered O_2 (histotoxic **hypoxia**). Cyanide is slowly converted to thiocyanate in the liver by the enzyme rhodanese; a small amount binds to methaemoglobin and a small amount to hydroxocobalamin.
- Features:
    - non-specific: dizziness, headache, confusion. Apnoea may follow initial tachypnoea.
    - reduced **arteriovenous O_2 difference**, due to reduced uptake of O_2 by tissues. Metabolic **acidosis** with increased **lactate** results from tissue hypoxia.
    - **convulsions** and cardiorespiratory collapse may occur.
    - chronic poisoning causes **peripheral neuropathy**, ataxia and optic atrophy.

Measurement of plasma levels is technically difficult and may be unreliable unless performed rapidly.
- Treatment:
    - general measures as for **poisoning and overdoses**. **O_2 therapy** is particularly important. Staff must avoid self-contamination.
    - **gastric lavage** may be helpful.
    - dicobalt edetate 300 mg iv over 1 min, repeated if necessary. Combines with cyanide to form inert compounds. May itself cause vomiting, hypertension and tachycardia; reservation for severe cases has been suggested. Given with 50% glucose (50 ml per dose).
    - sodium thiosulfate 50%, 25 ml iv over 10 min. Converts cyanide to thiocyanate. Used together with:

- sodium nitrite 3%, 10 ml iv over 3 min. Converts haemoglobin to methaemoglobin, which binds cyanide. More efficacious than inhaled amyl nitrite. Methaemoglobin together with carboxyhaemoglobin if present should not exceed 40% total haemoglobin.
- hydroxocobalamin 70 mg/kg iv over 20 min. Forms cyanocobalamin with cyanide. Has been used in cyanide poisoning and to reduce nitroprusside toxicity, but not widely used in the UK.

MacLennan L, Moiemen N (2015). Burns; 41: 18–24

Cyanosis. Blue discoloration of tissues due to increased concentration of reduced **haemoglobin** in the blood. Clinically detectable at less than 50 g/l reduced haemoglobin, although this value is often quoted as the minimum. Peripheral cyanosis, e.g. of fingernails, may result from impaired peripheral perfusion. Central cyanosis, typically affecting the tongue, may result from heart or lung disease, including right-to-left shunts. **Methaemoglobinaemia** and **sulfhaemoglobinaemia** may also cause bluish discoloration. Cyanosis may be further mimicked by grey or blue discoloration of skin caused by heavy metals (e.g. iron, gold and lead) or drugs (e.g. amiodarone and phenothiazines).

Cyclic AMP, *see Adenosine monophosphate, cyclic*

Cycling of ventilators, *see Ventilators*

Cyclizine hydrochloride/tartrate/lactate. **Antiemetic drug**, with antihistamine and anticholinergic actions. Available alone or combined with **opioid analgesic drugs** and ergotamine. **Half-life** is about 8 h.
- Dosage: 50 mg orally/im/iv qds.
- Side effects include drowsiness, blurred vision, movement disorders/oculogyric crisis/paralysis. Painful if given iv/im. Rapid injection may cause tachycardia.

Cyclodextrins. Cyclic oligosaccharides, studied for their ability to encapsulate lipophilic molecules. **Sugammadex** is a cyclodextrin with optimal affinity for **rocuronium**, and has been shown to reverse the neuromuscular blockade produced by the latter, even if given within a few minutes of paralysis. Cyclodextrins have also been studied as vehicles for drugs (e.g. **propofol**) in an attempt to avoid the use of emulsifiers and other carriers.

Cyclo-oxygenase (COX). **Enzyme** acting on **arachidonic acid** to produce prostaglandin H_2, from which other **prostaglandins, prostacyclin** and **thromboxanes** are formed. Exists in two forms:
- COX-1 ('constitutive'): present in many tissues and responsible for the maintenance of normal physiological functions of prostaglandins, e.g. **renal blood flow**, gastric mucosal protection.
- COX-2 ('inducible'): found in few resting cells (including brain, kidney, gravid uterus); induced during inflammation.

Most **NSAIDs** inhibit COX-1 more than (e.g. **aspirin, indometacin, naproxen, piroxicam**) or the same as (e.g. **ibuprofen, diclofenac**) COX-2. NSAIDs that preferentially inhibit COX-2 (e.g. **parecoxib**, celecoxib) have been developed in an attempt to minimise their side effects (e.g. upper GI bleeding). Selective COX-2 inhibitors are associated with a slight increased risk of MI and stroke (rofecoxib was withdrawn in 2004 for this reason). The mechanism is thought to be unequal inhibition of prostacyclin and thromboxane synthesis.

Kam P (2000). Anaesthesia; 55: 442–9

Cyclophosphamide. **Immunosuppressive** and **cytotoxic drug** used in organ **transplantation** (especially **bone marrow transplantation**), **autoimmune disease** and **malignancy**. An alkylating agent, it binds to DNA and is toxic to both resting and dividing cells. Exerts its greatest effect on B lymphocytes, thus inhibiting antibody production. Also suppresses delayed hypersensitivity reactions. **Bioavailability** is 90% after oral dosage, with peak levels at 1 h. Metabolised in the liver with a **half-life** of 6 h.
- Dosage: 100–300 mg/day orally or 80–300 mg/m²/day iv.
- Side effects: nausea, vomiting, hair loss, dose-related cardiac toxicity, haemorrhagic cystitis (caused by a metabolite, acrolein), increased risk of infection and malignancy. Levels are increased by concurrent administration of allopurinol and cimetidine. May prolong **suxamethonium**'s duration of action by decreasing **cholinesterase** activity.

Cyclopropane $(CH_2)_3$. **Inhalational anaesthetic agent**, first used in the early 1930s and used up until the mid/late 1980s. Its main advantages were very rapid onset of anaesthesia (blood/gas **partition coefficient** 0.45) and maintenance of BP and cardiac output (largely due to sympathetic activity) despite direct myocardial depression. Extremely flammable (explosive in O_2 at 2.5%–60% and in air at 2.5%–10%), it also caused marked respiratory depression and reduced renal and hepatic blood flow. Commonly used for paediatric induction using 50% in O_2 (**MAC** of 9.2%). Supplied in orange size B **cylinders** (containing 180 l, partly as liquid) at a pressure of 5 bar.

Cycloserine. **Antibacterial** and **antituberculous drug**, used in **TB** resistant to first-line drugs. Contraindicated in renal impairment, epilepsy and porphyria.
- Dosage: 250–500 mg orally bd.
- Side effects: rash, headache, dizziness, seizures, psychological changes, hepatic impairment.

Cyclosporin, *see Ciclosporin*

Cylinders. Traditionally made of molybdenum or chromium steel; newer cylinders are made of aluminium alloy and are much lighter. Composite cylinders usually comprise a metal liner to prevent leakage of gas, with a carbon or glass fibre overwrap to provide extra strength.

Provide medical gases either directly to an output (e.g. attached to an **anaesthetic machine**) or from a bank of cylinders (manifold) via pipelines.
- The valve block screws into the open end of the cylinder and has the following features:
  - marked with:
    - serial number.
    - tare (weight of the empty cylinder and valve block; used for calculation of contents by weight).
    - pressure of the last hydraulic test.
    - symbol of the contained gas.
  - the valve is opened by turning a longitudinal spindle, set within a gland screwed tightly into the valve block. Compression of a nylon ring around the spindle prevents leakage of gas along the spindle shaft.
  - bears the **pin index system** on the same face as the gas outlet.

Table 18 Colour-coding of cylinders

	UK			Recommended international system	
Gas	Shoulder	Body	USA	Shoulder	Body[a]
O_2	White	Black	Green	White	White
N_2O	Blue	Blue	Blue	Blue	White
CO_2	Grey	Grey	Grey	Grey	White
Entonox	Blue/white quarters	Blue		White/blue quarters	White
Helium	Brown	Brown	Brown	Brown	White
O_2 21%/helium	Brown/white quarters	Black	Brown/yellow	Brown/white quarters	White
Air	Black/white quarters	Grey	Yellow	Black/white quarters	White

[a]Use of white body agreed within Europe.

- a safety outlet is fitted to the valve block (USA) or between the block and cylinder neck (UK); it melts at low temperatures, allowing escape of gas in case of fire.
- a testing collar is attached (*see later*).

Colour-coding (UK): shoulder colour(s) represent the predominant gas(es) in the cylinder. US colour-coding is different. An international colouring system has been recommended, taking one of the colours from the UK system (Table 18). European standards initially followed this scheme but only applied to the cylinders' shoulders, the suppliers being able to paint the body as they chose. In 2000 it was suggested that all medical gas cylinders should be identified by having white bodies, and this was agreed within most of Europe over the next decade (including the UK, in 2010, with all cylinders complying with the new colour scheme by 2025).

- Bodies are labelled with:
  - name and symbol of the gas.
  - volume and pressure of contained gas.
  - information and warnings about explosions and flammability where appropriate. When the gas supply is turned on suddenly, compression of the gas within the valves and pipes causes a rise in temperature. Oil or grease in the system may ignite, hence the warning against these lubricants.
- Testing:
  - every hundredth cylinder is cut into strips and tested at manufacture.
  - each cylinder is tested 5-yearly to withstand high hydraulic pressures (about 200–250 **bar**). Cylinders are filled with water under pressure, within a water jacket. Expansion and elastic recoil of the metal are then measured.
  - internal inspection with an endoscope.
  - a plastic disc is placed around the valve block neck; its colour and shape are coded for the date of the last test. The year in which testing is due is stamped on the disc, and a hole punched to indicate the quarter of the year.
- Cylinder pressures (maximal values at 15°C, as marked on the cylinders):
  - **O_2**: 137 bar.
  - **N_2O**: 40 bar.
  - **CO_2**: 50 bar.
  - **air**: 137 bar.
  - O_2/**helium**: 137 bar.
  - O_2/N_2O: 137 bar.

Modern pressure gauges are marked in kPa × 100 (1 bar = 100 kPa).

N_2O and CO_2 cylinders contain liquid; as such a cylinder empties, pressure is maintained by evaporation of liquid (although a slight drop in pressure does occur as temperature falls) until the liquid is depleted. Pressure then falls rapidly with further emptying. Gas-filled cylinders (e.g. containing O_2) provide gas whose pressure is proportional to cylinder contents.

Large **Entonox** cylinders contain connecting tubes from the valve block to the lower part of the cylinder, to reduce risk of hypoxic gas delivery if separation of gases occurs below the **pseudocritical temperature**.

- Sizes of cylinders are denoted by capital letters, E being the usual size on anaesthetic machines:
  - O_2: C (gas content – 170 l), D (340 l), E (680 l).
  - N_2O: C (450 l), D (900 l), E (1800 l).

See also, Filling ratio; Piped gas supply

Cystic fibrosis. Autosomal recessive genetic disease; the commonest lethal inherited illness in white people affecting 1 in 1500 live births. Causes impaired production of cystic fibrosis transmembrane conductance regulator (CFTR) protein, a complex channel that regulates passage of water and ions across cell membranes. Primarily affects exocrine gland function resulting in abnormally viscous secretions.

- Features:
  - repeated respiratory infection, usually by staphylococcus and pseudomonas, leading to **bronchiectasis**, **pulmonary fibrosis** and eventually **pulmonary hypertension** and **cor pulmonale.** Nasal polyps are common. **Pneumothorax** may occur. **$\dot{V}/\dot{Q}$ mismatch**, restrictive and obstructive defects and increased residual capacity often result in **hypoxaemia.** Arterial $P\text{CO}_2$ is usually reduced unless lung disease is severe. **Laryngospasm** and coughing are common during anaesthesia.
  - pancreatic insufficiency with malabsorption, intestinal obstruction (e.g. meconium ileus in the newborn) and **diabetes mellitus.** Obstructive **jaundice** may occur.
  - renal impairment and amyloidosis may occur. Survival beyond the second and third decade is now common with intensive **physiotherapy**, antibiotic therapy and pancreatic supplementation. Heart–lung and lung transplantation is increasingly being performed because the disease seems not to recur in transplanted lungs.
- Anaesthetic management:
  - careful **preoperative assessment** and continuation of physiotherapy. **Coagulation** may be impaired.

Opioid premedication is usually avoided. **Anticholinergic drugs** may increase secretion viscosity but are commonly used to reduce the incidence of bradycardia; they may be given on induction.
- regional techniques, where appropriate.
- inhalational induction is prolonged because of $\dot{V}/\dot{Q}$ mismatch. **Ketamine** increases bronchial secretions.
- usual technique: tracheal intubation and IPPV, with tracheobronchial suction as required. **Bronchoalveolar lavage** may be beneficial. Extubation is performed awake. **Humidification** of gases is important.
- careful fluid balance to avoid dehydration.
- postoperative observation, physiotherapy, analgesia and humidified O_2 administration are important.

Elborn JS (2016). Lancet; 388: 2519–31

Cystic hygroma. Congenital multiloculated cystic mass arising from the jugular lymph sac, the embryonic precursor of part of the thoracic duct. Contains lymph; characteristically transilluminates very well. Usually presents soon after birth. Sometimes sclerosant treatment is used; surgery is difficult because of widespread cystic tissue throughout neck. The tongue and pharynx may be involved. Main anaesthetic problems are related to **airway obstruction** and difficult intubation. Manual IPPV via a facemask may be impossible; therefore spontaneous ventilation is usually maintained until intubation is achieved.
See also, Intubation, difficult

Cytochrome oxidase system. Series of iron-containing **enzymes** within mitochondrial inner membranes. Electron transport from oxidised nicotinamide adenine dinucleotide (NADH) or succinate proceeds via sequential cytochromes, the iron component becoming alternately reduced and oxidised as the electron is passed to the next in line. Their structure and arrangement within the membrane are thought to be crucial to their function. Electron flow is coupled to **ATP** formation; 3 molecules of ATP are formed per NADH and 2 ATP per succinate molecule. Cytochrome oxidase itself is the cytochrome binding to molecular O_2 to form water, and is inhibited in **cyanide poisoning** and **carbon monoxide poisoning**.

Similar enzymes exist in other membranes, e.g. cytochrome P_{450} isoenzymes ('P' for pigment, 450 nm for enzymes' absorption peak), found in smooth endoplasmic reticulum; these are responsible for phase I metabolism of many drugs. Genetic polymorphism of the various enzymes partly explains interindividual variability in drug metabolism, e.g. **codeine**.

Cytokines. Protein mediators released by many cells, including monocytes, lymphocytes, macrophages, **mast cells** and endothelial cells. Involved in regulating the activity, growth and differentiation of many different cells of the immune and haemopoietic systems. The cytokines tumour necrosis factor-α (TNFα; cachectin), interleukin (IL)-1 and IL-6 are thought to be central to the pathophysiology of **SIRS** and **sepsis**; TNFα and IL-1 produce the systemic and metabolic features of SIRS, while IL-6 causes the acute-phase protein response. All three are released in response to **endotoxin** and other stimuli. In sepsis, high blood concentrations of IL-6 especially have been associated with poor outcome. Therapies for sepsis have been developed directed against the actions of IL-1 and TNFα (e.g. using antibodies or antagonists), although encouraging results in animal experiments have generally not been reproduced in humans. Anti-TNFα therapies are now established in certain immunologically mediated diseases, e.g. inflammatory bowel disease, **rheumatoid arthritis**.

Other cytokines include additional interleukins, and interferons. Interferon-γ interacts with other cytokines and has been investigated as a target for the treatment of sepsis.

Cytomegalovirus (CMV). Herpes group virus usually acquired subclinically during childhood; by 50 years of age, 50% of individuals have anti-CMV antibodies. May be transmitted by **blood transfusion**, hence the requirement for screening before transfusion to at-risk groups. May cause major morbidity and mortality during pregnancy (resulting in cytomegalic inclusion disease: small infant with jaundice, hepatosplenomegaly, microcephaly, mental retardation) and in patients with **immunodeficiency** (clinical features include fever, interstitial pneumonia, enteritis, hepatitis, carditis, chorioretinitis, leucopenia and thrombocytopenia). Treatment includes **antiviral drugs** such as **ganciclovir** or **foscarnet sodium**.

Cytotoxic drugs. Used in the treatment of **malignancy** and as **immunosuppressive drugs**. All may cause nausea and vomiting and bone marrow suppression; most are teratogenic and require careful preparation by trained personnel. Extravasation of iv drugs may cause severe tissue necrosis. Some have side effects of particular anaesthetic/ICU relevance:
- alkylating agents (act by damaging DNA and impairing cell division): **cyclophosphamide** may prolong the effect of **suxamethonium**; **busulfan** may cause **pulmonary fibrosis**. Chlorambucil may rarely cause severe skin reactions.
- cytotoxic antibiotics: doxorubicin may cause **cardiomyopathy**; **bleomycin** may cause pulmonary fibrosis.
- antimetabolites: **methotrexate** may cause pneumonitis.
- vinca alkaloids: vincristine and vinblastine may cause **autonomic** and **peripheral neuropathy**.
- others: cisplatin may cause nephrotoxicity, ototoxicity and peripheral neuropathy; procarbazine has **monoamine oxidase inhibitor** effects; **azathioprine** may cause hepatic impairment, nephritis and rarely pneumonitis.

O_2 therapy has been implicated in exacerbating the pulmonary fibrosis caused by cytotoxic drugs.

Specific guidelines (issued by the Committee on the Review of Medicines) exist for the handling of cytotoxic drugs. These include the necessity for trained staff to administer drugs, designated areas for drug reconstitution, protective clothing, eye protection, safe disposal of waste material and avoidance of handling cytotoxics by pregnant staff.

Accidental intrathecal (instead of intravenous) injection of vincristine during combination chemotherapy almost inevitably results in death; in the UK, anaesthetists have been involved in such errors. Totally incompatible intrathecal/intravenous connections have been developed as a result.

δ wave, *see Wolff–Parkinson–White syndrome*

DA examination (Diploma in Anaesthetics). First specialist examination in anaesthetics; first held in 1935 in London. Originally intended for anaesthetists with at least 2 years' experience and 2000 anaesthetics, later reduced to 1 year's residence in an approved hospital. A two-part examination was introduced in 1947, becoming the **FFARCS examination** in 1953; the single-part DA remained separate until 1984, when the DA (UK) became the first part of the new three part FFARCS. Replaced by the new **FRCA examination** in 1996.

Dabigatran etexilate. Direct **thrombin inhibitor**; prevents the conversion of fibrinogen to fibrin, thereby impairing **coagulation** and **platelet** activation. Prolongs the activated partial thromboplastin time (APTT). A **prodrug**, rapidly metabolised to active metabolite (dabigatran) by non-specific esterases; oral **bioavailability** is 6.5%. Onset of action is 0.5–2 h, with steady state achieved within 3 days. 80% of drug is renally excreted unchanged; **half-life** is 8–14 h, increased to >24 h in severe **renal failure**. Also metabolised by the liver and excreted in the bile.

Recommended as a treatment option for **DVT** prophylaxis in adults undergoing total knee or hip replacement surgery, for prevention of **stroke** in patients with **AF** with certain risk factors, for the prophylaxis and treatment of recurrent DVT/**PE** in **acute coronary syndromes** when patients cannot tolerate **antiplatelet drugs**.

Developed as an alternative to **warfarin**, over which it has several advantages:

- no therapeutic monitoring required.
- fixed dosage (modified according to age, indication, renal function and **drug interactions**).
- faster onset and shorter duration of action.
- stable, predictable **pharmacokinetics**, with fewer drug interactions.

Disadvantages include: higher cost; unsuitable for patients with severe renal impairment (**GFR** <30 ml/min) and liver dysfunction.

- Dosage:
  - DVT prophylaxis in adults undergoing knee/hip replacement: 110 mg orally 1–4 h after surgery followed by 220 mg daily, reduced to 75 mg followed by 150 mg daily in renal impairment and the elderly.
  - stroke prophylaxis in patients with AF: 150 mg orally bd, reduced to 75 mg in renal impairment.
- Drug interactions: potentiated by concomitant **verapamil** and **amiodarone**; reduced dosing regimen is used. Inhibited by **rifampicin**, **ketoconazole** and **quinidine**.

Main side effect is bleeding; risk is lower than equivalent treatment with warfarin. A specific antidote, idarucizumab, is available for life-threatening haemorrhage or those needing urgent surgery.

Becatinni C, Agnelli G (2016). J Am Coll Cardiol; 67: 1941–55

Dalfopristin, *see Quinupristin/dalfopristin*

Dalteparin sodium, *see Heparin*

Dalton's law. The pressure exerted by a fixed amount of a gas in a mixture equals the pressure it would exert if alone. Thus, the pressure exerted by a mixture of gases equals the sum of the partial pressures exerted by each gas.
[John Dalton (1766–1844), English chemist]

Damage control resuscitation. Approach to major **trauma**, developed in modern military settings. Aims to reduce the incidence and severity of the combination of acute coagulopathy, **hypothermia** and **metabolic acidosis** that commonly accompany major **haemorrhage**. Consists of:

- 'permissive hypotension': restricted fluid resuscitation to maintain a radial pulse rather than a normal or near-normal BP, accepting a period of organ hypoperfusion (except in **TBI** or spinal injuries, where maintenance of **cerebral perfusion pressure** and spinal perfusion pressure is thought to be vital). This temporary period (up to 60 min) usually starts prehospital, allows control of any haemorrhage and is followed by normotensive resuscitation.
- 'haemostatic resuscitation': early use of **blood products** to prevent/treat acute coagulopathy, including **platelets** (in a 1:1 ratio with packed red cells [1 pool of platelets for every 5 units of red cells]), fresh frozen plasma (in a 1:1 ratio) and cryoprecipitate; **tranexamic acid**, recombinant **factor VIIa** and **calcium** have also been advocated. Use of more recently donated packed red cells rather than older units may be beneficial.
- aggressive warming to reduce hypothermia.
- 'damage-control surgery': restriction of early surgery to the minimum possible, e.g. clamping/packing/suturing major defects, rather than prolonged, definitive procedures.

Bogert JN, Harvin JA, Cotton BA (2016). J Intens Care Med; 31: 177–86

Damping. Progressive diminution of amplitude of oscillations in a resonant system, caused by dissipation of stored energy. Important in recording systems such as direct **arterial BP measurement**. In this context, damping mainly arises from viscous drag of fluid in the cannula and connecting tubing, compression of entrapped air bubbles, blood clots within the system and kinking. Excess damping causes a flattened trace that may be distorted (**phase shift**). The degree of damping is described by the damping factor (D); if a sudden change is imposed on a system, $D = 1$ if no overshoot of the trace occurs (critical damping; Fig. 50a). A marked overshoot followed by many oscillations occurs if $D \ll 1$ (Fig. 50b), and an excessively delayed

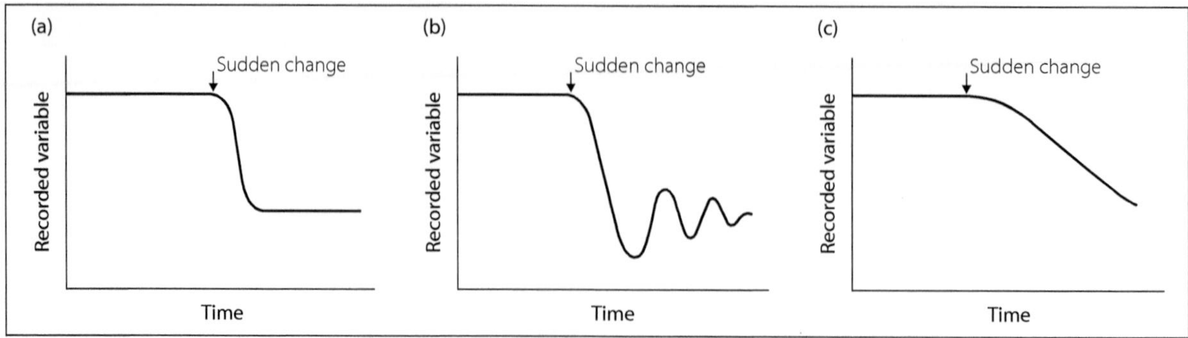

Fig. 50 Damping: (a) $D = 1$; (b) $D \ll 1$; (c) $D \gg 1$

response occurs if $D \gg 1$ (Fig. 50c). Optimal damping is 0.6–0.7 of critical damping, and produces the fastest response without excessive oscillations. D depends on the properties of the liquid within the system and the dimensions of the cannula and tubing.

Danaparoid sodium. **Heparinoid** mixture, containing no **heparin**, used for the prophylaxis of **deep vein thrombosis**. Useful as a heparin alternative in cases of **heparin-induced thrombocytopenia**.

- Dosage:
  - prophylaxis: 750 units sc bd for 7–10 days.
  - parenteral anticoagulation: 1250–3750 units (depending on body weight) iv, followed by 800 units over 2 h, 600 units over 2 h, then 200 units/h for 5 days.
- Side effects: as for heparin. Contains sulfite, which may trigger bronchospasm and hypotension in susceptible patients. Anti-Xa activity should be monitored in renal impairment or obese patients.

Dandy–Walker syndrome, *see Hydrocephalus*

Dantrolene sodium. Hydantoin skeletal **muscle** relaxant that acts by binding to the ryanodine receptor and limits entry of **calcium** into myocytes. Used to treat spasticity, **neuroleptic malignant syndrome** and **MH**.

- Dosage:
  - 25–400 mg orally od for muscle spasm.
  - 1 mg/kg iv for treatment of MH, repeated up to 10 mg/kg. The solution is irritant with pH 9–10, and is best infused into a large vein. Presented in bottles of 20 mg orange powder with 3 g mannitol and sodium hydroxide, each requiring mixing with 60 ml water. Preparation of a therapeutic dose is therefore time-consuming. Once prepared, the solution lasts 6 h at 15°–30°C. Dry powder has a shelf-life of 9 months.
- Side effects: hepatotoxicity may occur after prolonged oral use; muscle weakness and sedation may follow iv injection. The high pH of the iv solution may cause venous thrombosis following prolonged infusion, and tissue necrosis following extravasation.

Krause T, Gerbershagen MU, Fiege M, et al (2004). Anaesthesia; 59: 364–73

Darrow's solution. Isotonic solution designed for **iv fluid** replacement in children suffering from gastroenteritis. Composed of sodium 122 mmol/l, chloride 104 mmol/l, lactate 53 mmol/l and potassium 35 mmol/l.

[Daniel Darrow (1895–1965), US paediatrician]

Data. In **statistics**, a series of observations or measurements.

- Data may be:
  - continuous: e.g. length in metres; the difference between 2 and 3 m is the same as that between 35 and 36 m. Although they may be treated in the same way, there are two types of continuous data:
    - interval: does not include zero, e.g. Celsius **temperature** scale: the 'zero' is an arbitrary point in the scale; thus 10°C does not represent half as much heat as 20°C, and zero degrees does not equate to the absence of heat.
    - ratio: includes zero value, e.g. Kelvin temperature scale: 0 K equates to the absence of heat, and 10 K represents half as much heat as 20 K (i.e., the ratio of two measurements holds meaning).

    If they have a **normal distribution**, continuous data may be described by the **mean** and **standard deviation** as indicators of central tendency and scatter, respectively (described as for ordinal data if not normally distributed).
  - non-continuous:
    - ordinal, e.g. **ASA physical status**. The difference between scores of 2 and 3 does not equal that between scores of 4 and 5, and a score of 4 is not 'twice as unfit' as a score of 2. Ordinal data are described by the **median** and **percentiles** (plus range).
    - nominal (categorical), e.g. diagnosis, hair colour. May be dichotomous, e.g. male/female; alive/dead. Nominal data are described by the **mode** and a list of possible categories.

Different kinds of data require different **statistical tests** for correct analyses and comparisons: parametric tests for normally distributed continuous data; and non-parametric tests for non-continuous and non-normally distributed continuous data. The latter may often be 'normalised' by mathematical transformation, allowing application of the more sensitive parametric tests.

See also, Clinical trials; Statistical frequency distributions

Davenport diagram. Graph of plasma **bicarbonate** concentration against **pH**, useful in interpreting and explaining disturbances of **acid–base balance**. Different lines may be drawn for different arterial $P\text{CO}_2$ values, but for each line, bicarbonate falls as pH falls and increases as pH increases (Fig. 51).

- Can be used to demonstrate what happens in various acid–base disorders:
  - line BAD represents part of the titration curve for blood.

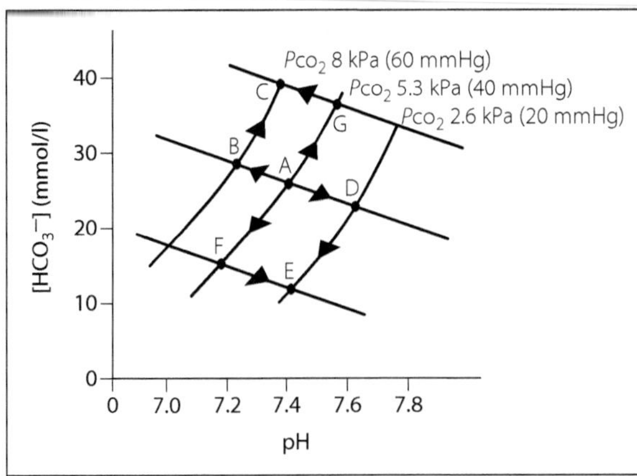

Fig. 51 Davenport diagram (see text)

- point A represents normal plasma.
- point B represents respiratory **acidosis**; i.e., a rise in arterial PCO_2, reducing pH and increasing bicarbonate. To return pH towards normal, compensatory mechanisms (e.g. increased renal reabsorption) increase bicarbonate; i.e., move towards point C.
- point D represents respiratory **alkalosis**; compensation (increased renal bicarbonate excretion) results in a move towards point E.
- point F represents metabolic acidosis; respiratory compensation (hyperventilation with a fall in arterial PCO_2) causes a move towards point E.
- point G represents metabolic alkalosis; compensatory hypoventilation causes a move towards point C.

The same relationship may be displayed in different ways, e.g. the **Siggaard–Andersen nomogram**, which contains more information and is more useful clinically

[Horace W Davenport (1912–2005), US physiologist]

Davy, Sir Humphrey (1778–1829). Cornish-born scientist, inventor of the miner's safety lamp. Discovered sodium, potassium, calcium and barium. Suggested the use of $\mathbf{N_2O}$ (which he named 'laughing gas') for analgesia in 1799, while director of the Medical Pneumatic Institution in Bristol. Later became President of the Royal Society.

Riegels N, Richards MJBM (2011). Anesthesiology; 114: 1282–8

Day-case surgery. Surgery in which the patient presents to hospital and returns home on the day of operation. Increasingly performed, as it has many advantages over inpatient surgery:

- reduced psychological upheaval for patients, especially children.
- reduced requirement for nursing care and hospital services, and thus cheaper.
- allows larger numbers of patients to be treated.
- reduced risk of hospital-acquired infection.

Standards of anaesthetic and surgical care and equipment (including preoperative preparation, **monitoring** and **recovery** facilities) are as for inpatient surgery.

- Patients may be managed within:
  - separate dedicated day-case units within hospitals: provide geographical, staffing and some administrative independence from the main hospital, but allow access to hospital facilities if needed, e.g. x-ray, laboratories, wards, ICU.
  - traditional inpatient lists.
  - completely separate units.
- Patient selection: traditional rigid criteria (e.g. relating to age, **ASA physical status**, **BMI**) are now generally considered unnecessary, three main criteria being:
  - social situation, e.g. willing patient, access to a telephone, responsible adult to collect the patient and stay at home for 24 h.
  - medical condition: patient should be fit or any chronic disease should be stable/controlled.
  - planned procedure: low risk of complications, which should be mild; mild expected pain/PONV. Operations expected to last less than 60 min are preferable. Operations previously considered unsuitable are increasingly performed on an outpatient basis, e.g. tonsillectomy, laparoscopic cholecystectomy.

Patients must be informed of the requirements for fasting and home arrangements; information leaflets are widely used for this purpose.

- Anaesthetic technique:
  - patients are fully assessed preoperatively (often using a questionnaire). Anaesthetic outpatient clinics are widely used.
  - **premedication** is usually omitted, although short-acting drugs (e.g. **temazepam**) are sometimes used.
  - general principles are as for any anaesthetic, but rapid recovery is particularly desirable. Short-acting drugs are usually used (e.g. **propofol**, **fentanyl**, **alfentanil**); **sevoflurane** and **desflurane** are commonly selected volatile agents because of their low blood gas solubility and rapid recovery. Tracheal intubation is acceptable but is usually avoided if possible. **Suxamethonium** is often avoided as muscle pains are more common in ambulant patients.
  - regional techniques may be suitable (often combined with general anaesthesia to provide postoperative analgesia).
  - facilities for admission to an inpatient ward must be available in case of complications (occur in <5% of cases).
- Postoperative assessment must be performed before discharge; the following are usually required:
  - full orientation and responsiveness.
  - ability to walk, dress, drink and pass urine.
  - adequately controlled pain and nausea/vomiting.
  - controlled bleeding and swelling.
  - stable vital signs.

Written and verbal instructions are given to the patient not to take sedative drugs or alcohol, or participate in potentially dangerous activities (e.g. operating machinery, driving, frying food), usually for 24–48 h.

AAGBI, BADS (2011). Anaesthesia; 66: 417–34

DDAVP, D-Amino-8-D-arginine-vasopressin, *see Desmopressin*

D-dimer, *see Fibrin degradation products*

Dead space. Volume of inspired gas that takes no part in gas exchange. Divided into:

- anatomical dead space: mouth, nose, pharynx and large airways not lined with respiratory epithelium. Measured by **Fowler's method**.
- alveolar dead space: ventilated lung normally contributing to gas exchange, but not doing so because of impaired perfusion. Thus represents one extreme of $\dot{V}/\dot{Q}$ **mismatch**.

Physiological dead space equals anatomical plus alveolar dead space. It is calculated using the **Bohr equation**. Assessment may be useful in monitoring $\dot{V}/\dot{Q}$ mismatch in patients with extensive respiratory disease, especially when combined with estimation of **shunt** fraction. Normally equals 2–3 ml/kg; i.e., 30% of normal tidal volume. In rapid shallow breathing, **alveolar ventilation** is reduced despite a normal minute ventilation, because a greater proportion of tidal volume is dead space.

- Increased by:
  - increased lung volumes.
  - bronchodilatation.
  - neck extension.
  - **PE/gas embolism.**
  - old age.
  - hypotension.
  - haemorrhage.
  - pulmonary disease.
  - general anaesthesia and **IPPV**.
  - **atropine** and **hyoscine**.
  - apparatus (*see later*).
- Decreased by:
  - tracheal intubation and **tracheostomy**.
  - supine position.

Apparatus dead space represents 'wasted' fresh gas within anaesthetic equipment. Minimal lengths of tubing should lie between the fresh gas inlet of a T-piece and the patient, especially in children, whose tidal volumes are small. **Facemasks** and their connections may considerably increase dead space.

Death. Defined as the irreversible loss of the capacity for consciousness and the capacity to breathe. Anaesthetists and intensivists may face several issues surrounding the death of patients:

- practical:
  - **mortality/survival prediction** and allocation of resources; **triage**.
  - relief of symptoms, e.g. **pain management, palliative care**.
  - **CPR**.
  - diagnosis of **brainstem death**.
  - **organ donation.**
- ethical:
  - informed **consent** before treatments (i.e., the risk of death).
  - withdrawing treatment or resisting aggressive interventions when they are likely to be futile.
  - **advance decisions.**
  - **do not attempt resuscitation orders.**
  - **euthanasia.**
- medicolegal:
  - reporting of deaths to the **coroner**.
  - claims of **negligence, manslaughter** or murder.
- psychological:
  - adequate preparation and support of patients, relatives and staff.
  - counselling of staff after a patient's death, especially when unexpected.
  - organisational/educational: **audit**; surveys of ICU and **anaesthetic morbidity and mortality**; **risk management**.

See also, Ethics; Medicolegal aspects of anaesthesia

Debrisoquine sulfate. **Antihypertensive drug**, acting by preventing **noradrenaline** release from postganglionic adrenergic neurones. Similar in effects to **guanethidine**, but does not deplete noradrenaline stores. No longer available in UK.

Decamethonium dibromide/diiodide. Depolarising **neuromuscular blocking drug**, introduced in 1948 and no longer available. Blockade lasts 15–20 min.

Decerebrate posture. Abnormal posture resulting from bilateral midbrain or pontine lesions (below the level of the red nucleus). Composed of internal rotation and hyperextension of all limbs, with hyperextension of neck and spine, and absent righting reflexes. Similar posturing may be seen in severe structural brain damage or **coning**.
See also, Decorticate posture

Declamping syndrome, *see Aortic aneurysm, abdominal*

Decompression sickness (Caisson disease). Syndrome following rapid passage from a high atmospheric pressure environment to one of lower atmospheric pressure (e.g. surfacing after underwater diving), especially if followed by air transport at high altitude. Caused by formation of **nitrogen** bubbles as the gas comes out of solution, which it does readily because of its low solubility. Bubbles may embolise to or form in various tissues, giving rise to widespread symptoms in: the joints ('the bends'); the CNS ('the staggers'); the skin ('the creeps'); the lungs ('the chokes'). Treated by immediate recompression followed by slow, controlled depressurisation.
[Caisson: pressurised watertight chamber used for construction work in deep water]
Mahon RT, Regis DP (2014). Compr Physiol; 4: 1157–75

Decontamination of anaesthetic equipment, *see Contamination of anaesthetic equipment*

Decorticate posture. Abnormal posture resulting from lesions of the cerebral cortex, internal capsule and thalamus with preservation of basal ganglia and brainstem function. Composed of leg extension, internal rotation and plantar flexion, with moderate arm flexion. Passive rotation of the head to one side causes extension of the ipsilateral arm, with full flexion of the contralateral arm, due to intact tonic neck reflexes. The contralateral leg may flex. Occurs in severe structural brain damage.
See also, Decerebrate posture

Decrement, *see Fade*

Decubitus ulcers (Pressure sores). May result from several factors:

- inadequate peripheral perfusion, e.g. peripheral vascular disease, use of vasopressor drugs, hypotension.
- **malnutrition**, including mineral deficiency.
- predisposing conditions, e.g. **diabetes mellitus, immunodeficiency**.
- reduced sensation.
- **diarrhoea** or urinary incontinence.
- poor support of limbs, with infrequent turning.

All may coexist in critically ill patients. May cause pain or be a source of infection. Prevention includes: identification of patients at risk (e.g. with the Waterlow pressure sore assessment tool); regular inspection of pressure points and turning; support of pressure points to spread the weight

of the body over a wider area; attention to nutrition; and use of air-fluidised mattresses that vary the pressure points continuously. Once present, ulcers are managed by raising the affected limb/area, regular dressings and cleaning, and negative-pressure dressings ('vac dressings') where indicated. Other strategies used include radiant heat dressings and electromagnetic therapy.
[Judy Waterlow, British nurse]
Levine SM, Sinno S, Levine JP, Saadeh PB (2013). Ann Surg; 257: 603–8

Deep vein thrombosis (DVT). Thrombus formation in the deep veins, usually of the leg and pelvis. A common postoperative complication, especially following major joint replacement, colorectal surgery and surgery for cancer. The true incidence is unknown but may exceed 50% in high-risk patients. Carries high risk of **PE**. May rarely cause systemic embolisation via a patent foramen ovale (present in 30% of the population at autopsy).
- Triad of predisposing factors described by Virchow in 1856:
  - venous stasis, e.g. low cardiac output (e.g. **cardiac failure**, **MI**, **dehydration**), pelvic venous obstruction, prolonged immobility.
  - vessel wall damage, e.g. direct trauma, inflammation, varicosities, infiltration.
  - increased blood coagulability, e.g. trauma, **malignancy**, **pregnancy**, oestrogen or antifibrinolytic administration, hereditary hypercoagulability, **smoking** (*see Coagulation disorders*).

More common in old age, sepsis and **obesity**. Increased risk after surgery is thought to be related to increased **platelet** adhesiveness and activation of the **coagulation** cascade caused by tissue trauma, exacerbated by possible venous damage and immobility.

Clinical diagnosis is unreliable but suggested by tenderness, swelling and increased temperature of the calf, and pain on passive dorsiflexion of the foot (Homan's sign). The two-level Wells test (Table 19) may help estimate the clinical probability of DVT. If DVT is suspected and is accompanied by a 'likely' two-level Wells score, a proximal leg vein **Doppler** ultrasound scan should be performed within 4 hours. If negative, measurement of **fibrin degradation products** (i.e., D-dimer) should be carried out (a normal level excluding DVT). If there is a delay of >4 h in obtaining an ultrasound scan, an interim 24-h dose of parenteral anticoagulant should be given.

Treatment consists of systemic anticoagulation with low-molecular-weight **heparin** (LMWH) or **fondaparinux**; patients with severe renal impairment or with an increased risk of bleeding should be treated with unfractionated heparin, the dose adjusted based on **coagulation studies**. **Warfarin** is started within 24 h of diagnosis and heparin discontinued when a prothrombin time of 2–3 times normal is achieved. Long-term interruption of leg blood flow may not be prevented, and prevention of PE has never been proven. Initial bed rest, leg elevation and analgesia are also prescribed, although there is no evidence that these measures affect outcome. Duration of warfarin therapy ranges from 3 to 6 months, depending on underlying risk factors. Direct factor Xa inhibitors (e.g. **rivaroxaban**) and direct **thrombin inhibitors** (e.g. **dabigatran**) are also used for the acute treatment of DVT and as an alternative to warfarin in the longer-term management. Catheter-directed thrombolytic therapy may be offered for iliofemoral DVT if symptoms have been present for <14 days, and if the patient has good functional status, a life expectancy >1 year and a low risk of bleeding. Temporary inferior vena caval filters should be considered in patients who cannot receive anticoagulants or those with recurrent DVT despite adequate anticoagulation.

Table 19 Two-level DVT Wells score. DVT is described as 'likely' for a total score ≥2, and 'unlikely' for a total ≤1

Active cancer	+1
Paralysis, paresis or recent plaster immobilisation	+1
Recently bedridden for >3 days or major surgery within last 12 weeks	+1
Local tenderness along distribution of deep venous system	+1
Entire leg swollen	+1
Calf at least 3 cm larger than asymptomatic side	+1
Pitting oedema of affected side	+1
Collateral superficial veins	+1
Previously documented DVT	+1
An alternative diagnosis is at least as likely as DVT	−2

- Prophylaxis should be considered for all but minor surgery, and in all immobile patients. Methods used:
  - reduction of stasis:
    - heel cushion to prevent pressure on calf veins and a cushion under the knees to prevent hyperextension, leading to popliteal vein occlusion.
    - elevation of legs.
    - intermittent pneumatic compression of the calves peri- and postoperatively.
    - graduated compression stockings.
    - encouragement of postoperative leg exercises and early mobilisation.
  - reduction of intravascular coagulation:
    - fibrinolytic drugs: not shown to prevent DVT.
    - **antiplatelet drugs**: have been shown to prevent DVT and PE.
    - heparin and warfarin anticoagulation: effective but with risk of haemorrhage. Low-dose heparin is widely used (5000 units sc 2 h preoperatively then bd/tds) and has been shown to be effective in reducing DVT and fatal PE. Low-molecular-weight heparin reduces DVT with reduced haemorrhagic side effects (*for doses, see Heparin*). Dihydroergotamine has been used together with heparin, and is thought to reduce the incidence further, possibly via venous vasoconstriction.
    - discontinuation of oral **contraceptives** preoperatively.
    - **epidural/spinal anaesthesia** is thought to be associated with increased **fibrinolysis** and reduced risk of DVT.
    - **statins** reduce the incidence of DVT.

LMWH, pneumatic calf compression and compression stockings are most commonly used.
[Rudolph LW Virchow (1821–1902), German pathologist; John Homans (1877–1954), US surgeon; Philip Wells, Canadian physician]
Di Nisio M, van Es N, Büller HR (2016). Lancet; 388: 3060–73
See also, Coagulation studies

Defibrillation. Application of an electric current across the heart, to convert (ventricular) fibrillation to sinus rhythm. Use of electricity was described in the late 1700s/early 1800s (e.g. by **Kite**), but modern use arose from experiments in the 1930s–1950s, largely by Kouwenhoven.

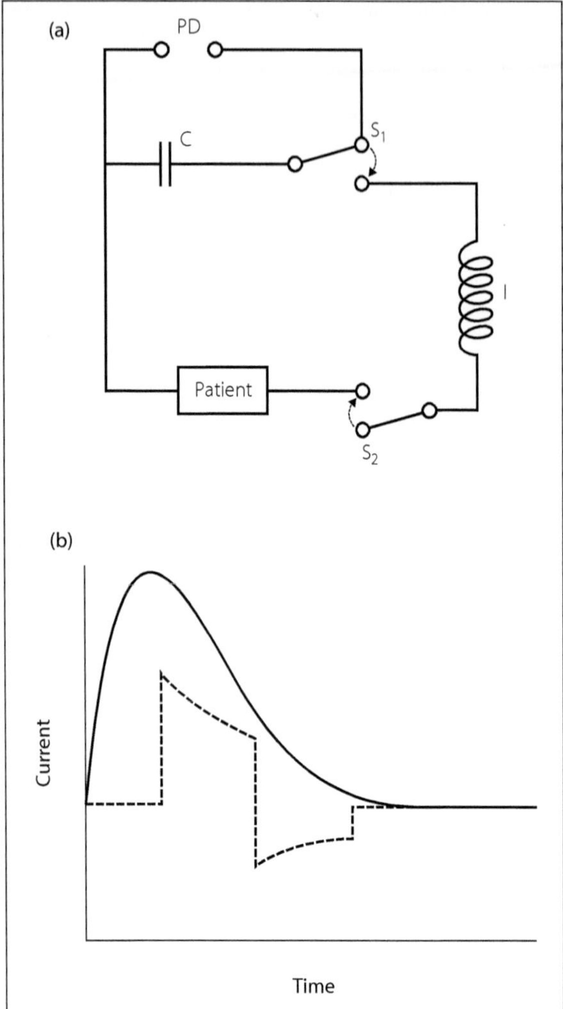

Fig. 52 Defibrillator. (a) Circuit diagram for basic model. *C*, Capacitor; *I*, inductor; *PD*, potential difference (5000–8000 V); S_1 and S_2, switches. (b) Comparison of currents delivered by monophasic *(solid)* and biphasic *(dashed)* types (N.B. the latter varies in current strength and duration according to settings and/or measured transthoracic impedance)

The first successful resuscitation of a patient from VF was by Beck in 1947. A portable debrillator was first used by Pantridge in 1966. Direct current is more effective and less damaging than alternating current.

Modern defibrillators contain a **capacitor**, with potential difference between its plates of 5000–8000 V (Fig. 52a). Stored charge is released during discharge; the energy released is proportional to the potential difference. An **inductor** controls the shape and duration of the delivered electrical pulse. With traditional monophasic defibrillation up to 400 J is used for external defibrillation (360 J actually delivered to the patient because of energy losses), and 10–50 J for internal defibrillation. The current pulse (up to 30 A) causes synchronous contraction of the heart muscle followed by a refractory period, thus allowing sinus rhythm to occur. Modern devices deliver lower-energy biphasic waveforms, which are more effective at terminating VF; current is delivered in one direction followed immediately by a second current in the opposite direction (Fig. 52b). More sophisticated developments include the ability to measure and correct for the transthoracic impedance by varying the shock delivered.

Table 20 North American Society of Pacing and Electrophysiology/ British Pacing and Electrophysiology Group generic implantable defibrillator code

Position 1: chamber shocked	*Position 2: chamber paced*	*Position 3: monitoring modality*	*Position 4: antibradycardic chamber paced*
0 = None	0 = None	E = ECG	0 = None
A = Atrium	A = Atrium	H = Haemodynamic	A = Atrium
V = Ventricle	V = Ventricle		V = Ventricle
D = Dual	D = Dual		D = Dual

Firm application of paddles (one to the right of the sternum, the other over the apex of the heart—taking care to avoid any implanted devices) using conductive jelly increases efficiency, although self-adhesive pads are now preferred. They may also be placed on the front and back of the chest. Thoracic **impedance** is reduced by the first shock, so a second discharge at the same setting will deliver greater energy to the heart. For children, 4 J/kg is used. Lower energy levels and R-wave synchronisation are used in **cardioversion.** Repeated shocks may result in myocardial damage.

Hazards include **electrocution** of members of the resuscitation team and fire. Standing clear of the patient and disconnection of the patient's oxygen supply (moving it 1 m from his/her chest) during defibrillation is mandatory.

Automatic external defibrillators (AEDs) identify life-threatening arrhythmias, prompt medical personnel on how to proceed, and deliver shocks with the operator's approval. They are increasingly available in public areas for use by non-medical staff.

Implantable cardioverter defibrillators (ICDs) are used for recurrent VF/VT or predisposing conditions (*see Defibrillators, implantable cardioverter*).

[William Kouwenhoven (1886–1975), US engineer; Claude S Beck (1894–1971), US thoracic surgeon; Frank Pantridge (1916–2004), N. Irish cardiologist]

See also, Individual arrhythmias; Cardiac pacing; Cardiopulmonary resuscitation

Defibrillators, implantable cardioverter (ICD). Specialised **pacemakers** designed to detect and treat potentially life-threatening **arrhythmias.** Have similar principles to pacemakers but are described by a different coding system (Table 20). Depending on the patient's arrhythmia, they may respond with anti-tachycardia pacing, anti-bradycardia pacing, a low-energy synchronised shock (<5 J) or a high-energy unsynchronised shock. Have been shown to improve survival in patients with **cardiomyopathy** and those with left ventricular ejection fraction <35%, e.g. in **cardiac failure.** Of particular concern during surgery is the potential for electromagnetic interference (e.g. from surgical **diathermy**) to be misinterpreted as **VF** or **VT**, causing inappropriate discharge of the defibrillator. Defibrillator function may be disabled either by preoperative reprogramming of the ICD or intraoperative application of a magnet. The latter may have unpredictable effects on the ICD and this should be confirmed with the ICD manufacturer before use.

Anaesthetic management for insertion is similar to that for pacemakers.

Stone ME, Salter B, Fischer A (2011). Br J Anaesth; 107 (suppl 1): i16–26

Deflation reflex. Stimulation of inspiration by lung deflation, initiated by **pulmonary stretch receptors.** Of uncertain significance in humans.
See also, Hering–Breuer reflex

Degrees of freedom. In **statistics**, the number of observations in a sample that can vary independently of other observations. For *n* observations, each observation may be compared with *n* – 1 others; i.e., degrees of freedom = *n* – 1. For chi-squared analysis, it equals the product of (number of rows – 1) and (number of columns – 1).

Dehydration. Reflects loss of water from **ECF**, alone or with **intracellular fluid** (ICF) depletion. Sodium is usually lost concurrently, giving rise to **hypernatraemia** or **hyponatraemia**, depending on the relative degrees of loss. If ECF **osmolality** rises, water passes from ICF into ECF by **osmosis**. A predominant water loss is shared by both ICF and ECF; water and sodium loss is borne mainly by ECF if osmolality is not greatly affected. Thus fever, lack of intake, **diabetes insipidus** and osmotic diuresis (mainly water loss) may be tolerated for longer periods than severe vomiting, diarrhoea, intestinal obstruction and diuretic therapy (water and sodium loss), although reduced water intake often accompanies the latter conditions.

The physiological response to dehydration includes increased thirst, **vasopressin** secretion and **renin/angiotensin system** activation, and CVS compensation for **hypovolaemia** via **osmoreceptor** and **baroreceptor** mechanisms.

Children are particularly prone to dehydration, as they exchange a greater proportion of body water each day.

- Clinical features are related to the extent of water loss:
  - 5% of body weight: thirst, dry mouth.
  - 5%–10% of body weight: decreased intraocular pressure, peripheral perfusion and skin turgor, **oliguria**, orthostatic hypotension. **JVP/CVP** are reduced.
  - 10%–15%: shock, coma.

Blood **urea** and **haematocrit** are increased, and urine has high osmolality (over 300 mosmol/kg) and low sodium content (under 10 mmol/l), assuming normal renal function.

Treatment includes oral and **iv fluid administration**; in the latter, dextrose solutions are favoured for combinations of ICF and ECF losses and electrolyte solutions for ECF losses alone. Dehydration should be corrected preoperatively.
See also, Fluid balance; Fluids, body

Delirium in the ICU, *see Confusion in the intensive care unit*

Delirium tremens (DTs). **Alcohol withdrawal syndrome** seen in chronic heavy drinkers. Occurs in about 5% of cases. Thought to be caused by reduction in both inhibitory **$GABA_A$** activity and presynaptic sympathetic inhibition; **hypomagnesaemia** and **hypocalcaemia** may contribute to CNS hyperexcitability. Characterised by:

- tremor, agitation.
- fluctuating disturbance of attention and cognition, disorientation, hallucinations (usually visual).
- sweating, tachycardia, hypertension.
- **dehydration.**

Usually occurs 2–3 days after withdrawal of alcohol, and lasts 3–4 days. May thus occur perioperatively.

Treatment includes: rehydration; correction of hypoglycaemia and electrolyte imbalance; and sedation. **Benzodiazepines** are the agents of choice, although **carbamazepine** and **phenobarbital** have also been used. Prevention is important and is achieved with the same drugs.
Schuckit MA (2014). N Engl J Med; 371: 2109–13

Demand valves. Valves that allow self-administration of **inhalational anaesthetic agents**; they may form part of **intermittent-flow anaesthetic machines**, or be used to administer **Entonox**. The standard Entonox valve was developed from underwater breathing apparatus, and contains a two-stage **pressure regulator** within one unit that fits directly to the **cylinder**. The first-stage regulator is like those on anaesthetic machines. At the second stage, gas flow is prevented by a rod that seals the valve. The patient's inspiratory effort moves a sensing diaphragm and tilts the rod, opening the valve. Very small negative pressures are required to produce gas flow of up to 300 l/min. The mouthpiece/mask elbow piece incorporates an expiratory valve and a safety (overpressure) valve. Other demand valves for use with Entonox have the second-stage (demand) regulator attached to the patient's mask.

Demeclocycline hydrochloride. Tetracycline, used as an **antibacterial drug** and to treat the **syndrome of inappropriate ADH secretion** (SIADH), possibly by blocking the renal action of **vasopressin.**

- Dosage:
  - infection: 150 mg qds or 300 mg bd orally.
  - SIADH: 600–1200 mg/day in divided doses, orally.
- Side effects: as for tetracycline.

Demyelinating diseases. Heterogeneous group of diseases in which damage to the **myelin** sheath of **neurons** results in defective **nerve conduction**. May affect the CNS or the peripheral nervous system.

- CNS demyelinating diseases:
  - myelinoclastic disorders (myelin is damaged by inflammatory or immune factors):
    - multiple sclerosis (MS):
      - most common demyelinating disease. Affects women 2–3 times more commonly than men. Exact aetiology is unknown but it is considered an autoimmune condition in which autoreactive T-lymphocytes infiltrate the **blood–brain barrier** resulting in inflammation and destruction of myelin. Genetic factors play a role, as members of families affected by MS are more likely to develop the disease. Environmental factors include geography (MS becomes more common the further away from the equator), leading to the suggestion that vitamin D deficiency may play a role. Viral factors implicated include the Epstein–Barr and measles viruses.
      - characterised by plaques of demyelination occurring throughout the CNS, with preservation of axon continuity. Optic nerve, brainstem and spinal cord are particularly affected, with sparing of peripheral nerves. Lesions are separated temporally and spatially, producing a variable clinical picture. Common presentations include limb weakness, spasticity, hyperreflexia, visual disturbances, paraesthesia and incoordination. Progression is variable, with relapses associated with trauma, infection, stress and rise in body temperature.
      - diagnosed clinically, supported by gadolinium-enhanced MRI findings and the presence of

oligoclonal IgG bands in the CSF. **Evoked potential** testing may support the diagnosis.
    - treatment is supportive, but often includes **corticosteroids**. Disease-modifying therapies include interferon beta, glatiramer, natalizumab and fingolimod.
    - anaesthetic implications are unclear, because effects of stress, surgery and anaesthesia cannot be separated from the spontaneity of new lesion formation. Thus case reports are often conflicting in their conclusions. Increases in body temperature should be avoided; avoidance of **anticholinergic drugs** has been suggested. An abnormal response to **neuromuscular blocking drugs**, including **hyperkalaemia** following **suxamethonium**, has been suggested but without direct evidence. Prolonged muscle spasms may occur, but epilepsy is rare. Increased tendency to **DVT** has been suggested. Impairment of respiratory and autonomic control has been reported. Although not contraindicated, **epidural** or **spinal anaesthesia** has sometimes been avoided for medicolegal reasons, although it is increasingly used as the preferred method of **obstetric analgesia and anaesthesia**.
  - a variety of similar conditions, including forms of neuromyelitis, encephalomyelitis and optic neuritis (some may be considered variants of MS).
- leukodystrophic disorders (myelin not properly produced):
  - **vitamin** $\mathbf{B_{12}}$ deficiency.
  - **central pontine myelinolysis**.
  - progressive multifocal leukoencephalopathy.
  - leukodystophies.
- Peripheral nervous system demyelinating diseases:
  - **Guillain–Barré syndrome** and chronic inflammatory demyelinating polyneuropathy.
  - Charcot–Marie–Tooth disease: a hereditary sensorimotor neuropathy.

[M Anthony Epstein, British pathologist; Yvonne Barr (1932–2016), British virologist; Jean M Charcot (1825–1893), French neurologist; Pierre Marie (1853–1940), French neurologist; Henry Tooth (1856–1925), English physician]

Denervation hypersensitivity. Increased sensitivity of denervated skeletal **muscle** to **acetylcholine**. Develops approximately 4–5 days after denervation, and is due to proliferation of extrajunctional acetylcholine receptors over the entire muscle membrane, instead of being restricted to the **neuromuscular junction**. Thought to be the mechanism underlying the exaggerated hyperkalaemic response to **suxamethonium** seen after peripheral nerve injuries. Its cause is unclear. Also occurs in smooth muscle.

Density. For a substance, defined as its **mass** per unit volume. Relative density (**specific gravity**) is the mass of any volume of substance divided by the mass of the same volume of water.

Dental injury, *see Teeth*

Dental nerve blocks, *see Mandibular nerve blocks; Maxillary nerve blocks*

Dental surgery. Anaesthesia may be required for tooth extraction, conservative dental surgery or **maxillofacial surgery**.

- For outpatient ambulatory surgery, the following may be used:
  - **mandibular** and **maxillary nerve blocks**.
  - **relative analgesia**.
  - iv **sedation**.
  - **inhalational anaesthetic agents**, including $\mathbf{N_2O}$ and/or volatile agents. Traditionally administered from **intermittent-flow anaesthetic machines**, using **nasal inhalers**, although continuous-flow machines are increasingly used. **Quantiflex apparatus** is also used. Occupational exposure to N_2O is a hazard, especially in small dental surgeries.
  - **iv anaesthetic agents**.

The use of general anaesthesia for dental surgery is declining, with local anaesthetic techniques becoming more common, especially for conservative dentistry. General anaesthesia is usually reserved for patients who have learning difficulties or extreme anxiety, children, those undergoing multiple extractions and those with local infection (infiltration is less effective, and may spread infection). Because of safety concerns, general anaesthesia is now provided by anaesthetists within hospitals, in the UK.

- General anaesthetic principles are as for **day-case surgery**; main problems:
  - high proportion of children, usually anxious and unpremedicated.
  - shared airway as for **ENT surgery**. **Airway obstruction**, mouth breathing during nasally administered anaesthesia, airway soiling and breath-holding may occur. For these reasons the traditional nasal inhaler (masklike device held over the nose from behind the patient's head) is now rarely used by hospital anaesthetists.
  - the risk of hypotension in the sitting position must be weighed against that of airway soiling if supine; the semi-sitting position with the legs raised is often used as a compromise.
  - **arrhythmias** may arise from use of **adrenaline** solutions, stimulation of the trigeminal nerve, anxiety and hypercapnia.

Mouth packs may be employed to prevent airway soiling. They should be placed under the tongue, pushing the tongue back to seal the mouth from the airway. **Mouth gags** or props are often used to hold the mouth open.

Dental surgery is performed on an inpatient surgery basis if airway obstruction, cardiac or respiratory disease, **coagulation disorders** or extreme **obesity** is present. Nasotracheal intubation is usually performed, and a throat pack placed. Use of concentrated adrenaline solutions (e.g. 1:80 000) by dentists is still common, despite anaesthetists' objections.

Depolarising neuromuscular blockade (Phase I block). Follows depolarisation of the postsynaptic membrane of the **neuromuscular junction** via activation of **acetylcholine receptors**, but with only slow repolarisation. Effect of depolarisation of presynaptic receptors is unclear, but may be partially responsible for the **fasciculation** seen. **Suxamethonium** is the most commonly used and widely available drug; previously used drugs include **decamethonium** and **suxethonium**.

- Features of depolarising blockade:
  - may be preceded by fasciculation.
  - does not exhibit **fade** or **post-tetanic potentiation**.
  - increased by **acetylcholinesterase inhibitors**.
  - potentiated by respiratory **alkalosis**, **hypothermia**, **hyperkalaemia** and **hypermagnesaemia**.

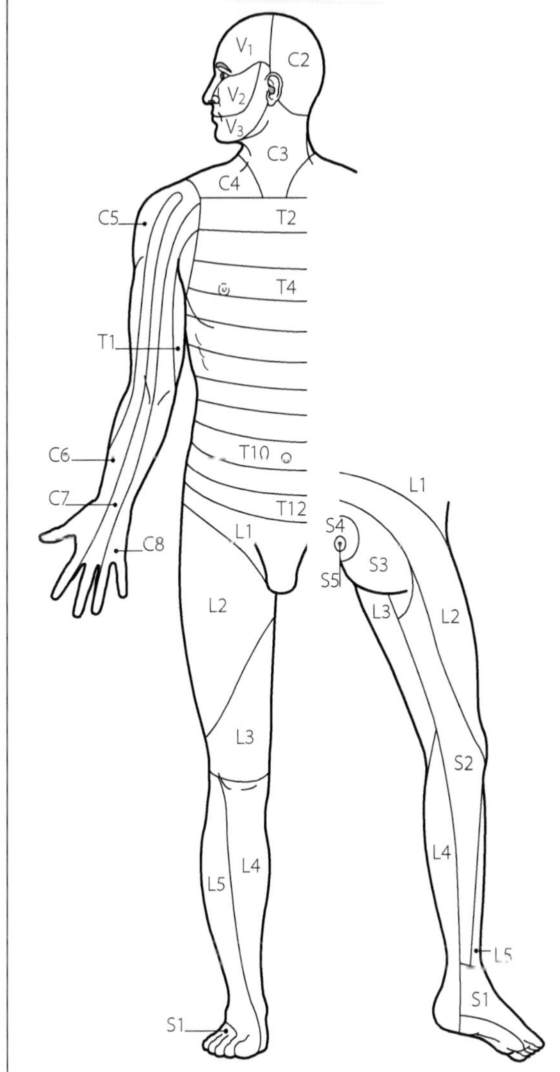

Fig. 53 Dermatomal nerve supply

- antagonised by non-depolarising neuromuscular blocking drugs.
- development of **dual block** with excessive dosage of drug.

See also, Neuromuscular blockade monitoring; Non-depolarising neuromuscular blockade

Depth of anaesthesia monitoring, *see Anaesthesia, depth of*

Dermatomes. Lateral walls of somites (segmental units appearing longitudinally early in embryonic development), which form the skin and subcutaneous tissues. Cutaneous sensation retains the somatic distribution, corresponding to segmental spinal levels. Thus, areas of skin are supplied by particular **spinal nerves**; useful in determining the extent of regional anaesthetic blocks and localising neurological lesions (Fig. 53).
See also, Myotomes

Dermatomyositis, *see Polymyositis*

Desensitisation block, *see Dual block*

```
      F   H         F
      |   |         |
  F — C — C — O — C — H
      |   |         |
      F   F         F
```

Fig. 54 Structure of desflurane

Desferrioxamine mesylate. **Chelating agent** used in the treatment of **iron poisoning** and iron overload (e.g. following repeated transfusions in **thalassaemia** major). Also used in aluminium poisoning. Deferiprone and deferasirox are alternative chelating agents.

- Dosage: 15 mg/kg/h iv to a maximum of 80 mg/kg/24 h. For iron overload: 20–50 mg/kg/day given over 8–12 h, 3–7 times per week.
- Side effects: anaphylaxis, hypotension, tachycardia, thrombocytopenia, visual and hearing loss.

Desflurane. 1-Fluoro-2,2,2-trifluoroethyl difluoromethyl ether. **Inhalational anaesthetic agent**, synthesised in the 1960s but only introduced in the UK in 1994. Chemical structure is the same as **isoflurane**, but with the chlorine atom replaced by fluorine (Fig. 54).

- Properties:
  - colourless liquid with slightly pungent vapour.
  - mw 168.
  - boiling point 23°C.
  - **SVP** at 20°C 88 kPa (673 mmHg).
  - **partition coefficients**:
    - blood/gas 0.42.
    - oil/gas 19.
  - **MAC** 5%–7% in adults; 7.2%–10.7% in children.
  - non-flammable, non-corrosive.
  - supplied in liquid form with no additive.
  - may react with dry **soda lime** to produce **carbon monoxide** (*see Circle systems*).
  - requires the use of an electrically powered **vaporiser** due to its low boiling point.
- Effects:
  - CNS:
    - rapid induction (although limited by its irritant properties) and recovery.
    - EEG changes as for isoflurane.
    - may increase **cerebral blood flow**, although the response of cerebral vessels to CO_2 is preserved.
    - **ICP** may increase due to imbalance between the production and absorption of **CSF**.
    - reduces **CMRO$_2$** as for isoflurane.
    - has poor analgesic properties.
  - RS:
    - causes airway irritation; not recommended for induction of anaesthesia because respiratory complications (e.g. laryngospasm, breath-holding, cough, apnoea) are common and may be severe.
    - respiratory depressant, with increased rate and decreased tidal volume.
  - CVS:
    - vasodilatation and hypotension may occur, similar to isoflurane. May cause tachycardia and hypertension via sympathetic stimulation, especially if high concentrations are introduced rapidly.
    - myocardial ischaemia may occur if sympathetic stimulation is excessive, but has cardioprotective effects in patients undergoing cardiac surgery.

- arrhythmias uncommon, as for isoflurane. Little myocardial sensitisation to catecholamines.
- renal and hepatic blood flow generally preserved.
- other:
  - dose-dependent uterine relaxation (although less than isoflurane and sevoflurane).
  - skeletal muscle relaxation; **non-depolarising neuromuscular blockade** may be potentiated.
  - may precipitate **MH**.

Only 0.02% metabolised.

3%–6% is usually adequate for maintenance of anaesthesia, with higher concentrations for induction. Uptake and excretion are rapid because of its low blood gas solubility; thus it has been suggested as the agent of choice in **day-case surgery**, although this is controversial. Although more expensive than isoflurane, less drug is required to maintain anaesthesia once equilibrium is reached, and equilibrium is reached much more quickly; it may therefore be more economical for use during longer procedures.

Desmopressin (1-desamino-8-D-argininevasopressin; DDAVP). Analogue of **vasopressin**, with a longer-lasting antidiuretic effect but minimal vasoconstrictor actions. Used to diagnose and treat non-nephrogenic **diabetes insipidus**. May also be used to increase factor VIII and von Willebrand factor levels by 2–4 times in mild **haemophilia** or **von Willebrand's disease**. Has also been used to improve platelet function in **renal failure** and to reduce blood loss in **cardiac surgery**.

- Dosage:
  - diabetes insipidus: 10–20 μg od/bd, intranasally; 100–200 μg orally tds; or 1–4 μg/day iv/sc/im.
  - to increase factor VIII levels: 0.4 μg/kg in 50 ml saline iv 1 h preoperatively, repeated at 4 and 24 h.
- Side effects: fluid retention, **hyponatraemia**, pallor, abdominal cramps, and angina in susceptible patients.

Dew point. Temperature at which ambient air is saturated with water vapour. As air containing water vapour cools (e.g. when it is in contact with a cold surface) condensation occurs when the dew point is reached (e.g. misting on the surface of spectacles on entering a warm room from the cold). This process may be used to measure **humidity**.

Dexamethasone. Corticosteroid with high **glucocorticoid** but minimal mineralocorticoid activity and long duration of action, thus used where sustained activity is required but when water retention would be harmful, e.g. **cerebral oedema**. Also used in congenital adrenal hyperplasia, to reduce oedema following ENT surgery, in **meningitis** and in the diagnosis of **Cushing's disease**. Other uses include prevention and treatment of **PONV**, and stimulation of fetal lung maturation in premature labour.

- Dosage:
  - 0.5–10 mg orally od.
  - 0.5–20 mg iv (10 mg followed by 4 mg qds in cerebral oedema; 4 mg to prevent PONV).
- Side effects: as for corticosteroids.

Dexmedetomidine hydrochloride. Selective **α-adrenergic receptor agonist**, with about 1300–1600 times the affinity for α_2-receptors as for α_1. Rapidly distributed after iv injection (**half-life** about 6 min) with an elimination half-life of 2–2.5 h. **Volume of distribution** is about 1.3 l/kg. 94% protein-bound. Inactivated mainly to glucuronides with 80%–90% excreted in the urine. Has similar effects to **clonidine** but more predictable and easier to titrate, e.g. for **sedation** in ICU. Has also been used via the intranasal route for anxiolytic premedication in children. Effects can be reversed by **atipamezole**.

- Dosage:
  - sedation: 0.7 μg/kg/h iv, adjusted according to response (usual range 0.2–1.4 μg/kg/h).
  - anxiolytic premedication: 1–2 μg/kg intranasally, ~30 minutes before surgery.
- Side effects: as for clonidine. May cause hypertension at high doses via peripheral vasoconstriction. May also reduce renal blood flow. Has little direct effect on respiration.

Dextrans. Group of branched polysaccharides of 200 000 glucose units, derived from the action of bacteria (*Leuconostoc mesenteroides*) on sucrose. Partial hydrolysis produces molecules of average mw 40 kDa, 70 kDa and 110 kDa (dextrans 40, 70 and 110, respectively). Dextran 40 is used to promote peripheral blood flow, e.g. in arterial insufficiency and in prophylaxis of **DVT**. Dextrans 70 and 110 are used mainly for plasma expansion; the latter is now rarely used and is unavailable in the UK. Dextrans increase peripheral blood flow by reducing **viscosity**, and may coat both endothelium and cellular elements of blood, reducing their interaction. They reduce **platelet** adhesiveness, possibly impair factor VIII activity and may have anti-inflammatory properties.

Size of dextran molecules is directly proportional to the degree of plasma expansion produced and the molecules' circulation time. **Half-life** ranges from 15 min for small molecules to several days for larger ones. Major route of excretion is via the kidneys.

Supplied in 5% dextrose or 0.9% saline, as 6% (dextrans 70 and 110) or 10% (dextran 40) solutions. Dextran 70 is also supplied as a 6% solution in hypertonic saline (7.5%); 250 ml given over 2–5 min should be followed immediately by isotonic fluids.

- Side effects:
  - **renal failure** caused by tubular obstruction by dextran casts; mainly occurs with dextran 40 when used in **hypovolaemia**; concurrent water and electrolyte administration should be provided.
  - **anaphylaxis**: thought to result from previous cross-immunisation against bacterial antigens. Its incidence is reduced from 1:4500 to 1:84 000 by pretreatment with 3 g dextran 1 (mw 1000), to occupy and block antigen binding sites of circulating antibodies to dextran.
  - interference with **blood compatibility testing**.
  - bleeding tendency. Initial administration should be limited to 500–1000 ml, and the total amount administered restricted to 10 (dextran 40) and 20 (dextran 70) ml/kg/day.
  - osmotic diuresis.

See also, Colloids

Dextromoramide tartrate. Opioid analgesic drug, related to **methadone**. Introduced in 1956. Less sedating, and shorter acting (duration 2–3 h) than **morphine**, but with similar effects. No longer available in the UK.

Dextropropoxyphene hydrochloride/napsilate. Opioid analgesic drug, related to **methadone**. Synthesised in 1953. Poorly effective alone, but effective when combined with **paracetamol** (as co-proxamol). Overdose of this combination is particularly dangerous; initial respiratory depression and coma (due to dextropropoxyphene) may be treated correctly but later liver failure (due to **paracetamol poisoning**) may occur if appropriate prophylaxis is not given. Safety concerns, even at or just above normal doses, led to the phased withdrawal of co-proxamol from the UK in 2005.

Dextrose solutions. **Intravenous fluids** available as 5%, 10%, 20%, 25% and 50% solutions in water (50, 100, 200, 250 and 500 g/l, respectively). Once administered, the glucose is rapidly metabolised and the water distributed to all body fluid compartments. Thus used in **hypoglycaemia**, and to replace water losses. Also used with **insulin** to treat acute hyperkalaemia.

Excess administration may result in **hyponatraemia**. Solutions of higher concentrations are increasingly hypertonic, acidic and viscous; they may cause thrombophlebitis if infused peripherally. Osmolality of 5% dextrose solution is 278 mosmol/kg; of 10% solution 523 mosmol/kg. pH of 5% solution is approximately 4.0. May cause haemolysis of stored erythrocytes when infused iv immediately before stored blood without first flushing the line with saline, presumably because the dextrose is taken up and metabolised by the cells to leave a hypo-osmotic solution.

See also, Fluids, body; Intravenous fluid administration

Dezocine. Synthetic **opioid analgesic drug**, related to **pentazocine**; available in the USA until 2011. Comparable in potency, onset and duration of action to **morphine**. Has some **opioid receptor antagonist** activity, less than that of **nalorphine** but greater than that of **pentazocine**.

Diabetes insipidus. Polyuria and polydipsia associated with reduced **vasopressin** activity, either because secretion by the **pituitary gland** is reduced (cranial/neurogenic) or the kidneys are unresponsive (nephrogenic):

- cranial: occurs in **head injury**, **neurosurgery** (especially post-pituitary surgery), intracranial tumours. Rarely familial.
- nephrogenic: caused by drugs, e.g. **lithium**, **demeclocycline** and **gentamicin**; a rare X-linked recessive form may also occur.

Characterised by inappropriate production of large volumes of dilute urine, with raised plasma **osmolality**. Patients cannot concentrate their urine in response to water deprivation. The two types are distinguished by their response to administered vasopressin.

- Treatment:
  - cranial: **desmopressin** (synthetic vasopressin analogue) 10–20 µg od/bd intranasally; 100–200 µg orally tds; or 1–4 µg/day iv/sc/im.
  - nephrogenic: **thiazide diuretics**.

Anaesthetic considerations are related to impaired **fluid balance** with **hypovolaemia**, **dehydration**, **hypernatraemia** and other electrolyte imbalance. Careful attention to **fluid balance**, with monitoring of urine and plasma osmolality and electrolytes, is required.

Diabetes mellitus. Disorder of **glucose** metabolism characterised by relative or total lack of **insulin** or insulin resistance. This results in lipolysis, gluconeogenesis and glycogenolysis, with hepatic conversion of fatty acids to **ketone bodies**, and **hyperglycaemia**. The resultant glycosuria causes an osmotic diuresis, with polyuria, polydipsia and excessive sodium and potassium loss.

Affects 6%–7% of the UK population and about 10%–15% of the hospital inpatient population.

- May be:
  - primary: thought to be related to genetic, infective and immunological factors, but the aetiology is unclear.
  - secondary:
    - pancreatic disease, e.g. **pancreatitis**, malignancy.
    - insulin antagonism, e.g. **corticosteroids**, **Cushing's syndrome**, **acromegaly**, **phaeochromocytoma**.
    - drugs, e.g. **thiazide diuretics**.

Classically divided into type 1 (insulin-dependent; IDDM), presenting in children or young adults, and type 2 (non–insulin-dependent; NIDDM), presenting in adults (and occasionally children) who are usually obese. Type 1 DM is an autoimmune disease, with 85% of patients having antibodies against pancreatic islet cells, and results in low or absent circulating insulin; treatment is with exogenous insulin. Type 2 DM is due to a relative lack of insulin and insulin resistance and is caused by excessive calorie intake and obesity in genetically susceptible individuals, it is treated with diet control, oral hypoglycaemic drugs (**sulfonylureas**, **biguanides**, **acarbose**, **thiazolidinediones** and **meglitinides**), a combination of oral hypoglycaemic drugs and insulin, or insulin alone.

The World Health Organization suggests the following diagnostic criteria:

- symptoms + plasma glucose concentration >11.1 mmol/l,
- or two fasting glucose concentrations >7.0 mmol/l,
- or glucose concentration >11.1 mmol/l, 2 h after ingestion of glucose in a **glucose tolerance test**.

Since 2011, a glycated haemoglobin (HbA1c) level >6.5% (48 mmol/mol) can be used to diagnose type 2 DM (but not in children/young people, patients with symptoms <2 months, those requiring hospital admission, those taking drugs known to increase glucose levels e.g. steroids, or those with acute pancreatic damage). However, patients with a level below this may still fulfil other criteria for DM.

- Complications:
  - renal impairment, caused by glomerulosclerosis, vascular insufficiency, infection and papillary necrosis.
  - arteriosclerosis causing **ischaemic heart disease**, peripheral vascular insufficiency and **stroke**. Microvascular involvement may cause **cardiac failure** and impaired ventricular function. **Hypertension** is more common than in non-diabetic subjects.
  - **autonomic** and **peripheral neuropathy**, the latter sensory or motor. Single nerves may also be affected, including **cranial nerves**.
  - retinopathy and cataract formation.
  - skin: collagen thickening, blisters, necrobiosis lipoidica.
  - increased susceptibility to infection and delayed wound healing.
  - **diabetic coma**.
  - syndrome of stiff joints may occur: suggested by the 'prayer sign' (inability to press the palmar surfaces of the index fingers fully flat against one another when pressing the palms together). Has been associated with difficult tracheal intubation and reduced compliance of the epidural space.
- Anaesthetic management:
  - all patients: perioperative management is related to the complications mentioned earlier and to the control of blood sugar. Patients should be assessed for fitness and diabetic control in the pre-anaesthetic assessment clinic and medication optimised (confirmed with HbA1c levels). Where possible, day surgery should

be performed (thus reducing the chances of iatrogenic harm, infection, etc.) and self-medication promoted because many patients have a better knowledge of their medication needs than medical or nursing staff. Insulin sliding scale infusions should be avoided unless there is poor glycaemic control or a period of prolonged starvation (i.e., missing two meals) is anticipated. Patients should be scheduled for surgery at the beginning of the operating list. The aim is to avoid hyperglycaemia, **ketoacidosis**, **hypoglycaemia** and electrolyte imbalance, all of which are associated with worse outcomes.

- NIDDM: for minor surgery, monitoring of blood sugar levels is usually all that is required. Chlorpropamide is withheld for 48 h before surgery; shorter-acting sulfonylureas and biguanides are withheld on the morning of surgery. A glucose level of 4–12 mmol/l is acceptable, although tighter control, aiming for 6–10 mmol/l, is considered ideal. Patients are treated as for IDDM when undergoing major/emergency surgery. Oral medication is restarted when oral calorie intake is resumed postoperatively.
- IDDM: patients are starved preoperatively, with morning insulin omitted. They should receive insulin and dextrose iv throughout the perioperative period, to avoid hyper- and hypoglycaemia and maintain plasma glucose between 6 and 10 mmol/l. Dextrose and insulin infusions should be through the same iv cannula, to reduce risk of accidental overdose of one infusion should the other infusion cease running. Several regimens are used:
  - Alberti regimen: 1000 ml 10% dextrose + 10 units soluble insulin + 10 mmol potassium infused at 100 ml/h. The infusion is changed to contain more or less insulin according to regular testing with **glucose reagent sticks**. The preoperative insulin regimen is restarted when the patient is drinking and eating normally.
  - the total daily insulin requirement is divided by four, adding the result to 500 ml 5% dextrose + 5–10 mmol potassium. The bag is infused at 100 ml/h, with regular checking of blood glucose levels.
  - variable-rate iv insulin infusions: generally preferred for patients who will miss more than one meal, those with poor control, and those undergoing emergency surgery. The rate of infusion is adjusted according to a sliding scale, with dextrose (e.g. 5% 500 ml + 5–10 mmol potassium at 100 ml/h) given concurrently.

Because the symptoms of hypoglycaemia are masked by general anaesthesia, regular perioperative monitoring of plasma glucose is required. Lactate-containing solutions are often avoided as they may increase plasma glucose levels, although actual increases are small unless large volumes are given.

Regional techniques are often preferred because they interfere less with oral intake. Insulin requirements may be increased after major surgery as part of the **stress response to surgery**.

Emergency surgery is particularly hazardous, especially if diabetes is poorly controlled. Adequate resuscitation must be performed, with treatment of ketoacidosis if present. Hyperglycaemia may present with abdominal pain, and abdominal surgery may reveal no abnormality.

Pregnancy may precipitate or worsen diabetes, and close medical supervision is required. During labour, regimens usually involve iv infusions of 5% dextrose (e.g. 500 ml/8 h) with iv insulin rate adjusted accordingly. **Epidural anaesthesia** is usually suggested, because it reduces acidosis in labour and facilitates **caesarean section** if indicated.

Although glucose level variability in ICU patients is associated with increased morbidity and mortality, the suggested benefits of 'tight' glucose control (4.4–6.2 mmol/l) have been negated by the NICE-SUGAR study, which showed increased mortality related to an increased incidence of hypoglycaemia. More permissive levels of blood sugar (i.e., up to 10 mmol/l) are now considered appropriate.

[K George MM Alberti, Newcastle physician]

Barker P, Creasey PE, Dhatariya K, et al (2015). Anaesthesia; 70: 1427–40

Diabetic coma. **Coma** in diabetes mellitus may be caused by:

- **hypoglycaemia**: caused by overdose of hypoglycaemic agent, excessive exertion or decreased food intake. Treatment includes iv glucose; iv/im **glucagon** may occasionally be useful in out-of-hospital situations.
- diabetic **ketoacidosis** (DKA): more common in insulin-dependent diabetics. Diagnostic triad consists of: ketonaemia (>3 mmol/l) or significant ketonuria; blood glucose >11 mmol/l or known diabetes mellitus; and bicarbonate <15 mmol/l and/or venous pH <7.3. Glucose levels may be normal in those chronically undernourished. May be the first presentation of diabetes but is usually due to underlying infection or illness (e.g. **MI**) or missed **insulin** dose in a known diabetic. Accounts for 2% of admissions to UK ICUs. Mortality is >5%, higher in old age.
  - features:
    - of **dehydration**, e.g. hypotension, tachycardia.
    - of **acidosis**, e.g. hyperventilation (**Kussmaul breathing**).
    - vomiting, diarrhoea, abdominal pain; the last may simulate an acute surgical emergency, requiring careful review of the diagnosis.
    - smell of acetone on the breath.
  - management:
    - measurement of urea and electrolytes, glucose, arterial blood gases, full blood count. Urine dipstick for ketones and nitrites. CXR and blood cultures.
    - general management: O_2 and airway control if required; nasogastric tube (gastric dilatation is common); urinary catheter; **CVP** measurement; ECG and other standard monitoring. Antibiotics are administered if infection is suspected. Prophylactic low-molecular-weight **heparin** is routinely given.
    - fluid therapy: up to 6–8 l may be required. Suitable starting regimen: 1l of 0.9% saline over 30 min, then hourly for 2 h, then 2-hourly, then 2–4-hourly. This is changed to 5% dextrose when blood glucose is 10–15 mmol/l (180–270 mg/dl). Hypotonic saline is used in hyperosmolar coma (see later).
    - potassium supplementation is required despite any initial **hyperkalaemia**, because the body potassium deficit will be revealed once tissue uptake is stimulated by insulin. Suitable starting regimen: 10–20 mmol in the first litre of fluid; 10–40 mmol thereafter, depending on the plasma potassium after 1 h (repeated every few hours).

Table 21 Features of different types of diabetic coma

Type	*Blood glucose (mmol/l)*	*Dehydration*	*Ketones*
Hypoglycaemia	<2	0	0
Ketoacidosis	>14	+++	++
Hyperosmolar non-ketotic	>14	+++	0
Lactic acidosis	Variable	+	0 to +

- insulin should be given using a fixed-rate iv infusion, which results in a safer and faster resolution of DKA than the classical variable rate. A rate of 0.1 units/kg/h is given, aiming for a reduction of blood ketone levels by >0.5 mmol/l/h (or an increase of venous bicarbonate by 3 mmol/l/h).
- **hypophosphataemia** may require replacement, e.g. with potassium phosphate, 5–20 mmol/h.

- hyperosmolar non-ketotic coma: typically seen in elderly patients with type 2 diabetes mellitus and presents with slow onset with polyuria and progressive dehydration. Focal neurological features may occur. Blood glucose levels and osmolality are very high, with little or no ketonuria. Treatment includes small doses of insulin and 0.45% saline administered slowly iv. **Cerebral oedema** and **convulsions** may occur if rehydration is too rapid; both are more common in children.
- **lactic acidosis**: usually occurs in elderly patients taking **biguanides**. Blood glucose may be normal, with little or no ketonuria.

Clinical distinction between different types of diabetic coma is unreliable. Features aiding the diagnosis are shown in Table 21.

Van Ness-Otunnu R, Hack JB (2013). J Emerg Med; 45: 797–805

Diagnostic peritoneal lavage, *see Peritoneal lavage*

Dialysis. Artificial removal of water and solutes from the blood by selective **diffusion** across a semipermeable membrane. Indications include **renal failure** and severe **cardiac failure** unresponsive to diuretic therapy; may also remove drugs from the circulation in **poisoning and overdoses**, although only effective for smaller, non-protein-bound, water-soluble molecules. Collectively termed renal replacement therapy; many variants exist but they may be classified into:

- **peritoneal dialysis**.
- intermittent **haemodialysis**.
- continuous **haemodiafiltration**.

All techniques rely on the diffusion of water and solutes across a semipermeable membrane; this passage may be manipulated by altering the hydrostatic or osmotic gradients across the membrane to optimise removal. In **haemoperfusion**, unwanted molecules (including lipid-soluble protein-bound ones) are adsorbed onto activated charcoal or an ion exchange resin, thus involving a different principle from that of dialysis. Both dialysis and adsorption techniques have been used to remove circulating toxins in **hepatic failure**, such techniques usually being termed **liver dialysis**.

Gemmell L, Docking R, Black E (2017). BJA Educ; 17: 88–93

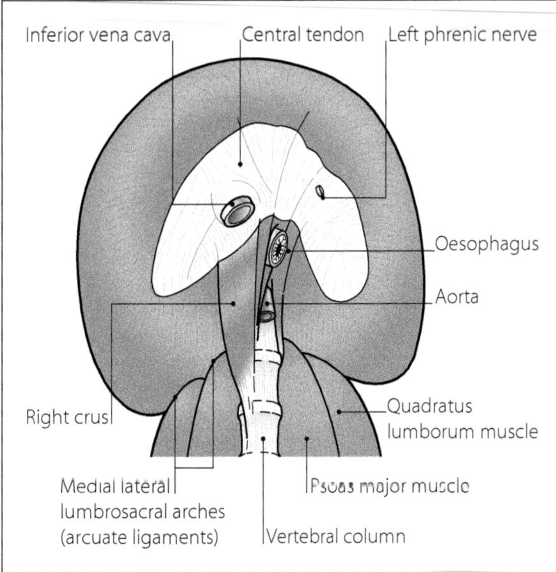

Fig. 55 Inferior aspect of diaphragm

Diamorphine hydrochloride (Diacetylmorphine; Heroin). **Opioid analgesic drug**, introduced in 1898; said to cause less constipation, nausea and hypotension than **morphine**, but more likely to cause addiction. Also suppresses coughing to a greater extent. Used especially in **palliative care**. Inactive prodrug that is rapidly hydrolysed by plasma **cholinesterase** to 6-monoacetylmorphine (responsible for the rapid onset of action), which is then slowly metabolised to morphine in the liver. Unavailable in the USA, Australia and parts of Europe (e.g. Germany) because of its reputation as a drug of addiction, although there is no evidence that medical use increases its abuse.

- Dosage: 5 mg is equivalent to 10 mg morphine. It may be given im, iv, sc, orally, epidurally (1–5 mg) or intrathecally (100–300 μg); also effective given intranasally.

See also, Spinal opioids

Diaphragm. Fibromuscular sheet separating the thorax from the abdomen. The main **respiratory muscle**, it flattens and descends vertically during inspiration, expanding the thoracic cavity. During expiration, it relaxes; in forced expiration, contraction of the anterior abdominal muscles pushes the diaphragm upwards.

- Consists of (Fig. 55):
  - central tendon, attached to the pericardium above.
  - peripheral muscular part. Attachments:
    - posteriorly via the medial and lateral lumbosacral arches (arcuate ligaments), to fascia covering psoas and quadratus lumborum muscles, respectively. The right and left crura attach to vertebrae L1–3 and L1–2, respectively; between them lies the median lumbosacral arch (median arcuate ligament).
    - to the lower six ribs, costal cartilages and xiphisternum anteriorly.
- Has three main openings transmitting the following structures:
  - inferior vena cava and right **phrenic nerve** at the level of T8.
  - **oesophagus**, vagus and gastric nerves and branches of the left gastric vessels at the level of T10.

- aorta, thoracic duct and azygos vein at the level of T12.

The diaphragm is also pierced by the left phrenic nerve and splanchnic nerves.

The sympathetic chain passes behind the medial lumbosacral arch.

- Nerve supply: from C3–5 via the phrenic nerves, with some sensory supply to the periphery via the lower intercostal nerves.
- Development:
  - originally in the neck; descends during development, retaining its cervical nerve supply.
  - formed from:
    - oesophageal mesentery dorsally.
    - right and left pleuroperitoneal membranes laterally.
    - septum transversum anteriorly (forming the central tendon).
    - small peripheral contribution from body wall.

Defects in development may produce **diaphragmatic herniae.**

See also, Hiatus hernia

Diaphragmatic hernia. Herniation of abdominal viscera through the **diaphragm** into the thorax. Congenital herniae occur in approximately 1 in 4000 live births (1 in 2500 of all births), are often familial and are caused by failure of fusion of the various components of the diaphragm, e.g.:

- foramen of Bochdalek: through a defective pleuroperitoneal membrane, usually left-sided. The most common form (80%).
- foramen of Morgagni: between xiphoid and costal origins; more common on the right side.
- through the central tendon or oesophageal hiatus.

Usually diagnosed during routine antenatal ultrasound. Other congenital defects may be present (e.g. cardiac anomalies found in 50%).

Causes respiratory distress, cyanosis, scaphoid abdomen and bowel sounds audible in the thorax. Diagnosed clinically and by x-ray. The lung on the affected side is often hypoplastic, with decreased **compliance** and increased **pulmonary vascular resistance** (PVR). Arterial **hypoxaemia** reflects immature lung tissue and impaired ventilation caused by presence of thoracic bowel, and persistent **fetal circulation** caused by the raised PVR. PVR is further increased by **hypoxic pulmonary vasoconstriction.**

Immediate management includes gastric decompression, improving oxygenation and decreasing PVR. PVR may be reduced by: avoiding **hypocapnia** and **hypothermia**; treating **acidosis**; use of inhaled **nitric oxide** and iv **vasodilator drugs** (e.g. **sodium nitroprusside** 1–2 µg/kg/min, **prostacyclin** 5–10 ng/kg/min).

IPPV by facemask may increase gastric distension and should be avoided. IPPV is best performed via a tracheal tube, avoiding excessive inflation pressures because **pneumothorax** and **ALI** may easily occur. Surgery is usually delayed until respiratory stability is achieved. **High-frequency ventilation** and **extracorporeal membrane oxygenation** have been used. Mortality is high if pneumothorax occurs and lung compliance is low.

Anaesthesia for surgical correction is as for **paediatric anaesthesia.** N_2O is avoided because of distension of thoracic bowel. Excessive inflation of the hypoplastic lung at the end of the procedure should be avoided, because pneumothorax may occur. Abdominal closure may be difficult once the bowel is returned to the abdomen; postoperative IPPV may be required. The hypoplastic lung slowly re-expands, usually within a few days/weeks.

Acquired acute herniae may follow blunt or penetrating **trauma** or surgery. They may impair ventilation, or only cause symptoms if strangulation or obstruction occurs. **Hiatus hernia** is gradual in onset.

[Giovanni B Morgagni (1682–1771), Italian anatomist; Victor A Bochdalek (1801–1883), Czech anatomist]

Bösenberg AT, Brown RA (2008). Curr Opin Anesthesiol; 21: 323–31

See also, Cardiopulmonary resuscitation, neonatal

Diarrhoea. Defined as three or more loose stools per day. Common problem in the ICU and contributes to increased mortality; may result in **dehydration**, electrolyte imbalance, urinary catheter-related infection and skin excoriation, and is upsetting to the patient and relatives. Also increases the burden of nursing care. There are many causes, including:

- infection (e.g. norovirus, *Clostridium difficile*, salmonella, campylobacter species).
- **inflammatory bowel disease.**
- **malabsorption.**
- **bowel ischaemia.**
- drugs (e.g. **antibacterial drugs**, **antifungal drugs**).
- enteral **nutrition.**

Spurious ('overflow') diarrhoea may occur in severe **constipation**. Non-infectious diarrhoea tends to occur without blood or mucus. Stools usually return to normal after the causal agent is removed.

Management includes appropriate investigation (stool cultures and microscopy, sigmoidoscopy; more invasive endoscopy or imaging may be required) and maintenance of fluid and electrolyte balance. Probiotic agents may be useful. Specific causes are managed accordingly. Symptomatic treatment (e.g. with **codeine** or loperamide) may be indicated, although they are generally avoided in children and in infective diarrhoea.

Tirlapur N, Zudin AP, Cooper JA, et al (2016). Sci Rep; 6: 24691

See also, Clostridial infections

Diastole, *see Cardiac cycle; Diastolic interval*

Diastolic blood pressure. Lowest **arterial BP** during diastole. Contributes to **MAP** and represents the pressure head for **coronary blood flow.**

Diastolic BP has been used to guide therapy in **hypertension**, treatment being advocated if it exceeds 90 mmHg.

Diastolic interval. Duration of diastole. Shortened when **heart rate** is increased; e.g. equals about 0.62 s at 65 beats/min, but only 0.14 s at 200 beats/min.

Short diastolic intervals reduce **coronary blood flow** and ventricular filling.

Diastolic pressure time index (DPTI). Area between tracings of left ventricular pressure and aortic root pressure during diastole (*see Fig. 62;* **Endocardial viability ratio**). Represents the pressure head and time available for **coronary blood flow**; used to calculate endocardial viability ratio.

See also, Cardiac cycle

Diathermy (Bovie machine). Device used to coagulate blood vessels and cut/destroy tissues during surgery, using the heating effect of an electric current. Alternating current with a frequency of 0.5–1 MHz is used; a sine wave pattern is employed for cutting and a damped or pulsed sine wave pattern for coagulation. Electrical stimulation of skeletal and cardiac muscle is negligible at these high frequencies. The **current density** is kept high at the site of intended damage by using small electrodes at this site, e.g. forceps tips.

- Diathermy may be:
  - unipolar (monopolar):
    - forceps or 'pencil-point', act as one electrode.
    - large plate strapped to the patient's leg acts as the other electrode, often at earth potential. Current density at this site is low because of the large area of tissue through which current passes, thus little heating occurs.
  - bipolar: current is passed across tissue held between the two tips of a pair of forceps. The power used is small and the current dispersal through other tissues is negligible; thus used for more delicate surgery, e.g. eye surgery and neurosurgery. No plate electrode is required.
- Hazards:
  - interference with **monitoring** equipment.
  - incorrect attachment of the plate may cause burns, e.g. if contact is only made over a small surface area.
  - burns may occur if the surgeon activates the diathermy accidentally, or if the forceps are touching the patient or lying on wet drapes. When not used, the forceps should be kept in a protective non-conducting holder. An audible buzzer warns that the device is operating.
  - if the plate electrode is earthed, and connections are faulty, current may take other routes to reach earth. Thus current may flow through any earthed metal conductor the patient touches (e.g. drip stands, ECG leads), causing burns at the site of contact. In addition, the mains (50 Hz) current may flow through the system. A capacitor within the circuit will prevent the latter, while allowing the diathermy current to flow. Risks from flow of current to earth are reduced if the circuit is completely isolated from earth ('floating'), because current will no longer take these other routes.
  - may act as an ignition source of flammable substances, e.g. anaesthetic agents, bowel gases, alcohol skin preps.
  - may interfere with implantable cardioverter **defibrillators** and **pacemaker** function.

[William T Bovie (1882–1958), US biophysicist]

See also, Cardiac pacing; Electrocution and electrical burns; Explosions and fires

Diazepam. **Benzodiazepine**, widely used for **sedation**, anxiolysis and as an **anticonvulsant drug**. Has been used for premedication, and to supplement or induce anaesthesia. Insoluble in water; original preparations caused pain on injection and thrombophlebitis. These are rare with emulsions of diazepam in soya bean oil.

May cause respiratory depression, especially in the elderly. Reduced cardiac output and vasodilatation occur with large doses. Drowsiness and confusion, especially in the elderly, may persist for several hours. Absorption after im injection is unreliable and the injection is painful.

Half-life is 20–70 h, with formation of active metabolites (that are renally excreted) including nordiazepam (half-life up to 120 h), desmethyldiazepam, oxazepam and **temazepam**. Thus, repeated doses (e.g. in ICU) may lead to delayed recovery.

- Dosage:
  - 10–30 mg orally for premedication (0.5 mg/kg in children, up to 10 mg).
  - 5–10 mg iv for sedation or anticonvulsant effect, repeated as necessary. Rectal administration is also effective.

Diazoxide. **Vasodilator drug**, used for emergency treatment of severe **hypertension**. Acts directly on blood vessel walls by activating potassium channels. Previously indicated in hypertensive crisis, but the risk from sudden reduction in BP has resulted in its indication for iv use being restricted to severe hypertension associated with renal disease. Increases blood **glucose** level by increasing **catecholamine** levels and by reducing **insulin** release; may be used orally to treat chronic **hypoglycaemia** (e.g. in insulinoma).

- Dosage: 1–3 mg/kg (up to 150 mg) iv for hypertension, repeated after 5–15 min if required. **MI** and **stroke** have followed larger doses. For hypoglycaemia, 5 mg/kg/day orally.
- Side effects: tachycardia, **hyperglycaemia**, fluid retention.

Dibucaine, *see Cinchocaine*

Dibucaine number. Degree of inhibition of plasma **cholinesterase** by dibucaine (**cinchocaine**). Sample plasma is added to a benzoylcholine solution, and breakdown of the latter is observed using measurement of light absorption. This is repeated using plasma pretreated with a 10^{-5} molar solution of dibucaine; the percentage inhibition of benzoylcholine breakdown by the enzyme is the dibucaine number. Abnormal variants of cholinesterase are inhibited to lesser degrees, with dibucaine numbers less than the normal 75%–85%. Thus useful in the analysis and typing of different abnormal variants, which may give rise to prolonged paralysis following **suxamethonium** administration.

Similar testing may be performed using inhibition by fluoride, chloride, suxamethonium itself and other compounds.

DIC, *see Disseminated intravascular coagulation*

Dichloroacetate, *see Sodium dichloroacetate*

Dichlorphenamide. **Carbonic anhydrase** inhibitor, used to treat **glaucoma** but also to stimulate respiration, possibly by lowering CSF pH. Actions are like those of **acetazolamide**, but longer lasting. Has been used to assist **weaning** in ICU.

Diclofenac sodium. **NSAID**, commonly used for **postoperative analgesia**, reducing opioid requirements. Also used for musculoskeletal pain and renal colic. Extensively (>99%) protein-bound in plasma; **half-life** is 1–2 h. 60% excreted via urine, the rest passing into the faeces.

- Dosage:
  - 1 mg/kg (up to 75 mg) via deep im injection bd for up to 2 days.
  - 75 mg iv qds for up to 2 days. Should be diluted immediately before use with 100–500 ml 0.9% saline or 5% glucose, which should then be buffered with 0.5 ml 8.4% or 1 ml 4.2% sodium bicarbonate solution. A new preparation, able to be given without buffering or diluting, was introduced in the UK in

2008 but was withdrawn 2 years later because vials were found to contain particulate material.
  - 75–150 mg/day orally/pr in divided doses (1–3 mg/kg in children). A case involving a misplaced diclofenac suppository inserted vaginally and subsequent claims of rape have led to recommendations that all planned suppository insertions should be discussed beforehand with the patient.
- Side effects: as for NSAIDs. Considered to be an intermediate-risk NSAID for gastric side effects and to have the same cardiovascular side effect profile as selective COX-2 inhibitors and high-dose (2.4 g/day) **ibuprofen.** Should be used with caution in renal impairment and asthma. Muscle damage after im injection has been indicated by increased plasma creatine kinase levels. Sterile abscesses have occurred after superficial injection.

Dicobalt edetate, *see Cyanide poisoning*

Dicrotic notch, *see Arterial waveform*

Diethyl ether. $C_2H_5OC_2H_5$. **Inhalational anaesthetic agent**, first prepared in 1540. **Paracelsus** described its effects on chickens in the same year. Produced by heating concentrated sulfuric acid with ethanol. First used for anaesthesia in 1842 by **Clarke** and **Long**, who did not publish their work until later. Introduced publicly by **Morton** in the USA in 1846; used in London by **Boott** and in Dumfries in the same year. Classically given by **open-drop techniques**, and more recently using a **draw-over technique** (e.g. using the EMO **vaporiser**), or by standard plenum vaporiser. Inspired concentrations of up to 20% may be required during induction of anaesthesia.

No longer generally available in the UK, although widely considered one of the safest inhalational agents, largely because respiratory depression is late and precedes cardiovascular depression. Still used worldwide, because of its safety and low cost.

Its many disadvantages include flammability, high blood/gas **partition coefficient** resulting in slow uptake and recovery, respiratory irritation causing coughing and **laryngospasm**, stimulation of salivary secretions, high incidence of nausea and vomiting, and occurrence of convulsions postoperatively, typically associated with pyrexia and **atropine** administration. Sympathetic stimulation maintains BP with low incidence of arrhythmias, but **hyperglycaemia** may occur.

Has been used in severe **asthma** because of its bronchodilator properties.

10%–15% metabolised to alcohol, acetaldehyde and acetic acid.

Differential lung ventilation (DLV). Performed when the requirements of each lung are so different that conventional **IPPV** cannot maintain adequate gas exchange, e.g. because the poor **compliance** of one lung diverts the delivered tidal volume to the other, more compliant, lung. Thus reserved for when lung pathology is unilateral or much worse on one side, e.g. following **aspiration of gastric contents** or irritant substances, unilateral pneumonia, **bronchopleural fistula**. May be performed using two conventional ventilators, each connected to one lumen of a double-lumen **endobronchial tube**. The settings of each (including the ventilatory mode) are adjusted independently to achieve adequate lung expansion and gas exchange; synchronised inflation/deflation is usually not necessary, although sideways motion of the mediastinum (if one lung inflates just as the other deflates) may cause haemodynamic disturbance in susceptible patients. In some circumstances, it may be possible to ventilate the better lung while applying only **CPAP** to the diseased one.

Difficult intubation, *see Intubation, difficult*

Diffusing capacity (Transfer factor). Volume of a substance (usually carbon monoxide [CO]) transferred across the alveoli per minute per unit alveolar partial pressure. CO is used because it is rapidly taken up by **haemoglobin** in the blood; thus its transfer from alveoli to blood is limited mainly by diffusion across the alveolar membrane.
- Measurement:
  - a single breath of gas containing 0.3% CO and 10% helium is held for 10–20 s. Initial alveolar partial pressure of CO is derived by measuring the dilution of helium that has occurred. Expired partial pressure of CO is measured.
  - continuous breathing of gas containing 0.3% CO, for up to a minute. Rate of uptake of CO is measured when steady state is reached.
- Normal value: 17–25 ml/min/mmHg.

Reduction in pulmonary diseases (e.g. **pulmonary fibrosis**) has been traditionally attributed to increased alveolar membrane thickness, although **$\dot{V}/\dot{Q}$ mismatch** may be more important. Also reduced when alveolar membrane area is reduced, e.g. after pneumonectomy (corrected for by calculation of diffusing coefficient: diffusing capacity per litre of available lung volume).

The term 'transfer factor' is sometimes used because the measurement refers to overall measurement of gas transfer, which may be affected by ventilation, perfusion and diffusion defects distributed unevenly throughout the lung. Correlation with clinical examination is not always reliable for these reasons.

Diffusion. Movement of a substance from an area of high concentration to one of low concentration, resulting from spontaneous random movement of its constituent particles. May occur across **membranes**, e.g. from alveoli to bloodstream.
- Rate of diffusion across a membrane is proportional to:
  - available area of membrane.
  - concentration gradient across the membrane (**Fick's law**).
  - $\frac{1}{\sqrt{\text{mw of the substance}}}$ (**Graham's law**).

For diffusion of a gas across a membrane into a liquid (e.g. across the alveolar membrane), concentration gradient is proportional to the pressure gradient, and is maintained if the gas is soluble in the liquid; i.e., rate of diffusion is proportional to **solubility**.

Diffusion hypoxia, *see Fink effect*

Digital nerve block. Each digit is supplied by two palmar and two dorsal digital nerves. A fine needle is introduced from the dorsal side of the base of the digit, and 2–3 ml **local anaesthetic agent** (without **adrenaline**) injected on each side, between bone and skin.

Digoxin. Most widely used **cardiac glycoside**, used to treat **cardiac failure** and supraventricular **arrhythmias**, e.g. **AF**,

atrial flutter and **SVT**. Described and investigated by Withering in 1785 in his *Account of the Foxglove*. Slows atrioventricular conduction and increases **myocardial contractility**. Current indications include the treatment of systolic cardiac failure with an ejection fraction <25% in patients who have failed to respond to first-line agents, and as an adjunct for rate control of AF and atrial flutter. Reduces hospitalisation rates and symptoms due to severe cardiac failure refractory to first-line treatment, but has no effect on mortality. **Volume of distribution** is large (700 l) and **half-life** long (36 h); elimination is therefore lengthy after termination of treatment. Dosage must be reduced in renal impairment and in the elderly. Therapeutic plasma levels: 0.8–2 ng/ml (blood is taken 1 h after an iv dose, 8 h after an oral dose).

Contraindicated in **Wolff–Parkinson–White syndrome**, because atrioventricular block may encourage conduction through accessory pathways with resultant arrhythmia.

- Dosage:
  - loading dose for rapid digitalisation:
    - 1.0–1.5 mg orally in divided doses over 24 h (250–500 mg/day if less urgent).
    - 0.75–1.0 mg iv over at least 2 h. Fast injection may cause vasoconstriction and coronary ischaemia.
  - maintenance: 62.5–500 µg daily (usual range 125–250 µg).
- Side effects and toxicity:
  - more common in **hypokalaemia**, **hypercalcaemia** or **hypomagnesaemia**.
  - nausea, vomiting, diarrhoea.
  - headache, malaise, confusion. Blurred or yellow discoloration of vision (xanthopsia) occurs early; the presence of **hyperkalaemia** suggests severe toxicity.
  - any cardiac arrhythmia may occur; bradycardia, heart block and ventricular ectopics, including bi- and trigemini, are commonest.
  - ECG findings:
    - prolonged **P–R interval** and **heart block**.
    - **T wave** inversion.
    - **S–T segment** depression (the 'reverse tick').
  - life-threatening arrhythmias and hyperkalaemia should be treated promptly with digoxin-specific antibody fragments. Potassium replacement may also be required. Electrical **cardioversion** may result in severe arrhythmias, and should be avoided. **Magnesium** is the drug of choice for digoxin-induced ventricular arrhythmias.

[William Withering (1741–1799), English physician]

Stucky MA, Goldberg ZD (2015). Postgrad Med J; 91: 514–8

Dihydrocodeine tartrate. **Opioid analgesic drug**, of similar potency to **codeine**. Prepared in 1911. Causes fewer side effects than **morphine** or **pethidine** at equivalent analgesic doses. Also has a marked antitussive effect. Commonly used in combination with **paracetamol** as co-dydramol (500 mg/10 mg per tablet).

- Dosage: 30 mg orally or up to 50 mg sc/im, 4–6-hourly; 0.5–1 mg/kg in children.

Diltiazem hydrochloride. Class III **calcium channel blocking drug** and class IV **antiarrhythmic drug**, used to treat angina and hypertension, especially when **β-adrenergic receptor antagonists** are contraindicated or ineffective. Causes vasodilatation and prolonged atrioventricular nodal conduction. Causes less myocardial depression than **verapamil** but may cause severe bradycardia. After single oral dosage, 90% absorbed but **bioavailability** is only 45% because of extensive **first-pass metabolism**. About 65% excreted via the GIT. An iv preparation is available in the USA for treatment of **AF**, **atrial flutter** and **SVT**.

- Dosage:
  - 60–120 mg orally tds (90–180 mg bd, or 120–360 mg od for sustained-release preparations).
  - 0.25 mg/kg iv over 2 min, followed by 0.35 mg/kg over 2 min, then 5–15 mg/h if required.
- Side effects: bradycardia, hypotension, malaise, headache, GIT disturbances; rarely, impaired liver function.

Dilution techniques. Used for measuring body compartment volumes (e.g. **blood**, plasma, **ECF** and **lung volumes**). A known quantity of tracer substance is introduced into the space to be measured, and its concentration measured after complete mixing:

$$C_1 \times V_1 = C_2 \times (V_1 + V_2)$$

where C_1 = initial concentration of indicator
C_2 = final concentration of indicator
V_1 = volume of indicator
V_2 = volume to be measured

Tracer substances include dyes and **radioisotopes**; the latter may be injected as radioactive ions or attached to proteins, red blood cells, etc. Gaseous markers may be used to study lung volumes, e.g. helium to measure **FRC**.

The principle may be extended for **cardiac output measurement**, where radioisotope, dye or cold crystalloid solution is injected as a bolus proximal to the right ventricle, and its concentration measured distally, e.g. radial or pulmonary artery. A concentration–time curve is plotted to enable calculation of cardiac output. A double indicator dilution technique has been used to measure **extravascular lung water**.

Dimercaprol (BAL; British Anti-Lewisite). **Chelating agent** previously used in the treatment of heavy metal poisoning, especially antimony, arsenic, bismuth, mercury and gold. Now superseded by newer agents. Following im injection, peak levels occur within 1 h, with elimination in 4 h. Contraindicated in liver disease and **glucose 6-phosphate dehydrogenase deficiency**.

- Dosage: 2.5–3.0 mg/kg im 4-hourly for 2 days, bd/qds on day 3 and od/bd thereafter.
- Side effects: haemolytic anaemia, transient hypertension and tachycardia, agitation, paraesthesia, headache, tremor, nausea and vomiting, erythema and pain on injection. Contains peanut oil as a solvent.

[Lewisite: a potent arsenic-based chemical weapon used in World War II (Winford Lee Lewis (1878–1943), US chemist)]

Dimethyl tubocurarine chloride/bromide (Metocurine). Non-depolarising **neuromuscular blocking drug**, derived from **tubocurarine**; introduced in 1948 and no longer available. More potent and longer-lasting than tubocurarine, causing less ganglion blockade and **histamine** release. Almost entirely renally excreted.

Dinoprost/dinoprostone, *see Prostaglandins*

2,3-Diphosphoglycerate (2,3-DPG). Substance formed within red blood cells from phosphoglyceraldehyde, produced during **glycolysis**. Binds strongly to the β chains of deoxygenated **haemoglobin**, reducing its affinity for O_2

and shifting the **oxyhaemoglobin dissociation curve** to the right, i.e., favours O_2 liberation to the tissues. Binds poorly to the γ chains of **fetal haemoglobin**.

- Levels are increased by:
  - **anaemia**.
  - **alkalosis**.
  - chronic **hypoxaemia**, e.g. in cyanotic heart disease.
  - high **altitude**.
  - **exercise**.
  - **pregnancy**.
  - **hyperthyroidism**.
  - **hyperphosphataemia**.
  - certain red cell enzyme abnormalities.
- Levels are decreased by:
  - **acidosis**, e.g. in stored blood; requires 12–24 h for levels to be restored.
  - **hypophosphataemia**.
  - **hypothyroidism**.
  - **hypopituitarism**.

Diphtheria. Infection caused by *Corynebacterium diphtheriae*, a gram-positive rod. Now rare in the Western world due to immunisation, but formerly a major cause of death, particularly in children. Mortality is 5%–10%.

- Features:
  - symptoms of upper respiratory infection with fever (>38°C), sore throat and painful dysphagia.
  - a thick exudative pseudomembrane forms across the posterior pharynx/larynx, causing **croup**-like breathing and may result in complete obstruction. This may be aggravated by neck lymphadenopathy ('bull neck').
  - diphtheria toxin may cause **myocarditis** and **arrhythmias. Cranial nerve** and peripheral nerve palsies may occur.
- Treatment:
  - as for **airway obstruction**.
  - antitoxin administration.
  - **metronidazole, erythromycin** or **penicillin** G are the antibacterial drugs of choice.

Both L, Collins S, de Zoysa A, et al (2015). J Clin Microbiol; 91: 514–8

Dipipanone hydrochloride. Opioid analgesic drug, similar to **methadone** and **dextromoramide**. Developed in 1950. Available in the UK for oral use as tablets of 10 mg combined with **cyclizine** 30 mg.

- Dosage: 1–3 tablets qds. Anticholinergic effects of cyclizine may limit its use.

Diploma in Intensive Care Medicine (DICM). Instituted in 1997/8 to permit identification of doctors trained to an adequate standard to undertake a career with a large commitment to intensive care medicine in the UK. Aimed to test knowledge and its application, and the ability to communicate with medical and nursing staff, patients and their relatives. Candidates for the Diploma had to possess a postgraduate qualification in their primary specialty (e.g. FRCA, MRCP, FRCS), have completed the stipulated periods of training (*see Intensive care, training in*), and submitted a dissertation. Replaced in 2013 by the Fellowship of the **Faculty of Intensive Care Medicine** exam (FFICM).

Dipyridamole. Antiplatelet drug, used to prevent **stroke** and as an adjunct to oral anticoagulation, e.g. in patients with prosthetic heart valves. Modifies **platelet** aggregation, adhesion and survival by inhibiting adenosine uptake. Also given iv for stress testing during diagnostic cardiac imaging; causes marked vasodilatation. May cause **coronary steal**.

- Dosage: 100–150 mg orally tds/qds (slow-release: 200 mg bd).
- Side effects: may be hazardous in severe coronary and aortic stenosis due to its vasodilation effects. Nausea, vomiting and headache may also occur.

Disaster, major, *see Incident, major*

Disequilibrium syndrome. Syndrome comprising nausea, vomiting, headache, restlessness, visual disturbances, tremor, coma and convulsions, associated with **dialysis**. More common in patients with pre-existing intracranial pathology, severe acidosis or uraemia. The cause is uncertain, although increased brain water is suggested by CT scanning. Rapid changes in **osmolality** or CSF pH have been suggested. Reduced by gradual institution of dialysis, especially if plasma urea is very high, and by careful management of sodium balance. Management is supportive.

Disinfection of anaesthetic equipment, *see Contamination of anaesthetic equipment*

Disodium pamidronate, *see Bisphosphonates*

Disopyramide phosphate. Class Ia **antiarrhythmic drug**, used to treat **SVT** and **VT**. Also used in the treatment of hypertrophic **cardiomyopathy**. **Half-life** is 7 h.

- Dosage:
  - 300–800 mg/day orally in divided doses.
  - 2 mg/kg up to 150 mg iv over at least 5 min, followed by 0.4 mg/kg/h infusion or 200 mg orally tds; maximum 300 mg in the first hour and 800 mg/day.
- Side effects: myocardial depression, hypotension, anticholinergic effects, e.g. urinary retention, atrioventricular block.

Disseminated intravascular coagulation (DIC). Syndrome caused by systemic activation of **coagulation**, generating intravascular fibrin clots leading to organ hypoperfusion and failure. The concomitant consumption of clotting factors and **platelets** and secondary **fibrinolysis** results in bleeding.

- May be precipitated by:
  - **sepsis** and severe infection/inflammatory conditions (including **pancreatitis**).
  - **trauma**.
  - malignancy, e.g. leukaemia
  - obstetric conditions: **pre-eclampsia**, **amniotic fluid embolism**, **placental abruption**.
  - **hepatic failure**.
  - toxins e.g. snake venoms, transfusion reactions, recreational drugs.
- Effects:
  - may occur chronically, with little clinical abnormality.
  - bruising, bleeding from wounds, venepuncture sites, GIT, lung, urinary tract and uteroplacental bed.
  - capillary microthrombosis may cause **MODS**.
  - shock, **acidosis** and **hypoxaemia** may occur.

Diagnosis is supported by **thrombocytopenia** (platelet count <100 × 10^9/l), prolonged prothrombin, partial thromboplastin and thrombin times, elevated D-dimer and **fibrin degradation products** and fibrinogen level <1 g/l.

- Treatment:
  - directed at underlying causes.
  - platelet transfusion should be reserved for bleeding patients with a platelet count <50 × 10^9/l. If the patient is not bleeding, platelet counts of 10–20 × 10^9/l can be tolerated.
  - correction of clotting factor deficiency with fresh frozen plasma (superior to **prothrombin complex concentrate**, which lacks factor V).
  - if fibrinogen levels are low despite fresh frozen plasma, fibrinogen concentrate or cryoprecipitate should be given.
  - if thrombosis is prominent, treatment with **heparin** should be considered. Prophylactic heparin is recommended in non-bleeding patients.

Wada H, Thachil J, Di Nisio M, et al (2013). J Thromb Haemost; 11: 761–7

See also, Blood products; Coagulation disorders; Coagulation studies

Disseminated sclerosis, *see Demyelinating diseases*

Dissociation curves, *see Carbon dioxide dissociation curve; Oxyhaemoglobin dissociation curve*

Dissociative anaesthesia, *see Ketamine*

Distigmine bromide. **Acetylcholinesterase inhibitor**, used in urinary retention and intestinal atony.

- Dosage: 5–20 mg orally od.
- Side effects: as for **neostigmine**.

Distribution curves, statistical, *see Statistical frequency distributions*

Disulfiram. Drug used in the treatment of **alcoholism**; inhibits the metabolism of **alcohol** by alcohol dehydrogenase with increased production of acetaldehyde, the latter causing unpleasant effects (flushing, headache, palpitations, nausea and vomiting) when alcohol is ingested. Arrhythmias and hypotension may follow large intakes of alcohol. Similar but lesser reactions may occur in patients taking **metronidazole** who ingest alcohol.

- Dosage: 200 mg orally od initially, increased up to 500 mg.
- Side effects: drowsiness, nausea, vomiting, psychosis, peripheral neuritis, hepatic impairment. Causes **enzyme inhibition**, thus enhancing the actions of many drugs, including **tricyclic antidepressant drugs**, **benzodiazepines**, **warfarin**, **theophylline** and **phenytoin**.

Diuresis, forced, *see Forced diuresis*

Diuretics. Drugs increasing the rate of urine production by the kidney.

- Divided into:
  - **thiazide diuretics**: act at the proximal part of the distal convoluted tubule of the **nephron**, and at the proximal tubule. Have low ceilings of action; i.e., maximal effects are produced by small doses. May cause **hypokalaemia**, **hypomagnesaemia**, hyperuricaemia, **hyperglycaemia** and hypercholesterolaemia.
  - osmotic diuretics, e.g. **mannitol**: increase **renal blood flow** by plasma expansion, then draw water into the renal tubules by osmosis. Other small molecules that are filtered but not reabsorbed may have similar osmotic diuretic actions, e.g. glucose, urea and sucrose.
  - potassium-sparing diuretics, e.g. triamterene, amiloride, **spironolactone**: act at the distal convoluted tubule, where most potassium is normally lost; spironolactone acts by **aldosterone** receptor antagonism. May cause **hyperkalaemia** and **hyponatraemia**.
  - loop diuretics, e.g. **furosemide**, **bumetanide**, ethacrynic acid: act at the ascending loop of Henle. More potent, with high ceilings of action. Immediate benefit in fluid overload/cardiac failure is thought to be due to vasodilatation. May cause hypokalaemia, hyperuricaemia, hypomagnesaemia and hyperglycaemia. Ototoxicity may occur following rapid iv injection and with concurrent **aminoglycoside** therapy.
  - other substances causing diuresis:
    - **carbonic anhydrase** inhibitors, e.g. **acetazolamide**.
    - **xanthines**, e.g. **aminophylline**: reduce sodium excretion and increase **GFR**.
    - **dopamine**: increases renal blood flow and GFR; also reduces sodium absorption.
    - water and ethanol: inhibit **vasopressin** secretion.
    - acidifying salts, e.g. ammonium chloride: increase hydrogen ion and sodium excretion.
    - **demeclocycline**: blocks the action of vasopressin on the distal tubule and collecting duct; used in the **syndrome of inappropriate ADH secretion**.

Anaesthesia for patients taking diuretics: **hypovolaemia** and electrolyte disturbances are possible, especially in the elderly. Hypokalaemia may represent severe body potassium depletion; conversely, potassium supplements and potassium-sparing diuretics may cause hyperkalaemia. Severe hyponatraemia may follow treatment with potassium-sparing diuretics. Combinations of different types of diuretic tend to be synergistic.

[Friedrich GJ Henle (1809–1885), German anatomist]

Diving reflex. Decreased respiration, vagal bradycardia and splanchnic and muscle bed vasoconstriction following immersion of the face in cold water. Cerebral and cardiac circulations are preserved. Occurs in mammals, birds and reptiles; it has been suggested that it may aid survival in humans, e.g. in boating and skiing accidents.

Panneton WM (2013). Physiology (Bethesda); 28: 284–97

Divinyl ether. **Inhalational anaesthetic agent**, introduced in 1933 and no longer used. Similar in potency and explosiveness to **diethyl ether**, but less irritant. Liver damage resulted from prolonged use. Combined 1:4 with ether as Vinesthene Anaesthetic Mixture.

DLV, *see Differential lung ventilation*

DNAR orders, *see Do not attempt resuscitation orders*

DNR orders, Do not resuscitate orders, *see Do not attempt resuscitation orders*

$\dot{D}O_2$, *see Oxygen delivery*

Do not attempt resuscitation orders (DNAR orders; Do not resuscitate orders; DNR orders). Instructions in a patient's records that **CPR** is not to be performed should cardiorespiratory arrest occur. Generally reserved for patients in whom quality of life is currently so poor, or the likelihood of success so low, that active resuscitation is not indicated. Patients with capacity to participate in discussions regarding resuscitation must be consulted before a DNAR order is issued unless the clinician considers that the discussion will cause physical or psychological harm to the patient, or the patient states that he or she does not wish to discuss resuscitation. If the patient lacks capacity, the order should be discussed with the patient's legal proxy (e.g. someone with a lasting power of attorney). If none is available, the decision should be discussed with the patient's family and friends. If there is disagreement with the clinician's decision, a second opinion should be sought.

Discussions regarding DNAR should be in plain language and understandable to the patient.

DNAR/DNR orders are often suspended perioperatively, as the fact that surgery is taking place implies that active treatment is worthwhile; also the results of resuscitation during anaesthesia are often better than those of CPR on the wards. Similar considerations may apply to patients nursed in the ITU.

Any discussion and decision regarding DNAR/DNR orders should be clearly documented and, more importantly, all staff involved in the patient's care must be made aware of any changes in DNAR/DNR status. The use of standard forms is becoming more widespread.

Etheridge Z, Gatland E (2015). Br Med J; 350: h2640.

See also, Advance decisions; Ethics

Dobutamine hydrochloride. Synthetic **catecholamine**, used as an **inotropic drug**, e.g. in cardiac stress testing, after **cardiac surgery**, and in **septic** or **cardiogenic shock**. Stimulates **β_1-adrenergic receptors**, with weak stimulation of β_2- and α-receptors. Does not affect **dopamine receptors**. Increases myocardial contractility, with less increase in myocardial O_2 consumption than other catecholamines. Causes less tachycardia than **dopamine** or **isoprenaline**, probably because of a reduced effect on the sinoatrial node, and less activation of the **baroreceptor reflex**. Reduces **left ventricular end-diastolic pressure** if raised.

Plasma **half-life** is about 2 min. Excreted via the urine. Supplied as a solution for dilution with saline or 5% dextrose before use.

- Usual dosage: 2.5–10 µg/kg/min by infusion; higher rates may be required.
- Side effects: hypotension (due to β_2-receptor agonism), tachycardia and ventricular arrhythmias at high doses.

Dog bites, *see Bites and stings*

Dolasetron mesylate. $5\text{-}HT_3$ receptor antagonist, used as an **antiemetic drug** in chemotherapy-induced and **PONV**. Discontinued in the UK in 2009.

Doll's eye movements (Oculocephalic reflex). Reflex elicited in unconscious patients by quickly turning the patient's head to one side and holding it there. The eyes move conjugately to the right when the head is turned to the left, and vice versa; i.e., they continue to point in the original position in relation to the body, as if fixed on a distant object. They then move to the mid-position. The reflex involves bilateral vestibular apparatus and nerves, brainstem and oculomotor nerves; it is therefore absent in **brainstem death** or dysfunction. Normally absent because of cerebral activity influencing eye movement; i.e., it becomes apparent if cerebral activity is suppressed or interrupted.

Domperidone maleate. Antiemetic and **prokinetic drug** related to **metoclopramide**, and with similar actions. Less able to penetrate the **blood–brain barrier**, thus less likely to cause sedation and **dystonic reactions** than other antiemetic drugs. No longer available for iv use, because of associated ventricular arrhythmias. Contraindicated in heart disease and patients with **prolonged Q–T syndromes** or hepatic impairment

- Dosage: 10 mg tds orally, for up to a week.

Donepezil, *see Acetylcholinesterase inhibitors*

Donnan effect (Gibbs–Donnan effect). Effect of charged particles on one side of a membrane on the distribution of other charged particles, when the former cannot diffuse through the membrane but the latter can. For example, the cell membrane is largely impermeable to negatively charged intracellular proteins, whereas it is relatively permeable to K^+ and Cl^- ions. The distribution of these ions on either side of the membrane is therefore affected by the electrical gradient produced by the proteins, as well as their own concentration gradients. There is a fixed ratio between the concentration of diffusible ions on one side of the membrane and the concentration of those on the other. This ratio is the same for all the ions distributed about a particular membrane under the same conditions.

[Frederick Donnan (1870–1956), English chemist; Josiah Gibbs (1839–1903), US physicist]

Dopamine. Naturally occurring **catecholamine** and **neurotransmitter**, found in postganglionic sympathetic nerve endings and the adrenal medulla. A precursor of **adrenaline** and **noradrenaline**. Used as an **inotropic drug**, e.g. in **cardiogenic** or **septic shock**. Formerly used to provide 'renal protection' in situations when kidney function is compromised but no evidence exists for its efficacy and reports of bowel hypoperfusion have led to diminishing use of low-dose ('renal') dopamine in ICU.

Supplied as the hydrochloride in a concentrated solution for dilution in saline or 5% dextrose, or as a ready-made iv solution in dextrose. Inactivated by alkali.

- Effects depend on the dose used:
  - up to 5 µg/kg/min: traditionally believed to stimulate **dopamine receptors**, causing renal and mesenteric vasodilatation and increasing **renal blood flow**, **GFR**, urine output and sodium excretion. However, it is now thought that these so-called renal effects of dopamine are actually a non-specific response to increased **cardiac output**.
  - 5–15 µg/kg/min: stimulates **β_1-adrenergic receptors**; **myocardial contractility**, cardiac output, BP and O_2 consumption are increased. **Pulmonary capillary wedge pressure** may paradoxically increase, possibly because of increased venous return secondary to venoconstriction. Some α_2-stimulation also occurs.
  - over 15 µg/kg/min: stimulates α_1-receptors, causing peripheral vasoconstriction.

Rapidly taken up by tissues and metabolised by dopamine β-hydroxylase and **monoamine oxidase** pathways, with renal excretion of metabolites. Plasma **half-life** is about 1 min. Dosage must be reduced if the patient is taking **monoamine oxidase inhibitors**.

- Side effects: tachycardia and ventricular arrhythmias are common at higher doses. Severe tissue necrosis may follow peripheral extravasation; it should thus be administered into a large vein (preferably central). May cause gastric stasis and suppress release of oxytocin and other pituitary hormones. Has also been implicated in reducing T-cell responsiveness and reducing GIT oxygenation via shunting of blood at mucosal level.

Dopamine receptors. Family of **G protein-coupled receptors** found peripherally and in the CNS. Subdivided into:

- central:
  - D_1 receptors: stimulation results in increased intracellular **cAMP**. Related to D_5 receptors.
  - D_2 receptors: receptor found in pathways involving the basal ganglia and hypothalamus, concerned with coordination of locomotion, reward behaviour and inhibition of prolactin release. Also present in the **chemoreceptor trigger zone** where stimulation results in **vomiting**, and in the spinal cord. **Butyrophenones** are the classical antagonists; others include **phenothiazines** and **metoclopramide**. Bromocriptine is an agonist. Related to D_3 and D_4 receptors.
- peripheral:
  - DA_1 receptors: postsynaptic; thought to be analogous to central D_1 receptors. Stimulation causes vasodilatation in renal and mesenteric vascular beds.
  - DA_2 receptors: presynaptic; stimulation inhibits **noradrenaline** release via negative feedback. Inhibition of cAMP formation may be involved. May also be present at cholinergic nerve endings. Inhibited by butyrophenones, i.e., thought to be analogous to central D_2 receptors.

Further subclasses of **dopamine** receptors may also exist.
Beaulieu J-M, Gainetdinov RR (2011). Pharmacol Rev; 63: 182–217

Dopexamine hydrochloride. Synthetic analogue of **dopamine**, used as an **inotropic drug** in **cardiac failure**, e.g. after **cardiac surgery**. Has been used to maintain renal perfusion in critically ill patients but with little evidence of its efficacy. Stimulates peripheral **dopamine receptors** and **β_1-adrenergic receptors**, with indirect stimulation of β_1-adrenergic receptors via inhibition of neuronal reuptake of **catecholamines**. Causes peripheral (including renal) vasodilatation with reduced BP and increased cardiac output. 40% bound to red blood cells. **Half-life** is 7 min.

- Dosage: 0.5–6.0 μg/kg/min.
- Side effects include tachycardia (usually mild) and arrhythmias, nausea, vomiting and tremor.

Doppler effect. Change in observed frequency of a signal when the signal source moves relative to the observer; increasing as the source approaches, decreasing as it moves away. For example, the wavefronts in front of a moving car horn will be closer together than when the horn is stationary, because when each wavefront is emitted, the horn moves forward before emitting another. Similarly, the wavefronts behind the horn are further apart. To the observer, the tone of the horn changes from higher-pitched to lower-pitched as the horn approaches and passes, although the actual frequency emitted has not changed.

The principle is used clinically to determine velocities and flow rates of moving substances, e.g. in **cardiac output measurement**. An **ultrasound** beam may be directed along the path of flow; the sound waves reflect from the surfaces of the blood cells as they approach or move away. Analysis of the reflected frequencies allows determination of blood velocity. Doppler probes contain both emitter and detector in the probe tip.

May also be used to detect arterial wall movement in **arterial BP measurement**; onset of movement occurs at systolic pressure, and cessation at diastolic pressure, as the cuff is deflated from high pressure. The ultrasonic beam is directed across the artery.

[Christian Doppler (1803–1853), Austrian physicist]
See also, Transcranial Doppler ultrasound

Doripenem. Broad-spectrum **carbapenem** and **antibacterial drug**. Previously licensed for treatment of **nosocomial pneumonia** (including **ventilator-associated pneumonia**) and complicated intra-abdominal and urinary tract infections. Withdrawn from the European Union for commercial reasons.

Dorsal column stimulation, *see Spinal cord stimulation*

Dorsal root entry zone procedure (DREZ procedure). Production of destructive lesions in the DREZ; has been used to treat pain following spinal cord injury, brachial plexus avulsion and **postherpetic neuralgia**. Thought to interrupt the site of integration of **pain pathways** via the lateral spinothalamic and spinoreticulothalamic tracts. A microelectrode is inserted into the spinal cord at each level of the pain and radiofrequency lesions induced to destroy the abnormally active dorsal horn neurones.
Kanpolat Y, Tuna H, Bozkurt M, Elhan AH (2008). Neurosurgery; 62 (suppl 1): 235–42

Dorsalis pedis artery. Continuation of the anterior tibial artery, itself a branch of the popliteal artery. Passes along the dorsum of the foot to the space between the first and second metatarsal bones, where it enters the sole of the foot to anastomose with the lateral plantar artery. May be used as a site for **arterial cannulation**, lateral to extensor hallucis longus tendon with the foot flexed. Cannulation may be difficult in peripheral vascular disease.

Dose–response curves. Curves describing the relationship between dose of a drug or physiological agent and the resultant response. If a logarithmic scale is used for the abscissa the curve is sigmoid-shaped, with increasing response as dose is increased until a plateau is reached (Fig. 56).

- Different curves are characterised by their:
  - position on the abscissa (related to **potency**).
  - maximal height (**efficacy**).

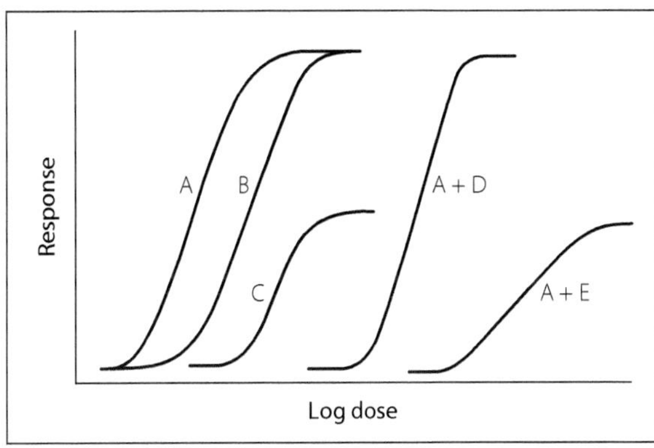

Fig. 56 Dose–response curves (see text)

- slope (influenced by the number of receptors that must be activated before a drug has an effect).

Drugs A and B are both **agonists**, but A is more potent. Drug C is less efficacious and is therefore a partial agonist. Addition of a competitive **antagonist**, D, to A shifts the curve to the right (i.e., reduced potency) but without altering its height (i.e., same efficacy). A non-competitive antagonist, E, shifts the curve to the right, reduces its height and alters its slope.

The curves are affected by individual variability in response, related to differences in **pharmacokinetics** and **pharmacodynamics**. The dose of drug required to produce a certain response in a given percentage of the population (n%) is described as the effective dose, ED_n.
See also, Receptor theory

Dosulepin hydrochloride (Dothiepin). **Tricyclic antidepressant drug**, similar to **amitriptyline**. Used in endogenous depression and in chronic **pain management**.
- Dosage: 50–75 mg orally, increased up to 225 mg/day. 25–50 mg is used in pain management.
- Side effects: as for amitriptyline.

Double-blind studies, *see Clinical trials*

Double-lumen tubes, *see Endobronchial tubes*

Down's syndrome. Syndrome resulting from presence of an extra chromosome 21 (trisomy 21). Usually due to non-dysjunction of chromosomes during germ cell formation, and rarely due to translocation in parental cells. Incidence is ~1:700 overall, increasing with maternal age. 45% of patients live to 60 years.
- Features:
  - round head and face, slanting eyes with prominent and wide epicanthic folds. Ears are low-set; the mouth is small with a large tongue.
  - broad, short hands, with a single transverse palmar crease; the gap between first and second toes is large.
  - respiratory involvement includes obstructive **sleep apnoea** (in 60%), abnormal central respiratory drive, tracheal stenosis and a tendency to develop chest infections.
  - congenital heart disease is common, especially **ASD** and **VSD** (and atrioventricular septal defect), **Fallot's tetralogy** and patent **ductus arteriosus**.
  - duodenal atresia and other congenital abnormalities are common, as is **gastro-oesophageal reflux**.
  - acute myeloid leukaemia is common.
  - hypotonicity.
  - learning difficulties (IQ 20–60); epilepsy (in 10%). Dementia is common, as is postoperative agitation.
  - hypothyroidism and insulin-dependent **diabetes mellitus** are common.
- Anaesthetic problems:
  - cardiac abnormalities (see earlier).
  - airway difficulties, including difficult tracheal intubation due to macroglossia and subglottic stenosis; obstructive sleep apnoea. Excessive secretions are common.
  - hypotonia.
  - atlantoaxial subluxation and instability.

[John Down (1828–1896), English physician]

Lewanda AF, Matisoff A, Revenis M, et al (2016). Paediatr Anaesth; 26: 356–62

Doxacurium chloride. Non-depolarising **neuromuscular blocking drug**, introduced in 1991. Unavailable in the UK. Has similar features to **pancuronium**, but without cardiovascular effects. Dose range: 25–80 μg/kg; intubation may be performed 4–6 min after the initial dose. Effects last 1–3 h, depending on dosage. Excreted unchanged via the kidneys and liver. Causes **histamine** release only at much higher doses than required clinically. Used for prolonged surgery where cardiovascular stability is required, e.g. neurosurgery or cardiac surgery.

Doxapram hydrochloride. **Analeptic drug**, used for its respiratory stimulant properties. Acts on peripheral **chemoreceptors**, increasing tidal volume more than respiratory rate. Increases work of breathing and therefore oxygen demand. Used to reverse postoperative respiratory depression, without reversing opioid-induced analgesia. Formerly used in type 2 **respiratory failure** in patients with **COPD**, to avoid the need for IPPV; however, it has been superseded by **non-invasive positive pressure ventilation. Half-life** is 2–4 h.
- Dosage:
  - 1–1.5 mg/kg iv over 30 s; repeated hourly.
  - 1.5–4 mg/min by infusion, according to response.
- Side effects: hypertension, tachycardia (resulting from vasomotor stimulation), restlessness, confusion, dizziness, sweating, nausea, salivation. Convulsions may occur with high doses.

Contraindicated in coronary artery disease, severe hypertension, thyrotoxicosis, asthma and epilepsy. Effects are said to be potentiated by **monoamine oxidase inhibitors**.

2,3-DPG, *see 2,3-Diphosphoglycerate*

DPL, Diagnostic peritoneal lavage, *see Peritoneal lavage*

Draw-over techniques. Anaesthesia in which the patient's inspiratory effort draws room air (with or without added O_2) over a volatile agent with each breath. Similar to **open-drop techniques**, but more sophisticated. There should be minimal resistance in the breathing system and **vaporiser**. Incorporation of **bellows** or a **self-inflating bag** into the breathing system allows IPPV, and provides a reservoir if continuous flow of O_2 is added. **Non-rebreathing valves** prevent exhalation back into the vaporiser; a unidirectional valve is necessary upstream of the bellows or bag, if used, to allow IPPV (Fig. 57).

Mainly used where there is a shortage of compressed gas supplies, e.g. battlefields, accident sites, developing countries. Was also used for inhalational analgesia in obstetrics. A simplified draw-over device has recently been introduced for analgesia via self-administration of **methoxyflurane**.

Dreaming, *see Awareness*

Dressler's syndrome, *see Myocardial infarction*

DREZ, *see Dorsal root entry zone procedure*

Dronedarone, *see Antiarrhythmic drugs*

Droperidol. **Butyrophenone**, discontinued in the UK in 2001 because of cases of prolonged **Q–T interval** but reintroduced in 2009 at a lower recommended dosage and licensed only for use as an **antiemetic drug**. A powerful

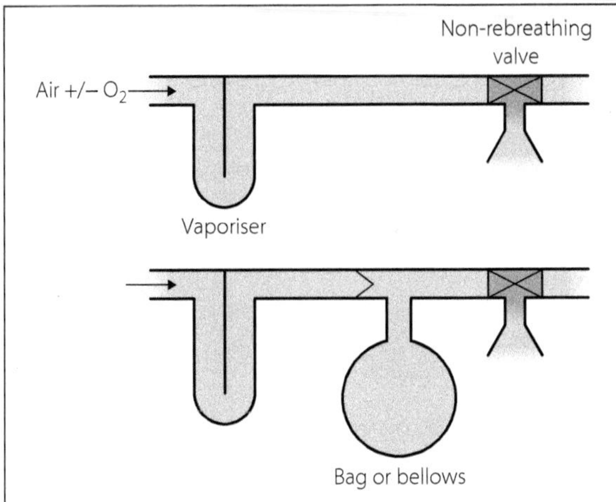

Fig. 57 Draw-over systems

dopamine antagonist, related to **haloperidol** but of shorter duration of action (6–12 h; cf. haloperidol 24–48 h). Typically caused apparent outward sedation but internal distress.

- Dosage: 0.625–1.25 mg iv 30 min before end of surgery, repeated up to qds. Has also been added to morphine **PCA** (15–50 µg per 1 mg morphine, up to 5 mg droperidol per day).

Drotrecogin alfa (alpha), *see Protein C*

Drowning, *see Near-drowning*

Drug absorption, distribution, metabolism and excretion, *see Pharmacokinetics*

Drug addiction, *see Substance abuse*

Drug development. New drugs or indications for old drugs may arise from:
- incidental observation, e.g. antiplatelet action of aspirin.
- modification of the structure of known natural substances, e.g. H_2 receptor antagonists.
- modification of existing drugs, e.g. opioid analgesics.
- screening of natural compounds.
- computer-assisted modelling of new molecules.

- Stages of development:
  - identification of the substance.
  - in vitro studies.
  - animal studies:
    - effects, interactions, **pharmacokinetics**, etc.
    - toxicology: acute/chronic (usually up to 2 years) effects, **therapeutic index**; use of different animals, routes, doses. Includes histological/biochemical effects on organs, bacterial mutagenicity, teratogenicity, carcinogenicity, and effects on fertility.

    Doubts have been expressed over the ethics of animal experiments and problems caused by species differences (e.g. thalidomide was free of teratogenicity in mice and rats but had devastating effects in humans). In the UK, undertaking animal studies requires a Home Office licence.
  - chemical aspects, e.g. formulation, manufacture, quality, storage.
  - human studies:
    - phase I (clinical pharmacology): 20–50 subjects, usually healthy volunteers. Pharmacokinetic and pharmacodynamic effects, safety, etc.
    - phase II (clinical investigation): 50–300 patients. Further information as mentioned earlier, plus effective dose ranges and regimens.
    - phase III (formal **clinical trials**): 250–1000+ patients. Comparison with other treatments. Frequent side effects are noted.
    - phase IV (postmarketing surveillance): 2000–10 000+ patients. Rare side effects are noted, e.g. oculomuco-cutaneous syndrome following oral practolol therapy. Techniques used:
      - cohort studies: large numbers are observed over long periods, noting side effects when they occur. May detect rare effects (less than 1:500), but costly and difficult to organise. May examine specific groups (e.g. the elderly) previously excluded.
      - case–control studies: records of patients with a suspected side effect are analysed for previous drug exposure. Easier and cheaper than cohort studies, but less precise and more susceptible to bias. May detect side effects with frequency up to 1:500. Prove association, not causation; give relative risk.
      - voluntary reporting (yellow card system in UK). Specific anaesthetic cards are available.
      - general statistics, e.g. recording sudden changes in disease incidence.

Statutory regulatory bodies are concerned with drug development from the animal study stage onwards: the **Medicines and Healthcare products Regulatory Agency** in the UK, the **Food and Drug Administration** in the USA (the **European Medicines Agency** coordinates such activities in Europe). A product licence is granted after phase III trials, and reviewed every 5 years in the UK. Financial costs of new drug development are considerable and often prohibitive.

Drug interactions. Common cause of morbidity and mortality, especially in hospital, although some interactions are beneficial.
- May be:
  - **pharmacokinetic**:
    - outside the body, e.g. precipitation of **thiopental/atracurium** mixture.
    - at site of absorption, e.g. effect of opioids and **metoclopramide** on **gastric emptying**, use of vasoconstrictors to delay local anaesthetic drug absorption, **second gas effect**.
    - affecting distribution, e.g. displacement of **warfarin** from protein-binding sites by **salicylates**.
    - affecting metabolism (e.g. concurrent administration of carbidopa inhibiting peripheral conversion of levodopa to dopamine), **enzyme induction/inhibition**, e.g. by **cimetidine** (inhibition) or **barbiturates** (induction).
    - affecting elimination, e.g. decreased **penicillin** excretion caused by probenecid.
  - **pharmacodynamic**:
    - additive:
      - summation: net effect equals the sum of individual drug effects.
      - synergism: net effect exceeds the sum of individual effects.

- potentiation: one drug increases the effect of another. Examples: decreased requirement for anaesthetic agents when opioids and other sedatives are used, and the increase in **non-depolarising neuromuscular blockade** caused by aminoglycosides and phenytoin.
- **antagonism**: may be competitive, physiological, etc.
- indirect effects, e.g. **hypokalaemia** induced by **diuretics** increases **digoxin** toxicity; **pethidine** interaction with **monoamine oxidase inhibitors**; sensitisation of the myocardium to catecholamines by **halothane**.

See also, Adverse drug reactions; Dose–response curves

Drug labels, *see Syringe labels*

Dual block (Phase II block). Phenomenon seen when large doses of **suxamethonium** or related drugs are administered, in which features of **non-depolarising neuromuscular blockade** gradually replace those of **depolarising neuromuscular blockade**. More commonly seen with concurrent administration of **acetylcholinesterase inhibitors** and in **myasthenia gravis**.

Typically, tachyphylaxis to suxamethonium develops after administration of 400–500 mg by infusion or repeated doses, although individual variation is wide. This is followed by non-depolarising neuromuscular blockade, which may be reversed by **neostigmine**, although reversal is inconsistent. In doubtful cases, **edrophonium** 10 mg has been suggested as a test; the block worsens if depolarising, reverses if non-depolarising. Use of nerve stimulators has largely superseded this test.

Has also been termed desensitisation block, and sometimes subdivided into different phases. The mechanism is unclear; depolarisation is thought not to persist despite continued presence of the drug. Pre- or postjunctional receptor modulation may be involved.

See also, Neuromuscular blockade monitoring

Ductus arteriosus, patent (Arterial duct). Accounts for 5%–10% of **congenital heart disease**. More common in premature babies. The duct normally closes within a few days of birth; bradykinin, **prostaglandins** and a rise in $P\text{O}_2$ are thought to be involved, although the precise mechanism is unclear. If it remains open, significant left-to-right **shunt** may occur.

- Features:
  - neonates/infants: **cardiac failure**, **respiratory failure**.
  - older patients:
    - may be symptomless; cardiac failure or bacterial **endocarditis** may occur.
    - signs: continuous murmur heard at the left sternal edge, louder on expiration; may be systolic only, if the shunt is large. A pulmonary regurgitant murmur may be present.
    - pulmonary plethora and cardiomegaly on CXR.
  - **pulmonary hypertension** may develop.

Usually diagnosed using colour-flow Doppler mapping.

- Treatment:
  - medical (in the first 10–14 days of life): indometacin 200 µg/kg iv, then two doses of 100 µg/kg (up to 8 h old), 200 µg/kg (2–7 days old) or 250 µg/kg (over 7 days old) at 12–24 h intervals. Ibuprofen is equally effective.
  - transcatheter occlusion if duct is small.
  - surgical: ligation/division of duct; left thoracotomy is usually performed. Haemorrhage, recurrent laryngeal nerve or thoracic duct damage may occur. Postoperative IPPV may be required, especially in babies.
- Anaesthesia: as for congenital heart disease.

Prostaglandin E_1 is used to prevent ductal closure in babies with congenital heart disease awaiting surgery, e.g. permitting right-to-left shunting to allow perfusion of the legs in severe aortic coarctation, or left-to-right shunting to allow pulmonary perfusion in **Fallot's tetralogy** with severe right ventricular outflow obstruction.

See also, Fetal circulation

Duloxetine. Antidepressant drug acting via inhibition of uptake of **5-HT** and **noradrenaline**. Licensed for depression, generalised anxiety disorders and stress incontinence in women. Also a first-line treatment for **neuropathic pain**.

- Dosage: 30–120 mg orally per day in divided doses.
- Side effects: nausea, abdominal pain, insomnia, dry mouth, visual disturbances.

Dumping valve. Device preventing application of excessive negative pressure to patients' airways, used in **scavenging** systems and some breathing attachments. Usually opens at –0.5 cmH_2O, allowing air to be drawn in.

Dural tap. Accidental puncture of the dura while performing **epidural anaesthesia**; the term usually refers to puncture by the epidural needle, although the epidural catheter may rarely enter the subarachnoid space, especially if there has been a partial dural tear during insertion. Important because it may interfere with the planned anaesthetic technique and because of the risk of **post-dural puncture headache**. Said to occur in 1% of cases in UK hospitals, although most authorities believe this is too high, with an incidence of 0.5% or lower being attainable with good training.

- Predisposing factors:
  - inexperienced operator.
  - unfamiliar equipment, e.g. sharper or blunter needles than one is used to.
  - faulty equipment, e.g. blocked needles, sticking syringes.
  - use of air instead of saline for loss of resistance has been implicated but strong evidence is lacking.
- Diagnosis is usually obvious because a stream of **CSF** flows from the needle hub, although flow may be slow and lead to confusion if saline has been used. Testing the fluid for pH (CSF >7), temperature (CSF is warm), glucose and protein content (CSF contains both) will reliably distinguish saline from CSF.
- Management options:
  - remove needle/catheter and abandon the procedure.
  - convert the block into single-shot or continuous spinal anaesthesia (the presence of a subarachnoid catheter has been suggested as causing inflammation of the dural edges, leading to more rapid healing and closure of the hole with a reduced incidence of severe headache, although strong evidence for this is lacking).
  - resite the catheter in an adjacent interspace:
    - cautious administration of test dose and subsequent doses (fractionated injection may be safer, as partial subarachnoid injection may occur).
    - 1 l saline may be given over 12–24 h through the catheter to reduce the incidence of post-dural

puncture headache. 50–60 ml boluses of saline over 10–20 min have also been used. Avoid dehydration. Use of laxatives has been suggested as a means of reducing straining; abdominal binders have also been suggested as reducing the incidence of headache but neither method is commonly used.
    - in obstetrics, instrumental delivery has been suggested to avoid straining during the second stage of labour, but this is controversial.
    - prophylactic **blood patch** via the epidural catheter at the end of the case/labour is controversial because it may be less successful than one performed later; it also exposes patients to a treatment that not all will require.
  - inform the patient and nursing/midwifery staff.
  - management of headache if it occurs (*see Post-dural puncture headache*).

Post-dural puncture headache may rarely occur without suspected dural puncture, possibly via a small breach of the dura (with or without the subarachnoid), that then extends.

Durrans's sign. Increased rate and depth of breathing following rapid injection of solution into the epidural space. More common in unconscious patients.
[Sidney F Durrans, Dorset anaesthetist]
See also, Epidural anaesthesia

DVT, *see Deep vein thrombosis*

Dye dilution cardiac output measurement, *see Cardiac output measurement*

Dynamic hyperinflation (DHI). Progressive accumulation of gas ('gas trapping') within the lung due to incomplete exhalation of the inspired volume. Occurs in patients with increased airway resistance (e.g. in **asthma** and **COPD**), when expiratory time is insufficient to allow the lungs to return to a normal **FRC**. Gas trapping continues until a new equilibrium is reached; at this higher FRC, increased small airway diameter and elastic recoil forces compensate for the airflow obstruction such that expired and inspired volumes equalise (this state is termed static hyperinflation).

Pressure exerted by trapped gas at end-expiration (termed intrinsic or auto-**PEEP**), combined with increased lung volumes, may result in the following:
  - increased **work of breathing** and **dyspnoea** (in spontaneously breathing patients).
  - reduced **venous return** and increased **pulmonary vascular resistance**; this may impair **cardiac output** and cause significant hypotension.
  - patient–ventilator asynchrony and impaired pressure-contolled ventilation.
  - **barotrauma** (e.g. **pneumothorax**).
- Methods of assessing DHI include:
  - assessment of cardiac output with the ventilator disconnected; dramatic improvement suggests significant DHI.
  - measurement of the plateau airway pressure ($P_{Plateau}$), the airway pressure measured after transient expiratory occlusion at end-inspiration.
  - measurement of intrinsic PEEP.

Modern ICU **ventilators** are usually able to perform the last two measurements. DHI during mechanical ventilation may be mitigated by ensuring prolonged expiratory times (>4 s) and low tidal volumes (e.g. 5–7 ml/kg).

Marini JJ (2011). Am J Respir Crit Care Med; 184: 756–62

Dyne. **Unit** of **force** in the **cgs system of units.** 1 dyne is the force required to accelerate a mass of 1 gram by 1 centimetre per second per second. 1 newton = 100 000 dyne.

Dynorphins. Endogenous opioid peptides; dynorphin 1–8 (8 amino acids) is found in the CNS, especially hypothalamus and posterior pituitary; dynorphin 1–17 (17 amino acids) is found in the duodenum. Thought to act as **neurotransmitters** in **pain pathways**; more active at κ than at μ **opioid receptors**.

Dysaesthesia. Abnormal unpleasant sensation, whether spontaneous or evoked; e.g. **hyperalgesia**, **allodynia**.

Dysequilibrium syndrome, *see Disequilibrium syndrome*

Dyspnoea. Feeling of breathlessness, with sensory and affective components. Mechanism is unclear, but may involve 'neuromechanical dissociation', a mismatch between central ventilatory drive and the magnitude of ventilation produced (as reflected by ongoing sensory afferent signalling). Sensory afferents originate in chest wall stretch receptors, pulmonary vagal receptors and chemoreceptors.
- May occur in:
  - increased respiratory drive, e.g. due to **hypoxaemia**, **hypercapnia**, **acidosis**, pulmonary receptor activity.
  - increased work of breathing.
  - impaired neuromuscular function of respiratory muscles.

Dyspnoea related to exercise tolerance is useful as a means of assessing respiratory/cardiovascular function, e.g. during **preoperative assessment.** Certain patterns are characteristically associated with certain disease processes, e.g. orthopnoea (left ventricular failure, severe restrictive lung disease, paralysis of the **diaphragm**) or paroxysmal nocturnal dyspnoea (left ventricular failure).
Nishino T (2011). Br J Anaesth; 106: 463–74
See also, Breathing, control of

Dyspnoeic index. Difference between **maximal voluntary ventilation** and maximum minute ventilation reached during exercise, as a percentage of maximal voluntary ventilation. Has been used to try to relate the subjective feeling of breathlessness to an objective measure of cardiorespiratory function.

Dysrhythmias, *see Arrhythmias*

Dystonic reaction. Acute side effect of dopamine antagonist drugs, e.g. many **antiemetic drugs.** May follow oral therapy, but particularly common after parenteral administration. More common after **phenothiazine** administration (e.g. **prochlorperazine** and **perphenazine**) than after **metoclopramide**, but the latter is especially likely to cause it in children and young women.

Consists of involuntary muscle contraction, especially involving the face. Oculogyric crisis (involuntary conjugate deviation of the eyes, usually upwards) may also occur.
- Treatment: **diazepam** 5–10 mg iv; **benzatropine** 1–2 mg iv/im; **procyclidine** 5–10 mg iv/im.

Dystrophia myotonica. Most common of the **myotonic syndromes**, with prevalence of 1 in 20 000. Multisystem disease with autosomal dominant inheritance; patients present at 15–35 years old.

- Features:
  - myotonia (increase in muscle tone following contraction). Exacerbated by cold.
  - **cardiomyopathy** and conduction defects.
  - respiratory muscle weakness and poor central control of respiration; may lead to **respiratory failure**.
  - central and obstructive **sleep apnoea**.
  - cognitive defects.
  - cataracts, frontal balding, sternomastoid and temporal muscle wasting, ptosis.
  - weakness of forearm and calf muscles.
  - testicular atrophy.
  - thyroid and adrenal impairment.
  - poor bulbar function and delayed **gastric emptying**.
- Anaesthetic problems:
  - related to poor cardiorespiratory reserve.
  - increased risk of **aspiration of gastric contents**.
  - increased sensitivity to **iv anaesthetic agents, opioids** and **non-depolarising neuromuscular blocking drugs**.
  - **suxamethonium** and **acetylcholinesterase inhibitors** may cause prolonged muscle contraction that may hinder laryngoscopy and ventilation.

Russell SH, Hirsch NP (1994). Br J Anaesth; 72: 210–16

See also, Myotonia congenita

Ear, nose and throat surgery (ENT surgery). Procedures vary from minor **day-case surgery** (e.g. myringotomy) to major head and neck dissections. Anaesthetic considerations:

- preoperatively:
  - **airway obstruction** may be present (often worse on lying flat), particularly in adults presenting with known or suspected tumours. Assessment of the airway in clinic using flexible nasendoscopy provides useful information. Potential difficulty with intubation/mask ventilation should be assessed.
  - obstructive **sleep apnoea** (with features of chronic hypoxaemia) may be present.
  - specific emergencies include bleeding **tonsil**, inhaled **foreign body**, **epiglottitis** and peritonsillar abscess.
  - good communication with the surgeon allows selection of airway techniques that are both safe and provide adequate surgical access.
  - anxiolytic, analgesic or antisialagogue **premedication** may be useful depending on the clinical context and intended anaesthetic technique.
- perioperatively:
  - induction appropriate to the patient's age, comorbidities, anticipated airway difficulty, etc.
  - techniques for securing the airway in potentially difficult cases include:
    - direct laryngoscopy under deep inhalational anaesthesia.
    - **fibreoptic intubation** (awake or anaesthetised).
    - **videolaryngoscopy**.
    - **tracheostomy** or **cricothyrotomy** performed under local anaesthesia.
  - options for airway maintenance:
    - **tracheal tube**: traditionally used for most procedures, with a throat pack if bleeding or debris is anticipated. Preformed tubes are useful. Oral intubation is suitable for many procedures, including laryngectomy and tonsillectomy. Nasal intubation provides better surgical access to the oral cavity; topical **local anaesthetic agents** and **vasopressor drugs** (e.g. **cocaine**) are used to reduce nasal bleeding (*see Nose*). A small-diameter (5 mm) tube, passed orally or nasally, is usually suitable for microlaryngoscopy.
    - **SAD**: avoids problems associated with intubation/extubation but may impair surgical access and be more prone to displacement.
    - facemask anaesthesia: suitable for minor ear operations (e.g. myringotomy/grommets).
    - **injector techniques**: often used for bronchoscopy, laryngoscopy, tracheal surgery.
  - access to the airway during surgery is restricted, therefore **monitoring** is particularly important. Obstruction of the airway is possible, especially during tonsillectomy if a **mouth gag** is used.
  - N_2O is usually avoided in middle ear surgery, because of expansion of gas-filled cavities.
  - surgery involving the face and neck may damage the facial and **laryngeal nerves**, respectively (*see Hyperthyroidism*). Absence of neuromuscular blockade may be requested by the surgeon to allow identification of nerves by electrical stimulation. Spontaneous ventilation, or IPPV using opioids (e.g. **remifentanil**), a volatile agent and induced hypocapnia, may be employed.
  - hypotensive anaesthesia is sometimes used, especially for major reconstructive surgery, laryngectomy, mastoidectomy and middle ear surgery.
  - thoracotomy is occasionally required, e.g. mobilisation of the stomach for anastomosis.
  - **laser surgery** is common, especially for laryngeal surgery.
  - **adrenaline** solutions are often used by the surgeon.
  - if used, the throat pack must be removed before the patient wakes. The pharynx may be inspected and suctioned to ensure absence of bleeding and blood clot, especially behind the soft palate ('coroner's clot').
  - tracheal **extubation** is performed with the patient deeply anaesthetised or awake (but not in-between, because of the risk of **laryngospasm**) and in the head-down, lateral position to reduce airway soiling.
- postoperatively: as for any surgery. Major procedures may require postoperative ICU/IPPV.

See also, Intubation, difficult; Mandibular nerve blocks; Maxillary nerve blocks

Early warning scores. Simple scoring systems used to aid identification of critically ill patients or those at risk of further clinical deterioration. Several different systems have been described, employing different groups of physiological parameters (e.g. systolic BP, heart rate, respiratory rate, temperature, **AVPU scale** and urine output) that are weighted according to their deviation from a 'normal' range. Early warning schemes may be used to 'trigger' calls for assistance from the patient's primary team, a **medical emergency team**, an **outreach team** or others. In the UK, the **modified early warning score** is most commonly used. Although widely adopted, demonstration of the efficacy of such scoring systems (e.g. reduction in mortality, admission to ICU, etc.) is hampered by the lack of standardisation.

Alam N, Hobbelink EL, van Tienhoven AJ, et al (2014). Resuscitation; 85: 587–94

See also, Acute life-threatening events—recognition and treatment

Earth-leakage circuit-breaker, *see Current-operated earth-leakage circuit-breaker*

Eaton–Lambert syndrome, *see Myasthenic syndrome*

Ebstein's anomaly. Congenital heart defect characterised by apical displacement of the posterior and septal leaflets of the tricuspid valve, causing 'atrialisation' of the right ventricle. Results in:
- right heart failure and cyanosis (due to right-to-left shunting).
- tricuspid valve regurgitation.
- **ASD** is often present.

May lead to **arrhythmias**, conduction defects (especially the **Wolff–Parkinson–White** syndrome) and sudden death. Surgical repair may be indicated in severe cases.
[Wilhelm Ebstein (1836–1912), German physician]
See also, Congenital heart disease; Tricuspid valve lesions

$ECCO_2R$, *see Extracorporeal carbon dioxide removal*

ECF, *see Extracellular fluid*

ECG, *see Electrocardiography*

Echocardiography. Cardiac imaging using reflection of **ultrasound** pulses from interfaces between tissue planes. A single beam may be studied as it passes through the heart, displaying movement of tissue planes over time, usually recorded on moving paper (M mode). Alternatively, beams are directed in different directions from the same point, covering a sector of tissue; a moving cross-section may then be displayed on a screen. Analysis of the frequencies of reflected pulses may provide information about the velocity of moving structures and blood flow (**Doppler effect**); flow characteristics may be colour-coded and superimposed on sector images. The passage of injected saline may be studied as it travels through the heart, probably due to entrainment of small air bubbles.

Useful in diagnosing and quantifying **valvular heart disease**, **congenital heart disease**, patent foramen ovale, myocardial and pericardial disease, and in assessing myocardial function. Techniques for the latter involve measurement of left ventricular dimensions and provide information about **ejection fraction** and **cardiac output**. Doppler techniques may be used to estimate pressure gradients across valves, as the gradient is related to the difference in velocities across the stenosis. Abnormalities of ventricular wall movement may occur in the early stages of **myocardial ischaemia**, before ECG changes occur.

'Focused' echocardiography consists of an abbreviated examination using limited views; increasingly performed by non-cardiologists to guide immediate management in emergency or critical care environments.

Transoesophageal echocardiography gives a good view of much of the heart, and has been used perioperatively and in ICU.

Barber RL, Fletcher SN (2014). Anaesthesia; 69: 764–76

Eclampsia. Convulsions associated with **pre-eclampsia**. Incidence is 2–3 cases per 10000 births in the UK. Occurs antepartum in 45% of cases, intrapartum in 20% and postpartum in 35% (usually under 2–4 days postpartum but eclampsia has been reported up to 2–3 weeks afterwards). Only 40% of cases have hypertension and proteinuria in the preceding week, and in many cases premonitory signs of headache, photophobia and hyperreflexia do not precede convulsions, which may recur if untreated. Mortality is almost 2% in the UK, usually from **stroke**; perinatal mortality is 5%–6%. Maternal mortality is up to 25% in developing countries.

Complications include **cerebral oedema** due to loss of cerebral autoregulation, stroke, **cerebral venous thrombosis, aspiration of gastric contents, cardiac failure** and **pulmonary oedema**.
- Treatment:
  - O_2 administration with the head-down, left lateral position if the trachea is unprotected. Tracheal intubation and IPPV may be required; the former may be difficult because of airway oedema.
  - **anticonvulsant drugs**; iv **magnesium sulfate** is the most effective drug for treating and preventing recurrence of eclamptic seizures. If seizures persist, **benzodiazepines** or **phenytoin** should be considered. If **status epilepticus** occurs, tracheal intubation and general anaesthesia will be required.
  - lowering of BP as for pre-eclampsia.
  - delivery of the fetus.
  - admission to ICU is often required.

ECMO, *see Extracorporeal membrane oxygenation*

Ecothiopate iodide. Organophosphorus compound, used as eye drops to treat severe **glaucoma**. Plasma **cholinesterase** levels may be reduced for 3–4 weeks following its use, prolonging the action of **suxamethonium**.

Ecstasy, *see Methylenedioxymethylamfetamine*

ECT, *see Electroconvulsive therapy*

Ectopic beats, *see Atrial ectopic beats; Junctional arrhythmias; Ventricular ectopic beats*

ED_{50}, *see Dose response curves; Therapeutic ratio/index*

Edema, *see Oedema*

Edetate, *see Cyanide poisoning; Sodium calcium edetate*

EDRF, Endothelium-derived relaxing factor, *see Nitric oxide*

Edrophonium chloride. Acetylcholinesterase inhibitor, used to reverse **non-depolarising neuromuscular blockade**, and in the diagnosis of **myasthenia gravis** and **dual block**. Has also been used to treat **SVT**. Binds reversibly to **acetylcholinesterase**, with onset of action 30 s and duration of about 5 min. Of faster onset than **neostigmine**, and with fewer muscarinic side effects.
- Dosage:
  - reversal of neuromuscular blockade: 0.5–0.7 mg/kg iv with **atropine**.
  - diagnosis of myasthenia gravis: 2 mg iv, followed by 8 mg iv, if no adverse reaction has occurred. Improvement in muscle strength occurs in myasthenia gravis. The test has low sensitivity and specificity.
  - diagnosis of dual block: 8 mg iv; causes transient improvement in muscle power.
  - treatment of SVT: 5–20 mg iv.
- Side effects: bradycardia, hypotension, nausea, vomiting, diarrhoea, abdominal cramps, increased salivation, muscle fasciculation. Convulsions and bronchospasm may also occur. The **ECG** should always be monitored when edrophonium is administered, and atropine must always be available.

EEG, *see Electroencephalography*

Efficacy. Maximal effect attainable by a drug; e.g. **morphine** is more efficacious than **codeine**. A pure antagonist has an efficacy of zero.
See also, Dose–response curves; Potency

EGTA, Esophageal gastric tube airway, *see Oesophageal obturators and airways*

Eicosanoids. Collective term used for products of **arachidonic acid** metabolism involved in inflammation, immunity and cell signalling. Include:
- prostanoids: produced by the **cyclo-oxygenase** pathway, e.g. **prostaglandins**, **prostacyclin** and **thromboxanes**.
- **leukotrienes** produced by the lipoxygenase pathways.

Eisenmenger's syndrome. Right-to-left cardiac **shunt** developing after long-standing left-to-right shunt; shunt reversal occurs because increased pulmonary blood flow results in increased **pulmonary vascular resistance** and **pulmonary hypertension**. Prognosis is poor, because pulmonary hypertension is not affected by surgical correction of the shunt. May follow any left-to-right shunt, although the original description referred to **VSD**. May occur late in **ASD** and patent **ductus arteriosus**.
- Features:
  - dyspnoea, effort syncope, angina, haemoptysis.
  - supraventricular **arrhythmias**, right ventricular failure, features of pulmonary hypertension.

Anaesthesia is tolerated poorly; reduction in peripheral resistance increases the shunt with worsening hypoxaemia, which in turn further increases pulmonary vascular resistance. Factors that decrease pulmonary blood flow also exacerbate the right-to-left shunt, e.g. **IPPV**. Risk of systemic **gas embolism** following iv injection of bubbles is high.

Pregnancy is also tolerated badly; maternal mortality is 30%–50%. Very cautious **epidural anaesthesia** has been suggested if pregnancy progresses to term.

Heart–lung transplantation is the only definitive treatment.

[Victor Eisenmenger (1864–1932), German physician]

Ejection fraction. Left ventricular **stroke volume** as a fraction of end-diastolic volume.

$$\text{equals: } \frac{\text{end-diastolic vol.} - \text{end-systolic vol.}}{\text{end-diastolic volume}} \times 100\%$$

Useful as an indication of the heart's ability to eject stroke volume. Measured using **nuclear cardiology**, **echocardiography**, **pulmonary artery catheterisation** or contrast angiography. Normally 50%–75%. May also be determined for the right ventricle.

Ejector flowmeter. Device used for **scavenging** from **anaesthetic breathing systems**. O_2 or air passing through the ejector causes entrainment of waste gases by the **Venturi principle**. The rate of removal is adjusted using a **flowmeter** until it equals the rate of fresh gas supply. Several litres of driving gas may be required per minute, at a pressure of at least 1 bar.

EKG, *see Electrocardiography*

Elastance. Reciprocal of **compliance**. Total elastance for lungs + chest wall is approximately 10 cmH_2O/l.

Elbow, nerve blocks. Used for surgery to the hand and wrist; useful for supplementation of a **brachial plexus block**. May be performed using surface anatomy landmarks, a peripheral nerve stimulator and/or **ultrasound** guidance.
- The following nerves are blocked (Fig. 58):
  - **median** (C5–T1): lies immediately medial to the brachial artery in the **antecubital fossa**. A needle is inserted with the elbow extended, level with the epicondyles, to approximately 5 mm, and 5 ml **local anaesthetic agent** injected. Subcutaneous infiltration blocks cutaneous branches.
  - **radial** (C5–T1): lies in the antecubital fossa in the groove between biceps tendon medially and brachioradialis muscle laterally. A needle is inserted level with the epicondyles with the elbow extended, and directed proximally and laterally to contact the lateral epicondyle. 2–4 ml solution is injected, and a further 5 ml during withdrawal to skin. This is repeated with the needle directed more proximally.
  - lateral cutaneous nerve of the forearm (C5–7): lies alongside the radial nerve. It is a continuation of the musculoskeletal nerve of the **brachial plexus**. May be blocked by subcutaneous infiltration between biceps and brachioradialis, using the same puncture site as for the radial nerve.
  - **ulnar** (C6–T1): passes through the ulnar groove behind the medial humeral epicondyle. With the elbow flexed to 90 degrees, a fine needle is inserted 1–2 cm proximal to the groove, pointing distally. At 1–2 cm depth, 2–5 ml solution is injected. Neuritis may follow injection into the nerve, or block within the ulnar groove.

See also, Brachial plexus block; Wrist, nerve blocks

Elderly, anaesthesia for. Increasingly common as the population ages. Mortality and morbidity are higher in older patients.
- Anaesthetic considerations, compared with younger patients:

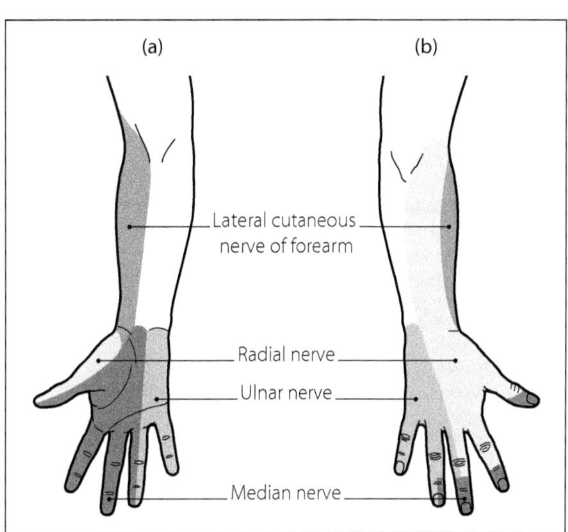

Fig. 58 Cutaneous distribution of nerves blocked at the elbow: (a) anterior; (b) posterior

- CVS:
  - **ischaemic heart disease** is more likely, with reduced ventricular compliance and contractility, and cardiac output.
  - decreased blood flow to vital organs.
  - widespread **atherosclerosis** with a less compliant arterial system. **Hypertension** is common.
  - veins are more tortuous, thickened and fragile.
  - **DVT** is more common.
- RS:
  - decreased lung **compliance** and alveolar surface area.
  - increased **closing capacity**, therefore more airway collapse with resultant increase in **alveolar–arterial O_2 difference**. Normal alveolar PO_2 is approximately:

$$13.3-\frac{\text{age}}{30}\text{ kPa}\left(100-\frac{\text{age}}{4}\text{ mmHg}\right)$$

  - decreased response to **hypercapnia** and **hypoxaemia.**
  - higher incidence of postoperative **atelectasis, PE** and **chest infection.**
- pharmacology:
  - increased sensitivity to many drugs, especially CNS depressants.
  - drug distribution, metabolism and elimination are altered. A greater proportion of body weight is fat, due to a decrease in total body water. Plasma proteins are reduced with altered drug binding.
  - **half-lives** of many drugs are increased.
- metabolic:
  - metabolic rate is lower.
  - impaired renal function, thought to be due to decreased renal blood flow and decreased number of glomeruli; suggested decrease in GFR is 1% per year over 20.
  - **fluid balance** is more critical with reduction in total body water; **dehydration** is common following trauma and illness.
  - **diabetes mellitus** and **malnutrition** are more common.
- nervous system:
  - cerebrovascular disease is common.
  - **confusion** and **postoperative cognitive dysfunction** are more likely, and may be caused by hypoxia, **hyperventilation**, drugs, hospitalisation and any illness.
  - autonomic nervous system dysfunction is common.
  - impaired hearing, vision and memory loss are common.
- other considerations:
  - **heat loss during anaesthesia** is more likely, due to impairment of both central control and compensatory mechanisms.
  - **hiatus hernia** is more common, with risk of regurgitation and aspiration.
  - systemic diseases and multiple drug therapy are more common.
  - cervical spondylosis is common, with reduced neck movement. Pain from arthritis may cause great discomfort, e.g. during local anaesthetic techniques. Ligaments are often calcified and tough.

In general, patients are frailer, with greater likelihood of perioperative complications and slower healing. Attention to detail (e.g. fluid balance) is more important than with younger patients because physiological reserves are reduced. Smaller doses of most agents are required, and **arm–brain circulation time** is prolonged.

Warming blankets, adequate **humidification** and appropriate monitoring (e.g. of urine output) should be provided. Postoperative O_2 therapy should be instituted immediately and possibly continued for 1–3 days, because hypoxaemia may readily occur.

The 'physiological age' of the patient is usually more relevant than the chronological age: e.g. fit 90-year-olds may present less risk than frail 70-year-olds.

Griffiths R, Beech F, Brown A, et al (2014). Anaesthesia; 69: 81–98

Electrical symbols. Used to denote components of electrical circuits. Specific symbols are also used on electrical equipment to indicate the safety features or other characteristics or instructions (Fig. 59).

See also, Electrocution and electrical burns

Electroacupuncture, *see Acupuncture*

Electrocardiography (ECG). Recording and display of cardiac electrical activity. First performed through the intact chest in 1887 by Waller. Used for investigation of cardiac disease, particularly **ischaemic heart disease** and **arrhythmias**, also for **monitoring** cardiac rhythm.

Standard modern ECG recordings are obtained from different combinations of chest and limb electrodes, each set recording along a different vector, thus providing information about a different part of the heart. A 'lead' refers to the recorded voltage difference between two electrodes; one acts as the positive electrode, the other as the negative (or reference) electrode. The limb leads (I–III, aVR, aVL, aVF) record in the frontal plane, the chest leads ($V_{1–6}$) in the transverse plane. The leads may be represented on the chest and heart as in Fig. 60a. Thus abnormalities of the inferior portion of the heart will be demonstrated in the 'inferior' leads (i.e., aVF, II and III), and abnormalities of the anterolateral heart in aVL, I, II, etc. $V_{1–2}$ demonstrate electrical activity from the right side of the heart, $V_{3–4}$ from the septum and front, and $V_{5–6}$ from the left side. Depolarisation towards a positive electrode (or repolarisation away) results in a positive deflection; depolarisation away (or repolarisation towards) causes negative deflection.

- standard bipolar limb leads:
  - I: between left arm (positive electrode) and right arm (negative).
  - II: between left leg (positive electrode) and right arm (negative).
  - III: between left leg (positive electrode) and left arm.

  Einthoven's triangle is the imaginary inverted equilateral triangle centred on the heart, whose sides are formed by the axes of the standard limb leads.
- augmented unipolar limb leads: combinations of reference electrodes are used that 'augment' the signal along the desired vector:
  - aVR: right arm.
  - aVL: left arm.
  - aVF: left leg.

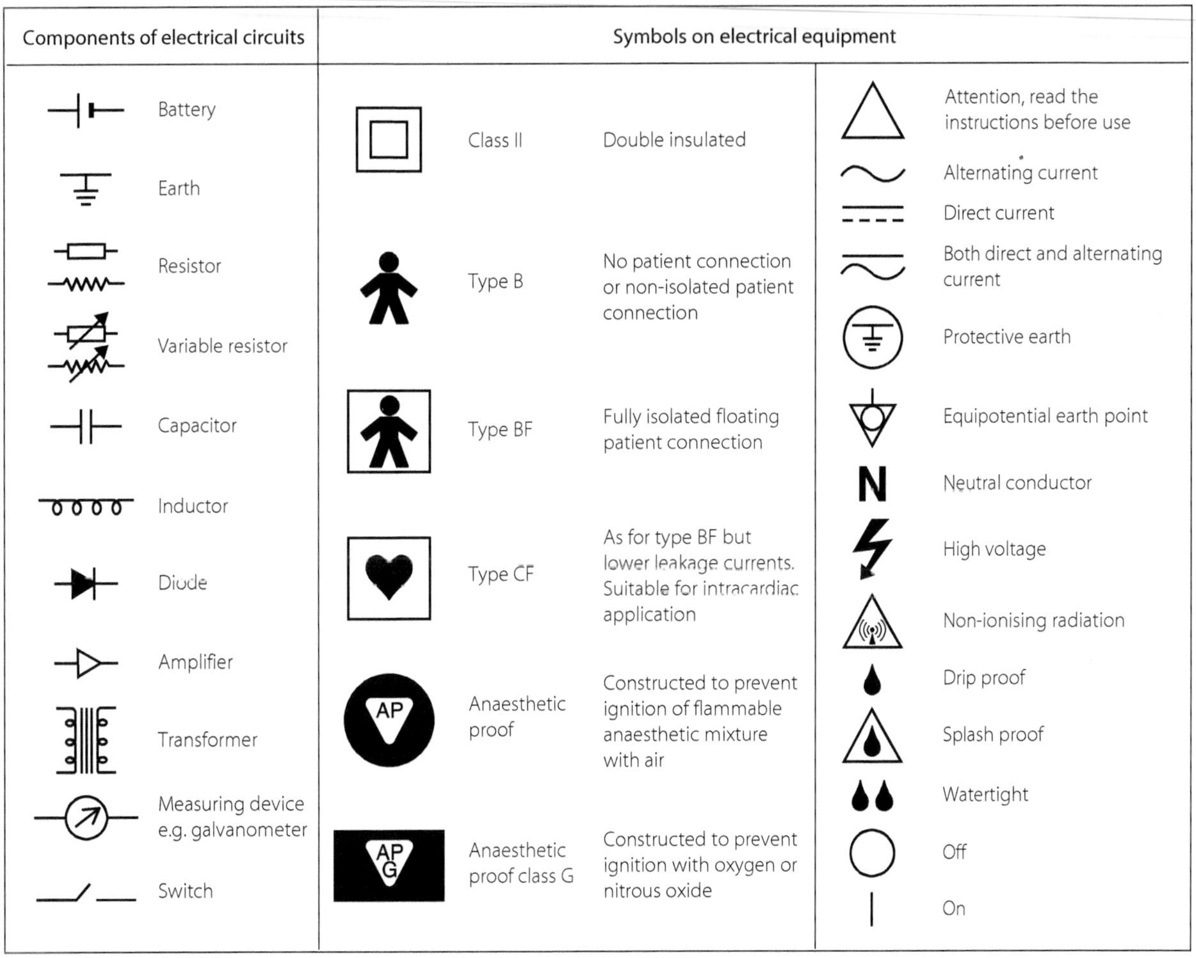

Components of electrical circuits
Symbols on electrical equipment
Battery
Earth
Resistor
Variable resistor
Capacitor
Inductor
Diode
Amplifier
Transformer
Measuring device e.g. galvanometer
Switch
Class II
Double insulated
Type B
No patient connection or non-isolated patient connection
Type BF
Fully isolated floating patient connection
Type CF
As for type BF but lower leakage currents. Suitable for intracardiac application
AP
Anaesthetic proof
Constructed to prevent ignition of flammable anaesthetic mixture with air
AP G
Anaesthetic proof class G
Constructed to prevent ignition with oxygen or nitrous oxide
Attention, read the instructions before use
Alternating current
Direct current
Both direct and alternating current
Protective earth
Equipotential earth point
N
Neutral conductor
High voltage
Non-ionising radiation
Drip proof
Splash proof
Watertight
Off
On

Fig. 59 Electrical symbols

(a)
(b)
(c)
aVR
aVL
I
V leads
III
aVF
II
1
2
3
4
5
6
R
P
T
U
Q
S
P–R
QRS
S–T
Q–T
aVR
–90°
aVL
±180°
0°
I
III
+90°
II
aVF

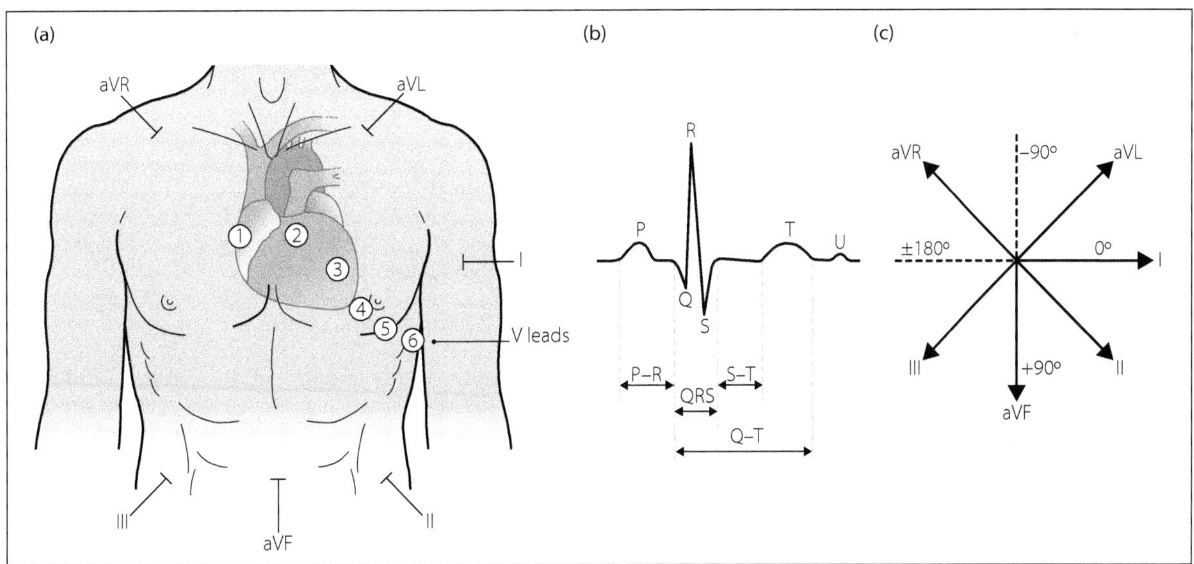

Fig. 60 The ECG: (a) arrangement of leads; (b) normal ECG; (c) electric axis

- electrode placement for unipolar chest leads (reference electrode is formed by the combined limb leads, such that the reference point is mid-chest):
  - V_1: fourth intercostal space, right sternal edge.
  - V_2: fourth intercostal space, left sternal edge.
  - V_3: midway between V_2 and V_4.
  - V_4: fifth intercostal space, left midclavicular line.
  - V_5: fifth intercostal space, left anterior axillary line.
  - V_6: fifth intercostal space, left midaxillary line.

Output is displayed on an **oscilloscope** or recorded on moving paper. Frequency range is 0.5–80 Hz. Magnitude of deflection is proportional to the amount of heart muscle, but reduced by passage through the chest. Skin resistance is reduced by cleaning with alcohol and skin abrasion. Electrodes are usually silver/silver chloride with chloride conducting gel, to reduce generation of potentials in the electrode by the recorded potential, and reduce **impedance** variability. Electrodes of differing compounds may generate potential by a battery-like effect. Interference may result from muscle activity, radiofrequency waves from **diathermy** and other equipment and **inductance** by electrical equipment. Differential **amplifiers** with common-mode rejection (elimination of signals affecting both input terminals of a recording system) are used to reduce interference.

- Plan for the interpretation of standard ECG, with normal values (Fig. 60b):
  - patient's name, clinical context, date.
  - usual speed of recording is 25 mm/s; usual calibration is 1 mV/cm (usually confirmed on each recording with a calibration mark).
  - rate: **heart rate** in beats/min is calculated by dividing the number of 5-mm squares between successive **QRS complexes** into 300, assuming a recording speed of 25 mm/s.
  - rhythm:
    - regular or irregular. An irregular rhythm may be regularly (e.g. missing every third QRS) or irregularly irregular (e.g. completely random in **AF**).
    - presence/absence of **P waves**, flutter waves in **atrial flutter**, **ventricular ectopic beats**, pacing spikes, etc.
  - axis: summation of electrical potentials from the standard and aV leads, plotted as vectors. The normal axis lies between −30 degrees and +90 degrees (Fig. 60c). Simple method of determination: because leads I and aVF are at right angles to each other, they can be used alone; e.g. if the QRS deflection is positive in both, the axis lies between 0 and 90 degrees. If I is positive and aVF negative, the axis lies between 0 and −90 degrees.

    Left axis deviation (<−30 degrees) may occur in:
    - normal subjects (especially if pregnant), ascites, etc.
    - left **bundle branch block**, left anterior hemiblock.
    - left ventricular hypertrophy.

    Right axis deviation (>90 degrees) may occur in:
    - normal subjects.
    - right ventricular hypertrophy.
    - right bundle branch block, left posterior hemiblock.
  - P wave (atrial depolarisation):
    - positive in I, II, and V_{4-6}; negative in aVR, because depolarisation moves downwards and to the left.
    - height <2.5 mm.
    - width <3 mm.
    - shape.
  - **P–R interval**: normally 0.12–0.2 s (3–5 mm squares).
  - QRS complex (ventricular depolarisation):
    - usually positive in I, II and V_{4-6}; negative in aVR and V_{1-2}, because most left ventricular depolarisation moves downwards and to the left. Progresses smoothly across the chest leads, e.g. stepwise increase in height from V_1 to V_4; either increases or decreases in V_{5-6}.
    - duration is 0.04–0.12 s (1–3 mm squares).
    - amplitude in I + II + III >5 mm. Left ventricular hypertrophy exists if the **R wave** in V_6 + **S wave** in V_1 >35 mm. In right ventricular hypertrophy the R:S ratio >1 in V_{1-2}.
    - shape; presence of **Q waves**.
    - abnormal waves, e.g. J and δ waves in **hypothermia** and **Wolff–Parkinson–White syndrome**, respectively.
  - **S–T segment**:
    - level within 1 mm of baseline.
    - shape.
  - **T wave** (ventricular repolarisation):
    - orientation as for QRS complexes.
    - height <5 mm.
    - shape.
  - **Q–T interval**: corrected Q–T

$$= \left(\frac{\text{measured Q–T}}{\sqrt{\text{cycle length}}} \right) \text{Normal range } 0.35\text{–}0.43\text{ s}$$

  - **U wave**.

During anaesthesia/intensive care, a three-electrode system (allowing recording of the three standard limb leads) is often used and lead II is selected for continuous rhythm monitoring. A five-electrode system incorporating a right leg and a precordial electrode (in addition to the right arm/left arm/left leg electrodes) enables recording of an anterior chest lead; useful when monitoring left ventricular **myocardial ischaemia**. The CM_5 lead configuration (central manubrium V_5) also 'looks at' the left ventricle:

- right arm electrode in suprasternal notch.
- left arm electrode over apex of heart (V_5 position).
- left leg electrode on left shoulder or leg serves as ground.

Other lead configurations are also used, e.g. CH_5, CC_5 and CS_5, with right arm electrode on the patient's head, right side of chest and subscapular regions, respectively. The CB_5 configuration with electrode over the right scapula is better for demonstrating arrhythmias.

24-hour ambulatory ECG monitoring is performed for assessing arrhythmias and their therapy, and detecting myocardial ischaemia. Some devices run continuously while others are activated by the patient when he or she experiences symptoms. 24-hour tapes have been used to investigate arrhythmias and ischaemia perioperatively.

[Augustus Desiré Waller (1856–1922), French-born British physiologist; Willem Einthoven (1860–1927), Dutch physician and physiologist]

See also, Cardiac cycle; Heart block; His bundle electrography; Myocardial infarction

Electroconvulsive therapy (ECT). Passage of electric current, usually alternating, across the skull to produce convulsions; used to treat severe depressive psychosis. 30–45 J is usually given over 0.5–1.5 s; it may also be given as repeated ultra-short bursts. Usually given in courses over a few weeks. First used in the late 1930s.

Brief general anaesthesia is required; partial neuromuscular blockade is usually provided, to allow assessment of resultant convulsions while reducing the risk of vertebral fractures and other trauma.

- Anaesthetic considerations:
  - preoperatively:
    - patients should be prepared, starved and investigated as for any anaesthetic procedure. Particular care is required if cardiovascular disease or intracranial pathology coexists.

   - concurrent drug therapy may include **antidepressant drugs**, including **monoamine oxidase inhibitors, lithium**.
   - premedication is usually omitted.
- perioperatively:
   - **monitoring** is required as for any procedure.
   - a single induction dose of iv agent is usually given. **Methohexital** was traditionally used because of its short action and proconvulsant properties. **Propofol** (at 1 mg/kg) provides greater haemodynamic stability and more rapid post-ictal recovery while having the same therapeutic benefit as methohexital and has become the induction agent of choice.
   - **suxamethonium** 0.5 mg/kg is commonly given, although smaller doses have been used.
   - a soft mouth guard is inserted to protect the teeth and gums.
   - the lungs are ventilated with O_2 by facemask after induction of anaesthesia, because seizure threshold is reduced by hypocapnia. Oxygenation is usually continued during and after the convulsions, although the need for the former has been questioned.
   - intense parasympathetic discharge may follow passage of current, and may be followed by increased sympathetic activity. **Atropine** should always be available; routine administration has been suggested.
- **recovery** facilities: as normal. Confusion may follow.

Electrocution and electrical burns. Hazard of using electrical equipment; during anaesthesia, malfunction or improper use of **diathermy**, **monitoring** equipment or infusion devices may cause sudden **cardiac arrest** or burns.

Current flows between opposite poles for direct current, or from live wire to earth for alternating current, e.g. mains power. Mains voltage is 240 V at 50 Hz in the UK and 110 V at 60 Hz in the USA. Current flows via the path of least resistance; if this path includes a person (e.g. patient or doctor) via earthed equipment, ECG lead or floor, electrocution occurs.

- Effects:
   - heat production due to high resistance of tissues. Amount of heat is related to **current density**. May produce burns at sites of current entry/departure.
   - nerve and muscle stimulation; e.g. effect of current across chest (approximate values):
      - 1 mA: tingling.
      - 5 mA: pain.
      - 15 mA: tonic muscle contraction, i.e., 'can't let go' threshold.
      - 50 mA: respiratory arrest.
      - 100 mA: VF.
      - >5 A: tonic contraction of the myocardium (used in **defibrillation**).

   Magnitude of current depends on the resistance to flow, which is reduced if contacts are wet or have large surface area. Current density at the myocardium is important; thus 100 μA is sufficient to cause VF if delivered directly to the heart (microshock). Other important factors include:
      - frequency of alternating current: 50–60 Hz is particularly dangerous but cheap to provide.
      - timing of shock (e.g. **R on T phenomenon**).
- Methods of protection:
   - regular checking and maintenance of electrical equipment.
   - use of batteries only (impractical).
   - connection of equipment casing to earth (defined as class I equipment). Accidental contact between the live wire and casing then causes a large current to flow to earth, with melting of protective fuses and breakage of the circuit. Fuses are made of thin wire that melts at certain current loads; they serve to protect equipment in case of faults, but do not melt quickly enough to prevent dangerous currents flowing. Fuses are usually placed in live and neutral wires and mains plugs.
   - double insulation of all conducting wires within equipment (class II).
   - use of isolated circuits, e.g. in diathermy, ECG: patients are not connected directly to earth via plates and electrodes, but via transformers within each piece of apparatus. Current thus cannot reach earth through the patient if contact with a live supply occurs. Class III equipment uses internal transformers to reduce voltage, e.g. to under 24 V. Internal transformers are cheaper and more practical than large external transformers, e.g. one for an operating suite.
   - reduction of stray leakage currents, e.g. due to drops in potential along the length of conductors, caused by **capacitance** between casing and innards or **inductance**. Leakage currents may be sufficient to produce microshock. Earth conductors are connected to each other to reduce differences between them. **Current-operated earth-leakage circuit breakers** may be used. Standards for leakage currents are defined, e.g. 10 μA maximum from the casing or delivered to the patient for intracardiac equipment; 100–500 μA for other equipment, depending on usage.
   - reduction of the risk of microshock by avoiding conducting solutions (e.g. saline) in intracardiac lines such as CVP manometers. Needle electrodes are also avoided, because their resistance is low.
   - electrical equipment, plugs, etc., should not be placed on the floor where solutions may fall on them.

Medical electrical equipment is marked with the appropriate **electrical symbols** to indicate its level of safety features (*see Fig. 59*).

Electroencephalography (EEG). Recording of electrical activity of the brain. Signals from different combinations of 20–22 scalp electrodes are presented as 16 continuous traces. Shape, distribution, incidence and symmetry of waves are analysed to give information about underlying brain activity, in conjunction with clinical details. Concealed abnormalities may be revealed during voluntary hyperventilation.

- Different rhythms:
   - alpha: normal 8–13 Hz waves. Prominent at the parieto-occipital area during the awake but resting state, with the eyes closed.
   - beta: normal 13–30 Hz waves. Prominent over the frontal area during the awake and active state.
   - delta: <4 Hz waves; normal during adult slow-wave **sleep**.
   - theta: 4–8 Hz waves; present during the transition between wakefulness and sleep, and during meditative states.

As age increases, infantile beta activity is slowly replaced by adult alpha activity. Characteristic patterns occur in normal sleep. During anaesthesia, alpha rhythms become depressed, and are replaced by theta and delta rhythms. Slow rhythms may reappear at deeper levels of anaesthesia, followed by periods of little or no activity separated by bursts of activity (burst suppression). The pattern differs with different agents used. Perioperative use is limited by electrical interference and difficult interpretation. Modified forms of EEG have therefore been developed, e.g. **cerebral function monitor**, **cerebral function analysing monitor**, **power spectral analysis**, **bispectral index monitor**. Used to investigate intracranial activity in, e.g. **TBI**, **epilepsy**, cerebrovascular disease, coma, encephalopathies, surgery. Similar principles are involved in measuring **evoked potentials**.

Purdon PL, Sampson A, Pavone KJ, Brown EN (2015). Anesthesiology; 123: 937–60

See also, Anaesthesia, depth of

Electrolyte. Compound that dissociates in solution to produce ions, allowing conduction of electricity; also refers to the ions themselves. **Sodium**, **potassium**, **calcium**, **magnesium** and **hydrogen ions** are the most important cations in the body; chloride and **bicarbonate** ions the most important anions.

See also, Fluids, body; Intravenous fluids

Electrolyte imbalance, *see individual disorders*

Electrolyte solutions, *see Intravenous fluids*

Electromagnetic flow measurement. Relies on the principle that a moving conductor within a magnetic field induces current that is proportional to the rate of movement (Faraday's law). Relationship of movement, field and current is described by Fleming's right-hand rule, with thumb, forefinger and middle finger of the right hand extended at mutual right angles (e.g. forefinger pointing forward, thumb upward and middle finger medially). If the forefinger points in the direction of the field, and thumb in the direction of movement, the middle finger will point in the direction of the induced current.

Electromagnets within a semicircular probe are placed around an artery, and the moving blood is the conductor. The potential difference between the walls of the vessel is measured and average velocity of blood flow determined. Alternating current is used for magnetic field generation, to avoid the effect of induction of current in the detector electrode circuit.

[Michael Faraday (1791–1867), English chemist; Sir John Fleming (1849–1945), English electrical engineer]

Electromechanical dissociation (EMD). Term used to describe a cardiac state in which organised electrical depolarisation occurs throughout the myocardium, but there is no synchronous shortening of the myocardial fibres and mechanical contractions are absent. Part of the spectrum of **pulseless electrical activity**, though the latter also includes mechanical contractions too weak to produce a detectable cardiac output.

See also, Cardiac arrest

Electromyography (EMG). Recording of spontaneous or evoked electrical activity from skeletal muscle; usually combined with nerve conduction studies that measure the velocity of nerve conduction following stimulation at different sites along a nerve pathway. Thus useful in distinguishing between disorders of muscle, isolated or generalised nerve disease or lesions, and disorders affecting the **neuromuscular junction**.

In anaesthesia, it has been used to determine frontalis muscle tone to monitor depth of anaesthesia. Also used in **neuromuscular blockade monitoring**; nerve stimulation and muscle action potential recording are achieved using surface skin electrodes, although needle electrodes have been used. Less convenient than devices measuring mechanical muscle response, it may detect electrical activity when mechanical contraction is undetectable.

Also used to investigate **critical illness polyneuropathy/myopathy.**

See also, Anaesthesia, depth of

Electron capture detector. Device used in the analysis of gas mixtures that have been separated by, for example, **gas chromatography**; particularly useful in detecting halogenated compounds. Electrons within an ionisation chamber pass from cathode to anode, but are 'captured' by the halogenated substance blown through the chamber. The current passing across the chamber is therefore reduced, depending on how many electrons are captured. Used to quantify the amount of known substances, not to identify unknown ones.

See also, Gas analysis

Embryo, *see Environmental safety of anaesthetists; Fetus, effect of anaesthetic agents on*

EMD, *see Electromechanical dissociation*

Emergence phenomena. Usually consist of agitation and **confusion**, with laryngospasm, breath-holding, etc.; may be equivalent to the second stage of anaesthesia seen on induction, or be due to other causes of confusion, including the **central anticholinergic syndrome** and **dystonic reactions**. Hallucinations and frightening dreams are common after **ketamine**.

Emergency surgery. Usually refers to surgery occurring within 24 h of admission or diagnosis; i.e., includes those cases where surgery follows resuscitation, and those where surgery and resuscitation proceed simultaneously (e.g. ruptured aortic aneurysm).

- Problems may be related to:
    - inadequate preparation of patients for surgery:
        - full stomach, i.e., risk of **aspiration of gastric contents**.
        - untreated pre-existing disease, electrolyte imbalance, etc.
        - appropriate investigations and cross-matching of blood not performed or not ready.
    - the presenting complaint:
        - **haemorrhage** and **hypovolaemia.**
        - intestinal obstruction/intra-abdominal pathology: **dehydration** and hypovolaemia, electrolyte imbalance, etc. Further risk of aspiration due to delayed gastric emptying and vomiting/haematemesis.
        - **trauma**: haemorrhage, **head injury**, **chest trauma**, etc.
        - **airway obstruction**/inhaled **foreign body**.
        - related to specialist surgery, e.g. **cardiac surgery**, **neurosurgery**.

The balance between the need for preoperative optimisation and urgency of surgery is sometimes difficult, but inadequate preoperative correction of fluid and electrolyte disturbance is consistently associated with increased perioperative mortality. Treatment of **cardiac failure** is also important whenever possible. Careful **preoperative assessment** and discussion with the surgeon are vital. Anaesthetic management is as for routine surgery but with the previous considerations. Thus smaller doses of drugs than usual are given initially. Rapid sequence induction is usually employed. Measures against **heat loss** are important. Invasive monitoring and postoperative HDU/ICU and IPPV should be considered.

Regional techniques are particularly useful for limb surgery, but **epidural/spinal anaesthesia** is hazardous if hypovolaemia is present.

Special Issue (2013). Anaesthesia; 68 (suppl s1): 1–124

See also, specific procedures; Anaesthetic morbidity and mortality

Emesis, *see Vomiting*

Emetic drugs. Given to empty the stomach, e.g. following **poisoning**, or preoperatively to reduce risk of **aspiration pneumonitis**. Now rarely used, because of poor efficacy and the risk of causing aspiration; particularly dangerous after ingestion of corrosive or petroleum derivatives, or in unconscious patients. Include **apomorphine** and **ipecacuanha**; copper sulfate and sodium chloride are no longer used.

EMG, *see Electromyography*

EMLA cream (Eutectic mixture of local anaesthetics). Mixture of **prilocaine** base 2.5% and **lidocaine** base 2.5% as an oil–water emulsion. The melting point of each local anaesthetic agent is lowered by the presence of the other; the resultant mixture has a melting point of 18°C and is effective in providing analgesia of the skin 60–90 min after topical application and covering with an occlusive dressing. May continue to be released from skin depots even after removal of surface cream. Particularly useful in children. May produce blanching of the skin; increases in methaemoglobin have been reported several hours after application. Systemic toxicity has also been reported.

Uses include analgesia for venepuncture, venous and arterial cannulation, lumbar puncture, epidural injection, superficial skin surgery and relief of tourniquet pain during IVRA.

EMMV, Extended mandatory minute ventilation, *see Mandatory minute ventilation*

EMO inhaler, *see Vaporisers*

Emphysema, *see Chronic obstructive pulmonary disease*

Emphysema, subcutaneous. Presence of gas in subcutaneous tissues.

May be caused by:
- trauma, including surgery (hence the term 'surgical emphysema'); gas arises from the atmosphere, viscera or air sinuses.
- **pneumothorax** or rupture of a viscus, e.g. oesophagus.
- **barotrauma.**
- infection with gas-producing organisms, e.g. **gas gangrene.**
- rarely, deliberate self-injection of subcutaneous air in disordered mental states.

Often palpable under the skin, and may be visible on x-ray. The gas is slowly absorbed once the cause is treated. Multiple skin puncture has been performed to allow escape of gas, and high F_IO_2 suggested to increase absorption (O_2 being more soluble than nitrogen), but the value of these measures is unknown.

Empyema. Collection of pus within the pleural cavity. A complication of **chest trauma** (especially if haemothorax was present), pneumonia, chest drainage, **thoracic surgery** and subdiaphragmatic abscess. Clinical features include pyrexia, chest pain and productive cough. **CXR** features are those of a pleural effusion; if encapsulated it may resemble a pulmonary cyst. Diagnosis is confirmed by imaging and aspiration of pus. Treatment depends on aetiology but includes **antibacterial drugs, chest drainage** (sometimes requiring **ultrasound** or **CT scan** guidance) and surgery. May rarely lead to **bronchopleural fistula.**

Lee SF, Lawrence D, Booth H, et al (2010). Curr Opin Pulm Med; 16: 194–200

Enalapril maleate. Angiotensin converting enzyme inhibitor, used to treat hypertension and **cardiac failure** (including following **MI**). A **prodrug**, it is converted to enalaprilat by hepatic metabolism. Longer acting than **captopril**, with onset of action within 2 h; **half-life** is up to 35 h via active metabolites.
- Dosage: 2.5–40 mg orally od.
- Side effects: hypotension following the first dose or following induction of anaesthesia, cough, dizziness, weakness, nausea, diarrhoea, rash, renal impairment.

Encephalitis. Acute infection of the **brain** parenchyma, usually caused by a virus, that results in diffuse inflammation affecting the **meninges**. Usually presents with the triad of fever, headache and altered mental status. Other clinical features include neck stiffness, lethargy, **confusion, coma, encephalopathy**, focal neurological signs and **epilepsy.**
- Causes:
  - viral infection: viruses gain entry to the CNS via the haematological route or retrograde neuronal spread. Viruses include herpes simplex (most commonly), varicella zoster, cytomegalovirus and Epstein–Barr virus.
  - immunologically mediated para-infectious phenomenon following a variety of infections or vaccinations.
  - autoimmune encephalitis (including anti-**NMDA** receptor encephalitis and anti-voltage-gated potassium channel encephalitis) is being increasingly recognised; presents with psychiatric, epileptic and movement disorder features.
  - neoplastic or paraneoplastic encephalitis.

Differential diagnosis includes **meningitis** and **cerebral abscess**. Investigations include **CSF** examination (mild increase in protein, lymphocytosis, normal glucose in viral encephalitis), **CT** and **MRI scanning, EEG** and viral titres/cultures from blood and CSF. Treatment is largely supportive, with tracheal intubation and IPPV for patients with depressed consciousness. **Aciclovir** should be given to all cases of suspected viral encephalitis while a definitive diagnosis is sought.

[M. Anthony Epstein, British pathologist; Yvonne Barr (1932–2016), British virologist]

Solomon T, Michael BD, Smith PE, et al (2012). J Infect; 64: 347–73

Encephalopathy. Diffuse disorder of cerebral function with or without focal neurological deficit. Usually results in delirium, stupor and **coma.** Aetiology is as for coma.

Endobronchial blockers (Bronchial blockers). Used in **thoracic surgery** to isolate a portion of lung, e.g. to avoid air leaks during IPPV or prevent contamination of normal lung with secretions, pus or blood. Less often used now, except for paediatric surgery, **endobronchial tubes** being more popular and versatile. Previous versions were made of red rubber; modern versions are thin plastic catheters with an inflatable distal cuff, usually inserted under direct vision via a bronchoscope, either before tracheal intubation with a standard tracheal tube or after intubation with a specific tube–blocker combination.

Endobronchial tubes. Used in **thoracic surgery** to allow sleeve resection of the bronchus, or to isolate infected lung or potential air leak, e.g. in **bronchopleural fistula** or emphysematous lung cysts. Other pulmonary surgery (e.g. pneumonectomy/lobectomy, pleural, aortic, oesophageal and mediastinal surgery) is possible with conventional tracheal tubes, although surgery may be made easier by collapsing one lung. Also used in ICU in patients with severe, unilateral lung injury or bronchopleural fistula. Risks of **one-lung anaesthesia** should be considered before use.

Different tubes, usually made of red rubber, were developed in the 1930s–1950s, and included single-lumen and double-lumen designs, for insertion into the left (most commonly) or right main bronchus. Modern double-lumen tubes are usually plastic, with thinner walls and low-pressure cuffs, and have the following features (Fig. 61):

- cuffed endobronchial portion, curved to the left or right as appropriate (the latter's cuff is deflected around a slot for the right upper bronchus). The bronchial cuff and inflation port on single-use tubes are blue by convention.
- cuffed tracheal portion.
- oropharyngeal portion, concave anteriorly.

The main problem with right-sided tubes is related to the short length of the right main bronchus before giving off the upper lobe bronchus. Hence left-sided tubes are usually preferred, even for right-sided surgery, because of the risk of inadequate ventilation of the right upper lobe if incorrectly positioned. Right-sided tubes are often preferred if the left main bronchus is compressed by aortic aneurysm, to prevent traumatic haemorrhage.

- Insertion:
    - as for tracheal tubes initially, with the bronchial curve concave anteriorly to aid passage through the pharynx.
    - rotated 90 degrees when the tip is through the larynx, to direct the endobronchial part to the appropriate side.
    - connected to the breathing system via a double catheter mount, each lumen connected via a capped connector and compressible tubing. Cuff inflation:
        - the tracheal cuff is inflated until the air leak stops; both sides of the chest are checked for ventilation.
        - the catheter mount to the tracheal lumen is clamped, and the tracheal lumen opened to air.
        - the lung is inflated via the bronchial lumen only, inflating the bronchial cuff until no air leak is heard from the tracheal lumen. Only the selected side of the chest should now move.
        - the tracheal lumen is reconnected and both sides of the chest are checked as before.
        - both lungs should now be able to be ventilated separately, by inflating via one lumen only and opening the other to air.

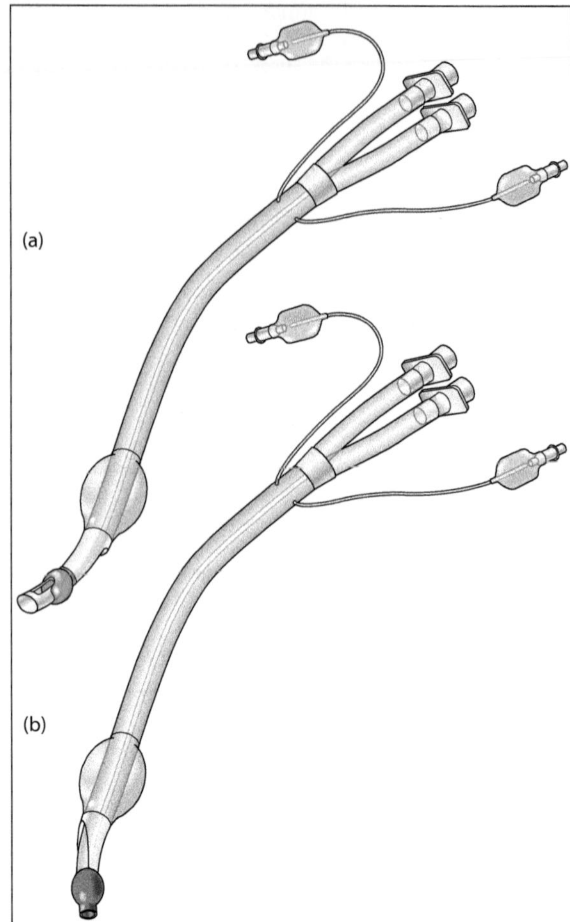

Fig. 61 Double-lumen endobronchial tubes: (a) right-sided; (b) left-sided

Fibreoptic endoscopy is essential to confirm correct positioning as clinical assessment may not be reliable; it is also useful to check for bronchial cuff herniation causing tube or bronchial obstruction.

Complications are as for tracheal intubation (*see Intubation, complications of*). Bronchial rupture may occur if excessive volumes are used for cuff inflation. Incorrect positioning, or movement during positioning of the patient, may result in uneven ventilation and impaired gas exchange.

See also, Tracheobronchial tree

Endocardial viability ratio (EVR). Ratio of **diastolic pressure time index** to **tension time index**, obtained by recording left ventricular and aortic root pressure tracings (Fig. 62). May indicate myocardial O_2 supply/demand ratio and likelihood of **myocardial ischaemia** (thought to be likely when the ratio is under 0.7).

Endocarditis, infective. Infective colonisation and inflammation of the endocardial lining of the heart and valves, most commonly the aortic valve (previously the mitral valve). Incidence is 3–10 per 100 000 population. Rheumatic heart disease is the main risk factor in low-income countries, accounting for 65% of cases; it usually affects young adults and is caused by streptococci entering the oral cavity. In high-income countries, most common >70 years; major risk factors are degenerative valve disease, **diabetes**

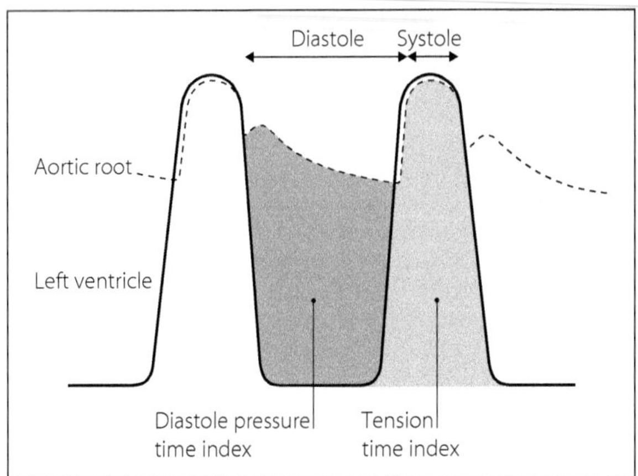

Fig. 62 Left ventricular and aortic root pressure tracings

mellitus, malignancy, iv drug abuse and **congenital heart disease**. Approximately 50% of cases involve normal valves. Nosocomial infection (usually with staphylococci) accounts for 25% and is associated with **catheter-related sepsis** and invasive procedures (e.g. endoscopy, dental procedures), especially in the presence of cardiac **pacemakers** and prosthetic valves, which act as nidi for infection. Results in tissue destruction and vegetations of platelets, macrophages and organisms, with systemic embolisation. Systemic immune complex deposition may also occur. Overall mortality is ~25% at 6 months and is worse with old age, prosthetic valve endocarditis, heart failure, **stroke** and infection with *Staphylococcus aureus*.

The traditional classification into acute, subacute and chronic endocarditis has been replaced with descriptions of the valve involved (i.e., whether native or prosthetic), the source of infection and the organism responsible.

- Microbiology:
  - staphylococcal, streptococcal and enterococcal infection account for 80%–90% of cases. *S. aureus* is responsible in 25%, coagulase-negative staphylococci in 10%, oral and non-oral streptococci in 35% and enterococci in 11%.
  - candida infection occurs in 1%–2% and is more commonly seen in iv drug users and more commonly affects the tricuspid valve.
- Features:
  - often non-specific; diagnosis should be considered in all patients with **sepsis** of unknown origin or fever in those with known risk factors.
  - fever (90%), malaise, weight loss, night sweats, anaemia.
  - **heart murmurs** (85%), **cardiac failure**, valve lesions.
  - peripheral embolisation/vasculitic phenomena, e.g. splinter haemorrhages in nail beds, conjunctivae and retina (Roth spots), painful fingertip swellings (Osler's nodes), painless haemorrhagic lesions on palms and soles (Janeway lesions), kidneys (causing haematuria), CNS (causing **stroke**). Splenomegaly and clubbing may occur.
- Diagnosis:
  - blood cultures: three sets will detect bacteraemia in 96%–98% of cases and should be taken before antibacterial agents are started. Positive cultures with typical organisms are highly suggestive of the condition. Bacteraemia is continuous with endocarditis so timing of cultures around peaks of temperature is unnecessary.
  - **echocardiography** (initially transthoracic then transoesophageal if the former is equivocal or negative).
  - serological testing is performed if cultures are negative (e.g. if the patient is already on antibiotics).
  - tissue culture of skin lesions may be helpful.

Treatment is supportive, with antimicrobial therapy depending on the infecting organism and whether a prosthetic valve is involved. Treatment usually lasts 4–6 weeks. Cardiac valve replacement is necessary in 40%–50%; indications include cardiac failure associated with valve destruction, persistent fever despite prolonged antimicrobial therapy, presence of highly resistant organisms, prosthetic valve involvement and large vegetations with embolic potential. Prophylaxis in structural disease is as for congenital heart disease.

[Moritz Roth (1849–1914), Swiss physician; Sir William Osler (1849–1919), Canadian-born US and English physician; Theodore Caldwell Janeway (1872–1917), US physician]

Cahill TJ, Prendergast BD (2016). Lancet; 387: 882–93

Endocrine disorders, *see individual diseases*

Endomorphins. Endogenous opioid peptides for μ **opioid receptors**. Produce spinal and supraspinal analgesia experimentally; have been found in the human brain, although their role is uncertain.

Endorphins. Endogenous opioid peptides derived from β-lipotropin, secreted by the anterior pituitary and hypothalamus. β-Endorphin (31 amino acids) is the most potent endogenous opioid, active mainly at μ and δ **opioid receptors**. Also inhibits **GABA** and promotes **dopamine** secretion. Derived from pro-opiomelanocortin (99 amino acids), from which **ACTH** is derived. Involved in central **pain pathways**, endorphins are released in response to painful stimuli but also during aerobic exercise and during laughter. May also be involved in haemorrhagic and **septic shock**; thought to reduce SVR, cardiac output and BP, while decreasing GIT motility and sympathetic activity and enhancing parasympathetic activity. This may explain why **naloxone** sometimes improves cardiovascular variables in shock.

Endothelial glycocalyx, *see Glycocalyx*

Endothelin. Vasoconstrictor peptide derived from vascular endothelium, involved in regulation of basal vascular tone and BP. Produced from an inactive precursor, it acts at specific endothelin receptors to cause vasoconstriction (type A receptors). Type B receptor activation may also result in production of **nitric oxide** and **prostacyclin**. Involved in regulation of local blood flow and in various cardiovascular disorders, notably **cardiac failure** and **pulmonary hypertension**. **Endothelin receptor antagonists** are used in the treatment of the latter.

Endothelin receptor antagonists. Group of drugs that inhibit **endothelin** receptors and cause vasodilatation. May be selective for type A receptors, e.g. ambrisentan, or non-selective (i.e., types A and B), e.g. bosentan, macitentan. Used to treat **pulmonary hypertension** (bosentan is also indicated in systemic sclerosis with ongoing digital ulcers). Side effects include GIT upset, hypotension, palpitations, oedema, headache, anaemia, blood dyscrasias and hepatic impairment.

Endothelium-derived relaxing factor, *see Nitric oxide*

Endotoxins. Lipopolysaccharides (LPS) present on the surface of gram-negative bacteria. LPS consist of: a lipid chain (lipid A), responsible for the biological effects; a core polysaccharide; and oligosaccharide side chains specific to each strain. Released when the bacteria die, and extremely toxic, probably via release and activation of many inflammatory substances, including **cytokines**. Endotoxaemia may be involved in the aetiology of **sepsis**, although it may occur in the absence of infection, and proven gram-negative sepsis may not be accompanied by endotoxaemia. Translocation of GIT organisms or their endotoxins into the bloodstream across the gut wall has been suggested to occur in critical illness. Attempts have been made to prevent endotoxaemia by killing GIT organisms (**selective decontamination of the digestive tract**), and to treat established endotoxaemia with **anti-endotoxin antibodies**.
Tan Y, Kagan JC (2014). Mol Cell; 54: 212–23
See also, Bacterial translocation

Endotracheal tubes, *see Tracheal tubes*

Endovascular aneurysm repair, *see Aortic aneurysm, abdominal*

End-plate potentials. Depolarisation potentials produced at the postsynaptic motor end-plate of the **neuromuscular junction** by binding of **acetylcholine** (ACh) to receptors. Their size and duration depend on the amount of ACh released, the number of ACh receptors free and the activity of **acetylcholinesterase**. Miniature end-plate potentials (under 1 mV) are thought to be produced by random release of ACh from single vesicles (**quantal theory**), and are too small to initiate **muscle contraction**. Simultaneous release of ACh from many vesicles follows depolarisation of the presynaptic membrane; the resultant large end-plate potential causes depolarisation of adjacent muscle membrane, and muscle contraction.
See also, Neuromuscular transmission

End-tidal gas sampling. Gives the approximate composition of alveolar gas, unless major $\dot{V}/\dot{Q}$ **mismatch** exists or tidal volume is very small. Useful for estimating alveolar and hence arterial $P\text{CO}_2$, e.g. for monitoring adequacy of ventilation. Alveolar concentrations of inhalational anaesthetic agents may also be monitored. May also indicate extent and rate of uptake of inhalational agents, if expired and inspired concentrations are compared, and the state of O_2 supply/demand. Online multiple gas monitors are now routine, providing breath-by-breath measurements. Because the gas sampled by these is not strictly end-tidal, the sampling line being placed some distance away from the patient's airway, the term 'end-expiratory' is more accurately applied. Mixing of end-expiratory gas with fresh gas may lead to inaccuracy, especially if samples are taken between the breathing system filter and the anaesthetic machine.
See also, Carbon dioxide, end-tidal; Gas analysis

Energy. Capacity to perform **work**, whether mechanical, chemical or electrical. Kinetic energy is the energy of a body due to its motion; potential energy is the energy of a body due to its state or position. Thus a body on a table has potential energy due to the effect of gravity; when it falls, this is converted to kinetic energy. Similarly, the potential energy of a stretched spring is converted to kinetic energy as it recoils. The law of conservation of energy states that energy cannot be destroyed or created, but only converted to other forms of energy, e.g. heat, light, sound. Molecules within a body have potential energy due to their chemical composition and forces between them, and kinetic energy due to their movement. SI unit is the **joule**, although the **Calorie** (Cal; equals 1000 cal) is widely used for dietary energy estimations.

Energy is liberated in the body by breakdown of metabolic substrates, e.g. approximately 4 Cal/g **carbohydrate** and **protein**, 9 Cal/g **fat**, 7 Cal/g **alcohol**. It may be stored in high phosphate bonds, e.g. in **ATP**, and in other compounds, e.g. **glycogen**.
See also, Basal metabolic rate; Energy balance; Metabolism

Energy balance. Difference between **Calorie** intake and **energy** output. If intake is less than expenditure, energy balance is negative and endogenous energy stores are used; if it is greater, balance is positive and the individual gains weight. Many critically ill patients (e.g. those with **trauma**, **sepsis**) have increased **catabolism** and glycogenolysis, **insulin** resistance with resultant lipolysis and increased **basal metabolic rate**. To provide adequate nutrition in these patients it is possible to estimate energy expenditure, e.g. with indirect calorimetry using bedside devices ('metabolic carts'). This allows measurement of O_2 and CO_2 exchange and thus **respiratory exchange ratio**; however, such techniques are not widely used because of inaccuracies related to gas leaks from the patient/ventilator circuit and the effect of water vapour.

Normal subjects require about 25 Cal/kg/day; most critically ill patients require about 25–40 Cal/kg/day.
Ridley E, Gantner D, Pellegrino V (2015). Clin Nutr; 34: 565–71
See also, Nitrogen balance

Enflurane. 2-Chloro-1,1,2-trifluoroethyl difluoromethyl ether (Fig. 63). **Inhalational anaesthetic agent**, introduced in 1966. No longer commonly used, and unavailable in the UK.

- Properties:
  - colourless volatile liquid with ether-like smell; vapour is 7.5 times denser than air.
  - mw 184.5.
  - boiling point 56.5°C.
  - **SVP** at 20°C 24 kPa (175 mmHg).
  - **partition coefficients**:
    - blood/gas 1.9.
    - oil/gas 98.
  - **MAC** 1.7% (middle age); 1.9% (young adults); 2.4%–2.5% in children/teenagers.
  - flammable and non-corrosive. Stable without additives and unaffected by light.
- Effects:
  - CNS:
    - smooth and rapid induction and recovery.

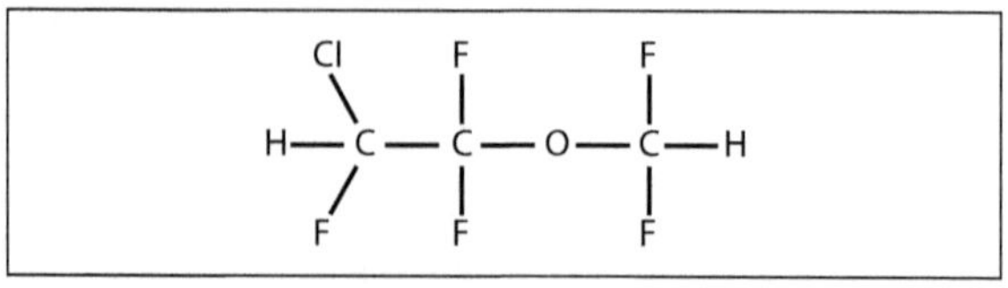

Fig. 63 Structure of enflurane

- epileptiform EEG activity may occur (typically a three per second spike and wave pattern), especially at doses >2 MAC with coexisting **hypocapnia**. **Convulsions** may occur postoperatively.
- increased **cerebral blood flow** but reduced **intraocular pressure**.
- weak analgesic properties.

- RS:
  - depresses airway reflexes less than **halothane** and therefore tracheal intubation is more difficult when the patient is breathing spontaneously.
  - causes greater respiratory depression than halothane or **isoflurane**; an increased respiratory rate is common, with decreased tidal volume.
  - bronchodilatation.
- CVS:
  - causes greater myocardial depression than halothane. SVR is reduced, with compensatory tachycardia. Hypotension is common.
  - causes fewer arrhythmias than halothane, and less sensitisation of the myocardium to catecholamines.
- other:
  - dose-dependent uterine relaxation.
  - nausea and vomiting are uncommon.
  - muscle relaxation and potentiation of non-depolarising neuromuscular blocking drugs is greater than that seen with halothane or isoflurane.
  - may precipitate **MH**.

About 2% metabolised, the rest excreted via the lungs. Although **fluoride ions** may be produced by metabolism, toxic levels are usually not reached, although they have been reported in obese patients after prolonged anaesthesia. Patients with pre-existing renal impairment or receiving other nephrotoxic drugs or enzyme-inducing drugs, e.g. isoniazid, are also thought to be at risk.

Hepatitis has been reported following enflurane; cross-sensitivity with halothane has been suggested, but this is disputed.

Inspired concentrations of 1%–3% are usually adequate for anaesthesia, with higher concentrations for induction.

Enhanced recovery, *see Recovery, enhanced*

Enkephalins. Endogenous opioid peptides found in the CNS, especially:

- periaqueductal grey matter.
- periventricular grey matter.
- limbic system.
- medullary raphe nucleus.
- spinal cord, especially laminae II and III (substantia gelatinosa) of the dorsal horn.

Methionine enkephalin and leucine enkephalin (each 5 amino acids) are derived from proenkephalin; they are thought to be involved in the modulation of **pain pathways**, e.g. **gate control theory of pain**. Active mainly at δ and μ **opioid receptors**.

See also, Endorphins

Enoxaparin, *see Heparin*

Enoximone. Selective (PDE III) **phosphodiesterase inhibitor** unrelated to **catecholamines** or **cardiac glycosides**. Used as an **inotropic drug**, particularly in cardiogenic or other types of **shock**, in which there is an element of **heart failure** (e.g. after **cardiac surgery**, and in patients awaiting heart transplants). Increases cardiac contractility and stroke volume with minimal tachycardia, and without increasing myocardial O_2 demand. Also causes vasodilatation (reducing both **preload** and **afterload**), thereby decreasing ventricular filling pressures. BP may fall.

Acts directly on cardiac muscle rather than via adrenergic (or other) receptors.

Preparation contains alcohol, propylene glycol and sodium hydroxide (pH 12). Crystal formation may occur with glass syringes, etc., and if mixed with other drugs and dextrose solutions.

Undergoes hepatic metabolism to partially active metabolites, excreted renally.

- Dosage: 90 μg/kg/min over 10–30 min iv, followed by continuous or intermittent infusion of 5–20 μg/kg/min, up to 24 mg/kg/day.
- Side effects: hypotension, nausea and vomiting, insomnia, headache.

ENT surgery, *see Ear, nose and throat surgery*

Enteral nutrition, *see Nutrition, enteral*

Entonox. Trade name for gaseous N_2O/O_2 50:50 mixture, supplied in **cylinders** at a pressure of 137 bar. Invented by Tunstall in 1962. Cylinders are blue with blue/white quartered shoulders. May also be supplied by pipeline. Formed by bubbling O_2 through liquid N_2O (**Poynting effect**).

Cylinders must be kept above −7°C (**pseudocritical temperature**) to prevent liquefaction of the N_2O (a process called lamination). If this occurs and gas is drawn from the top of the cylinder, O_2 will be delivered first, followed by almost pure N_2O. In the large cylinders used for connection to a pipeline system via a manifold, gas is therefore drawn first from the bottom of the cylinder by a tube; should liquefaction of N_2O now occur, N_2O containing about 20% O_2 is delivered first. Warming and repeated inversion of the cylinders will reconstitute the gaseous mixture.

Widely used for inhalational analgesia for trauma and minor procedures, e.g. physiotherapy or change of dressings; most commonly used with a **demand valve** for self-administration. Onset of analgesia is rapid, with minimal cardiovascular, respiratory or neurological side effects. Should sedation occur, the patient reduces the intake and recovery rapidly occurs. Caution is required if the patient has an undrained **pneumothorax**, as N_2O may increase its size.

Also widely used in the UK for inhalational analgesia during labour, although there is little evidence that pain scores are reduced.

Continuous use (e.g. in ICU) has declined because of interaction of N_2O with the **methionine** synthase system.

[Michael Tunstall (1928–2011), Scottish anaesthetist]

See also, Obstetric analgesia and anaesthesia

Envenomation, *see Bites and stings*

Environmental impact of anaesthesia. Has attracted increasing attention through two main areas:

- direct effects of inhalational agents:
  - reaction of chlorine and bromine atoms from atmospheric volatile agents, released by the action of ultraviolet radiation, with ozone, depleting the latter.
  - acting as 'greenhouse gases', preventing the escape of infrared radiation from the earth. N_2O is less

potent in this regard than sevoflurane (which is less potent than isoflurane and especially desflurane), but lasts longer in the atmosphere so is thought to have a greater overall effect. In addition, it is used in much higher concentrations, thus thought to account overall for >99% of the climate impact potential of anaesthetic gases (with medical N_2O accounting for ~1% of atmospheric N_2O).
- increasing use of disposable equipment that must be incinerated at high temperature, generating further CO_2 and releasing toxins (e.g. dioxins, plasticisers) into the atmosphere, as well as generation of large amounts of waste from packaging.

Suggested measures to minimise the above include:
- reduction of waste, e.g. reduced packaging, reuse where possible, dilution of drugs from iv fluid bags already in use rather than fresh saline/water ampoules.
- increased recycling, including glass from ampoules.
- incineration only for contaminated material, and high-temperature incineration only for truly sharp objects.
- power-saving strategies, e.g. turning off equipment not in use.
- avoidance of N_2O, use of low-flow systems.
- consideration of transportation costs when ordering equipment/drugs.

Sneyd JR, Montgomery H, Pencheon D (2010). Anaesthesia; 65: 435–7

Environmental safety of anaesthetists. Hazards faced may be due to:
- inhalational agents: fears were expressed, especially in the 1960s, because of reported high incidence of lymphoid tumours in anaesthetists. Chronic exposure to low concentrations of volatile agents was thought to be responsible, hence attempts to remove it from the immediate atmosphere by adsorption or **scavenging**. Such an association was not supported by subsequent studies, and effects of breathing small amounts of volatile agents are thought to be minimal, if any. Effects of **N_2O** are now considered potentially more harmful; increased incidence of spontaneous abortion and possibly congenital malformation in theatre workers or their spouses is suspected but has never been conclusively proven. This may be via **methionine** synthase inhibition.

  Effect on performance is controversial; there is no conclusive evidence that the low atmospheric concentrations measured are deleterious. Any risks are reduced using **circle systems**, scavenging, avoiding spillage, monitoring contamination levels and testing apparatus for leaks. Workplace exposure limits set out in **COSHH regulations** for Great Britain and Northern Ireland are 100 ppm N_2O, 50 ppm enflurane/isoflurane and 10 ppm halothane (each over an 8-h period). In the USA, the National Institute for Occupational Safety and Health has recommended an 8-h time-weighted average limit of 2 ppm for halogenated anaesthetic agents in general (0.5 ppm together with exposure to N_2O).
- infection, e.g. with **hepatitis** or **HIV** infection. Risks are reduced by immunisation against hepatitis B, wearing gloves and goggles, avoidance of needles wherever possible, and careful disposal of contaminated equipment. Needles should never be resheathed by holding their cover in one's hand. Devices for safe handling of used needles (e.g. non-removable caps/sheaths or cannulae/syringes with self-retracting needles) became mandatory in the USA in 2001; a European Directive was issued in 2010 and implemented in the NHS via new regulations in 2013. In case of accidental needlestick injuries:
  - wash with soap and water. Do not scrub the site or use other antiseptic agents.
  - gently encourage bleeding. The source patient should be risk-assessed (ideally by a doctor other than the person who sustained the injury), with a view to considering post-exposure prophylaxis (PEP) for HIV infection.
  - testing for HIV and hepatitis infection requires informed patient consent and counselling, a cause of much controversy should a healthcare worker suffer a needlestick injury from an unconscious patient. If considered necessary, PEP with 2–3 antiretroviral agents (including **zidovudine**) started within 72 h after exposure and continued for 28 days is recommended. PEP reduces the risk of infection by 80%. Follow-up HIV serology testing should be performed at 1, 3 and 6 months. Risk of infection after accidental exposure of healthcare workers is estimated at 1 in 300 for HIV (needlestick; higher risk after conjunctival inoculation), 1 in 30 for hepatitis C and 1 in 3 for hepatitis B. Risk is affected by the number of viral particles inoculated and the route. Other more contagious infections: deaths were reported following exposure to patients infected with **severe acute respiratory syndrome**.
- risk of **electrocution and burns**, **explosions and fires**, **radiation** exposure, back injury, stress and fatigue. Access to addictive drugs makes **abuse of anaesthetic agents** easier. **Alcohol** abuse is common among doctors. Increased risk of suicide is suspected, but not proven.
- personal injury during interhospital transfer of patients.

Similar concerns exist for staff on the ICU.

Andersen MP, Nielsen OJ, Wallington TJ (2012). Anesth Analg; 114: 1081–5

See also, Contamination of anaesthetic equipment

Enzyme. Protein accelerating a specific chemical reaction, i.e., a biological catalyst. Sensitive to pH and temperature.
- Classified according to the reaction catalysed:
  - oxidoreductases: oxidation/reduction, e.g. metabolism of many drugs.
  - transferases: transfer of groups between molecules, e.g. transaminases.
  - hydrolases: hydrolytic cleavage or reverse, e.g. **acetylcholinesterase**.
  - lyases: cleavage of C–C, C–N, etc., without oxidation, reduction or hydrolysis, e.g. decarboxylases.
  - isomerases: intramolecular rearrangements, e.g. mutases.
  - ligases: reactions involving high-energy bonds, e.g. **ATP**, and formation of C–C, C–N, etc.

Reactions involve formation of intermediate structures, with formation of reaction products and reformation of enzyme.

See also, Enzyme induction/inhibition; Michaelis–Menten kinetics

Enzyme induction/inhibition. Certain drugs may alter the activity of **enzymes** involved in their metabolism, most importantly, in the liver. Induction is an increase in the amount of enzyme, caused by increased synthesis or decreased breakdown. It is usually related to the duration and extent of drug exposure. The cytochrome P_{450} system is often involved (*see Cytochrome oxidase system*). Inhibition is a reduction in the amount of enzyme or impairment of its activity.

- May affect metabolism of the original drug and other drugs, leading to **drug interactions**:
  - enzyme induction:
    - **barbiturates** increase metabolism of **warfarin, phenytoin** and **chlorpromazine**.
    - phenytoin increases metabolism of digitoxin, thyroxine, **vecuronium, pancuronium** and **tricyclic antidepressants**.
    - **alcohol** increases metabolism of warfarin, barbiturates and phenytoin.
    - **smoking** increases metabolism of vecuronium, pancuronium, **morphine, aminophylline**, chlorpromazine and phenobarbital.
  - enzyme inhibition:
    - **ecothiopate** reduces metabolism of **suxamethonium**.
    - **metronidazole** reduces metabolism of acetaldehyde produced by alcohol metabolism.
    - **cimetidine** reduces metabolism of **lidocaine**, morphine, **pethidine, labetalol, propranolol** and **nifedipine**.

Sweeney BP, Bromilow J (2006). Anaesthesia; 61: 159–77

EOA, Esophageal obturator airway, *see Oesophageal obturators and airways*

Ephedrine hydrochloride. **Sympathomimetic** and **vasopressor drug**, mainly used to treat hypotension (especially in **spinal** and **epidural anaesthesia**). Sometimes used in the treatment of **bronchospasm** and **autonomic neuropathy**.

- Actions:
  - directly stimulates α- and β-**adrenergic receptors**.
  - releases **noradrenaline** from nerve endings.
  - inhibits **monoamine oxidase**.
- Effects:
  - increased heart rate, **myocardial contractility** and BP.
  - vasoconstriction.
  - bronchodilatation.
  - CNS arousal and pupillary dilatation.
  - increased sphincter tone.
  - placental and uterine blood flow is maintained; thus it has been traditionally considered the agent of choice in obstetric regional anaesthesia.
- Dosage:
  - 3–6 mg repeated as required up to 30 mg.
  - 15–60 mg orally/im tds.

Tachyphylaxis occurs with repeated administration. May cause restlessness and palpitations in overdose.

Epidural anaesthesia. Introduction of **local anaesthetic agent** into the epidural space to induce loss of sensation adequate for surgery (the term 'epidural analgesia' refers to provision of pain relief, e.g. during labour). Can be divided anatomically into cervical, thoracic, lumbar and caudal. **Caudal analgesia** was first performed in 1901; lumbar blockade was performed by Pages in 1921 and popularised by Dogliotti in the 1920s–1930s, although it was probably introduced by **Corning** following his initial experiments. Continuous catheter techniques were introduced in the late 1940s.

Following injection, local anaesthetic may act at epidural, paravertebral or subarachnoid nerve roots, or directly at the **spinal cord**. Systemic effects may also occur.

Indications are as for **spinal anaesthesia**; main advantages are avoidance of dural puncture, and those related to catheter technique, i.e., allows control over onset, extent and duration of blockade. Thus used for peri- and **postoperative analgesia**, analgesia following **chest trauma**, **obstetric analgesia and anaesthesia**, and treatment of chronic **pain**. However, blockade is less intense than spinal anaesthesia, with greater chance of missed segments, and the dose of drug injected is potentially dangerous if incorrectly placed.

Opioid analgesic drugs may be injected into the epidural space to provide analgesia.

(For anatomy, path taken by needle, etc., *see Epidural space*.)

- Technique (lumbar block):
  - performed with the patient in the lateral or sitting position. Preparation of patient is as for spinal anaesthesia. Full aseptic technique, including sterile gown and hat/mask, is usual in the UK, especially when a catheter is inserted.
  - median/paramedian approaches are used as for spinal anaesthesia. Easier catheter insertion, with less risk of dural or vascular puncture, is claimed for the latter approach. It may also be easier in the elderly, particularly if back flexion is difficult or the ligaments are calcified.
  - deep and superficial infiltration with local anaesthetic is performed.
  - 16–19 G Tuohy **needles** are usually employed, especially for catheter insertion. The curved blunt tip reduces the risk of dural puncture and facilitates catheter direction (Fig. 64). The needle is usually marked at 1-cm intervals (Lee markings), and may be winged. The Crawford needle (straight tipped with an oblique bevel) is sometimes used. The stylet is removed when the needle tip is gripped by the interspinous ligament (*see Vertebral ligaments*). Less damage to the longitudinal ligamentous fibres has been claimed if the needle is inserted with the bevel facing laterally; the needle may then be rotated 90 degrees once the space is entered. However, insertion with the bevel facing cranially is usually advocated, because this avoids the risk of dural puncture during rotation of the needle.

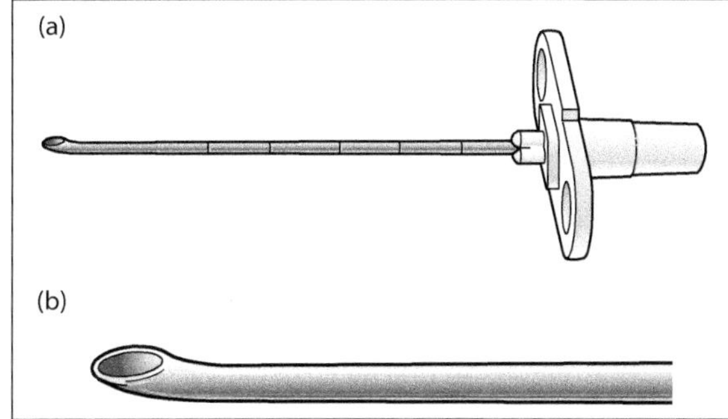

Fig. 64 (a) Winged Tuohy needle. (b) Detail of tip

- the epidural space is identified by exploiting the negative pressure that is usually present within it. Methods:
  - passive techniques, e.g. **hanging drop technique**; a bubble indicator placed at the needle hub; collapsing drums or balloons (e.g. **Macintosh**'s); syringe devices with spring-loaded plungers.
  - 'loss of resistance' technique: the most commonly used method:
    - a low-resistance syringe device is attached to the needle (after checking first to ensure a smooth action). It may be filled with:
      - saline: minimal 'give' when compressed, thus easier to judge resistance to injection. May be confused with **CSF** if dural puncture occurs (differentiated by detection of glucose/protein in CSF but not in saline, using reagent strips). The most common method in the UK nowadays.
      - air: avoids confusion with CSF but compressible in the syringe, i.e., 'bounces'; judgement of loss of resistance is therefore harder. Neck ache is common and thought to be caused by small air emboli (may be detected by sensitive **Doppler** ultrasound). Pneumocephalus has been reported.
      - local anaesthetic: has been described but risks iv or subarachnoid injection.
    - continuous pressure is applied to the plunger as the needle is advanced, until a sudden 'give' is felt. Alternatively, pressure is applied intermittently after each (small) advance of the needle. The former technique is thought to be more likely to push the dura away from the needle when the epidural space is entered. In either case, the operator's other hand controls advancement, e.g. by placing the back of the hand against the patient's back and gripping the needle firmly between thumb and fingers.
    - high resistance to injection is encountered while the needle tip is in the ligamentum flavum; sudden loss of resistance with easy injection occurs when the epidural space is entered.
- injection of a **test dose** through the needle is controversial and rarely performed, especially if a catheter is to be inserted.
- injection through the needle may be 'single shot' or fractionated; faster onset and higher block are claimed for the former but better control and safety claimed for the latter.
- catheter technique:
  - a 16–18 G catheter is inserted through the needle and directed usually upwards within the epidural space. Incidence of bloody tap is thought to be reduced if saline is injected before the catheter is inserted. If insertion is difficult, injection of 5–10 ml saline or slight straightening of the legs may help. The catheter should never be pulled back through the needle, as its tip may be sheared off. Smaller needles are available for children.
  - the needle is removed over the catheter. 3–5 cm of the latter is usually left in the space; too little may increase the risk of falling out; too much may increase the risk of inadequate block, e.g. by passing through an intervertebral foramen. After aspiration and confirmation of the absence of CSF or blood in the catheter, it is fixed to the patient's back.
  - catheter types:
    - single end hole: thought to be more likely to obstruct, and to produce incomplete blockade, e.g. if the tip is near an intervertebral foramen.
    - closed end with (usually three) side holes: the most common type in the UK. May account for development of extensive blockade, e.g. if the distal hole is in the subarachnoid space and the proximal hole is in the epidural space. Solution injected slowly is thought to leave via the proximal hole with epidural block as expected; rapid injection may produce subarachnoid injection. Similar events may occur with iv placement of the tip.
  - a 0.2-μm filter is attached to the proximal end of the catheter to reduce bacterial contamination and injection of fragments of glass from ampoules.
  - test doses of 2–3 ml local anaesthetic (or bigger volumes if low concentrations are used) are commonly used to detect accidental subarachnoid or intravascular placement of the catheter, although their use is controversial.
  - single or fractionated injections are controversial, as earlier.
  - assessment and management of blockade: as for spinal anaesthesia.
- Thoracic block:
  - especially useful for postoperative analgesia and following trauma. Allows selective blockade of required thoracic segments with sparing of lower segments.
  - general principles are as earlier. The paramedian approach is often employed as thoracic spinous processes are angled more steeply caudally, making the median approach difficult. The negative pressure is of greatest magnitude in the thoracic region; this may aid identification of the epidural space.
  - the needle is inserted lateral to the interspace below that to be blocked, and directed slightly medially to encounter the lamina. It is then walked off cranially to enter the ligamentum flavum.
  - a catheter technique is almost always used.
- Cervical block: has been performed for pain therapy, and for carotid artery, thyroid and arm surgery. General principles are as above.
- Solutions used:
  - **bupivacaine**, levobupivacaine or **ropivacaine** 0.25%–0.75%, and lidocaine 1%–2%, are most commonly used in the UK. Onset with bupivacaine is about 15–30 min; effects last about 1.5–2.5 h. Lower concentrations of bupivacaine (≤0.1%), especially combined with opioids, e.g. **fentanyl** 2–4 μg/ml, are commonly used to provide analgesia while allowing mobility, particularly in obstetrics and for postoperative analgesia (*see Spinal opioids*). Infusions (≤15–20 ml/h) or boluses (≤20 ml) may be used; the former are especially common postoperatively because the duration of action is shorter than with concentrated solutions. Onset with lidocaine is about 5–15 min; effects last about 1–1.5 h if 1:200 000 adrenaline is added. Higher concentrations are used if muscle relaxation is required. Alkalinised solutions produce faster onset of denser blockade.
  - lumbar blockade: 10–30 ml is usually adequate. Rough guide: 1.5 ml/segment to be blocked, including sacral segments; 1.0 ml/segment if over 50 years or in **pregnancy**; 0.75 ml/segment if over 80 years.

Reduction of requirement with age is thought to be due to decreased leakage, e.g. through intervertebral foramina. The above scheme does not take into account body size or site of injection/catheter insertion.

Effect of gravity: the dependent side tends to experience faster and denser block.

- thoracic block: 3–5 ml is used to block 2–4 segments at the required level.
- cervical block: 6–8 ml is usually used.
- tachyphylaxis is common; it may be related to local pH changes but the precise mechanism is unclear.

- Effects: similar to spinal anaesthesia, but block (and hypotension) are slower in onset. Density of block and muscle relaxation are less, with greater incidence of incomplete block. Motor block may be assessed using the **Bromage scale**.
- Contraindications: as for spinal anaesthesia.
- Complications:
  - related to insertion of needle/catheter:
    - trauma:
      - local bruising/pain.
      - neurological damage is rare, although restriction of the technique to awake patients is common practice, especially for thoracic or cervical block.
    - bloody tap: if bleeding occurs through the needle, it should be withdrawn and a different space used. If blood is obtained through the catheter (vigorous aspiration is avoided as it may collapse the veins), withdrawal of the catheter 1 cm following saline flushing may be performed. If blood is still obtained, the catheter should be removed and a different space used. If no further flow of blood occurs, the catheter may be fixed. Subsequent injection of local anaesthetic is performed with care in case the catheter still lies (at least partially) within a vein.
    - epidural haematoma: as for spinal anaesthesia. Recommendations for patients receiving low-molecular-weight heparin (LMWH): in fully anticoagulated patients an interval of 24 h should be allowed between the last dose and insertion/removal of an epidural catheter; this is reduced to 12 h in those receiving lower-dose LMWH for DVT prophylaxis. The first dose of LMWH may be given 3–4 h after removal of the catheter (e.g. immediately postoperatively).
    - **dural tap**: usually obvious if caused by the epidural needle, as CSF flows back. Puncture by the epidural catheter may be harder to detect; flow of CSF may not be obvious, especially if saline was used to identify the epidural space.
    - shearing of the catheter tip: should be documented and the patient informed. Thought not to have adverse effects.
    - knotting of the catheter is possible if excessive lengths are inserted.
  - following injection of drug:
    - hypotension as for spinal anaesthesia.
    - local anaesthetic toxicity due to systemic absorption or iv injection.
    - extensive blockade:
      - accidental spinal (subarachnoid) blockade: onset is usually within a few minutes. May lead to total spinal block if a large amount of drug is injected, with rapidly ascending motor and sensory blockade, respiratory paralysis and central apnoea, **cranial nerve** involvement with fixed dilated pupils and loss of consciousness. Management includes oxygenation with tracheal intubation and IPPV, and cardiovascular support. Recovery without adverse effects is usual if hypoxaemia and hypotension are avoided.
      - subdural blockade: piercing by the catheter of the dura but not arachnoid. Onset is typically within 20–30 min; blockade may be unilateral and include cranial nerve lesions. The arachnoid may rupture if large volumes are injected, leading to high or total spinal block.
      - unexplained, with correct epidural placement of the catheter. Partial subarachnoid or subdural catheter placement is thought to be responsible for the many patchy blocks encountered in practice. Catheter migration may occur during prolonged blockade, e.g. in obstetrics.
      - isolated cranial nerve palsies (e.g. fifth and sixth) and **Horner's syndrome** have been reported.

      Extensive blocks may develop after top-up injections during apparently normal epidural blocks.
    - incomplete blockade: missed segments/unilateral block. Management: as for obstetric analgesia and anaesthesia.
    - nerve damage due to injection of incorrect drugs/solutions. In addition, preservatives in certain preparations of local anaesthetics are suspected to be neurotoxic, as are skin cleansing solutions.
    - **shivering**.
    - prolonged blockade: uncommon; has lasted up to 8–12 h after the last injection.
    - **anterior spinal artery syndrome**: thought to be related to severe hypotension, not to the technique itself.
    - **adverse drug reactions** to agents used: rare.
  - late:
    - **arachnoiditis, cauda equina syndrome**.
    - abscess formation/meningitis: thought to be rare if aseptic techniques are used.

[Fidel Pages (1886–1923), Spanish surgeon; Achilles Dogliotti (1897–1966), Italian surgeon; Edward B Tuohy (1908–1959), US anaesthetist; John Alfred Lee (1906–1989), Southend anaesthetist; Oral B Crawford (1921–2008), US anaesthetist]

Epidural opioids, *see Spinal opioids*

Epidural space. Continuous space within the vertebral column, extending from the foramen magnum to the sacrococcygeal membrane of the **sacral canal**. The **vertebral canal** becomes triangular in cross-section in the lumbar region, its base anterior; the epidural space is that part external to the spinal dura. It is very narrow anteriorly, and up to 5 mm wide posteriorly.

- Boundaries:
  - internal: dura mater of the **spinal cord** (at the foramen magnum, reflected back as the periosteal lining of the vertebral canal).
  - external:
    - posteriorly: ligamenta flava, and periosteum lining the vertebral laminae.
    - anteriorly: posterior longitudinal ligament.
    - laterally: intervertebral foramina, and periosteum lining the vertebral pedicles. The space may extend through the intervertebral foramina into the paravertebral spaces.

Contains epidural fat, epidural veins (**Batson's plexus**), lymphatics and spinal nerve roots. Connective tissue layers have been demonstrated by radiology and endoscopy within the epidural space, in some cases (rarely) dividing it into right and left portions.

- Pressure in the epidural space is found to be negative in most cases, occasionally positive. Postulated explanations include:
  - artefactual or transient negative pressure:
    - anterior dimpling of the dura by the needle.
    - anterior indentation of the ligamentum flavum by the needle, followed by its sudden posterior recoil when punctured.
    - back flexion causing stretching of the dural sac, and/or squeezing out of **CSF**.
  - true negative pressure:
    - transmitted negative intrapleural pressure via thoracic paravertebral spaces.
    - relative overgrowth of the vertebral canal compared with the dural sac.
    - true positive pressure: bulging of dura due to pressure of CSF.
- Passage taken by an epidural needle when entering the epidural space (median approach):
  - 1: skin.
  - 2: subcutaneous tissues.
  - 3: supraspinous ligament (along the tips of spinous processes from C7 to sacrum).
  - 4: interspinous ligament (between spinous processes of adjacent vertebrae).
  - 5: ligamentum flavum (between laminae of adjacent vertebrae).
  - 6: epidural space.

The normal distance between the skin and the epidural space varies between 2 and 9 cm.

For the paramedian approach: 1, 2, 5, 6.

See also, Epidural anaesthesia; Vertebrae; Vertebral ligaments

Epidural volume expansion, *see Combined spinal–epidural anaesthesia*

Epiglottis, *see Larynx*

Epiglottitis. Infective inflammation of the epiglottis, often resulting in upper **airway obstruction**. Caused by *Haemophilus influenzae* type b in over 50% of cases. Most common in children aged 2–5 years but may also occur in adults (usually aged 20–40 years); the incidence in the UK has fallen since a specific vaccine was introduced. Classically follows an acute course, with fever, marked systemic upset, **stridor** and adoption of the sitting position with the jaw thrust forward and an open, drooling mouth. These features, plus absence of cough, help distinguish it from croup. Epiglottitis may progress to complete airway obstruction, which may be provoked by pharyngeal examination and anxiety (e.g. due to iv cannulation). Although lateral x-rays of the neck may reveal epiglottic enlargement, they may also provoke obstruction, and clinical assessment is sufficient in severe cases. **Pulmonary oedema** may occur if obstruction is severe.

- Management:
  - assessment:
    - general state: exhaustion, fever, etc.
    - respiratory distress: stridor, use of accessory **respiratory muscles**, including flaring of the nostrils, intercostal and suprasternal recession, tachypnoea, cyanosis.
  - experienced anaesthetic, paediatric and ENT help should be sought.
  - humidified O_2 administration.
  - nebulised **adrenaline** (0.4 ml/kg [400 µg/kg] of a 1:1000 racemic solution to a maximum of 5 ml [5 mg]).
  - **iv fluids** and **antibacterial drugs** are required, although iv cannulation should not be attempted before relief of the airway obstruction. Third-generation **cephalosporins** are the drugs of choice because of increasing resistance to the traditionally used **chloramphenicol** or **ampicillin**.
  - anaesthesia is as for airway obstruction; commonly inhalational induction using **sevoflurane** in O_2 with the patient sitting until tracheal intubation is possible. Induction is usually slow. Apparatus for difficult intubation plus facilities for urgent tracheostomy must be available. Atropine may be given once an iv cannula is sited. An oral tracheal tube is passed initially, and is changed for a nasal tube to allow better fixation and comfort.
  - intubation is usually required for less than 24 h. Spontaneous ventilation is usually acceptable. **Humidification** is essential. **Sedation** may not be required, but care must be taken to avoid accidental extubation.
  - extubation is performed when the clinical condition has improved, and a leak is present around the tube.
  - members of the patient's household should receive prophylactic antibacterial agents.

See also, Paediatric anaesthesia

Epilepsy. Tendency to epileptic seizures, associated with abnormal or excessive hypersynchronous neuronal activity within the brain. Affects 1% of the population.

- Traditionally classified into:
  - generalised:
    - grand mal (tonic–clonic **convulsions**): tonic (sustained muscle contraction) followed by clonic (jerking) phases lasting about 30 s each, with loss of consciousness. May be preceded by prodromal symptoms hours or days before, and an aura minutes before.
    - petit mal (absence seizures): characterised by 3 Hz synchronised spikes on the EEG. May present as inattentive staring or head-banging; despite appearances, the patient is not conscious during these seizures.
    - other types of generalised seizures include atonic and myoclonic.
  - partial (focal):
    - may occur with (complex partial) or without (simple partial) derangement of consciousness.
    - classic presentations:
      - temporal: associated with auditory, visual or olfactory hallucinations and emotional or mood changes.
      - Jacksonian: clonic movements spreading from an extremity (e.g. single digit) to involve the whole body.

Definition of disease is difficult because certain stimuli will induce convulsions in normal subjects, e.g. hypoxia, hypo/hyperglycaemia. Usually idiopathic, especially in childhood; intracranial lesions and infections (e.g. **encephalitis**) must be excluded in adults presenting with a single seizure. Pyrexia is a common cause in children; other causes are as for convulsions.

Treatment is with **anticonvulsant drugs**, and is directed at any underlying cause.

- Anaesthetic considerations:
  - **preoperative assessment**: frequency of seizures, date of last seizure, drug therapy (including measurement of blood levels where appropriate). Identification of cause if known.
  - therapy is continued throughout the perioperative period; **benzodiazepines** are often used for premedication because of their anticonvulsant activity.
  - anaesthetic drugs associated with convulsions are avoided, e.g. **enflurane, ketamine.** Although **propofol** may activate the EEG at low concentrations and may cause myoclonic jerks, it is used successfully to treat **status epilepticus. Thiopental, halothane** and **isoflurane** have anticonvulsant properties and have been the traditional drugs of choice. **Doxapram, naloxone** and **tramadol** are avoided. **Hypocapnia** lowers the seizure threshold.
  - anticonvulsant therapy is restarted as soon as possible postoperatively.

[John Hughlings Jackson (1835–1911), English neurologist]

Perks A, Cheema S, Mohanraj R (2012). Br J Anaesth; 108: 562–71

Epinephrine, *see Adrenaline*

Epistaxis. Nasal bleeding. May occur from:

- veins of the nasal septum (younger patients).
- arterial anastomoses of the lower part of the nasal septum (Little's area), especially in older patients. May be associated with **hypertension**.

Usually follows trauma, but predisposing conditions include bleeding disorders, hereditary telangiectasia and raised venous pressure. Bleeding may be caused by nasal intubation or passage of a nasal airway, especially if a vasoconstrictor (e.g. **cocaine**) is not used first.

Usually managed by nasal packing but may require ligation of the maxillary or anterior ethmoidal arteries, the former via the neck or oral route, the latter from the front of the **nose**.

Anaesthetic management is similar to that of the bleeding tonsil (*see Tonsil, bleeding*).

[James L Little (1836–1885), US surgeon]

EPLS, *see European Paediatric Life Support*

Epoprostenol, *see Prostacyclin*

EPSP, Excitatory postsynaptic potential, *see Synaptic transmission*

Eptacog alfa, *see Factor VIIa, recombinant*

Eptifibatide. Antiplatelet drug, used in **acute coronary syndromes.** Acts by reversibly inhibiting activation of the glycoprotein IIb/IIIa complex on the surface of **platelets.**

- Dosage: 180 µg/kg iv followed by 2 µg/kg/min for up to 72 h (96 h if **percutaneous coronary intervention** performed).
- Side effects are related to increased bleeding. Platelet function takes up to 2–4 h to return to normal after discontinuation of therapy.

Equivalence. Amount of a substance divided by its **valence.** Equivalent weight (gram equivalent) is the weight of substance combining with or chemically equivalent to 8 g O_2, or 1 g hydrogen.

Electrical equivalence is the number of moles of ionised substance divided by valence.

ERAS, Enhanced recovery after surgery, *see Recovery, enhanced*

Erg. Unit of **work** in the **cgs system.** 1 erg = work done by a force of 1 dyne acting through a distance of 1 centimetre.

Ergometrine maleate. Smooth muscle constrictor, with potent effects on uterine and vascular tone; used to reduce postpartum or post-termination uterine bleeding. Often given routinely combined with synthetic **oxytocin** at the end of the second stage of labour. Uterine contraction occurs 5 min after im injection and 1 min after iv injection and lasts up to an hour. Its CVS effects result from vasoconstriction, with increased CVP exacerbated by autotransfusion of blood from the **uterus**, and lasting up to several hours. Therefore hazardous in patients with cardiovascular disease, particularly pre-eclampsia.

- Dosage: 0.1–0.5 mg im/iv; 0.5–1.0 mg orally.
- Side effects: nausea, vomiting, abdominal/chest pain, hypertension, arrhythmias, dyspnoea, headache, tinnitus.

See also, Uterus

Error, fixation, *see Fixation error*

Errors, statistical. In **statistics**, may lead to incorrect conclusions because of inadequate test design and analysis.

- May be:
  - type I (α; false positive): acceptance of a result as not due to chance when it is (i.e., false rejection of the **null hypothesis**). Represented by the *P* value (**probability**); a value of 0.05 is traditionally accepted as the maximum acceptable. Commonly arises if multiple statistical tests are performed, when the chance of a 'significant' difference occurring due to chance alone increases, unless adjustments are made to account for multiple testing.
  - type II (β; false negative): rejection of a result as due to chance when it is not (i.e., false acceptance of the null hypothesis). A value of 0.1–0.2 is traditionally considered the maximum acceptable. Commonly arises if the sample size is too small, or if the difference between the groups is small.

As the required *P* value for 'significance' is made smaller, the risk of rejecting a real result (i.e., type II error) increases (assuming a constant sample size). Errors may limit the usefulness of an investigation described by its **sensitivity, specificity** and **predictive value.**

See also, Power

Ertapenem. Broad-spectrum **carbapenem** and **antibacterial drug**, active against gram-positive organisms and anaerobes, but not against pseudomonas or acinetobacter species, unlike **imipenem** or **meropenem.**

- Dosage: 1 g iv od.
- Side effects: as for imipenem.

Erythrocytes (Red blood cells). Biconcave discs, about 2 µm thick and 8 µm in diameter and without nuclei. Produced by red bone marrow. Contain **haemoglobin,**

maintained in an appropriate state for **O_2 transport** (i.e., containing iron in the reduced state, in the presence of **2,3-DPG**). Also have an integral role in **carbon dioxide transport**. Maintenance of structural integrity and osmotic stability is via membrane pumps; the main energy source is aerobic **glycolysis**.

Circulating lifespan is about 120 days; they are removed by the reticuloendothelial system and broken down, with salvage and reuse of iron and amino acids from haemoglobin.

- Normal laboratory findings (adult):
  - red cell count (RBC): 4.5–6.0 × 10^{12}/l blood (male); 4.0–5.2 × 10^{12}/l blood (female).
  - reticulocyte count: <2% of red cells. Increased in red cell loss from **haemolysis** or **haemorrhage**, signifying a normal bone marrow response. Also increased in treatment of deficiency **anaemias**.
  - mean corpuscle volume (MCV): 80–100 fl. Decreased in iron deficiency or defective haemoglobin synthesis. Increased when reticulocyte count is increased, or due to megaloblastic cell formation (e.g. vitamin B_{12}/folate deficiency). Also increased in **alcoholism**.
  - mean corpuscle haemoglobin (MCH): 26–34 pg.
  - mean corpuscle haemoglobin concentration (MCHC): 320–360 g/l. Decreased in iron deficiency or defective haemoglobin synthesis.
  - erythrocyte sedimentation rate (ESR): <10 mm/h. Measure of the rate at which red cells settle when a column of blood is left for 1 h. High values indicate reduced settling. Increased in many inflammatory, autoimmune and infective diseases, malignancy, old age and pregnancy.

Examination of the peripheral blood film gives information about haematological disease, e.g. abnormally shaped erythrocytes (**sickle cell anaemia**, hereditary spherocytosis, target cells in impaired haemoglobin production or liver disease).

See also, Erythropoiesis

Erythromycin. **Macrolide**-type **antibacterial drug** with similar spectrum to **penicillin**; thus a useful alternative in penicillin allergy. Especially useful in respiratory infections (including **Legionnaires' disease** and **mycoplasma infections**) and **staphylococcal infections**. Also promotes GIT activity via stimulation of GIT motilin receptors; used as a **prokinetic drug** in **ileus** (given iv or via nasogastric tube).

- Dosage:
  - 250 mg–1 g orally qds.
  - 50 mg/kg/day by iv infusion or in divided doses.
- Side effects: nausea, vomiting, abdominal pain, diarrhoea, rash, reversible hearing loss, arrhythmias, pain on iv injection.

Erythropoiesis. Formation of **erythrocytes**, usually restricted to the vertebrae, sternum, ribs, upper long bones and iliac crests in adults. Requires iron, vitamin B_{12} and folate, and possibly other vitamins and minerals. Stepwise differentiation from stem cells includes **haemoglobin** synthesis and nuclear extrusion to form reticulocytes, taking about 7 days. Regulated by **erythropoietin**.

Erythropoietin. Glycoprotein hormone secreted mainly by the kidneys, but also by the liver. Secretion is increased by **haemorrhage** and **hypoxia** (possibly via **prostaglandin** synthesis), and inhibited by increased numbers of circulating **erythrocytes**. Causes increased **erythropoiesis**. Erythropoietin receptors are present in erythrocytes, bone marrow and on central and peripheral neurones; the latter are involved in neuronal development and repair although erythropoietin has not been shown to be beneficial in **TBI**. Infusion of erythropoietin produced by recombinant genetic engineering is used to correct **anaemia** and avoid transfusions in patients with **renal failure** receiving **haemodialysis**. It has also been used to increase the yield of blood collected for autologous **blood transfusion**, e.g. 300 U/kg thrice weekly, reducing to 100 U/kg after 2 weeks. The first dose given iv produces higher levels; subsequent sc dosage produces a more sustained effect. Red cell aplasia has been reported following its sc use in renal failure.

Escape beats. On the **ECG**, complexes arising from sites other than the sinoatrial node, when the latter does not discharge (i.e., sinus arrest or severe bradycardia). Distinct from ectopic beats, which arise prematurely in the cardiac cycle.

Esmolol hydrochloride. Cardioselective **β-adrenergic receptor antagonist**, with no **intrinsic sympathomimetic activity**. Hydrolysed by red blood and other esterases, with a **half-life** of 9 min. Used to treat **AF**, atrial flutter and **SVT**, and during anaesthesia to prevent/treat tachycardia and hypertension, e.g. associated with tracheal intubation. Has been used in **hypotensive anaesthesia**.

- Dosage:
  - SVT, etc.: 500 μg/kg/min loading dose iv for 1 min, then 50–150 μg/kg/min maintenance titrated to effect.
  - perioperative use: 0.5–1.0 mg/kg iv over 15–30 s, followed by 50–300 μg/kg/min infusion.
- Side effects: bradycardia, hypotension, sweating, nausea, confusion, thrombophlebitis, pain on injection. Bronchospasm may occur in susceptible patients.

ESR, Erythrocyte sedimentation rate, *see Erythrocytes*

Etamsylate (Ethamsylate). Haemostatic drug, thought to reduce bleeding by correcting abnormal platelet adhesion. Does not affect fibrinolysis. Has been used to prevent and treat periventricular haemorrhage in premature babies (12.5 mg/kg im/iv qds). Also used orally in menorrhagia.

Ethambutol hydrochloride. **Antituberculous drug** added to triple therapy (**isoniazid**, **rifampicin**, **pyrazinamide**) if resistance is suspected.

- Dosage: 25 mg/kg orally od for 2 months, then 15 mg/kg daily for 6 months.
- Side effects: visual disturbances, peripheral neuritis, rash, thrombocytopenia. Requires monitoring of plasma levels (peak 2–6 mg/l; trough <1 mg/l).

Ethamsylate, *see Etamsylate*

Ethanol, *see Alcohols*

Ethanol poisoning, *see Alcohol poisoning*

Ether, *see Diethyl ether*

Ethics. Principles of moral behaviour; often translated into medical practice by reference to four basic principles ('principlism'):

- respect for autonomy: the right of an individual to choose a course of action (or inaction).

- beneficence: the obligation to do good; may not necessarily lie in preserving life if that life is of such poor quality (e.g. because of pain or severe disability) that it is considered less beneficial for the patient than death.
- non-maleficence: the obligation to avoid doing harm (*primum non nocere*). Difficulties may arise if beneficial medical interventions also cause harm (recognised in the doctrine of 'double effect'), e.g. administration of morphine to a terminally ill patient to relieve pain, even though it may hasten death.
- justice: the right to receive what is deserved. Although easy in certain circumstances (e.g. requirement for dialysis in acute kidney injury), other situations may be less clear (e.g. liver transplantation in chronic alcoholism). Overlaps with equity (fairness), manifested in arguments over rationing of healthcare.

The principles underlying ethical practice are not mutually exclusive and may even oppose one another, e.g. withholding blood from a **Jehovah's Witness** respects his/her autonomy while not practising beneficence/non-maleficence.

Principlism is favoured by many because it is relatively simple and easy to understand, though there are many other systems for judging the moral value of medical decisions, such as consequentialism (judgement according to the outcomes of decisions) and rights-based approaches.

- Anaesthetic/ICU implications include:
  - informed **consent.**
  - patients' rights to confidentiality, including non-disclosure of records without permission, although the doctor has statutory duties that may override this (e.g. reporting of **notifiable diseases**, births and deaths).
  - **HIV infection**: there is a moral duty to treat infected patients as well as taking steps to protect oneself. A doctor who has reason to believe that he/she is infected has a duty to seek advice and testing.
  - the duty to seek Research Ethics Committee approval and informed consent for research.
  - the duty to protect patients from sick and incompetent medical colleagues (*see Sick Doctor Scheme*).
  - **do not attempt resuscitation orders** and **advance decisions.**
  - admission criteria for, and rationing of, intensive care.
  - withholding or **withdrawal of treatment** (including surgery) in cases of medical futility.
  - management of terminal and **palliative care.**
  - **euthanasia.**

Waisel DB, Truog RD (1997). Anesthesiology; 87: 411–17

Ethmoidal nerve block, anterior, *see Ophthalmic nerve blocks*

Ethosuximide. Anticonvulsant drug used as first-line treatment of absence attacks in petit mal **epilepsy**; also used for myoclonic seizures. Thought to block T-type calcium channels in thalamic neurones.

- Dosage: 500 mg–1.5 g orally daily. Therapeutic plasma concentration 40–100 mg/l.
- Side effects: GIT disturbance, drowsiness, psychiatric disturbance, rash, hepatic and renal impairment, blood dyscrasias.

Ethyl alcohol, *see Alcohol poisoning; Alcohol withdrawal syndromes; Alcoholism; Alcohols*

Ethyl chloride. Inhalational anaesthetic agent, first described in 1848; popular in the 1920s particularly for induction of anaesthesia because of its rapid action. Extremely volatile (boiling point 13°C) and difficult to control; also inflammable. Now used solely for its cooling action when sprayed on to skin, to cause anaesthesia before minor procedures or to test the extent of regional blockade.

Ethylene. Inhalational anaesthetic agent, first used clinically in 1923. A gas of similar blood/gas solubility to $\mathbf{N_2O}$, but more potent. Also extremely explosive and unpleasant to inhale. Cylinder body and shoulder are coloured violet.

Ethylene glycol poisoning, *see Alcohol poisoning*

Ethylene oxide, *see Contamination of anaesthetic equipment*

Etidocaine hydrochloride. Local anaesthetic agent introduced in 1972, derived from **lidocaine**. Onset is rapid, and duration of action is similar to that of **bupivacaine**. Produces motor blockade that may exceed sensory blockade. Used in 1%–1.5% solutions. Maximal safe dose is 2 mg/kg. Not available in the UK.

Etomidate. Intravenous anaesthetic agent, introduced in 1973. A carboxylated imidazole (five-membered ring containing three carbon atoms and two nitrogen atoms) compound (Fig. 65), presented in 35% **propylene glycol**; pH is 8.1. 75% bound to plasma proteins after injection. Methoxycarbonyl-etomidate (MOC-etomidate) is a new etomidate analogue that undergoes rapid ester metabolism and does not cause adrenocortical suppression (*see later*).

- Effects:
  - induction:
    - rapid onset of anaesthesia, lasting up to 8 min after a single dose.
    - myoclonus is common; reduced by use of opioids.
    - pain is common when injected into small veins; reduced by mixing with 1–2 ml 1% lidocaine. Thrombosis is rare.
  - CVS/RS:
    - causes less hypotension than **propofol** and **thiopental**; thus often used in shocked patients, the elderly and those with cardiovascular disease.
    - respiratory depression is less than with thiopental.
  - CNS:
    - not analgesic.
    - not associated with epileptiform discharges.
    - reduces **cerebral blood flow** and **intraocular pressure.**

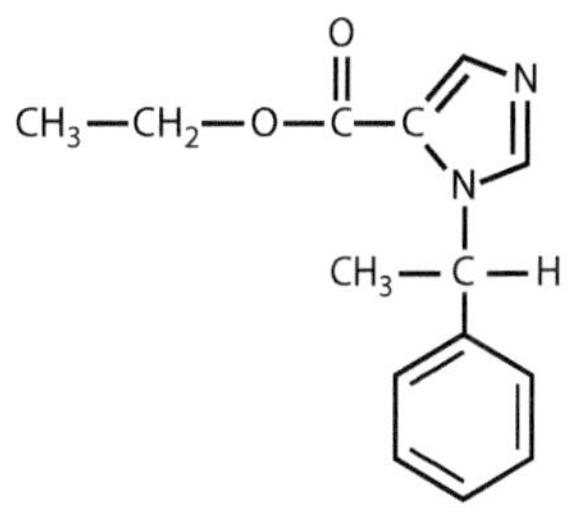

Fig. 65 Structure of etomidate

- other:
  - increases the incidence of **PONV**.
  - does not cause **histamine** release.
- Metabolism:
  - rapidly metabolised by plasma esterases and liver enzymes; elimination **half-life** is about 70 min. Largely excreted via the urine. Not cumulative.
  - interferes with adrenal corticosteroid synthesis by inhibiting 11-β-hydroxylase and 17-α-hydroxylase. IV infusion for sedation on ICU increases mortality; it is now contraindicated for this purpose. Following a single induction dose, the rise in plasma cortisol normally seen after surgery is delayed for up to 6 h. The significance of this is disputed.
- Dose: 0.2–0.3 mg/kg.

Forman SA (2011). Anesthesiology; 114: 695–707

Etorphine hydrochloride. Analogue of thebaine, a naturally occurring **opioid.** 1000–3000 times as potent as **morphine.** Used to immobilise large animals.

European Academy of Anaesthesiology (EAA). Founded in 1978 to improve standards, training and research in anaesthesia. Organises the **European Diploma in Anaesthesiology and Intensive Care.** Amalgamated with the **European Society of Anaesthesiologists** and the **Confederation of European National Societies of Anaesthesiologists** to form the **European Society of Anaesthesiology** in 2005.

Thomson D (1995). Acta Anaesth Scand; 39: 442–4

See also, European Federation of Anaesthesiologists

European Board of Anaesthesiology (EBA). Governing body for specialist anaesthetic training within the European Union, under the auspices of the European Union of Medical Specialties, which was founded in 1958. Works with the various anaesthetic bodies in member states.

Scherpereel P (1995). Acta Anaesth Scand; 39: 438–9

European Diploma in Anaesthesiology and Intensive Care (EDAIC). Examination held since 2005 by the **European Society of Anaesthesiology**, having taken over this function from the **European Academy of Anaesthesiology**, which ran it from 1984. Available in multiple languages; consists of two parts (written and oral), each covering basic science and clinical topics. Pass rates are in the order of 60% and 80%, respectively. There is also an optional in-training assessment part.

European Diploma in Intensive Care Medicine (EDIC). Organised by the **European Society of Intensive Care Medicine** since 1989. Consists of an English written (multiple choice) examination and an oral/clinical one (usually in the country and language of the examinee), together with a requirement for a basic medical specialty and 2 years' intensive care medicine training.

European Federation of Anaesthesiologists (EFA). Umbrella organisation formed in 2001 to coordinate the activities of and encourage cooperation between the **European Academy of Anaesthesiology, European Society of Anaesthesiologists** and **Confederation of European National Societies of Anaesthesiologists.**

Adopted the ***European Journal of Anaesthesiology*** as its official journal.

European Journal of Anaesthesiology. Established in 1984. The official journal of the **European Society of Anaesthesiology**, having been the official journal of the **European Academy of Anaesthesiology**, the **European Society of Anaesthesiologists**, the **Confederation of European National Societies of Anaesthesiologists, Fondation Européenne d'Enseignement en Anaesthésiologie** and **European Union of Medical Specialties** (since 1999) and the **European Federation of Anaesthesiologists** (since 2001).

European Medicines Agency (EMA). Body established in 1995 as the European Agency for the Evaluation of Medicinal Products (EMEA) to regulate the introduction and investigation of new drugs throughout Europe, and to ease communication between the various national regulatory bodies. Thus acts as a link between the **Medicines and Healthcare products Regulatory Agency** (previously **Committee on Safety of Medicines**) in the UK and similar bodies in other countries.

European Paediatric Life Support (EPLS). Collaboration between the **European Resuscitation Council** and the **Resuscitation Council (UK).** The EPLS course provides training in the recognition of the child in respiratory or circulatory failure and the prevention of respiratory or cardiorespiratory arrest.

European Resuscitation Council (ERC). Formed in 1989 with a mandate to produce guidelines and recommendations appropriate to Europe for the practice of basic and advanced cardiopulmonary and cerebral resuscitation. Composed of elected representatives from the participating European countries. Held its first major international conference in 1992. Regularly produces guidelines regarding basic and advanced **CPR.** *Resuscitation* is its official journal.

See also, Resuscitation Council (UK); International Liaison Committee on Resuscitation

European Society of Anaesthesiologists. Formed in 1993 to provide continuous education and promote research. Amalgamated with the **European Academy of Anesthesiology** and the **Confederation of European National Societies of Anaesthesiologists** to form the **European Society of Anaesthesiology** (ESA) in 2005.

European Society of Anaesthesiology (ESA). Formed in 2005 by the amalgamation of the **European Society of Anaesthesiologists,** the **European Academy of Anaesthesiology** and the **Confederation of European National Societies of Anaesthesiologists.** Seeks to provide all the educational and regulatory activities of the three component organisations. Adopted the ***European Journal of Anaesthesiology*** as its official journal. Representation of different nationalities within the organisation is via individual members (who are all eligible to join the ESA's various committees) and the National Anaesthesia Societies Committee (NASC).

Priebe HJ (2005). Eur J Anaesth; 22: 1–3

European Society of Intensive Care Medicine (ESICM). Founded in 1982 in Geneva to advance knowledge, research and education in intensive care medicine, and subsequently to improve facilities for intensive care medicine in Europe. Holds an annual congress, organises the **European Diploma in Intensive Care Medicine** and administers several multicentre and multinational surveys, e.g. the European Consortium for Intensive Care Data (ECICD). Also administers the educational programme PACT. ***Intensive Care Medicine*** is its official journal.

European Society of Paediatric and Neonatal Intensive Care (ESPNIC). Founded and based in Brussels to advance and promote paediatric and neonatal intensive care. Has medical and nursing branches. Holds an annual congress and has ***Intensive Care Medicine*** as its official journal.

European Union of Medical Specialties (Union Européenne des Médecins Spécialistes; UEMS), *see European Board of Anaesthesiology*

Euthanasia. Intentional ending of a patient's life for his or her benefit, e.g. to relieve intolerable and incurable suffering. May be voluntary if administered to a competent person in response to his or her informed request, or non-voluntary if administered to an incompetent person. Distinction is also made between active euthanasia, in which medical intervention hastens death, and passive euthanasia, in which life-sustaining treatment (e.g. enteral feeding) is withheld or withdrawn. Assisted suicide differs in that the physician provides the mechanism for death but the patient administers the lethal agent. Euthanasia remains illegal throughout the world except in the Netherlands, where it was legalised in 2000, Belgium (2002), Luxembourg (2009) and Colombia (2015), all with formal guidelines laid down for its use. Assisted suicide is legal in Switzerland (since 1941), Germany, Japan, Canada, and the states of Washington, Oregon, Colorado, Vermont, Montana, and California in the USA.

Emanuel EJ, Onwuteaka-Philipsen BD, et al (2016). JAMA; 316: 79–90

EVAR, Endovascular aneurysm repair, *see Aortic aneurysm, abdominal*

EVE, Epidural volume expansion, *see Combined spinal–epidural anaesthesia*

Evoked potentials (EPs). Electrical activity recorded from the CNS or peripherally following peripheral or central stimulation. Used to investigate demyelinating disease, neuropathies and in monitoring of **TBI** and coma. Also used to assess depth of anaesthesia and CNS integrity during surgery.

Requires complex equipment to increase recording sensitivity and reduce interference. Recorded potentials are small (usually 1–2 μV) compared with background electrical activity (over 100 μV); the signal is amplified and (random) background activity eliminated using computer averaging. Filters reduce noise. Displayed as a plot of voltage against time; a stimulation spike occurs within 1 ms, followed by a composite pattern representing potentials from near and distant structures along the conduction pathway, depending on the sites of stimulation and recording. Upward peaks represent negative potentials by convention. Latency is the time between the stimulation spike and the first major peak; amplitude is the height from this peak to the following trough.

- Different types:
  - sensory EPs:
    - somatosensory (SEPs):
      - supramaximal stimulation of the posterior tibial or median nerves. Direct spinal cord stimulation may be performed to monitor cord integrity during spinal surgery.
      - recording from:
        - scalp EEG electrodes, e.g. one over the sensory area appropriate to the site of stimulus plus a reference electrode elsewhere. May also examine transmission between different sites along the conduction pathway, e.g. central conduction time (CCT) between activity at the level of C5 to cortical activity.

          In general, most anaesthetic agents increase latency and decrease amplitude (**etomidate** consistently increases amplitude) in a dose-related manner. Amplitude increases following tracheal intubation or skin incision, suggesting that SEPs represent magnitude of stimulus rather than anaesthetic depth. The technique has also been used to monitor function during craniotomy, e.g. measuring CCT: impaired conduction may represent physical damage, hypoxia or ischaemia.
        - epidural space in spinal surgery; e.g. bipolar electrodes placed via an epidural needle at the lower cervical level. Electrodes may also be placed in the subdural space if the dura is opened. Skin/vertebral recording is less reliable.

          Anaesthetic agents have minimal effects on spinal evoked potentials; the technique is useful for investigating spinal conduction at any anaesthetic depth. Each side is tested individually; amplitude reduction greater than 50% during surgery is likely to indicate postoperative neurological deficit. Used for surgery for **kyphoscoliosis**, tumours, vascular lesions, etc., also for surgery to the brachial plexus, aortic arch, etc.
    - auditory (AEPs):
      - stimulation of the eighth cranial nerves with audible clicks, usually at 6–10 Hz.
      - recording from scalp electrodes (e.g. vertex/mastoid), and reference on the forehead.
      - recorded pattern represents brainstem, and early and late cortical responses. Brainstem EPs are little affected by anaesthetics; early cortical EPs are most consistently affected as for SEPs.
    - visual (VEPs):
      - stimulation of optic nerves using swimming goggles incorporating light-emitting diodes; 2 Hz is usually employed.
      - recording from the occiput.
      - thought to be less reliable than SEPs or AEPs, but have been used to monitor function during surgery for lesions involving the optic nerve and chiasma, and pituitary gland.
  - motor EPs:
    - stimulation of the scalp using large voltages, or the motor cortex directly. Induction of potential using magnetic fields has been used.
    - recording from the median or posterior tibial nerve, or EMG of limb muscles. Very sensitive to volatile anaesthetic agents, thus **TIVA** is needed during intraoperative use. Recording from the epidural space is less affected by anaesthetics, and has been used for spinal surgery.

Shils JL, Sloan TB (2015). Int Anesthesiol Clin; 53: 53–73

See also, Anaesthesia, depth of

Exercise. Produces physiological changes that increase **oxygen flux** and removal of waste products from active tissues:

- cardiovascular:

  - increased **cardiac output** mainly due to increased **heart rate** (to a maximum rate of about 195 beats/min in adults). **Stroke volume** increases slightly in normal individuals, although it can double in trained athletes. The increase in cardiac output starts before exercise due to cortical activation of the **sympathetic nervous system**. Following initiation of exercise, CVS reflexes are activated following stimulation of **muscle** mechanoreceptors, **baroreceptors** and joint receptors.
  - BP increases (systolic > diastolic), reflecting increased cardiac output despite decreased **SVR** due to vasodilatation in exercising muscles.
  - increased **venous return** due to increased skeletal muscle pump activity and thoracic pump action.
  - blood flow is diverted to skin and actively contracting muscles at the expense of renal and splanchnic blood flow. Muscle blood flow may increase 30-fold as a result of accumulation of local metabolites (e.g. K^+, lactic acid), a decrease in arterial PO_2 and an increase in PCO_2. Arteriovenous O_2 difference may increase threefold due to a shift of the **oxyhaemoglobin dissociation curve** to the right secondary to the **acidosis**, raised temperature in muscles and raised **2,3-DPG** levels found during exercise.
  - **coronary blood flow** may increase to up to five times the resting level.
- respiratory:
  - increased minute ventilation due to increase in respiratory rate and **tidal volume**. The increase is proportional to the rise in oxygen demand and is due to cortical stimulation and afferent impulses from proprioceptors in muscles, tendons and joints.
  - pulmonary blood flow increases up to sixfold. Thus oxygen uptake by the lungs can reach 4000 ml/min, which exceeds cardiac oxygen delivery capacity.
  - CO_2 excretion can reach 8000 ml/min.
- **temperature regulation**: the heat produced is dissipated by increased sweating, skin vasodilation and heat loss through expired air.

If extreme exercise continues, exhaustion follows; BP falls, cutaneous vasoconstriction occurs, body temperature rises and accumulation of lactic acid and CO_2 results in increasing acidosis. Muscle cramps and fatigue occur. Exertional **myoglobinuria** may be seen.

Exercise testing. Most commonly, involves **ECG** recording while performing **exercise**, e.g. using a treadmill or bicycle, with workload increased in steps.

Testing is used to investigate chest pain or breathlessness, and to indicate prognosis in **ischaemic heart disease**, especially following **MI**. S–T depression is the most significant sign during exercise, but other changes, e.g. S–T elevation, Q waves, may occur. Chest pain, hypotension and arrhythmias may also be provoked. Testing may be combined with other measurements, e.g. arterial BP, respiratory rate, tidal volume, O_2 consumption, CO_2 output, arterial blood gases and **cardiac output**. Reduced **ejection fraction** (e.g. demonstrated by **echocardiography**) or cardiac output may suggest reversible ischaemia that may persist after cessation of exercise (myocardial stunning).

Inotropic drugs (e.g. **dobutamine**) may also be used to provoke similar changes to those caused by exercise (dobutamine stress test).

Traditionally, the patient's own exercise tolerance (e.g. maximum walking distance or stairs climbed) has been used as a general indicator of cardiorespiratory function. More recently, formal **cardiopulmonary exercise testing** has been used to predict outcomes after major surgery, using the work at which maximal O_2 consumption is reached, or the work at which anaerobic energy metabolism (**anaerobic threshold**) starts, as markers of cardiopulmonary reserve.

Albouaini K, Egred M, Alahmar A, Wright DJ (2007). Heart; 93: 1285–92

Exomphalos, *see Gastroschisis and exomphalos*

Exotoxins. High-molecular-weight, heat-labile and antigenic proteins produced by micro-organisms. Although some bacteria produce only one significant kind of exotoxin (e.g. clostridia), others produce several (e.g. streptococci and staphylococci). Exotoxins and **endotoxins** contribute to the pathogenesis of **sepsis**. Some are used clinically, e.g. **botulinum toxins**.

Expert systems. Computerised systems consisting of databases of knowledge and rules that are connected to the user via an interface. The latter takes data from the database and delivers inferences to the user. A facility for adding knowledge to the database allows the system to 'learn' continually. Expert systems may be:
- diagnostic, e.g. for interpretation of arterial blood gases, ECG.
- therapeutic, e.g. for providing optimal ventilator settings.

Expiratory flow rate, *see Forced expiratory flow rate*

Expiratory pause, *see Inspiratory:expiratory ratio*

Expiratory reserve volume (ERV). **FRC** minus **residual volume**. Normally 1–1.2 l. Reduced ERV is usually the cause of reduced FRC.
See also, Lung volumes

Expiratory valve, *see Adjustable pressure-limiting valve*

Expired air ventilation. Component of **CPR** said to be referred to in the Bible (2 Kings 4: 34–5). Reported in the 1700s and 1800s, but only became medically accepted practice in the 1950s, following demonstration that it was effective in apnoea during anaesthesia. Adequate oxygenation may be maintained with expired air of O_2 concentration 15%–16%.

Having cleared the airway of debris, and with the patient supine, the neck is extended and the jaw held forward. In adults, the nose is pinched closed and the operator's mouth placed firmly over that of the patient (mouth-to-mouth respiration). Slow, deep exhalations are made while observing the patient's chest for expansion. Exhalation is passive. May also be performed through the patient's nose (mouth-to-nose respiration). In children, the operator's mouth is placed over the patient's nose and mouth.

Regurgitation of gastric contents may occur during expired air ventilation; this may be reduced by application of **cricoid pressure** if another person is available.

Various devices, some with valves, are available for avoidance of direct mouth-to-mouth contact, to improve aesthetic acceptability and reduce risk of cross-contamination; most hinder efficient ventilation. An anaesthetic facemask is suitable. Expired air ventilation may be performed through a correctly placed tracheal tube or **SAD**.

Explosions, *see Burns; Chest trauma; Explosions and fires; Incident, major; Smoke inhalation; Trauma*

Explosions and fires. Occur when a substance combines with O_2 or another oxidising agent, with release of **energy**. **Activation energy** is required to start the process, with utilisation of energy produced to maintain combustion. If the reaction proceeds very quickly, large amounts of heat, light and sound are given out, i.e., an explosion occurs. Speed of reaction is greatest for **stoichiometric mixtures**.

- The following are required for explosions to occur:
  - combustible substance (fuel):
    - anaesthetic agents, e.g. **cyclopropane, diethyl ether**. C–C bonds are susceptible to breakdown; C–F bonds are resistant, hence the non-**flammability** of modern **inhalation anaesthetic agents**.
    - alcohol used to clean skin.
    - gases, e.g. methane and hydrogen in the patient's GIT.
    - grease/oil in anaesthetic pressure gauges (*see Adiabatic change*).
  - gas to support combustion: O_2 is standard in most anaesthetic techniques. **N_2O** breaks down to O_2 and nitrogen with heat, producing further energy; thus reactions may be more vigorous with N_2O than with O_2 alone.
  - energy source: About 1 µJ is required for most reactions with O_2; about 100 µJ with air. Sources include:
    - sparks from:
      - build-up of static electricity.
      - electrical equipment, e.g. **diathermy**, monitors, switches.
    - naked flames, cigarettes, hot wires, diathermy, light sources.
    - lasers (*see Laser surgery*).

May result in **burns**, direct **trauma** and **smoke inhalation**. Although uncommon now with modern techniques, explosions and fires continue to be reported.

- Precautions during anaesthesia include:
  - avoidance of flammable agents. If used, a zone of risk (within which no potential source of ignition should be placed) has been defined, e.g. extending 25 cm from any part of the apparatus or patient's airways that contain the anaesthetic mixture.
  - **antistatic precautions**, e.g. conductive rubber, floor.
  - checking and maintenance of all electrical equipment. Use of spark-free switches.
  - use of air instead of N_2O.
  - use of **circle systems**.
  - air conditioning and **scavenging**, to reduce levels of anaesthetic agents. Sparks are reduced by maintaining relative humidity above 50%, and temperature above 20°C.

Fire-fighting equipment should be present in every operating department.

Non-combustion explosions may occur if **cylinders** are faulty or internal pressure is excessively high.

See also, Ignition temperature

Exponential process. A process in which the rate of change of a quantity at a given time is in constant proportion to the amount of the quantity at that time.

- Different types:
  - exponential decay (negative exponential), e.g. passive lung deflation after a breath, radioactive decay, **washout curves** (Fig. 66a). Similar curves are obtained in **pharmacokinetics**, in which several curves may be superimposed. For exponential decay:

    $A = A_0 b^{-kt}$

    where A = value of variable at a given time
    A_0 = A at time zero
    b = a particular base, usually e (2.718) because mathematical manipulations are easier
    k = a constant (the rate constant)
    t = time

    The rate constant (k) is the constant of proportionality linking the rate of the change of the quantity to its value (i.e., k = rate/quantity). Its reciprocal is the **time constant** (τ), and is also defined as the time required for completion of the process at the initial rate of change. Substituting τ for k (and e for b):

    $A = A_0 e^{-t/\tau}$

    At time τ: $A = A_0\, e^{-1}$
    Thus:
    - at time = τ, $A = e^{-1}$ of its original value = 37% (63% complete);
    - at 2τ, $A = e^{-2}$ of its original value = 13.5% (86.5% complete);
    - at 3τ, $A = e^{-3}$ of its original value = 5% (95% complete).

    The duration of the process is also indicated by **half-life** (time taken for original value to fall by half; Fig. 66b).
  - build-up exponential (wash-in curve), e.g. lung inflation with a constant-pressure generator ventilator, or uptake of inhalational anaesthetic agents (Fig. 66c).

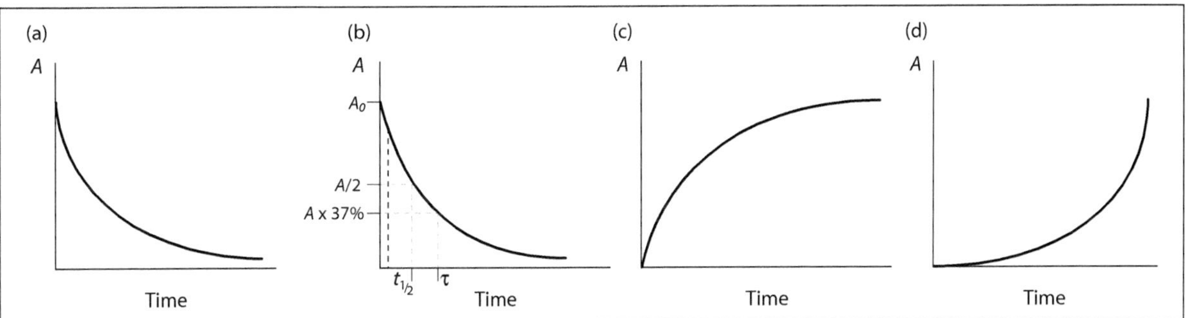

Fig. 66 Types of exponential processes: (a) and (b) exponential decay; (c) exponential build-up; (d) positive exponential

- positive exponential (breakaway function), e.g. growth of bacteria (Fig. 66d).

Plotted on semilogarithmic paper, exponential processes assume straight lines, e.g. used in the analysis of washout curves.

Extended mandatory minute ventilation, *see Mandatory minute ventilation*

External jugular venous cannulation. The external **jugular vein** passes posteriorly over the sternomastoid muscle from the angle of the jaw and joins the subclavian vein behind the midpoint of the clavicle (*see Fig. 90;* **Internal jugular venous cannulation**). It is often visible and thus easier to locate than the internal jugular vein, although valves may hinder cannulation and misplacement is common. In some individuals the vessel is not a distinct structure but is replaced by a venous plexus. The technique of cannulation involves placing the patient slightly head down with the arms by the side and the head turned to the contralateral side. After cleaning the skin, the skin is punctured well above the clavicle and the needle advanced immediately over the vein at about 20 degrees to the frontal plane. A J-wire may help the catheter negotiate the valves at the junction with the subclavian vein.

Extracellular fluid (ECF). Body fluid compartment; volume is about 14 l (20% of body weight). Consists of **interstitial fluid** and **plasma.** Transcellular fluid (approximately 1 l, composed of **CSF**, synovial fluid, etc.) and fluid within dense connective tissue, bone, etc., are usually excluded from the definition because these fluids are not readily exchangeable.

Measurement by **dilution techniques** is difficult because of eventual exchange with the above compartments, and because the substance used must remain extracellular. Substances used include inulin labelled with carbon-14, mannitol, sucrose, chloride-36 ions, bromide-82 ions, sulfate and thiosulfate. Slightly different values are obtained with each.

Compositions of plasma and interstitial fluid are different (*see Fluids, body*).
See also, Dehydration; Fluid balance

Extracorporeal carbon dioxide removal ($ECCO_2R$). Method of respiratory support in which CO_2 is removed via a venovenous extracorporeal circuit and oxygenation is maintained by either **apnoeic oxygenation** or IPPV at very slow rates (1–4 breaths/min). Facilitates lung-protective ventilation strategies by preventing respiratory acidosis. The extracorporeal circuit runs at only 1–2 l/min; thus lung ischaemia is less likely than with **extracorporeal membrane oxygenation.** There is currently a lack of evidence as to its efficacy.

Practical considerations and complications are as for **cardiopulmonary bypass.**
Camporota L, Barrett N (2016). Biomed Res Int: 9781695

Extracorporeal circulation, *see Cardiopulmonary bypass; Extracorporeal carbon dioxide removal; Extracorporeal membrane oxygenation; Haemodiafiltration; Haemodialysis; Haemofiltration; Haemoperfusion; Plasma exchange; Ultrafiltration*

Extracorporeal membrane oxygenation (ECMO). Method of cardiorespiratory support for patients with end-stage heart or lung failure. Used as a 'bridge' to transplant or recovery (depending on the underlying disease process). An arteriovenous extracorporeal circuit may be used to provide complete cardiorespiratory support (i.e., oxygenation and removal of CO_2 with arterial flow); venovenous circuits may be used for respiratory support only. Very successful in specific groups (e.g. neonates with **respiratory distress syndrome** due to meconium aspiration). Has been used successfully in **respiratory failure** e.g. caused by **influenza** in recent **pandemics.** Also used to provide temporary support after **cardiac surgery.**

Problems include cannula misplacement, infection and complications of anticoagulation. Other practical considerations and complications are as for **cardiopulmonary bypass.**
Leligdowicz A, Fan E (2015). Curr Opin Crit Care; 21: 13–19

Extracorporeal shock wave lithotripsy. Non-invasive treatment of renal and biliary calculi using an acoustic pulse. Early technology used shock waves generated by the underwater discharge of a spark plug (18–24 000 V), focused on the calculus by a computer-controlled reflector, with the patient suspended in a water bath on a hydraulic supportive cradle. The newest lithotriptors do not require immersion of the patient in water. At the interface between tissue fluid and calculus, energy released from the shock wave fragments the stone. Approximately 1000–2000 shocks are required to disintegrate an average stone, taking about 30–60 min. Contraindications include cardiac pacemakers unless reprogrammed (timing may be modified), aortic calcification, pregnancy and presence of orthopaedic prostheses.

Energy may be released at any interface and cause pain, e.g. at water/skin interfaces. General anaesthesia, sedation and regional techniques have been used. IV fluid administration is usually required to produce a good diuresis, to wash away calculi fragments. Renal bleeding may occur if coagulation is impaired.

Plasma lactate dehydrogenase concentrations may be increased postoperatively. **PONV** is common.

Extraction ratio (ER). Measure of the amount of removal of drug by an organ, e.g. liver:

$$ER = \frac{C_i - C_o}{C_i}$$

where C_i = drug concentration in blood entering the organ,
C_o = drug concentration in blood leaving the organ.

Factors affecting ER include enzyme activity and drug protein-binding.

Drugs with high ER (e.g. **lidocaine** and **propranolol**) undergo significant **first-pass metabolism** in the liver after oral administration. The rate of elimination is thus more dependent on hepatic blood flow than hepatic function; **clearance** of drugs with a low ER is more sensitive to changes in hepatic function (e.g. **enzyme induction/inhibition**) than blood flow.

Drugs with low ER include **diazepam**, **digoxin** and **phenytoin.**

Extradural (epidural) haemorrhage. Haemorrhage between the periosteum and dura.
- May be:
  - intracranial: may occur from meningeal vessels (classically the middle meningeal artery), dural sinuses or fractured bone. Features are as for **TBI**; typically, depressed consciousness, contralateral hemiparesis

and ipsilateral pupillary dilatation follow a **lucid interval** of a few hours after recovery from relatively minor trauma. CT shows a biconvex hyperintense lesion. Management: as for head injury, with urgent evacuation of the clot.

- spinal: may occur spontaneously in patients with impaired coagulation, or following lumbar puncture, and **spinal** or **epidural anaesthesia**. Marked haemorrhage with haematoma formation may cause **spinal cord**/nerve compression that may be masked by regional blockade.

Extravascular lung water (EVLW). Volume of water contained within the pulmonary interstitium and alveolar space. Usually 4–5 ml/kg. Measurement of EVLW has attracted attention as a possible means of detecting **pulmonary oedema** before it becomes apparent, although its usefulness in clinical practice is controversial. Determined by **Starling forces** and integrity of the pulmonary capillary and alveolar epithelium. Disruption of the former (e.g. by left ventricular failure) or the latter (e.g. in **ALI**) may result in increased EVLW.

Measured by the double indicator dilution technique in which cold indocyanine dye is injected into the right atrium. The dye is contained within the intravascular space and its dilution curve allows calculation of the intravascular compartment. In contrast, the heat (measured by a thermistor placed in the aorta) from the solution is dissipated into the surrounding lung tissue and its dilution curve represents the sum of the intravascular and extravascular compartments. Subtraction of the curves allows calculation of the EVLW. Other methods of assessing EVLW include **CXR**, **CT** and **MRI scanning** and **positron emission tomography** techniques.

See also, Cardiac output measurement; Dilution techniques

Extubation, tracheal. Problems that may occur include the following:

- cardiovascular response: similar to tracheal intubation but usually somewhat reduced.
- coughing and **laryngospasm**: the latter is especially likely to occur at light planes of anaesthesia and in children.
- regurgitation and **aspiration of gastric contents**.
- **airway obstruction.**
- laryngeal trauma caused by the **cuff** if still inflated.

At the end of anaesthesia, tracheal extubation is performed with the patient either deeply anaesthetised or awake. While the former avoids complications such as coughing and hypertension, the latter option allows return of the patient's respiratory and laryngeal reflexes and is therefore recommended in patients particularly at risk of complications. These include those in whom access to the airway is impaired and those at risk of airway obstruction or aspiration (in whom extubation may be performed in the lateral position).

In patients in whom deep extubation is unsuitable but when smooth emergence from anaesthesia is particularly important (e.g. **neurosurgery**, **maxillofacial surgery**), alternative techniques include exchanging the tracheal tube for a **SAD** (in the Bailey manoeuvre, an **LM** is placed behind the tracheal tube before the latter is removed) or use of a **remifentanil** infusion.

Extubation should be preceded by suction to the pharynx and larynx, preferably under direct vision, to remove secretions and blood that might otherwise be inhaled. Secretions are particularly marked in unpremedicated patients and following **neostigmine**. Inflation of the lungs with O_2 immediately before and during extubation provides an O_2 reserve in case of laryngospasm and helps expel sputum from the upper airway. Facilities for reintubation should be available.

In patients in whom reintubation is predicted to be difficult, a bougie, fibrescope or **airway exchange catheter** may be placed into the trachea before extubation. In this group of patients high-dose corticosteroids may be given to prevent post-extubation laryngeal oedema. After extubation, adequate ventilation should be confirmed and supplemental oxygen administered during transfer to a **recovery room.**

Similar considerations apply to patients in ICU after successful **weaning from ventilators.**

[Peter L. Bailey, US anaesthesiologist]

Popat M, Mitchell V, Dravid R, et al (2012). Anaesthesia; 67: 318–40

Eye, anatomy, *see Cranial nerves; Skull*

Eye care. Important during both anaesthesia and intensive care because the eye is at risk for several reasons:

- the cornea is susceptible to hypoxia because it is usually covered by the eyelid when unconscious, thus preventing diffusion of O_2 from the atmosphere. Hypoxaemia may thus lead to corneal oedema that in turn may cause sloughing and corneal abrasion. The latter may also occur with direct trauma during anaesthesia and surgery.

  Paraffin-based ointments reduce the incidence of abrasions but may impair vision for several hours. Methylcellulose or saline drops may also be efficacious but require regular administration (e.g. hourly). Routine taping of the eyes is the simplest method of preventing corneal abrasions.
- rarely, postoperative blindness (in one or both eyes) can occur in patients with normal preoperative vision and may be the result of damage to the retina and/or the optic nerve. Suggested causative factors include hypotension, microemboli in retinal vessels and increased pressure on the eyeball. Risk factors include:
  - spinal surgery in the prone position especially if surgery lasts >6 h and involves major haemorrhage.
  - **cardiopulmonary bypass** (CPB).
  - bilateral neck dissection.
  - patient factors: cardiovascular disease (e.g. **hypertension**, **stroke**, previous **MI**), **diabetes mellitus**, polycythaemia.

Overall risk of blindness following GA is 1 in 60–125 000; risk following spinal surgery is 1 in 1330 and CPB 1 in 1100.

Roth S (2009). Br J Anaesth; 103: i31–40

Eye, penetrating injury. Anaesthetic considerations:

- as for any intraocular **ophthalmic surgery**.
- risk of expulsion of intraocular contents should **intraocular pressure** (IOP) rise.
- may present as an acute emergency following **trauma**, for eye or other surgery, i.e., with risk of **aspiration of gastric contents.**

- Management:
  - preoperatively:
    - general assessment, particularly of airway and risk of difficult intubation.

- delaying surgery should be considered if possible, to allow **gastric emptying**. Risk of **aspiration pneumonitis** may be reduced by **metoclopramide**, **H_2 receptor antagonists**, etc.
- perioperatively: choice to be made, if surgery cannot wait:
  - to risk the rise in IOP caused by **suxamethonium** while performing rapid sequence induction. Risks may be reduced by:
    - methods used to reduce the rise in IOP, although not always reliable:
    - 'generous' dose of induction agent, or a supplementary dose before intubation, especially using **propofol**.
    - iv **β-adrenergic receptor antagonists**, **lidocaine**, opioids, acetazolamide, and non-depolarising neuromuscular blocking drug pretreatment have been studied, with mixed results.

    Some centres have reported that use of suxamethonium need not result in loss of intraocular contents.
  - to use alternative means of achieving tracheal intubation (although laryngoscopy and intubation themselves raise IOP):
    - rapid sequence induction using high-dose **rocuronium**.
    - inhalational induction/awake intubation: however, coughing and straining increase IOP.
    - the above may be combined with measures to reduce risk from aspiration.

The individual patient's medical condition and severity of injury, and the skill of the anaesthetist, should be carefully considered before deciding on the most appropriate technique. Ultimately, safe tracheal intubation must take precedence over protection of the eye. Other drugs known to increase IOP (e.g. **ketamine**) should be avoided.

F wave, *see Atrial flutter.*

Facemasks. The traditional black antistatic rubber anaesthetic masks, with soft edges or inflatable rims, have largely been replaced by clear, disposable, plastic masks. Ideally, they should have minimal **dead space** and make an airtight seal with the patient's face. Some are malleable to improve fit. Damage may be caused to eyes, nose and face if excessive pressure is used. Dead space may be measured using water, and may be up to 200 ml if the elbow attachment is included. Paediatric facemasks may be small versions of adult ones or specially designed to minimise dead space, e.g. Rendell-Baker's (anatomically moulded to fit the face). Others are specifically designed for delivery of CPAP or non-invasive ventilation.
[Leslie Rendell-Baker (1917–2008), British-born US anaesthetist]
See also, Open-drop techniques

Facet joint injection. Injection of the posterior facets of the intervertebral joints, performed in patients with mechanical low back pain not associated with leg symptoms or signs of root irritation/compression. The posterior primary ramus of each **spinal nerve** divides into lateral and medial branches; the latter supplies the lower portion of the facet joint capsule at that spinal level and the upper portion of the capsule below. Thus two posterior primary rami must be blocked to anaesthetise one facet joint.

With the patient prone, the joint is located using image intensification radiography, and a needle inserted under local anaesthesia. It is walked medially and superiorly off the transverse process of the vertebra to reach the angle where the lateral edge of the facet joint meets the superomedial aspect of the transverse process. **Local anaesthetic agent** may be injected, or longer-lasting relief obtained by destroying the facet joint nerve using radiofrequency rhizolysis.
Cohen SP, Raja SN (2007). Anesthesiology; 106: 591–614

Facial deformities, congenital. Patients may present for radiological assessment and corrective cosmetic surgery.
- Anaesthetic considerations are usually related to:
  - airway difficulties, including difficult intubation.
  - other congenital abnormalities, e.g. CVS, renal, CNS.
  - general problems of **paediatric anaesthesia** and **plastic surgery**, e.g. fluid balance, heat and blood loss during prolonged procedures. Topical vasoconstrictor solutions are used to reduce bleeding. **Tranexamic acid** is routinely given if major haemorrhage is anticipated.
  - repeat anaesthetics.
- Common conditions:
  - cleft lip and palate: incidence is about 1 in 600; it may involve the lip (right, left or bilateral), palate, or combinations thereof. Other abnormalities are present in up to 15% of cases. Swallowing abnormalities may be present, with risk of **aspiration pneumonitis**. Surgery for cleft lip is usually performed at 3–6 months, for cleft palate at 6–12 months. Induction of anaesthesia is as for standard paediatric anaesthesia, but tracheal intubation may be difficult if the **laryngoscope blade** slips into the cleft. To prevent this the cleft may be packed with gauze or the Oxford blade used. Preformed or rigid **tracheal tubes** are usually employed, with a throat pack. Further surgery may be required in later years.
  - mandibular hypoplasia (micrognathia): e.g. in Pierre Robin syndrome (macroglossia, cleft palate and cardiac defects) and Treacher Collins syndrome (**choanal atresia**, downwards sloping eyes, deafness, low-set ears and cardiac defects). The small mandible leaves little room for the tongue, the larynx appearing anterior. Intubation may be extremely difficult; deep inhalational anaesthesia, awake or blind nasal intubation, **cricothyrotomy** and **tracheostomy** have been employed.
  - hypertelorism (increased distance between the eyes): associated with many other abnormalities or syndromes, including airway abnormalities. Corrective surgery may include mandibular or maxillary osteotomies, craniotomy and multiple rib grafts; it is often prolonged with significant haemorrhage.
  - other deformities that may produce airway problems include macroglossia, **cystic hygroma** and branchial cyst. Raised **ICP** may occur with **hydrocephalus** and craniosynostosis (premature closure of the cranial sutures).

[Edward Treacher Collins (1862–1919), English ophthalmologist; Pierre Robin (1867–1950), French paediatrician]
See also, Intubation, difficult

Facial nerve block. Performed to prevent blepharospasm during ophthalmic surgery, under regional anaesthesia.
- Methods:
  - local anaesthetic infiltration between muscle and bone along the lateral and inferior margins of the orbit.
  - injection of 5 ml solution over the condyloid process of the mandible, just anterior to the ear and below the zygoma.

Facial trauma. Anaesthetic and resuscitative considerations include: possible **airway obstruction** and difficult tracheal intubation; risk of **aspiration of gastric contents**; postoperative management of the airway; and the presence of other **trauma** (especially to head, eyes, chest and neck).
- Classification of facial injuries:
  - maxillary fractures: often more serious, and associated with significant head injury. Classified by Le Fort after dropping heavy objects on to the faces of cadavers:
    - I: transverse fractures of mid-lower maxilla.
    - II: triangular fracture from top of the nose to base of the maxilla.

- III: severe fractures involving the orbit, with disruption of facial bones from the skull. Cribriform plate disruption and CSF leak are common.
  - zygomatic fractures: may hinder mouth opening.
  - nasal fractures: may require reduction under anaesthesia; tracheal intubation and insertion of a throat pack may be required if epistaxis occurs. If the latter is severe, a nasal compression device may be necessary.
- Anaesthetic management:
  - preoperatively:
    - assessment for the above factors. Airway obstruction and major haemorrhage are more likely with bilateral fractures.
    - risk of aspiration of **gastric contents**, including swallowed blood. Fractures rarely require immediate surgery; preoperative fasting is usually possible.
    - the patient should be warned about postoperative inability to open the mouth if the jaw is wired.
  - perioperatively:
    - rapid sequence induction may be indicated. Other techniques may be required if airway obstruction or cervical instability is present (e.g. awake fibreoptic tracheal intubation, **tracheostomy**).
    - nasal tracheal intubation is usually required. Oral intubation may be performed first to secure the airway.
    - procedures often involve wiring of jaw segments together, and splinting of the mandible to the upper jaw. Silk threads are sometimes used. Plates may be applied, with wiring 1–2 days later.
  - postoperatively:
    - tracheal **extubation** should be performed when the patient is awake and in the lateral position. If severe oedema is anticipated, the tracheal tube is left in place postoperatively until it has subsided. Oral suction may be impossible. Dexamethasone is often given intraoperatively to reduce oedema.
    - the tracheal tube may be withdrawn into the pharynx to act as a nasal airway or an **airway exchange catheter** placed.
    - postoperative care should be on HDU/ICU, because the airway must be closely monitored. Wire cutters should be next to the patient at all times.

[René Le Fort (1829–1893), French surgeon]

See also, Dental surgery; Maxillofacial surgery; Induction, rapid sequence; Intubation, difficult

Facilitation, post-tetanic, *see Post-tetanic potentiation*

Factor VIIa, recombinant (Eptacog alfa). Recombinant activated **coagulation** factor VIIa. Prohaemostatic agent that activates the coagulation cascade mainly via factors IX and X. Licensed for use in patients with **haemophilia** A/B who have developed antibodies to administered factor IX or X. Has also been used 'off-label' to prevent and treat haemorrhage in cardiac surgery, liver transplantation, trauma, obstetric haemorrhage and spontaneous intracranial haemorrhage. Not shown to improve mortality in these situations and therefore not currently recommended. Use is also associated with an increased incidence of thromboembolic complications.

- Dosage: 90–120 µg/kg iv over 3–5 min, repeated 2–6-hourly.
- Side effects: hypersensitivity, arterial and venous thrombosis.

Lin Y, Moltzan CJ, Anderson DR (2012). Transfus Med; 22: 383–94

Factor Xa inhibitors. Class of direct oral **anticoagulant drugs** that inhibit coagulation factor Xa, thus preventing conversion of prothrombin to thrombin. Have rapid onset and offset of action and do not require routine monitoring with **coagulation studies**. Studies suggest equal efficacy as vitamin K antagonists such as **warfarin** in the prevention of recurrent **DVT** and **PE** and a safer alternative for patients with non-valvular **AF**. Examples include **apixaban** and **rivaroxaban**. **Fondaparinux** is a parenteral factor Xa inhibitor. Andexanet is under investigation as a class-specific antidote.

Faculty of Anaesthetists, Royal College of Surgeons of England. Founded in 1948 at the request of the **Association of Anaesthetists**, to manage the academic side of anaesthesia while the latter body concentrated on general and political aspects. Administered and regulated the **FFARCS examination** and training of junior anaesthetists, until it became the **College of Anaesthetists** in 1988 and thence the **Royal College of Anaesthetists** in 1992. The corresponding Faculty in Ireland was founded in 1959, becoming a College in 1998.

Faculty of Intensive Care Medicine, Royal College of Anaesthetists. Established in 2010 by seven parent Colleges, its remit is to define and promote standards of education and training in critical care. Replaced the Intercollegiate Board for Training in Intensive Care Medicine. Responsible for developing a primary specialty training programme for intensive care medicine and runs the Final FFICM examination.

Faculty of Pain Medicine, Royal College of Anaesthetists. Established in 2007, to promote education, training and excellence in the delivery and management of pain medicine. Also administers the Fellowship of the Faculty of Pain Medicine (FFPMRCA) examination, a mandatory requirement for admission.

Fade. Progressive reduction in strength of **muscle contraction** during tetanic or intermittent stimulation (e.g. train-of-four), exaggerated in **non-depolarising neuromuscular blockade**. Thought to be caused partly by inadequate mobilisation of **acetylcholine** in presynaptic nerve endings at the **neuromuscular junction** compared with the rate of release. Block of prejunctional **acetylcholine receptors**, which normally increase mobilisation by a positive feedback mechanism, is thought to be involved during neuromuscular blockade. Thus patterns of fade vary between blocking drugs, reflecting their differing affinities for prejunctional receptors (e.g. greater with **tubocurarine** than with **pancuronium**).

Feldman S (1993). Anaesthesia; 48: 1–2

Failed intubation, *see Intubation, failed*

Fallot's tetralogy. Commonest cause of cyanotic heart disease (65%), accounting for approximately 10% of **congenital heart disease**. 25% of patients have associated abnormality of chromosome 22.

- Consists of:
  - **VSD**.
  - pulmonary stenosis (ranges from subvalvular stenosis to pulmonary atresia).

- overriding aorta.
- right ventricular hypertrophy.

Blood flow from right ventricle to pulmonary artery is reduced, with right-to-left shunting through the VSD and aortopulmonary collaterals.

- Features:
  - **hypoxaemia** and cyanosis, usually from birth, with secondary **polycythaemia**. Dyspnoea occurs on effort.
  - acute exacerbations of shunt are attributed to infundibular spasm and increased **pulmonary vascular resistance** secondary to hypoxia. Features include worsening cyanosis, syncope and metabolic acidosis. Symptoms are relieved by squatting; thought to increase SVR and encourage pulmonary blood flow.
  - supraventricular **arrhythmias**; right heart failure in adults.
  - a loud pulmonary murmur suggests mild stenosis. A large VSD may be unaccompanied by a murmur.

Corrective surgery is usually performed within the first year of life. The VSD and right ventricular outflow are repaired with patches; right ventricular pressure measurement indicates whether there has been adequate relief of obstruction. Shunt procedures are performed for palliation if marked polycythaemia or pulmonary arterial hypoplasia is present.

- Anaesthetic management:
  - as for congenital heart disease, VSD, **cardiac surgery**, **paediatric anaesthesia**.
  - infundibular spasm is provoked by fear and anxiety, and may be treated with **β-adrenergic receptor antagonists**. Sedative **premedication** is often given.
  - avoidance of air bubbles in iv injectate, because of the risk of systemic embolisation.
  - peripheral vasodilatation worsens shunt and cyanosis. **Vasopressor drugs** (e.g. **phenylephrine**) are used to increase SVR and therefore pulmonary blood flow.

[Etienne-Louis Fallot (1850–1911), French physician]

Twite MD, Ing RJ (2012). Semin Cardiothorac Vasc Anesth; 16: 97–105

False negative/false positive, *see Errors*

Familial periodic paralysis. Rare group of autosomal dominant myopathies due to defects in sodium and calcium channels in skeletal **muscle**; characterised by episodes of severe weakness, often precipitated by extremes of temperature, physical activity, fasting and large carbohydrate loads. Although classified into hypo- or hyperkalaemic variants, the condition may be associated with normal plasma potassium levels. Diagnosis may be difficult, but exercise EMG has a high level of sensitivity; detection of known gene mutations can be helpful. Treatment of the hypokalaemic variant consists of avoiding carbohydrate-rich meals and strenuous exercise and the use of **carbonic anhydrase inhibitors** (e.g. **acetazolamide**); oral potassium supplements are given if paralysis occurs. Treatment of the hyperkalaemic variant includes a carbohydrate-rich, low potassium diet and avoidance of strenuous exercise and fasting. Dichlorphenamide helps prevent attacks.

Suxamethonium use may result in severe myotonia and must be avoided. Careful use of non-depolarising **neuromuscular blocking drugs** is required, with close monitoring of perioperative potassium levels. **Arrhythmias** may accompany potassium changes. Glucose-containing **intravenous fluids** should be avoided in the hyperkalaemic form of the disease. Normothermia should be maintained as cooling may lead to flaccid muscle weakness. Increased susceptibility to **MH** is considered unlikely.

Bandschapp O, Iaizzo PA (2013). Paediatr Anaesth; 23: 824-33

Fascia iliaca compartment block. Injection of local anaesthetic solution deep to the fascia iliaca into a compartment between the iliacus and psoas muscles, through which the femoral nerve runs (Fig. 67). The lateral cutaneous nerve of the thigh pierces the fascia iliaca behind the inguinal ligament and is usually blocked too. The obturator nerve may also be blocked. Primarily used to provide analgesia for surgery to the hip, anterior thigh and knee; increasingly performed in emergency departments by non-anaesthetists to provide analgesia for **fractured neck of femur**.

A needle is inserted 0.5 cm caudal to the junction of the lateral third of the inguinal ligament with the medial two-thirds. A click or 'give' (the latter if continuous pressure is applied to the plunger of the syringe) is felt as the needle passes through the fascia lata, followed by a second click as the fascia iliaca is pierced. An ultrasound-guided in-plane approach may also be used. 30–40 ml **local anaesthetic agent** (e.g. 0.25% **bupivacaine**) is then injected.

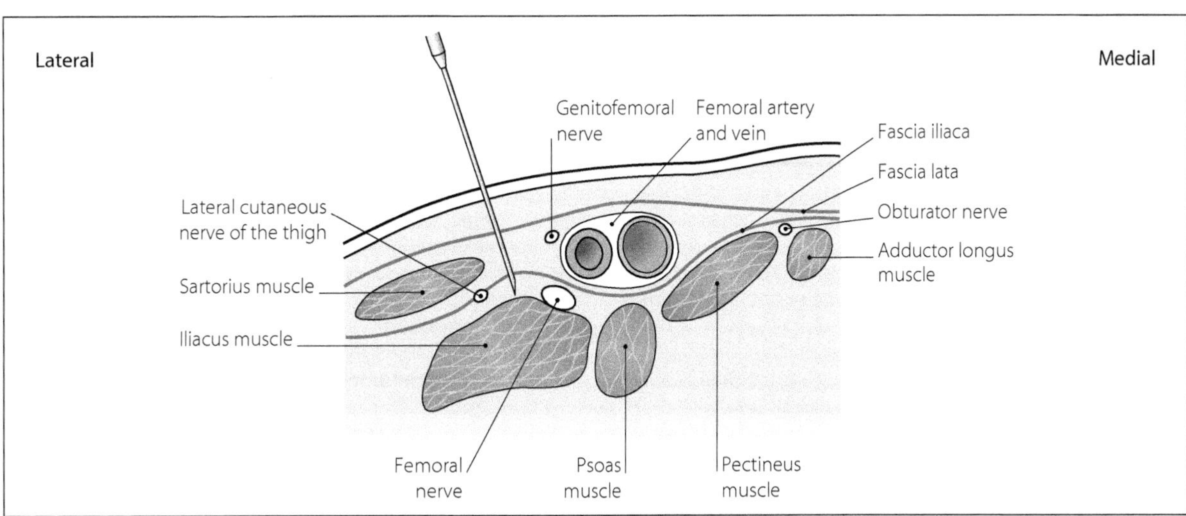

Fig. 67 Fascia iliaca compartment block

Addition of **magnesium sulfate** may enhance the block. Distal pressure is advocated to encourage cranial extension of the solution. A catheter may be inserted to allow continuous infusion of local anaesthetic.

Dalens B, Vanneuville G, Tanguy A (1989). Anesth Analg; 69: 705–13

See also, individual nerve blocks

Fascicular block, *see Bundle branch block*

Fasciculation. Visible contraction of skeletal muscle fasciculi, seen following use of **suxamethonium** and other depolarising **neuromuscular blocking drugs**. Possible damage to fibres is suggested by increased serum myoglobin and creatine kinase following suxamethonium; it may also be partly responsible for the raised potassium that occurs. Implicated in post-suxamethonium myalgia, because measures that reduce the latter often reduce visible fasciculation.

Also occurs with excess **caffeine** ingestion, in spinocerebellar degeneration, in **motor neurone disease**, in **hyperparathyroidism** and following **neostigmine** and **isoniazid** administration. Muscle fibre fibrillation (e.g. occurring after denervation injury) is invisible.

Fasciitis, necrotising, *see Necrotising fasciitis*

Fat, brown, *see Brown fat*

Fat embolism. Dispersion of fat droplets into the circulation, usually following major **trauma**. Also occurs in acute **pancreatitis**, **burns**, **diabetes mellitus**, joint reconstruction (possibly related to **bone cement implantation syndrome**), **cardiopulmonary bypass**, liposuction, **bone marrow harvest/bone marrow transplantation** and parenteral infusion of lipids. Postmortem evidence of fat embolism is found in 90% of fatal trauma cases. The mechanical (infloating) theory proposes that fat liberated from fractured bone enters the venous system and impacts in pulmonary capillaries, resulting in pulmonary dysfunction. Systemic embolism may occur via pulmonary arteriovenous shunts or a patent foramen ovale. The biochemical theory suggests that free fatty acids released following trauma induce an inflammatory response that causes pulmonary dysfunction, possibly mediated via an increase in plasma lipase. Both processes may be responsible.

The fat embolism syndrome occurs after fewer than 10% of trauma cases, typically 12–36 h after long bone fractures. Early fixation of fractures reduces its incidence fivefold.

- Features:
    - confusion, restlessness, **coma**, **convulsions**, cerebral infarction.
    - dyspnoea, cough, haemoptysis. **Hypoxaemia** is almost inevitable. **Pulmonary hypertension** and **pulmonary oedema** may occur. Typically, gives a 'snowstorm' appearance on the CXR, but radiography may be normal. May contribute to development of **ALI**.
    - petechial rash, typically affecting the trunk, pharynx, axillae and conjunctivae.
    - tachycardia, hypotension, pyrexia.
    - **platelets** are reduced in 50%; **hypocalcaemia** is also common. **Coagulation disorders** may occur.
    - fat droplets are detected in cells obtained by **bronchopulmonary lavage** in 70% of cases. The presence of fat droplets in the urine is a non-specific finding following trauma. Retinal examination may reveal intravascular fat globules.
- Management:
    - O_2 therapy; IPPV may be required.
    - supportive therapy. Fluid restriction has been advocated for reducing lung water.
    - **corticosteroids** have been shown to reduce mortality in several small studies, but optimum dosage, timing and patient selection remain unclear.
    - **heparin**, **aspirin**, clofibrate, **prostacyclin**, **dextran** and alcohol infusion have all been tried, without conclusive benefit.

Prognosis is variable and unrelated to initial severity. Mortality is 10%–20%.

Akhtar S (2009). Anesthesiol Clin; 27: 533–50

Fats (Lipids). Four main classes are present in plasma and cells:

- triglycerides:
    - composed of glycerol and fatty acids. Formed in the GIT, liver and adipose tissue.
    - the main source of dietary fat; digested in the small bowel. Initially emulsified by bile salts and broken down to monoglycerides, free fatty acids (FFAs) and glycerol by lipases within the GIT. Undigested triglycerides are only minimally absorbed but glycerol and FFAs are taken up readily. Short-chain fatty acids pass directly into the portal vein and circulate as FFAs; long-chain FFAs (over 10–12 carbon atoms) are reconstituted with glycerol to reform triglycerides before incorporation into chylomicrons.
    - endogenous triglycerides are synthesised in the liver and secreted as very-low-density lipoproteins (VLDLs). These are hydrolysed in the blood by lipoprotein lipase; the FFAs released are taken up by tissues for resynthesis of triglycerides or remain free in the plasma. During starvation, intracellular hormone-sensitive lipase breaks down adipose triglycerides to FFAs and glycerol (increased by β-adrenergic stimulation; decreased by **insulin**).
- sterols:
    - include corticosteroids, bile salts and cholesterol (from which the former two are derived).
    - plasma cholesterol is esterified with fatty acids, or circulates within low-density, high-density and intermediate-density lipoproteins (LDLs, HDLs and IDLs, respectively) and VLDLs, especially the first. Unesterified cholesterol forms a major component of cell **membranes**.
    - cholesterol is either synthesised, mainly in the liver, or absorbed from the GIT and delivered to the liver in chylomicrons.
- phospholipids:
    - mainly synthesised in the liver and small intestine mucosa.
    - circulate in the plasma in lipoproteins and constitute important cellular components, but not part of the depot fats. Present in **myelin** and cell membranes.
- fatty acids:
    - may be saturated (no double bonds between carbon atoms) or unsaturated (variable number of double bonds). Deficiency of certain polyunsaturated fatty acids may impair capillary, hepatic, immune and GIT function; hence they are termed essential. A change in intake from omega-6 to omega-3 essential fatty acids (the latter found in fish oils

and plant oils) has been suggested as reducing production of inflammatory mediators and thereby various cardiovascular and inflammatory disorders.
- esterified with triglycerides, cholesterol or phospholipids, or bound to circulating albumin as FFAs.
- FFAs are used as an energy source by most tissues.

Lipoproteins are classified according to their size: chylomicrons, 80–500 nm; VLDLs, 30–80 nm; IDLs, 25–40 nm; LDLs, 20 nm; HDLs, 7.5–10 nm. LDLs and IDLs are formed from VLDLs; HDLs are formed in the liver. High levels of cholesterol, LDLs and VLDLs are associated with **ischaemic heart disease**, although the role of each is controversial. HDLs may be protective.

Fazadinium bromide. Obsolete non-depolarising **neuromuscular blocking drug**, introduced in 1972. Acts within 60 s and marketed as an alternative to **suxamethonium**. Withdrawn because of marked cardiovascular effects due to ganglion and vagal blockade.

FDA, *see Food and Drug Administration*

FDPs, *see Fibrin degradation products*

FEEA, *see Fondation Européenne d'Enseignement en Anaesthésiologie*

Felypressin. Synthetic analogue of **vasopressin**, used as a locally acting vasoconstrictor. Has minimal effects on the myocardium; therefore safer than **adrenaline** during anaesthesia with **halothane**. Available in combination with **prilocaine** for local infiltration.

Femoral artery. Continuation of the external iliac artery; enters the thigh below the inguinal ligament midway between the anterior superior iliac spine and symphysis pubis, where it lies between the femoral vein medially and femoral nerve laterally. Descends through the **femoral triangle** and enters (and runs in) the subsartorial canal. Ends by piercing adductor magnus 10 cm above the knee joint where it becomes the popliteal artery.

May be cannulated for **arterial BP measurement**, **dialysis**, **extracorporeal membrane oxygenation** and use of the **intra-aortic counter-pulsation balloon pump**, as well as providing access for angiography.

Femoral nerve block. Useful as an adjunct to general anaesthesia for operations involving the anterior thigh, hip, knee and medial lower leg. May be combined with **sciatic nerve block** and/or **obturator nerve block** for more extensive surgery to the lower limb. Also used for analgesia in **fractured neck of femur**.

- Anatomy:
  - the **femoral nerve** (L2–4) arises from the **lumbar plexus**, passing under the inguinal ligament to enter the **femoral triangle** lateral to the **femoral artery**. Divides into terminal branches within 3–6 cm.
  - supplies hip and knee joints and muscles of the anterior thigh. Also supplies skin of the anterior thigh and knee, and medial lower leg and foot via the saphenous branch (Fig. 68).
- Block:
  - the femoral artery is palpated below the mid inguinal point (i.e., halfway between the superior anterior iliac spine and pubic tubercle); the femoral vein lies medially and the nerve laterally.

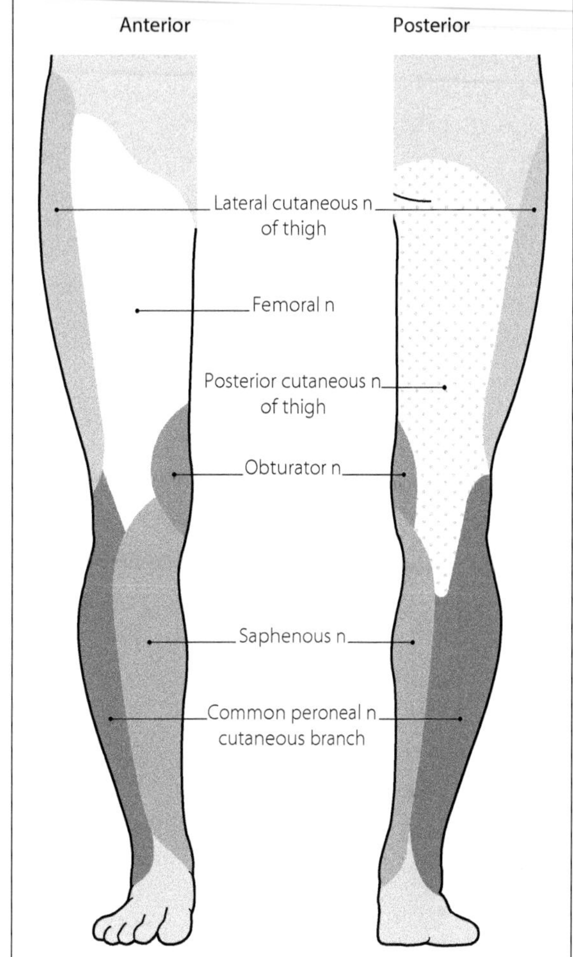

Fig. 68 Nerve supply of leg (*for nerve supply of ankle and foot, see Fig 11* **Ankle, nerve blocks**)

  - a needle is introduced through a wheal 1–2 cm lateral to the pulsation, and directed slightly cranially, to a depth of 3–4 cm. Ultrasound guidance or a nerve stimulator (looking for contraction of the quadriceps muscle) may be used to aid needle placement.
  - after aspiration to exclude vascular puncture, 10–15 ml **local anaesthetic agent** is injected. A further 5–10 ml is injected in a fan laterally as the needle is withdrawn, in case cutaneous branches arise higher than normal.
  - injection of 30–40 ml solution at the initial site, with distal compression, has been claimed to force solution cranially to the lumbar plexus, lying between psoas and quadratus lumborum muscles (three-in-one block). In fact, a continuous femoral 'sheath' probably does not exist as a separate entity; the 'three-in-one block' is thought to represent combined femoral and lateral cutaneous nerve blocks below the inguinal ligament due to non-specific spread. **Fascia iliaca compartment block** is a more reliable and anatomically sound method of producing block of the three nerves.

May also be blocked via the **adductor canal block**.

Femoral triangle. Compartment of the anterior upper thigh; its borders are the inguinal ligament superomedially,

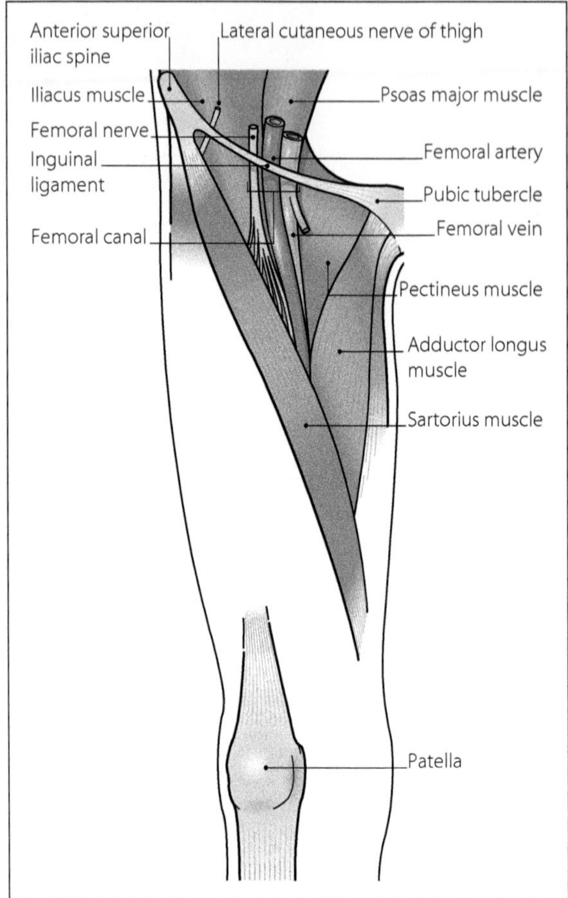

Fig. 69 Right femoral triangle (N.B. The spermatic cord emerging through the external inguinal ring superolateral to the pubic tubercle is not shown)

the medial border of adductor longus medially and the medial border of sartorius laterally (Fig. 69). Its floor is formed by adductor longus, pectineus, psoas and iliacus muscles, and its roof by the fascia lata of the thigh. Contains the **femoral artery**, vein and canal within the femoral sheath; the **femoral nerve** and **lateral cutaneous nerve of the thigh** lie laterally.

Femoral venous cannulation. The femoral vein is the continuation of the popliteal vein and accompanies the **femoral artery** in the **femoral triangle**, ending medial to the latter at the inguinal ligament, where it becomes the external iliac vein. The patient's leg is extended and slightly abducted at the hip. The femoral vein lies 1–1.5 cm medial to the femoral artery, 2–3 cm below the inguinal ligament. After the skin is cleaned, the needle is inserted here and advanced at an angle of 45–60 degrees to the frontal plane. When venous blood is aspirated, the syringe is lowered to lie flat on the skin. A **Seldinger technique** is usually employed thereafter. Ultrasound guidance is often used.

May be performed for **central venous cannulation**; traditionally avoided if other routes are available because of (probably unfounded) fears of infection or thrombosis. May be useful in **superior vena caval obstruction**.

Femur, fractured neck, *see Fractured neck of femur*

Fenoldopam mesylate. Selective D_1-**dopamine receptor** partial agonist, introduced in the USA in 1998 as an iv **vasodilator drug**. Also has mild α_2-adrenergic agonist properties. Causes increased renal blood flow, diuresis and sodium excretion. Given as an infusion for hypertensive crisis, its short **half-life** of 5 min results in rapid offset of action. Metabolised in the liver to inactive compounds. Not available in the UK.

Fenoterol hydrobromide. **β-Adrenergic receptor agonist**, used as a **bronchodilator drug**. Similar in action to **salbutamol** and **terbutaline** but less β_2-selective. Now only available in the UK as part of a compound aerosol formulation.
- Dosage: 200–400 μg by aerosol inhalation tds as required.
- Side effects: as for salbutamol.

Fentanyl citrate. Synthetic **opioid analgesic drug**, derived from **pethidine**. Developed in 1960. 100 times as potent as **morphine**. Widely used for perioperative analgesia, **sedation** (e.g. on ICU) and in chronic **pain**. Onset of action is within 1–2 min after iv injection; peak effect is within 4–5 min. Duration of action is about 20 min, terminated by redistribution initially as plasma **clearance** is less than for morphine. Postoperative respiratory depression is possible if large doses are used, especially in combination with opioid premedication and other depressant drugs. Causes minimal **histamine** release or cardiovascular changes, although may cause bradycardia.
- Dosage:
  - to obtund the pressor response to laryngoscopy: 7–10 μg/kg iv.
  - as a co-induction agent/during anaesthesia: 1–3 μg/kg iv with spontaneous ventilation; 5–10 μg/kg with IPPV. Up to 100 μg/kg is used for **cardiac surgery**. Muscular rigidity and hypotension are more common after high dosage. Has been used in **neuroleptanaesthesia**.
  - by infusion: 1–5 μg/kg/h, e.g. for sedation. For **patient-controlled analgesia**: 20–100 μg bolus with 3–5 min lockout.
  - 25, 50, 75 or 100 μg/h transdermal patch placed on the chest or upper arm and replaced (using a different site) every 72 h. A patch employing **iontophoresis** has been developed for postoperative patient-controlled analgesia but is not currently marketed.
  - 100–800 μg by sublingual lozenges, buccal tablets or intranasal spray for breakthrough cancer pain or short, painful procedures (e.g. burns dressing change).

Commonly used for epidural and spinal anaesthesia (*see Spinal opioids*).

Fetal circulation. Oxygenated blood from the **placenta** passes through the single umbilical vein and enters the inferior vena cava, about 50% bypassing the liver via the ductus venosus. Most of it is diverted through the foramen ovale into the left atrium, passing to the brain via the carotid arteries (Fig. 70). Deoxygenated blood from the brain enters the right atrium via the superior vena cava, and passes through the tricuspid valve to the right ventricle. Because the resistance of the pulmonary vessels within the collapsed lungs is high, the blood passes from the pulmonary artery trunk through the ductus arteriosus to enter the aortic arch downstream from the origin of the carotid arteries. Thus relatively O_2-rich blood is reserved for the brain, and the rest of the body is perfused with the less oxygenated blood. Deoxygenated blood reaches the placenta via the two umbilical arteries, arising from the internal iliac arteries; they receive about 60% of cardiac output.

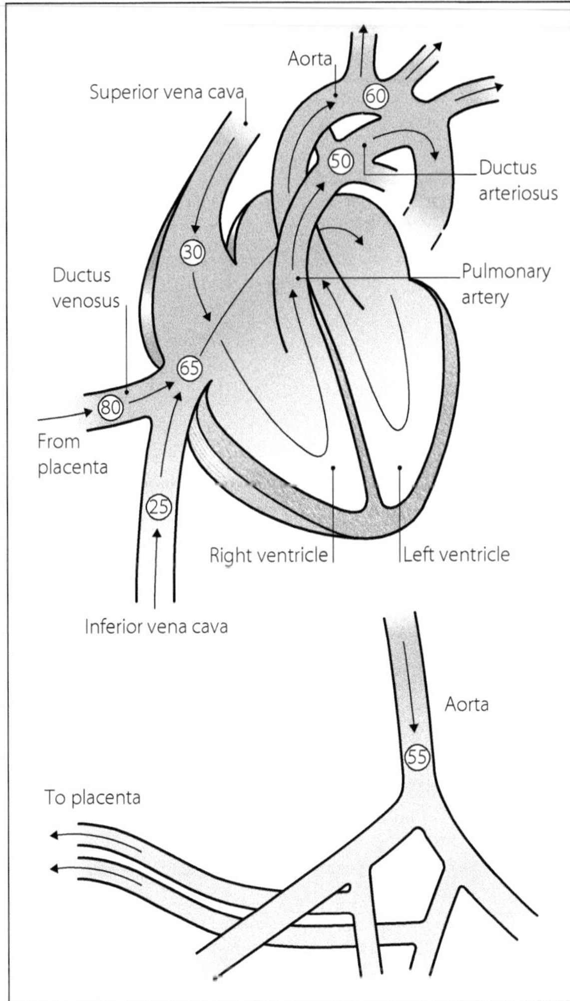

Fig. 70 Diagram of fetal circulation; *arrows* denote flow of blood. *Numbers* refer to the approximate oxygen saturation

- Approximate values:
  - umbilical vein:
    - Po_2 4 kPa (30 mmHg).
    - Pco_2 6 kPa (45 mmHg).
    - pH 7.2
  - umbilical artery:
    - Po_2 2 kPa (15 mmHg).
    - Pco_2 7 kPa (53 mmHg).

At birth, placental blood flow ceases, and peripheral resistance increases. Lung expansion lowers **pulmonary vascular resistance**, both directly and via reduction of **hypoxic pulmonary vasoconstriction.** Thus pulmonary and right heart pressures fall, and aortic and left heart pressures rise. Pulmonary blood flow increases and flow through the ductus arteriosus and foramen ovale ceases. The ductus arteriosus usually closes within 48 h due to the high Po_2. Pulmonary artery pressure, pulmonary vascular resistance and pulmonary blood flow approach adult values by 4–6 weeks.

Neonates may revert to persistent fetal circulation, with decreased pulmonary blood flow and right-to-left **shunt** through the ductus arteriosus, foramen ovale, or both. This may occur if pulmonary vascular resistance is increased, e.g. by **hypoxia**, **hypothermia**, **hypercapnia**, **acidosis** or polycythaemia. It may occur during surgery if anaesthesia is too light or if the patient strains on the tracheal tube. Right-to-left shunt increases with worsening hypoxia and further reflex vasoconstriction. Ductal shunting may be demonstrated clinically by measuring O_2 saturation (e.g. by pulse **oximetry**) in the arm and leg simultaneously; a large difference (higher saturation in the arm) represents significant ductal blood flow (i.e., pulmonary artery pressure exceeds aortic pressure). If the right ventricle fails, right atrial pressure exceeds left atrial pressure, increasing shunt through the foramen ovale.

Treatment of persistent fetal circulation includes: O_2 therapy; correction of acidosis, hypercapnia and hypothermia; and inotropes and fluid administration. Drugs that lower pulmonary vascular resistance (e.g. inhaled **nitric oxide**) may be given. **Extracorporeal membrane oxygenation** has been used.

See also, Ductus arteriosus, patent

Fetal haemoglobin. Consists of two α chains and two γ chains, the latter differing from β chains by 37 amino acids. Binds **2,3-DPG** less avidly than **haemoglobin** A (adult), thus shifting the **oxyhaemoglobin dissociation curve** to the left (P_{50} is 2.4 kPa [18 mmHg]) and favouring O_2 transfer from mother to fetus. At the low fetal Po_2, it gives up more O_2 to the tissues than adult haemoglobin would, because its dissociation curve is steeper in this part. Forms 80% of circulating haemoglobin at birth; replaced by haemoglobin A normally within 3–5 months. May persist in the **haemoglobinopathies** (e.g. **thalassaemia**). Reactivation of production of fetal haemoglobin using hydroxyurea has been used in the treatment of **sickle cell anaemia.**

A variety of embryonic haemoglobins are present up to 2–3 months of gestation.

Fetal monitoring. Methods include:
- presence of meconium in amniotic fluid: usually represents fetal compromise, and presents risk of meconium aspiration on delivery.
- heart rate, especially related to uterine contractions. May be performed intermittently using a trumpet-shaped stethoscope (Pinard) or portable **ultrasound** machine, or continuously using a cardiotocograph (CTG), a device that measures heart rate by external ultrasonography or fetal scalp electrode, and contractions by external transducer or intrauterine probe:
  - normal baseline heart rate is 110–160 beats/min, with beat-to-beat variability of 5–25 beats/min, related to autonomic activity. Increased baseline and reduced variability may indicate compromise, although they may also be caused by administration of depressant drugs to the mother or maternal pyrexia.
  - accelerations usually indicate reactivity and wellbeing.
  - decelerations; usual significance:
    - early (type I), i.e., with contractions: vagally mediated, due to head compression.
    - late (type II), i.e., after contractions: represent hypoxia, although not always with acidosis.
    - variable: usually due to cord compression; they may indicate compromise if severe.
    - Prolonged decelerations are more sinister, and may represent severe fetal compromise.

  Recent **NICE** guidelines classify the CTG according to the baseline rate, variability, accelerations and decelerations as being 'normal' (all four criteria are normal), 'suspicious' (one of the four is 'non-reassuring') or 'pathological' (two or more of the four are non-reassuring or one is 'abnormal'). Predictive value of cardiotocography is poor in low-risk patients; hence its routine use is controversial. Combination with fetal electrocardiography (S–T waveform analysis) is thought to increase its sensitivity.

Signs of fetal compromise may be related to treatable conditions, e.g. uterine hypertonicity associated with excessive oxytocin administration, maternal hypotension. **Aortocaval compression** should always be considered, especially if regional analgesia has been provided.

- fetal blood sample: pH under 7.2 represents severe acidosis. May be measured serially to observe trends.
- fetal scalp oximetry, EEG, ECG and continuous pH measurement have been investigated but are not routinely available.

Post-delivery, cord **blood gas interpretation** (pH represents degree of acidosis at time of delivery), **Apgar scoring, time to sustained respiration** and **neurobehavioural testing of neonates** may be assessed; these may be useful prognostically.

[Adolphe Pinard (1844–1934), French obstetrician]

Stout MJ, Cahill AG (2011). Clin Perinatol; 38: 127–42

Fetus, effects of anaesthetic drugs on. The fetus is usually defined as such from the ninth week of gestation. Most major organ structures develop earlier than this.

- Main anaesthetic considerations:
  - effect of anaesthetic drugs on fetal development and spontaneous abortion:
    - animal studies consistently show that general anaesthetic agents are potentially toxic to the developing brain and may have an impact on neurocognitive function later in life. However, the 2016 General Anaesthesia compared to Spinal Anaesthesia (GAS) study did not demonstrate differences in neurodevelopmental outcome at 2 years between infants given general anaesthesia and those receiving spinal anaesthesia for inguinal hernia repair, suggesting that a single exposure to anaesthesia is safe (although multiple or prolonged exposures may still have adverse effects).
    - animal studies suggest increased fetal loss and abnormalities following prolonged exposure to high concentrations of volatile agents and **N_2O**. Human studies have produced conflicting results. It is generally accepted that general anaesthesia should be avoided where possible during pregnancy, particularly during the first trimester.
    - N_2O has been implicated (but not proven) as increasing the incidence of spontaneous abortion in health workers chronically exposed; current opinion holds that its use is not contraindicated in pregnant patients.
    - new drugs should be avoided during early pregnancy, until more information becomes available.
  - effect of anaesthetic drugs given during labour on the **neonate**:
    - indirect effects:
      - reduced uteroplacental blood flow (e.g. due to oxytocin) or hypotension following regional blockade or general anaesthesia.
      - maternal hypoxia (e.g. due to drug-induced respiratory depression, total spinal block, convulsions).
      - increased maternal catecholamine levels during inadequate general anaesthesia with **awareness**; uteroplacental vasoconstriction and fetal acidosis may result. Levels are reduced in labour following epidural block; this may reduce fetal acidosis.
    - direct effects related to fetal plasma levels, affected by:
      - uteroplacental blood flow.
      - placental, maternal and fetal protein concentrations and drug binding. For example, **diazepam** binds to albumin and is extensively transferred to the fetus; **bupivacaine** binds to α_1-acid glycoprotein (present in lower concentrations in the fetus) and is transferred to a lesser extent.
      - peak maternal plasma drug levels and their duration.
      - **diffusion** of drug across the **placenta**, depending on membrane thickness, molecular size and shape, degree of ionisation and lipid solubility.
      - reduced fetal hepatic and renal function. Most drugs bypass the fetal liver via the ductus venosus.
      - umbilical vein drug levels: reduced by dilution with blood from the rest of the body. Thus umbilical vein levels may not reflect fetal levels.
      - fetal hypoxia and acidosis: cause trapping of basic drugs (e.g. opioids and **local anaesthetic agents**) and increase blood flow to vital centres, e.g. brain. Thus brain levels may be increased.
  - specific drugs:
    - **opioid analgesic drugs:**
      - fetal respiratory and CNS depression are well recognised.
      - fetal opioid levels are increased by acidosis. Peak levels occur 2–5 h after im **pethidine**, 6 min after iv injection.
      - **half-life** in the fetus is prolonged; e.g. pethidine: up to 20 h; that of norpethidine is longer.
      - **naloxone** crosses the placenta easily, but its administration is usually reserved for the fetus.
    - **iv anaesthetic agents:**
      - all cross the placenta rapidly, but have usually redistributed by the time of delivery. **Thiopental** selectively accumulates in fetal liver.
      - neurobehavioural depression has been shown following their use, although the effect is small.
    - **inhalational anaesthetic agents:**
      - at low inspired concentrations, any effect is small.
      - benefits of their use include uteroplacental vasodilatation and prevention of maternal awareness.
    - **neuromuscular blocking drugs:**
      - very little transfer follows normal use.
      - **gallamine** and **alcuronium** cross the placenta to a slightly greater extent than the others.
    - local anaesthetic agents:
      - transfer varies according to dose, site of injection (e.g. high fetal levels following **paracervical block**), use of vasoconstrictors and different plasma protein-binding characteristics of the fetus and mother for certain drugs; e.g. umbilical vein:maternal blood levels:
        - **prilocaine:** >1.
        - **lidocaine:** 0.5.
        - bupivacaine: 0.3.
        - **etidocaine:** 0.2.

- subtle neurobehavioural effects have been shown; initial fears about adverse effects of lidocaine compared with bupivacaine are now thought to be unfounded.
- fetal **methaemoglobinaemia** may follow excessive doses of prilocaine.
- **procaine** and **chloroprocaine** are metabolised by esterases in maternal and fetal plasma.

- others, e.g. benzodiazepines, phenothiazines:
  - all cross the placenta to some extent.
  - diazepam is more strongly bound to fetal than to maternal protein, and has been associated with neonatal hypotonia and hypothermia. Umbilical vein:maternal blood ratio is 2.0.
  - all drugs that significantly cross the blood–brain barrier may cross the placenta to similar extents, e.g. atropine, propranolol.

See also, Environmental safety of anaesthetists; Fetal monitoring; Neurobehavioural testing of neonates

FEV$_1$, *see Forced expiratory volume*

Fever, *see Pyrexia*

FFARCS examination (Fellowship of the Faculty of Anaesthetists at the Royal College of Surgeons of England). First held in 1953; became the FCAnaes examination in 1989 following the founding of the **College of Anaesthetists** and the **FRCA examination** upon granting of a royal charter to the College in 1992. The Irish equivalent exam (FFARCSI) was first held in 1961.

FFP, Fresh frozen plasma, *see Blood products*

Fibreoptic instruments. First use of a fibreoptic instrument (a choledochoscope) for tracheal intubation was in 1967 by Murphy. Fibreoptic bronchoscopes were introduced in 1968. Flexible fibreoptic intubating bronchoscopes as thin as 3–4 mm diameter are now widely available.

- Features:
  - rely on total internal reflection of light within bundles of glass fibres about 20 μm diameter.
  - each fibre is encased in glass of different refractive index, the interface acting as the reflective surface.
  - fibres are lubricated and flexible; the instrument's tip can be flexed using controls at the proximal end.
  - each instrument contains bundles for passage of light for illumination, and bundles for passage of the image back to the proximal end. The arrangement of the image-bearing bundles is identical at each end of the instrument (coherent), allowing accurate spatial representation of the object.
  - a lens at each end allows focusing. A camera may be attached to the eyepiece at the proximal end, allowing the operator and others to observe the view on a screen.
  - may contain channels for suction, passage of gas, liquid and forceps.
  - very delicate instruments; easily damaged, e.g. by teeth. Careful cleaning is required; passage of disinfectant into the 'scope may disrupt lubrication between fibres.

With improved miniaturisation it is now possible to place a small video chip directly at the distal end of the instrument, so that there is no need for fragile optical bundles to be contained within its shaft (which now contains electrical wires carrying the digital image instead).

- Apart from diagnosis (e.g. biopsy) and therapy (e.g. removal of secretions and foreign bodies), they have been used for:
  - tracheal intubation, with the patient awake or anaesthetised. Especially useful in cases of known difficult intubation. The endoscope may be passed through a tracheal tube, and then guided via the mouth or nose into the larynx. Lidocaine may be sprayed through a side port. The tube is passed over the 'scope into the trachea. May also be guided through various **airways** that act as conduits. Has been used to place endobronchial tubes.
  - checking the position of tracheal and endobronchial tubes. Also used to aid placement of percutaneous **tracheostomy**. May be passed through special connectors with rubber ports, thus allowing undisturbed delivery of O_2 and anaesthetic gases.
  - assessment/diagnosis, sputum clearance and lavage, e.g. during/after thoracic surgery or in ICU.

Considerable practice is required to achieve adequate skill in their use, which has been suggested as being essential during anaesthetic training but widely acknowledged as being too difficult for many UK units to achieve.

Rigid **laryngoscopes** incorporating fibreoptic channels may also be used for tracheal intubation.

Fibreoptic sensors have also been used for clinical measurement of, for example, pressure, flow and chemical concentrations.

[Peter Murphy, US anaesthetist]

See also, Intubation, awake; Intubation, difficult; Intubation, endobronchial; Intubation, tracheal

Fibrin degradation products (FDPs). Products of fibrin breakdown by plasmin; thus blood levels reflect the rate of **fibrinolysis** (e.g. increased levels occur in **DIC**). **Half-life** is about 9 h. May inhibit clot formation by competing for fibrin polymerisation sites. Also interfere with **platelet** function and thrombin; excess fibrinolysis may impair further **coagulation**. May possibly damage vascular endothelium.

Non-specific testing for FDPs has been replaced in many centres by testing for the D-dimer portion of fibrin, which is released only during fibrinolysis and is not present on fibrinogen or released during the latter's breakdown.

Measurement of FDPs (especially D-dimer) has been used to aid diagnosis of **DVT**, a normal value excluding thrombosis; however, levels may also be raised in many other conditions (e.g. **trauma**, **malignancy**, **pregnancy**, recent surgery and chronic inflammatory diseases). Thus D-dimer testing for thrombotic events has a sensitivity of about 90% and a specificity of 50%.

Normal levels: <10 mg/l (FDPs); <500 ng/ml (D-dimer).

See also, Coagulation studies

Fibrinogen, *see Coagulation*

Fibrinolysis. Dissolution of fibrin; occurs following clot formation, allowing blood vessel remodelling, and also after wound healing. Fibrinolytic and **coagulation** pathways are in equilibrium normally, each composed of a series of plasma precursor molecules.

Plasminogen, a globulin, is activated to form plasmin, a fibrinolytic enzyme. Activation involves clotting factors XII and XI, **kallikrein** and **kinins**, and leucocyte products.

Activation of tissue plasminogen is caused by products released by endothelial cells. Plasminogen activators and plasminogen itself bind to fibrin, with plasmin formation thus localised to the site of fibrin formation. Fibrin is degraded to **fibrin degradation products**, with **complement** and **platelet** activation. Fibrinolysis may be decreased by physiological stress, including surgery; effects are greatest 2–3 days postoperatively. It may be increased by **fibrinolytic drugs**, and following **DIC** as a response to the large amount of fibrin formed. Also increased by venous occlusion, **catecholamines**, and possibly **epidural** and **spinal anaesthesia**. Primary fibrinolysis may occur in certain malignancies.

Fibrinolytic drugs. Drugs causing **fibrinolysis** by activating plasminogen. Used iv and intra-arterially to prevent thrombosis, and to break up established thrombi, e.g. **PE**. Reduce mortality in acute **MI** when given iv within 12 h. Also reduce morbidity when given within 4.5 h after acute ischaemic **stroke**. **Streptokinase** acts by binding to plasminogen, the resultant complex activating other plasminogen molecules. Allergic reactions are common. **Urokinase** cleaves a specific peptide bond in plasminogen, converting it to plasmin; it is used mainly for thrombolysis in the eye and arteriovenous shunts. **Alteplase**, **reteplase** and **tenecteplase** bind to fibrin and activate plasminogen, converting it to plasmin; like streptokinase, they are used as thrombolytics in MI. The major side effect is haemorrhage; nausea, vomiting and back pain may also occur.

Fibrocystic disease, *see Cystic fibrosis*

Fibronectin. Glycoprotein, involved in the removal of intravascular debris and foreign substances via interaction with circulating **leucocytes**, enabling the opsonisation process. May become depleted in critical illness, especially **trauma** and **sepsis**; resultant impairment of opsonisation is thought to contribute to organ hypoperfusion and **MODS**. Fibronectin level has been suggested as an additional indicator of disease progression in critical illness. Present in **cryoprecipitate**; replacement has been used therapeutically but with conflicting results.

Fick principle. Blood **flow** to an organ in unit time =

$$\frac{\text{amount of a marker substance taken up by the organ in that time}}{\text{concentration difference of the substance in the vessels supplying and draining the organ}}$$

The amount of a substance given up by an organ can also be used, e.g. CO_2 (*see following*).

May be used to determine blood flow to individual organs, e.g. **cerebral blood flow** (**Kety–Schmidt technique**) or **renal blood flow**.

May also be used to determine **cardiac output**, using O_2 or CO_2 as the substance measured, and the whole body as the organ concerned:

- Using O_2: cardiac output

$$= \frac{O_2 \text{ consumption (ml/min)}}{\text{arterial} - \text{mixed venous } O_2 \text{ concentration (ml/l)}}$$

$$= \frac{250 \text{ ml/min}}{200 - 150 \text{ ml/l}}$$

$$= 5 \text{ l/min}$$

- Using CO_2: cardiac output

$$= \frac{CO_2 \text{ output (ml/min)}}{\text{mixed venous} - \text{arterial } CO_2 \text{ concentration (ml/l)}}$$

$$= \frac{200}{540 - 500 \text{ ml/l}}$$

$$= 5 \text{ l/min}$$

[Adolf Fick (1829–1901), German physiologist]

Fick's law of diffusion. Rate of **diffusion** across a **membrane** is proportional to the concentration gradient across that membrane.
See also, Fick principle

Filgrastim, *see Granulocyte colony-stimulating factor*

Filling ratio. Describes the extent to which **cylinders** containing liquefied gases (e.g. N_2O and CO_2) are filled; defined as the weight of substance contained in the cylinder, divided by the maximum weight of water it could contain. The presence of gas above the liquid reduces the pressure increase caused by any temperature rise, reducing the risk of pressure build-up and rupture.

- Applicable to substances at temperatures below their **critical temperatures**, e.g.:
  - N_2O:
    - 0.75 (temperate climate).
    - 0.67 (tropical climate).
  - CO_2: as for N_2O.
  - **cyclopropane**:
    - 0.51 (temperate climate).
    - 0.48 (tropical climate).

Filters, breathing system. Devices routinely used for reducing **contamination of anaesthetic equipment**. Two main types of filter exist:

- pleated: resin-bonded ceramic or glass fibres in a densely packed, pleated sheet. Also known as hydrophobic filters as they do not absorb water.
- electrostatic: flat layer of electrostatically charged material, with lower fibre density than pleated filters.

In vitro evidence suggests that pleated filters are more effective at preventing transmission of water-borne pathogens (e.g. **hepatitis** C); because **circle systems** often contain condensation their use with electrostatic filters is not recommended. Filtration efficiency varies non-linearly with particle size; most modern filters are minimally efficient at particle sizes <0.3 µm in diameter. Testing involves challenging the filter with an aerosol of sodium chloride particles at the most penetrating particle size, using gas flow of 30 l/min for adult filters (15 l/min for paediatric). Modern filters usually incorporate a **heat–moisture exchanger**.

Can be placed anywhere in the breathing system, although most commonly placed between the patient and the breathing system; require changing between cases. All devices increase dead space and resistance to spontaneous ventilation, and are vulnerable to blockage with fluid.

Wilkes AR (2011). Anaesthesia; 66: 31–9, 40–51

Filtration fraction. Ratio of **GFR** to renal plasma flow (RPF). As RPF falls, GFR remains fairly constant because of efferent arteriolar constriction, causing filtration fraction to rise. Normally 0.16–0.2.

Fink effect. Reduced alveolar concentration of a gas resulting from its dilution by another gas leaving the bloodstream and entering the alveoli. Analogous but opposite to the **second gas effect.** Originally described (as 'diffusion anoxia') in 1955 as the underlying cause of **hypoxaemia** seen at the end of anaesthesia, when N_2O leaving the bloodstream dilutes alveolar O_2. Since recognised as having little clinical importance, the effect of **hypoventilation** and $\dot{V}/\dot{Q}$ **mismatch** being much more important.
[Bernard Raymond Fink (1914–2000), Seattle anaesthetist]

F_IO_2. Fractional inspired concentration of O_2. By convention, expressed as a decimalised fraction, e.g. 0.21, 0.5, although commonly still expressed as a percentage.

First-pass metabolism. Metabolism of a substance once absorbed, occurring before it reaches the systemic circulation. Active metabolites may be formed. Most commonly refers to metabolism by the liver following oral administration of drugs, e.g. **propranolol, morphine, lidocaine** and **GTN** (i.e., drugs with a high hepatic **extraction ratio**). Drugs may be given by alternative routes to bypass the liver, e.g. parenterally, sublingually or rectally. May also occur in the intestinal mucosa following oral administration (e.g. **methyldopa, chlorpromazine, midazolam**), and in the bronchial mucosa following inhalation (e.g. **isoprenaline**).

Fixation error. Form of disordered situation awareness in which individuals distort available information so that it 'fits' with their notion of what is happening, rather than revise their assessment. Typically divided into: not appreciating the problem or its solution despite evidence to the contrary ('everything but that'); persisting with one diagnosis or plan despite evidence that it is wrong ('this and only this'); or continuing to believe that there is no problem despite a worsening situation ('everything is all right'). Anaesthetic examples include: repeated topping up of an epidural during labour that has ceased to function, not accepting that it might have become dislodged; giving repeated doses of sedation to an agitated patient without appreciating that the cause is urinary retention; and dealing with a worsening pulse oximeter reading by repeatedly cleaning and repositioning the probe instead of addressing the hypoxaemia. Typically, a 'fresh' practitioner can rapidly diagnose the fixation when introduced to the scene, highlighting the value of involving colleagues early when crises occur.

Flail chest. Disruption of chest wall integrity, where a portion of the thoracic cage becomes detached from the bony structure of the rest. The flail segment no longer moves outwards on inspiration, but is free to be drawn inwards by negative intrathoracic pressure; it is pushed out during expiration while the rest of the thorax contracts. Occurs in severe **chest trauma** with multiple fractures involving several **ribs** and usually accompanied by significant pulmonary contusion. May also result from surgery.

- Features:
  - **hypoventilation**, with reduced tidal volume and vital capacity. **Pendelluft** is now thought not to occur; mediastinal shift results in air entry to both lungs, although overall hypoventilation may be severe. Hypoventilation is further exacerbated by pain. Ability to cough is reduced due to mechanical impairment and pain.
  - underlying lung contusion/**atelectasis/pneumothorax** with resultant **shunt** and $\dot{V}/\dot{Q}$ **mismatch**; thought to be more important than hypoventilation.
  - associated injuries, e.g. to mediastinum, head, abdomen.
  - mediastinal shift may affect cardiac output.
- Management is as for chest trauma, i.e.:
  - O_2 administration.
  - analgesia (e.g. systemic opioids/**intercostal nerve block/epidural analgesia**).
  - treatment of hypovolaemia and associated injuries.
  - **chest drainage** if required.
  - **physiotherapy**.
  - nasogastric drainage helps prevent gastric distension.
  - if arterial blood gases are acceptable, no further treatment may be required. Improved oxygenation and chest wall splinting may be achieved by **CPAP**.
  - tracheal intubation and IPPV. May be continued until the underlying lung improves or surgical fixation of the flail segment (i.e., up to several weeks).
  - early fixation of rib fractures is preferred by some surgeons.

Vana PG, Neubauer DC, Luchette FA (2014). Am Surg; 80: 527–35

Flame ionisation detector. Device used in analysis of gas mixtures, separated, e.g. by **gas chromatography**. A potential difference is applied across a flame of hydrogen gas burning in air. Addition of organic vapour to the gas stream causes a change in current flow across the flame, the amount of change proportional to the amount of substance present. Used only to quantify the amount of a known substance, not to identify unknown ones.
See also, Gas analysis

Flammability. Ability to support combustion. Dependent on molecular structure; e.g. C–C bonds readily break down with heat and O_2 to form carbon monoxide/dioxide, whereas C–F bonds are resistant. Flammability limits refer to concentrations of a substance that will support combustion; e.g.:

- **cyclopropane:**
  - 2.5%–60% in O_2.
  - 2.5%–10% in air.
  - 1.5%–30% in **N_2O**.
- **diethyl ether:**
  - 2%–82% in O_2.
  - 2%–35% in air.
  - 1.5%–24% in N_2O.

Ranges for explosive mixtures occur within these limits, especially with high O_2 concentration. The **stoichiometric mixture** lies within the explosive range. Flammability is greater in N_2O than in O_2, because the former decomposes to produce O_2 with release of energy. Addition of water vapour reduces flammability.

Modern, non-flammable agents will ignite only at higher concentrations than occur during anaesthesia, and require much greater amounts of energy to initiate ignition (**activation energy**).
See also, Explosions and fires

Flash-point. Lowest temperature at which a saturated vapour of a liquid ignites when exposed to a flame, in the presence of one or more other gas(es).

Flecainide acetate. Class Ic **antiarrhythmic drug.** Slows impulse conduction by blocking sodium channels, thus prolonging phase 0 of the cardiac **action potential** (in both the conducting system and myocardial cells). Used for severe **VT** and extrasystoles, and **SVT**, especially those involving accessory pathways (e.g. **Wolff–Parkinson–White syndrome**). Should not be given to patients with known ischaemic or structural heart disease.

- Dosage:
  - 2 mg/kg up to 150 mg, over 10–30 min iv (with ECG monitoring).
  - by infusion: 1.5 mg/kg/h for 1 h; 0.1–0.25 mg/kg/h thereafter.
  - 100 mg orally bd for VT (50 mg for SVT) up to 300–400 mg/day.
- Side effects:
  - dizziness, visual disturbances, corneal deposits.
  - myocardial depression, **proarrhythmias.**
  - resistance to endocardial pacing.
  - increased plasma levels in hepatic/renal failure (levels should be monitored).
  - has been associated with increased risk of cardiac arrest after MI; therefore reserved for life-threatening **arrhythmias.**

Flow. Volume of **fluid** moving per unit time. Flow through a tube may be:
  - laminar: flow is smooth and without eddies. Flow velocity reduces towards the tube's sides (approaching zero at the edge); flow at the centre is greatest, at approximately twice the mean (Fig. 71a). Described by:

    laminar flow

    $$= \frac{\text{pressure gradient alone tube} \times \text{radius}^4 \times \pi}{\text{tube length} \times \text{viscosity of fluid} \times 8}$$

    (**Hagen–Poiseuille equation**).
  - turbulent (Fig. 71b): caused when the tube is unevenly shaped, or when the fluid flows through an orifice or around sharp edges. Also occurs from laminar flow when flow velocity is high, exceeding the **critical velocity. Reynolds' number** describes the relationship between tube and fluid characteristics and velocity at which turbulent flow occurs. Turbulent flow is proportional to:
    - radius^2.
    - $\sqrt{\text{pressure gradient}}$.
    - 1/length.
    - 1/density of fluid.

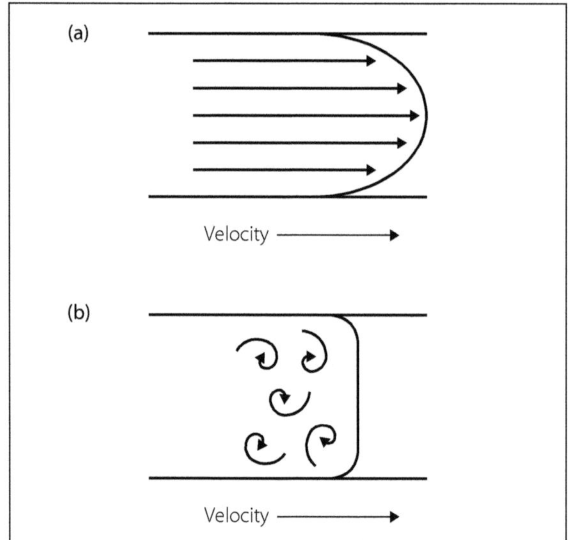

Fig. 71 Flow profiles: (a) laminar with parabolic profile; (b) turbulent with flat profile

Flow in the airways and blood vessels is a mixture of laminar and turbulent, but behaves approximately according to the above principles.
- Measurement:
  - gas: **flowmeters.**
  - liquid: **dilution techniques, electromagnetic flow measurement, Fick principle.** Similar flowmeters to those used for gases may also be used.
  - measurement of volume over a certain time.

Flow-directed balloon-tipped pulmonary artery catheters, *see Pulmonary artery catheterisation*

Flow generators, *see Ventilators*

Flowmeters. Devices for measuring **flow**, usually referring to **gas flow**, e.g. from cylinders and anaesthetic machines, or in breathing systems.
- May be:
  - constant orifice, variable pressure. Because flow through an orifice is proportional to the pressure difference across it, flow may be deduced by measuring the pressure difference across a fixed orifice. In the first two examples, only the downstream pressure is measured, because the pressure upstream of the orifice is constant:
    - simple pressure gauge downstream from the outlet of an O_2 cylinder. The gauge may be calibrated directly for flow, e.g. l/min.
    - water depression flowmeter. The pressure is measured with a simple water manometer.
    - **pneumotachograph.** Pressure is measured electronically using transducers.
  - constant pressure, variable orifice. If the pressure across a variable orifice remains constant, the size of the orifice depends on the gas flow. Examples:
    - **rotameter**, simple ball flowmeter and dry bobbin flowmeter. The size of the orifice is determined by the height of the bobbin in its tube: the greater the height, the larger the orifice. In the rotameter and ball flowmeter, the tube is of tapered bore, being wider at the top than at the bottom. The dry bobbin flowmeter tube is of uniform diameter, with small holes arranged longitudinally. The variability of the effective orifice size is provided by the number of holes below the bobbin, i.e., the bobbin's height.
    - Heidbrink flowmeter. The 'bobbin' is extended vertically to form a rod; its bottom end sits in a tapered tube while its top end lies opposite a linear scale above the tapered part. It functions in a similar way to the rotameter, but without rotating.
    - **peak-flow meters.**
  - variable pressure, variable orifice. In the watersight flowmeter, gas passes through a tube with holes along its length, immersed into water. At low gas flows, gas bubbles from the upper holes only; at higher flow rates, from the lower holes as well. The holes are marked with according flow rates. Orifice variability results from the different number of holes

through which gas may pass; pressure variability arises because pressure is higher at greater depth of water.
- constant pressure, constant orifice. Bubble flowmeters may be used for calibration at low flow rates. Gas passes along a uniform tube, carrying a thin soap film with it. Flow is deduced by measuring the velocity of the film along the tube using a timer.

- Other flowmeters include:
  - thermistor flowmeter: the cooling effect of a gas stream on a thermistor varies with flow rate.
  - ultrasonic flowmeter: turbulent eddies are formed around a rod in the gas path. The frequency of oscillation of the eddies, measured by **Doppler** probe, is proportional to flow rate. Alternatively, ultrasound beams may be projected diagonally across the gas, and transit time measured.

Flow can also be determined by measuring the volume of gas per unit time, e.g. using a **respirometer**.
[Jay A Heidbrink (1875–1957), US anaesthetist]

Flow–volume loops. Curves resulting from simultaneous measurement and plotting of air flow and lung volume during a maximal forced expiration. If **residual volume** is known, lung volume may be determined by measuring expired volume. Characteristic loops are obtained in certain conditions, although the loops obtained in practice are rarely as easily distinguishable (Fig. 72). Also useful for assessing the efficacy of bronchodilator therapy in **COPD**.

Much of the information from studying forced expiration may be obtained from flow–volume loops, e.g. forced expiratory flow rate, forced expiratory volume and peak expiratory flow rate.
Miller MR, Hankison J, Brusasco V (2005). Eur Resp J; 26: 319–38
See also, Lung function tests

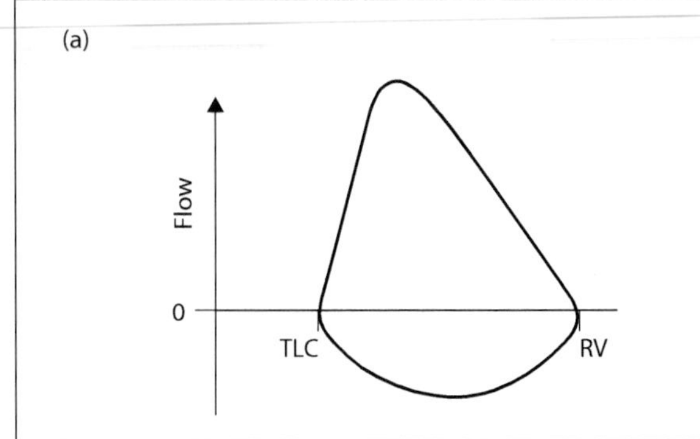

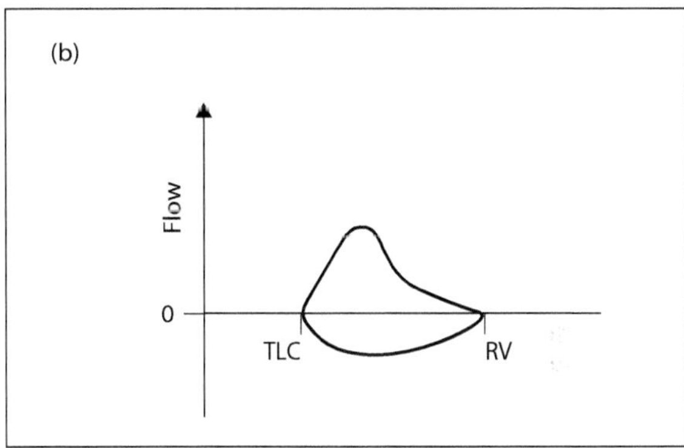

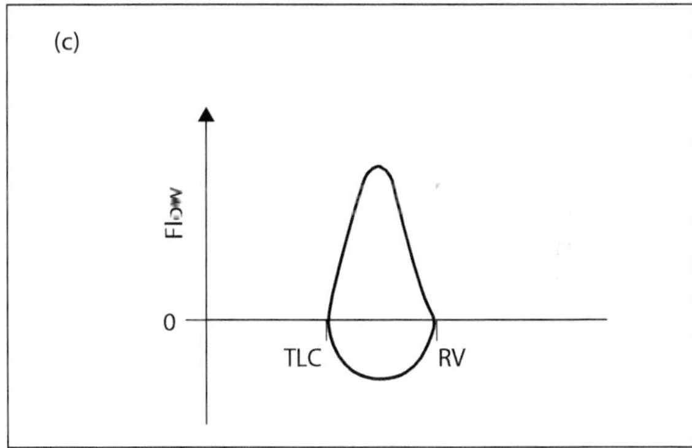

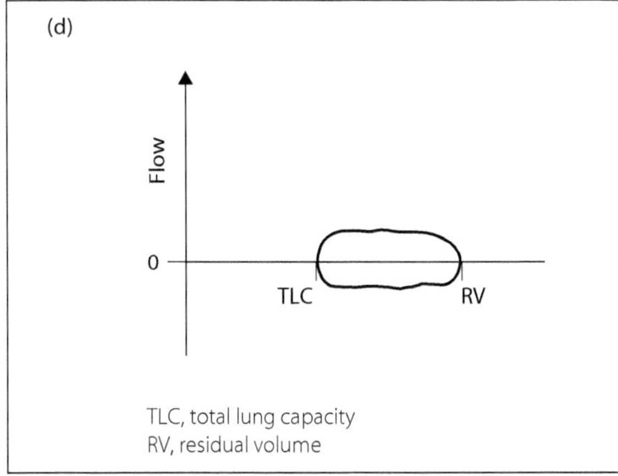

Fig. 72 Characteristic flow–volume loops: (a) normal; (b) obstructive lung disease; (c) restrictive lung disease; (d) tracheal/laryngeal obstruction

Flucloxacillin. Penicillinase-resistant **penicillin** used to treat **staphylococcal infections**. Peak levels occur within an hour of administration. 90% protein-bound; although metabolised in the liver, 50% appears unchanged in the urine.
- Dosage:
  - 250–500 mg orally/im qds.
  - 250 mg–2.0 g slowly iv qds.
- Side effects: as for **benzylpenicillin**. Acute cholestatic jaundice may occur even after stopping therapy.

Fluconazole. Triazole **antifungal drug** used to treat local and systemic candidiasis and cryptococcal infection (including meningitis), especially associated with **HIV infection**. Well absorbed orally, with peak levels within 6 h. Elimination **half-life** 30 h.
- Dosage: 50–400 mg orally/iv daily.
- Side effects: nausea, vomiting, rashes, allergic reactions, toxic epidermal necrolysis, hepatic impairment. May increase blood levels of the antihistamines terfenadine and astemizole, resulting in **prolonged Q–T syndrome** and fatal ventricular arrhythmias, including **torsade de pointes**.

Flucytosine. **Antifungal drug** used to treat systemic candidiasis and cryptococcal infections; it is a relatively weak agent and susceptible to resistance so it is often used together with **amphotericin** or **fluconazole**, with which it is synergistic.

- Dosage: 50 mg/kg qds iv over 20–40 min, usually for no more than 7 days (prolonged therapy needed for cryptococcal infection). Trough plasma levels of 25–50 mg/l (200–400 μmol/l) are optimal.
- Side effects: nausea, vomiting, diarrhoea, rashes, confusion, hepatitis, blood dyscrasias. Weekly blood counts are required in prolonged treatment.

Unlicensed tablets are available on a 'special-order' basis.

Fludrocortisone acetate. **Mineralocorticoid** used for replacement therapy in **adrenocortical insufficiency**, congenital adrenal hyperplasia and postural hypotension associated with **autonomic neuropathy**. Has similar actions to **aldosterone**; also has mild **hydrocortisone**-like actions.

- Dosage: 50–300 μg od orally.
- Side effects: hypertension, sodium and water retention, hypokalaemia. May also produce **glucocorticoid** effects.

Fluid. Form of matter that continuously deforms when subjected to a shearing force, i.e., gas or liquid. Continuous shearing force results in **flow**; resistance to flow is proportional to **viscosity**. For a Newtonian fluid (e.g. water) viscosity is constant for different shear rates and flows; for a non-Newtonian fluid (e.g. blood), it varies with shear rates and flows.

[Sir Isaac Newton (1642–1727), English scientist]

See also, Fluidics

Fluid balance. Important component of human **homeostasis**. For a normal 70-kg adult, approximate daily fluid balance comprises:

- intake:
  - 1500 ml liquid.
  - 750 ml in food.
  - 250 ml from **metabolism** within the body.

  Total therefore 2500 ml.
- output:
  - 1500 ml **urine**.
  - 100 ml in faeces.
  - 900 ml **insensible water loss**.

  Total therefore 2500 ml.

Loss in sweat is normally negligible but may exceed several litres in hot environments. Insensible losses are also increased in high temperatures. About 5% of body water is exchanged per day in adults, 15% in infants; hence the increased risk of **dehydration** in the latter.

Balance is normally regulated to maintain **ECF** volume and **osmolality**; changes are detected by **baroreceptors** and **osmoreceptors**, with resultant compensatory mechanisms:

- water intake is regulated by thirst; increased by **hypovolaemia** and **hyperosmolality**.
- cardiovascular compensation for hypovolaemia.
- urinary output is regulated by **vasopressin**, **atrial natriuretic peptide** and the **renin/angiotensin system**.

- Causes of fluid imbalance in patients presenting for anaesthesia, perioperatively and in ICU:
  - reduced intake, e.g. coma, dysphagia, nausea, fasting instructions.
  - increased intake, e.g. excessive iv administration.
  - redistribution, e.g. to **third space**.
  - reduced output, e.g. **syndrome of inappropriate antidiuretic hormone secretion**.
  - increased output, e.g. sweating, polyuria, vomiting, diarrhoea.

Perioperative fluid management is increasingly recognised as an important aspect of enhanced recovery after surgery (*see Recovery, enhanced*). Fluid overload is associated with increased morbidity (demonstrated in GIT and thoracic surgery), increased incidence of postoperative ileus and delayed hospital discharge; relative fluid restriction decreases postoperative complications. In addition, excessive dextrose administration may lead to **hyperglycaemia** and **hyponatraemia**, while excessive salt solution administration may cause peripheral and pulmonary **oedema**. Improved recovery with reduced **PONV** has been claimed following fluid administration during minor surgery compared with no fluids.

Intravenous fluid administration should be guided by the following:

- maintenance requirements: 40 ml/kg/day (1.6 ml/kg/h). Requirements are greater in **paediatric anaesthesia**.
- replacement of **blood loss** (*see Haemorrhage*).
- third-space losses: with perioperative evaporative losses, approximately 10–15 ml/kg/h during major abdominal surgery.
- other losses, e.g. nasogastric aspirate.

The aim is to achieve a well-hydrated, euvolaemic patient throughout the pre- and operative periods while ensuring the patient can eat and drink postoperatively, preferably without the need for iv infusions.

Gupta R, Gan TJ (2016). Anaesthesia; 71(suppl 1): 40–5

See also, Colloid/crystalloid controversy; Fluids, body

Fluid responsiveness. An increase in baseline **stroke volume** by 10%–15% following a 500-ml bolus of crystalloid or following a passive leg-raising (PLR) manoeuvre, i.e., a measure of a patient's response to a change in **preload** in, e.g. haemorrhage, sepsis. PLR is favoured as it avoids the potentially deleterious effects of a fluid challenge and is reversible. Although traditionally **CVP** and pulmonary capillary wedge pressure have been used to assess fluid responsiveness, they are poor predictors and have been superseded by dynamic measures such as systolic pulse and stroke volume variation, Doppler measurement of stroke volume and filling time and echocardiographic measurement of inferior vena cava calibre and distensibility.

Ansari BM, Zochios V, Falter F, Klein AA (2016). Anaesthesia; 71: 94–105

Fluid therapy, *see Intravenous fluids*

Fluidics. Technology of operating control systems by utilising flow characteristics of gases or liquids. Has been used in control mechanisms of ventilators, e.g. employing the **Coanda effect**. The direction of a jet of gas in a valve may be switched by 'signal' jets of driving gas across the main jet. Combinations of signal jets allow complex manipulation of the valve output, without moving parts.

Pneumatic spool valves may contain moving shuttles, driven by gas from either end. The valve chamber is divided into segments by seals through which the shuttle passes; the valve output depends on the lining up of ports and channels in the shuttle and valve wall. The output may be used to drive cylinders that may be driven from either end.

Fluids, body. Approximately 60% of male body weight is water; 50%–55% in females (greater proportion of fat). Total body water may be measured using a **dilution technique** with deuterium oxide (heavy water). Its main constituent compartments are **intracellular fluid** (ICF), **ECF**, **plasma** and **interstitial fluid** (Fig. 73). Approximately

Table 22 Approximate composition of body fluid compartments (mmol/l)

Compartment	Na^+	K^+	HCO_3^-	Cl^-	Ca^{2+}	Mg^{2+}	SO_4^{2-}	$HPO_4^{2-} + PO_4^{3-}$
Intracellular fluid	10	150	10	3	3	30	20	100
Interstitial fluid	140	5	30	110	5	3	1	2
Plasma	140	5	28	110	5	3	1	2

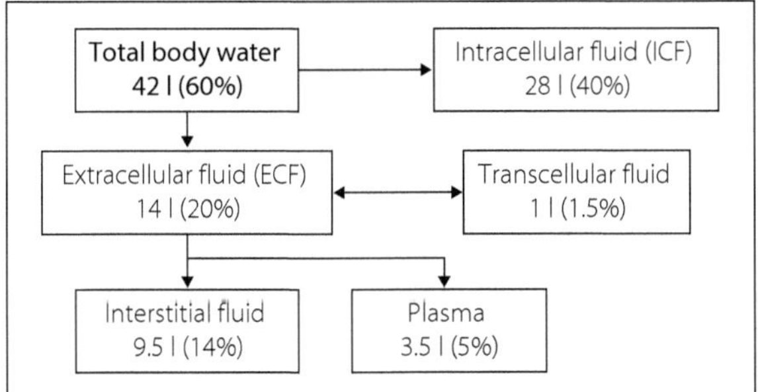

Fig. 73 Composition of body fluids, with volumes for an average 70-kg man (% body weight)

1 l is contained within the GIT and CSF (transcellular fluid).

In **neonates**, ECF exceeds 30% (but plasma is still 5%), and ICF is less than 40%. These differences are greatest in premature babies, when ECF exceeds ICF. During childhood, the adult situation slowly develops.
Composition of fluid compartments is shown in Table 22.
- Modes of movement of ions and molecules between compartments:
  - **diffusion.**
  - facilitated diffusion: carrier molecules transport substances from high to low concentrations, requiring no energy.
  - **active transport.**
  - filtration.

Movement of substances is also affected by other substances, e.g. **Donnan effect.**
Water moves across **membranes** from solutions of low concentrations to those of high concentrations (**osmosis**). Depending on their constitution, different **iv fluids** will fill certain compartments more than others.
See also, Blood volume; Fluid balance

Flumazenil. Benzodiazepine antagonist, structurally related to **midazolam** and introduced in 1987. A competitive inhibitor of benzodiazepines at the central **GABA$_A$**/benzodiazepine receptor complex. Used to reverse excessive sedation due to benzodiazepines, e.g. following attempted suicide, prolonged sedation with benzodiazepines in ICU and iatrogenic overdose. Has also been used as a diagnostic tool for delirium in **alcohol withdrawal syndromes**. Benzodiazepine metabolism is unaffected. 50% protein-bound.
- Dosage: 0.2–0.3 mg iv, repeated as necessary up to 1–2 mg. May also be given by infusion (0.1–0.4 mg/h).
- Side effects: nausea, vomiting, dizziness, headache, confusion, pulmonary oedema. Has caused excessive excitement and convulsions, especially in patients maintained on long-term benzodiazepines, e.g. for epilepsy. Because of its short **half-life** (less than 1 h), its effects may wear off with recurrence of sedation.

Fluoride ions. Nephrotoxic ions implicated in the high-output renal failure seen following **methoxyflurane** administration. Evidence for their role:
  - degree of renal impairment is proportional to plasma concentration:
    - subclinical evidence of renal impairment occurs above 50 μmol/l.
    - polyuria, decreased urinary osmolality and increased plasma sodium and osmolality occur above 80–100 μmol/l.
  - infusion of fluoride ions into rats produces similar renal effects.

Mechanism of renal damage is unclear but may involve impairment of both renal Na/K/ATPase systems and **vasopressin** action.
- Levels are highest after methoxyflurane, but may be raised after other halogenated volatile agents:
  - methoxyflurane: 50–60 μmol/l after 2.5 MAC hours; 90–120 μmol/l after 5 MAC hours.
  - **enflurane**: up to 30 μmol/l after prolonged use (over 9 h). Plasma levels are highest in obese patients. **Enzyme induction** with isoniazid is thought to increase levels.
  - **isoflurane**: under 5 μmol/l even after prolonged surgery. Levels of up to 90 μmol/l have been reported after several days' use for sedation in ICU.
  - **halothane**: minimal production of fluoride ions.
  - **sevoflurane**: up to 40 μmol/l after prolonged surgery (unaffected by obesity).
  - **desflurane**: minimal production of fluoride ions.

Fluotec vaporiser, *see Vaporisers*

Flupirtine maleate. Non-opioid, non-**NSAID**, centrally acting **analgesic drug**. Indirectly blocks **NMDA receptors** by activating potassium channels thus preventing glutamate-induced rise in intracellular calcium. Also causes muscular relaxation via enhancement of **GABA**-mediated spinal inhibition. Available in many European countries since the mid-1980s but unavailable in the UK.

Flurbiprofen. NSAID available for oral and pr administration; has been used for **postoperative analgesia**.
- Dosage: 50–100 mg 4–6-hourly up to 300 mg/day (100 mg suppositories available).
- Side effects: as for NSAIDs.

Fluroxene (Trifluoroethyl vinyl ether). Obsolete **inhalational anaesthetic agent**, introduced in 1954. The first fluorine-containing volatile agent. Explosive, possibly mutagenic, and toxic to experimental animals due to biotransformation to trifluoroethanol.

Flying squad, obstetric. Mobile team including anaesthetist, obstetrician and midwife; first suggested in 1929, and organised in Glasgow in 1933. The usual problems of obstetric anaesthesia and neonatal resuscitation are

compounded by the unfamiliar environment, limitation of facilities, requirement for portable equipment and lack of patient preparation. Commonest emergency is **post-partum haemorrhage** caused by retained placenta. Use of a flying squad has become largely obsolete in the UK as the number of home deliveries has decreased and emphasis has shifted towards rapid transfer of sick patients to hospital for treatment.
See also, Cardiopulmonary resuscitation, neonatal; Obstetric analgesia and anaesthesia

Foetal, *see Fetal*

Fomepizole (4-Methylpyrazole). Competitive inhibitor of alcohol dehydrogenase, available on a named-patient basis for methanol or ethylene glycol poisoning. A loading dose of 15 mg/kg iv over 30 min is followed by 10 mg/kg every 12 h for four doses, then 15 mg/kg every 12 h until methanol or ethylene glycol concentrations are <4–6 mmol/l, and the patient is asymptomatic with normal pH. Undergoes hepatic metabolism and excreted in the urine.
Brent J (2009). N Engl J Med; 360: 2216–23
See also, Alcohol poisoning

Fondaparinux sodium. Synthetic **factor Xa inhibitor**; sulfated pentasaccharide derived from the factor Xa-binding moiety of unfractionated **heparin**. Licensed for treatment of **acute coronary syndromes** and prophylaxis and treatment of venous thromboembolism in adults.

- Dosage:
  - treatment of unstable angina/non-S–T segment elevation MI and **DVT** prophylaxis in immobilised patients: 2.5 mg sc od (in surgical patients, first dose 6 h after skin closure).
  - treatment of DVT and **PE**: 5, 7.5 or 10 mg sc od (for body weight <50 kg, 50–100 kg and >100 kg, respectively) until oral anticoagulation established.
  - treatment of S–T segment elevation MI: 2.5 mg iv, followed by 2.5 mg sc od for 8 days or until hospital discharge or **percutaneous coronary intervention**.
- Side effects: haemorrhage, purpura, thrombocytopenia, GIT upset, rash.

Fondation Européenne d'Enseignement en Anaesthésiologie (Foundation for European Education in Anaesthesiology; FEEA). Organisation founded in 1986 (with financial support from the European Union) to provide continuous medical education in anaesthesiology throughout Europe. Acts in agreement with national anaesthetic societies and organises courses throughout Europe, South America, Africa and Asia.

Food and Drug Administration (FDA). US organisation, involved in testing new drugs and reviewing test results. Also controls imports, and regulates foods and cosmetics. Companies must apply to the FDA before initiating **clinical trials**. Evolved after World War II from the 1938 Food, Drug and Cosmetics Act, restricting labelling and advertising of drugs; amended in 1968 to require that drugs be shown to be efficacious as well as safe. Thus enforces laws enacted by US Congress. Previously, the Pure Food and Drugs Act of 1906 and subsequent amendments attempted to prevent improper labelling and fraudulent claims by manufacturers.
Borchers AT, Hagie F, Keen CL, Gershwin ME (2007). Clin Ther; 29: 1–16
See also, Medicines and Healthcare products Regulatory Agency

Foot, nerve blocks, *see Ankle, nerve blocks; Digital nerve block*

Force. That which changes a body's shape or state of motion. Derived SI **unit** of force is the **newton**; in base units this is equivalent to m·kg/s^2.

Forced diuresis. Method of increasing renal excretion of certain drugs using iv fluids or **diuretics** to increase urinary volume. Sometimes used in **poisoning and overdoses**. Further drug removal is achieved by manipulating urinary pH, thereby 'trapping' the ionised fraction of the drug and preventing its diffusion back into the bloodstream, because charged molecules diffuse poorly across biological membranes.

- Forced alkaline diuresis:
  - used in poisoning with acid drugs, e.g. **salicylates** and barbiturates.
  - 500 ml/h of the following fluids are administered in rotation:
    - 500 ml 1.26% sodium bicarbonate.
    - 500 ml 5% dextrose.
    - 500 ml 0.9% saline.
  - CVP, urine output and pH, blood gases and plasma electrolytes (especially potassium) must be closely monitored. Infusion rate is reduced in the elderly.
- Forced acid diuresis:
  - used in poisoning with alkaline drugs, e.g. **amfetamines**, phencyclidines.
  - 1000 ml/h of the following fluids are administered in rotation:
    - 500 ml 5% dextrose + 1.5 g ammonium chloride.
    - 500 ml 5% dextrose.
    - 500 ml 0.9% saline.
  - monitoring as above.

Severe metabolic upset and circulatory overload may occur. The technique is rarely used now, since it has been superseded by **haemodialysis** and **haemofiltration**.

Forced expiration. Means of investigating lung function, from which may be measured: **forced expiratory flow rate** ($FEF_{25\%-75\%}$), **FEV**, **FVC** and **peak expiratory flow rate**. Other suggested measurements exclude the first 200 ml of expiration, or analyse the flow rate at 50% of vital capacity.

Flow–volume loops and data from **spirometers** (e.g. the Vitalograph) may be analysed (Fig. 74). Repetition following bronchodilator therapy may indicate the extent of reversible airway obstruction.

At lung volumes of up to 60% of vital capacity, maximal expiratory flow rate is independent of effort; increasing effort raises intrathoracic pressure, increasing the pressure difference across the airways and leading to airway collapse.
Miller MR, Hankison J, Brusasco V (2005). Eur Resp J; 26: 319–38
See also, Lung function tests

Forced expiratory flow rate ($FEF_{25\%-75\%}$). Average flow rate measured at between 25% and 75% of forced maximal expired volume (Fig. 74). Highly dependent on **FVC** and level of expiratory effort, it has a wider spread of normal values.

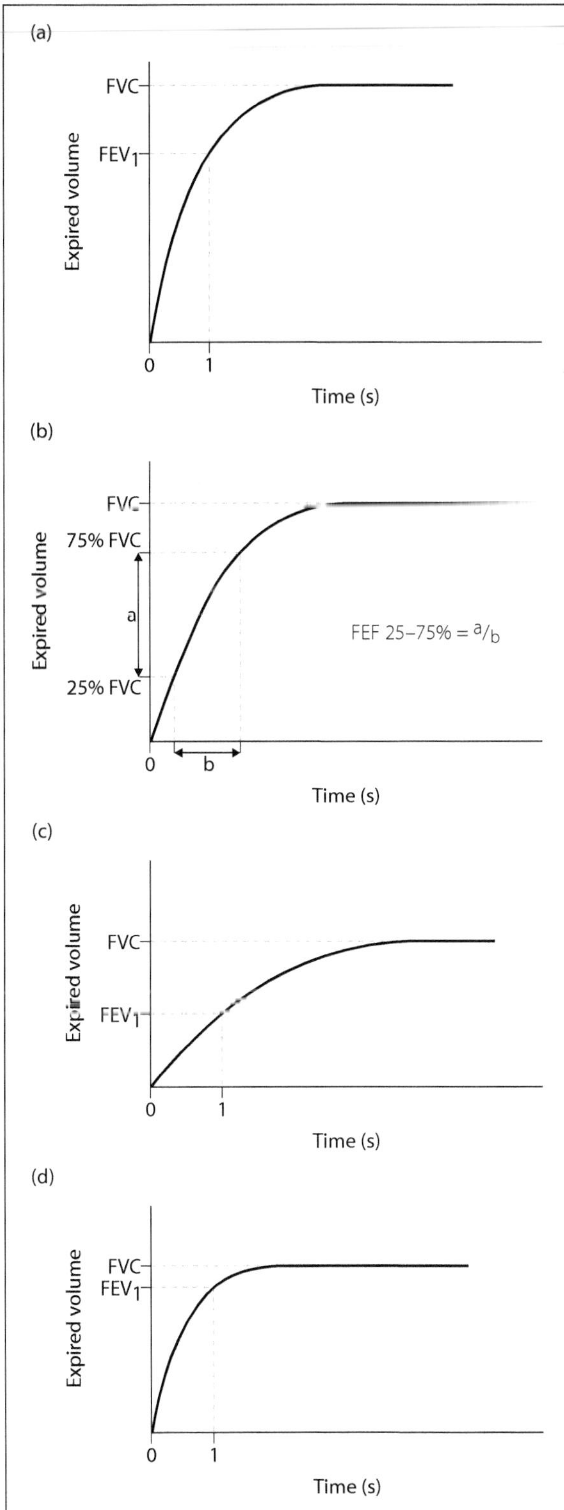

Fig. 74 Typical forced expiratory patterns: (a) normal; (b) showing calculation of FEF (25%–75%); (c) obstructive lung disease; (d) restrictive lung disease

See also, Forced expiration; Lung function tests; Peak expiratory flow rate

Forced expiratory volume (FEV). Volume of gas forcibly exhaled from full inspiration, in a set period of time (normally 1 s; the volume is then called FEV_1). Normally 80% of **FVC**, which may be measured at the same time using a **spirometer**. Reduced in obstructive lung disease, as is the FEV_1/FVC ratio. In restrictive disease, FEV_1 may be normal, but FVC is reduced. FEV_6 (forced expiratory volume in 6 s) has been used a surrogate measure of FVC.

Easier and more comfortable to measure than **maximal voluntary ventilation.**

See also, Forced expiration; Lung function tests

Forced vital capacity (FVC). **Vital capacity** measured when expiration is forced. Closure of some airways may occur when intrathoracic pressure is high, causing air-trapping. FVC thus may be less than 'true' vital capacity. Reduced in restrictive disease, the supine position, the elderly, muscle weakness, abdominal swelling, pain, and when premature airway closing occurs during forced expiration, e.g. emphysema.

Miller MR, Hankison J, Brusasco V (2005). Eur Resp J; 26: 319–38

See also, Forced expiration; Lung function tests; Lung volumes

Forceps. Many varieties may be used by anaesthetists, for example (Fig. 75):

- **Magill** forceps: introduced in 1920 to assist placement of gum-elastic bougies for insufflation anaesthesia. Used to guide tracheal tubes into the larynx, or nasogastric tubes into the oesophagus, under direct vision. May damage the tracheal tube cuff if grasped. Also used to place pharyngeal packs or to remove foreign bodies. The operator's hand is held out of the line of vision by the angled handles. Adult and paediatric sizes are available; disposable, single-use versions are normally used. Many modifications have been described.
- Krause forceps: used to hold local anaesthetic-soaked pledgets in the piriform fossae for blocking the superior laryngeal nerves for awake intubation. They bear a spring catch and spiked jaws.
- several tongue forceps exist; formerly used to pull the tongue forward to relieve airway obstruction, but now more likely to be used for fixing tubing and drapes.

[Herman Krause (1848–1921), German laryngologist; Berkley GA Moynihan (1865–1936), English surgeon]

See also, Mouth gags

Foreign body, inhaled. Leading cause of accidental death in children less than 4 years old. May obstruct upper or lower airways. Should be considered in any child with **stridor** or persistent cough and chest infections. Diagnosis is based on history, clinical findings and imaging (although only 11% of aspirated objects are radio-opaque). Most small objects lodge in the right main bronchus, because of its more vertical angle of origin and greater width. Organic matter (e.g. peanuts) may cause intense bronchial inflammatory reactions within a few hours, with oedema and possibly bronchial obstruction. **Bronchiectasis** may be a late complication. Other features may include:

- distal **atelectasis.**
- distal air-trapping if the object acts as a ball-valve. CXR at end-expiration may reveal unilateral hyperinflation.
- features of **airway obstruction.**
- infection.

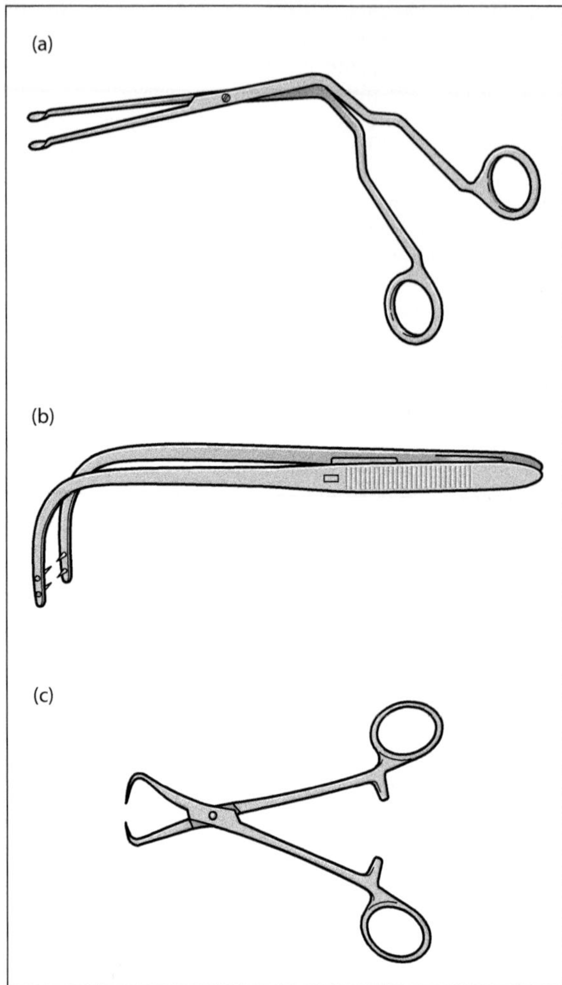

Fig. 75 Types of forceps used in anaesthesia: (a) Magill; (b) Krause; (c) Moynihan tongue forceps

- Removal is via **bronchoscopy** (rigid most commonly). Anaesthetic management:
  - preoperatively:
    - assessment for: type of object aspirated; timing of aspiration; and severity of airway obstruction. Preoperative fasting is appropriate if possible.
    - **premedication** with **atropine**. Anxiolytic drugs may be helpful.
  - perioperatively:
    - an experienced anaesthetist's presence is mandatory, as is good communication with the surgeon.
    - classic technique is inhalational induction of anaesthesia; **sevoflurane** is usually the modern drug of choice (replacing **halothane**). **N_2O** is avoided in case of distal air-trapping, and to raise F_IO_2. Induction may be slow.
    - cautious intravenous induction while attempting to maintain spontaneous ventilation is an alternative.
    - **lidocaine** spray to the vocal cords may reduce risk of perioperative **laryngospasm.**
    - intraoperatively, both spontaneous and controlled ventilation can be used, although IPPV is often avoided because of the risk of blowing the object distally. Adequate depth of anaesthesia and oxygenation may be difficult to maintain with an inhalational agent and spontaneous ventilation, without excessive hypercapnia. **TIVA** (e.g. with **remifentanil** and **propofol**) may provide more reliable and constant depth of anaesthesia, and can be titrated to allow spontaneous ventilation.
  - postoperatively:
    - close monitoring is required in case of bronchospasm or laryngospasm.
    - humidified O_2 administration by mask.

Major complications occur in 1% of cases, and include cardiorespiratory arrest (most commonly due to hypoxaemia), bronchial rupture, pneumothorax or pneumomediastinum, laryngeal oedema and failed bronchoscopy requiring thoracotomy.

Fidowski CD, Zheng H, Firth PG (2010). Anesth Analg; 111: 1016–25

Forward failure, *see Cardiac failure*

Foscarnet sodium. **Antiviral drug**, reserved for treatment of **cytomegalovirus** retinitis in AIDS (when **ganciclovir** is contraindicated) or for herpes simplex virus infections that are unresponsive to **aciclovir.**

- Dosage: 60 mg/kg iv tds, reduced to 60 mg/kg od after 2–3 weeks. For resistant herpes simplex virus infections, 40 mg/kg iv tds for 2–3 weeks.
- Side effects: nausea, renal failure, GIT upset, hypocalcaemia, convulsions, paraesthesiae, genital ulceration.

Fosphenytoin sodium. Water-soluble **prodrug**, completely converted to **phenytoin** after parenteral administration, with a conversion **half-life** of 15 min. Used to treat acute partial and generalised tonic–clonic seizures, especially **status epilepticus** and seizures associated with **neurosurgery** or **head injury**. 1.5 mg of fosphenytoin is equivalent to 1 mg of phenytoin; should be prescribed in terms of phenytoin equivalent (PEq). Can be administered iv or im with good absorption. Following its administration, monitoring of phenytoin levels is not recommended until conversion to phenytoin is complete (i.e., within 2 h after iv infusion and 4 h after im injection).

- Dosage:
  - status epilepticus: 20 mg (PEq)/kg followed by 50–100 mg (PEq)/min.
  - neurosurgery/head injury: 10–15 mg (PEq)/kg followed by 50–100 mg (PEq)/min.
- Side effects: paraesthesia, hypotension, nystagmus, ataxia, skin reactions, pruritus. Severe hypotension and arrhythmias, including heart block, VF and asystole have been described following its use; monitoring of ECG, BP, pulse rate and respiratory function is recommended for 30 min after the end of the infusion.

Fospropofol. Water-soluble phosphorylated **prodrug** of **propofol**; converted to the latter by plasma alkaline phosphatases within a few minutes of iv injection. Licensed in the USA for **sedation** in adults during endoscopic procedures (but not for general anaesthesia). Presented as a clear, colourless solution of 3.5% concentration. Initial iv bolus dose is 6.5 mg/kg followed by supplemental doses of 1.6 mg/kg titrated to effect. Dose is modified in patients >65 years, with **ASA physical status** >3 and weight >90 kg. Onset of action and recovery are slower than with propofol. Does not cause pain on injection but frequently (>50% incidence) causes unpleasant perineal paraesthesia (e.g. burning, stinging) and pruritus. Other adverse effects (e.g. hypotension, respiratory depression) are as for propofol.

Table 23 FOUR coma score

Activity	*Best response*	*Score*
Eye response	Eyelids open or opened, tracking or blinking to command	4
	Eyelids open but not tracking	3
	Eyelids closed but open to loud voice	2
	Eyelids closed but open to pain	1
	Eyelids remain closed with pain	0
Motor response	Thumbs-up, fist or peace sign to command	4
	Localising to pain	3
	Flexion response to pain	2
	Extensor posturing	1
	No response or generalised myoclonic status epilepticus	0
Brainstem reflexes	Pupillary and corneal reflexes present	4
	One pupil dilated and fixed	3
	Pupillary *or* corneal reflexes absent	2
	Pupillary *and* corneal reflexes absent	1
	Absent pupillary, corneal and cough reflexes	0
Respiration	Not intubated, regular breathing pattern	4
	Not intubated, Cheyne-Stokes respiration	3
	Not intubated, irregular breathing pattern	2
	Breathes above ventilator rate	1
	Breathes at ventilator rate or apnoea	0

FOUR score (Full Outline of Unresponsiveness score). **Coma scale** devised in 2005. Unlike the **Glasgow coma scale**, it does not rely on the patient's verbal response and is therefore more appropriate for assessing patients whose tracheas are intubated. Four activities (eye response, motor response, brainstem reflexes and respiration) are assessed and a maximum of 16 points may be scored (Table 23). Studies have shown good inter-rater reliability and comparability with the Glasgow coma scale in predicting outcome after **TBI**, **cardiac arrest** and medical **emergency** admissions.

Bruno MA, Ledoux D, Lambermont B, et al (2011). Neurocrit Care; 15: 447–53

Fourier analysis. Mathematical breakdown of **waveforms** into simple sine wave constituents. Any complex waveform consists of sine waves of different frequencies: the slowest (fundamental) frequency and **harmonics** thereof. Used in analysis and reconstruction of waveforms, e.g. transmission of electrical signals. The higher the frequencies analysed, the more accurate the reproduction.

[Baron Jean-Baptiste Fourier (1768–1830), French mathematician]

Fournier's gangrene. *see Necrotising fasciitis*

Fowler's method (Single-breath nitrogen washout). Method of investigation of **lung volumes**, described in 1948. The subject breathes air normally, and takes a maximal breath of O_2 (i.e., to **vital capacity**) from the end of normal expiration (i.e., **FRC**). Exhaled nitrogen concentration is measured during maximal slow expiration (i.e., to **residual volume**), and plotted against volume of expired gas. A rapid-response nitrogen meter is required.

- Four phases are described (Fig. 76):
  - phase 1: O_2 from the conducting airways (anatomical **dead space**), containing no nitrogen.
  - phase 2: mixture of dead-space gas and alveolar gas.

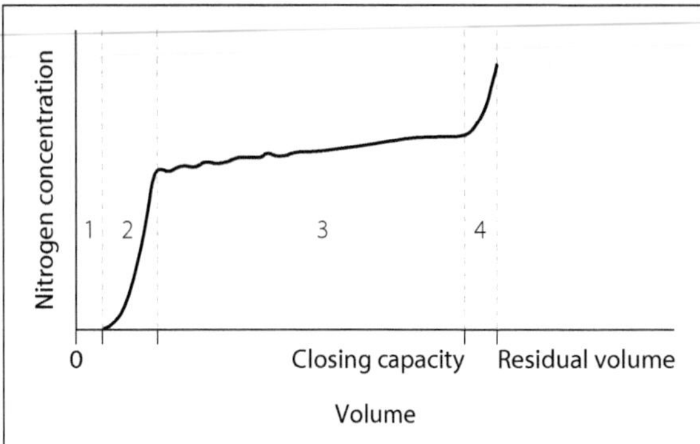

Fig. 76 Fowler's method of estimating anatomical dead space and closing capacity (*see text*)

  - phase 3: alveolar gas, containing the nitrogen present in the alveoli before the O_2 breath started. There is a slight upward slope normally, increased in lung disease.
  - phase 4: at **closing capacity**, lower alveoli and airways collapse; thus the exhaled gas comes from upper airways only. At the onset of the O_2 inspiration, the upper airways were already considerably expanded (with nitrogen-containing air) compared with lower ones, because most ventilation is of upper lung regions at normal tidal volume. Most of the inspired O_2 therefore entered the lower alveoli, because they started off smaller. When they collapse, nitrogen-rich gas from the upper alveoli is exhaled, giving rise to phase 4.

Anatomical dead space is measured to the mid-point of phase 2.

CO_2 measurement may be used in a similar way, using **capnography**.

[Ward S Fowler, US physiologist]

Fractional shortening, *see Left ventricular fractional shortening*

Fractured neck of femur. The most common serious injury affecting the elderly, with ~70 000 fractures per year in the UK; represents a major burden in terms of cost and use of beds and other resources. Addressed by increasing attempts to prevent falls, and to co-ordinate and standardise treatment when fractures occur. The main problems relate to the underlying health of the population at risk, the associated physiological disruption following injury, and general challenges of surgery in the elderly population (*see Elderly, anaesthesia for*).

- Fractures may be (see Fig. 77):
  - intracapsular: ~50% of fractures. Typically associated with little local blood loss because of the relatively poor blood supply and tamponade within the capsule. Treated by internal fixation with hip screw(s) if undisplaced, and hemiarthroplasty (total arthroplasty in younger patients) if displaced.
  - extracapsular (trochanteric or subtrochanteric): typically associated with more blood loss (e.g. 500–1500 ml depending on the size and number of bone fragments). Treated by screws, or intramedullary femoral nail if subtrochanteric.
- National audits have revealed considerable variation in management, at all stages of the patient's journey, from admission through to discharge. Best practice is considered to include:

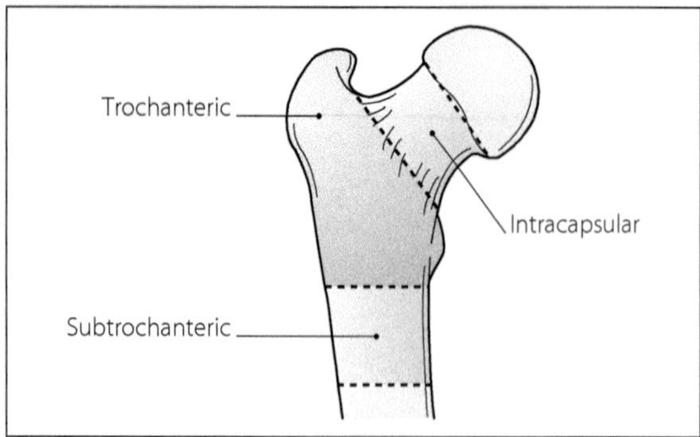

Fig. 77 Types of fractured neck of femur

- surgery within 1–2 days of admission.
- immediate assessment and management of pain with or without use of early nerve block (usually **fascia iliaca block**).
- appropriately senior medical/orthogeriatric input into **preoperative assessment** and management, and postoperative care.
- use of dedicated **trauma** lists, staffed by appropriately senior anaesthetic and surgical staff.
- use of **spinal anaesthesia** is strongly recommended over general anaesthesia by several authorities, but there is no clear evidence of definite benefit because randomised trials are few, and those that do exist are small. The advantages of a standardised approach have been highlighted as possibly being more important, whatever the technique used.
- careful attention to **monitoring** and maintaining intraoperative blood pressure, with both general and spinal anaesthesia (for which small doses may be associated with less hypotension); invasive monitoring may be indicated depending on the patient's condition and stability.
- awareness of the risk of **bone cement implantation syndrome**.
- attention to **postoperative analgesia**, with use of intraoperative nerve blocks and minimal use of long-acting opioids if possible.
- early postoperative mobilisation and rehabilitation.

Components of enhanced recovery have been developed into specific 'integrated care pathways' for fractured neck of femur, which incorporate the above. Total length of hospital stay in the UK is ~20 days, with 30-day mortality ~8%. Up to a third of patients die within the year after injury.

Association of Anaesthetists of Great Britain and Ireland (2012). Anaesthesia; 67: 85–98

Frankenhauser's plexus block, *see Paracervical block*

FRC, *see Functional residual capacity*

FRCA examination (Fellowship of the Royal College of Anaesthetists). Predated by the **FFARCS examination** (1953–1989) and the FCAnaes examination (1989–1992). Since 1985 (as the FFARCS examination) it consisted of three parts: I, relating to the fundamentals of clinical anaesthesia; II, relating to the basic sciences; III, relating to the practice of anaesthesia as a whole. Replaced in 1996 by a two-part examination: the Primary, relating to basic sciences and clinical safety; and the Final, relating to applied basic sciences and the practice of anaesthesia/intensive care. Pass rates have fluctuated over the years but are currently in the order of 60%–70% for each part.

Free radicals. Atoms or molecules with unpaired electrons, produced as intermediaries during certain biological reactions. For example, the reduction of molecular O_2 to oxide ions produces oxygen-derived free radicals including superoxide ($O\bullet_2^-$), hydroxyl (OH•) and hydroperoxy ($HO\bullet_2$) radicals, the latter two being particularly reactive.

Involved in normal phagocyte function and host defence; released into phagosomes to destroy bacteria. May also be produced by radiation and certain chemicals, and increased production has been implicated in many disease processes, e.g. pulmonary **O_2 toxicity**, **halothane hepatitis**, **ALI**, **paracetamol poisoning**, **burns**, carcinogenesis and **bowel ischaemia**. Defence mechanisms against normal free radical formation may be overwhelmed, resulting in oxidation of tissue components. Reactions with free radicals may liberate further free radicals.

Defence mechanisms include the enzymes superoxide dismutase (SOD) and catalase, and antioxidants (free radical scavengers), e.g. ***N*-Acetylcysteine**, glutathione and vitamin E. Increasing these substances indirectly, or administering them directly, reduces tissue injury in some experimental models, but extrapolation to clinical use is unclear.

Free water clearance, *see Clearance, free water*

Freud, Sigmund (1856–1939). Austrian neurologist and psychiatrist, the inventor of psychoanalysis. Postulated that **cocaine** might be a treatment for morphine addiction, and a stimulant for psychoneurotic patients. Investigated the drug with his friend **Koller**, who introduced it as the first local anaesthetic drug. Fled from Vienna to London in 1938 to escape the Nazis.

Friedreich's ataxia. Hereditary (autosomal recessive) condition consisting of progressive degeneration of spinocerebellar and pyramidal tracts and dorsal root ganglia, mainly affecting the legs. Onset is in childhood or teens.

- Features:
  - upper **motor neurone** weakness, with upgoing plantar reflexes (if present).
  - ataxia, dysarthria and nystagmus.
  - impaired joint position, vibration and touch sense. Reflexes may be absent.
  - **kyphoscoliosis** and pes cavus.
  - **diabetes mellitus** occurs in 20% of patients.
  - **cardiomyopathy** in over 50% of patients, with risk of **cardiac failure** and **arrhythmias**.
- Anaesthetic precautions:
  - **preoperative assessment** of neurological, cardiovascular and respiratory systems.
    - cautious use of **neuromuscular blocking drugs**.
    - risk of respiratory failure postoperatively; physiotherapy, O_2 therapy and adequate analgesia are required.

[Nikolaus Friedreich (1825–1882), German neurologist]

Frontal nerve block, *see Ophthalmic nerve blocks*

Frusemide, *see Furosemide*

Fuel cell, *see Oxygen measurement*

Fuller's earth. Soft, claylike substance containing silica and clay minerals; found naturally in many parts of the world. Used for pressing and cleaning cloths and fleeces ('fulling') and in the purification of oils. Used as an adsorbent in **paraquat poisoning**.

Functional imaging. The study of changes in cerebral haemodynamic and metabolic status. Techniques include **positron emission tomography**, which provides maps of regional blood flow and oxygenation; functional **MRI**, which produces high-resolution oxygenation maps; and **near infrared spectroscopy**, which provides a continuous measure of tissue oxygenation.

Functional residual capacity (FRC). **Lung volume**, equivalent to the volume of gas present in the lung after a normal expiration (the sum of **residual volume** and **expiratory reserve volume**). Normally 2.5–3.0 l for an average male.

- Measurement:
  - helium dilution: breathing of air with a known concentration of helium from a **spirometer**, starting from the end of normal expiration. CO_2 is absorbed using soda lime, and O_2 replaced as it is used. The helium distributes between spirometer, tubing and the subject's lungs, with minimal uptake by the bloodstream. After equilibrium is reached, the new concentration of helium is measured:

    total amount of helium in the system
    = initial concentration × volume of apparatus
    = new concentration × volume of (apparatus + lungs)
  - **nitrogen washout**: the subject breathes 100% O_2 from end of normal expiration, and total volume of expired gas over several minutes is analysed for nitrogen content. This amount of nitrogen was originally contained in the FRC to give a concentration of 79%; thus FRC may be calculated.
  - **body plethysmograph.**

  The helium dilution and nitrogen washout techniques do not include collapsed portions of lung, or those with poor air entry (if not enough time is allowed for equilibration). Measurements using the body plethysmograph include these areas, which may not participate in gas exchange. Comparison of the tests may indicate the degree of airway collapse/hypoventilation.
- FRC is important because **hypoxaemia** may result if it is reduced:
  - if **closing capacity** (CC) exceeds FRC, airway closure occurs with quiet breathing, causing $\dot{V}/\dot{Q}$ **mismatch.** Hypoxaemia of old age is thought to result from this, because CC rises with age.
  - FRC serves as an O_2 reserve; thus a reduced FRC holds less O_2, e.g. if airway obstruction occurs. The FRC O_2 store helps prevent large swings in arterial PO_2 during respiration.

  Reduced FRC may also reduce lung **compliance** and increase **pulmonary vascular resistance.**
- Reduced by:
  - supine position.
  - **obesity.**
  - **pregnancy.**
  - anaesthesia, even with IPPV (thought to involve decreased muscle tone and shift of thoracic and peripheral blood to the abdomen).
  - restrictive lung disease, e.g. **pulmonary fibrosis**; it may also be reduced in **pulmonary oedema**, infection, **atelectasis** and **ALI.**
- Increased by:
  - **PEEP** and **CPAP.**
  - increased airway resistance, e.g. **asthma.**
  - **exercise** due to sustained inspiratory muscle tone.

Fungal infection in the ICU. The incidence of **nosocomial infection** involving fungi is increasing in ICU practice, largely due to the increasing population with **immunodeficiency** (either present before the presenting illness or acquired during it) and the increasing use of antibacterial drugs.

- Specific risk factors:
  - high risk: neutropenia, allogenic stem cell transplant, haematological malignancy.
  - medium risk: **corticosteroid** treatment, **bone marrow transplantation**, **COPD**, **cystic fibrosis**, **HIV**, liver disease.
  - lower risk: solid organ **transplantation**, **diabetes mellitus**, prolonged ICU stay, **malnutrition**, **burns**, intravascular and urinary catheters.

Diagnosis of invasive (systemic) fungal infection is notoriously difficult and requires a high degree of suspicion as symptoms are non-specific; these include pyrexia, tachycardia and end-organ damage (e.g. **endocarditis**, hypoxaemia, confusion). Diagnostic techniques include microscopy and culture of sputum, urine and other body fluids, antigen testing on blood or CSF and assays for fungal cell wall components (e.g. glucan, mannan). Liaison with microbiologists is essential.

- Fungal organisms seen in ICU include:
  - candida species (especially *Candida albicans*): responsible for 10% of ICU bloodstream infections in the UK, and the third most commonly isolated bloodstream pathogen. Mortality is up to 40%. Other non-albicans species (e.g. *Candida glabrata* and *Candida krusei*) are seen in different geographical areas and are associated with worse outcomes; their incidence seems to be increasing, possibly due to increased resistance to fluconazole. Candidaemia often occurs following colonisation of urinary and intravascular catheters and may result in endocarditis and retinitis. Treatment consists of early removal of indwelling devices and **antifungal drug** treatment (fluconazole as first-line therapy, **amphotericin** for drug-resistant candida species).
  - aspergillus infection: normally confined to the lungs and results in a range of conditions from a simple fungal ball (aspergilloma) to cavitating and necrotising lung damage. Most common species is *Aspergillus fumigatus*. Uncommonly, cerebral involvement may occur following haematogenous spread or direct spread through nasal sinuses. Treatment is with **voriconazole** or amphotericin.
  - cryptococcus infection: seen in patients with **HIV infection** and is typically respiratory (pneumonia, pulmonary infiltrates, effusions, hilar lymphadenopathy) and/or meningoencephalitis, often with non-specific symptoms (e.g. headache, cranial nerve palsies, hydrocephalus, coma, etc.). Common species include *Cryptococcus neoformans* and *Cryptococcus gattii*. Treatment consists of amphotericin and **flucytosine** followed by fluconazole.
  - histoplasmosis: primarily a respiratory disease caused by *Histoplasma capsulatum* (present in soil and bird faeces). Causes non-specific respiratory symptoms that can mimic **TB.** Spread from the lungs may cause mediastinitis and subsequent fibrosis. Disseminated histoplasmosis is seen in immunocompromised

individuals (especially with HIV) and may affect any organ but especially the heart (endocarditis) and CNS (causing headache, visual and gait disturbance, confusion, seizures, coma, etc.). Treatment is with **itraconazole** or amphotericin.
- **pneumocystis pneumonia**.
- others, e.g. zygomycosis, blastomyces, coccidioides: occur sporadically and in endemic areas.

De Pascale G, Tumbarello M (2015). Curr Opin Crit Care; 21: 421–9

Furosemide (Frusemide). Loop **diuretic**, derived from sulfonamides. Decreases renal sodium and water reabsorption, with potassium loss. IV injection causes vasodilatation, with diuresis within 30 min.
- Dosage:
  - depends on renal function and response: 5–10 mg may cause considerable diuresis given orally or iv (less than 4 mg/min) to healthy patients. Up to 500 mg may be given in severe renal impairment.
  - suitable starting dose in fluid retention or cardiac failure: 0.5–1.0 mg/kg.
  - often given as an infusion, e.g. on ICU: 1–4 mg/h, although evidence suggests that **renal failure** is not prevented by this strategy.
- Side effects:
  - ototoxicity, especially after rapid iv injection.
  - **hypokalaemia**.
  - raised creatinine, urea and uric acid.
  - rash, thrombocytopenia and leucopenia rarely.

Fusidic acid (Sodium fusidate). Steroidal **antibacterial drug**, chemically related to the **cephalosporins**. Used to treat **penicillin**-resistant **staphylococcal infections**, especially endocarditis and osteomyelitis (achieves high levels in bone). Well absorbed from the GIT and metabolised in the liver to inactive metabolites. **Half-life** 5–6 h; 98% protein-bound.
- Dosage: 0.5–1.0 g orally or iv tds.
- Side effects include nausea, vomiting, rashes, jaundice (with high doses).

Fuzzy logic. Method of describing and controlling systems in which various qualities are described in terms of degrees, rather than absolutes, e.g. varying shades of grey instead of merely black and white. Allows finer control than yes/no systems because, even if the latter are made more discerning by defining many divisions (e.g. black, very dark grey, dark grey, medium grey), there will always be a 'step' between adjacent categories. In fuzzy logic, each division (or shade) overlaps its neighbours, and thus any point may be defined according to the extent to which it 'belongs' to each shade. Has been used in various systems, e.g. control of iv infusions.

FVC, *see Forced vital capacity*

G protein-coupled receptors (GPCRs). Family of transmembrane receptors with a broad range of ligands, including **neurotransmitters** and hormones. The target receptors of many drugs, including **adrenaline** and other **catecholamines**, **opioids** and **antihistamine drugs**. Consist of seven membrane-spanning helices bound on the inner surface of the membrane to a G protein, so called because they bind guanine diphosphate (GDP) and triphosphate (GTP). G proteins consist of three subunits: Gα, Gβ and Gγ. In the inactive state, Gα has GDP on its binding site (Fig. 78a). Activation of the GPCR by a ligand causes an allosteric change in the Gα subunit, resulting in the displacement of GDP and replacement by GTP; the Gβ and Gγ subunits dissociate from the complex (Fig. 78b). The activated Gα subunit in turn activates an effector molecule, e.g. adenylate cyclase (*see Fig. 5;* **Adenylate cyclase**). Activated Gα is a GTPase that rapidly reconverts GTP to GDP, thus restoring the G protein to its inactive state.

Many types of Gα subunit exist, including:

- Gα_s: stimulates adenylate cyclase, increasing intracellular **cAMP** levels, e.g. β-adrenergic agonists and glucagon are Gα_s-coupled.
- Gα_i: inhibits adenylate cyclase, e.g. α_2-adrenergic receptor agonists are Gα_i-coupled.
- Gα_q: activates phospholipase C, generating inositol triphosphate (IP_3), e.g. α_1-adrenergic receptor agonists are Gα_q-coupled.

In addition to **second messenger** systems, G proteins can also be directly coupled to ion channels.

Hollmann MW, Strumper D, Herroeder S, Durieux ME (2005). Anesthesiology; 103: 1066–88

See also, Receptor theory

G proteins, *see G protein-coupled receptors*

G6PD deficiency, *see Glucose-6-phosphate dehydrogenase deficiency*

GABA, *see γ-Aminobutyric acid*

GABA receptors, *see γ-Aminobutyric acid receptors*

Gabapentin. Oral **anticonvulsant drug**, also used in chronic **pain management**. Used perioperatively to reduce acute postoperative pain, opioid requirement and **PONV**. May also reduce the incidence of chronic post-surgical pain. Although structurally related to **GABA**, it has no activity at GABA receptors; action is thought to be via modulation of presynaptic voltage-gated calcium channels in the CNS, thereby inhibiting glutamatergic pain transmission and **'wind-up'**. Peak plasma levels occur within 2–3 h of administration, with **half-life** of 5–7 h. Absorption can be significantly impaired by **antacids**. Excreted renally with minimal metabolism.

- Dosage: 300 mg orally on the first day; bd then tds on successive days, then titrated to response up to 3600 mg/day. For perioperative use (though not currently licensed): 600–1200 mg preoperatively plus 200–300 mg tds postoperatively.
- Side effects include sedation, dizziness, ataxia, nystagmus, tremor, diplopia, nausea, convulsions, cough. Severe respiratory depression has been reported; possible risk factors include use of CNS depressants and respiratory, neurological or renal impairment.

Schmidt PC, Ruchelli G, Mackey SC, Carroll IR (2013). Anesthesiology; 119:1215–21

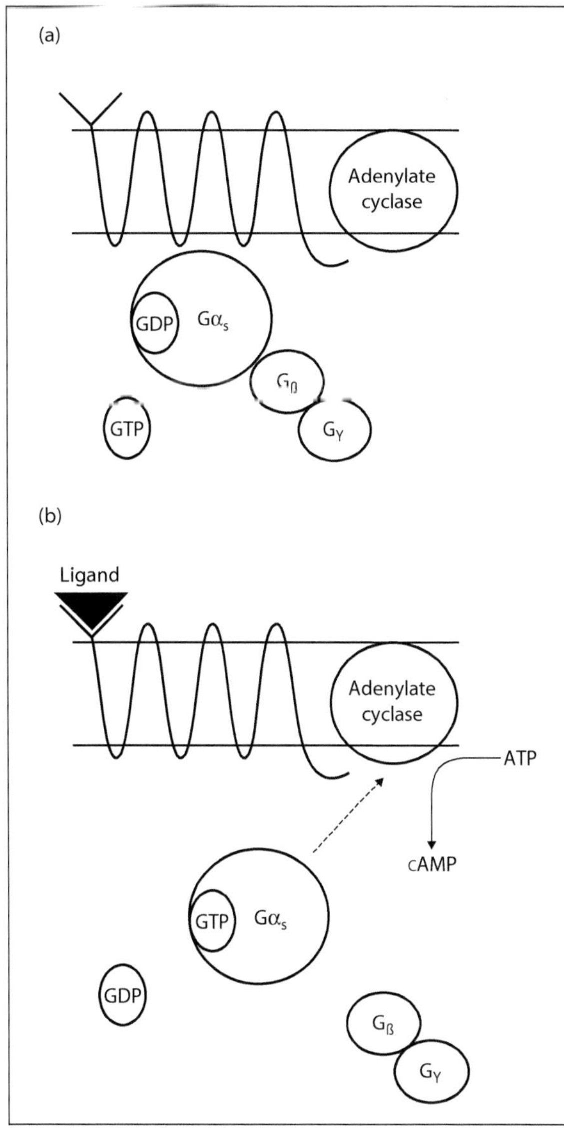

Fig. 78 G protein-coupled receptor in (a) inactive and (b) activated states (*see text*)

Gabexate mesylate. Synthetic serine protease inhibitor; has been studied as a protective and therapeutic agent in **pancreatitis**, as a neuroprotective agent in **spinal cord injury**, and as a treatment for **DIC**. Not available in the UK.

Gag reflex. Elevation and constriction of the pharynx following stimulation of the posterior pharyngeal wall. The afferent pathway is via the glossopharyngeal nerve; the efferent is via the vagus. Elevation of the soft palate when it is touched relies on afferent fibres in the maxillary division of the trigeminal nerve; often the two reflexes are elicited together. The gag reflex is abolished following local anaesthesia and lesions of the pharynx, lesions of the vagal nuclei in the medulla, and deep anaesthesia or coma. Absence of the gag reflex may indicate that the airway is at risk, e.g. from aspiration of vomit. The reflex is assessed as part of testing for **brainstem death**.
See also, Cranial nerves

Gain, electrical. Ratio of output signal amplitude to input signal amplitude. Thus a measure of amplification of signal, e.g. in **monitoring** equipment. May be specified as voltage, current or power gain; expressed as a simple ratio, or for power gain, also expressed as logarithm (base 10) of the ratio (e.g. in bels or decibels).
[Alexander Bell (1847–1922), Scottish-born US inventor]
See also, Amplifiers

Gallamine triethiodide, *see Neuromuscular blocking drugs*

Galvanic skin response (Skin conductance response; Sympathogalvanic response). Measurement of the skin's electrical conductivity, which varies with its moisture level. Test of sympathetic afferent, efferent and spinal interconnecting pathways, used to assess the effects of **sympathetic nerve blocks**. Has also been used to assess other regional blocks in which sympathetic blockade occurs, e.g. **epidural anaesthesia, brachial plexus block**.

Skin electrodes are placed on dorsal and ventral surfaces of the hand/foot, with a reference electrode elsewhere. Opposite sides of the body are normally compared. The output is displayed on an **oscilloscope** (e.g. ECG machine); a steady line results. With intact sympathetic pathways, pinching the skin causes altered skin conductance via changes in sweat gland secretion, displayed as a deflection lasting under 5 s. Deflection is abolished by successful blockade. The response may be diminished by use of **atropine**, repeated testing and in the elderly.

Baseline deflection amplitude may be used to assess suitability for subsequent sympathetic block.

Ganciclovir. **Antiviral drug**, related to **aciclovir** but more active against **cytomegalovirus** and more toxic, thus reserved for severe infections associated with poorly controlled and advanced **HIV** disease and to prevent infection during immunosuppression following organ transplantation. Valganciclovir, a **prodrug**, is available for oral use.

- Dosage: 5 mg/kg iv bd for 2–3 weeks (treatment) or 1–2 weeks (prophylaxis), followed by 5–6 mg/kg daily.
- Side effects: many, including blood dyscrasias, rash, hepatorenal impairment, GIT upset, arrhythmias, coma. Contraindicated in pregnancy. May cause severe myelosuppression in combination with **zidovudine**.

Ganglion blocking drugs. Nicotinic **acetylcholine receptor** antagonists acting at autonomic ganglia. The first **antihypertensive drugs**, now rarely used because of widespread side effects caused by sympathetic blockade (postural and exertional hypotension, decreased sweating) and parasympathetic blockade (constipation, urinary retention, impotence, dry mouth, blurred vision). May first stimulate then block receptors (e.g. **nicotine**) or exhibit competitive antagonism (e.g. **hexamethonium, pentolinium, trimetaphan**). None is generally available in the UK.

Because of the similarity between neuromuscular and ganglionic nicotinic receptors, ganglion blockers (e.g. hexamethonium) may cause neuromuscular blockade, and **neuromuscular blocking drugs** (e.g. **tubocurarine**) may cause ganglion blockade.

Gangrene. Death and decay of body tissues; usually a consequence of ischaemia ± bacterial decomposition but may be caused by micro-organisms in well-perfused tissue (e.g. **gas gangrene**). Traditionally described according to the causative insult and clinical appearances, even though some terms are now obsolete: traumatic gangrene (resulting from direct injury); gas gangrene (associated with gas formation within the tissues); Fournier's gangrene (affecting the perineum); wet gangrene (associated with venous congestion and oedema); dry gangrene (affected tissue is blackened and shrunken). Many terms have been superseded by more specific ones, e.g. **necrotising fasciitis.**
[Jean A Fournier (1832–1914), Paris dermatologist]

Gas. Form of matter whose constituent particles (molecules or atoms) are constantly moving, and whose mean positions are far apart. Tends to expand in all directions and mix with other gases. Governed by the gas laws under specified conditions. Formed when a **liquid** exceeds its **critical temperature**. The constituent particles are sufficiently far apart for the forces (e.g. **van der Waals forces**) between them to be negligible unless the gas is compressed. Pressure exerted by a gas is proportional to the number of collisions of particles against the container's walls, which is proportional to the number of gas molecules in the container.
See also, Boyle's law; Charles' law; Ideal gas law

Gas analysis. Possible methods:

- chemical:
  - gas reacts chemically with other substances to form non-gaseous compounds, with reduction of overall volume (e.g. **Haldane apparatus**) or pressure (e.g. **van Slyke apparatus**). Alternatively, the reaction results in emission of light that is measured by a photodetector, e.g. chemiluminescence nitric oxide analysis (NO + ozone $\rightarrow O_2 + NO_2$ + light).
  - electrochemical: gas reacts with other substances, the number of electrons transferred during the reaction being proportional to the concentration of gas in the sample. Used in nitric oxide analysers (NO being converted to NO_2).
- physical:
  - **spectroscopy** (e.g. infrared).
  - adsorption of vapours on to surfaces:
    - rubber strips, e.g. in the Dräger Narkotest. Tension of the strips is reduced by volatile agents; the extent is proportional to their concentration. Temperature compensated using a bimetallic strip. Adjustable for use with different agents and in the presence of N_2O, to

which it is also sensitive. Has a slow response; now rarely used.
  - silicone polymer coating a vibrating quartz crystal, e.g. in the Engström Emma. Passing alternating current through a crystal can cause it to vibrate at its resonant frequency (the piezoelectric effect); change in resonant frequency is proportional to the concentration of volatile agent dissolved in the polymer coating.
- interferometer: a light beam is split and passed through two chambers, one for reference and the other for samples. The beams are delayed to different extents; thus the emergent beams are out of phase. The resultant interference pattern is viewed through a telescope, and is displaced when gas is drawn into the sample chamber. Degree of change is related to the sample concentration. Used for calibration, e.g. of vaporisers, not for perioperative monitoring.
- **mass spectrometry**.
- **gas chromatography** and detectors, e.g. **katharometer**, **flame ionisation detector**, **electron capture detector**.
- fuel cell, and paramagnetic and polarographic analysers, used for **O_2 measurement**.
- other methods (e.g. depending on different viscosities of gases or velocity of sound through gases) are rarely used now.

[Heinrich Dräger (1847–1917), German engineer; Carl-Gunnar Engström (1912–1987), Swedish physician]

See also, Carbon dioxide measurement

Gas chromatography. Technique used for **gas analysis**. The sample mixture is injected into a stream of inert carrier gas (the mobile phase) that passes through a column of silica–alumina particles coated in oil or wax (the stationary phase). Separation of the sample component gases occurs along the column's length, depending on their relative solubilities in the two phases. Temperature of the column is carefully controlled. Liquids may also be analysed. Suitable detectors (e.g. **katharometer, flame ionisation detector** or **electron capture detector**) are required.

Gas embolism. Introduction of bubbles into the circulation, usually of air into veins (although arterial air embolism has been caused by prolonged flushing of arterial lines in neonates). A potential risk when venous pressure is lower than atmospheric pressure. It may occur during any surgery when an open vein is raised above the heart; it is particularly likely in **neurosurgery** with the patient in the sitting position because the skull's diploic veins and dural sinuses do not collapse. May also occur during insertion or removal of a CVP line (minimised by tilting the patient head-down during the former and using occlusive dressings as opposed to gauze in the latter). Procedures involving insufflation or injection of gas, e.g. **laparoscopy**, **epidural anaesthesia** using loss of resistance to air, laser surgery with gas-cooled probes, may also lead to embolism. **N_2O** diffuses into air bubbles, increasing their volume and exacerbating their effects. Morbidity and mortality are dependent on the volume of the gas entrained and the rate of accumulation.

Gas in the heart is compressed with each beat and not expelled, causing foaming and interruption of blood flow. Pulmonary vessels may become obstructed. Small bubbles may have little effect. Paradoxical gas emboli pass to the systemic circulation via the pulmonary vascular bed or cardiac septal defects (a probe-patent foramen ovale exists in 20%–30% of patients at autopsy). The bubbles may obstruct the coronary or cerebral vessels.

- Clinical features:
  - reduced cardiac output.
  - tachycardia.
  - cyanosis.
  - bronchospasm and pulmonary oedema may occur. Dyspnoea, coughing and chest pain are common in the awake patient.
  - tinkling sounds on auscultation, e.g. with an oesophageal/precordial stethoscope; large amounts of gas may cause a 'mill-wheel' murmur. May be detected by a precordial **Doppler** probe or **transoesophageal echocardiography**, although the extreme sensitivity of these techniques may reveal many tiny bubbles of disputed clinical significance.
  - sudden reduction of end-tidal CO_2 due to decreased cardiac output and possibly a contribution from increased **dead space**. End-tidal nitrogen monitoring has also been used to monitor gas embolism.
  - raised pulmonary artery resistance and pressure.
  - signs of right ventricular strain on the ECG; ventricular ectopics or fibrillation may occur.
- Treatment:
  - to prevent further embolism:
    - seal veins.
    - flood the wound with fluid.
    - increase venous pressure using head-down tilt, iv fluids, jugular venous compression, **PEEP**. The latter and the **antigravity suit** have been advocated for prevention of air embolism in neurosurgery in the traditional sitting position. The use of the modified sitting position with the legs placed horizontally may decrease the incidence.
  - once gas has entered the circulation:
    - **CPR** if required.
    - stop N_2O.
    - the head-down, left lateral position is said to increase the likelihood of gas remaining in the right atrium but may be difficult or impossible during certain types of surgery e.g. neurosurgery.
    - remove gas from the right atrium or ventricle via a central line. Special wide-bore, multiholed catheters are available for this purpose, although whether these are necessary is controversial.
    - hyperbaric O_2 has been used to reduce the size of the embolism and improve oxygenation.

Mirski MA, Lele AJ, Fitzsimmons L, Toung TJK (2007). Anesthesiology; 106: 164–77

Gas flow. Principles of **flow** are as for any **fluid**. Clinical applications:
  - flow is turbulent in the upper airway, trachea and bronchi, especially during forceful breathing; i.e., gas **density** has greater impact on flow than **viscosity**. Thus in upper **airway obstruction**, flow is increased if low-density gas is used, e.g. **helium**–oxygen mixture.
  - flow is laminar in small bronchioles; i.e., viscosity is more important; although tube radius is very small, velocity is also very low. Helium has traditionally been considered of no use in improving gas flow in asthma, primarily a disease of small airways, but some evidence suggests that helium–oxygen may be useful in severe asthma, suggesting an element of turbulent flow.
  - flow may be mostly laminar during quiet breathing, with turbulence at branches in the trachea and

bronchi. Turbulence is more likely at mid-inspiration/expiration, when flow rate is highest (e.g. up to 50 l/min).

- turbulence usually occurs in **anaesthetic breathing systems** during peak flow, especially if sharp-angled bends are present, e.g. at connections between components. Turbulence is more likely with narrow tubing and tubes.
- other applications include the **Venturi principle**, **fluidics**, **flow–volume loops** and **flowmeters**.

See also, Airway resistance

Gas gangrene. Infection due to clostridium species, usually *C. perfringens*, a spore-forming gram-positive anaerobic bacillus found in soil and faeces. Classically associated with deep war wounds, especially those contaminated with dirt or foreign bodies, but may follow any **trauma**, e.g. surgery. The incubation period is under 4 days, usually under 1 day.

The organism produces gas within tissues, often detectable clinically as subcutaneous emphysema. Local spread is rapid, with oedema, pain and tissue necrosis; **endotoxin** production often results in **sepsis** with **MODS**.

Prevented and treated by wound debridement and cleaning. **Penicillin** is an effective adjunct. Hyperbaric O_2 therapy has been used to increase local tissue O_2 content; antitoxin therapy is more controversial.

See also, Clostridial infections; Gangrene; Oxygen, hyperbaric

Gas laws, *see Avogadro's hypothesis; Boyle's law; Charles' law; Dalton's law; Henry's law; Ideal gas law*

Gas transport, *see Carbon dioxide transport; Oxygen transport*

Gasp reflex. Production of a deep slow breath following a large positive pressure inflation of the lungs. Originally described in cats and dogs, but may be seen in newborn babies; during neonatal resuscitation, it may occur within primary **apnoea**. A similar response may also be seen after opioid administration in anaesthetised patients.

Head's paradoxical reflex, although similar, is produced under different experimental conditions.

See also, Cardiopulmonary resuscitation, neonatal

Gasserian ganglion block. Block of the trigeminal ganglion, which lies medially in the middle cranial fossa within a dural reflection (Meckel's cave), lateral to the internal carotid artery and cavernous sinus. Results in anaesthesia of the face, forehead and anterior scalp (Fig. 79). Used mainly for treatment of **trigeminal neuralgia**, but also for surgery to the face.

- Technique:
    - usually performed under fluoroscopic, CT or ultrasound guidance. With the patient supine and looking straight ahead, a 22-G, 10-cm needle is introduced 3 cm lateral to the angle of the mouth, level with the second upper molar. Aiming at the pupil from the front, and the midpoint of the zygoma from the side, it is inserted until it contacts bone (greater wing of sphenoid, anterior to the foramen ovale). It is redirected posteriorly 1–1.5 cm deeper, passing through the foramen. Correct positioning is confirmed by electrical stimulation of the needle, which elicits paraesthesia in the distribution of the appropriate branch of the trigeminal nerve.

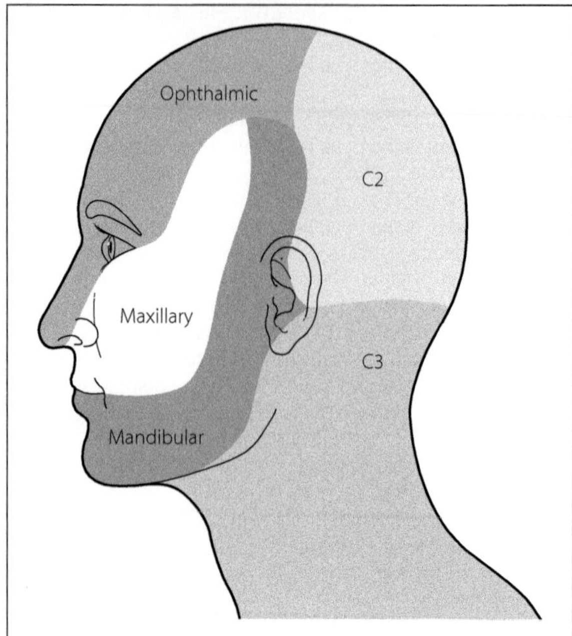

Fig. 79 Innervation of the face

    - after careful aspiration, 1–2 ml solution, e.g. 1% **lidocaine**, is injected. Glycerol or phenol injection or thermocoagulation may follow if ablative therapy is required. Accidental subarachnoid injection may occur.

Often painful; general anaesthesia or sedation is required, with waking up or reversal to confirm paraesthesia, followed by resedation for ablation. Complications include **anaesthesia dolorosa**.

[Johann Gasser (1723–1765), Austrian anatomist; Johann Meckel (1714–1774), German anatomist]

See also, Mandibular nerve block; Maxillary nerve block; Ophthalmic nerve block

Gastric contents. Anaesthetic importance:

- absorption of orally administered drugs; e.g. related to **gastric emptying**, pH and **drug interactions** within the stomach.
- **aspiration of gastric contents**; severity of **aspiration pneumonitis** is related to the pH, volume and particulate nature of the aspirate.

- Gastric secretion is increased by:
    - presence of food in the mouth (vagal reflex).
    - anger, stress.
    - presence of food in the stomach (local reflex).
    - protein meal, via duodenal gastrin secretion.
    - **hypoglycaemia**.
    - **alcohol**, **caffeine**.
- Gastric secretion and acidity are decreased by:
    - vagotomy.
    - **H_2 receptor antagonists**.
    - **proton pump inhibitors**.
    - drinking water.

Gastric acidity is decreased by **antacids**.

Gastric volume is related to gastric emptying and intake and may be assessed by gastric ultrasound. Volume is reduced by H_2 antagonists and protein pump inhibitors, but increased by antacids.

Gastric emptying. Normally results from peristaltic waves of contraction passing through the cardia, antrum, pylorus and duodenum, occurring up to three times/minute after a meal. Small amounts of liquid traverse the pylorus, which closes as the contraction wave reaches it, redirecting most of the propelled (solid) material back into the proximal stomach for further mixing. Thus liquids transit faster than solids. Carbohydrates leave faster than proteins and fats are slowest, due to inhibitory feedback mechanisms involving duodenal hormone secretion.

- Slowed by:
  - lying down.
  - increased **sympathetic nervous system** activity (e.g. anxiety, fear, pain).
  - mechanical obstruction and duodenal distension.
  - drugs, e.g. **opioid analgesic drugs**, **anticholinergic drugs**, **alcohol**, **dopamine**.
- Increased by:
  - gastric distension.
  - drugs, e.g. **metoclopramide**, **domperidone** (opioid-induced gastric stasis is not reversed; cf. **cisapride**).

Rate of emptying is important because of the risks of nausea, vomiting, regurgitation and **aspiration of gastric contents**. Emptying also affects absorption of orally administered drugs. A commonly used preoperative starvation guideline is 6 h for solid food/milk and 2 h for water in all but life-threatening emergencies; this is an estimate and **gastric contents** may be considerable even after fasting if gastric emptying is delayed. Small volumes of water (150 ml) given 2–3 h preoperatively have been shown to reduce the volume and acidity of gastric contents. Recent guidelines call for withholding of all solid food on the day of surgery, unrestricted clear fluids up to 3 h preoperatively and consideration of **H_2 receptor antagonists** for patients at risk.

- Measurement:
  - measurement of plasma levels of orally administered substance, e.g. paracetamol (absorbed from the small intestine, not from the stomach).
  - serial nasogastric aspiration, with measurement of orally administered marker substance.
  - measurement of **impedance** across the lower chest/upper abdomen; alters as composition of tissues, i.e., gastric contents, changes.
  - oral administration of radioisotope, with measurement of radioactivity over the stomach.
  - gastric ultrasonography has been used in the acute setting.
  - x-ray imaging following oral contrast medium.

Emptying can be aided by naso- or orogastric aspiration. The latter is more effective, using a wide-bore tube with multiple holes and lumina, but is unpleasant and rarely used except for emptying the stomach intraoperatively. **Emetic drugs** are no longer used.

Gastric intramucosal pH, *see Gastric tonometry*

Gastric lavage. Previously performed following **poisoning and overdose**; now has a very limited role, as evidence suggests the risk of harm outweighs potential benefits in the majority of cases.

Previously performed up to 4 h after ingestion (longer if gastric emptying is delayed, e.g. by anticholinergic drugs, aspirin), or at any time if the patient is unconscious. Involves passage of a wide-bore orogastric tube, with aspiration to ensure the trachea has not been entered accidentally. 300–600 ml warm water is introduced and allowed to drain under gravity; this is repeated until the aspirate is clear. Pulmonary aspiration may occur; the patient should be placed in the head-down lateral position with suction available. Tracheal intubation is required if laryngeal reflexes are absent. Lavage is contraindicated if petroleum derivatives have been ingested, because pulmonary aspiration is particularly harmful. Oesophageal/gastric perforation is also likely if caustic substances have been ingested.

Benson BE, Hoppu K, Troutman WG, et al (2013). Clin Toxicol; 51: 140–6

Gastric tonometry. Indirect method of measuring gastric intramucosal pH, which in turn is used as an indicator of gastric (and therefore GIT) mucosal O_2 balance. Intramucosal acidosis may indicate impaired GIT **O_2 delivery** or utilisation, and has been proposed as a useful indicator of poor splanchnic perfusion and mortality; may be used to guide vasoactive drug therapy in the ICU and during major surgery.

A tonometer incorporating a saline-filled balloon is placed via the **oesophagus** into the stomach, and luminal $P\text{CO}_2$ (which approximates to intramucosal $P\text{CO}_2$) inferred by measuring $P\text{CO}_2$ in the saline. A gas-filled balloon has also been used, with recirculation of gas into and out of the balloon with continuous measurement of $P\text{CO}_2$ at the distal end of the system. **H_2 receptor antagonists** eliminate the error caused by gastric acid (which combines with pancreatic **bicarbonate** to produce intraluminal CO_2). Direct measurement is also possible but involves mucosal trauma and is less reliable. Arterial bicarbonate concentration is measured simultaneously and approximates to mucosal concentration, allowing calculation of intramucosal pH (pH_i).

Although there is some evidence of benefit, its use has not been shown to reduce ICU or hospital mortality or length of stay; furthermore, it is not widely used due to cost, unfamiliarity with the technique and poor specificity.

Zhang X, Xuan W, Yin P, et al (2015). Crit Care; 19: 22

Gastrointestinal haemorrhage. May arise from any part of the GIT, although most acute bleeds are caused by **peptic ulcer disease**. May result in the need for resuscitation, surgery and/or ICU management. Mortality is 5%–10% (higher in some contexts, e.g. 30% in **oesophageal varices**). Features range from gross haematemesis to vomiting of small amounts of 'coffee grounds' (blood altered by gastric acid) or the passage of melaena.

- Main considerations:
  - of the underlying cause, e.g.: oesophageal/gastric varices associated with **alcoholism**; **NSAID**-induced ulceration associated with arthritic disease; **anticoagulant drugs** or **coagulation disorders**; systemic effects of **malignancy** or chronic illness.
  - **haemorrhage** and **hypovolaemia**.
  - presence of a full stomach and the risk of **aspiration of gastric contents**.
  - difficulty securing the airway while there is copious haematemesis.
- Management:
  - O_2, volume resuscitation, correction of coagulation disorders.
  - upper GIT bleeding:
    - assessment of risks using:
      - Blatchford score: defines the need for urgent endoscopy and intervention based on clinical observations (systolic BP, heart rate, presentation

with melaena or syncope, presence of hepatic or cardiac disease), haemoglobin level and blood urea.
    - Rockall score: calculated following endoscopy and based on age, presence of shock, co-morbidity and endoscopic findings; it allows assessment of risk of death and rebleeding.
  - management as for oesophageal varices, i.e., endoscopy immediately after resuscitation in unstable patients; all other patients should have endoscopy within 24 h. Treatment includes:
    - non-variceal bleeding: clipping of vessels (with or without the use of **adrenaline**), thermocoagulation with adrenaline or the use of fibrin or thrombin with adrenaline. **Proton pump inhibitors** are given following endoscopy.
    - variceal bleeding: endoscopic variceal band ligation (oesophageal) or injection of cyanoacrylate (gastric).
- lower GIT bleeding: tends to be less acute, although may occasionally present with severe bleeding and hypovolaemia. May be associated with effects of chronic **anaemia** and other features of systemic disease. Usually managed conservatively initially, with lower GIT endoscopy ± imaging as appropriate. Abdominal surgery may be required.
- prevention of rebleeding may involve alteration of antiplatelet therapy (including stopping NSAIDs) and anticoagulant treatment, depending on evaluation of individual patients' risk/benefits.

GIT haemorrhage associated with **stress ulcers** may occur in critically ill patients on the ICU.

[Oliver Blatchford, Glasgow epidemiologist; Timothy Rockall, British surgeon]

Dworzynski, K., Pollit, V., Kelsey, A., et al. (2012). *Br Med J, 344*, e3412.

Gastro-oesophageal reflux. Normally prevented by the **lower oesophageal sphincter** and anatomical arrangement of the **oesophagus** and stomach. Occurs in 10%–20% of the population but especially common in **hiatus hernia**, **obesity** and **obstructive sleep apnoea**. May cause burning retrosternal pain and regurgitation of bitter fluid into the mouth, especially on stooping/lying. Associated oesophagitis may cause pain after meals. Medical treatment is as for **peptic ulcer disease**/hiatus hernia, including weight loss and avoidance of the supine/head-down position. Anaesthetic management is as for hiatus hernia.

Iwakiri K, Kinoshita Y, Hubo Y, et al (2016). J Gastroenterol; 51: 751–67

Gastro-oesophageal sphincter, *see Lower oesophageal sphincter*

Gastroschisis and exomphalos. Congenital malformations of the abdominal wall, associated with protrusion of abdominal contents:
- gastroschisis: abdominal wall defect, not associated with the midline or umbilicus, causing herniation of abdominal contents without a covering sac. Incidence is 1:5000; overall mortality is up to 10%.
- exomphalos: midline defect, related to the umbilicus. Bowel and other abdominal organs (with a covering sac) fail to return to the abdominal cavity during fetal development. Incidence is 1:10000; overall mortality is 10%–20%, depending on the presence of other abnormalities.

- Associated with:
  - Prematurity, particularly with gastroschisis.
  - other congenital abnormalities (e.g. cardiac defects, other GIT malformations and genitourinary abnormalities), especially with exomphalos.
- Initial problems:
  - damage to exposed organs.
  - fluid and electrolyte balance.
  - heat loss.
  - infection.
- Treatment:
  - the bowel is covered with a dry towel/plastic bag.
  - primary surgical closure is preferable to delayed closure if possible.
- Anaesthetic considerations: as for **paediatric anaesthesia** plus the above considerations. In addition:
  - **N_2O** diffuses into the bowel, increasing its size, and is avoided.
  - postoperative IPPV is frequently required, particularly with primary closure. Staged closure using a Silastic pouch may be performed if adverse effects of primary closure (e.g. impaired ventilation) are excessive.
  - postoperative nutrition and prevention/treatment of infection are important.

Raghavan M, Montgomerie J (2008). Paediatr Anaesth; 18: 731–5

Gate control theory of pain. Proposed in 1965 by Melzack and Wall to account for the influence of psychological and physiological factors on **pain** transmission. Although incompletely understood, the theory forms the basis for understanding **spinal cord** modulation of pain.

Nociceptive impulses flow along nociceptive nerve fibres from the periphery, via the spinal cord neurons to the brain. However, pain is regulated by activity from other myelinated afferents that do not transmit nociceptive information. The balance between nociceptive and non-nociceptive afferent activity determines the pain experience.
- Has four components (Fig. 80):
  - primary afferent axons: synapse with interneurones and projection neurones (see later):
    - small-diameter Aδ (myelinated) and C (unmyelinated) fibres that function as nociceptors and terminate in laminae I and II (substantia gelatinosa) of the dorsal horn.

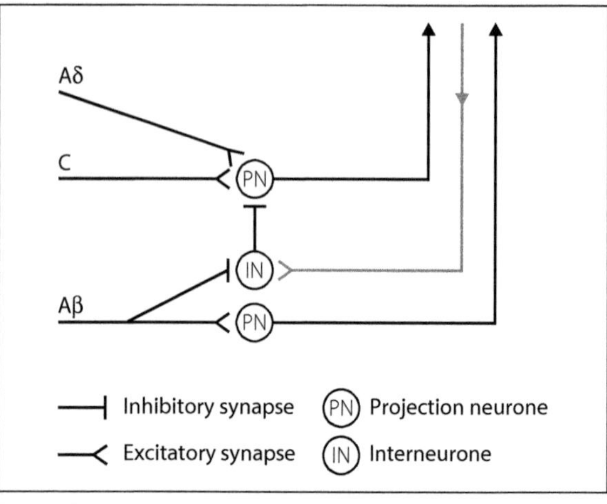

Fig. 80 Gate control theory of pain

- larger, myelinated Aβ fibres convey innocuous mechanical information (touch/proprioception/vibration) and terminate in laminae III–V of the dorsal horn.
- projection neurones: synapse with primary afferent fibres and have axons that travel directly to the brain.
- interneurones: have axons remaining in the spinal cord and synapse presynaptically with primary afferent fibres and postsynaptically with projection neurones, to influence neuronal transmission to the brain. May be excitatory (**glutamate**-mediated facilitation of nociceptive transmission) or inhibitory (**GABA**- or **glycine**-mediated inhibition of further nociceptive transmission).
- descending axons from the main descending pathways from the brain: monoaminergic systems that originate from the raphe nuclei of the medulla (serotonergic) and locus coeruleus and adjacent regions of the pons (noradrenergic), and can further modulate interneurons and projection neurons.

Interneurones, stimulated by either non-nociceptive fibres (e.g. Aδ fibres) or descending pathways, can inhibit or facilitate transmission of nociceptive stimuli to the brain (Fig. 80). They act by closing the 'gate' to nociceptive transmission at the spinal level. For example, in **TENS** treatment a vibratory stimulus activates large-diameter Aβ fibres, which stimulate inhibitory interneurones that 'close the gate' and prevent transmission of nociceptive impulses to the brain.
[Patrick D Wall (1925–2001), English neuroscientist; Ronald Melzack, Montreal psychologist]
Mendell LM (2014). Pain; 155: 210–16
See also, Sensory pathways

Gauge. Measure of thickness/width; applied in medicine to cannulae, **needles** and catheters. Common systems include wire gauges used for needles and cannulae, and the French gauge (Charrière), originally applied to urinary catheters and which equals external circumference in mm (approximately 3 × external diameter).
[Joseph FB Charrière (1803–1876), Paris instrument-maker]

Gay-Lussac's law, *see Charles' law*

GCSF, *see Granulocyte colony-stimulating factor*

Gelatin solutions. **Colloid** solutions derived from animal gelatin, a derivative of collagen. Commonly used forms contain urea-linked (Haemaccel) or succinylated (Gelofusine) gelatin components (Table 24); average mw is about 35 kDa. Solutions containing physiological concentrations of sodium and chloride are also available (Isoplex). Although extensively used in the past as plasma substitutes, e.g. in **haemorrhage** and **shock**, current concerns regarding their safety have reduced their popularity (*see Colloid*). Cheaper than **albumin** solutions and starch solutions, but with shorter plasma **half-life** (about 4 h). Only 1% metabolised with no accumulation in reticuloendothelial system. **Adverse drug reactions** including **anaphylaxis** have occurred, especially to Haemaccel (said to be reduced in its current form); usually mild but occasionally severe. The incidence of reactions is less than 0.15%.

Renal function and **blood compatibility testing** are unaffected. Gelatin solutions may interfere with platelet function and coagulation (via reduction in von Willebrand factor activity), and restriction of their administration in major haemorrhage has been suggested, although this is controversial. The calcium in Haemaccel may coagulate stored blood if infused through the same giving set without first flushing with saline.

Table 24 Components of gelatin solutions

Solution	*Gelatin (g/l)*	*Sodium (mmol/l)*	*Chloride (mmol/l)*	*Calcium (mmol/l)*	*Potassium (mmol/l)*
Haemaccel	35 urea-linked	145	145	6.26	0.4
Gelofusine	40 succinylated	154	120	0	0
Isoplex	40 succinylated	145	105	0	4.0

Gelofusine, *see Gelatin solutions*

Gender differences and anaesthesia. Many factors may contribute to differences in responses to anaesthetic and analgesic drugs between genders, for example:
- **pharmacokinetics**:
  - absorption and drug binding: some differences but little evidence relating to anaesthetic drugs. Alcohol is absorbed more rapidly in women because it is metabolised less in the gastric mucosa than in men.
  - distribution: greater fat/water ratio in women; thus **volume of distribution** of water-soluble drugs (e.g. **vecuronium**) is reduced, and of fat-soluble drugs (e.g. **diazepam**) is increased. It has been suggested that women recover more quickly after **propofol** anaesthesia than men.
  - metabolism: e.g. greater metabolism of **morphine** to the active 6-glucuronide than the antagonistic 3-glucuronide in women, compared with men. Other differences may relate to sex-specific isoenzyme systems but experimental results are often conflicting.
  - excretion: renal excretion is affected by body weight and composition.
- **pharmacodynamics**: women are thought to be more susceptible to the analgesic effects of **opioid analgesic drugs** and **neuromuscular blocking drugs** and, although different pharmacokinetics may contribute, pharmacodynamic factors have also been suggested. Reduced sensitivity and earlier waking of women after propofol may also be a pharmacodynamic phenomenon.

Further differences may result from cyclical changes in body fluid and hormonal status during the menstrual cycle (e.g. **PONV** may be affected by phase of menstrual cycle). There are also significant effects of **pregnancy**. Psychological factors and the reported greater incidence of adverse effects in women may also contribute to apparent differences between the sexes.
Buchanan FF, Myles PS, Cicuttini F (2011). Br J Anaesth; 106: 823–9

General Medical Council (GMC). Independent regulator for medical doctors in the UK, funded largely through registration fees. Its remit is to promote and protect patient safety by: fostering good practice; promoting and regulating education and training; and dealing with doctors whose fitness to practise is in question. Sets standards of ethical and professional conduct through its guidance document,

Table 25 Glasgow coma scale for adults and infants

Glasgow coma scale for adults			*Glasgow coma scale for infants*		
Activity	*Best response*	*Scale*	*Activity*	*Best response*	*Scale*
Motor	Obeys commands	6	Motor	Obeys commands	6
	Localises pain	5		Localises pain	5
	Withdraws from pain	4		Withdraws from pain	4
	Flexes in response to pain	3		Flexes in response to pain	3
	Extends in response to pain	2		Extends in response to pain	2
	No response	1		No response	1
Verbal	Fully orientated	5	Verbal	Coos or babbles	5
	Confused	4		Irritable cries	4
	Inappropriate words	3		Cries to painful stimuli	3
	Incomprehensible sounds	2		Moans to painful stimuli	2
	No response	1		None	1
Eye opening	Eyes open spontaneously	4	Eye opening	Spontaneous	4
	Eyes open to command	3		To speech	3
	Eyes open in response to pain	2		To pain	2
	Eyes remain closed	1		None	1

Good Medical Practice. Assumed the role of the Postgraduate Medical Education and Training Board in 2010, and so sets and approves all postgraduate medical curricula, assessment systems and training programmes.

All practising doctors in the UK must be on the publicly available GMC List of Registered Practitioners. Doctors referred to the GMC may undergo a fitness to practise assessment consisting of investigation and adjudication processes, which may result in: acceptance of the doctor's actions; issuance of a warning; imposition of conditions on practice; or suspension/removal from the register ('striking off').

Since 2003, the GMC has itself been accountable to the Council for Healthcare Regulatory Excellence (now Professional Standards Authority for Health and Social Care), which audits the performance of the GMC and other regulators, and may challenge outcomes of fitness to practise investigations.

Genitofemoral nerve block, *see Inguinal hernia field block*

Gentamicin. Broad-spectrum **antibacterial drug** of the **aminoglycosides** group, especially active against gram-negative organisms, but poorly active against haemolytic streptococci, haemophilus and anaerobes; thus often given with **penicillin** ± **metronidazole** when given empirically. <10% protein-bound and excreted renally, with plasma **half-life** of 2–3 h with normal renal function.

- Dosage: 3–5 mg/kg daily in three divided doses slowly iv or im. Less frequent administration is required in renal impairment. One-hour (peak) plasma levels should not exceed 10 mg/l; trough levels should not exceed 2 mg/l. A single daily iv dose of 5–7 mg/kg over 30–60 min provides an equally good response to tds dosing, with fewer complications (including renal impairment). Monitoring is also easier.
- Side effects: as for aminoglycosides.

Geriatric patient, *see Elderly, anaesthesia for*

GFR, *see Glomerular filtration rate*

GHBA, *see γ-Hydroxybutyric acid*

Gland/gland nut, *see Cylinders*

Glasgow coma scale (GCS). Scoring system originally devised in 1974 for assessment of patients with **TBI** but now widely applied to other causes of **coma**. Validated as useful predictor of outcome after head injury, intracranial haemorrhage, subarachnoid haemorrhage, poisonings and cardiac arrest. Originally described for adults, it has been modified for use in infants. A maximum of 15 points may be scored (Table 25), expressed as a total or, more usefully, separated into the three categories (e.g. 'M_3, V_2, E_2' gives more information than 'GCS 7'). Changes in scores over time are more useful than single values. Despite its limitations in assessing patients unable to speak (e.g. aphasia, intubation), it remains the most widely used **coma scale** and is a component of the **APACHE scoring system**.

Teasdale G, Maas A, Lecky F (2014). Lancet Neurol; 13: 844–54

See also, FOUR score; Trauma scales

Glaucoma. Damage to the eye associated with raised **intraocular pressure** (IOP).

- Anaesthetic considerations:
  - related to IOP:
    - avoidance of drugs that raise IOP, e.g. **ketamine**. Systemic **atropine** is safe; topical use may cause mydriasis and obstruct drainage of aqueous humour.
    - IOP increases following tracheal intubation and extubation.
    - avoidance of: trauma to the eye; steep head-down position; coughing and straining.
    - IOP may be reduced by specific measures, e.g. iv **mannitol**, **acetazolamide**.
  - related to concurrent drug therapy:
    - timolol drops and related drugs: systemic absorption and β-blockade may occur.
    - **ecothiopate** drops: may prolong action of **suxamethonium**.
    - pilocarpine and **physostigmine** drops: systemic absorption and bradycardia may occur.
    - acetazolamide: electrolyte imbalance may occur.
    - **cannabis** may be used by patients with glaucoma.

Glomerular filtration rate (GFR). Volume of plasma filtered by the **kidneys** per unit time. Normally ~120 ml/min (173 l/day).

- Depends on:
  - effective glomerular surface area: reduced by contraction of mesangial cells within the glomerulus, e.g. in response to angiotensin II, **vasopressin, noradrenaline, leukotrienes, histamine** and certain **prostaglandins. Dopamine** and **atrial natriuretic peptide** cause relaxation.
  - permeability of the capillary wall, basement membrane and glomerular epithelium. Increased in certain diseases.
  - hydrostatic gradient across the capillary walls. Affected by:
    - **renal blood flow** and arteriolar tone (e.g. noradrenaline constricts the afferent arterioles predominantly, whereas angiotensin II constricts the efferent arterioles). **Autoregulation** is thought to involve afferent arteriolar vascular tone.
    - ureteric obstruction/renal oedema.
  - osmotic gradient: rarely clinically important.

Measured by iv infusion of a substance that is freely filtered and neither reabsorbed nor secreted by the renal tubules. It must also be non-toxic, not metabolised and have no effect on GFR. At steady state, the **clearance** of the substance is calculated. The volume of plasma cleared per minute then equals the volume filtered per minute, i.e.:

$$\text{GFR} = \frac{\text{urine concentration} \times \text{urinary volume/min}}{\text{plasma concentration}}$$

Inulin, a carbohydrate derived from plant tubers, is usually used. Radioactive chromium-labelled EDTA may also be used.

Provides an indication of renal function, but is difficult to measure routinely. **Creatinine clearance** approximates to GFR, and is commonly measured instead. Creatinine is actually secreted by the renal tubules to a small degree, but measurement of plasma levels overestimates by a small amount, tending to cancel any error.

The MDRD (Modification of Diet in Renal Disease) equation allows an estimated value (eGFR) to be calculated from the serum creatinine concentration, adjusted for sex (creatinine concentration lower in women), age (creatinine concentration lower in older people) and race (creatinine concentration higher in African Americans than Caucasians). The eGFR is more accurate than a 24-h urine collection for creatinine clearance but is not applicable to the extremes of age or body size, muscle disease, vegetarian diet or pregnancy.

See also, Nephron; Renin/angiotensin system

Glomerulonephritis. Renal disease of varied aetiology, but often involving immune complex deposition or antibodies against glomerular basement membrane. Histological classification is unrelated to clinical presentation, which may include:

- oliguria, salt and water retention, hypervolaemia and **hypertension** due to impaired glomerular filtration (**nephritic syndrome**). Classically follows streptococcal infection.
- proteinuria, causing **hypoproteinaemia** and marked **oedema** if severe (**nephrotic syndrome**).
- others: hypertension, haematuria, loin pain, **renal failure** (acute and chronic).

- Anaesthetic considerations:
  - impaired renal function.
  - oedema and hypoproteinaemia.
  - hypertension.
  - drug therapy: may include antihypertensive drugs and corticosteroids.

Floegl J, Amann K (2016). Lancet; 387: 2036–48

See also, Goodpasture's syndrome

Glomus tumours. Rare benign tumours arising from glomus bodies (arteriovenous anastomoses adjacent to blood vessels, receiving rich sympathetic tone and involved in regulating local blood flow and skin temperature). More common in the limbs, but may arise from the glomus jugulare (tympanic body) in the upper jugular bulb. The latter may extend into the cerebellum and brainstem, middle ear, internal jugular vein or laterally into the neck. Thus associated with neurological lesions, including of lower **cranial nerves**. May rarely secrete **catecholamines** or **5-HT**. Anaesthetic concerns include length of surgery and blood loss, and those of **neurosurgery**.

Glossopharyngeal nerve block. Used to supplement topical anaesthesia and/or superior laryngeal nerve block, e.g. in awake intubation. Also used for tonsillectomy and **glossopharyngeal neuralgia**. Acute **airway obstruction** has followed its use.

- Techniques:
  - internal:
    - posterior: having applied topical anaesthesia to the tongue, it is depressed and an angled needle inserted behind the middle of the posterior tonsillar pillar, to 1 cm depth. After aspiration, 3 ml **local anaesthetic agent** is injected. Blocks the sensory pharyngeal, lingual and tonsillar branches, and the motor branch to stylopharyngeus. Carotid puncture is more likely using this approach than with the anterior.
    - anterior: after topical anaesthesia, the tongue is displaced away from the side to be blocked, revealing a gutter between the tongue and the teeth. A needle is inserted 0.25–0.5 cm at the posterior end of the gutter, and 2 ml local anaesthetic is injected. Blocks the lingual branch primarily.
  - external: 5–6 ml solution is injected just behind and deep to the styloid process, found 2–4 cm deep, midway between the tip of the mastoid process and angle of the jaw. Internal carotid and jugular vessels lie very close.

Glossopharyngeal neuralgia. Recurrent, sudden, stabbing **pain** in the distribution of the glossopharyngeal nerve. May result from nerve compression by vertebral or posterior inferior cerebellar arteries, local musculoskeletal anomalies or trauma. May be relieved by topical local anaesthetic to oropharyngeal trigger areas. Treatment includes **glossopharyngeal nerve block** using local anaesthetic at weekly intervals; alcohol injection or surgical decompression of the glossopharyngeal nerve may be required.

Glottis, *see Larynx*

Glucagon. Polypeptide hormone secreted by the A (α) cells of pancreatic islets. Acts on the glucagon receptor (a **G protein-coupled receptor**), resulting in hepatic adenylate cyclase stimulation, leading to **glycogen** breakdown and release of **glucose** (hence its emergency use in **hypoglycaemia**). Also increases hepatic gluconeogenesis from amino acids, and breakdown of **fats** to form **ketone bodies**. Stimulates secretion of **growth hormone**, **insulin** and **somatostatin**. Has positive inotropic and chronotropic effects on the heart, unrelated to **adrenergic receptors**. Thought to increase **calcium** transport into myocardial cells, possibly via adenylate cyclase activation; has also been used in the treatment of **β-adrenergic receptor antagonist poisoning** and resistant **anaphylaxis**. **Half-life** is less than 10 min.

Secretion is increased by β-adrenergic stimulation, stress, exercise, amino acids, gastrin, cholecystokinin and starvation. It is decreased by **hyperglycaemia**, somatostatin, ketone bodies, fatty acids, insulin and α-adrenergic stimulation.

- Dosage:
  - severe hypoglycaemia: 0.5–1 mg sc/im/iv.
  - (unlicensed use) β-receptor antagonist overdose: 2–10 mg iv (child: 50–150 μg/kg up to 10 mg) then 50 μg/kg/h; resistant anaphylaxis: 1–5 mg iv then 5–15 μg/min.

Glucocorticoids. Hormones secreted by the adrenal cortex; consist mainly of cortisol and corticosterone. Diffuse through cell membranes and act on intracellular receptors, causing changes in gene transcription, protein synthesis and cell function. Secretion is increased by **ACTH**.

- Actions:
  - increased **glycogen** and **protein** breakdown, and **glucose** synthesis, with increased blood glucose levels.
  - required for normal effects of **catecholamines** on **metabolism**, bronchi, CVS and fluid balance. This may explain the hypotension seen in **adrenocortical insufficiency**.
  - required for efficient **muscle contraction** and **nerve conduction**; also involved in inflammatory/immunological responses.
  - mild **aldosterone**-like activity.

Large doses of glucocorticoids suppress inflammation, and are used in many inflammatory and immunological diseases.

See also, Adrenal gland; Corticosteroids

Glucose. **Carbohydrate**, of central importance as an **energy** source within the body.

- Main metabolic pathways (Fig. 81):
  - production:
    - from breakdown of carbohydrate foodstuffs.
    - from **glycogen**, **protein** and **fats** via intermediate steps in glucose metabolism; occurs in the liver during **starvation** and **exercise**. Produces glucose 6-phosphate, which is converted by hepatic glucose-6-phosphatase to glucose, which enters the bloodstream. Other tissues (e.g. muscle) lack this enzyme, and glucose 6-phosphate is catabolised directly via the glycolytic pathway.
  - uptake:
    - from the GIT via an **active transport** mechanism for sodium ions. Thus indirectly utilises energy.
    - from the bloodstream into cells by the action of **insulin**.
  - utilisation for energy production: via conversion into glucose 6-phosphate and subsequent breakdown (**glycolysis**).

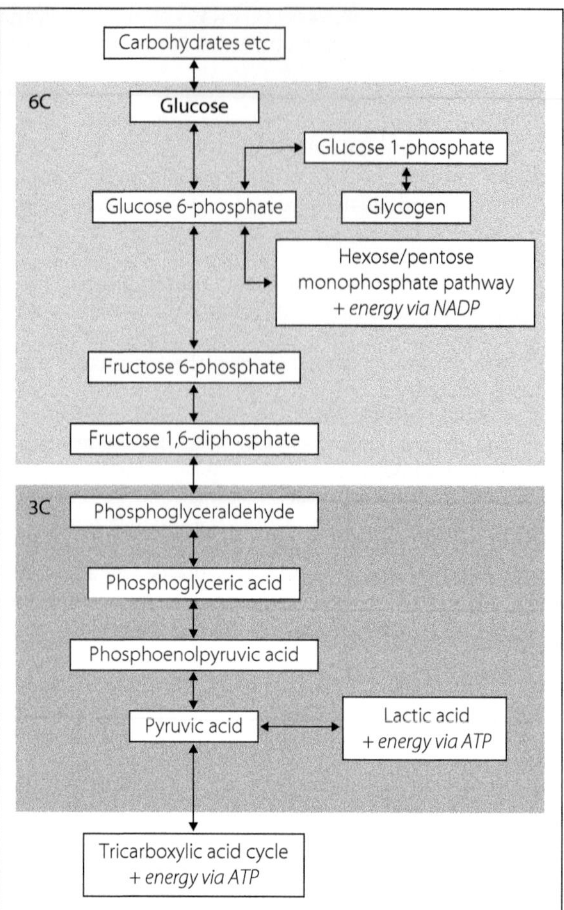

Fig. 81 Main metabolic pathways of glucose

  - conversion to glycogen via glucose 6-phosphate and glucose 1-phosphate.
  - hexose/pentose monophosphate shunt: alternative energy-producing pathway from glucose 6-phosphate, with reduction of nicotinamide adenine dinucleotide phosphate (NADP).
  - conversion to fats and proteins.

Fasting plasma levels are maintained at 4–6 mmol/l (72–108 mg/dl) by the action of various hormones, mainly on the liver; e.g. insulin decreases blood glucose, whereas **glucagon**, **catecholamines**, **growth hormone**, **glucocorticoids** and thyroid hormones increase it.

Filtered and reabsorbed in the proximal tubules of the kidneys; renal capacity for reabsorption is exceeded above plasma levels of about 10 mmol/l (180 mg/dl). Congenital inability to reabsorb glucose results in renal glycosuria at normal plasma levels. The renal threshold may also be reduced in **pregnancy** and tubular damage.

See also, Catabolism; Diabetes mellitus; Glycaemic control in the ICU; Metabolism; Nutrition

Glucose–insulin–potassium infusion. Infusion regimen used in an attempt to reduce the size of **MI**, increase cardiac output and reduce arrhythmias. First used in the 1960s. Current evidence does not support routine use, although standard management of hyperglycaemia via titrated **insulin** infusion ('sliding-scale') is recommended.

Glucose-6-phosphate dehydrogenase deficiency (G6PD deficiency). X-linked recessive inherited disorder of red blood cell metabolism, common in Mediterranean, African, Middle Eastern and South-East Asian populations. Impairs the hexose monophosphate shunt of **glucose** metabolism, required for cell protection against products of oxidation. Results in **haemolysis**, which may be chronic or associated with acute illness (especially typhoid and viral hepatitis infection), drugs (e.g. antimalarials, sulfonamides, aspirin and related drugs, methylthioninium chloride [methylene blue]), and ingestion of broad beans (favism). Reduction of **methaemoglobin** is impaired, thus avoidance of **prilocaine** has been suggested.

Classified according to degree of enzyme activity; class 1 is severely deficient; class 2 has 1%–10% normal activity; class 3 has 10%–60% normal activity; classes 4 and 5 have increased activity. Provides some protection against falciparum **malaria**.

Chronic haemolysis is also associated with other **inborn errors of metabolism**, e.g. pyruvate kinase deficiency.

Glucose reagent sticks. Used to measure **glucose** concentration, e.g. in blood or urine. Glucose is converted by glucose oxidase to gluconic acid and hydrogen peroxide, the latter oxidising a dye to produce a colour change. Accuracy is increased by using reflectance colorimeters to quantify the colour change, and may be reduced by use of alcohol swabs for cleaning the skin. They are less accurate at lower (hypoglycaemic) glucose levels. Useful as a bedside test, and for home monitoring of glucose levels.

Glucose tolerance test. Investigation used in the diagnosis of **diabetes mellitus**. Diabetes is usually diagnosed on random and fasting blood **glucose** estimations alone; the tolerance test is mainly used to investigate diabetes in pregnancy, or when the fasting glucose level is equivocal (e.g. 5.6–7 mmol/l). Also used in the diagnosis of **acromegaly**.

Involves administration of glucose either orally or iv, usually the former. 1.75 g/kg is given orally up to 75 g, in at least 250 ml water. Blood glucose normally rises from fasting levels to a peak at 10–60 min, declining thereafter. Fasting and 2-h levels are used for diagnosis:

- venous plasma glucose under 7.8 mmol/l (140 mg/dl) fasting and at 2 h: normal.
- venous plasma glucose over 11.1 mmol/l (200 mg/dl) at 2 h: diabetic.
- intermediate values: 'impaired glucose tolerance'.

α-Glucosidase inhibitors. Saccharide **hypoglycaemic drugs** that compete with saccharidases in the small intestine, thus slowing the breakdown of poly- and disaccharides to monosaccharides in the gut. Used alone or in combination with other drugs to improve glycaemic control, especially post-prandial hyperglycaemia. Include acarbose, miglitol and voglibose.

Glue-sniffing, *see Solvent abuse*

Glutamate. **Amino acid** and major excitatory **neurotransmitter** throughout the CNS, especially brain. Released presynaptically, it activates various specific receptors:

- **α-Amino-3-hydroxy-5-methyl-4-isoxazolepropionic acid receptors**: involved in rapid neurotransmission.
- kainate (a neurotoxin) receptors: similar effects to those of AMPA receptors.
- **NMDA receptors**: slower response; thought to be involved in long-term potentiation, including modulation of pain and memory formation.
- others, linked to **G protein-coupled receptors**: less clearly understood.

Manipulation of glutamate pathways is currently an active area of research because it is thought to be involved in pain perception, wakefulness and memory, post-injury or ischaemic neurotoxicity (via glutamate-mediated intracellular **calcium** accumulation) and spinal cord neurotransmission.

Glutamine, *see Amino acids; Glutamate*

Glycaemic control in the ICU. Mostly relates to management/avoidance of **hyperglycaemia**, which is common in critical illness, although **hypoglycaemia** may also require prevention/control.

- Causes of hyperglycaemia in ICU include:
  - pre-existing diabetes mellitus.
  - **stress response to surgery** and critical illness resulting in release of inflammatory **cytokines**, **catecholamines** and cortisol, which inhibit **insulin** release and increase insulin resistance.
  - administration of exogenous catecholamines and **corticosteroids**.
  - iv infusion of glucose-containing solutions.
  - **parenteral nutrition**.
  - immobility resulting in decreased uptake of glucose into muscle.

Hyperglycaemia is associated with worse outcomes in critically ill patients although this is now thought to be a marker of severity of disease rather than a causal factor. The 2001 Leuven Surgical Trial suggested that ICU mortality fell from 8% to 4.6% with tight glucose control (blood sugar levels 4.5–6.5 mmol/l). The 2006 Leuven Medical Trial found that tight glucose control in medical ICU patients improved morbidity but not mortality. Although both trials were flawed (single-centre studies, open label, differences seen with subgroup analysis), tight glucose control was adopted widely. The 2009 NICE-SUGAR trial (randomised controlled trial of 6000 ICU patients) found increased mortality in those whose glucose was tightly controlled; the increase was largely due to an increased frequency of hypoglycaemia. Current practice is to initiate insulin infusion only for blood sugar levels >8.3 mmol/l, with a goal of maintaining levels <10 mmol/l.

A particular hazard of glycaemic control in ICU is the use of arterial line samples for analysis of glucose concentrations; if glucose is present in the arterial flush solution this may cause high measured concentrations and inappropriate administration of insulin, leading to severe and sustained hypoglycaemia. Arterial flush solutions should therefore not contain glucose, and the labels of flush solutions should always be visible (and checked regularly) to protect against accidental use.

Mesotten D, Preiser JC, Kosiborod M (2015). Lancet Diabetes Endocrinol; 3: 723–33

Glyceryl trinitrate (GTN; Nitroglycerin). **Vasodilator drug**, used to treat **myocardial ischaemia** and **cardiac failure**, and to lower BP, e.g. in severe **hypertension** and **hypotensive anaesthesia**. Acts via **nitric oxide** release to relax vascular smooth muscle (mainly venous), lowering **preload** and reducing **SVR** and **pulmonary vascular resistance**. Also increases **coronary blood flow**. A cutaneous slow-release patch may be applied preoperatively in patients with **ischaemic heart disease**, and these have also been applied to sites of **iv fluid administration**, reducing infusion failure by up to 60%. Has also been used to reduce uterine contraction, e.g. in premature rupture of membranes (cutaneous patch) or as an acute **tocolytic drug** (iv or sublingual).

- Dosage:
  - sublingually 0.3–1.0 mg, repeated as required. Lasts 20–30 min. Available as 0.3-mg or 0.5-mg tablets, and as a 0.4-mg/dose spray.
  - orally as slow-release tablets: 2–5 mg tds.
  - cutaneously: 5–10 mg/day applied to the chest; 5 mg 3–4-hourly to infusion sites.
  - iv: 0.2–5 μg/kg/min. Effects occur within 2–5 min and last 5–10 min after stopping the infusion. Some preparations contain 30%–50% **propylene glycol** and alcohol. GTN is adsorbed on to PVC; polyethylene and rigid plastic/glass infusion sets are acceptable.
- Side effects: headache, flushing, hypotension, tachycardia. Tachyphylaxis is common.

Glycine. **Amino acid**, thought to be active as an inhibitory **neurotransmitter** at spinal interneurones. Increases membrane chloride conductance, causing postsynaptic hyperpolarisation. May also be involved in inhibitory pathways within the **ascending reticular activating system**. Also acts as a co-agonist with **glutamate** at **NMDA receptors**. Used as an irrigating solution for **TURP**. Systemic absorption is thought to be associated with CNS symptoms, e.g. transient blindness, via either central inhibitory pathways or transamination to serine, which is then deaminated to produce ammonia.

Glycocalyx. Complex layer of glycoproteins and proteoglycans that coats all intact vascular endothelium, varying in thickness between 0.1 and 1 μm. Facilitates binding of endothelial cells to cellular **adhesion molecules** (e.g. integrins, **immunoglobulins**), which in turn mediate interactions with **platelets** and leucocytes. Plays a critical role in **coagulation**, fibrinolytic and inflammatory systems; dysfunction (e.g. due to ischaemia, hyperglycaemia, hypervolaemia) may lead to capillary leak, hypo- or hypercoagulability, and accelerated inflammation. Several agents have been shown to reverse glycocalyx damage in animal models (e.g. **corticosteroids**, **heparin**, **nitric oxide**); these findings are yet to be replicated in human studies.

Alphonsus CS, Rodseth RN (2014). Anaesthesia; 69: 777–84

Glycogen. Storage form of **glucose**; consists of glucose molecules linked together into a branched polymer. Found mainly in liver and skeletal muscle, and formed from glucose 1-phosphate, derived from glucose 6-phosphate. Glycogenolysis provides glucose for **glycolysis**, and is increased by **adrenaline** via liver β-receptors (via **cAMP**) and α-receptors (via intracellular **calcium**). Defects in the various storage and breakdown pathways result in the **glycogen storage disorders**.

Glycogen storage disorders. **Inborn errors of metabolism** affecting **glycogen** and **glucose** metabolism. All are rare, and almost all are autosomal recessive. Classified according to the deficient enzyme and the site of abnormal glycogen storage; over 12 types have been described. Most lead to susceptibility to **hypoglycaemia** and **acidosis** with hepatomegaly; cardiac, mental and renal impairment may also occur. Perioperative principles include minimisation of fasting times, avoidance of hypoglycaemia, and maintenance of **acid–base balance**.

- The following are of particular concern:
  - type I: von Gierke's disease: glucose-6-phosphatase deficiency; i.e., cannot convert glucose to glycogen. Hypoglycaemia, acidosis, mental and growth retardation, hepatomegaly, platelet dysfunction and renal impairment may occur, with death within early childhood.
  - type II: Pompe's disease: acid maltase deficiency results in glycogen deposition in skeletal, cardiac and smooth muscle. **Cardiac failure** and generalised muscle weakness are common. Diaphragmatic weakness and hypertrophic **cardiomyopathy** also occur. The tongue may be enlarged. Enzyme replacement therapy is under investigation.
  - type V: McArdle's disease: skeletal muscle phosphorylase deficiency, impairing glycogenolysis. Muscle weakness and **myoglobinuria** may occur following **suxamethonium**. Muscle atrophy may follow use of tourniquets for surgery. Hypoglycaemia and acidosis are common.

[Edgar von Gierke (1877–1945), German pathologist; Joannes C Pompe (1901–1945), Dutch pathologist; Brian McArdle (1911–2002), English physician]

Glycolysis. Breakdown of **glucose** (six carbon atoms) to pyruvic acid or **lactate** (three carbon atoms). Each step in the pathway (*see Fig. 81*; **Glucose**) is catalysed by a specific enzyme. **Energy** released during the process is used to produce **ATP**. Reactions are anaerobic, with a net gain of 2 moles of ATP per mole glucose. Under aerobic conditions, pyruvic acid enters the **tricarboxylic acid cycle**, with a net gain of 36 more moles of ATP. Anaerobic energy production is therefore less efficient; formation of lactate from pyruvate limits ATP production to 2 moles per mole glucose. This may occur in exercising muscle and red blood cells.

Other pathways may branch from the glycolytic pathway, e.g. the hexose monophosphate shunt from glucose 6-phosphate in red blood cells. Protein and fat derivatives may enter the glycolytic chain and **glycogen** may be broken down to glucose 6-phosphate via glucose 1-phosphate.

Glycopeptides. Group of **antibacterial drugs**; include **vancomycin** and **teicoplanin**. Both are true antibiotics because they are derived from micro-organisms. Have bactericidal activity against aerobic and anaerobic gram-positive organisms, including meticillin-resistant *Staphylococcus aureus*.

Glycoprotein IIb/IIIa inhibitors, *see Antiplatelet drugs*

Glycopyrronium bromide (Glycopyrrolate). **Anticholinergic drug**, used as **premedication** and pre- and perioperatively to prevent or treat bradycardia. Also used to prevent muscarinic effects of **acetylcholinesterase inhibitors** used to reverse neuromuscular blockade. A quaternary ammonium compound, it does not cross the blood–brain barrier and therefore has minimal central effects, as opposed to **atropine** and **hyoscine**. Also less likely to cause tachycardia, mydriasis and blurred vision, but markedly reduces production of sweat and saliva. Its action persists for longer than that of atropine, reducing postoperative bradycardia. Dry mouth may persist postoperatively.

- Dosage:
  - 4–5 μg/kg im/iv.
  - with acetylcholinesterase inhibitors: 10–15 μg/kg.

'Golden hour'. Period following **trauma** in which active intervention is thought to be crucial in preventing the development of severe organ (especially brain) injury or death. The concept has arisen from the observation that many trauma victims die shortly after the insult; many of the survivors have evidence of persisting brain injury; and experimental brain injury may be considerably exacerbated by subsequent aggravating factors such as **hypoxaemia** and **hypotension** (and these two factors in particular are common after severe trauma). Similar considerations are likely to apply to other organs, although to less dramatic or significant extents.

Recognition of the importance of the first hour or so after trauma has fuelled the debate on whether it is better to resuscitate and stabilise victims at the scene of the accident before transfer to a hospital, or take them at once ('scoop and run'). The former approach is now generally accepted as being preferable in most cases for the above reasons, although controlled studies are rare and there are situations in which 'scoop and run' is favoured, e.g. penetrating cardiac trauma and close proximity of an appropriate hospital. In practice, the emphasis is on maintenance of oxygenation, stabilisation of major fractures and control of external haemorrhage, before undertaking as rapid a transfer as possible.

Rogers FB, Rittenhouse KJ, Gross BW (2015). Injury; 46: 525–7

See also, Head injury; Transportation of critically ill patients

Goldman cardiac risk index, *see Cardiac risk index*

Goldman constant-field equation. Equation used to calculate the **membrane potential** of a cell. Similar in concept to that of the **Nernst equation**, utilises the concentrations of sodium, potassium and chloride ions on either side of the membrane, and membrane permeability to each:

$$V = \frac{RT}{F}\ln\frac{P_{K^+}[K_o^+]+P_{Na^+}[Na_o^+]+P_{Cl^-}[Cl_i^-]}{P_{K^+}[K_i^+]+P_{Na^+}[Na_i^+]+P_{Cl^-}[Cl_o^-]}$$

where V = membrane potential
R = gas constant
F = Faraday constant
T = absolute temperature
$P_{K^+}, P_{Na^+}, P_{Cl^-}$ = permeability to potassium, sodium and chloride, respectively
$[K_o^+], [Na_o^+], [Cl_o^-]$ = outside concentration of ions
$[K_i^+], [Na_i^+], [Cl_i^-]$ = inside concentration of ions

[David E Goldman (1910–1998), US physiologist; Michael Faraday (1791–1867), English chemist]

Goodpasture's syndrome. Combination of **glomerulonephritis**, rapidly progressive pulmonary haemorrhage and antibodies against glomerular basement membrane (the first two may also occur without these antibodies, e.g. in systemic **vasculitides** and **connective tissue disease**, and strictly, do not constitute Goodpasture's syndrome). The antibodies react against a specific antigen present in both basement and alveolar membranes, hence the association. Often follows an upper respiratory tract infection or exposure to certain chemicals (e.g. glue sniffing), presumably via formation of new antigenic molecules, resulting in autoantibody production. Usually responds well to aggressive immunosuppressive therapy if treated early (i.e., before significant renal impairment). **Plasma exchange** has been used.

[Ernest W Goodpasture (1886–1960), US pathologist]

Greco A, Rizzo MI, DeVirgilio A, et al (2015). Autoimmun Rev; 14: 246–53

Graft-versus-host disease (GVHD). Potentially life-threatening condition affecting recipients of organ or tissue transplants in which donor inflammatory cells recognise host cells as being 'foreign' and mount an inflammatory response against them. Particularly problematic and aggressive when the transplanted cells are immunologically active, e.g. **bone marrow transplantation.** Acute GVHD typically occurs within 2–3 months of transplantation; affects mainly the skin, liver and GIT, causing rash, hepatic impairment, diarrhoea with sloughing of gut mucosa, and, in severe cases, death. A chronic form may also occur, affecting the same organ systems. Occurs to some extent in up to two-thirds of bone marrow recipients. Thought to be caused by transplanted T lymphocytes, GVHD may be prevented by various **immunosuppressive drugs** (and anti-T-cell antibodies) and removal of T cells from donor preparations, e.g. with radiation treatment. Activation of **cytokines** and other inflammatory mediators is also thought to be involved.

Treatment is with immunosuppressive drugs (typically **ciclosporin** and **prednisolone**), although the response may be poor unless started early. If survived, GVHD may protect against subsequent relapse of leukaemia. GVHD has also been described after intestinal, **heart–lung** and **liver transplantation.**

May also follow **blood transfusion**, especially in immunocompromised recipients or when first-degree relatives donate blood (involves close mismatch of leucocyte antigen haplotypes); prevented by transfusing irradiated blood products. Typically occurs up to a month post-transfusion; features are similar to those above.

Zeiser R, Blazar BR (2017). New Engl J Med; 377: 2167–79

Graham's law. Rate of **diffusion** of a gas is inversely proportional to the square root of its mw.

[Thomas Graham (1805–1869), Scottish chemist]

Gram-negative/positive bacteria, *see Bacteria*

Granisetron hydrochloride. **5-HT_3 receptor antagonist,** licensed as an **antiemetic drug** in postoperative and radiotherapy/chemotherapy-induced nausea and vomiting. Similar to **ondansetron.**

- Dosage:
  - nausea/vomiting following radiotherapy or chemotherapy: 1–2 mg orally, followed by 2 mg/day in 1–2 doses, or 10–40 µg/kg (up to 3 mg iv), diluted in 5 ml saline per 1 mg and given over 30 s or as iv infusion over 5 min, repeated up to twice in 24 h. A maximum of 9 mg/day should be given by any route.
  - **PONV:** 1 mg slowly iv as above, repeated up to 2 mg/day.
- Side effects: GI upset, headache, Q–T prolongation, arrhythmias.

Granulocyte colony-stimulating factor (G-CSF). Substance used to stimulate neutrophil production, especially in febrile neutropenic patients receiving chemotherapy. Has also been studied as a possible treatment of **MODS, SIRS** and **sepsis.** Various recombinant human preparations are available:

- filgrastim (unglycosylated G-CSF) and lenograstim (glycosylated G-CSF): similar effects on neutrophils.

- Side effects include musculoskeletal pain (especially sternum and iliac crests), hypotension, allergic reactions, hepatosplenomegaly, hepatic impairment.
- molgramostim (GM-CSF): stimulates production of all granulocytes and macrophages. Has more side effects than the preparations discussed earlier.

Estcourt LJ, Stanworth SJ, Hopewell S, et al (2016). Cochrane Database Syst Rev; 4: CD005339

Gravity suit, *see Antigravity suit*

Greener, Hannah (1832–1848). Fifteen-year-old girl, traditionally accepted as being the first recorded death under anaesthesia, although this is probably not the case (*see later*). She was having a toenail removed under open **chloroform** anaesthesia in Newcastle in January 1848, when she suddenly collapsed and died, despite attempted revival with brandy.

A report published in England in March 1848 referred to the death in July 1847 of a 55-year-old man, Alexis Montigny, in Auxerre, France. He died during removal of a breast tumour under ether anaesthesia, possibly because of airway obstruction ± aspiration or pulmonary oedema. Other reports from 1847 described early postoperative deaths associated with ether anaesthesia, although the causes are unclear.

Knight PR, Bacon D (2002). Anesthesiology; 96: 1250–3

Griffith, Harold Randall (1894–1985). Canadian anaesthetist in Montreal; famous for the use of **curare** in anaesthesia in 1942. None of the patients described apparently required respiratory assistance. Active in many other areas of anaesthetic research, including the properties of **cyclopropane**. Of world renown, he received many honours and medals.

Seldon TH (1986). Anesth Analg; 65: 1051–3

Growth hormone. Polypeptide hormone released from the anterior **pituitary gland**. Release is increased by:

- **hypoglycaemia**, sleep and exercise.
- stress; i.e., produced as part of the **stress response to surgery**.
- protein meal and **glucagon**.
- dopamine receptor agonists.

Growth hormone-releasing and inhibiting hormones (the latter is **somatostatin**) are released by the hypothalamus; growth hormone inhibits its own secretion.

- Effects:
  - increased skeletal growth and cell division.
  - increased protein synthesis, lipolysis and gluconeogenesis (anti-insulin effect). Oversecretion causes gigantism before puberty, **acromegaly** thereafter.

G-suit, *see Antigravity suit*

GTN, *see Glyceryl trinitrate*

GTT, *see Glucose tolerance test*

Guanethidine monosulfate. Antihypertensive drug, depleting adrenergic neurones of **noradrenaline** and preventing its release. Rarely used for hypertension now, but sometimes useful in **complex regional pain syndrome**; e.g. 10–25 mg in 20 ml saline injected iv into the exsanguinated arm (30–40 mg in 40 ml for leg), and the tourniquet kept inflated for 10–20 min. Close cardiovascular observation is required afterwards; hypotension may be delayed. A small amount of lidocaine is sometimes added. The procedure may be repeated, e.g. on alternate days for a number of weeks, often with long-lasting results.

May cause diarrhoea and postural hypotension.

Guedel, Arthur Ernest (1883–1956). US anaesthetist, practising in Indiana, then California. Considered a pioneer of modern anaesthesia; published extensively on many subjects, including tracheal tube **cuffs**, **divinyl ether**, **cyclopropane**, his pharyngeal airway (*see Airways*) and a classic description of the stages of anaesthesia. Received many honours and medals.

Baskett TF (2004). Resuscitation; 63: 3–5

Guillain–Barré syndrome (Acute inflammatory/postinfectious polyneuropathy). Acute inflammatory polyneuropathy described in 1916, although previously reported by Landry in 1859. Commonest cause of acute paralysis in the Western world. A number of variants are described. 95% of cases have a demyelinating polyneuropathy; in the remainder the axon itself is affected. The Fisher variant is characterised by ophthalmoplegia, ataxia and areflexia. Incidence is 1–2 per 100 000. 60% of cases follow an infective process (usually an upper respiratory tract infection or diarrhoeal illness) within the previous 6 weeks. Infectious agents implicated include campylobacter, mycoplasma, cytomegalovirus and **HIV**. May occasionally follow vaccination.

Thought to be an autoimmune condition. Antiganglioside antibodies are associated with the axonal variant, although no specific antibodies have been identified in the commoner demyelinating form.

- Features:
  - weakness, usually bilateral and symmetrical; typically ascending from the legs but may affect any region first. Cranial nerve involvement is common. Weakness typically develops over 1–7 days and reaches a nadir in 4 weeks. Areflexia is invariable. 30% require mechanical ventilation. Recovery takes from several weeks to months, and up to years if axonal damage has occurred. 10%–15% are left with residual disability; 5% relapse.
  - sensory disturbance: paraesthesia occurs in 50%, usually with glove and stocking distribution. Reduced touch, sensation and joint position sense may also occur. Pain (e.g. in the calves and back) is common and may be a presenting feature.
  - features autonomic disturbance include hypotension or hypertension, tachy- and bradyarrhythmias, ileus and urinary retention.

Diagnosed by history/clinical features. CSF protein is raised (without an increase in white cell count) in >90% of patients after a few days. Nerve conduction studies help to differentiate demyelination from axonal damage.

Differential diagnosis is extensive and includes **myasthenia gravis**, **poliomyelitis**, **porphyria**, lead and solvent poisoning, **botulism** and other causes of **peripheral neuropathy**.

- Management:
  - supportive:
    - turning/nursing care/physiotherapy.
    - prophylaxis against **DVT**.
    - adequate **nutrition**.
    - prompt treatment of infection, e.g. urinary, respiratory.

- appropriate treatment of haemodynamic abnormalities.
- respiratory: close monitoring of **vital capacity**; 15 ml/kg is usually taken as the minimum before IPPV is instituted, together with other features of **respiratory failure**. However, earlier tracheal intubation may be necessary if bulbar failure coexists. **Tracheostomy** is often necessary because prolonged respiratory support may be required.

- immunoglobulin therapy (IVIg) is now the specific treatment of choice: 0.4 g/kg/day iv over 3–5 days (*see Immunoglobulins, intravenous*).
- **plasma exchange** is equally effective as IVIg at speeding recovery and is most beneficial if performed within the first 2 weeks, and before ventilatory support is required. Usually performed daily for 4–5 days. Combining plasma exchange and IVIg has no additional benefit.
- **corticosteroids** have no role.
- **CSF filtration** has been used occasionally in severe, resistant cases.

[Georges Guillain (1876–1961), Jean A Barré (1880–1967) and Octave Landry (1826–1865), French neurologists; Charles Miller Fisher (1913–2012), Canadian-born US neurologist]

Willison HJ, Jacobs BC, van Doorn PA (2016). Lancet; 388: 717–27

GVHD, *see Graft-versus-host disease*

H_2 receptor antagonists. Competitive antagonists of H_2 **histamine** receptors. Used to reduce histamine-mediated gastric acid secretion in: **peptic ulcer disease**; **gastro-oesophageal reflux**; those at risk of **aspiration of gastric contents**; and to reduce gastric/duodenal bleeding in patients in ICU. Their routine use in critically ill patients receiving enteral feeding is declining because they increase the risk of nosocomial chest infections. Have also been used with **antihistamine drugs** to reduce the severity of **adverse drug reactions** and other allergic responses involving histamine.

- Drugs include:
  - **cimetidine**: introduced first. Cheapest, but with more side effects. Inhibits hepatic microsomal enzymes.
  - **ranitidine**: fewer side effects than cimetidine and does not inhibit hepatic enzymes. Longer duration of action.
  - **nizatidine**: similar to ranitidine.
  - famotidine: similar to ranitidine. Available for oral use only. Half-life is 2–3 h and duration of action about 10 h.

Marik PE, Vasu T, Hirani A, Pachinburavan M (2010). Crit Care Med; 38: 2222–8

Haemaccel, *see Gelatin solutions*

Haematocrit (Hct). Total red cell volume as a proportion of **blood volume**. Slightly higher in venous than arterial blood because of entry of chloride ions (**chloride shift**) into red cells with accompanying water entry. An easily measured index of O_2-carrying capacity of the blood, assuming normal red cell **haemoglobin** concentration and function. Normal values: 0.4–0.54 (male); 0.37–0.47 (female). **Haemodilution** to a Hct of 0.3–0.35 may be beneficial for tissue O_2 delivery (e.g. in critically ill patients) because of reduced blood **viscosity** and increased **flow**; a value below this level is thought to compromise **O_2 delivery**.

- Useful as a guide to adequate fluid replacement therapy, e.g.:
  - **blood loss**: indicates relative need for red cells/colloid.
  - plasma loss, e.g. **burns**: plasma deficit may be determined:

$$\text{fall in plasma volume (\%)} = 100 \times \left[1 - \left(\frac{1 - \text{new Hct}}{\text{new Hct}} \times \frac{\text{original Hct}}{1 - \text{original Hct}}\right)\right]$$

See also, Investigations, preoperative

Haemoconcentration. Increase in **haematocrit** and **haemoglobin** concentration following **dehydration** or plasma loss. Degree of haemoconcentration may indicate the extent of fluid deficiency. Does not occur immediately after **haemorrhage**, because red cells and plasma are lost together; compensatory mechanisms restoring blood volume cause subsequent **haemodilution**. In prolonged severe **shock**, however, fluid shifts into the interstitium with resulting haemoconcentration.

Haemodiafiltration. Modification of continuous arteriovenous or venovenous **haemofiltration** (CAVHD or CVVHD, respectively) in order to improve efficiency and solute clearance rate. Circuitry and other aspects are identical to those for haemofiltration except that 1–2 l/h of dialysate fluid is allowed to run counter-current to the blood flow on the filtrate side of the haemofilter (Fig. 82). Solute is cleared by a combination of diffusion and convection.

Haemodialysis. Technique for removal of solutes and water from blood by their passage across a semipermeable membrane into dialysis fluid (dialysate). Indications include **renal failure**, fluid overload and **pulmonary oedema**, electrolyte disturbances, severe **acidosis** and some cases of drug **poisoning and overdoses**.

- Principles:
  - vascular access: usually via a: 'single-needle', single-lumen catheter (through which blood is withdrawn into the dialyser and then returned to the patient in an alternating cycle); double-lumen central venous catheter (or two single ones); Silastic arteriovenous shunt connecting adjacent vessels, e.g. radial artery/cephalic vein (Scribner shunt); or permanent arteriovenous fistula (*see Shunt procedures*).
  - passage of blood via an extracorporeal circuit to a semipermeable membrane or hollow fibre system. Traditional cellulose-based membranes may be associated with **complement** activation and subsequent inflammatory cascade; thus newer synthetic membranes (e.g. polyacrylonitrile, polysulfone) are increasingly used, although more expensive. Dialysate may be passed on the other side of the membrane, usually in a counter-current fashion. Blood flow is usually 150–300 ml/min. The following are exchanged:
    - solutes: pass by diffusion from blood to dialysate, depending on the concentration gradient, size (mw) of solute, membrane porosity and duration of dialysis. Thus fluids of different composition may be used to remove different amounts of solute as required. Most dialysis fluids contain sodium, chloride, calcium, magnesium, acetate or bicarbonate (as an alkali source; bicarbonate itself cannot be added directly because it may precipitate calcium and magnesium) and variable amounts of glucose and potassium. Solutes may also pass across the membrane by applying a hydrostatic pressure across the membrane, thereby removing water (**ultrafiltration**); solutes that can pass through the membrane pores are swept along with the water (solvent drag).
    - water: removed by ultrafiltration. The amount of water extracted depends on the pressure gradient;

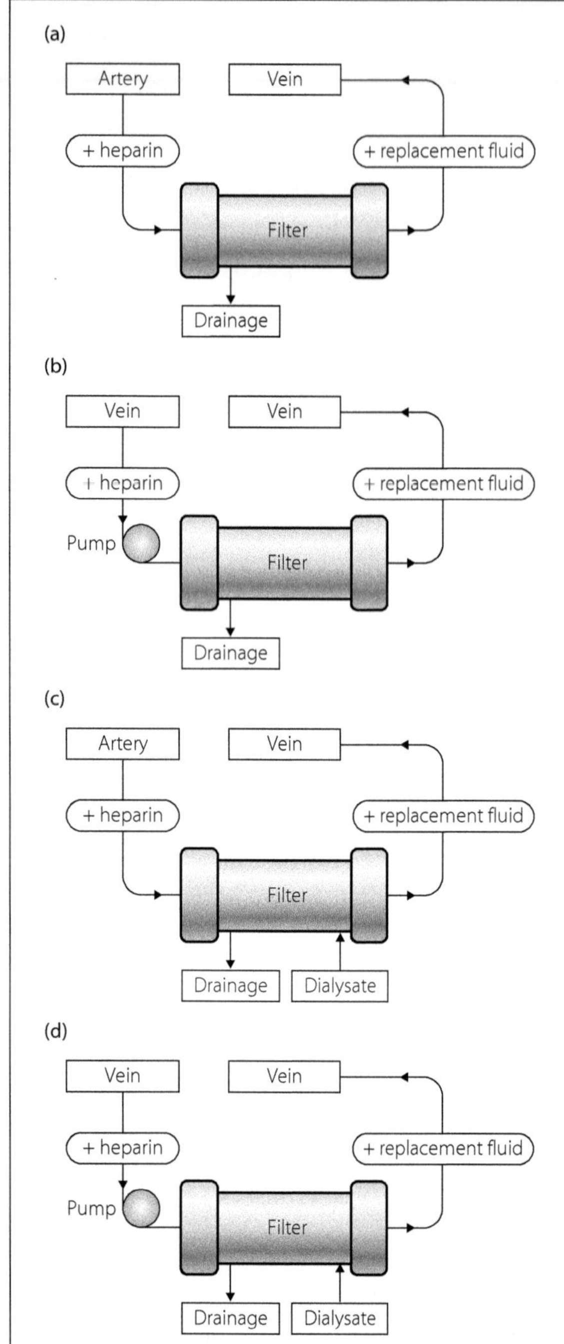

Fig. 82 Circuits used for (a) continuous arteriovenous haemofiltration (CAVH); (b) continuous venovenous haemofiltration (CVVH); (c) continuous arteriovenous haemodiafiltration (CAVHD); (d) continuous venovenous haemodiafiltration (CVVHD). Replacement fluid is often given pre-filter (termed pre-dilution) in order to prolong life of the filter

positive pressure may be applied to the blood side of the membrane, or negative pressure to the dialysate side.
- anticoagulation of the extracorporeal circuit is required, e.g. with **heparin** or **prostacyclin** infused into the line upstream to the dialysis machine. Control of coagulation with infusion of **protamine** to the downstream line has been used but may be difficult.
- return of blood to the patient.

Performed intermittently, e.g. for 4–6 h daily/weekly as required.
- Complications:
  - technical, e.g. related to vascular access and bleeding, **gas embolism**, clotting within the circuit. Modern machines usually incorporate alarms and monitors for air bubbles.
  - hypotension: may be related to **hypovolaemia**, **disequilibrium syndrome** or acetate in the dialysate (thought to cause vasodilatation and cardiac depression; replacement with bicarbonate has been suggested, although it is more complex to achieve).
  - increased susceptibility to infection, especially pneumonia secondary to bacteraemia; blood-transmitted viral infections (e.g. **hepatitis** B and C, **HIV** disease) may also occur.
  - hypoxaemia: mechanism is unclear.
  - electrolyte and acid–base disturbances.
  - increased rate of removal of many therapeutic drugs including salicylates, phenobarbital, disopyramide, methyldopa, lithium, theophylline, and many antibacterial drugs.

[Belding H Scribner (1921–2003), Seattle nephrologist]

Ricci Z, Romagnoli S, Ronco C (2016). F1000 Res; F1000 Faculty Rev: 103

See also, Dialysis; Haemodiafiltration; Haemofiltration

Haemodilution. Lowering of **haematocrit** and **haemoglobin** concentration due to fluid shift, retention or administration. May follow compensatory restoration of blood volume after **haemorrhage**, or iv fluid therapy with only partial replacement of red cell losses. Also occurs as a physiological process in **pregnancy**. Reduction of haematocrit lowers blood **viscosity** and increases **blood flow**, although O_2 content falls. Optimal haematocrit following acute blood loss is thought to be about 0.3; in addition to improved tissue blood flow, hazards of **blood transfusion** and risk of **DVT** are reduced. Animal studies of **cerebral ischaemia** have suggested reduced infarct size if early haemodilution is achieved, although human evidence (e.g. in **subarachnoid haemorrhage**) is lacking.

Haemofiltration. Common form of renal replacement therapy used in the ICU. First described in 1977; its main benefit over **haemodialysis** is cardiovascular stability. Initially described as continuous arteriovenous haemofiltration (CAVH; Fig. 82a) using an extracorporeal circuit via a surgically performed arteriovenous shunt (*see Shunt procedures*) or using large-bore arterial and venous cannulae. Blood flow through the circuit relies upon the arterial–venous pressure difference.

Now more frequently employs a continuous venovenous circuit (CVVH; Fig. 82b) using a large-bore double-lumen venous cannula and a peristaltic roller pump that incorporates monitors to detect **gas embolism** and extremes of circuit pressure. Blood is pumped at 100–200 ml/min. Anticoagulation of the extracorporeal circuit, but not the patient, is achieved using **heparin** (200–1000 U/h) or **prostacyclin** (2–10 ng/kg/min). Anticoagulation is not usually necessary if the patient has a coagulopathy.

Both CAVH and CVVH rely on the passage of blood through a filter containing a highly permeable membrane (polysulfone, polyamide or polyacrylonitrile; surface area 0.6–1.0 m^2) that acts as an artificial glomerulus. **Ultrafiltration** occurs by virtue of the hydrostatic pressure gradient between the blood and ultrafiltrate sides of filter; solute removal occurs because of convection. Water and solutes lost from the plasma are replaced by haemofiltration fluid containing water and electrolytes. Ultrafiltration can be slow and titrated to the patient response. Replacement fluid is infused into the 'arterial' limb of the circuit (pre-dilution) or, more usually, into the 'venous' limb after the filter (post-dilution). Pre-dilution may be useful when there is a high filtrate removal rate (>10 l/day) or a high **haematocrit** (>35%) as it decreases **viscosity** and subsequent clotting in the circuit. However, pre-dilution decreases the efficiency of the system as the blood being filtered contains a lower concentration of waste products.

Both CAVH and CVVH require an exchange of 12–20 l/day to achieve adequate solute clearance. Filtration can be increased by applying a negative pressure to the filtrate side of the filter or by increasing the distance between the filter and filtrate collecting chamber. In **haemodiafiltration**, dialysate fluid is passed through the filter to improve efficiency and solute clearance rate (Fig. 82c, d).

Complications relate to the extracorporeal circuit and vascular access (gas embolism, clotting, haemorrhage, **complement** activation, infection), ultrafiltration (**hypovolaemia**), electrolyte loss (**hyponatraemia, hypocalcaemia**), **hypothermia**, **metabolic alkalosis** (use of large volumes of lactate-rich replacement fluid) and removal of therapeutic drugs, including parenteral nutrition.

It has been suggested that CAVH and CVVH have a beneficial effect in **sepsis** by removing proinflammatory cytokines but no improvement in survival has been demonstrated.

See also, Haemodialysis; Renal failure

Haemoglobin (Hb). Red pigment in **erythrocytes**, composed of:
- globin: four polypeptide subunits, in two pairs. Different types of haemoglobin contain different types of polypeptide:
  - Hb A (adult): two α chains, two β chains.
  - Hb A_2 (usually 2%–3%): two α chains, two δ chains.
  - Hb F (fetal): two α chains, two γ chains.

  There are 141 amino acid residues in α chains; 146 in β, δ and γ chains.

  Fetal Hb is normally replaced by Hb A within 6 months of birth, unless polypeptide chain production is abnormal, e.g.:
  - **thalassaemia**: reduced synthesis of normal chains.
  - **haemoglobinopathies**, e.g. **sickle cell anaemia**: abnormal β chains are synthesised.
- haem: porphyrin derivative containing iron in the ferrous (Fe^{2+}) state. One haem moiety, containing one iron atom, is conjugated to each polypeptide. Oxidation of the iron to the ferric (Fe^{3+}) state forms methaemoglobin (high levels cause **methaemoglobinaemia**).

● Reactions of **Hb**:
- the iron atom in each haem moiety (remaining in the ferrous state but sharing one of its electrons) can reversibly bind one O_2 molecule, forming oxyhaemoglobin. Thus each Hb molecule can bind four O_2 molecules. In its deoxygenated form, the Hb molecule exists in a 'taut' configuration. Binding of one O_2 molecule breaks salt linkages between α- and β-globin chains and produces a more 'relaxed' configuration. This results in increased affinity for further binding ('cooperativity'), resulting in the sigmoid-shaped **oxyhaemoglobin dissociation curve**. Affinity is reduced by increasing $P\text{CO}_2$ (**Bohr effect**), acidity, temperature and amount of **2,3-DPG** present. Fetal Hb has greater affinity for O_2 than has adult Hb.
- CO_2 may bind reversibly to amino groups of the polypeptide chains, forming carbamino compounds ($RNH_2 + CO_2 \rightarrow RNHCO_2H$). Deoxygenated Hb has a greater affinity for CO_2 than oxygenated Hb (**Haldane effect**).
- imidazole groups of histidine residues act as **buffers** in the blood and provide a large buffering capacity owing to their abundance. Deoxygenated Hb is a weaker acid and better buffer than oxygenated.
- others:
  - with carbon monoxide, forming carboxyhaemoglobin.
  - formation of methaemoglobin.
  - causing **sulfhaemoglobinaemia**.
  - prolonged exposure to raised glucose levels in **diabetes mellitus**, forming glycosylated Hb.

Normal blood Hb concentration is 130–170 g/l (men), 120–160 g/l (women).

Hb is split into globin and haem portions when erythrocytes are destroyed. The iron is extracted and reused; the porphyrin ring opened to form biliverdin. The latter is converted to bilirubin and excreted via bile.

Hsia CCW (1998). N Engl J Med; 338: 239–47

See also, Anaemia; Carbon dioxide transport; Carbon monoxide poisoning; Methaemoglobinaemia; Myoglobin; Oxygen transport; Polycythaemia

Haemoglobinopathies. Diseases of abnormal **haemoglobin** production (cf. **thalassaemias**: impaired production of normal haemoglobin). Over 300 variants have been described, mostly due to single amino acid substitutions. Originally named after letters of the alphabet, then after the place of origin of the first patient described. Most are clinically insignificant, but some may lead to acute or chronic **haemolysis**, and some are associated with impaired O_2 binding and secondary **polycythaemia**. **Sickle cell anaemia** is the most important; it may be combined with other abnormalities, e.g. haemoglobin C. The latter on its own may cause mild haemolytic **anaemia** and splenomegaly. The only curative treatment of haemoglobinopathies is **bone marrow transplantation** although genetic therapy (e.g. gene editing) is under investigation.

Haemolysis. Abnormal destruction of **erythrocytes**. Normal red cell survival is about 120 days; bone marrow compensation may restore red cell volume if the lifespan is shortened. **Anaemia** may result if haemolysis is excessive, bone marrow abnormal, or haematinics (e.g. iron) are deficient. Haemolysis may result in **jaundice**, decreased **haptoglobin** concentration (*see later*) and reticulocytosis.

● Caused by:
- genetic red cell abnormalities:
  - membrane abnormalities, e.g. hereditary spherocytosis, elliptocytosis.
  - **haemoglobinopathies, thalassaemia**.
  - enzyme deficiencies, e.g. **glucose-6-phosphate dehydrogenase deficiency**, pyruvate kinase deficiency.
- acquired disorders:
  - immune:
    - autoimmune:
      - primary.
      - secondary to:
        - connective tissue diseases.
        - **malignancy**.

- infection, e.g. viral, mycoplasma.
- drugs, e.g. **penicillins, methyldopa, rifampicin, sulfonamides**.
- incompatible **blood transfusion** (including **rhesus blood group** incompatibility).

Antibodies bound to red blood cells may be detected by the direct Coombs' test; those circulating in the blood may be detected by the indirect Coombs' test.

- non-immune:
- infection, e.g. **malaria**, generalised **sepsis**.
- drugs, e.g. sulfonamides, phenacetin.
- lead poisoning.
- **renal** and **hepatic failure**.
- hypersplenism.
- trauma, e.g. prosthetic heart valves, extracorporeal circuits. Also associated with red cell damage following contact with vasculitic endothelium (e.g. **haemolytic–uraemic syndrome**).
- burns.
- **paroxysmal nocturnal haemoglobinuria**.

- Haemolysis may be:
  - extravascular: most common type; involves sequestration of red cells from the circulation.
  - intravascular, e.g. haemolytic–uraemic syndromes, paroxysmal nocturnal haemoglobinuria, incompatible blood transfusion. In the last example, renal damage results from immune complex and red cell stroma deposition. Haemoglobin is released into the plasma and binds to haptoglobulin; the resultant complex is rapidly removed by the liver. Thus the amount of plasma haptoglobulin is inversely related to the degree of haemolysis. If haemolysis is severe, free haemoglobin may appear in glomerular filtrate; if proximal tubular reabsorption is exceeded, haemoglobinuria and haemosiderinuria may result.

[Robin RA Coombs (1921–2006), Cambridge immunologist]

Haemolytic–uraemic syndrome. Acquired condition involving **thrombocytopenia**, a microangiopathic haemolytic **anaemia** and endothelial injury to the renal vasculature, leading to **acute kidney injury**. Usually occurs in children, especially following diarrhoea (usually due to Shiga toxin-producing *Escherichia coli*) or upper respiratory infection, but may occur in adults. Atypical forms may occur in cancer, infections and during chemotherapy administration. Closely related to **thrombotic thrombocytopenic purpura**, but neurological features such as **stroke** that characterise the latter are uncommon. A similar condition may occur postpartum or in women taking the contraceptive pill.

Treatment is mainly supportive. Although **heparin** and **prostacyclin** have been used, their benefit is unproven. **Plasma exchange** and **immunosuppressive drugs** have also been used.

Fakhouri F, Zuber J, Frémeaux-Bucchi V, Loirat C (2017). Lancet; 390: 681–96

See also, Haemolysis

Haemoperfusion. Removal of toxic substances from plasma by adsorption on to special filters, e.g. amberlite resin, activated **charcoal** granules coated in acrylic gel or cellulose. Performed in **poisoning and overdoses**, and **hepatic failure**. Modern devices are extremely efficient; complete removal of toxin from the body is limited by tissue binding. Thus haemoperfusion is most effective for poisons with small **volumes of distribution**, e.g. **barbiturates**, **disopyramide**, **theophylline** and methaqualone; these are rarely taken in overdose. **Tricyclic antidepressant drugs** are not removed. Requires vascular cannulation (e.g. femoral vein), extracorporeal circuit and heparinisation. Blood flow of 100–200 ml/min is employed, continued for several hours according to the clinical condition or plasma toxin levels.

Complications: as for **dialysis**. Thrombocytopenia was common with earlier adsorption columns.

Ghannoum M, Bouchard J, Nolin TD, et al (2014). Semin Dial; 27: 350–61

Haemophilia. X-linked recessive **coagulation disorder** with an incidence (type A) of 1:5000–10 000. One-third of cases are new mutations. Predominantly affects males, although female carriers may exhibit mild disease. Female homozygotes almost always die in utero. Results in deficiency of factor VIII (haemophilia A) or IX (haemophilia B; Christmas disease; one-tenth as common), leading to increased bleeding into muscles, joints and internal organs. The intrinsic **coagulation** pathway is slowed, with activated partial thromboplastin time prolonged; prothrombin and bleeding times are normal. Specific factor VIII/IX assay reveals reduced activity, and von Willebrand factor assay is normal.

- Intensive care/anaesthetic considerations:
  - risk of haemorrhage:
    - spontaneous bleeding may occur at factor VIII levels below 5%; prolonged bleeding may follow surgery or trauma at 5%–15%. At 15%–35%, bleeding is likely only if surgery or trauma is major; it is unlikely if levels exceed 35%, but over 50% is suggested for surgery where possible.
    - factor VIII is given as a concentrate (preferred), as cryoprecipitate, or as fresh frozen plasma, with haematological advice and monitoring of blood levels. **Half-life** is 8–12 h; adequate levels are required for at least a week postoperatively. About 15% of patients have circulating antibodies to factor VIII or IX, making control more difficult; **recombinant factor VIIa** may be useful in such cases.
    - **desmopressin** 0.4 μg/kg iv may transiently increase levels of factor VIII by 3–6 times in mild cases, and **tranexamic acid** 1 g orally may also be given.
    - im injections are avoided.
    - care should be taken with any invasive procedure, including venesection or arterial blood sampling.
    - **NSAIDs** and **antiplatelet drugs** should be avoided.
  - high risk of **HIV infection** in haemophiliacs given pooled factor VIII before the availability of recombinant factor VIII in the mid/late 1980s and of recombinant factor IX in 1997.

[Stephen Christmas (1947–1993); name of British patient in whom the disease was first described]

Mensah PK, Gooding R (2015). Anaesthesia; 70(suppl 1): 112–20

See also, Coagulation studies; von Willebrand's disease

Haemorrhage. Physiological effects of acute haemorrhage:
- **blood volume** is reduced, leading to reduced **venous return** and **cardiac output**.
- arterial BP falls, with activation of the **baroreceptor reflex**, reduced parasympathetic activity and increased sympathetic activity. Tachycardia, peripheral arterial vasoconstriction (to skin, viscera and kidneys) and venous constriction restore BP, initially. Classified in **ATLS** guidelines as follows:

- I: up to 15% of blood volume lost (usually little physiological change).
- II: 15%–30% lost (tachycardia, peripheral vasoconstriction, postural hypotension).
- III: 30%–40% lost (hypotension, mental confusion, maximum tachycardia).
- IV: >40% lost (cardiovascular collapse and **shock**). Bradycardia and hypotension may occur with over 20%–30% loss; thought to be vagally mediated, due to cardiac afferent C-fibre discharge caused by ventricular distortion and underfilling.

- increased **vasopressin** secretion and **renin/angiotensin system** activity causes vasoconstriction, sodium and water retention and thirst.
- **catecholamine** and corticosteroid secretion increase as part of the **stress response**.
- increased movement of interstitial fluid to the intravascular compartment and **third space**.

- Long-term effects:
  - increased **2,3-DPG** production, increasing tissue O_2 delivery.
  - increased plasma protein synthesis.
  - increased **erythropoietin** secretion and **erythropoiesis**.

Volume restoration takes 1–3 days after moderate haemorrhage, with reduction of **haematocrit** and plasma protein concentration.

- Features: as for **hypovolaemia**.
- Management:
  - local pressure over bleeding points/pressure points, supine position, raising the feet, O_2 therapy, military antishock trousers, specific haemostatic measures.
  - large-bore intravenous cannulae and **iv fluid administration**:
    - blood: cross-matched blood is best, but the test requires 45–60 min to complete. In time-critical life-threatening haemorrhage ABO-compatible blood can usually be issued within 10–15 min. If immediate transfusion is required and the options discussed earlier are unavailable, O Rhesus-negative blood is used.
    - **colloid** maintains intravascular expansion for longer than **crystalloid**.
    - crystalloid: saline is more effective than dextrose.
    - **CVP**, **urine** output and **cardiac output measurement** are useful for monitoring volume replacement and **fluid responsiveness**.

See also, Blood loss, perioperative; Blood transfusion; Colloid/crystalloid controversy; Damage control resuscitation; Trauma

Haemostasis, *see Coagulation*

HAFOE, High air-flow oxygen enrichment, *see Oxygen therapy*

Hagen–Poiseuille equation. For laminar **flow** of a **fluid** of **viscosity** η through a tube of length L and radius r, with pressure gradient P across the length of the tube:

$$\text{Flow} = \frac{Pr^4\pi}{8\eta L}$$

Originally derived by observing flow of liquid through rigid cylinders of different dimensions, with different driving pressures. Applied to **blood flow** through blood vessels, and **gas flow** through breathing systems and airways, although these tubes are neither rigid nor perfect cylinders.

[Jean Poiseuille (1797–1869), French physiologist; Gotthilf HL Hagen (1797–1884), German engineer]

Haldane apparatus. Burette for measuring gas volumes before and after removal of CO_2 by reaction with potassium hydroxide. The volume percentage of CO_2 in the original gas mixture may thus be determined. Similar determination of O_2 concentration may be performed, using pyrogallol as the absorbant.

[John Haldane (1860–1936), Scottish-born English physiologist]

See also, Carbon dioxide measurement; Gas analysis

Haldane effect. Increased capacity of deoxygenated blood for **CO_2 transport** compared with oxygenated blood.

- Results from:
  - increased binding of reduced **haemoglobin** to CO_2, forming carbamino groups (accounts for 70% of the effect).
  - increased buffering ability of reduced haemoglobin, allowing more CO_2 to be transported as bicarbonate.

Teboul J-L, Scheeren T (2017). Int Care Med; 43: 91–3

See also, Haldane apparatus

Half-life ($t_{1/2}$). The time taken for a substance undergoing decay to decrease by half. Commonly used to describe an **exponential process** (in which the half-life is constant), but may also refer to a non-exponential process (in which the half-life varies).

- Examples:
  - radioactive half-life (time taken for half the number of atoms to disintegrate).
  - drug half-life (time taken for drug concentration to fall by half, whether resulting from redistribution or **clearance**).

In **pharmacokinetics**, context-sensitive half-life refers to the time for plasma concentration of a drug to decrease by 50% after terminating an iv infusion that has maintained steady-state plasma concentration. For example, for **propofol** it is approximately 20 min after 2 h infusion, 30 min after 6 h infusion and 50 min after 9 h infusion. Corresponding figures for **midazolam** and **alfentanil** are in the order of 40 min, 70 min and 80 min; for **fentanyl**: 40 min, 4 h and 5 h. Ultra-short-acting drugs are less affected by 'context' (i.e., duration of infusion); for example, for **remifentanil** it is approximately 3 min, irrespective of the duration of the infusion.

See also, Time constant

Hall, Richard, *see Halsted, William Stewart*

Haloperidol. Butyrophenone used as a sedative and **antipsychotic drug.** Acts by blocking central (D_2) **dopamine receptors**. Also acts on cholinergic, serotonergic, histaminergic and **α-adrenergic receptors**. Has tranquillising effects without impairing consciousness; used to treat **confusion in the intensive care unit. Half-life** is approximately 20 h.

- Dosage:
  - psychosis and schizophrenia; 2–20 mg orally per day or 2–5 mg im/iv 4–8-hourly, up to 12 mg per day. A depot preparation, haloperidol decanoate, is given by deep im injection for long-term therapy (50–300 mg 4-weekly).
  - agitation in the elderly; 0.75–1.5 mg orally bd/tds.

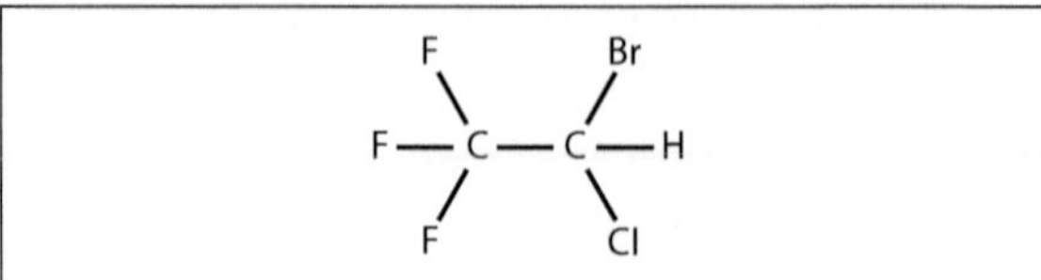

Fig. 83 Structure of halothane

- Side effects include **prolonged Q–T syndromes** (especially with higher doses and/or iv administration), extrapyramidal symptoms (parkinsonism, dystonia, tardive dyskinesia); may trigger the **neuroleptic malignant syndrome**. Other side effects are similar to those of **chlorpromazine**, but with less sedation and fewer antimuscarinic effects.

Halothane. 2-Bromo-2-chloro-1,1,1-trifluoroethane (Fig. 83). **Inhalational anaesthetic agent**, introduced in 1956. Its use rapidly spread because of its greater potency, ease of use, non-irritability and non-inflammability compared with **diethyl ether** and **cyclopropane**. Risks of **arrhythmias** and liver damage on repeated administration (halothane hepatitis) and introduction of newer agents (e.g. **sevoflurane**, which has replaced halothane as the agent of choice for inhalational induction) have led to a decline in its use. Discontinued for human use in the UK in 2007 and unavailable from 2013.

- Properties:
  - colourless liquid; vapour has characteristic pleasant smell and is 6.8 times denser than air.
  - mw 197.
  - boiling point 50°C.
  - SVP at 20°C 32 kPa (243 mmHg).
  - **partition coefficients**:
    - blood/gas 2.5.
    - oil/gas 225.
  - **MAC** 0.76%.
  - non-flammable.
  - supplied in liquid form with **thymol** 0.01%; decomposes slightly in light.
- Effects:
  - CNS:
    - smooth rapid induction, with rapid recovery.
    - anticonvulsant action.
    - increases **cerebral blood flow** but reduces **intraocular pressure**.
  - RS:
    - non-irritant. Pharyngeal, laryngeal and cough reflexes are abolished early, hence its value in difficult airways.
    - respiratory depressant, with increased respiratory rate and reduced tidal volume.
    - bronchodilatation and inhibition of secretions.
  - CVS:
    - myocardial depression and bradycardia. Has ganglion blocking and central vasomotor depressant actions. Hypotension is common.
    - myocardial O_2 demand decreases.
    - **arrhythmias** are common, e.g. bradycardia, nodal rhythm, ventricular ectopics/bigemini.
    - sensitises the myocardium to catecholamines, e.g. endogenous or injected **adrenaline**.
  - other:
    - dose-dependent uterine relaxation.
    - nausea/vomiting is uncommon.
    - may precipitate **MH**.

Up to 20% is metabolised in the liver. Metabolites include bromine, chlorine and trifluoroacetic acid; negligible amounts of **fluoride ions** are produced. Repeat administration after recent use may result in hepatitis.

0.5%–2.0% is usually adequate for maintenance of anaesthesia, with higher concentrations for induction. Tracheal intubation may be performed easily with spontaneous respiration, under halothane anaesthesia.
See also, Vaporisers

'Halothane shakes', *see Shivering, postoperative*

Halsted, William Stewart (1852–1922). US surgeon, pioneer of local anaesthetic nerve blocks with Hall and others. He and Hall described blocks of most of the nerves of the face, head and limbs, experimenting on each other and becoming **cocaine** addicts in the process. Chief of surgery and professor at Johns Hopkins University, where he started the first formal surgical training programme in the USA. Pioneer of aseptic technique, introducing use of rubber gloves during surgery.
[Richard J Hall (1856–1897), Irish-born US surgeon]
Osborne MP (2007). Lancet Oncol; 8: 256–65

Hamburger shift, *see Chloride shift*

Hanging drop technique. Method of identifying the **epidural space**, e.g. during **epidural** or **spinal anaesthesia**, described by Guitierrez in 1933. A drop of saline is placed at the hub of a needle that is advanced towards the epidural space; when the space has been entered the drop is drawn into the needle by the negative pressure within the space. Not always reliable, because negative pressure is not always present.
[Alberto Guitierrez (1892–1945), Argentinian surgeon and anaesthetist]
Aldrete AJ, Auad O, Guitierrez VP, Wright AJ (2005). Reg Anesth Pain Med; 30: 397–404

Haptoglobin. Alpha-globulin synthesised by the liver, that binds free **haemoglobin** in the blood. Normal serum level is 30–190 mg/dl; this usually binds 100–140 mg free haemoglobin per 100 ml plasma. Haptoglobin–haemoglobin complex is rapidly removed from the circulation by the reticuloendothelial system; if the liver is unable to produce new haptoglobin quickly enough, the plasma haptoglobin level falls. Although the reduction in haptoglobin is used mainly as a sensitive indicator of intravascular **haemolysis**, it may also occur if haemolysis is extravascular.

Haptoglobin is an acute-phase protein, but may also be raised in carcinoma and inflammatory disease and after trauma or surgery.
See also, Acute-phase response

Harmonics. Related sine waveforms; the frequency of each is a multiple of the fundamental frequency of the first harmonic, the slowest component of the series. Complex **waveforms** may be produced by adding higher harmonics to the first (fundamental) harmonic. **Monitoring** equipment must be able to reproduce harmonics of high enough frequency for the signal recorded; e.g. up to the 10th harmonic for many recorders. More harmonics are required for more complex waveforms with higher frequencies, increasing the required frequency response of the monitor concerned, e.g. **ECG** 0.5–80 Hz, **EEG** 1–60 Hz, **EMG** 2–1200 Hz.
See also, Fourier analysis

Harnesses. Used to secure breathing attachments or facemasks to the patient. May damage soft tissues around the face, and **airway obstruction** may still occur.

- Examples:
    - Clausen harness: triangular back placed behind the head, with straps at each corner for attachment to hooks around the facemask.
    - Connell harness: square back placed behind the head, with attachments at each end for the sides of the facemask.
    - Hudson harness (for dental surgery): long strap for fixation of the catheter mount from the nasotracheal tube; binds around the patient's forehead.

Formerly widely used during 'mask' anaesthesia, their use has declined with increasing use of **SADs**, though many modern facemasks are still supplied with plastic hooks for attachment. Their disposable silicone/rubber equivalents are used for **non-invasive positive pressure ventilation** or **CPAP**.

[RJ Clausen (1890–1966), English anaesthetist; Karl Connell (1873–1941), US surgeon; Maurice WP Hudson (1901–1992), London anaesthetist]

Hartmann's solution (Ringer's lactate; Compound sodium lactate). **Intravenous fluid** containing sodium 131 mmol/l, potassium 5 mmol/l, calcium 2 mmol/l, chloride 111 mmol/l and sodium **lactate** 29 mmol/l. pH is 5–7. Originally formulated from **Ringer's solution** for fluid replacement and treatment of metabolic acidosis in children, using an isotonic solution containing more sodium than chloride. Lactate is metabolised to **glucose** and **bicarbonate** by the liver within a few hours, and the hazards of bicarbonate administration avoided. Now widely used as the crystalloid of choice for **ECF** replacement, because it is more 'physiological' in make-up; however, its advantage over saline solutions for routine use has been questioned.

Often avoided in patients with renal failure because of the risk of **hyperkalaemia**, in sick patients or those with hepatic failure because of the risk of hyperlactataemia (although the relevance of this is unclear), and in diabetics because of the risk of hyperglycaemia (although significant increases in blood glucose are unlikely unless very large volumes are infused). Due to its calcium content, may cause clotting of stored blood when transfused through a line that has not first been flushed with saline.

[Alexis Hartmann (1898–1964), US paediatrician]

Lee JA (1981). Anaesthesia; 36: 1115–21

Hayek oscillator, *see Intermittent negative pressure ventilation*

Hb, *see Haemoglobin*

HBE, *see His bundle electrography*

Hct, *see Haematocrit*

HDU, *see High dependency unit*

Head injury. Common cause of morbidity and mortality in **trauma**, especially in young males; it should be suspected in all trauma cases, especially those involving the chest and neck. The most serious aspects are usually related to **TBI** but there may also be other important associated injuries, including **facial trauma**, upper **spinal cord injury** and **chest trauma**.

General management is as for the above, with an assumption that significant TBI and **cervical spine** injury have occurred until these can be ruled out.

Head's paradoxical reflex. Sustained diaphragmatic contraction, followed by shallow respiration, after a small passive lung inflation. A rare example of a positive feedback loop in the human nervous system; thought to be important in the first breaths of the neonate. May also be elicited in apnoeic anaesthetised patients.

[Sir Henry Head (1861–1940), English neurologist]

Widdicombe J (2004). J Physiol; 559: 1–2

See also, Gasp reflex

Health and safety issues, *see COSHH regulations; Environmental safety of anaesthetists; Scavenging*

Healthcare Commission, *see Care Quality Commission*

Healthcare Quality Improvement Partnership (HQIP). Body established in 2008 and contracted by the UK Department of Health to oversee national audits, registers and confidential enquiries. Led by a consortium including the Academy of Medical Royal Colleges, the Royal College of Nursing and patient representatives. Programmes of particular relevance to anaesthesia include audits/registers of various cancers, paediatric intensive care, cardiac surgery/cardiology, pain, carotid endartectomy, **fractured neck of femur**, and the **Confidential Enquiries into Maternal Deaths**.

Heart. Develops from a single tube that doubles up forming primitive atrium and ventricle; divided by septa into left and right sides (*see Atrial septal defect; Ventricular septal defect*). The primitive arterial outlet (truncus arteriosus) splits to form the aorta and pulmonary trunk; the venous inlet (truncus venosus) absorbs into the smooth-walled part of the right atrium.

- Surface anatomy:
    - right border: from third to sixth right costal cartilages, 1–1.5 cm from the right sternal edge.
    - left border: from second left costal cartilage, 1–1.5 cm from the left sternal edge, to the apex beat (usually at the fifth left intercostal space in the midclavicular line).
    - upper limit: level with the angle of Louis (T4–5).
    - base: level with the xiphisternum (T8–9).

The left border is composed mainly of left ventricle, the right border mainly of right atrium, and the base mainly of right ventricle, as on the **CXR**. Weighs about 300 g. Enclosed within **pericardium**.

- Chambers:
    - right atrium:
        - bears the right auricular appendage (broad and triangular).
        - receives superior and inferior venae cavae, and coronary sinus.
    - right ventricle:
        - crescent-shaped in cross-section, due to bulging of the left ventricle.
        - tendinous cords from the interventricular septum and papillary muscles attach to the tricuspid valve.
        - pulmonary valve: composed of three cusps.
    - left atrium: bears the left auricular appendage (narrow and tubular) and receives four valveless pulmonary veins.

- left ventricle:
  - thick-walled.
  - the bicuspid mitral valve is anchored by tendinous cords as for the tricuspid valve. The anterior cusp is larger.
  - aortic valve: composed of three semilunar cusps, one anterior and two posterior.
- Blood supply: *see Coronary circulation*
- Nerve supply: from **vagus** and **sympathetic nervous system** from upper thoracic and cervical ganglia; mainly T1–4. The cardiac plexus receives branches from both components of the autonomic nervous system.

[Antoine Louis (1723–1792), French surgeon]

See also, Action potential; Atrial …; Cardiac …; Coronary …; Heart …; Left ventricular …; Myocardial …; Ventricular ….

Heart, artificial. Device used to replace or assist the heart in end-stage **cardiac failure** when **heart transplantation** is unavailable, or following **cardiac surgery**.

- Main types:
  - left ventricular assist devices (LVAD): previously used solely as a 'bridging' therapy pending heart transplant, now increasingly used as a definitive (or 'destination') therapy. First-generation pneumatic pumps provided pulsatile flow but involved interaction between multiple moving parts (including valves) and thus had a high failure rate. Newer, non-pulsatile flow devices do not require valves and are more reliable; they utilise either a spinning 'impeller' within a conduit, drawing blood in a continuous stream from the left ventricular apex and delivering it to the descending aorta, or more recently, a centrifugal pump. Significant reduction in mortality and morbidity (compared with medical therapy alone) is achievable, but requires adequate right ventricular function.
  - total artificial heart: indicated in patients with biventricular failure awaiting heart transplant (i.e., not currently licensed as a definitive therapy). Consist of two pneumatically driven pumps with tilting disc valves. Patients must remain in hospital.

Main problems are related to infection, thromboembolism, and reliability and flexibility of the devices.

Yaung J, Arabia FA, Nurok M (2017). Anesth Analg; 124: 1412–22

Heart block. Usually refers to atrioventricular (AV) block, i.e., interruption of impulse propagation between atria and ventricles. **Bundle branch block** refers to interruption distal to the atrioventricular node.

- Classification:
  - first-degree (Fig. 84a): delay at the AV node:
    - **P–R interval** >0.2 s at normal heart rate.
    - usually clinically insignificant.
    - caused by:
      - ageing.
      - **ischaemic heart disease.**
      - increased vagal tone.
      - drugs, e.g. **halothane, digoxin.**
      - **cardiomyopathy, myocarditis.**
  - second-degree: occasional complete block. May be:
    - Mobitz type I (Wenckebach phenomenon) (Fig. 84b):
      - AV delay; P–R interval lengthens with successive **P waves** until complete AV block occurs, i.e., no **QRS complex** follows the P wave. The cycle then repeats.

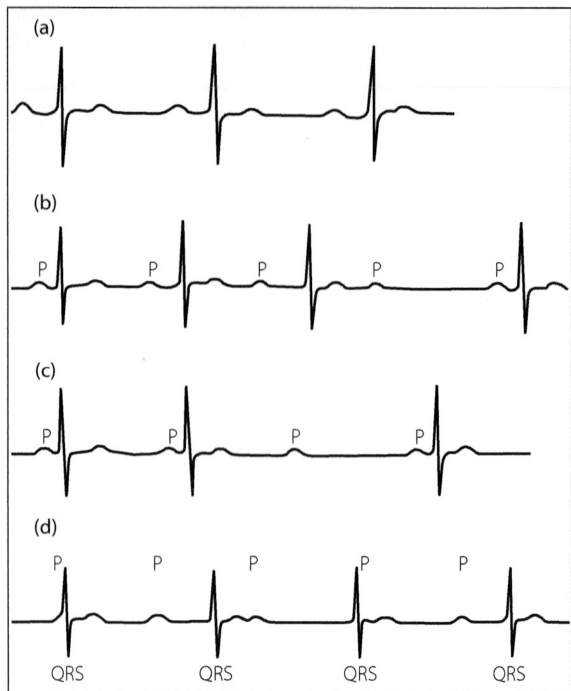

Fig. 84 Heart block: (a) first-degree; (b) second-degree, Mobitz I; (c) second-degree, Mobitz II; (d) third-degree

      - usually due to AV conduction delay.
      - rarely proceeds to complete heart block.
    - Mobitz type II (Fig. 84c):
      - sudden block below the AV node; i.e., P–R interval may be normal. May occur regularly, e.g. every second or third complex (termed 2:1 or 3:1 block, respectively).
      - at risk of developing complete heart block, particularly if it occurs regularly.
  - third-degree (Fig. 84d): complete heart block, at the AV node or below:
    - **ECG** demonstrates independent atrial and ventricular activity, the latter arising from an ectopic site. The ventricular rate is usually slow, especially if the ectopic site is far from the AV node (wide QRS complexes; rate <45/min).
    - clinical findings:
      - hypotension is common.
      - wide pulse pressure (large stroke volume).
      - cannon waves in the **JVP.**
      - escape ventricular arrhythmias may occur.
    - caused by:
      - old age.
      - ischaemic heart disease.
      - myocarditis/cardiomyopathy.
      - **cardiac surgery.**
      - increased vagal tone.
      - **β-adrenergic antagonists**, digoxin.
      - **hyperkalaemia.**
      - congenital abnormality.

Preoperative insertion of a **pacemaker** or pacing wire should be considered in those with symptomatic first-degree/Mobitz type I, or Mobitz type II/complete heart block (with or without symptoms). In emergency situations, transcutaneous pacing or **isoprenaline** 0.02–0.2 μg/kg/min may be used to increase ventricular rate in complete heart

block. **Antiarrhythmic drugs** that suppress ventricular activity should be avoided.
[Karl Wenckebach (1848–1904), Dutch physician; Woldemar Mobitz (1889–1951), German cardiologist]
See also, Pacemakers

Heart, conducting system. Composed of:
- sinoatrial node: at the junction of the superior vena cava and right atrium. Normally discharges more rapidly than the rest of the heart, thus setting the rate of contraction, although all cardiac muscle is capable of depolarising spontaneously.
- atrioventricular node (AV node): lies in the atrial septum, above the coronary sinus opening. Normally the only means of conduction between atria and ventricles; the bundle of Kent is an abnormal accessory conduction pathway that bypasses the AV node, and is present in **Wolff–Parkinson–White syndrome**.
- bundle of His: divides into left and right bundle branches above the interventricular septum, passing down on either side subendocardially:
  - the left bundle branch divides into anterior and posterior fascicles.
  - Purkinje fibres spread from the ends of bundle branches/fascicles to the rest of the ventricles.

Impulses pass from node to node through normal atrial muscle, then via specialised cardiac muscle cells, insulated from the rest of the myocardium by connective tissue sheaths. Conduction through each of the following takes about 0.1 s:
- atria.
- AV node.
- bundle of His/Purkinje system.

Vagal and sympathetic innervation is directed to both nodes; conduction through the AV node is slowed by the former and speeded by the latter.

Ventricular depolarisation begins at the heart's apex and spreads outwards and upwards, causing the ventricles to shorten in a spiral fashion, encouraging upward expulsion of blood into the great arteries.

Interruption of impulse conduction may result in **bundle branch block** or **heart block**.
[Wilhelm His (1863–1934), German anatomist; Albert Kent (1863–1958), English physiologist and radiologist; Johannes von Purkinje (1787–1869), Czech physiologist]

Heart failure, *see Cardiac failure*

Heart–lung transplantation. First performed in 1968 with poor results; outcomes have steadily improved since the 1980s, although rates have declined due to limited organ availability and evolving indications (e.g. isolated **lung transplantation** can now provide similar outcomes for **cystic fibrosis**). Worldwide ~50 are performed each year, with 1-year survival ~70%.
- Indications include: **pulmonary hypertension**, **Eisenmenger's syndrome**, **pulmonary fibrosis**, cystic fibrosis and emphysema.
- Donor:
  - as for **heart transplantation**, with normal CXR, minimal sputum and no history of aspiration or pulmonary oedema. Arterial $P\text{O}_2$ should exceed 13.3 kPa (100 mmHg) with $F_I\text{O}_2$ 0.4.
  - the heart and lungs are placed into a bag and immersed in cold electrolyte solution, with IPPV at low rates and perfusion of the coronary arteries with donor blood. Whole body transfer using cardiopulmonary bypass has also been used.
- Recipient:
  - immunosuppression and general management as for heart transplantation.
  - the trachea is divided above the carina. Damage to vagi, phrenic and recurrent laryngeal nerves is possible.
  - **PEEP** and inotropes are usually required; **isoprenaline** is particularly useful because of its ability to reduce **pulmonary vascular resistance**. Pulmonary oedema and sputum retention are common. The cough reflex is destroyed and **ciliary activity** impaired.
  - **weaning** from IPPV is as for cardiac surgery.
  - lung rejection may occur without heart rejection, and may be difficult to detect. **Graft-versus-host disease** may also occur.

Idrees JJ, Petterrson GB (2016). Curr Cardiol Rep; 18: 36 (1–9)

Heart murmurs. General principles:
- caused by turbulent flow of blood, including abnormal flow through a normal valve or normal flow though an abnormal valve or orifice.
- systolic murmurs may be physiological; diastolic murmurs are always pathological.
- low murmurs are heard best with the stethoscope bell, high-pitched ones with the diaphragm.
- left-sided murmurs are heard best at end-expiration; right-sided ones best at end-inspiration.
- murmurs radiate usually in the direction of turbulent flow.
- when auscultating the heart, murmurs are best described by:
  - time of occurrence.
  - site and radiation.
  - character including relation to respiration. Loudness is usually expressed as a score of 1–5, where 1 = only just audible; 5 = audible without a stethoscope.
  - associated **heart sounds**.
- Classification:
  - systolic:
    - pansystolic:
      - **VSD**.
      - **mitral regurgitation**.
      - tricuspid regurgitation.
    - ejection:
      - **aortic stenosis** or sclerosis (although severe disease can produce a pansystolic murmur).
      - pulmonary stenosis.
      - **ASD**.
  - diastolic:
    - **mitral stenosis**.
    - **aortic regurgitation**.
  - continuous:
    - patent **ductus arteriosus**.

(N.B. Venous hum: due to kinking of major neck veins, especially in children. Abolished by pressure on the neck.)
See also, Cardiac cycle; Preoperative assessment; Pulmonary valve lesions; Tricuspid valve lesions

Heart rate. Normal range in adults is usually defined as 60–100 beats/min, but it may be less than 50 beats/min in fit young subjects, and increase up to 200 beats/min on **exercise**. Rate is ~100 beats/min in the denervated heart. In children, heart rate decreases with age from 110–160 beats/min during infancy, reaching adult values at about 12 years.

- Rate is increased by:
  - sympathetic activity, e.g. secondary to **hypotension, hypoxaemia, hypercapnia, pain, fear, anger, exercise.**
  - hormones, e.g. **catecholamines**, thyroxine.
  - infection and fever.
  - **Bainbridge reflex** and inspiration.
  - drugs, e.g. **salbutamol.**
- Rate is decreased by:
  - parasympathetic activity via the **vagus nerve**, e.g. secondary to the **baroreceptor reflex**, fear, pain, raised **ICP**, expiration.
  - hypoxaemia.
  - drugs, e.g. **neostigmine, β-adrenergic receptor antagonists.**

Critically ill children often respond to handling, tracheobronchial suction, hypoxaemia and acidosis with a profound bradycardia.

See also, Arrhythmias; Pacemaker cells; Sinus arrhythmia; Sinus bradycardia; Sinus rhythm; Sinus tachycardia

Heart sounds. The first sound is due to closure of the tricuspid and mitral valves; it lasts 0.15 s with frequency 25–45 Hz. The second is due to closure of the aortic and pulmonary valves; it lasts 0.12 s with frequency 50 Hz. Valve opening is normally silent.

- Intensity:
  - quiet in obese or muscular subjects, and in **pericarditis.**
  - second sound is quiet in **aortic stenosis**, because valve mobility is reduced.
  - first sound is quiet in **mitral regurgitation**, because valve closure is incomplete.
  - first sound is increased in **mitral stenosis**, because the valve is kept open right up to systole by increased left atrial pressure, instead of gradual closure at end of diastole.
- Splitting of the second sound:
  - heard at the left sternal edge.
  - the aortic component normally precedes the pulmonary component, because left ventricular emptying is faster than that of the right.
  - increased in inspiration, when right ventricular contraction is delayed by increased preload. Fixed in **ASD**; reversed in left **bundle branch block** and severe aortic stenosis, when left ventricular emptying is markedly prolonged.
- Extra sounds:
  - third heart sound (thought to be due to ventricular filling). Occurs shortly after the second sound. May occur in normal subjects, also in reduced ventricular compliance/increased volume, e.g. in **cardiac failure**, mitral regurgitation, **VSD.**
  - fourth heart sound (thought to be due to atrial contraction under pressure with forceful ventricular distension). Occurs shortly before the first sound. Always pathological, reflecting poor ventricular compliance; may occur in aortic stenosis, pulmonary stenosis, **hypertension.**
  - gallop rhythm: all four sounds, e.g. cardiac failure.
  - others, e.g. the late ejection click of aortic stenosis, the late systolic click of **mitral valve prolapse**, and the early diastolic opening snap of mitral stenosis.
  - **heart murmurs.**

See also, Cardiac cycle; Preoperative assessment

Heart transplantation. First performed in humans in 1967 by Barnard. Survival was initially severely limited by graft rejection. Interest resurged in the late 1970s with the introduction of **ciclosporin**; median survival after transplant is now ~11 years.

- Indications: mostly end-stage **ischaemic heart disease** and **cardiomyopathy**; also **congenital heart disease**, valvular disease and others.
- Contraindications include advanced age, insulin-dependent **diabetes mellitus**, active infection, and recent **PE/MI**; these contraindications have been relaxed in recent years.
- Donor:
  - normal past medical history/examination and ECG. A short period of cardiac arrest, and minimal requirements for inotropic support are acceptable.
  - initial management including **heparin** and **cardioplegia** is as for **cardiac surgery**. The heart is placed in cold crystalloid solution and both the atria opened; it is transported in ice.
- Recipient:
  - most patients are prepared for the possibility of emergency transplantation. By definition they are in poor general health, i.e., high-risk patients.
  - **immunosuppressive drugs** include **corticosteroids**, ciclosporin, **tacrolimus**, **mycophenolate** (which has superseded **azathioprine**), and antithymocyte immunoglobulin.
  - all iv lines, tracheal tube, laryngoscope, tubing, etc., are sterile to reduce infection.
  - general management is as for cardiac surgery. After **cardiopulmonary bypass** and aortic cross-clamping, the ventricles are removed, leaving most of the atria. The atria and aortas are anastomosed. The donor heart may also be piggy-backed next to the original heart (heterotopic transplantation, i.e. to a different site in the recipient's body from its position in the donor), anastomosing left atria, aortas, pulmonary arteries and venae cavae.
  - inotropes are usually required for over 24 h. The denervated **heart rate** is usually faster than that of the innervated heart, with no response to indirectly acting drugs, e.g. **atropine**. Drugs acting directly on the myocardium (e.g. **isoprenaline**) are used. The rate responds slowly to circulating catecholamines. Postoperative care is as routine, but barrier nursing is required.
  - rejection may be diagnosed by endocardial biopsy via the right internal jugular vein.
  - late complications include those of immunosuppression and cardiac allograft vasculopathy (obliterative vasculopathy that leads to late allograft failure).

For anaesthesia in a heart recipient, aseptic techniques and directly acting cardiovascular drugs are used, as discussed earlier. Otherwise, management is as for any high-risk cardiac case. 90% of recipients return to full activity and 40% to work 1 year after transplantation. However, current demand for hearts exceeds supply. Cardiac denervation during transplantation means that ~90% of patients do not suffer angina.

[Christian N Barnard (1922–2001), South African surgeon]

Davis MK, Hunt SA (2014). Trends Cardiovasc Med; 24: 341–9

See also, Heart–lung transplantation

Heat. Form of **energy** associated with movement of particles (e.g. molecules, atoms) within a substance or system; **temperature** describes the propensity for transfer of heat energy between systems.

- Heat is transferred by:
  - radiation: especially from bright, shiny bodies to dark, matt bodies.
  - convection: as air next to a warm body is warmed, it expands and becomes less dense, rising and being replaced by colder air.
  - evaporation: heat is transferred to liquid molecules, providing the energy required to break the bonds between them, thus forming a vapour.
  - conduction: especially via good conductors of heat, e.g. metals.

All these routes may be important in **heat loss during anaesthesia**.

See also, Temperature regulation

Heat capacity. Quantity of **heat** required to raise the **temperature** of a mass by 1 K (J/K). Specific heat capacity (*C*) is the quantity of heat required to raise the temperature of unit mass of substance by 1 K (J/kg/K). The total heat capacity of an object may be calculated from knowledge of the mass and values for *C* of its constituent parts.

- Examples of *C*:
  - human tissues, including blood: 3.5 kJ/kg/K.
  - water: 4.18 kJ/kg/K (1 Cal/kg/°C).

For a gas, C_p is specific heat capacity at constant pressure, and C_v is specific heat capacity at constant volume. For an ideal gas, $C_p - C_v = R$ (**universal gas constant**).

Because gases are much less dense than liquids, the energy required to heat unit volume is much less. Thus little energy is expended in heating inspired air (although significant energy is expended humidifying it).

See also, Latent heat

Heat loss, during anaesthesia. Prevention is important because of the adverse effects of **hypothermia** and the increased O_2 consumption (up to 5 times) caused by postoperative **shivering**. In addition, the duration of action of neuromuscular blocking drugs is prolonged and drug **clearance** delayed. Particularly important in **neonates** and children, and in the **elderly**, because of reduced reserves.

- **Temperature** may fall by several °C during surgery, via:
  - reduced heat production and impaired **temperature regulation**. Neuraxial anaesthesia and anaesthetic agents both lower the temperature thresholds for the onset of shivering and vasoconstriction; the latter results in rapid redistribution of heat from the core to the periphery, and accounts for the initial drop in core temperature during surgery.
  - increased loss of **heat**:
    - radiation (accounts for 40%–50% of loss): increased if the patient is uncovered and surrounded by cold objects. Also increased by vasodilatation.
    - convection (15%): increased if the patient is uncovered.
    - evaporation (30%–35%): increased if a body cavity is opened, especially if ambient humidity is low. Heat loss via evaporation in the trachea and airways may be considerable if inspired gases are not humidified.
    - conduction (3%): usually a less important route; increased by use of cold irrigating solutions.
- Prevention:
  - identification of high-risk patients:
    - extremes of age.
    - ill, malnourished patients.
    - prolonged surgery/open body cavity.
    - major blood loss.
    - **sickle cell anaemia**.
  - **temperature measurement** during anaesthesia.
  - covering during transfer to the operating suite.
  - maintenance of ambient temperature at 22°–24°C and **humidity** about 50% (compromise between patient temperature and staff comfort).
  - covering with drapes, reflective garments and head coverings (especially children).
  - warming of all skin cleansing solutions and iv fluids.
  - **humidification** of inspired gases.
  - warming blankets, e.g. using heated water or air.
  - warming of the bed/blankets postoperatively.

Sessler DI (2016). Lancet; 387: 2655–64

Heat–moisture exchanger (HME; Swedish nose; hygroscopic condenser). Passive humidifier device. Positioned between the breathing tubing and the facemask, tracheal/tracheostomy tube or other airway device. Originally contained material (e.g. sponges, paper or metal mesh) that acts as a screen that can absorb large amounts of water. During expiration, latent heat of the water is transferred to the mesh resulting in condensation; the heat and water produced warm and humidify inspiratory gases. Most models are disposable with single patient use. Minimum recommended moisture output is 20 g/m³ for anaesthesia and 30 g/m³ for intensive care.

Modern HMEs contain bacterial filters (HMEF) with a pore size of 0.2 µm, which trap >99% of bacteria. Filters are either high-density pleated or low-density electrostatic models.

Efficiency is reduced in the presence of large tidal volumes, drug nebulisers and copious secretions. All devices increase **dead space** and increase the **work of breathing**.

Wilkes AR (2011). Anaesthesia; 66: 31–9, 40–51

See also, Filters, breathing system; Humidification

Heat of vaporisation, *see Latent heat*

Heatstroke, *see Hyperthermia*

Heavy metal poisoning. Poisoning by exposure to any toxic metal (regardless of its molecular weight), including lead, mercury, arsenic, cadmium, bismuth, aluminium, antimony, chromium, cobalt, copper, gold, manganese, nickel, thallium, vanadium and zinc. Renal, hepatic, neurological and gastrointestinal damage are common following ingestion; **ALI** often follows inhalation of fumes. Antidotes (**chelating agents**) include **dimercaprol** (for antimony, arsenic, bismuth, gold, mercury, thallium and lead), **penicillamine** (copper and lead), ascorbic acid (chromium), succimer (arsenic, mercury), unithiol (arsenic, mercury, nickel) and **sodium calcium edetate** (lead, manganese, zinc).

Ibrahim D, Froberg B, Wolf A, Rusyniak DE (2006). Clin Lab Med; 26: 67–97

Hedonal. Obsolete anaesthetic agent, used iv (1905), rectally and orally.

Heidbrink valve, *see Adjustable pressure-limiting valve*

Heimlich manoeuvre. Method of relieving **choking** caused by a foreign body using forceful compression of

the upper abdomen. The resultant rise in intrathoracic pressure expels the object from the upper airway. The operator stands behind the subject with hands clenched over the subject's epigastrium, the operator's arms passing under the subject's. A sharp thrust is delivered inwards and upwards. A similar manoeuvre may be performed with the subject lying prone. Compression of the lower chest has been found to be as effective. Clearance of one's own airway by falling forwards on to the back of a chair has been reported.
[Henry J Heimlich (1920–2016), US surgeon]

Heimlich valve. Disposable device used in the treatment of **pneumothorax**. Consists of a flattened rubber tube within a clear plastic tube; attached to a thoracostomy tube, it allows the venting of air from within the chest and prevents the ingress of air. May block/malfunction if blood passes through valve. Useful during the prehospital phase of resuscitation or during interhospital transfer. Now infrequently used since the introduction of plastic underwater seal bottles and portable, disposable bag/valve assemblies.
See also, Chest drainage

Helium. Inert gas, present in natural gas and to a lesser extent in **air**. Less dense than nitrogen. Thus, if **flow** is turbulent, greater flow of a helium/O_2 mixture will occur than of a nitrogen/O_2 mixture, as turbulent flow depends on fluid density (and density of 21% O_2 in helium is 34% of that of 21% O_2 in nitrogen). Used therefore to increase alveolar O_2 supply in upper **airway obstruction**. Of less use in lower airway obstruction (e.g. **asthma**) because most peripheral flow is laminar and therefore depends on viscosity, which is greater for helium/O_2 mixtures than for nitrogen/O_2. However, some benefit may occur where flow is turbulent.

Supplied in **cylinders** with brown shoulders and body, at 137 bar. Also available with 21% O_2, in brown-bodied cylinders with brown and white quartered shoulders, at the same pressure.

Has also been used to investigate small airway resistance to flow, by comparing **flow–volume loops** breathing air and helium/O_2. The two curves are more similar in small airway obstruction than in normal lungs.

Because of its very low solubility, helium is also used in measurement of **lung volumes**.
Harris PD, Barnes R (2008). Anaesthesia; 63: 284–93

HELLP syndrome (Syndrome of haemolysis elevated liver enzymes and low platelets). Condition first recognised in 1982; thought to represent part of the spectrum of **pre-eclampsia** characterised primarily by abnormal blood tests rather than hypertension, proteinuria and oedema (although they may occur). Risk factors for HELLP syndrome include maternal age >34 years, multiparity and European descent. The syndrome is associated with significant maternal morbidity, including **DIC** (20%), **placental abruption**, **acute kidney injury** (7%), **pulmonary oedema** (6%) and hepatic rupture. Fetal morbidity and mortality are similarly increased. General principles of management are as for pre-eclampsia; in addition **corticosteroids**, plasma exchange, administration of fresh frozen plasma and **prostacyclin** have been used.
del-Rio-Vellosillo M, Garcia-Medina JJ (2016). Acta Anaesthesiol Scand; 60: 144–57

Hemo ..., *see Haemo...*

Henderson–Hasselbalch equation. Equation describing the relationship between the concentrations of dissociated and undissociated **acid** or **base**, acid or base dissociation constants (K_a and K_b, respectively) and **pH**. In its generic form for weak acids (e.g. carbonic acid, **thiopental sodium**):

$$\mathrm{pH} = \mathrm{p}K_a + \log\frac{[\mathrm{A}^-]}{[\mathrm{AH}]}$$

and for weak bases (e.g. **local anaesthetic agents**):

$$\mathrm{pH} = \mathrm{p}K_b + \log\frac{[\mathrm{B}]}{[\mathrm{BH}^+]}$$

Applicable to any **buffer** system; commonly illustrated using the **bicarbonate** buffer system. For the reaction of CO_2 with water to form carbonic acid, which dissociates to form bicarbonate and **hydrogen ions**:

$$CO_2 + H_2O \rightleftharpoons H_2CO_3 \rightleftharpoons H^+ + HCO_3^-$$

The acid dissociation constant K_a for the dissociation of H_2CO_3 then equals

$$\frac{[H^+][HCO_3^-]}{[H_2CO_3]}$$

Taking logarithms of both sides:

$$\log K_a = \log[H^+] + \log\frac{[HCO_3^-]}{[H_2CO_3]}$$

$$\text{therefore} - \log[H^+] = -\log K_a + \log\frac{[HCO_3^-]}{[H_2CO_3]}$$

$$\text{or, pH} = \mathrm{p}K_a + \log\frac{[HCO_3^-]}{[H_2CO_3]}$$

Because $[H_2CO_3]$ is related to $[CO_2]$ by the original reaction, and $[CO_2]$ is related to $P\text{CO}_2$ and a solubility factor (0.03 mmol/l/mmHg, or 0.23 mmol/l/kPa),

$$\mathrm{pH} = \mathrm{p}K_a + \log\frac{[HCO_3^-]}{P\text{CO}_2 \times 0.03}$$

with $P\text{CO}_2$ measured in mmHg

$$\text{or } \mathrm{p}K_a + \log\frac{[HCO_3^-]}{P\text{CO}_2 \times 0.23}$$

with $P\text{CO}_2$ measured in kPa.

Thus used to explain changes in pH, $P\text{CO}_2$ and $[HCO_3^-]$ in disturbances of **acid–base balance**.

Maximal efficiency of a buffering system occurs at pH values close to its $\mathrm{p}K_a$. $\mathrm{p}K_a$ for carbonic acid/bicarbonate is 6.1 at body temperature; its importance arises from the ability to excrete CO_2 via the lungs.

When applied to **pharmacokinetics**, the equation can be used to predict the effect of plasma/tissue pH on the fraction of unionised drug; e.g. **acidosis** reduces the unionised fraction of **lidocaine** hydrochloride, rendering it less effective in infected tissues.
[Lawrence Henderson (1878–1942), US biochemist; Karl Hasselbalch (1874–1962), Danish physiologist]
See also, Acid–base balance

Henry's law. Amount of **gas** dissolved in a solvent is proportional to the partial pressure of the gas when in equilibrium with the solvent, at constant temperature.
[William Henry (1744–1836), English chemist]

Heparin-induced thrombocytopenia (HIT). Immune-mediated destruction of **platelets** typically occurring 5–10 days after starting **heparin** treatment. Should be considered if the platelet count falls by >50% following administration. Clinical features are usually absent but may include fever, dyspnoea and chest pain following an iv bolus of the drug. More common with unfractionated heparin (0.75%) than low-molecular-weight preparations (<0.1%). Detection of antibodies against platelet factor 4 confirms the diagnosis.

Patients with HIT are susceptible to thrombotic events including **DVT**, **PE**, **stroke**, **MI** and limb arterial occlusion. Management consists of discontinuing heparin (including flushes), avoidance of platelet transfusion and anticoagulation with alternative agents (e.g. **hirudins**).
Warkentin TE (2015). Curr Opin Crit Care; 21: 576–85

Heparin sodium/calcium. **Anticoagulant drug**, used for secondary prevention in **acute coronary syndromes** and for the prophylaxis and treatment of thromboembolism. Has also been used in **DIC**. Discovered in 1916. A mucopolysaccharide, derived from animal lung and intestine. Strongly acidic and electronegative, binding strongly to proteins and amines.

- Actions:
  - potentiates the action of antithrombin III, a naturally occurring inhibitor of activated **coagulation** factors XII, XI, IX, X and thrombin.
  - inhibits **platelet** aggregation by fibrin.
  - activates lipoprotein lipase, involved in fat transport.
  - thought to be involved in immunological/inflammatory reactions, possibly via binding to **histamine** and **5-HT**. Contained within **mast cells**.

Fast onset but short-acting, with **half-life** of about 90 min; therefore most effectively given by iv infusion (heparin sodium). Effects persist for 4–6 h and are monitored by measuring the activated partial thromboplastin time (APTT), although thrombin and clotting times are also prolonged.

Low-mw heparins inhibit activated factor X (factor Xa) preferentially and thus cause fewer systemic anticoagulation effects, with less effect on platelet function. Also have longer half-lives. They do not require regular monitoring, may be given once daily and cause fewer haemorrhagic effects than unfractionated heparin when given for **DVT** prophylaxis. Several low-mw heparins exist, with varying properties according to the particular preparation (e.g. ratio of anti-Xa to anti-II activity).

Both unfractionated and low-mw heparin may be used for perioperative prophylactic 'bridging' in patients taking long-acting oral anticoagulants (e.g. **warfarin**, **dabigatran**). 'Therapeutic' doses are reserved for patients deemed moderate or high risk for thromboembolism. Most centres have local clinical guidelines regarding risk stratification and the preparation/dosages to be used (*see Warfarin sodium for example of bridging regimens*).

- Dosage:
  - unfractionated heparin:
    - prophylaxis of DVT: 5000 units sc 2 h preoperatively, then bd/tds until the patient is walking.
    - treatment of thrombosis: 5000 units iv, then 1000–2000 units/h (14–28 units/kg/h) by infusion, or 5000–10 000 units iv 4-hourly by bolus. APPT is kept at 1.5–2.5 times normal. Oral anticoagulation is usually commenced at the same time as heparin.
    - during arterial surgery, 100 units/kg iv; for **cardiac surgery**, 300–400 units/kg. Also used to anticoagulate extracorporeal circuits, e.g. **cardiopulmonary bypass**, **haemofiltration**.
  - low-mw heparin:
    - prophylaxis of DVT.
      - dalteparin sodium: 2500 units sc 1–2 h preoperatively (repeated after 12 h in high-risk patients), followed by 2500 units od (5000 units if high risk) for 5 days.
      - enoxaparin: 2000 units (20 mg) sc 1–2 h preoperatively (4000 units [40 mg] 12 h preoperatively in high-risk patients), followed by 2000 units od (4000 units if high risk) for 7–10 days.
      - tinzaparin: 3500 units sc 2 h preoperatively (4500 units 12 h preoperatively in high-risk patients), followed by 3500 units od (4500 units if high risk) for 7–10 days.
      - bemiparin sodium: 2500 units sc 2 h preoperatively or 6 h postoperatively, followed by 2500 units od (3500 units if high risk) for 7–10 days.
    - treatment of venous thrombosis: may be more effective than unfractionated heparin and does not require dose adjustment according to laboratory tests. Treatment should be continued for at least 5–6 days, during which time oral anticoagulants should also be given:
      - dalteparin: 200 units/kg od (100 units/kg bd in patients at risk of haemorrhage) (maximal daily dose 18 000 units).
      - enoxaparin 150 units/kg (1.5 mg/kg) od.
      - tinzaparin 175 units/kg od.
      - bemiparin: 115 units/kg od for 5–9 days.
    - treatment of acute coronary syndromes:
      - dalteparin: 120 units/kg bd (maximum 18 000 units bd).
      - enoxaparin 100 units/kg (1 mg/kg) bd.

  Higher doses are required in pregnancy.
- Side effects:
  - increased bleeding: cessation of infusion is usually adequate; **protamine** may be given but only partially reverses low mw heparin.
  - **heparin-induced thrombocytopenia**.
  - hypersensitivity.
  - osteoporosis following prolonged use.
  - inhibition of **aldosterone** secretion has been described and regular monitoring of plasma potassium concentration is recommended if the duration of therapy exceeds 7 days.

  Side effects are less frequent with low-mw heparins than with unfractionated heparin.

See also, Coagulation studies

Heparinoids. Heteropolysaccharide derivatives of **heparin**; used for the prevention and treatment of thromboembolism in patients with a history of **heparin-induced thrombocytopenia**. **Danaparoid** is the only preparation licensed for use in the UK.

Hepatic failure. May involve:
- chronic disease and cirrhosis:
  - chronic autoimmune **hepatitis**.
  - chronic viral hepatitis.
  - drugs, e.g. **methyldopa**, **alcohols**.
  - non-alcoholic fatty liver disease.
  - metabolic disease, e.g. haemochromatosis, Wilson's disease, α_1-antitrypsin deficiency, other **inborn errors of metabolism**.
  - biliary disease, e.g. primary biliary cirrhosis.
  - vascular lesions, e.g. venous occlusion, chronic **cardiac failure**.

- acute disease (fulminant hepatic failure):
  - drugs, e.g. **paracetamol** (commonest cause), **halothane**, **chloroform**, **chlorpromazine**, **monoamine oxidase inhibitors**, **phenytoin**, **isoniazid**.
  - acute viral hepatitis A, B and E.
  - others: less common, including:
    - poisons, e.g. carbon tetrachloride.
    - acute hepatic venous thrombosis (Budd-Chiari syndrome).
    - acute fatty liver of pregnancy (as part of the **HELLP syndrome**).
    - hypoxic hepatitis, e.g. due to **cardiac failure**, respiratory failure, **sepsis**.
    - **Reye's syndrome**.

- Features:
  - chronic liver disease:
    - malaise, GIT symptoms.
    - **jaundice**.
    - skin: spider naevi, palmar erythema, leukonychia, finger clubbing, Dupuytren's contracture, bruising, pigmentation, caput medusae (engorged paraumbilical veins).
    - hepatic fetor.
    - gynaecomastia and testicular atrophy, caused by decreased metabolism of circulating oestrogens.
    - **encephalopathy**: affects about 20% of patients with cirrhosis each year. Thought to be caused by reduced clearance of toxic waste products, e.g. **ammonia**, glutamine, methionine and fatty acids. May be provoked by physiological stress, including surgery, trauma and infection and worsened by electrolyte disturbance (e.g. **hyponatraemia**) and by muscle wasting (muscle is an alternative site for ammonia detoxification). Classification:
      - stage 1: altered personality or cognition. EEG is usually normal.
      - stage 2: confusion, abnormal sleep and drowsiness. Asterixis (flapping tremor especially affecting the hands/wrists) and increased reflexes, with plantar response up or down. EEG is abnormal.
      - stage 3: marked somnolence and confusion, with inability to perform fine movements. Responsive to painful stimuli.
      - stage 4: unresponsive; comatose with depressed reflexes.

      Treatment includes reduction of protein intake (e.g. to 1.2–1.5g/kg/day) and oral administration of lactulose (20–50 ml/day) and/or **neomycin** (1 g 4–6-hourly) to reduce ammonia-producing GIT bacteria and encourage nitrogen-utilising bacteria. Probiotics may have a role.
    - portal hypertension is caused by vascular occlusion, possibly due to fibrotic changes in cirrhosis. It may cause splenomegaly and enlargement of portal–systemic vascular anastomoses, e.g. oesophagogastric junction, retroperitoneal and umbilical vessels. **Oesophageal varices** may cause severe **GIT haemorrhage**. Haemorrhage may also be caused by gastric erosions or **peptic ulcer disease**. **Coagulation** factors and **platelets** may be reduced. **Anaemia** is common.
    - cirrhotic **cardiomyopathy** may be present, with features of cardiac failure, **arrhythmias** and reduced response to **inotropic drugs**.
    - **hypoproteinaemia**, with reduced plasma **oncotic pressure**, drug binding, **immunoglobulins**, **cholinesterase** and coagulation factors.
    - fluid retention: may cause **ascites**, **pleural effusion**, peripheral **oedema** and a hyperdynamic circulation. Treatment includes **spironolactone**, sodium restriction and drainage of ascites/pleural effusion.
    - hypoxaemia is common, caused by **$\dot{V}/\dot{Q}$ mismatch**, **atelectasis**, diaphragmatic splinting or pleural effusion. Portopulmonary hypertension may be present in end-stage disease due to accumulation of vasoactive substances normally cleared by the liver.
    - infection is common, especially bacterial.
    - renal impairment may occur.
    - metabolic and respiratory **alkalosis** may occur.

    Acute decompensation of stable chronic liver disease may be provoked by any acute illness, trauma or surgery.
  - acute fulminant hepatic failure: defined as hepatic failure occurring within 8 weeks of illness, in a previously normal liver. It presents with rapidly progressing encephalopathy, **coma** and **cerebral oedema**, **hypoglycaemia**, hyponatraemia, **hypokalaemia**, alkalosis, **hypothermia**, **ALI**, haemorrhage, coagulopathy and **renal failure**. Renal failure may be due to **hepatorenal syndrome** or acute tubular necrosis. Jaundice is uncommon initially. **DIC** and infection may occur.

Treatment is supportive and includes **O_2 therapy**, **IPPV**, neomycin/lactulose, **H_2 receptor antagonists/omeprazole**, prophylactic antibiotics and nutritional support with dextrose. Reversal of coagulopathy is now not routinely performed unless active bleeding occurs, as thrombotic complications are more common than haemorrhage. **ICP monitoring** may be useful and measures (e.g. head-up tilt, **mannitol**, hypertonic saline) employed to reduce ICP if raised. However, such monitoring has not been shown to reduce mortality. **Liver dialysis** techniques have been used and **liver transplantation** may be required. Experimental therapies include auxiliary liver transplantation, temporising hepatectomy, artificial liver systems (live liver cells within an extracorporeal circuit), intraperitoneal hepatocyte transplantation, use of liver growth factors and xenotransplantation.

- Anaesthetic management of patients with hepatic failure or chronic liver disease:
  - directed towards the complications discussed earlier, particularly **preoperative assessment** for, and optimisation of:
    - encephalopathy, and haematological and coagulation abnormalities. Vitamin K may be given if coagulation is abnormal, fresh frozen plasma if surgery is urgent.
    - pulmonary and renal function.
    - fluid, acid–base and electrolyte disturbance.
  - anaesthetic technique: increased doses of iv agents and neuromuscular blocking drugs may be required in cirrhosis, due to increased **volume of distribution**, but elimination may be prolonged; all sedative drugs require careful titration if encephalopathy is present. Opioids should be used cautiously. Drug metabolism is reduced; **isoflurane/desflurane** and **atracurium** are often preferred as reliance on metabolism is less than with other agents. **Hypocapnia** exacerbates the reduction in hepatic blood flow during general anaesthesia.
  - screening for infectious hepatitis should be performed.
  - maintenance of good peri- and postoperative renal function is important (*see Jaundice*).

Table 26 Scoring system for anaesthesia in hepatic failure

	Points scored		
	1	*2*	*3*
Bilirubin (µmol/l)	<25	25–40	>40
Albumin (g/l)	>35	28–35	<28
Prothrombin time prolongation (s)	<4	4–6	>6
Encephalopathy stage	0	1–2	3–4

A scoring system has been devised for assessment of risk, depending on preoperative blood tests and clinical assessment (Table 26). Good operative risk is suggested by <6 points, moderate risk by 7–9 points, and poor risk by >10 points.

[George Budd (1808–1882), English physician; Hans Chiari (1851–1916), Austrian pathologist; Baron Guillaume Dupuytren (1777–1835), French surgeon; Samuel AK Wilson (1878–1937), US-born English neurologist]

Singanayagam A, Bernal W (2015). Curr Opin Crit Care; 21: 134–41

Hepatitis. Acute hepatitis may be:
- viral:
  - hepatitis A:
    - RNA enterovirus, spread via the orofaecal route. Incubation period is 3–5 weeks.
    - causes fever, headache, GIT symptoms, impaired **liver function tests, jaundice** and hepatomegaly.
    - recovery is usually within 6 weeks, although malaise may persist longer.
    - pre-exposure vaccination with attenuated virus is effective in preventing the condition.
  - hepatitis B:
    - DNA virus, spread mainly via blood/blood products and body secretions, including sexual contact, tattooing, iv drug abuse and childbirth. Incubation period is 2–6 months.
    - features are as for hepatitis A but more severe. May lead to: recovery; acute fulminant **hepatic failure** (rarely); or a chronic infective state. The last includes asymptomatic carriage or chronic hepatitis that may lead to hepatocellular carcinoma or **hepatic failure**.
    - serological markers include surface (Australia) antigen (HBsAg), e antigen (HBeAg), corresponding antibodies (anti-HBs, anti-HBe) and antibody to core antigen (anti-HBc). Pattern:
      - HBsAg: increases 1 month after infection, peaks at 2–3 months, and falls at 4–5 months.
      - HBeAg: increases at 1 month, peaks at 2 months and falls at 3 months.
      - anti-HBc: increases at 2 months, peaks at 4 months and falls slowly thereafter.
      - anti-HBe: increases at 2–3 months, remaining elevated.
      - anti-HBs: increases at 6–7 months, remaining elevated.

      An asymptomatic carrier state is associated with HBsAg, HBeAg and anti-HBc expression. Its incidence is under 0.1% in the West, and up to 20% in Southeast Asia. Serum viral DNA levels may also be measured; they may distinguish between chronic hepatitis B (>10^5 copies/ml) and the inactive state (<10^5 copies/ml). Patients with chronic infection may receive interferon-α or lamivudine.
    - prevention:
      - active immunisation (against HBsAg) of medical workers and high-risk groups, e.g. homosexuals, drug abusers, multiple blood transfusion recipients, renal dialysis patients and babies of infected mothers.
      - passive immunisation using immunoglobulin; preferably performed within 24 h of exposure and certainly within 7 days.
      - treatment of existing infection involves long-term therapy with nucleotide analogues or interferon-based therapies.
      - screening of blood for transfusion, use of disposable needles, etc.; operating theatre precautions as for **HIV infection.** Pregnant women should be screened for HbsAg to reduce fetal transmission.
      - infected staff are allowed to return to work normally, including performing invasive procedures, if they have responded to treatment successfully and are considered low-risk for transmitting infection to patients (previously all affected staff were prevented from performing invasive procedures). Individuals about to start careers or training that would rely on the performance of exposure-prone procedures are still routinely tested.
  - hepatitis C (causes most cases of what was previously called non-A non-B hepatitis):
    - RNA virus, identified with a serological marker.
    - thought to be responsible for over 90% of post-tranfusion hepatitis in the developed world before screening. Also common in patients receiving renal dialysis.
    - acute infection is usually asymptomatic; however, about 85% become carriers, with 20%–40% developing chronic liver disease and cirrhosis. About 5% develop hepatocellular carcinoma. Patients with chronic infection may receive interferon-α and **ribavirin.**
    - screening of blood products began in the UK in 1991.
    - infected staff are allowed to work normally as for hepatitis B.
  - hepatitis D (delta): RNA virus, dependent on coexistent hepatitis B infection.
  - hepatitis E (enteral non-A non-B infection): RNA virus, spread by orofaecal route and usually causing mild illness.
  - other viral infections include **cytomegalovirus,** herpes simplex, varicella zoster and glandular fever.
- due to other infections, e.g. toxoplasmosis, **leptospirosis.**
- chemical:
  - idiosyncratic, e.g. **phenothiazines, monoamine oxidase inhibitors, tricyclic antidepressant drugs, chloroform, methyldopa, indometacin, erythromycin, rifampicin, chlorpropamide.** '**Halothane** hepatitis' was first described in 1958, with an estimated incidence of 1:6000 to 1:30000, typically following repeated exposure within a short period. The cause is uncertain but a direct toxic effect, an immune reaction to halothane or hepatocytes

altered by halothane, or halothane-induced hepatic hypoxia have all been implicated. Hepatitis has also followed exposure to more modern volatile anaesthetic agents, but a causative role is unclear, the incidence is thought to be extremely low, and repeated exposure is generally considered safe.
  - dose-related, e.g. **paracetamol**, carbon tetrachloride, **alcohol**.
- metabolic, e.g. Wilson's disease, or associated with pregnancy.
- associated with circulatory abnormalities, e.g. right ventricular failure, severe hypotension.

The cause of postoperative hepatitis is difficult to determine as many factors may be involved. 1 in 700 healthy patients have incidental impaired liver function tests preoperatively.
[Samuel AK Wilson (1878–1937), US-born English neurologist]
See also, Environmental safety of anaesthetists

Hepatorenal syndrome (HRS). Renal impairment secondary to severe hepatic dysfunction, usually cirrhosis. May coexist with or mimic other causes of **renal failure** (e.g. **hypovolaemia**, **glomerulonephritis**, urinary tract obstruction); therefore considered a diagnosis of exclusion.

- Diagnostic criteria:
  - cirrhosis with **ascites**.
  - serum **creatinine** >133 μmol/l and no improvement after 2 days of volume expansion with **albumin** and withdrawal of **diuretics**.
  - absence of **shock**.
  - no recent/current treatment with nephrotoxic drugs.
  - normal renal ultrasound and no evidence of renal parenchymal disease.

Patients with cirrhosis and ascites have a 20% 1-year probability of developing HRS. Mechanism involves renal hypoperfusion due to hypotension and intrarenal vasoconstriction; a functional aetiology is suggested by normal renal histology in HRS and the observation that kidneys donated by HRS patients function normally in their recipients.

Classified according to speed of onset and progression; type 1 is rapidly progressive (often with a precipitating cause, such as **infection**) and associated with **MODS**, while type 2 is associated with slowly worsening ascites and haemodynamic function. Median survival is 1 month and 6 months, respectively.

Prognosis is poor, even with renal replacement therapy, unless hepatic function improves or transplant is performed. Administration of albumin and **inotropic drugs** (e.g. terlipressin, **noradrenaline**) improves renal function in up to 50% of patients; early improvement in MAP predicts response to treatment.
Al-Khafaji A, Nadim MK, Kellum JA (2015). Chest; 148: 550–8

Herbal medicines. Taken by up to 20%–30% of patients presenting for surgery and often overlooked by medical staff. May have unpredictable physiological and pharmacological effects relevant to the perioperative period.

- Common examples include:
  - *Echinacea*: activates the immune system with reports of allergy (including **anaphylaxis**), decreased effectiveness of **immunosuppressive drugs** with short-term use and immunosuppression with long-term use.
  - *Ephedra* (ma huang): contains **ephedrine** and other sympathomimetic alkaloids. Causes dose-dependent tachycardia and hypertension with subsequent risk of **myocardial ischaemia** and **stroke**. Increases risk of **arrhythmias**. Haemodynamic instability may occur with concomitant use of **monoamine oxidase inhibitors**. Should be discontinued 24 h preoperatively.
  - garlic (ajo): inhibits **platelet** aggregation (sometimes irreversibly), increasing the risk of perioperative bleeding. Should be discontinued 7 days preoperatively.
  - ginkgo: inhibits **platelet-activating factor** with potential for increased bleeding. Should be discontinued 36 h preoperatively.
  - ginseng: may cause **hypoglycaemia** and inhibition of platelet aggregation. Should be discontinued 7 days preoperatively.
  - kava and valerian: cause sedation and may potentiate the effects of anaesthetic agents. Should be discontinued 24 h preoperatively.
  - St John's wort (*Hypericum*): causes **enzyme induction** of the **cytochrome oxidase system** (especially the cytochrome P_{450} family). Should be discontinued at least 5 days preoperatively.

Hodges PJ, Kam PCA (2002). Anaesthesia; 57: 889–900

Hereditary angio-oedema. Congenital deficiency and/or dysfunction of C1 esterase inhibitor, leading to **complement** activation with non-pruritic swelling of the face, mouth, skin and GIT. Of autosomal dominant inheritance, but new mutations account for 25% of cases; prevalence is 1 in 50 000. May occur spontaneously or after a trigger (e.g. trauma, infection, surgery, stress), possibly via activation of **kinins**, plasmins or other proteases. An acquired form may occur in lymphomas.

Attacks may mimic an acute surgical abdomen, with pain, diarrhoea and vomiting. May also cause upper **airway obstruction**, carrying a mortality of 25%–40%. Synthetic, partially purified C1 esterase inhibitor is the treatment of choice for the termination of acute attacks. It is effective within 30–45 min. Alternatives include recombinant C1 esterase inhibitor (conestat alfa) and fresh frozen plasma (which contains C1 esterase inhibitor). Unlike **anaphylaxis** or allergic angio-oedema, adrenaline, corticosteroids and antihistamines should not be used for the treatment of acute attacks, including those involving laryngeal oedema, as they are ineffective and may delay appropriate treatment.

Perioperative prophylaxis consists of 7 days' preoperative treatment with danazol or tranexamic acid, or administration of C1 esterase inhibitor 24 h in advance. Additional inhibitor or fresh frozen plasma should be immediately available. Upper airway instrumentation should be minimised and patients should be monitored in a critical care environment postoperatively.
Bhardwaj N, Craig TJ (2014). Transfusion; 54: 2989–96

Hereditary angioneurotic oedema, *see Hereditary angio-oedema*

Hering–Breuer reflex (Inflation reflex). Inhibition of respiratory muscles following lung inflation, leading to termination of inspiration. Afferent pathway is thought to be from **pulmonary stretch receptors** via the vagus. Bilateral vagotomy produces an increase in inspiratory amplitude and a longer duration of expiration. Of importance in neonates but less so in adults.
[Karl Hering (1834–1918), German physiologist; Josef Breuer (1852–1925), Austrian psychiatrist]
See also, Breathing, control of

Heroin, *see Diamorphine*

Hertz. SI **unit** of frequency. 1 Hz = 1 cycle per second. [Heinrich Hertz (1857–1894), German physicist]

Hetastarch, *see Hydroxyethyl starch*

Hewer, Christopher Langton (1896–1986). English anaesthetist, of major importance in the establishment and evolution of anaesthesia in the UK. Popularised the use of **trichloroethylene** in 1941. Edited ***Anaesthesia*** for its first 20 years, also *Recent Advances in Anaesthesia and Analgesia* for 50 years. Received many honours and medals.

Hewitt, Frederic (1857–1916). English anaesthetist, practised at St George's Hospital. Renowned for many contributions to anaesthesia, including the first fixed proportion N_2O/O_2 machine, inhalers, airways and other equipment. A strong advocate of teaching and high standards in anaesthesia. Knighted in 1911.
Howat DD (1999). J Med Biog; 7: 5–10 and 63–8

Hexafluorenium. Obsolete drug used to prolong the action of **suxamethonium** by inhibiting plasma **cholinesterase**. May cause arrhythmias and bronchospasm.

Hexamethonium. Obsolete **ganglion blocking drug** used in **hypotensive anaesthesia**.

Hexastarch, *see Hydroxyethyl starch*

Hexobarbital. Obsolete **iv anaesthetic agent**, introduced in 1932. Replaced by the safer and more predictable **thiopental**.

HFJV, HFPPV, HFO, HFV, *see High-frequency ventilation*

Hiatus hernia. Protrusion of stomach through the diaphragmatic crura into the thorax. May be sliding (type I), when the oesophagocardiac junction and upper stomach move into the thorax, or rolling (type II), when this junction remains intra-abdominal but part of the fundus herniates. The former is more common and more likely to cause gastro-oesophageal valve incompetence; the latter is more likely to strangulate.

More common in the elderly and in **obesity**.

- Symptoms:
  - epigastric pain, belching, indigestion.
  - regurgitation; may lead to stricture formation.
  - GIT bleeding may occur.
- Anaesthetic problems:
  - **aspiration of gastric contents**:
    - chronic pulmonary damage due to repeated aspiration.
    - risk of acute aspiration perioperatively.
  - chronic **anaemia**.
- Management:
  - medical: weight loss, **antacids, H_2 receptor antagonists**.
  - surgical: repair of the diaphragmatic defect and fundoplasty: the oesophagogastric junction is invaginated into a sleeve of fundus (Nissen's plication).

[Rudolph Nissen (1896–1981), Swiss surgeon]
See also, Diaphragmatic hernia; Gastro-oesophageal reflux; Lower oesophageal sphincter

Hiccups. Intense synchronous contraction of the **diaphragm** and inspiratory intercostal muscles lasting about 500 ms, followed approximately 30 ms after its onset by glottic closure. May involve phrenic or vagal efferents. Results in a characteristic inspiratory sound associated with discomfort. On average, occur at a rate of less than 30/min. Frequent in the newborn. Frequency is decreased by breath-holding or a raised arterial $P\text{CO}_2$ and increased by a lowered arterial $P\text{CO}_2$. Episodes may be terminated by a sudden shock. May occur recurrently with neurological disease (e.g. brainstem tumours, **encephalitis, meningitis**), metabolic disease (e.g. uraemia) and many thoracic, abdominal or cardiac conditions. During anaesthesia, hiccups may be provoked by airway manipulation or surgical stimulation, especially around the diaphragm, and particularly in the presence of inadequate paralysis or anaesthesia.

- Rarely troublesome, but the following have been suggested as treatment:
  - **hyperventilation.**
  - **metoclopramide, chlorpromazine, haloperidol, baclofen, anticonvulsant drugs.**
  - nasopharyngeal stimulation.
  - during anaesthesia, all the above have been used, as has deepening anaesthesia ± increasing analgesia and muscle relaxation.

Hickman, Henry Hill (1800–1830). English surgeon, practising in Ludlow and Shifnall, Shropshire. First described the production of insensibility in animals by exposure to a gas (CO_2) and suggested its use for painless surgery, in 1824. His efforts to publicise his experiments were unsuccessful, both in the UK and abroad.

Hickman line, *see Central venous cannulation, long-term*

High dependency unit (HDU). Area providing a level of care between that of a general ward and an **ICU** (i.e., level 2 care). Provides care for patients with a single failing organ system, those stepping down from ICU and high-risk patients requiring postoperative care. Costs and nursing requirements are less than for an ICU; they usually have a nurse:patient ratio of 1:2.
See also, Care of the critically ill surgical patient; Medical emergency team; Postoperative care team; Safe transport and retrieval team; Transportation of critically ill patients

High-frequency ventilation (HFV). Mechanism of respiratory support developed in the 1970s. Small tidal volumes (1–3 ml/kg) are delivered at high frequencies, maintaining gas exchange without **barotrauma** or other deleterious effects of **IPPV**. May be superimposed on spontaneous ventilation.

- Three modes are used:
  - high-frequency positive pressure ventilation (HFPPV): 60–150 cycles/min, delivered via an intratracheal insufflation catheter, bronchoscope or **tracheal tube**. Tidal volumes of 100–400 ml are used. Fluidic valves are often used, without moving parts. Possible using some conventional **ventilators**, especially paediatric ones.
  - high-frequency jet ventilation (HFJV): 60–600 cycles/min, delivered via a cannula inserted through the cricothyroid membrane, placed within a bronchoscope, or incorporated near the tip of a tracheal tube. Expiration is continuous through the open system. Principles of gas entrainment are as for **injector techniques**. Tidal volume is up to 150 ml.

Produces positive airway pressure of about 5 cmH_2O. Most ventilators employ electrical solenoid valves.
- high-frequency oscillation (HFO): 500–3000 cycles/min; the gas column is oscillated using a vibrating membrane (similar to a loudspeaker) applied directly to the gas column (thus providing active expiration). Mean airway pressure determines oxygenation, while oscillatory amplitude determines CO_2 removal.

The mechanism of gas exchange is unclear but is thought to involve continuous mixing of gases. HFJV is also used for ENT and thoracic procedures such as sleeve resection of the trachea/bronchi and tracheo-bronchial fistula, in which increased airway pressures and excessive movement may be especially detrimental. HFO has been used in **ALI** in all ages. Although it has been shown to be effective in the management of neonatal and paediatric patients with acute respiratory distress syndrome, it has no benefits over conventional ventilation in adult ALI; its routine use is currently not recommended for the latter group.

Maitra S, Bhattacharjee S, Khanna P, Baidya DK (2015). Anesthesiol; 122: 841–51

Hirudin. Peptide (65 amino acid) **thrombin inhibitor**, originally derived from leech saliva, now manufactured using recombinant techniques. Specifically inhibits the actions of thrombin in the **coagulation** pathway; unlike **heparin**, it does not require antithrombin III as a cofactor and is not inhibited by anti-heparin proteins. It also does not affect platelets directly and may also inhibit thrombin bound to a fibrin clot. Has been studied as a means of preventing primary and recurrent **MI** and **DVT**; initial studies have been encouraging, although bleeding may be a problem, as with heparin. **Lepirudin** and **bivalirudin** are recombinant forms available in the UK.

His bundle electrography. Electrophysiology study, used to investigate cardiac conduction defects and tachycardias, utilising transvenous intracardiac bipolar electrodes at various sites. Concurrent recording of a formal **ECG** is usually undertaken. Assesses conduction through different parts of the **heart conducting system**, identifying conduction defects and accessory pathways. May also be used to distinguish supraventricular from ventricular **arrhythmias**; ventricular complexes in the former are preceded by His bundle activity. The effects of pacing stimuli at different sites may also be observed, e.g. in assessment of refractory tachycardias. Often performed under **sedation** or general anaesthesia.

[Wilhelm His (1863–1934), German anatomist]

Histamine and histamine receptors. Histamine, an amine, is present in **mast cells**, basophils, gastric mucosa and the CNS. It is involved in the inflammatory response and gastric acid secretion, and is a **neurotransmitter** involved in cognition, arousal and control of **pituitary** function. Associated with many other inflammatory mediator pathways (e.g. **cytokines**, **complement**, **leukotrienes**) and with **coagulation** and other processes. Synthesised by decarboxylation of L-histidine, and broken down by deamination and/or methylation with renal excretion.

- Histamine receptor subtypes have been identified:
  - H_1:
    - cause smooth muscle contraction in the GIT and uterus, and bronchoconstriction via cholinergic pathways following stimulation of irritant pulmonary receptors.
    - cause vascular smooth muscle relaxation and dilatation, with increased vascular permeability.
    - cause stimulation and irritation of cutaneous nerve endings.
  - H_2:
    - cause some vasodilatation (but less than H_1 receptors).
    - have direct inotropic and chronotropic effects on isolated hearts, but hypotension usually results from vasodilatation.
    - increase acid, pepsin and intrinsic factor secretion from gastric mucosa.
  - H_3: present in the CNS and of uncertain clinical significance. Thought to inhibit histamine and acetylcholine release.
  - H_4: present in GIT and basophils and involved in chemotaxis.

All subtypes are **G protein-coupled receptors**; H_2 actions are mediated via **cAMP**, and H_1 via cyclic guanosine monophosphate.

Specific receptor antagonists have been developed; they are called **antihistamine drugs** (H_1) and **H_2 receptor antagonists** largely for historical reasons (the latter were designed many years after the former).

Histamine is released from mast cells following iv injection of certain drugs, e.g. **tubocurarine** and **morphine**. The amount released depends partly on the rate of injection. Skin wheals, hypotension and bronchospasm may occur.

See also, Anaphylaxis; Carcinoid syndrome

Histamine receptor antagonists, *see Antihistamine drugs; H_2 receptor antagonists*

HIT, *see Heparin-induced thrombocytopenia*

HIV, *see Human immunodeficiency viral infection*

HME, *see Heat–moisture exchanger*

Hofmann degradation. Spontaneous degradation of amides ($RCONH_2$) to amines (RNH_2), and quaternary ammonium salts to tertiary ones, under certain physical conditions. **Atracurium** (a quaternary ammonium compound) spontaneously degrades to **laudanosine** at body temperature and plasma pH.

[August von Hofmann (1818–1892), German chemist]

Alston TA (2003). Anesth Analg; 96: 622–5

Holmes, Oliver Wendell (1809–1894). US physician, poet and author; Professor of Anatomy at Harvard, Boston. Famous for his treatise on puerperal fever and its prevention, and for his non-medical writing. Suggested **anaesthesia** as a suitable term for ether narcosis in a letter written to **Morton** in 1846.

Homeostasis. Concept first proposed by **Bernard**, relating to maintenance of physiological variables within normal limits, allowing optimal functioning of tissues and cells. Includes maintenance of **acid–base balance**, **fluid balance**, **temperature regulation**, **arterial BP** and hormone secretion. Most mechanisms involve negative feedback; i.e., an increase of a substance or parameter causes direct inhibition of mechanisms that increase it, bringing about its restoration to normal.

Hormone replacement therapy (HRT). Use of oestrogen or oestrogen/progestogens to prevent menopausal symptoms (e.g. hot flushes, night sweats and vaginal dryness). Also protects against cardiovascular disease and osteoporosis but may increase the risk of stroke, MI and certain cancers (e.g. breast) and **DVT**, e.g. perioperatively. Perioperative precautions similar to those used for oral **contraceptives** have been suggested for women on HRT, although this is controversial because the risk is thought to be less.
Brighouse D (2001). Br J Anaesth; 86: 709–16

Horner's syndrome. Clinical picture results from interruption of sympathetic innervation to the head. Originally described with cervical lesions, it may be due to lesions anywhere along the sympathetic pathway, including **epidural anaesthesia**. Consists of partial ptosis, meiosis, apparent enophthalmos, lack of sweating and nasal congestion on the affected side.
[Johann Horner (1831–1886), Swiss ophthalmologist]

Hospital-acquired infections, *see Nosocomial infection*

HQIP, *see Healthcare Quality Improvement Partnership*

HRT, *see Hormone replacement therapy*

5-HT, *see 5-Hydroxytryptamine*

5-HT_3 receptor antagonists. Group of drugs including **ondansetron, granisetron, tropisetron, dolasetron** and **palonosetron**, used in the prevention and treatment of **PONV** and cytotoxic-induced nausea and vomiting. **5-HT** is released by the action of anticancer drugs on enterochromaffin cells in the gut mucosa, stimulating gut 5-HT_3 receptors and activating vagal afferents, resulting in vomiting. 5-HT_3 receptors are also thought to be involved centrally in the vagal reflex pathways; 5-HT_3 receptor antagonists therefore have both a central and a peripheral action. May also be useful in the treatment of opioid-induced **pruritus** (unlicensed use).

Hüfner constant. The volume of O_2 carried by 1 g **haemoglobin**; e.g. used in the calculation of **O_2 delivery** and **O_2 flux**. Figures vary, according to whether it is measured in vitro or in vivo; 1.39 and 1.34 ml are most commonly quoted, respectively. The latter value is the more relevant clinically.
[Carl von Hüfner (1840–1908), German physician]

Human immunodeficiency viral infection (HIV infection). First recognised in 1981 in the USA as the acquired immunodeficiency syndrome (AIDS) in otherwise healthy homosexual males. The retrovirus, human immunodeficiency virus type 1 (HIV-1) was first isolated in 1983. HIV-2 was identified in 1986, limited mainly to West Africa, where the disease is thought to have originated; most HIV disease worldwide is caused by HIV-1. The virus binds to CD4 receptors on T-helper lymphocytes, introducing its RNA genome into the cells; the viral enzyme reverse transcriptase generates a DNA copy that is then incorporated into the human DNA. It may then remain latent or produce viral copies; viral protease cleaves viral precursor proteins into their active forms, which are released from infected cells. T-cells are eventually destroyed in the process, leading to increased susceptibility to infection and malignancy.

The history and epidemiology of HIV are complex; however, a fall in new infections in the last decade has been offset by a reduction in AIDS-related deaths, causing global prevalence to stabilise at 0.8%. An estimated 1.2 million people are infected in the USA and 750 000 in western Europe, with over 40 million people infected worldwide (65% of them in sub-Saharan Africa); over 25 million deaths have occurred since the disease was first recognised.

- Transmitted mainly via semen and blood, i.e., via:
  - sexual contact (especially male–male).
  - transfusion of **blood products**.
  - infected needles, e.g. used by drug addicts.
  - transplacentally, at delivery or via breast milk.
  - spillage of infected blood on to broken skin, or into the eye.

The virus may be isolated from other body fluids, e.g. vaginal secretions, saliva, tears. Transmission by mouth-to-mouth contact (e.g. during **CPR**) is not thought to occur.

High-risk groups include the sexually promiscuous, iv drug abusers, haemophiliacs, Haitians and Central/West Africans.

- Features:
  - most infected people are thought to be asymptomatic.
  - an acute, flulike seroconversion illness may occur 1–3 weeks after infection. The incubation period may be as long as several years.
  - weight loss, diarrhoea, fever and thrush (AIDS-related complex) commonly progress to AIDS itself. Thrombocytopenic purpura and anaemia, dementia, encephalitis and psychosis may occur, related to HIV infection itself or secondary infection by other organisms.
  - AIDS: presence of indicator diseases, e.g. opportunistic infection (e.g. *Pneumocystis jirovecii* [formerly *P. carinii*] chest infection, pneumonia, candidiasis, cytomegalovirus), Kaposi's sarcoma, lymphoma, encephalopathy.

Classified using the CD4 count (≥500/μl; 200–499/μl, ≤200/μl), viral load and the World Health Organization Staging System for HIV infection:
  - stage 1: asymptomatic or lymphadenopathy only.
  - stage 2: minor mucocutaneous manifestations (e.g. oral ulceration, seborrhoeic dermatitis) and upper respiratory tract infections.
  - stage 3: chronic diarrhoea, weight loss, severe bacterial infections, hairy leucoplakia, pulmonary **tuberculosis**.
  - stage 4: presence of AIDS-defining illness as discussed earlier.
- Diagnosis, monitoring and progression:
  - testing for HIV is a two-step process consisting of initial screening for serum antibodies followed by confirmation of positive results with a more specific test, e.g. immunofluorescence assay.
  - seroconversion occurs on average 1 month after infection. Before HAART (*see later*) two-thirds progressed to AIDS within 10 years, with a 5-year survival of about 20% once AIDS was diagnosed. With current therapy, meticulous adherence to drug regimens and follow-up, many patients may live for several decades.
  - in Africa, due to poorer access to treatment, survival is shorter, with about 30% of HIV-positive cases progressing to death without passing through AIDS itself.
  - the CD4 count may fall gradually or suddenly; a count below 200/μl (normal 600–1500/μl) indicates increased risk of opportunistic infection. Plasma viral

load refers to the amount of viral RNA measurable in the plasma and correlates with speed of disease progression; current practice uses viral load with CD4 count to guide management.

- Treatment: previously reserved for AIDS, drug therapy is now commonly used before immunosuppression occurs. Typically consists of triple therapy (e.g. two nucleoside reverse transcriptase inhibitors and a protease inhibitor), termed highly active antiretroviral therapy (HAART). Indications for HAART in confirmed HIV infection:
  - stage 1 or 2 disease with CD4 count <200/μl.
  - stage 3 disease with CD4 count <350/μl.
  - stage 4 disease regardless of CD4 count.
- Treatment consists of:
  - supportive measures, e.g. nutrition, treatment of infection. **Co-trimoxazole** and **pentamidine** are usually used for **pneumocystis pneumonia**; the latter drug may be given iv, im or by nebuliser to reduce side effects (and as prophylaxis).
  - nucleoside reverse transcriptase inhibitors (NRTIs), e.g. **zidovudine**, didanosine, abacavir, zalcitabine, stavudine, lamivudine.
  - protease inhibitors, e.g. indinavir, ritonavir, lopinavir, nelfinavir, amprenavir, saquinavir. Inhibition of hepatic cytochrome P_{450} may give rise to interactions with other drugs.
  - non-nucleoside reverse transcriptase inhibitors (NNRTIs), e.g. efavirenz, nevirapine: used in combination therapy.
- Side effects and syndromes associated with HAART include:
  - **lactic acidosis**, particularly with NRTIs: due to mitochondrial toxicity. May be asymptomatic or progress to **MODS** and death. Treatment involves cessation of the triggering agent, **bicarbonate** and **haemofiltration** in severe cases.
  - hypersensitivity syndromes, including: **anaphylaxis**; interstitial **pneumonitis**; **hepatitis** and **toxic epidermal necrolysis**.
  - immune reconstitution syndromes (IRS): paradoxical worsening of inflammatory processes after initiation of HAART, due to improved immune response to infectious agents (especially **tuberculosis**). May result in **pericarditis**, **meningitis** and lymphadenitis; difficult to distinguish from infection.
  - lipodystrophy syndrome: redistribution of fat, insulin resistance and dyslipidaemia may occur after long-term HAART.
  - non-specific side effects include GIT upset, neuropathies, psychological disturbances, hepatotoxicity.
- Anaesthetic/ICU considerations:
  - features of illness and complications of drug therapy as above. Although patients still present to ICU with HIV-related illness such as pneumocystis pneumonia, these conditions are becoming less common. More common indications for ICU admission are respiratory failure, IRS and HAART-related toxicity. ICU mortality is approximately 30%; prognosis is worse for those with poor nutritional status and those requiring mechanical ventilation.
  - patients are at risk from infection as for **immunodeficiency**.
  - measures to protect staff and other patients from HIV infection:
    - avoidance of use of needles/parenteral medication.
    - wearing of gowns, goggles, gloves and overshoes.
    - careful disposal of sharps; needles should not be resheathed after use. Hospitals should have policies for management of accidental needlestick injuries, from which the risk of transmission is about 0.3% (*see Environmental safety of anaesthetists*).
    - use of disposable equipment where possible.
    - filters on breathing tubing if not disposable.
    - all non-disposable equipment is soaked in hypochlorite or glutaraldehyde solution after use; theatre equipment, walls, floors, etc., are washed down.
    - general considerations:
      - blood and its products are used increasingly sparingly; although donor blood is screened for anti-HIV antibodies, virus infection without seroconversion cannot be excluded.
      - iv equipment should not be used for more than one patient.
  - since 2014, staff with HIV infection are allowed to work normally, including performing invasive procedures, if they have responded to combination antiretroviral drug therapy and have an undetectable viral load (previously all affected staff were prevented from performing invasive procedures). Staff about to start careers or training that would rely on the performance of exposure-prone procedures are routinely tested.

[Moricz K Kaposi (1837–1902), Austrian dermatologist]

Akgün KM, Pisani M, Crothers K (2011). J Int Care Med; 26: 151–64

Human Rights Act. Introduced in the UK in 1998 (came into force in 2000), the Act incorporates the European Convention on Human Rights, ratified by the UK in 1951. Has 18 Articles, many of which have particular relevance to clinical anaesthesia/critical care:

- 2: right to life. Withdrawal/withholding of treatment is still permissible if it is in the patient's best interests.
- 3: prohibition of torture and inhuman or degrading treatment. This Article is absolute; i.e., there are no exceptions.
- 5: right to liberty and security. Relevant to treatment or restraint of patients against their will.
- 8: right to respect for private and family life. Relevant to disclosure of information. Requires qualification by balancing individuals' and society's interests.
- 9: freedom of thought, conscience and religion. Relevant to refusal of treatments for religious reasons.
- 14: prohibition of discrimination. Relevant to rationing of scarce resources on the grounds of age or race.

Other Articles may be relevant to doctors' rights as employees. All public authorities (including the NHS and its employees) must comply with the Convention.

White SM, Baldwin TJ (2002). Anaesthesia; 57: 882–8

Humidification. Inspired air is normally maximally humidified in the naso/oropharynx, becoming saturated by the time it reaches the trachea. Absolute **humidity** in the upper trachea is 34 g/m^3 (i.e., fully saturated at 34°C); in alveoli it is 43 g/m^3 (i.e., fully saturated at 37°C). Delivery of dry gases to the trachea (e.g. via a tracheal tube or tracheostomy) may cause drying of the respiratory mucosa with reduced **ciliary activity**, keratinisation and ulceration, increased tenacity of mucus with plugging of airways, atelectasis and reduced gas exchange. Humidification of inspired gases prevents this and reduces heat loss, partly by warming the gases (under 2% of total basal heat loss) but more importantly by avoiding the requirement for **latent heat** of vaporisation (10%–15% of total basal heat loss) within the trachea.

Humidification is thus mandatory during ventilation on ICUs and during prolonged general anaesthesia.

- Humidification of the patient's environment may be achieved (e.g. with an O_2 tent) but it is usually restricted to inspired gases only. Methods:
  - passive:
    - tracheal water/saline instillation; inefficient and potentially dangerous if large volumes are used.
    - bubbling inspired gas through cold water; simple but relatively inefficient (up to 10 g/m^3 produced). Vaporisation cools the water, decreasing efficiency further.
    - **heat–moisture exchanger** (HME): light, simple and highly efficient with a small dead space. Heat is conserved during expiration, allowing inspired gas to be heated and humidified. Most HMEs are hygroscopic, consisting of a foam or chemically coated (calcium or lithium chloride) paper membrane. Many HMEs are also filters. Efficiency is up to 90%. Useful for short-term IPPV provided secretions are not tenacious. Should be changed every 24–48 hours.
  - active, i.e., energy source required; commonly used in ICU because efficiency is high:
    - hot water bath: up to 60°C is employed in some, to reduce bacterial contamination. Inspired gas is passed over or through the water. Efficiency is increased by passing gas through a perforated screen to form tiny bubbles (cascade humidifier), or using absorbent wicks to increase surface area. Humidified gas is unsaturated at the working temperature, but becomes near-saturated as the temperature falls along the tubing to the patient. Condensation of water within the tubing may be reduced by heating wires within the tubing, giving closer control of the temperature drop between machine and patient. Risk of delivering excessively hot gases is reduced by monitoring the temperature within the humidifier and at the patient end of the tubing (usually kept at about 35°C), using thermostat controls and alarms.
    - other heated humidifiers, e.g. dropping water on to a heated element.
    - **nebulisers**.

Infection risks (typically with pseudomonas) are reduced by addition of antiseptic to the water, maintenance at high temperature where appropriate, and changing tubing and water daily. Condensation within tubing may provide foci for infection, obstruct ventilation or drain water into the patient's airways. The level of the water source should be kept below that of the patient. Overheating and **electrocution** may also occur.

Gross JL, Park GR (2012). Minerva Anestesiol; 78: 496–502

See also, Filters, breathing system

Humidity. Absolute humidity is the mass of water vapour per unit volume of gas at given temperature and pressure, in g/m^3 or mg/l. Relative humidity (%) is the absolute humidity divided by the amount present when the gas is fully saturated at the same temperature and pressure.

Maximal possible water content varies with temperature (Fig. 85). Thus heating a gas does not affect its absolute

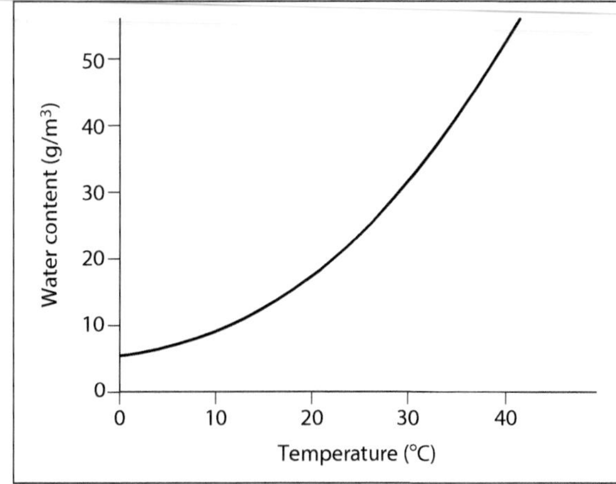

Fig. 85 Water content of saturated air at different temperatures

humidity, because the amount of water contained remains constant, but relative humidity is reduced, because warmer gas can contain more water vapour.

- Normal values of absolute humidity in:
  - upper trachea: 34 g/m^3 (fully saturated at 34°C).
  - alveoli: 43 g/m^3 (fully saturated at 37°C).

Usual value of relative humidity in operating theatres: 50%–60%. Higher values are too uncomfortable; lower values increase risk of sparks. Measured using a **hygrometer**.

See also, Humidification

Hunter's syndrome, *see Inborn errors of metabolism*

Huntington's disease. Rare autosomal dominant inherited proteinopathy, resulting in neurological degeneration in middle life. Ataxia, dementia and choreiform movements occur, with emaciation and death usually within 15 years. Anaesthetic considerations include the management of the unco-operative patient and interactions between anaesthetic and psychiatric medication.

[George Huntington (1850–1916), US physician]

Kwella JE, Sprung J, Southorn PA, et al (2010). Anesth Analg; 110: 515–23

Hurler's syndrome, *see Inborn errors of metabolism*

Hyaline membrane disease, *see Respiratory distress syndrome*

Hyaluronidase. **Enzyme** that reversibly depolymerises hyaluronic acid, a polysaccharide present in connective tissue. Aids dispersal and absorption of drugs and fluids, given sc or im. Has also been mixed with **local anaesthetic agents** to aid spread. Administration: 1500 IU in 1–2 ml water is injected into the absorption site, before, after or together with the drug. May be injected through sc cannula before administration of fluid (hypodermoclysis), allowing up to 1000 ml to be given into the thigh, calf, chest, abdomen or back regions.

Hydatid disease, *see Tropical diseases*

Hydralazine hydrochloride. **Vasodilator drug**, acting mainly on arterioles. Used to lower BP, e.g. in **hypertension**, **hypotensive anaesthesia** and **pre-eclampsia**. **Half-life** is 2–3 h; up to 16 h in renal failure. Certain patients acetylate the drug quickly, reducing half-life to under 1 h. Its onset of action may be up to 15 min after iv bolus, with effects lasting up to 90 min.

- Dosage:
  - 25–50 mg orally bd.
  - 5–10 mg increments iv.
  - 200–300 μg/min by infusion initially, then 50–150 μg/min.
- Side effects:
  - hypotension, tachycardia, fluid retention, nausea.
  - **systemic lupus erythematosus** syndrome, especially in slow acetylators and following prolonged oral therapy at doses greater than 100 mg/day.

Hydrocephalus. Increased **CSF** volume. May be caused by increased production or decreased drainage, usually the latter:

- non-communicating: blockage between the lateral ventricles and fourth ventricular outlets.
- communicating: blockage distal to the fourth ventricular outlets, e.g. at the basal cisterns.

- Causes:
  - congenital, e.g. narrowed aqueduct, obstruction of fourth ventricle outlet by a membrane (Dandy–Walker syndrome), herniation of the cerebellar tonsils through the foramen magnum (Arnold–Chiari syndrome).
  - acquired: **meningitis** with adhesions, surgery, **TBI**, **subarachnoid haemorrhage**, tumour, etc.

Usually accompanied by increased **ICP**; it may be acute, requiring urgent drainage. Pressure may be normal in some chronic forms, with slow ventricular enlargement. Head size is increased in children, with bulging of fontanelles. Cerebral or cerebellar atrophy may be present.

- Treatment:
  - surgery to the obstructive lesion.
  - shunt insertion: e.g. from the lateral ventricle to the peritoneum or right atrium.
- Anaesthetic considerations:
  - as for **neonates/paediatric anaesthesia**.
  - as for **neurosurgery**.
  - head enlargement may hinder tracheal intubation.

[Walter E Dandy (1886–1946) and Arthur E Walker (1907–1995), US neurosurgeons; Julius Arnold (1835–1915), German pathologist; Hans von Chiari (1851–1916), Austrian pathologist]

Hydrocodone bitartrate. Opioid analgesic drug, available in the USA together with other ingredients in oral preparations for cough and pain.

Hydrocortisone. Natural **corticosteroid**, with considerable **glucocorticoid** activity but little **mineralocorticoid** activity. Used therapeutically in **adrenocortical insufficiency**, hypopituitarism, acute immunological reactions (e.g. **anaphylaxis**) and various inflammatory/autoimmune conditions.

- Dosage:
  - acutely iv/im as the sodium succinate or sodium phosphate (iv injection of the latter may cause perineal irritation): 100–500 mg tds/qds.
  - orally in replacement therapy: 20–30 mg/day in two or three doses.
  - other routes: rectally, intra-articularly or topically as the acetate.

Hydrogen ions (H^+). About 12 500–13 000 mmol are produced in the body per day, mainly from the reaction of CO_2 (produced during respiration) with water. Also produced during metabolism of foodstuffs, etc. **Acid–base balance** requires buffering and excretion to maintain extracellular hydrogen ion concentration at 34–46 nmol/l, equivalent to **pH** of 7.34–7.46. Hydrogen ion **homeostasis** is required to maintain proper functioning of proteins (especially **enzymes**).

See also, Acidosis; Alkalosis; Buffers

Hydromorphone hydrochloride. Opioid analgesic drug, widely used in the USA but less so in the UK. 1.5 mg is equivalent to 10 mg **morphine**, from which it is derived. Action lasts 3–5 h. Available for rectal, oral and parenteral administration.

Hydrostatic pressure, *see Starling forces*

γ-Hydroxybutyric acid (GHBA). Drug related to **GABA** and used as an **iv anaesthetic agent** in the 1960s and 1970s. Present as a **neurotransmitter**, especially in the hypothalamus and basal ganglia. Causes slow onset of anaesthesia, lasting up to 90 min. Has been used for paediatric anaesthesia (especially cardiac catheterisation) because of its relative lack of cardiorespiratory depression, although bradycardia may occur. No longer available medicinally in the UK, although still used elsewhere in the world, e.g. certain other parts of Europe and Russia.

Has become a drug of abuse for bodybuilders (in an attempt to increase **growth hormone** production) and as a recreational drug ('liquid ecstasy'). Has also been used by criminals to induce unconsciousness in victims because the drug is difficult to detect when added to drinks. Overdose results in confusion, ataxia, visual disturbances, hallucinations, coma and convulsions; effects are increased when combined with alcohol. Treatment is largely supportive; gastric lavage and activated charcoal are of little value because absorption from the GIT is rapid. Classified in the UK as a class C **controlled drug** from 2003.

Snead OC 3rd, Gibson KM (2005). N Engl J Med; 352: 2721–32

Hydroxydione. Obsolete corticosteroid **iv anaesthetic agent**, introduced in 1955. Produced slow induction of anaesthesia and delayed recovery, with a high incidence of thrombophlebitis.

Hydroxyethyl starch (HES). Synthetic **colloid** component. Although previously widely used perioperatively and in critical care, recent evidence of increased mortality and renal impairment in some contexts has led to restriction of its licensed indications. Contraindications include: burns; sepsis; all critically ill patients; intracranial haemorrhage; dehydration/fluid overload; pulmonary oedema; and severe coagulopathy. They are now only indicated in patients with severe hypovolaemia due to acute haemorrhage, where crystalloid solutions are not considered sufficient.

Of similar structure to **glycogen**, consisting of chains of glucose molecules (>90% amylopectin), etherified with hydroxyethyl groups. Properties of each HES solution depend on:

- concentration: determines the initial volume expansion effect, e.g. 6% HES is isotonic with a given volume replacing the same volume of blood; 10% HES is hypertonic, drawing water from the interstitium into the vasculature, thus expanding the circulating volume by 145% of the infused volume.

- molar substitution (MS) ratio (degree of hydroxyethyl substitution): determines the **half-life** of the starch in plasma; the first HES solution had a high substitution ratio of 0.7 (i.e., 7 hydroxyethyl residues for every 10 glucose molecules—termed a hetastarch), resulting in extensive accumulation in tissues and persistence in plasma for >24 h.
- mean molecular weight (mw): may contribute to plasma half-life, although MS ratio is thought to be more important in vivo.
- carrier solution: either 0.9% saline or a 'balanced' electrolyte solution; the latter reduces the risk of hyperchloraemic metabolic **acidosis**, although the clinical relevance of this is unclear.

Thus, HES preparations are identified by three numbers, e.g. HES 6% 670/0.7 refers to 6% starch solution with a mean mw of 670 kDa and MS ratio of 0.7.

- Specific solutions:
  - hetastarch (0.7–0.75 MS): first HES product, introduced in the 1970s. Mean mw is 450–670 kDa. Elimination half-life of 17 days; moderate doses are associated with significant accumulation in tissues, coagulopathy and renal impairment, limiting its use.
  - hexastarch and pentastarch (0.6 and 0.5 MS ratios, respectively): development of hetastarch with a lower mean mw (200–250 kDa) and lower MS; half-life and accumulation are reduced as a result.
  - tetrastarch (0.4 MS ratio): mean mw is 130 kDa. Latest generation of HES solution, and the only form currently licensed in the UK. Degraded to smaller molecules (~70 kDa) at a constant rate, providing a more consistent concentration in the plasma that lasts ~ 4 h, with almost complete renal clearance and low risk of accumulation. May also have an anti-inflammatory effect in sepsis and after surgery. Available as 6% solutions in 0.9% saline or in a balanced electrolyte solution. Maximum recommended dose of 30 ml/kg/day, with a maximum treatment duration of 24 hr.

Myburgh JA (2015). J Intern Med; 277: 58–68

See also, Intravenous fluids

5-Hydroxytryptamine (5-HT, Serotonin). Monoamine neurotransmitter, abundant in GIT enterochromaffin cells (90%), smooth muscle, **platelets**, **mast cells** and peripheral and central nervous systems. Acts on at least seven receptor subtypes; all are **G protein-coupled receptors** except the 5-HT_3 receptor, which is a ligand-gated ion channel permeable to Na^+ and K^+.

- Involved in:
  - inflammatory mechanisms: increases vascular permeability and platelet aggregation, causes bronchoconstriction and modulates local vascular tone.
  - GIT function: increases motility, water and electrolyte secretion.
  - neurotransmission affecting arousal, muscle tone, hypothalamic/parasympathetic regulatory mechanisms, mood, memory and spinal modulation of pain.

Formed by hydroxylation and decarboxylation of tryptophan and stored in cytoplasmic vesicles. Taken up from synaptic clefts via the presynaptic membrane and metabolised mainly by **monoamine oxidase** to form 5-hydroxyindoleacetic acid (5-HIAA); urinary levels of the latter reflect the rate of metabolism.

- Drugs acting on 5-HT receptors:
  - serotonin reuptake inhibitors (e.g. fluoxetine and related **antidepressant drugs**).
  - 5-HT_{1D} receptor agonists (e.g. **sumatriptan**) used in **migraine**.
  - 5-HT_2 receptor antagonists (e.g. **ketanserin**) used in various vascular disorders, including **carcinoid syndrome**.
  - pizotifen and methysergide (also 5-HT_2 receptor antagonists) used in migraine prophylaxis.
  - **5-HT_3 receptor antagonists** used as **antiemetic drugs**.

Others are in development for use in hypertension and psychiatric or GIT disorders. Many other drugs also affect 5-HT as part of a wider spectrum of activity, e.g. **octreotide**, **reserpine**, **MAO inhibitors**, **tricyclic antidepressant drugs**.

Hygrometer. Device for measuring atmospheric **humidity**.

- Examples:
  - hair hygrometer: pointer attached to a hair whose length increases with increasing humidity. Human hair, animal tissue and paper have been used. Inaccurate but simple. The first hair hygrometer was built by da Vinci.
  - Regnault's hygrometer: silver tube containing ether; cooled by blowing air through it with a rubber bulb. When condensation appears on the outside, the air is saturated with water at that temperature (**dew point**). From a graph of water content of saturated air against temperature, water content at dew point and that at room temperature may be found. Relative humidity is the latter divided by the former.
  - wet and dry bulb hygrometer: consists of two thermometer bulbs: one dry, the other wrapped in a wet wick. The wet thermometer bulb loses heat due to water evaporation, which varies with atmospheric humidity. Humidity is read from tables, according to the temperatures measured by the two thermometers. Accuracy depends on adequate air movement.
  - humidity **transducers**: electrical properties of certain compounds (e.g. lithium chloride) alter as they absorb water. Electrical resistance or capacitance is usually measured.
  - **mass spectrometer**.
  - ultraviolet light absorption: depends on water content of air.

[Leonardo da Vinci (1452–1519), Italian polymath; Henri Regnault (1810–1878), French physicist]

Hygroscopic condensers, *see Heat–moisture exchanger*

Hyoscine hydrobromide. **Anticholinergic drug**, used mainly for **premedication** and in **palliative care**. Tertiary ammonium compound, an ester of tropic acid and scopine; found naturally in the henbane plant. Has greater sedative, antiemetic and antisialagogue action than **atropine**, but with less action on the heart and bronchial muscle. Also used to prevent motion sickness, and (as the quaternary ammonium compound, hyoscine butylbromide) to prevent or reduce gut and bladder spasm.

- Dosage:
  - 200–600 µg sc/im for premedication (15 µg/kg in children). Confusion is more likely in the elderly.
  - 300 µg, repeated 6-hourly for motion sickness (maximum 900 µg/day). Slow-release cutaneous patches are available, and have been used to reduce **PONV**.
  - 20 mg butylbromide orally qds for GIT/bladder spasm and excessive respiratory secretions.

- 20 mg butylbromide by slow iv injection for acute spasm during diagnostic procedures.
- Side effects:
  - sedation, **amnesia**, mydriasis, antiemetic action via the vomiting centre; may cause the **central anticholinergic syndrome**.
  - reduced bronchial and GIT secretions; reduced gut motility.
  - tachycardia (may follow bradycardia). The butylbromide has been associated with tachycardia, hypotension, myocardial infarction and **anaphylaxis** (all thought to be more serious in patients with underlying cardiac disease).

Hyperaesthesia. Increased sensitivity to a sensory stimulus, excluding the special senses. Includes **allodynia** and **hyperalgesia**.

Hyperaldosteronism. Excessive **aldosterone** secretion. May be:
- primary (Conn's syndrome):
  - causes include adrenal adenoma (95% of cases), hyperplasia and carcinoma. Twice as common in women.
  - causes **hypertension**, hypervolaemia, **hypokalaemia** and metabolic **alkalosis**. Plasma sodium level is usually at the upper end of the normal range.
  - **spironolactone** (aldosterone receptor antagonist) is used to treat hyperplasia. Some forms are corrected by dexamethasone. Adenomas are treated by surgery.
  - anaesthetic considerations are related to appropriate preoperative correction of electrolyte, fluid and acid–base imbalances. Spironolactone is useful preoperatively. Cardiovascular instability may occur peri- and postoperatively. Postoperative mineralocorticoid deficiency may be treated with **fludrocortisone** 50–300 µg/day orally.
- secondary: may occur in cardiac and hepatic failure, malignant hypertension and renal artery stenosis.

Measurement of plasma renin activity may aid diagnosis (low in primary disease, increased in secondary forms).
[Jerome Conn (1907–1981), US physician]
Gyamiani G, Headley CM, Naseer A, et al (2016). Am J Med Sci; 352: 391–8

Hyperalgesia. Increased **pain** from a normally painful stimulus. The term usually refers to a feature of chronic pain, but is similar to the **antanalgesia** seen with certain centrally depressant drugs (e.g. **thiopental**).
See also, Opioid-induced hyperalgesia

Hyperalimentation, *see Nutrition, total parenteral*

Hypercalcaemia. Effects are due to raised ionised **calcium** levels; symptoms are usually present when ionised calcium is >2.5 mmol/l (or when total calcium is >3.5 mmol/l).
- Caused by:
  - primary or secondary **hyperparathyroidism** (e.g. parathyroid adenoma or **renal failure**, respectively).
  - **malignancy**, due to secretion of a parathyroid hormone-related protein by the tumour and/or bony metastases.
  - less commonly:
    - increased intake, e.g. milk-alkali syndrome.
    - others: **hyperthyroidism, sarcoidosis, adrenocortical insufficiency**, immobilisation, thiazide diuretics.
- Features:
  - psychiatric disturbances.
  - **dehydration**, polyuria/polydipsia.
  - nausea/vomiting, constipation.
  - muscle weakness.
  - drowsiness, **coma**.
  - shortened **Q–T interval**; prolonged **P–R interval** on the **ECG**.
  - may lead to renal calculi/nephrocalcinosis and **renal failure**.
- Urgent treatment (before investigation) is required in severe hypercalcaemia:
  - of underlying cause (if known).
  - rehydration followed by induced diuresis to increase renal calcium loss, e.g. with **furosemide** and saline administration (caution with furosemide in renal impairment). Careful fluid balance and CVP monitoring are required.
  - if severe hypercalcaemia persists, the following may be used:
    - **bisphosphonates**, e.g.:
      - disodium pamidronate: 15–90 mg, given once or divided over 2–4 days, up to a maximum of 90 mg in total.
      - ibandronic acid: 2–4 mg by a single infusion.
      - sodium clodronate: 300 mg/day for 7–10 days or 1.5 g by a single infusion.
      - zoledronic acid: 4 mg over 15 min by a single infusion.
    - **corticosteroids** (e.g. **prednisolone** up to 120 mg/day). Act by inhibiting vitamin D.
    - **calcitonin** from 5–10 units/kg/day im/sc in 1–2 divided doses up to 400 units tds/qds. Reduces bone resorption.
    - **trisodium edetate** up to 70 mg/kg/day iv over 3 h; rapidly acting but may cause renal failure. Chelates circulating calcium.
  - others include enteral or parenteral phosphate (precipitates calcium phosphate into the tissues, including kidneys, thus no longer recommended); and plicamycin (mithramycin; a cytotoxic agent, no longer available in the UK). **Dialysis** has been used when drug treatment has failed or if calcium levels are life threatening.

Maier JD, Levine SN (2015). J Intensive Care Med; 30: 235–52

Hypercapnia. Arterial $P\text{CO}_2$ over 6 kPa (45 mmHg).
- Caused by:
  - increased production, e.g. **MH**, **TPN** using high carbohydrate content. Average normal production is approximately 200 ml/min.
  - reduced **alveolar ventilation**.
  - $\dot{V}/\dot{Q}$ **mismatch**, e.g. severe **COPD**.
  - increased inspired CO_2.
- Effects:
  - respiratory:
    - arterial O_2 saturation falls below about 90% at an alveolar $P\text{CO}_2$ over about 8 kPa (60 mmHg), breathing air.
    - increased respiratory drive via central/peripheral chemoreceptors. Tidal volume and respiratory rate increase; the extent varies with other factors (*see Breathing, control of*). Respiration is depressed at very high levels.
    - response to **hypoxaemia** is increased.
    - **oxyhaemoglobin dissociation curve** shifts to the right.

- cardiovascular:
  - increased sympathetic activity (causing increases in circulating catecholamine levels, heart rate and arterial BP), overriding the direct myocardial depressant effect of CO_2. **Arrhythmias** may occur.
  - increased **cerebral blood flow**, **ICP** and **intraocular pressure**.
- other:
  - dilated pupils, with sluggish response.
  - respiratory **acidosis** and **hyperkalaemia**. Initial **bicarbonate** increase is about 0.76 mmol/l per kPa rise above 5.3 if hypercapnia is acute (1 mmol/l per 10 mmHg above 40). Renal compensation includes bicarbonate retention and excretion of hydrogen ions; bicarbonate increase in chronic hypercapnia is about 3 mmol/l per kPa (4 mmol/l per 10 mmHg).
  - confusion, headache and coma may result (**CO_2 narcosis**).

The CNS may adjust to higher CO_2 levels in chronic hypercapnia.

Treated according to cause. If $P\text{CO}_2$ is reduced too rapidly, **alkalosis** and potassium shift may occur, causing convulsions, hypotension and arrhythmias. Recent animal data suggest that raised levels of carbon dioxide may be potentially protective in acute organ injury.

Hyperglycaemia. Plasma **glucose** over 6.0 mmol/l (108 mg/dl).
- Caused by:
  - pancreatic failure, e.g. **diabetes mellitus** (including gestational diabetes), **pancreatitis**, **sepsis**, pancreatectomy.
  - stress response, due to actions of **catecholamines**, **growth hormone**, **glucocorticoids**, **glucagon**. May occur following trauma, surgery, burns, etc (*see Stress response to surgery*).
  - administration of glucose, e.g. TPN.
  - drugs, e.g. **diethyl ether**, **thiazide diuretics**.
- Effects:
  - osmotic diuresis, causing **dehydration**, sodium and potassium loss.
  - **diabetic coma**, e.g. **ketoacidosis**.
  - increased blood **osmolality** and **viscosity**.
  - may impair **platelet** function, increase susceptibility to infection and exacerbate effects of **cerebral ischaemia**.
  - chronic effects of diabetes.
- Treatment:
  - of primary cause.
  - **hypoglycaemic drugs**.

See also, Glycaemic control in the ICU

Hyperkalaemia. Plasma **potassium** >5.3 mmol/l. Graded as mild (5.4–6.0 mmol/l), moderate (6.1–6.5 mmol/l) or severe (>6.5 mmol/l).
- Caused by:
  - increased intake, e.g. iv administration, rapid **blood transfusion**.
  - decreased renal excretion:
    - **renal failure** (accounts for 75% of severe cases of hyperkalaemia).
    - **adrenocortical insufficiency**.
    - drugs: e.g. **ciclosporin**, **angiotensin converting enzyme inhibitors**, **NSAIDs**, potassium-sparing **diuretics**, e.g. amiloride, **spironolactone**.
  - movement of potassium out of cells:
    - **trauma**, **crush syndrome**, **tumour lysis syndrome**, rhabdomyolysis, **MH**, severe **exercise**.
    - action of **suxamethonium**; exaggerated in **burns**, nerve injury, etc.
    - **acidosis**, including diabetic ketoacidosis (*See Diabetic coma*).
    - **familial periodic paralysis**.
  - artefactual, e.g. haemolysed blood sample, very high white cell counts.
- Effects:
  - nausea, vomiting, diarrhoea, muscle weakness, paraesthesiae.
  - myocardial depression, **ECG** changes (peaked **T waves**, absent **P waves**, widened **QRS complexes**, and slurring of **S–T segments** into T waves). Ventricular **arrhythmias** including **VF** are common at above 7 mmol/l. **Cardiac arrest** may occur.
- Treatment:
  - **calcium** 5–10 mmol iv repeated after 10 min if no effect (acts as a physiological antagonist of potassium). ECG changes are reversed within 1–3 min.
  - **insulin** 10 units in 50 ml of 50% dextrose iv over 5–15 min, repeated as necessary (drives potassium into cells).
  - nebulised (5 mg) or iv (50 µg bolus/5–10 µg/min infusion) **salbutamol** (increases cellular uptake of potassium).
  - **bicarbonate** 50 mmol iv if acidosis is present (exchanges potassium ions for hydrogen ions across cell membranes). Decreasing the $P_a\text{CO}_2$ by increasing minute ventilation (if artificially ventilated) has the same effect by reducing H^+ concentration.
  - **furosemide** if renal function is adequate.
  - **polystyrene sulfonate resins**: 15 g tds/qds orally; 30 g rectally. May take 6 h to achieve full effect.
  - **dialysis**.

Urgent iv treatment is required for potassium >6.5 mmol/l or if ECG changes are present. Hyperkalaemia should be corrected before anaesthesia and surgery, although the ratio of intracellular:extracellular potassium is more important than isolated plasma levels.

Kovesdy CP (2015). Am J Med; 128: 1281–7

Hypermagnesaemia. Plasma **magnesium** >1.05 mmol/l.
- Caused by:
  - **renal failure**.
  - magnesium administration.
  - laxative/antacid abuse.
  - **adrenocortical insufficiency**, **hypothyroidism**.
- Effects:
  - vasodilatation, hypotension, cardiac conduction defects (e.g. **heart block**).
  - sedation, coma, weakness, areflexia, respiratory depression. Potentiation of **non-depolarising neuromuscular blockade**.
- Treatment:
  - iv **calcium** (physiological antagonist).
  - **diuretics** and **haemodialysis**.

Hypernatraemia. Plasma **sodium** >145 mmol/l.
- Caused by:
  - sodium excess (urine sodium >20 mmol/l):
    - **hyperaldosteronism** (although it is rare for the sodium concentration to rise above the normal range).
    - **Cushing's syndrome**.

- iatrogenic, e.g. sodium **bicarbonate**, hypertonic saline administration.
  - water depletion (urine sodium variable):
    - renal loss, e.g. **diabetes insipidus**.
    - **insensible water loss**.
    - insufficient water intake.
  - sodium deficiency, with greater water deficiency:
    - renal loss (urine sodium >20 mmol/l), e.g. osmotic diuresis caused by **mannitol**, glucose, urea, etc.
    - other loss (urine sodium <10 mmol/l):
    - vomiting, diarrhoea.
    - sweating, wound losses.
- Effects:
  - features of **dehydration** if present.
  - thirst, drowsiness, confusion, coma. Cerebral dehydration, with ruptured vessels and intracranial haemorrhage, may occur.
  - ICU-acquired hypernatraemia occurs in ~30% of patients and is associated with increased mortality. Risk factors for development include **sepsis**, decreased level of consciousness, parenteral and enteral feeding, hypertonic iv infusions, osmotic and other **diuretics** and mechanical ventilation. Whether hypernatraemia itself or the underlying condition is responsible for the increased mortality is unclear.
  - preoperative hypernatraemia is also associated with increased 30-day perioperative mortality.
- Treatment:
  - of underlying cause.
  - oral water is given when possible, and/or diuretics in sodium excess. 0.9% saline may be given iv, hypotonic saline in severe water and sodium deficiency. Rapid correction may lead to cerebral oedema and convulsions, especially in hypernatraemia of >48 h duration. In these cases, rate of correction should not exceed 10 mmol/l/day (0.5 mmol/l/h in children).
  - correction of any accompanying **hypovolaemia**.

Sterns RH (2015). N Engl J Med; 372: 55–65

Hyperosmolality. Plasma **osmolality** >305 mosmol/kg. Features are as for **hypernatraemia**, which usually accompanies it. May also occur in **hyperglycaemia**, e.g. due to **diabetic coma**, TPN, and ingestion/administration of osmotically active substances, e.g. hypertonic **mannitol** solutions, **alcohol poisoning**. Detected by hypothalamic **osmoreceptors**, causing compensatory changes in water ingestion/excretion.

Hyperparathyroidism. Increased parathyroid hormone production:
  - primary: usually from a single adenoma; multiple adenomata and carcinoma may be responsible. May be associated with **multiple endocrine adenomatosis**.
  - secondary: hyperplasia arising from prolonged **hypocalcaemia**, e.g. in **renal failure**, vitamin D deficiency.
  - tertiary: secondary hyperparathyroidism where autonomous secretion develops, e.g. after renal transplantation. Hormone secretion may occur in certain tumours, e.g. **bronchial carcinoma** (pseudo-hyperparathyroidism). May be asymptomatic.
- Features:
  - those of **hypercalcaemia**; renal stones are common.
  - bony erosion and cystic changes may occur.
- Treatment:
  - as for hypercalcaemia.
  - surgery; primary adenomata may be difficult to find.
- Anaesthetic considerations:
  - preoperative hypercalcaemia, **dehydration** and renal impairment should be corrected before surgery.
  - decalcified bone is easily fractured, e.g. during positioning.
  - practical management of anaesthesia is as for **hyperthyroidism**.

Fraser WD (2009). Lancet; 374: 145–58

Hyperpathia. Increased sensation from a sensory stimulus, but with raised threshold of sensation. **Pain** may increase during stimulation, and linger afterwards.

Hyperphosphataemia. Plasma **phosphate** >1.46 mmol/l.
- Caused by:
  - factitious: **haemolysis**, prolonged contact of plasma with red blood cells.
  - increased intake: diet, iv administration, excess vitamin D, excessive use of phosphate-containing laxatives.
  - increased release from cells/bone: **diabetes mellitus**, starvation, rhabdomyolysis, **acidaemia**, **malignancy**, **renal failure**.
  - decreased excretion: renal failure (most common cause), **hypoparathyroidism**, **bisphosphonate** therapy, excess growth hormone secretion.
- Effects are related to the underlying condition and secondary **hyperparathyroidism** but acute hyperphosphataemia may result in signs of **hypocalcaemia**.
- Treatment: reduced protein intake; aluminium hydroxide or calcium carbonate orally (the latter contraindicated in **hypercalcaemia**); hypertonic **dextrose solutions** have been used to shift phosphate from the ECF into the cells; **haemodialysis**.

Hyperpyrexia, malignant, *see Malignant hyperthermia*

Hypersensitivity, *see Adverse drug reactions; Atopy*

Hypertension. Raised **arterial BP**; defined and graded by the British Hypertension Society, European Society of Hypertension and World Health Organization as follows, according to BP measured in the clinic (as opposed to ambulatory):
  - grade 1 (mild): systolic 140–159 mmHg; diastolic 90–99 mmHg.
  - grade 2 (moderate): systolic 160–179 mmHg; diastolic 100–109 mmHg.
  - grade 3 (severe): systolic ≥180 mmHg; diastolic ≥110 mmHg.
  - isolated systolic hypertension: >140 mmHg with diastolic <90 mmHg.
- In 5% of cases, hypertension is secondary to:
  - adrenal disorders, e.g. **hyperaldosteronism**, **Cushing's syndrome**, **phaeochromocytoma**.
  - unilateral or bilateral renal disease, e.g. renal artery stenosis, infection, reflux, **glomerulonephritis**, congenital abnormalities, **diabetes mellitus**, **connective tissue diseases**, obstruction, tumour.
  - others: **coarctation of aorta**, **pre-eclampsia**, drugs, e.g. **corticosteroids**, oral **contraceptives**.

  In the remaining 95% of cases, hypertension is termed primary or 'essential', i.e., has no apparent cause. Associated with family history and obesity, possibly alcohol and salt intake, diet and stress. Caffeine and smoking increase BP, as does age.

- Pathophysiological effects:
  - arteriolar wall thickening, with greater reduction in vessel radius for a given vasoconstrictive stimulus.
  - degenerative changes (e.g. fibrinoid necrosis and atheroma formation) lead to reduced blood flow and propensity to aneurysm formation and rupture.
  - **baroreceptor** sensitivity is reduced.
  - increased myocardial workload, with left ventricular hypertrophy. Increased end-diastolic pressure and coronary atheromatous plaques reduce **coronary blood flow** despite increased O_2 demand. Angina and/or **cardiac failure** may result.
- Features:
  - of **ischaemic heart disease**.
  - of cardiac failure.
  - **stroke**, encephalopathy.
  - due to renal impairment.
  - **hypertensive crisis** may occur.
  - hypertensive retinopathy: arteriovenous nipping, increased light reflex, increased tortuosity, cotton-wool exudates, haemorrhages and papilloedema.
  - **ECG** features include those of ischaemia and left ventricular hypertrophy. **CXR** features may include left ventricular dilatation and those of left ventricular failure.
- Treatment:
  - weight loss, cessation of smoking, exercise.
  - **NICE** guidelines (2011) suggest four sequential steps in the **antihypertensive drug** treatment of hypertension until BP is controlled (Fig. 86). Drugs used include **ACE inhibitors**, **Calcium channel blocking drugs** and thiazide **Diuretics**:

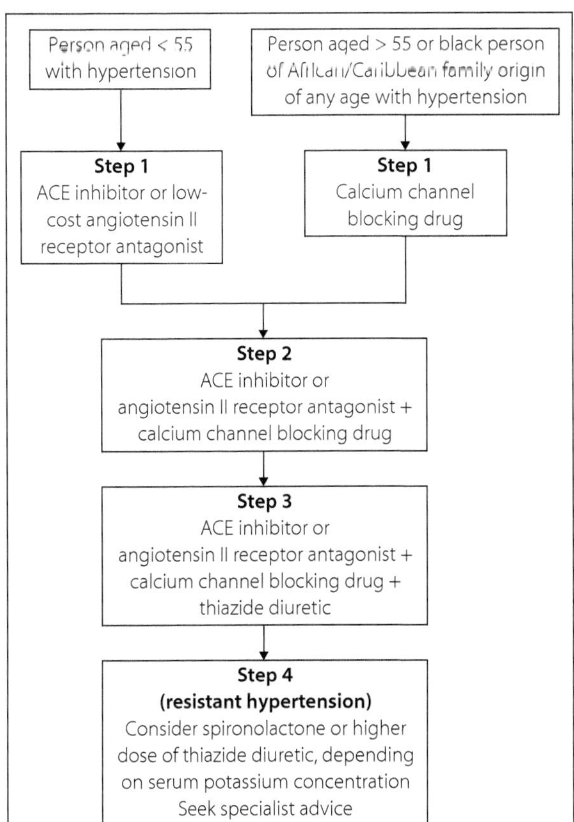

Fig. 86 NICE guidance on treatment of hypertension

    - Step 1: A (for patients <55 years) or C (for patients >55 years and all of African or Caribbean descent).
    - Step 2: A + C.
    - Step 3: A + C + D.
    - Step 4 (resistant hypertension): A + C + D + further diuretic or α- or **β-adrenergic receptor antagonists**.
  - benefits of treating severe hypertension are undoubted; those of treating milder forms are controversial. Recent guidance recommends maintaining BP <130/80 mmHg in patients at increased risk of ischaemic heart disease. The incidence of stroke is thought to be reduced if diastolic pressures >90 mmHg are treated. Recent guidelines recommend routine screening, investigation and optimal treatment of grade 2–3 hypertension in primary care, before referral for elective surgery.
- Anaesthesia for patients with hypertension:
  - preoperatively:
    - assessment for ischaemic heart disease, cardiac failure, cerebrovascular disease and renal impairment.
    - if not on treatment, surgery should be postponed unless it is an emergency. Patients with systolic pressure >180 mmHg and diastolic pressure above 110 mmHg should be investigated and hypertension treated before anaesthesia and surgery, because morbidity and mortality are greater if untreated. Antihypertensive drugs are continued up to the morning of surgery.
    - sedative **premedication** is often advocated to reduce endogenous catecholamine levels.
  - perioperatively:
    - induction and maintenance as for ischaemic heart disease. Swings in BP are more likely because of arteriolar hypertrophy; e.g. hypotension on induction and hypertension on intubation (*see Intubation, complications of*).
    - marked cardiovascular instability may accompany **spinal/epidural anaesthesia** if hypertension is uncontrolled.
  - postoperatively:
    - adequate analgesia is particularly important.
    - treatment of persistent hypertension may be required.
- Hypertension during anaesthesia may be due to:
  - inadequate anaesthesia/analgesia.
  - tracheal intubation/extubation.
  - inadequate paralysis.
  - underlying hypertensive disease.
  - aortic clamping.
  - **hypercapnia**, **hypoxaemia**.
  - **cerebral ischaemia**, stroke, raised **ICP**.
  - drugs, e.g. **ketamine**, **adrenaline**, **cocaine**.
  - rarely, **MH**, phaeochromocytoma, **thyroid crisis**, **carcinoid syndrome**.

  Management is directed towards the underlying cause. **Labetalol, hydralazine, nifedipine, sodium nitroprusside** and **GTN** are commonly used to control BP. Vasodilator therapy is less likely to be successful in atherosclerosis, because the arterial tree is relatively rigid; labetalol or other β-adrenergic antagonists may be more effective.

Postoperatively, urinary retention, residual neuromuscular blockade, pain and anxiety may cause hypertension, in addition to the above factors. In the ICU, hypertension is often due to inadequate **sedation**, but many of the factors above should also be considered.

Hartle A, McCormack T, Carlisle J, et al (2016). Anaesthesia; 71: 326–37

Hypertensive crisis. Severe **hypertension** (>180/120 mmHg) with or without acute end-organ damage. May occur as a feature of chronic hypertensive disease, postoperatively after cardiac/vascular surgery, or other conditions including **pre-eclampsia** and **phaeochromocytoma.** Features represent end-organ impairment:
- **acute coronary syndromes, cardiac failure** and **stroke.**
- **renal failure.**
- **encephalopathy**: confusion, headache, visual disturbances, convulsions, coma.
- retinal haemorrhage, papilloedema and **epistaxis.**

• Treatment:
- if not associated with end-organ damage, oral therapy is used (e.g. **atenolol, labetalol** or **nifedipine**), aiming to reduce BP cautiously to <160/100 mmHg over hours to days. Large loading doses or iv drugs may cause precipitous falls in BP, resulting in stroke/blindness, renal impairment or myocardial ischaemia.
- extreme hypertension (e.g. >220/130 mmHg) is usually associated with life-threatening end-organ damage, and requires admission to a critical care unit for invasive BP monitoring and prompt, titratable BP control (e.g. 15%–20% reduction in BP over the first hour then reduction to 160/110 mmHg over the next 2–6 h). Suitable agents include **sodium nitroprusside, esmolol** and **labetalol.** Patients commonly have sodium and volume depletion and require cautious loading with isotonic saline.

Rodriguez MA, Kumar SK, De Caro M (2010). Cardiol Rev; 18: 102–7

Hyperthermia. Defined as a core temperature >38°C. Fever is a type of hyperthermia caused by a resetting of thermoregulation (e.g. by infection) and defined as a core temperature >38.3°C. Hyperpyrexia is a temperature ≥40°C. Heatstroke is the clinical syndrome caused by exposure to excessively high environmental temperature, especially if unaccustomed, and if **temperature regulation** is impaired.

• Caused by:
- hypothalamic lesions, e.g. tumour, surgery, **stroke,** CNS infection.
- increased heat production:
  - occurs in 15%–50% of patients following surgery and represents a postoperative inflammatory response.
  - **sepsis.**
  - **exercise.**
  - drug-induced, e.g. **MH, neuroleptic malignant syndrome, salicylate poisoning, cocaine poisoning, methylenedioxymethylamfetamine** ingestion.
  - **hyperthyroidism.**
  - **phaeochromocytoma.**
  - **status epilepticus.**
  - **tetanus.**
- impaired heat loss:
  - **autonomic neuropathy.**
  - drug-induced, e.g. **anticholinergic drugs, phenothiazines,** neuroleptic malignant syndrome.
  - **dehydration.**
  - excessive warming during anaesthesia.

Features of heatstroke include confusion, headache, coma, anhydrosis and temperature >40.6°C. Hyperventilation may be followed by metabolic acidosis, convulsions, and cardiovascular and **MODS.**

• Treatment:
- specific, e.g. MH.
- cooling with tepid water; cold water may induce peripheral vasoconstriction with impairment of further heat exchange. Cooling blanket systems monitor the patient's core temperature and vary the temperature of the circulating water accordingly. Cold iv fluids and irrigation of body cavities may be used. Intravascular cooling may be necessary in refractory cases.
- drugs, e.g. **aspirin, paracetamol.**

Horseman MA, Rather-Conally J, Surani S (2013). J Intensive Care Med; 28: 334–40

Hyperthermia, malignant, *see Malignant hyperthermia*

Hyperthyroidism (Thyrotoxicosis). In 75% of cases, caused by primary thyroid overactivity produced by thyroid stimulating autoantibodies (Graves' disease) or toxic nodular goitre. Graves' disease is more common in women, those with other autoimmune diseases and smokers. Other causes include **pituitary** adenoma secreting thyroid stimulating hormone and drugs including **amiodarone, lithium** and highly active antiretroviral therapy.

• Features:
- malaise, anxiety, sweating, heat intolerance, tremor, psychological changes, myopathy (usually proximal).
- weight loss, increased appetite, diarrhoea.
- palpitations, tachycardia, **AF, cardiac failure.**
- goitre, oligomenorrhoea, gynaecomastia.
- eye features: usually lid retraction and mild proptosis; occasionally severe with visual disturbances. May be associated with pretibial myxoedema (pink/brown subcutaneous infiltration on the lower leg) and pseudoclubbing.
- **thyroid crisis** may occur, triggered by surgery, infection, etc.

• Investigation: measurement of plasma thyroxine and triiodothyronine (either or both of which may be raised), thyroid stimulating hormone, and, rarely, thyrotropin releasing hormone. Radioisotope and ultrasound scanning may be performed.

• Treatment:
- antithyroid drugs:
  - carbimazole or its active metabolite methimazole; propyluracil: prevent formation of thyroid hormones by acting as a substrate for iodination by thyroid peroxidase. Pruritus and rash are common; agranulocytosis may occur. Increase vascularity of the gland, therefore sometimes stopped 2 weeks preoperatively. Usually given for a course of 1–1.5 years. Act within at least 1–2 weeks.
  - iodine: temporarily inhibits hormone release; sometimes given for 2 weeks preoperatively to reduce glandular vascularity.
  - radioactive iodine: increasingly used as fears of subsequent sterility and tumours diminish.
- **β-adrenergic receptor antagonists**: act by reducing conversion of thyroxine to triiodothyronine and direct antagonism of the peripheral effects of hyperthyroidism. Act within 12–24 h.
- surgery: requires adequate medical control preoperatively, in order to prevent thyroid crisis.

• Anaesthetic management:
- preoperatively:
  - assessment of thyroid state, especially cardiovascular and neurological aspects. Emergency

treatment is as for thyroid crisis. Other **autoimmune disease** may be present, e.g. **myasthenia gravis**.
  - assessment for possible **airway obstruction**. **CXR** including **thoracic inlet** views is useful. Elective **tracheostomy** is sometimes performed if the goitre is very large. Indirect laryngoscopy is performed to assess vocal cord function in case of pre-existing damage to the **laryngeal nerves**.
- perioperatively:
  - tracheal intubation may be difficult. IPPV is usually used; reinforced tracheal tubes are sometimes preferred.
  - because of the risk of damage to the laryngeal nerves, special tracheal tubes are available through which the vocal cord muscle's electrical potentials may be monitored during surgery. The surgeon stimulates tissues electrically, allowing the nerves to be identified and thus avoided. Neuromuscular blocking drugs must be avoided if this technique is used.
  - the eyes should be protected from pressure.
  - operative bleeding may be reduced by infiltration with adrenaline solutions, head-up position and **hypotensive anaesthesia**.
  - **arrhythmias** may result from poor thyroid control or manipulation of the **carotid sinus**. Risk of **gas embolism** exists in the steep head-up position.
  - **pneumothorax** and tracheal trauma may occur.
  - regional anaesthesia may also be used in high-risk patients, using 0.5% **prilocaine** or **lidocaine** with adrenaline:
    - from the midpoint of the sternomastoid muscle on both sides, 10 ml is injected into the muscle body, 10 ml anteriorly and 10 ml infiltrated caudally and cranially.
    - 20 ml is injected sc to each side from the midline, below the thyroid gland.
- postoperatively:
  - assessment of the vocal cords' activity is often requested by the surgeon after extubation, although direct laryngoscopy may be difficult at this stage. Fibreoptic inspection, e.g. through a **SAD**, has been described.
  - airway obstruction may be caused by:
    - haemorrhage into the tissues of the neck. Skin sutures or clips must be easily removable.
    - tracheomalacia (floppy, collapsible trachea) if the goitre is large. Reintubation or tracheostomy may be required.
    - laryngeal nerve damage.
    - **hypoparathyroidism** causing **hypocalcaemia** and **tetany** may occur from several hours to several days later.
- thyroid crisis or subsequent **hypothyroidism** may also occur.

[Robert Graves (1796–1853), Irish physician]
De Leo S, Lee SY, Braverman LE (2016). Lancet; 388: 906–18
See also, Neck, cross-sectional anatomy; Thyroid gland

Hypertonic intravenous solutions. Intravenous solutions (typically **saline**) of high **osmolality**; have been used in small volumes (e.g. 250 ml boluses) for initial resuscitation in **shock** (e.g. due to **haemorrhage**). Also increasingly used as an alternative to **mannitol** to reduce **ICP** after **TBI** although current evidence does not suggest improved outcome. Effects include: expansion of the intravascular volume by drawing in fluid from the intracellular and interstitial spaces; reduced SVR and **afterload**; direct inotropy; and anti-inflammatory effects. Current evidence suggests that they are effective in improving BP and reducing ICP in these contexts; however, morbidity and mortality outcomes are similar when compared with conventional resuscitation fluids.

Various solutions have been used. Combinations of hypertonic 7.5% saline with colloid (usually 6% **dextran** 70) are thought to maximise the benefits of rapid and sustained plasma expansion by virtue of the saline and colloid components, respectively.
Lazaridis C, Neyens R, Bodie J, DeSantis SM (2013). Crit Care Med; 41: 1353–60

Hyperventilation. Abnormally increased pulmonary ventilation, resulting in increased excretion of CO_2. It may occur in both awake and anaesthetised spontaneously breathing patients, e.g. due to pain, **hypoxaemia**, **hypercapnia**, **acidosis** and **pregnancy**. Sometimes occurs in midbrain/pontine lesions. Commonly performed during **IPPV**, intentionally or unintentionally.

Its main effects are related to resultant **hypocapnia** (e.g. **tetany**), or the adverse cardiovascular effects of IPPV. Increases the work of breathing.

Hypnosis. Sleeplike state, with persistence of certain behavioural responses. The subject is susceptible to, and may respond to, the hypnotist's suggestions concerning behaviour, environment and memory, despite possible contradiction by actual stimuli and character. The effects may persist after return to normal consciousness, but possibly without recall of the hypnotic state.
- Has been used:
  - to help smoking cessation.
  - to aid recall of subconscious thoughts, e.g. psychiatric/psychological research and therapy, investigation of **awareness** under anaesthesia.
  - to modify pain perception, e.g. in obstetrics, perioperatively, and in chronic pain.
  - for entertainment.

Originally expounded as **mesmerism** in the mid/late 1700s, although evidence of similar techniques dates back thousands of years. The term was coined in the 1840s.

Whether hypnosis represents a separate physiological state, or an interpersonal social interaction (i.e., obeyer/commander) is controversial. Certainly suggestion is widely used, e.g. by doctors and dentists, to reduce fear, anxiety and use of drugs.
[Hypnos, Greek god of sleep]
Wobst AHK (2007). Anesth Analg; 104: 1199–208

Hypoadrenalism, *see Adrenocortical insufficiency*

Hypoaesthesia. Reduced sensitivity to a sensory stimulus, excluding special senses.

Hypoalgesia. Reduced **pain** from a normally painful stimulus. May be caused by: reduced afferent input e.g. sensory neuropathies, **NSAIDs**, **local anaesthetic drugs**; or altered central processing e.g. centrally acting **analgesic drugs**, exercise, heightened mental state.

Hypocalcaemia. Effects are usually present when total plasma **calcium** is under 2.0 mmol/l, and are due to decreased plasma ionised calcium. Although total calcium is reduced in **hypoproteinaemia**, the ionised portion is normal and clinical features are absent.

- Caused by:
  - decreased parathyroid hormone activity, e.g. **hypoparathyroidism, hypomagnesaemia.**
  - decreased vitamin D activity, e.g. the above, chronic **renal failure**, intestinal malabsorption, inadequate diet, liver disease.
  - increased calcium loss, e.g. **chelating agents**, calcification of soft tissues (e.g. rhabdomyolysis, **pancreatitis, hyperphosphataemia**).
  - decreased ionised calcium, e.g. **alkalosis.**
- Features (exacerbated by hypomagnesaemia):
  - paraesthesiae.
  - muscle cramps/spasm/**tetany**. **Stridor** may occur. Chvostek's sign is facial spasm following tapping over the facial nerve. Trousseau's sign is carpopedal spasm following inflation of a tourniquet around the arm.
  - mental excitability, **convulsions.**
  - prolonged **Q–T interval** on the **ECG**; decreased cardiac output.
- Treatment:
  - of predisposing cause.
  - supportive (airway, etc.).
  - iv calcium if severe, e.g. chloride 10% 5–10 ml or gluconate 10% 10–20 ml slow bolus, followed by infusion if required.
  - magnesium if deficient.

[Frantisek Chvostek (1835–1884), Austrian physician; Armand Trousseau (1801–1867), French physician]

Cooper MS, Gittoes NJL (2008). Br Med J; 1298–302

Hypocapnia. Arterial $P\text{CO}_2$ <4.7 kPa (35 mmHg).

- Caused by:
  - **hyperventilation**. May be iatrogenic (e.g. during **IPPV**), self-induced or a compensatory response to metabolic **acidosis.**
  - reduced CO_2 production, e.g. in **brainstem death.**
- Effects:
  - vasoconstriction; reduced **cerebral blood flow** may cause dizziness, light-headedness and confusion. Risk of convulsions if predisposed, e.g. if **enflurane** is used. Placental blood flow is reduced. If IPPV is employed, cardiovascular effects are increased.
  - **alkalosis, hypokalaemia** and **hypocalcaemia** may occur.
  - reduced respiratory drive; apnoea may occur postoperatively.
  - reduced requirement for anaesthetic agents has been inconsistently demonstrated.

If iatrogenic, corrected by reducing **alveolar ventilation**, e.g. by increasing **dead space** and rebreathing, or reducing minute volume. If compensatory, best not corrected until the underlying cause of acidosis is treated.

Hypoglycaemia. Low plasma **glucose** level; symptoms are uncommon until levels fall to 2–3 mmol/l (40–50 mg/dl); the threshold is lower in chronic hypoglycaemia and higher in chronic hyperglycaemia.

- Types:
  - fasting, i.e., only after several hours without food:
    - reduced glucose output from liver:
      - starvation (especially children).
      - alcohol ingestion.
      - **hepatic failure.**
      - **adrenocortical insufficiency.**
      - **renal failure, growth hormone** deficiency, **pregnancy.**
    - increased **insulin** activity:
      - insulin/**sulfonylurea** administration. Recognised as an important cause of increased morbidity and mortality in ICU patients treated with tight glucose control (*see Glycaemic control in ICU*).
      - insulinoma. Associated with increased C-protein levels.
      - sarcoma, hepatoma, adrenocortical and other tumours. Thought to be caused by secretion of an insulin-like factor.
      - **sepsis, malaria.**
  - reactive, i.e., 2–5 h post-prandially:
    - idiopathic.
    - gastric surgery; causes rapid glucose absorption and excessive insulin release (cf. dumping syndrome, due to sudden osmotic load and/or other gut hormone release).
    - may occur in **diabetes mellitus.**
    - **inborn errors of metabolism**, e.g. **glycogen storage disorders.**
  - rebound hypoglycaemia may follow sudden cessation of **TPN**, due to high levels of circulating insulin.
  - drug-induced e.g. ethanol, haloperidol, salicylates, sulfonamides, tramadol.
- Features:
  - secretion of hyperglycaemic hormones, e.g. **adrenaline, glucagon, growth hormone** and cortisol; the former causes tachycardia, sweating and pallor.
  - confusion, restlessness, dysarthria, diplopia, convulsions, coma. Permanent brain damage may occur with coma of increasing duration, but is rare if <4 h. May be exacerbated by hypoxaemia and hypotension. **Cerebral oedema** may contribute.
  - may be masked by anaesthesia, presenting only during recovery.
- Treatment:
  - 25–50 ml 50% glucose iv if unconscious, repeated as necessary. Risk of venous thrombosis is reduced by flushing the cannula with saline after injection. Oral glucose is given if able to drink.
  - glucagon 1 mg has been used im, but is ineffective in hepatic dysfunction and alcohol ingestion, and may exacerbate insulinoma-induced hypoglycaemia.

Hypoglycaemic drugs. Strictly, refers to all drugs used to lower plasma glucose concentration, although the term is often used to refer to oral drugs only. Used primarily in the treatment of **diabetes mellitus**, although **insulin** is also used in the treatment of **hyperkalaemia.**

- Divided into:
  - oral:
    - **biguanides** (e.g. metformin): decrease gluconeogenesis and increase peripheral glucose uptake.
    - **sulfonylureas** (e.g. glibenclamide): increase pancreatic secretion of insulin, and possibly increase peripheral glucose uptake.
    - **thiazolidinediones** (e.g. pioglitazone): increase peripheral sensitivity to insulin. Rosiglitazone has been withdrawn due to increased risk of cardiac events.
    - **meglitinides** (e.g. nateglinide): stimulate release of insulin from the pancreas.
    - α-glucosidase inhibitors (e.g. **acarbose**): inhibit absorption of carbohydrate from the GIT.

- parenteral, i.e., insulin and insulin analogues (e.g. glargine).

Novel agents undergoing evaluation:
- glucagon-like peptide-1 (GLP-1) receptor agonists (e.g. exenatide): stimulate insulin secretion, inhibit glucagon secretion, slow gastric emptying and suppress appetite.
- dipeptidyl peptidase-IV (DPP-4) inhibitors (e.g. sitagliptin): inhibit breakdown of GLP-1.

Thraser J (2017). Am J Med; 130 (Suppl 6): S4–17

Hypokalaemia. Plasma **potassium** <3.5 mmol/l. Symptoms usually occur below 2.5 mmol/l, although complications may occur at higher levels in predisposed patients (e.g. acute **MI**). Total deficit may be up to 500 mmol.

- Caused by:
  - reduced intake, e.g. iv fluid therapy without potassium supplementation.
  - excessive losses:
    - renal:
      - solute diuresis, e.g. saline, glucose, **mannitol**, urea.
      - **diuretic** therapy.
      - **hyperaldosteronism** and disorders of the **renin/angiotensin system.**
      - **Cushing's syndrome.**
      - diuretic phase of **acute kidney injury**.
    - GIT, e.g. diarrhoea, vomiting, fistulae.
  - movement of potassium into cells:
    - **alkalosis.**
    - drugs, e.g. **insulin**, **catecholamines**.
- Effects:
  - muscle weakness, ileus.
  - **arrhythmias, ECG** changes (**S–T segment** depression, **Q–T** and **P–R interval** prolongation, **T wave** inversion, **U wave**). **Cardiac arrest** may occur.
  - impaired renal concentrating ability.
  - increased sensitivity to non-depolarising **neuromuscular blocking drugs**.
  - increased adverse effects of **digoxin**.
  - may cause metabolic alkalosis.
- Treatment:
  - oral supplementation: up to 200 mmol (15 g)/day.
  - iv potassium chloride: up to 40 mmol (3 g)/l fluid peripherally, infused at up to 40 mmol/h. Excessively concentrated solutions may cause vascular necrosis, and too rapid administration may cause **VF**; in severe cases, the above limits may be exceeded with ECG monitoring.

Hypokalaemia should be corrected before anaesthesia and surgery, although the ratio of intracellular/extracellular potassium is more important than isolated plasma levels.

Unwin RJ, Luft FC, Shirley DG (2011). Nat Rev Nephrol; 7: 75–84

Hypomagnesaemia. Plasma **magnesium** <0.75 mmol/l. Because only 1% of magnesium is present in ECF, plasma levels may not correlate with clinical features.

- Caused by:
  - reduced magnesium intake, e.g. **TPN**, **alcoholism**, **malnutrition**, malabsorption (e.g. following gastric bypass surgery, chronic **pancreatitis**, **inflammatory bowel disease**)
  - increased loss, e.g. GIT (prolonged diarrhoea/vomiting), renal (diuretics, diabetes), **hypercalaemia**, **hyperaldosteronism.**
  - others e.g. **burns**, acute pancreatitis.
- Features:
  - arrhythmias (including **torsade de pointes**), **prolonged Q–T syndromes**.
  - neurological: nystagmus, confusion, irritability, tremor, convulsions.
  - exacerbation of the effects of **hypocalcaemia**.
- Treatment:
  - of primary cause.
  - acutely: 10–20 mmol $MgSO_4$ iv over 1–2 h, repeated as required with plasma monitoring, up to 50 mmol/day.

Hyponatraemia. Plasma **sodium** <135 mmol/l. Usually results in hypo-osmolar plasma (not always, e.g. **hyperglycaemia** or hypertonic **mannitol** infusion causing hyperosmolar plasma).

- Caused by:
  - water excess; relative euvolaemia:
    - excessive intake (urine sodium <10 mmol/l):
      - iv administration of sodium-deficient fluids.
      - **TURP syndrome.**
      - excessive drinking.
    - reduced excretion (urine sodium >20 mmol/l):
      - **syndrome of inappropriate antidiuretic hormone secretion** (SIADH).
      - drugs, e.g. chlorpropamide, oxytocin (have antidiuretic effect).
  - water excess with (smaller) sodium excess (urine sodium <10 mmol/l); hypervolaemia:
    - cardiac and hepatic failure.
    - **nephrotic syndrome.**
  - water deficiency with greater sodium deficiency; hypovolaemia:
    - renal loss (urine sodium >20 mmol/l):
      - **diuretic** therapy.
      - **adrenocortical insufficiency.**
      - **cerebral salt-wasting syndrome.**
      - salt-losing nephritis.
      - **renal tubular acidosis.**
      - post-relief of urinary obstruction.
    - other loss (urine sodium <10 mmol/l):
      - diarrhoea and vomiting.
      - **pancreatitis.**
  - redistribution of sodium/water:
    - sick cell syndrome in terminally ill patients: thought to be caused by impaired cell membrane sodium/potassium transport, resulting in sodium redistribution to the intracellular compartment.
    - water shift from intracellular to extracellular compartments, e.g. due to hyperglycaemia. Corrected plasma sodium concentration in hyperglycaemia: $[Na^+] + ([glucose] \div 4)$.
  - pseudohyponatraemia, e.g. in hyperlipidaemia: the sodium-poor lipid portion is analysed together with the aqueous portion. Modern equipment analyses only the aqueous portion.
- Features:
  - of **dehydration** and **hypovolaemia** in sodium deficiency.
  - symptoms attributed to water entering cells by osmosis include headache, nausea, confusion, coma and convulsions with possibly permanent neurological defects. Premenopausal women are especially at risk; the threshold for convulsions and/or respiratory arrest in this group may be as high as 130 mmol/l, compared with 115–120 mmol/l in men and postmenopausal women.

- Treatment:
  - of underlying cause.
  - as for SIADH: water restriction, **demeclocycline**.
  - iv hypertonic saline (3%) is used in severe cases of sodium and water deficiency (sodium <115 mmol/l). The optimal rate of plasma sodium increase is controversial, but correction should be slow, because subdural haemorrhage, **central pontine myelinolysis** and cardiac failure may occur if too rapid. 5–10 mmol/l/day has been suggested as the maximal safe rate; up to 2 mmol/l/h until a plasma sodium of 120 mmol/l is reached. Total sodium deficit (mmol) assuming distribution throughout total body water = (125 − measured sodium) × 60% of body weight (kg). Normal saline with **furosemide** has been used in less severe cases.
  - V_2 **vasopressin** receptor antagonists (e.g. tolvaptan): increase free water excretion; used in euvolaemic or hypervolaemic patients with SIADH.

Sterns RH (2015). N Engl J Med; 372: 55–65

Hypo-osmolality. Plasma **osmolality** <280 mosmol/kg. Features are as for **hyponatraemia**. Detected by hypothalamic **osmoreceptors**, causing compensatory changes in water ingestion and excretion.

Hypoparathyroidism. Most commonly occurs postoperatively, e.g. following parathyroid/thyroid/laryngeal surgery; may be acute or occur several years later. May also be idiopathic, sometimes familial.

Pseudohypoparathyroidism: same features, due to lack of peripheral response to parathyroid hormone; may be associated with **hypothyroidism**.

Pseudopseudohypoparathyroidism: features of pseudohypoparathyroidism but with normal **calcium** and **phosphate** levels.

- Features:
  - **hypocalcaemia**.
  - **hyperphosphataemia**.
- Treatment: calcium and vitamin D supplements. An injectable recombinant parathyroid hormone is available. Anaesthetic considerations are related to hypocalcaemia.

Clarke BL, Brown EM, Collins MT, et al (2016). J Clin Endocrinol Metab; 101: 2284–99

See also, Thyroid gland

Hypophosphataemia. Plasma **phosphate** <0.8 mmol/l.

- Caused by:
  - decreased intestinal absorption: e.g. **malnutrition**, vitamin D deficiency, **diarrhoea**, vomiting, nasogastric aspiration, **refeeding syndrome**, **TPN**, chronic **alcoholism**/withdrawal.
  - redistribution from extracellular to intracellular compartments: e.g. respiratory **alkalosis**, glucose/insulin therapy, **catecholamines**, recovery from diabetic ketoacidosis, **burns**.
  - increased excretion: e.g. **diuretics**, **corticosteroids**, **hyperparathyroidism**, **dialysis**.

Hypophosphataemia is common in ICU because of the presence of many of the above factors.

- Effects:
  - muscle weakness, myocardial depression.
  - irritability, dysarthria, encephalopathy, peripheral neuropathy, convulsions, coma.
  - rhabdomyolysis, haemolysis, platelet and leucocyte dysfunction.
- Treatment: sodium or potassium phosphate: 10–20 mmol orally or 5–20 mmol/h iv. Overtreatment and resultant hyperphosphataemia may cause **hypocalcaemia** and hypomagnesaemia.

Geerse DA, Bindels AJ, Kuiper MA, et al (2010). Crit Care; 14: R147

Hypopituitarism. Reduced secretion of anterior **pituitary gland** hormones (hyposecretion of posterior portion causes **diabetes insipidus**). Most commonly caused by pituitary tumour; may also follow surgery/radiotherapy, granulomatous disease, cysts or ischaemic necrosis of the pituitary during pregnancy (Sheehan's syndrome).

- Features:
  - absent axillary/pubic hair, breast and genital atrophy, pale skin, muscle wasting.
  - of **hypothyroidism** and **adrenocortical insufficiency**. Main anaesthetic considerations are related to the latter two features.
- Treatment:
  - of underlying cause.
  - hormone replacement, e.g. **hydrocortisone**, thyroxine and testosterone or oestradiol.

[Harold Sheehan (1900–1988), English pathologist]

Hypoproteinaemia. Plasma proteins <60 g/l. Most commonly due to low **albumin** levels (under 35 g/l). May occur in **malnutrition**, hepatic/**renal failure**, protein-losing nephropathy or enteropathy, and in severely ill catabolic patients, e.g. on ICU (where it correlates with poor respiratory outcome and increased mortality from **sepsis**).

- Anaesthetic significance:
  - for drugs that are largely protein-bound, reduced available binding sites increase the proportion of unbound drug, increasing the clinical effect; e.g. **opioid analgesic drugs**, **thiopental**, antibiotics. Effects are increased further if available binding sites are already occupied by other protein-bound drugs. Albumin is usually involved in **protein-binding**, but others are also involved, e.g. gammaglobulin and acid α_1-glycoprotein.
  - decreased plasma **oncotic pressure** may lead to tissue **oedema**.
  - specific protein deficiencies, e.g. **coagulation disorders**, plasma **cholinesterase** deficiency.

Hypotension. Because **MAP** = **cardiac output** (CO) × **SVR**, hypotension may result from reduction of:

- CO:
  - reduced **heart rate**:
    - vagal reflexes.
    - drugs, e.g. **halothane**, **β-adrenergic receptor antagonists**, **neostigmine**.
    - **arrhythmias**.
  - reduced **stroke volume**:
    - reduced **venous return**, e.g. **hypovolaemia**, **spinal/epidural/caudal anaesthesia**, head-up posture, **aortocaval compression**, **IPPV**, tension **pneumothorax**, **cardiac tamponade**.
    - arrhythmias.
    - increased **afterload**, e.g. **aortic stenosis**, **PE** (including **air** and **amniotic fluid embolism**), pneumothorax, tamponade.
    - reduced **myocardial contractility**, e.g. drugs, **hypoxia**, **hypercapnia**, **ischaemic heart disease**, **MI**, **cardiomyopathy**, **myocarditis**, **cardiac failure**, **acidosis**, **hypothermia**.

- SVR:
  - drugs, e.g. **vasodilator drugs**, volatile and iv anaesthetic agents.
  - **adverse drug reactions**.
  - spinal/epidural/caudal anaesthesia.
  - **sepsis**.

Reduction in blood flow to vital organs may result, with risk of permanent ischaemic damage, e.g. **stroke**, MI, **renal failure**. **Autoregulation** maintains **cerebral**, **coronary** and **renal blood flows** at systolic BP of approximately 70–80 mmHg.

Treatment consists of O_2 administration, raising the feet and specific treatment directed towards the cause.

Hypotensive anaesthesia. Usually defined as deliberate lowering of BP during anaesthesia by more than 30% of resting value. Techniques usually involve reduction of systolic BP to about 80 mmHg (**MAP** 50–60 mmHg), although levels of 60–70 mmHg (MAP 40 mmHg) have been employed. Performed in circumstances where surgery may be hindered by bleeding and to reduce **blood loss** (e.g. middle ear surgery, **neurosurgery**, **plastic surgery**) and extensive major surgery, e.g. cystectomy, pelvic clearance. Its use is controversial, because hypotension may cause organ ischaemia, dysfunction and infarction, particularly of heart, liver, kidneys, brain and spinal cord. Considered by some to be too dangerous for non–life-saving surgery, but by others to be routinely acceptable. Risks are lowest in fit young patients, but consequences of major infarction are more dramatic in this group.

- Contraindications are also controversial, but include:
  - impaired organ blood flow or function, e.g. **ischaemic heart disease**, renal disease, cerebrovascular disease, age (implies the foregoing).
  - **hypertension**.
  - **diabetes mellitus**: there may be increased sensitivity to hypotensive agents as autonomic function may be impaired already. Increased sensitivity to insulin has followed ganglion blockade.
  - severe respiratory disease. **Bronchospasm** may follow use of **ganglion blocking drugs** or **β-adrenergic receptor antagonists** in asthmatics.
  - **pregnancy**, **anaemia**, **hypovolaemia**.
  - anaesthetist and surgeon unfamiliar with the technique.

Originally achieved in the 1940s by deliberate hypovolaemia and/or high **spinal anaesthesia**. Now achieved by using:

- anaesthetic drugs/techniques that lower BP:
  - reduced **cardiac output**, e.g. **IPPV**, head-up **positioning of the patient**, volatile agents.
  - reduced **SVR**, e.g. **tubocurarine**, **isoflurane**, spinal/**epidural anaesthesia**.
- specific hypotensive drugs, e.g.:
  - β-receptor antagonists, including **labetalol**.
  - **vasodilator drugs**, e.g. **sodium nitroprusside**, **GTN**, **hydralazine**.
  - previously, **ganglion blocking drugs**.
- Management:
  - **preoperative assessment** with regard to contraindications.
  - **premedication** may be given to improve smoothness of induction. **Atropine** is avoided.
  - smooth induction of anaesthesia, with minimal coughing, straining, etc. Attempts may be made to reduce the hypertensive response to intubation (*see Intubation, complications of*). Drugs increasing heart rate or BP are avoided, e.g. atropine, **ketamine**, **pancuronium**.
  - tracheal intubation is usually performed. Spontaneous ventilation is preferred by some, because it may indicate adequacy of brainstem blood flow. IPPV is often employed to avoid **hypercapnia** and vasodilatation associated with spontaneous respiration; it also reduces venous return. **PEEP** has been used to augment the latter but may increase venous bleeding. **Dead space** and **$\dot{V}/\dot{Q}$ mismatch** are increased at low blood pressures, therefore F_IO_2 is usually increased to 0.5.
  - intra-arterial BP measurement is usually employed if profound hypotension or infusions of potent hypotensive agents are used; otherwise indirect methods of measurement are usually adequate. **CVP** measurement is useful in major surgery. A large-bore iv cannula is required. **EEG** and its derivatives have been used to monitor cerebral activity.
  - careful positioning of patient, with the site of surgery raised above the heart, and avoidance of venous kinking and obstruction. Head-up tilt is introduced gradually to avoid sudden severe hypotension. 20–30 degree tilt is usually sufficient; BP at the head is about 15–20 mmHg less than that at the heart.
  - a typical anaesthetic sequence consists of **thiopental** or **propofol**, IPPV, maintenance with volatile agent (e.g. isoflurane), with increments of labetalol or hydralazine. Infusions of nitroprusside, GTN and **remifentanil** may be used. Relative importance of BP over **blood flow** is controversial, e.g. whether use of vasodilators is better than reduction of cardiac output.
  - careful postoperative observation is important, because cardiovascular instability may persist.

Hypothalamus. Ventral part of the diencephalon, situated inferior to the thalamus and forming the floor of the third ventricle. Lies posterior to the optic chiasma and infundibular stalk attached to the posterior lobe of the **pituitary gland**. Important controlling area for **autonomic nervous system** activity; sympathetic mainly restricted to the posteromedial part, parasympathetic to the anterolateral part. Also involved in regulation of pituitary hormone secretion, **temperature regulation**, thirst, **sleep**, hunger, memory formation and sexual activity.

See also, Brain

Hypothermia. Defined as a core temperature <35°C. Described as mild (32°–35°C), moderate (28°–32°C) or severe (<28°C), although definitions vary in the literature. Primary hypothermia is uncommon and due to exposure to low environmental temperature with no underlying medical condition. The majority of patients presenting with hypothermia have an associated condition (secondary hypothermia).

- Caused by:
  - increased heat loss:
    - **trauma**: patients are exposed for long periods before and after admission to hospital. Hypothermia in major trauma triples mortality.
    - **coma** with obtunded **temperature regulation** (e.g. involving depressant drug overdose, **phenothiazine** therapy, etc.).
    - **near-drowning**: hypothermia is worsened by the high thermal conductivity of water and evaporative losses following rescue.
    - **burns**: associated with high evaporative losses.

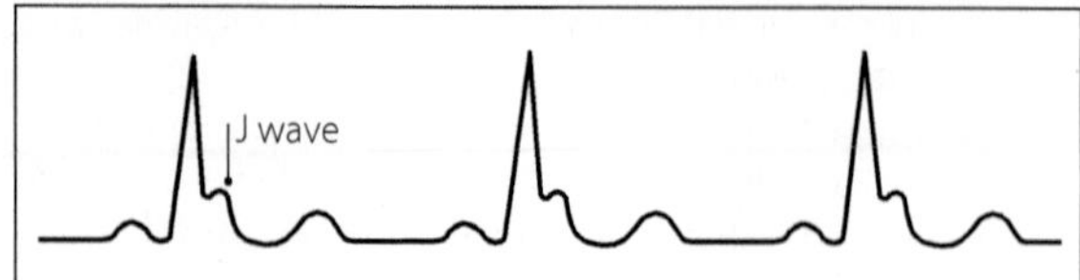

Fig. 87 ECG showing J waves

- **heat loss during anaesthesia**: hypothermia occurs in up to 70% of patients.
- impaired thermoregulation:
  - central failure, e.g. **stroke**, **TBI**, **hypothalamus** dysfunction, drug effects, **Parkinson's disease**, **subarachnoid haemorrhage**, etc.
  - peripheral failure, e.g. **spinal cord injury**, neuropathy.
  - endocrine dysfunction, e.g. **diabetic coma**, **hypothyroidism**, **adrenocortical insufficiency**, **hypopituitarism**.
  - extremes of age.
  - severe **malnutrition** and **hypoglycaemia**.
- deliberate measures:
  - for surgery, e.g. **cardiac surgery**.
  - therapeutic hypothermia (*see Targeted temperature management*).
- Effects:
  - cardiovascular:
    - reduced cardiac output (a 30% reduction at 30°C).
    - J waves (positive deflections at the end of **QRS complexes**) may appear on the ECG at 30°C (Fig. 87). They are clinically insignificant.
    - ventricular **arrhythmias** at 30°C, VF at 28°C.
    - vasoconstriction. Vasodilatation occurs below 20°C.
    - increased blood **viscosity**.
    - increased **haematocrit** below 30°C. **Thrombocytopenia** may be caused by sequestration, mainly hepatic. Fibrinolytic activity and prothrombin time increase. **DIC** may occur.
  - respiratory:
    - apnoea at 24°C.
    - reduced tissue O_2 delivery because of reduced cardiac output, vasoconstriction, increased viscosity and shift of the **oxyhaemoglobin dissociation curve** to the left, despite increased dissolved volume of O_2 in blood.
    - reduced O_2 demand and CO_2 production.
    - arterial blood gas tensions are measured at 37°C; values are traditionally corrected to body temperature but correction is now considered unnecessary.
  - neurological:
    - confusion below 35°C.
    - unconsciousness at 30°C.
    - reduced requirement for volatile agents.
    - cessation of all cerebral electrical activity below 18°C.
  - other:
    - diuresis due to inability to reabsorb sodium and water. GFR is reduced by 50% at 30°C.
    - respiratory and metabolic acidosis. Increased blood glucose and potassium.
    - metabolic rate increases initially, then decreases. **Hyperglycaemia** and increased fat mobilisation may occur.
- Management:
  - investigation: both routine and as for coma, in particular those causes mentioned earlier.
  - routine ICU monitoring.
  - treatment of hypoxia/hypoventilation/acidosis as required. Antiarrhythmic treatment may be ineffective at low temperatures.
  - rewarming methods; include:
    - heating blankets and baths.
    - radiant heaters.
    - warmed iv fluids.
    - irrigation of body cavities (e.g. bladder via catheter, peritoneal cavity via dialysis catheter, stomach via nasogastric tube) with warm solution.
    - **humidification** and warming of inspired gases.
    - **extracorporeal circulation** using heat exchangers.

    External warming may cause peripheral vasodilatation and hypotension, or subsequent rebound hypothermia if the core is relatively unwarmed. Rewarming should be gradual (e.g. 0.5°C//h) to allow equal body distribution of warmth.
  - treatment of the underlying cause.

Complications include **chest infection**, frostbite and **pancreatitis**. Residual hypothalamic damage may remain, especially in the elderly, with susceptibility for future episodes of hypothermia.

Brown DJA, Brugger H, Boyd J, Paal P (2012). N Engl J Med; 367: 1930–8

See also, Temperature regulation

Hypothesis testing, *see Null hypothesis*

Hypothyroidism. Usually follows thyroid disease (e.g. autoimmune) or treatment for **hyperthyroidism** (including surgery and radiotherapy). May also follow treatment with other drugs, e.g. **amiodarone** and **lithium**. Also occurs in **hypopituitarism**. Approximately 10 times more common in women; the incidence increases with age.

- Features:
  - severely impaired physical and mental development in children.
  - lethargy, slowed reactions, delayed relaxation of tendon reflexes (classically plantar reflex).
  - coarse skin and hair. Loss of the outer part of the eyebrows is classically described but is uncommon.
  - weight gain, reduced appetite, constipation.
  - hoarse voice, hypothermia.
  - **anaemia**: from menorrhagia or associated pernicious anaemia.
  - bradycardia, cardiomegaly and pericardial effusion may occur. Typical **ECG** findings include low-voltage complexes, bradycardia and T wave flattening/inversion. Hyperlipidaemia and **ischaemic heart disease** are common.
  - nerve entrapment, myopathy, confusion. **Coma** may occur (*see later*).
- Investigations: thyroxine (T_4) and triiodothyronine (T_3) levels are low. Thyroid stimulating hormone is high in primary thyroid failure, and low in pituitary failure.
- Treatment: thyroxine replacement (50–200 μg/day). Initial dosage is reduced in the elderly and those with heart disease, to reduce the risk of **myocardial ischaemia**.
- Hypothyroid coma (myxoedema coma):
  - particularly common during winter when **hypothermia** is common, especially in the elderly. May be precipitated by infection, stroke or anaesthesia.
  - mortality may exceed 50%.
  - treatment:
    - T_3 (liothyronine) 5–20 μg slowly iv, repeated 4–12-hourly depending on severity and response.

Alternatively, 50 µg iv may be followed by 25 µg tds, reducing to 25 µg bd. ECG monitoring is required.
    - hydrocortisone is often given but its place is uncertain if **adrenocortical insufficiency** is not present.
    - treatment of **hypoventilation**, hypothermia, hypotension, bradycardia, **acidosis**, **hyponatraemia**, **hypoglycaemia** and **convulsions** as required. Fluid restriction is usually advocated for treatment of hyponatraemia and prevention of cardiac failure.
- Anaesthetic considerations in hypothyroidism:
  - other **autoimmune diseases** may be present, e.g. **myasthenia gravis**.
  - patients show increased sensitivity to depressant drugs, especially opioids.
  - CO_2 and heat production, and drug metabolism/excretion are reduced.
  - hypoventilation and coma may occur.

Chakar L, Bianco AC, Jonklaast J, Peeters RP (2017). Lancet; 390: 1550–62

Hypoventilation. Reduced **alveolar ventilation**; it may result from reduction of respiratory rate and/or tidal volume.
- Caused by:
  - reduced central respiratory drive:
    - drugs, e.g. **opioid analgesic drugs**, **barbiturates**, **inhalational anaesthetic agents**.
    - **hypocapnia**, e.g. following IPPV. Also may occur in extreme **hypercapnia**.
    - metabolic disturbances, e.g. primary metabolic **alkalosis**, **hyperglycaemia**.
    - administration of high F_IO_2 to patients with **COPD** who rely on hypoxic respiratory drive.
    - intracranial pathology, e.g. **stroke**, tumour, infection, **head injury**, raised **ICP**.
    - **hypothermia**.
    - **alveolar hypoventilation** and **sleep apnoea** syndromes.
  - impaired peripheral mechanism of breathing:
    - **airway obstruction**.
    - restriction, e.g. due to pain, **obesity**, severe **ascites**, tight bandages, circumferential chest **burns**.
    - chest disease, e.g. COPD, **pneumothorax**, **asthma**, **flail chest**.
    - muscular weakness, e.g. electrolyte disturbances, **muscular dystrophy**, **dystrophia myotonica**, myopathy associated with critical illness.
    - **neuromuscular junction** impairment, e.g. **non-depolarising** and **depolarising neuromuscular blockade**, **myasthenia gravis**.
    - nerve lesions, e.g. **spinal cord injury**, **phrenic nerve** injury, **motor neurone disease**, **poliomyelitis**, **Guillain–Barré syndrome**, **critical illness polyneuropathy/myopathy**.
  - increased **dead space**, e.g. embolism, anaesthetic apparatus.

Effects are those of hypercapnia, respiratory **acidosis** and **hypoxaemia**. During anaesthesia, uptake and excretion of inhalational anaesthetic agents are slowed.
- Treatment:
  - **O_2 therapy**. Restores alveolar $P\text{O}_2$ as indicated by the **alveolar air equation**. Assisted or controlled ventilation may be required if arterial $P\text{CO}_2$ is high or rising.
  - directed at the cause. **Neuromuscular blockade monitoring** helps distinguish central from peripheral causes.
  - **doxapram** may be used to treat perioperative hypoventilation and acute exacerbations of COPD. **Naloxone** is used in opioid overdose.

See also, Breathing, control of

Hypovolaemia. Reduced circulating blood volume. May be caused by deficiency of:
  - blood; i.e., **haemorrhage**.
  - plasma; e.g. **burns**.
  - extracellular and/or intracellular fluid; e.g. **dehydration**, diuretic therapy, **haemodialysis/haemofiltration**, **third-space** losses (e.g. surgery, **sepsis**) and evaporative losses (e.g. **pyrexia**, during surgery).

'Relative hypovolaemia' refers to pooling of blood, e.g. during sepsis, as a result of drugs or following **spinal/epidural anaesthesia**. Less blood is available for circulation despite an unchanged blood volume.
- Results in increased sympathetic activity, reduced parasympathetic activity and other compensatory mechanisms, as in acute haemorrhage. Important clinically because:
  - many patients presenting with acute illness or for **emergency surgery** have a degree of hypovolaemia.
  - BP and perfusion of vital organs (e.g. heart, brain) are maintained largely by sympathetically mediated vasoconstriction and tachycardia. Drugs (e.g. sedatives, anaesthetic agents) that cause vasodilatation or reduce cardiac output may thus cause severe hypotension, as may spinal/epidural anaesthesia.
  - vital organs receive a greater proportion of cardiac output than normal, at the expense of other tissues, e.g. skin and GIT. Smaller doses of anaesthetic agents are therefore required to produce clinical effects, including side effects (e.g. myocardial depression).
  - **renal failure** may occur.

Hypovolaemia should therefore be detected and corrected whenever possible before induction of anaesthesia, and treated promptly when it occurs intra- and postoperatively.
- Features:
  - pallor (peripheral vasoconstriction).
  - tachycardia.
  - hypotension with low **CVP** and **pulmonary capillary wedge pressure**.
  - oliguria, thirst.
  - reduced O_2 delivery, e.g.:
    - to tissues: **lactic acidosis**.
    - to brain: confusion, restlessness.
    - to carotid/aortic bodies: breathlessness.
    - to heart: angina if susceptible.
  - haematocrit and urea and electrolyte abnormalities depending on aetiology.
- Treatment:
  - O_2 administration, supine position and raising the feet.
  - fluid replacement.
  - of the cause.

Hypoxaemia. Arterial $P\text{O}_2$ <12 kPa (90 mmHg).
- Caused by:
  - **hypoventilation** (*see Alveolar air equation*).
  - **diffusion** impairment, e.g. due to **pulmonary fibrosis**, **connective tissue diseases**; **$\dot{V}/\dot{Q}$ mismatch** is thought to be more significant.
  - **shunt**.
  - $\dot{V}/\dot{Q}$ mismatch.
  - reduced F_IO_2, e.g. due to high **altitude** or accidental hypoxic gas delivery during IPPV, resuscitation or anaesthesia.

In acute illness or during anaesthesia, hypoxaemia may occur because of respiratory depression, **airway obstruction**, **atelectasis** and $\dot{V}/\dot{Q}$ mismatch, including reduced FRC. It is especially common after upper abdominal surgery, due to the same factors plus hypoventilation caused by pain, depressant drugs and inability to cough. Impaired **ciliary activity** may also contribute. Hypoxaemia may persist for 2–3 days after upper abdominal surgery. All of these factors may be exacerbated by pre-existing **obstructive sleep apnoea**.

- Effects:
  - direct effects:
    - **cyanosis**.
    - confusion, drowsiness, agitation, headache, nausea. Unconsciousness, convulsions and death follow unless corrected.
    - myocardial depression, arrhythmias, bradycardia, coronary and cerebral vasodilatation.
    - **hypoxic pulmonary vasoconstriction** and **pulmonary hypertension**.
    - renal impairment.
  - effects of **carotid** and **aortic body** stimulation:
    - tachycardia, hypertension.
    - hyperventilation.

Acute hypoxaemia with 85% **haemoglobin** saturation may cause mental impairment, becoming severe at 75% saturation. Unconsciousness usually occurs at 65% saturation. Chronic hypoxaemia, e.g. at altitude, leads to adaptation.

- Treatment:
  - directed at the cause.
  - **O_2 therapy**: increases alveolar PO_2, resulting in increased arterial PO_2. The increase will be minimal if hypoxaemia is due to shunt.

See also, Breathing, control of; Hypoxia; Respiratory failure

Hypoxia. Reduced O_2 for tissue respiration.

- Classically divided into:
  - hypoxic hypoxia (**hypoxaemia**).
  - anaemic hypoxia: normal arterial PO_2 but reduced available **haemoglobin**, e.g. due to **anaemia**, **carbon monoxide poisoning**.
  - stagnant (ischaemic) hypoxia: normal arterial PO_2 and haemoglobin availability, but reduced tissue blood flow; may be due to reduced cardiac output or local interruption of blood flow.
  - histotoxic (cytotoxic) hypoxia: normal arterial PO_2, haemoglobin availability and blood flow, but inability of tissues to utilise O_2, e.g. due to **cyanide poisoning**, carbon monoxide poisoning.
- Effects:
  - aerobic metabolism at the **cytochrome oxidase system** is replaced by anaerobic metabolism, with increasing **lactate** production. Membrane pumps cease functioning, with impairment of normal intra/extracellular ion balance; irreversible cell damage may follow. Brain and heart are most susceptible. Other tissues may continue for long periods under hypoxic conditions. The critical value for intracellular O_2 tension is not known, but is thought to be about 0.3 kPa (2.3 mmHg) at the mitochondrial level (**Pasteur point**).
  - local stagnant hypoxia effects depending on the tissue involved.
  - general effects of hypoxia are as for hypoxaemia.

Stimulation of the **carotid** and **aortic bodies** occurs when arterial PO_2 falls; i.e., it may not occur in anaemic and histotoxic hypoxia.

See also, Oxygen cascade; Regional tissue oxygenation

Hypoxic pulmonary vasoconstriction. Reflex vasoconstriction of pulmonary arterioles in response to low PO_2 (under 11–13 kPa; 80–100 mmHg) in nearby alveoli. Does not rely on innervation of vessel walls, and is less dependent on PO_2 in blood; thus it occurs in isolated lung perfused with blood of high O_2 content and ventilated with gas of low O_2 content. Results in flow of blood away from poorly ventilated areas of lung, helping to reduce **$\dot{V}/\dot{Q}$ mismatch.**

Before birth, decreased pulmonary blood flow is caused by pulmonary vasoconstriction, relieved at birth when O_2 enters the lungs at the first breath.

Important in cardiac defects; **hypoxaemia** may cause a generalised increase in **pulmonary vascular resistance**, with increased right ventricular work and increased right-to-left shunting, particularly if SVR is lowered. Of major importance in the development of **pulmonary hypertension** and right heart failure (**cor pulmonale**) in patients with chronic lung disease.

- Increased by:
  - young age: greater in fetuses and neonates.
  - respiratory and metabolic **acidosis**.
  - increased temperature.
- Reduced by:
  - **hypocapnia** and alkalosis.
  - high serum iron levels.
  - increased distension of arterioles.
  - drugs including **acetazolamide**, **nitric oxide**, **dexamethasone**, **phosphodiesterase inhibitor** type 5 (sildenafil), **prostacyclin**, endothelin receptor antagonists (e.g. **bosentan**).
  - volatile anaesthetic agents in animal and laboratory experiments; the clinical relevance of this is controversial.

Lumb AB, Slinger P (2015). Anesthesiology; 122: 932–46

Hysteresis. A property of certain systems whose output variable depends on both the input variable and the internal state of the system, i.e., the output cannot be readily predicted simply by observing the recent history of the system. Commonly cited examples include elastic hysteresis and changes in lung **compliance** throughout the respiratory cycle and hysteresis as a source of error within measuring systems (e.g. direct **arterial blood pressure measurement**).

See also, Breathing, Work of

Ibandronic acid, *see Bisphosphonates*

Ibsen, Bjørn (1915–2007). Danish anaesthetist, considered by many to be the founding father of intensive care. Created a dedicated respiratory care unit for patients with poliomyelitis during the Copenhagen outbreak in 1952. Drastically cut mortality by employing positive pressure ventilation, mainly via tracheostomy. Opened the first general intensive care unit in 1953, a concept that was rapidly adopted worldwide.
Richmond C (2007). Br Med J; 335: 674
See also, Intensive care, history of

Ibuprofen. **NSAID** used to treat musculoskeletal pain, and for **postoperative analgesia**. Has weaker anti-inflammatory and analgesic properties than other NSAIDs, although has fewer GIT side effects.
- Dosage: 400–600 mg orally, tds/qds (max 2.4 g daily). A modified release preparation (1600 mg od or 300–900 mg bd), a topical gel and a combination preparation with codeine are also available.
- Side effects: as for NSAIDs. Up to 1.2 g/day is associated with a low risk of CVS side effects; 2.4 g/day is associated with the same risk as selective COX-2 inhibitors and **diclofenac**.

ICAM, intracellular adhesion molecules, *see Adhesion molecules*

Iceberg theory, *see Clathrates*

ICISS, *see International classification injury severity score*

ICNARC, *see Intensive Care National Audit and Research Centre*

ICP, *see Intracranial pressure*

ICU, *see Intensive care unit; Critical care*

ICU delirium, *see Confusion in the intensive care unit; Confusion, postoperative*

I–D interval. Time between induction of anaesthesia and delivery of the infant in **caesarean section**. Infant levels of **intravenous anaesthetic agent** may be high if the interval is very short. If very long, **inhalational anaesthetic agents** may accumulate in the infant. An I–D interval of less than 30 min is not thought to influence fetal acidosis if **aortocaval compression** and **hypoxaemia** are avoided.

Ideal gas law. For a perfect **gas**:

$$\frac{\text{pressure}, p \times \text{volume}, V}{\text{temperature}, T} = \text{constant}$$

rearranged as $PV = nRT$,

where n = number of moles of gas
R = **universal gas constant**

Thus a combination of **Boyle's law**, **Charles' law** and **Avogadro's hypothesis**.

IDICM, *see Intercollegiate Diploma in Intensive Care Medicine*

Idioventricular rhythm, *see Atrioventricular dissociation*

I:E ratio, *see Inspiratory:expiratory ratio*

Ignition temperature. Lowest temperature at which combustible mixtures ignite (energy required = **activation energy**). Lowest for **stoichiometric mixtures**.
See also, Explosions and fires

IHD, *see Ischaemic heart disease*

ILCOR, *see International Liaison Committee on Resuscitation*

Ileus. Small bowel atony (although the term is often used to describe gastric and colonic stasis).
- Causes include:
  - GIT pathology, e.g. surgery, haemorrhage, **peritonitis**.
  - drugs, e.g. **anticholinergic drugs**, **opioid analgesic drugs**.
  - severe **sepsis**.
  - autonomic failure (e.g. in Guillain–Barré syndrome, spinal cord injury)
  - others: acute kidney injury, diabetic coma, electrolyte imbalance, especially hyperkalaemia.

Clinical features include a distended and silent abdomen, with constant (usually mild) abdominal discomfort. Upright abdominal x-ray may reveal gas-filled loops of small intestine. If prolonged, fluid and electrolyte loss may occur. Distension may result in increased **intra-abdominal pressure** and **abdominal compartment syndrome**. It may also impair ventilation and contribute to **bacterial translocation** and **MODS**. The presence of colicky pain and increased bowel sounds suggests **intestinal obstruction**, which may follow paralytic ileus. Pseudo-obstruction of the colon occurs in bedridden patients with severe systemic illness and may present in a similar way. Abdominal x-ray however shows greatly dilated colonic loops.
- Management:
  - supportive: restriction of oral intake with free nasogastric drainage. Early oral administration of small amounts of clear fluids is becoming more common in uncomplicated cases. Fluid and electrolyte imbalance should be corrected.
  - **metoclopramide** and **erythromycin** are used to stimulate intestinal activity.

- **methylnaltrexone**, a peripherally acting mu **opioid receptor antagonist**, has been investigated as a treatment for postoperative ileus, which is thought to arise from a combination of endogenous endorphins and exogenous opioids given for pain relief.
- colonic tube placement following decompressive colonoscopy may be effective in reducing intestinal dilatation.

Reintam Blaser A, Starkopf J, Malbrain ML (2015). Anaesthesiol Intensive Ther; 47: 379–87

Iliac crest block. Blocks the ilioinguinal, iliohypogastric and lower 2–3 intercostal nerves, providing anaesthesia of the lower ipsilateral abdomen. An 8-cm needle is introduced 2–3 cm inferior and medial to the superior anterior iliac spine, and directed cranially and laterally to reach the inner ilium. 10 ml **local anaesthetic agent** is injected while the needle is withdrawn. Injection is repeated, directed more deeply.
See also, Inguinal hernia field block

Iliacus compartment block, *see Fascia iliaca compartment block*

Iliohypogastric nerve block/Ilioinguinal nerve block, *see Iliac crest block; Inguinal hernia field block*

ILS, *see Immediate Life Support*

Imaging in intensive care. Many modalities are available; usage depends on the body area involved and whether the patient is stable enough to be transferred to the radiology suite. In general, portable imaging equipment produces less clear images. Discussion with radiology staff is useful for making the correct choice of imaging.

- Techniques include:
  - conventional radiography:
    - **CXR**: demonstrates anatomical abnormalities of the lungs, tracheobronchial tree, pleura, diaphragm, heart and great vessels, chest wall, thoracic spine and soft tissues. May also detect foreign bodies, including invasive lines and tubes. Commonly performed every 1–3 days in the ICU (depending on the severity of illness; may require repeating several times per day) to check tubes, monitor progress and check for complications (e.g. **pneumothorax**) after invasive procedures.
    - abdominal x-ray: useful for demonstrating dilated loops of bowel and fluid levels in **intestinal obstruction**, free abdominal gas, kidney and gallstones.
    - others: include **cervical spine** and other bony structures, soft tissues for presence of gas in **gas gangrene**.
  - ultrasound:
    - abdomen:
      - general, e.g. in trauma, **intra-abdominal sepsis**.
      - renal tract in **acute kidney injury**; demonstrates renal size, obstructive nephropathy, vascular occlusion.
      - **biliary tract** (e.g. in **cholecystitis**, ascending **cholangitis**) and pancreas (**pancreatitis**).
    - chest:
      - **echocardiography** (and **transoesophageal echocardiography**).
      - both echocardiography and abdominal ultrasound may provide information about the lungs, diaphragm and pleura.
    - **central venous cannulation** using ultrasound devices.
  - **CT scanning**: remains the most sensitive and appropriate modality for critically ill patients with **head injury**, **cerebral oedema**, **subdural**, **subarachnoid** and **extradural haemorrhage** and **hydrocephalus**. Thoracic CT scanning gives detailed information of all structures, including lung pathology in **ALI**. Abdominal scanning is especially useful for imaging biliary tract, liver, pancreas and retroperitoneal structures. Portable bedside CT scanners are becoming available.
  - **MRI**: more sensitive than CT scanning for imaging cerebral and spinal structures, although logistical difficulties (including long scan times and problems with monitoring) limit its use in critically ill patients.
  - **positron emission tomography**: remains primarily a research tool in critically ill patients, although it has provided useful information about cerebral blood flow and metabolism in **TBI**.
  - **radioisotope scanning**: used to assess organ blood flow and perfusion, presence of infection and cardiac function.

Image guidance techniques may allow percutaneous drainage (e.g. of obstructed ureters, intra-abdominal abscesses, empyema) to be performed by radiologists, thereby avoiding the risks of surgery in critically ill patients.
See also, Functional imaging; Radiography in intensive care

Imipenem. Extremely broad-spectrum **carbapenem** and **antibacterial drug**, active against most pathogenic aerobic and anaerobic gram-negative and -positive organisms. Broken down in the kidney by dehydropeptidase, thus combined with cilastatin (1:1 ratio by weight), which inhibits the enzyme. Usually reserved for severe or mixed infections (excluding CNS infection).

- Dosage: 0.5–1.0 g iv qds.
- Side effects: GIT upset, blood dyscrasias, allergic reactions, convulsions, confusion, hepatic/renal impairment, red urine.

Imipramine hydrochloride. Tricyclic antidepressant drug, similar to **amitriptyline** but less sedating. Used in depression and panic disorders. Also used in nocturnal enuresis.

- Dosage: 75 mg/day orally, increased up to 300 mg/day (usually 50–100 mg/day). 25–50 mg is used in pain management.
- Side effects: as for amitriptyline.

Immediate Life Support (ILS). One-day course developed in 2002 by the **Resuscitation Council (UK)** in order to standardise much of the in-hospital training already undertaken by resuscitation officers. Trains healthcare personnel in recognition of sick patients, prevention of **cardiac arrest**, cardiac arrest rhythms, **basic life support** (BLS), simple airway management and safe **defibrillation** (manual and/or automatic). Aims to enable staff to manage patients in cardiac arrest until the arrival of a cardiac arrest team.

Soar J, Perkins GD, Harris S, Nolan JP (2003). Resuscitation; 57: 21–6

Immune system, anaesthesia and. Normal immune defences are:

- innate (non-specific), e.g. epithelial surface barriers, secreted **immunoglobulins**, local inflammatory

responses, including phagocytes and macrophages, **complement** system, pH of gastric juice, ciliary action.
- adaptive (specific):
  - humoral: B lymphocytes; under the influence of T-cell **cytokines**, form plasma cells that secrete specific immunoglobulins.
  - cellular: T lymphocytes conditioned in the thymus have killer activity and regulatory effects via helper/suppressor subsets.
  - natural killer cells.

- Main areas of anaesthetic importance:
  - patients with **immunodeficiency** (including those with **sepsis**).
  - **adverse drug reactions, blood compatibility testing.**
  - effects of anaesthesia on immunocompetence, especially against infection and malignancy. Difficult to study clinically, because of other factors (e.g. surgery, drugs, pre-existing disease, **stress response to surgery**), although phagocyte, monocyte and B-lymphocyte activity is reduced in vitro. **Ciliary activity** may be affected. Natural killer cell activity, lymphocyte proliferation and plasma cell formation are also reduced following anaesthesia with most inhalational agents. Lysosomal **free radical** formation may also be suppressed. Effects on spread and metastasis of malignancy are controversial, although spread in animals may be increased by anaesthesia and **blood transfusion** may be detrimental in colonic and ovarian cancer surgery and **renal transplantation**. A number of studies suggest that regional anaesthesia may be protective against recurrence of cancer.

Kurosawa S, Kato M (2008). J Anesth; 22: 263–77

Immunodeficiency. Results in increased susceptibility to infection and **malignancy**, the former a more common problem acutely. May result from deficient cell-mediated (T-cell lymphocyte) or antibody-mediated (B-cell lymphocyte) function, phagocytic activity or **complement** activity. Results in repeated and persistent infection, often with atypical organisms.

- May be:
  - primary, often inherited, e.g. B- or T-cell deficiency. Specific **immunoglobulin** types may be deficient. Neutrophil and complement disorders may also be inherited.
  - secondary to:
    - infection, e.g. **HIV infection, sepsis.**
    - drugs, e.g. **immunosuppressive drugs**, gold, penicillamine, cancer chemotherapy.
    - **connective tissue diseases.**
    - severe illness, **trauma, burns**; i.e., it may occur in any critically ill patient.
    - malignancy.
    - splenectomy.
- Management:
  - prevention of infection, e.g. meticulous aseptic technique, barrier nursing, prophylactic antibacterial therapy.
  - prompt diagnosis and treatment of infection.
  - treatment of the underlying cause.
  - immunoglobulin administration (*see Immunoglobulins, intravenous*).
  - immune-stimulant therapy may be indicated in certain contexts (e.g. **granulocyte colony-stimulating factor** in chemotherapy-induced neutropenic sepsis).

Immunoglobulins (Antibodies). Proteins secreted by plasma cells, involved in immunological defence systems. Each molecule consists of two heavy chains (that determine the class of immunoglobulin) and two light chains. The Y-shaped molecule presents two highly specific antigen-binding sites, each made up of portions of heavy and light chains, at one end (the Fab portion). The other end (the Fc portion) is made up of heavy chain only, and may bind to **complement**, or to the surface of mediator cells, e.g. **mast cells**, macrophages.

- Types of immunoglobulins:
  - IgG: the most abundant in plasma. Involved in complement fixation. The only one that crosses the placental barrier.
  - IgA: secreted from epithelial barriers, e.g. GIT.
  - IgM: comprises five joined molecules; involved in complement fixation.
  - IgD: involved in antigen recognition by lymphocytes.
  - IgE: on the surface of mast cells; involved in **histamine** release and **anaphylaxis.**

Most **adverse drug reactions** to anaesthetic drugs via immunoglobulins involve IgG and IgM (complement activation) or IgE (anaphylaxis).

- Immunoglobulins may be administered therapeutically, and are obtained from:
  - pooled human plasma:
    - from blood donated for transfusion (normal immunoglobulin): given im for prophylaxis of certain infections, e.g. measles, **hepatitis**, rubella in pregnant women. Certain forms may be given iv as replacement therapy in **immunodeficiency**, and in various other immune-related disorders (*see Immunoglobulins, intravenous*).
    - from donors who are convalescing, or whose antibody production has been boosted (specific immunoglobulins): given im and available against hepatitis B, tetanus, rabies, Rhesus D antigen and herpes viruses.

    Routinely screened for hepatitis and **HIV infection.**
  - monoclonal cell biology and recombinant genetic engineering: not yet widespread. Infliximab is a monoclonal antibody against tumour necrosis factor, used in rheumatoid arthritis.

Hypersensitivity reactions are more likely with immunoglobulins from pooled plasma. **Digoxin**-specific antibody fragments (Fab) derived from sheep immunoglobulins are used in digoxin toxicity.

See also, Autoimmune disease

Immunoglobulins, intravenous (IVIG). Obtained from a plasma pool of 1000–10000 donors and provide polyclonal immunoglobulins to a wide variety of pathogens. Originally used to treat idiopathic **thrombocytopenia** and congenital agammaglobulinaemia; also effective in **Guillain–Barré syndrome** and other **peripheral neuropathies, myasthenia gravis** and the **myasthenic syndrome.** Proposed mechanisms of action include an anti-inflammatory and **complement** effect, reduction in **cytokine** synthesis and blocking of IgG-binding Fc receptors on macrophages.

- Dosage varies widely according to indication: e.g. 0.4 g/kg iv daily for 5 days for Guillain–Barré syndrome; 1 g/kg iv weekly during pregnancy for gestational immune thrombocytopenia.
- Side effects: malaise, fever, acute meningism, **acute kidney injury, anaphylaxis.** Contraindicated in patients

with class-specific anti-IgA antibodies. Despite pre-donation testing, transmission of hepatitis C has been reported.

Immunosuppressive drugs. Used to treat inflammatory/ **autoimmune diseases** and **connective tissue diseases**, and to prevent rejection following **transplantation**.

- Types of drug used:
  - **cytotoxic drugs**, e.g. **cyclophosphamide, azathioprine**, chlorambucil, **mycophenolate**. All depress bone marrow haemopoiesis and increase susceptibility to infection.
  - **corticosteroids**.
  - anti-lymphocyte agents, e.g. **ciclosporin, tacrolimus**.
  - **immunoglobulins** or immuno-active receptor agonists/ antagonists, e.g. tumour necrosis factor (TNF) receptor–antibody complexes (e.g. etanercept), anti-TNF antibodies or interleukin-1 receptor antagonist, used to treat **rheumatoid arthritis**.

Impedance, electrical. **Resistance** to flow of an alternating **current** in an electrical circuit, dependent on the current's frequency. Represented by the letter Z, although measured in **ohms**. Different components within circuits (e.g. loudspeakers, monitor screens) should be matched for impedance to maximise efficiency. Amplifiers in **monitoring** equipment generally have high input impedance to minimise the effect of poor contact with the patient; any increased impedance because of the latter makes little difference to the overall input impedance.
See also, Impedance plethysmography

Impedance plethysmography. Method of determining changes in intrathoracic gas and fluid volumes by measuring transthoracic **impedance**, which varies according to the composition of thoracic contents.

- Used for:
  - **monitoring** respiration, e.g. on ICU: a small high-frequency current is passed between ECG electrodes; the changes in impedance between them represent ventilatory movements. Has been used to detect oesophageal intubation (produces a different impedance pattern to tracheal intubation).
  - **cardiac output measurement**: two sets of circular wire electrodes are placed around the chest and neck. Current is passed between the outer two, with measurement of potential difference between the inner two. Maximal rate of change of impedance occurs with peak aortic flow, although absolute values do not correlate well.
  - others, e.g. lung water measurement.

May also be applied to other parts of the body, e.g. leg veins to diagnose **DVT**.
See also, Inductance cardiography

IMV, *see Intermittent mandatory ventilation*

Inborn errors of metabolism. Group of disorders caused by inherited single **enzyme** defects. Over 200 are known; some are clinically insignificant and others fatal. Most are rare (1:20000–500 000), caused by autosomal recessive genes, and present in infancy/early childhood.

- Include disorders of:
  - porphyrin metabolism (*see Porphyrias*).
  - **carbohydrate** metabolism, e.g. **glycogen storage disorders**, galactosaemia and fructose metabolic disorders. Liver, brain, skeletal and cardiac muscle may be affected. **Hypoglycaemia** is common; also metabolic **acidosis** and electrolyte imbalance.
  - **amino acid** metabolism, e.g. phenylketonuria, homocystinuria, alcaptonuria. Mental handicap, neurological abnormalities and metabolic disturbances are common. Skeletal abnormalities may present difficulty with tracheal intubation in the latter two disorders. Hypoglycaemia may occur.
  - lysosomal storage; results in accumulation of macromolecules within lysosomes. Most conditions cause severe mental retardation and neurological abnormalities, with death in childhood. Include:
    - sphingolipidoses, e.g. Gaucher's disease; coagulation abnormalities and hepatosplenomegaly are common.
    - mucopolysaccharidoses, e.g. Hurler's and Hunter's syndromes (the latter is sex-linked recessive). CNS, skeleton and viscera are affected. Characteristic 'gargoyle' facies occur, with possible difficult intubation, and thoracic spinal deformities. Hurler's syndrome is more severe than Hunter's, with corneal clouding, valvular and **ischaemic heart disease**.
  - purine metabolism: may lead to gout, with tissue deposition of urate crystals, especially in the joints. This group includes Lesch–Nyhan syndrome, with mental and neurological abnormalities.
  - red blood cell metabolism, e.g. **glucose-6-phosphate dehydrogenase deficiency**. **Haemolysis** may also feature in other defects.
  - copper metabolism (Wilson's disease): impaired hepatic and central nervous motor function.
  - iron metabolism (haemochromatosis): hepatic and myocardial impairment are common; **diabetes mellitus** may occur.

Kloesel B, Holzman RS (2017). Anesth Anal; 125: 822–36
[Philippe Gaucher (1854–1918), French physician; Gertrud Hurler (1889–1965), German paediatrician; Charles Hunter (1872–1955), US physician; Michael Lesch (1939–2008), US cardiologist; William Nyhan, US paediatrician; Samuel Wilson (1878–1937), US-born English neurologist]

Incentive spirometry. Lung expansion technique designed to encourage deep breathing to reduce **atelectasis** and improve respiratory muscle function, e.g. postoperatively.

- Apart from verbal encouragement and teaching of breathing exercises, the following techniques have been used:
  - inspiration from bellows; when the preset tidal volume has been reached, a light illuminates.
  - inspiration or expiration through flowmeters, e.g. glass cylinders containing coloured balls; the patient attempts to reach preset targets.
  - inflation of a balloon on expiration.
  - expiration through a blow-bottle: the patient breathes out through a tube passing into a sealed jar containing water, which is displaced through a second tube into a second jar.

Evidence suggests that the technique is useful in reducing breathlessness in **COPD** but evidence for its efficacy in preventing postoperative pulmonary complications is lacking.
Overend TJ, Anderson CM, Lucy SD, et al (2001). Chest; 120: 971–8
See also, Physiotherapy

Incident, critical, *see Critical incidents*

Incident, major. Practical definition: any incident where the location, number, severity or type of live casualties requires extraordinary resources. May refer to transport accidents, riots, terrorist activities or natural disasters.

- Main problems:
  - large number of patients to be sorted (**triage**) for treatment and transfer, with their sudden arrival at hospital. Although there have been arguments over whether prehospital treatment is better than a 'scoop and run' policy, it is now generally accepted that certain interventions (e.g. airway management) should ideally be carried out before transfer to hospital if competent staff are available on site. Adequate record-keeping is difficult, e.g. patient identification, assessment, treatment given, location.
  - co-ordination of emergency services, with organisation of staff and resources at the scene of the incident and receiving (designated) hospitals.
  - clearing of non-urgent cases from wards and operating theatres.
  - communication between medical teams, hospitals, police, fire brigade and public. Telephone and computer networks may be non-functioning or disabled, and/or the volume of calls from the press, public and staff may be overwhelming.
  - sudden need for specific equipment (e.g. breathing apparatus, protective suits), drugs, blood products and other support services, e.g. x-ray.
  - dispersal of patients once initially treated; identification and holding of corpses.
- Major incident plans of most hospitals are similar:
  - affected hospitals are informed, and main receiving hospitals designated. Use is made of nearby specialist centres, e.g. thoracic, neurosurgical.
  - specific duties are assigned to each member of staff on duty, including formation of a mobile team. Assignment of a team leader and establishment of routes of communication in each area are vital.
  - duties of anaesthetists include triage and treatment at the scene of the incident, resuscitation in the receiving area, and anaesthesia for surgery.
  - duties of ICU staff include resuscitation and managing admissions to ICU.
  - pre-prepared emergency drug and resuscitation equipment boxes. **Triservice apparatus** has been suggested as suitable for field anaesthesia, but most anaesthetists' experience of this is limited, and anaesthesia is rarely required before transfer to hospital.

National Clinical Guideline Centre (2016). NICE Guideline NG39

See also, Biological weapons; Chemical weapons; Transportation of critically ill patients; Trauma

Incident, serious, *see Critical incidents*

Independent lung ventilation, *see Differential lung ventilation*

Indocyanine green. Strongly infrared absorbing and fluorescent agent, given iv as a marker substance to permit organ **blood flow**, liver function or **cardiac output measurement.** Has also been used to study cerebral perfusion using **near infrared spectroscopy**. Transported on proteins, it is exclusively eliminated by the liver but does not undergo enterohepatic circulation. Elimination is dependent on both liver blood flow and parenchymal cellular function.

Vos JJ, et al (2014). Anaesthesia; 69: 1364–76

Indometacin (Indomethacin). Analgesic **NSAID**, available for oral and rectal use. Also used to promote closure of a patent **ductus arteriosus** (PDA).

- Dosage:
  - 100 mg rectally od/bd.
  - 25–50 mg orally tds/qds.
  - for PDA closure: 200 μg/kg iv initially.
- Side effects: as for NSAIDs; in addition, dizziness and headache may occur.

Inductance. Capacity for an **inductor** to generate an electromotive force in opposition to a changing **current** flowing in that circuit, or in a neighbouring one. Flow of current induces a magnetic field, that in turn induces an electromotive force proportional to the rate of change of current. In effect, this acts as a store of energy within the circuit. May give rise to interference in electrical equipment, or occur intentionally in transformers. Has been used as a basis for measuring **cardiac output** and monitoring respiration, by using two coils placed on the chest, e.g. one anteriorly, one posteriorly.

Inductance cardiography (Thoracocardiography). Method for measuring changes in intrathoracic volume, and thus estimating **cardiac output**. An insulated electrical conductor placed around the chest, level with the heart, is connected to an alternating current, and changes in cross-sectional area detected via changes in its self-inductance (via changes in the oscillatory frequency of the induced current). Accuracy is generally not as good as other methods of measuring cardiac output; thus absolute values are less useful than trends.

Induction agents, *see Intravenous anaesthetic agents*

Induction of anaesthesia. Transition from the awake to the anaesthetised state, although the end-point is difficult to define. Has the potential for significant physiological derangement, during which the following may occur:

  - cardiovascular changes, e.g. **hypotension, arrhythmias.**
  - **hypoventilation/apnoea.** Particularly dangerous in patients with airway problems.
  - **aspiration of gastric contents.**
  - **laryngospasm, hiccups** and **vomiting** during the stage of excitement, particularly if disturbed, e.g. by movement, noise or pain.
  - adverse drug reactions, especially following iv injections.
  - others, e.g. involuntary movement/**convulsions, MH/masseter spasm.**
- Inhalational induction:
  - usually reserved for children, patients with **airway obstruction** and in difficult intubation. By allowing continuous spontaneous ventilation, the anaesthetist avoids being unable to ventilate an apnoeic patient. May also be used in patients with poor veins or needle phobia.
  - the anaesthetic agent is gradually introduced to the patient in increasing concentrations. The characteristics of induction depend on the **inhalational anaesthetic agent** used. More rapid induction has been achieved using maximal breaths of high percentage of volatile agent, e.g. 4%–8% **sevoflurane** ('single breath induction').
  - the progressive **stages of anaesthesia** may be seen, especially in unpremedicated patients.

- induction is slower than with iv agents. The stage of excitement may be prolonged.
- IV induction:
  - much faster, allowing rapid progression through the stage of excitement. Usually more pleasant for adults than an inhalational technique.
  - an estimated appropriate dose should be given slowly, and the patient observed for its effect before injecting more. Considerable time may be required if the **arm–brain circulation time** is prolonged, e.g. in the elderly and those with cardiovascular disease.
  - the characteristics of induction depend on the **iv anaesthetic agent** used.
  - carries risk of extravasation, intra-arterial or painful injection, thrombosis, chemical reaction with other drugs in the cannula, and adverse drug reactions.
  - movement and hiccupping may occur.
  - overdosage is more likely because induction is faster, especially if injection is given rapidly without titrating to effect.

Respiratory and cardiac depression may follow both methods of induction, but may be more sudden after iv induction. Use of other depressant drugs (e.g. for **premedication**) may reduce the amount of iv agent required and allow smoother induction. Respiratory depressants (e.g. opioids) may slow inhalational induction. Other routes of induction, e.g. rectal and im, are rarely used now.

Emergency drugs and equipment, a tipping trolley and skilled assistance should always be present before inducing anaesthesia. Equipment should always be checked before use.

See also, Anaesthesia, stages of; Checking of anaesthetic equipment; Induction, rapid sequence

Induction, rapid sequence ('Crash induction'). **Induction of anaesthesia** in which risks of regurgitation and **aspiration of gastric contents** are minimised by:

- presence of emergency drugs and equipment, a tipping trolley and skilled assistance (should be present before inducing anaesthesia in any patient, but especially important in rapid sequence induction, as is **checking of anaesthetic equipment**).
- **suction equipment** should be turned on before induction and within easy reach of the anaesthetist.
- aspiration of gastric tube if in place, before induction. Pre-induction passage of a stomach tube is rarely done routinely. A nasogastric tube is usually left in situ during induction.
- **preoxygenation** before induction of anaesthesia.
- use of a rapidly acting iv induction agent and **suxamethonium** to achieve rapid muscle relaxation. **Rocuronium** (1–1.2 mg/kg) is an alternative, particularly with the availability of **sugammadex** for immediate reversal should intubation fail. Regurgitation and aspiration have been reported during use of the **priming principle**. Other analgesic or sedative drugs should not precede the iv agent.
- application of **cricoid pressure**.
- traditionally, ventilation by facemask was avoided, to reduce gastric inflation and risk of regurgitation. Recent guidelines recommend gentle mask ventilation to maintain oxygenation before laryngoscopy.
- tracheal intubation and inflation of the cuff before cricoid pressure is released.

Spare laryngoscopes and tubes must be available, and a plan made in case of difficult or impossible intubation.

Rapid sequence induction should be performed in patients with:

- increased risk of regurgitation:
  - **obesity**.
  - incompetent lower oesophageal sphincter e.g. **hiatus hernia**, **pregnancy**.
  - full stomach e.g. inadequate fasting, delayed **gastric emptying** (e.g. due to **trauma**, pain, administration of opioids, acute abdomen, bowel obstruction etc.).
  - positioning e.g. lithotomy, head-down.
- increased risk of aspiration, e.g. impaired laryngeal reflexes due to reduced conscious level, anaesthesia, bulbar palsy.

Classical rapid sequence induction may not be possible in children, as effective preoxygenation may be impossible in an unco-operative child, iv access may be difficult and cricoid pressure can distort the airway. An alternative approach involves induction of anaesthesia in a 20-degree head-up position, the use of non-depolarising neuromuscular blocking drugs, avoidance of cricoid pressure until consciousness has been lost.

See also, Intubation, difficult; Intubation, failed; Nasogastric intubation

Inductor. Electrical component usually consisting of a conducting coil within a magnetic field. Applications include signal filtering, transformers and current dampening (e.g. in **defibrillation** equipment).

See also, Inductance

Inert gas narcosis. Loss of consciousness caused by inhalation of high partial pressures of inert gases, e.g. **xenon**, neon, argon and **nitrogen** (nitrogen narcosis). Nitrogen has no anaesthetic properties at sea level pressures, but impairs cognitive and motor function at partial pressures above 4–5 atmospheres, e.g. diving to depths greater than 30–40 metres while breathing air. Use of **helium** in breathing apparatus allows deeper dives.

Infection. Most common cause of disease worldwide. Anaesthetic and ICU implications may be related to:

- primary cause of illness, e.g. meningitis, chest infection, hepatitis.
- complication of surgery, anaesthesia, intensive care, trauma, e.g. nosocomial infection.
- treatment, e.g. side effects of antibacterial or antiviral drugs.
- risk of transmission to susceptible patients or from infected patients to staff.

Whatever its cause and site, infection may result in **sepsis** and/or **septic shock**.

See also, Infection control; individual infections and organisms

Infection control. Important in anaesthetic and ICU practice for prevention of **nosocomial infection**. Most hospitals have an infection control team (microbiologist, nurse and laboratory staff) with major responsibility for surveillance/investigation of infection, review of antibiotic therapy/resistance and education of staff.

- Measures include:
  - provision of isolation rooms for patients susceptible to infection or those who pose a cross-infection hazard to other patients. Barrier nursing is often necessary. Patients returning from ICUs to general wards should also be isolated until they are clear of

infections with organisms such as meticillin-resistant *Staphylococcus aureus* (MRSA) and **vancomycin-resistant enterococcus.**
- maintaining sufficient nurse:patient ratios to manage fluctuating workload.
- staff hygiene: often poor, it is the major controllable factor in cross-infection. Hands should be washed before and after each patient contact, watches/jewellery not worn, and meticulous aseptic technique used during medical and nursing procedures. Gloves (and, in ICU, aprons) should be worn during all procedures.
- early identification and treatment of infection. Immediate screening (e.g. for MRSA) with decolonisation of high-risk patients is essential when patients are admitted from other ICUs or hospitals. Regular culture of sputum and urine should continue for all patients on ICU.
- identification and avoidance of **catheter related sepsis**, and use of **care bundles**.
- use of bacterial **filters** on breathing systems and regular changing of disposable ventilator tubing (e.g. every 48 h).
- use of disposable syringes and pressure transducers, which should not be reused.
- safe use and disposal of sharps.
- restricting drug ampoules to single patients only and preparing syringes immediately before use.
- avoiding **contamination of anaesthetic equipment** by appropriate cleaning/disposal of equipment after each patient.
- appropriate management of patients with proven or possible **Creutzfeldt–Jakob disease**.
- joint daily ward rounds between microbiologists and the ICU team. Antimicrobial therapy should only be used when clinically necessary and the choice of agent informed by bacterial sensitivity.
- regular cleaning/decontamination of the ICU.
- better ward design to minimise environmental contamination, including air filtration and conditioning.

The routine use of **selective decontamination of the digestive tract** is controversial.

Gandra S, Ellison RT (2014). J Intensive Care Med; 29: 311–26

See also, Bacterial resistance; Staphylococcal infections

Infection, hospital-acquired, *see Nosocomial infection*

Infiltration anaesthesia. Commonly performed for minor surgery and suturing. Subcutaneous and intradermal infiltration is performed around the lesion, with further injection as required. May also be used for manipulations and more extensive surgery (e.g. **caesarean section**) in which the deeper tissues are also infiltrated. The maximal safe dose of **local anaesthetic agent** should not be exceeded. Dilute solutions are usually adequate. Excessive volumes of injectate containing adrenaline may cause skin necrosis. Adequate time must be allowed before starting surgery.

Inflammatory bowel disease. Chronic inflammatory GIT disease of uncertain aetiology. Comprises:
- Crohn's disease: transmural granulomatous disease; commonly affects the terminal ileum and ascending colon, although it may affect the GIT from mouth to anus.
- ulcerative colitis (UC): characterised by inflammation of the colonic and rectal mucosa.

Features include fever, malaise, weight loss, **anaemia**, **vitamin deficiencies**, **dehydration**, abdominal pain and tenderness and **diarrhoea** (often bloody). Chronic inflammation may lead to **intestinal obstruction**; Crohn's disease typically is associated with fistula formation. Non-intestinal manifestations include arthritis, sacroiliitis, **ankylosing spondylitis**, uveitis, skin involvement and liver/gallbladder disease. Diagnosis is confirmed by intestinal biopsy.
- Management:
    - medical: correction of nutritional deficiencies and anaemia; sulfasalazine, 5-aminosalicylic acid enemas; **corticosteroids**.
    - surgical: may be required for Crohn's disease (e.g. for obstruction, fistulae) or UC (e.g. in toxic megacolon when extensive disease is unresponsive to medical therapy, or in total colitis lasting more than 10 years when malignant change becomes more common).

Anaesthetic considerations encompass the above complications and the need for **emergency surgery**. Severe toxic megacolon may require admission to ICU for resuscitation.

[Burrill B Crohn (1884–1983), US physician]

Inflation pressure, *see Airway pressure*

Inflation reflex, *see Hering–Breuer reflex*

Influenza. Acute illness caused by influenza virus infection. Epidemiologically characterised by regular seasonal epidemics with a larger **pandemic** occurring every few decades; the latter arises when there is a major shift in viral antigenic type (against which the population has little immunity).

All strains are single-stranded RNA viruses classified according to their haemagglutinin and neuraminidase surface proteins (e.g. H1N1, H2N2). H1N1 influenza ('swine flu') was responsible for the pandemic of 2009, causing >375 000 infections worldwide with >4500 deaths (137 in the UK). While the majority of infections were self-limiting, a small proportion of patients (including previously well, young adults) developed severe/fatal complications. Pregnant women, the immunosuppressed, and those with respiratory co-morbidities were over-represented in those requiring ICU admission.

Vaccines are available against influenza (including pandemic H1N1) and may prevent 50%–80% of cases in healthy adults; their use is recommended in all at-risk groups (e.g. healthcare workers, pregnant women, the elderly).
- Features:
    - common symptoms: fatigue, fever, cough, sore throat, rhinitis, dyspnoea, headache, myalgia, diarrhoea and vomiting.
    - complications requiring ICU admission: **respiratory failure**, **ALI**, secondary bacterial infection, **septic shock** and **MODS**.
- Investigations:
    - general: CXR, arterial blood gases, routine blood tests.
    - diagnostic tests: antigen detection tests (e.g. 'rapid influenza detection test'); immunofluorescence assay; viral culture; RT-PCR (reverse transcription polymerase chain reaction). The latter two have the greatest **sensitivity** and **specificity**, and are able to

distinguish H1N1 pandemic influenza from other types.
- Treatment:
  - general measures: O_2, iv fluids, analgesia, isolation/infection control measures.
  - antiviral therapy for pandemic H1N1:
    - oseltamivir: 75 mg orally bd in adults; weight-adjusted dosage scale for children.
    - zanamivir: 10 mg bd via metered dose inhaler; first-line in pregnant patients as inhalational administration reduces fetal exposure.
- ICU management includes: early intubation and **IPPV** (interim non-invasive ventilation may worsen outcome); **high-frequency ventilation; extracorporeal membrane oxygenation** where available; fluid resuscitation and cardiovascular support with avoidance of overhydration.

The potential for pandemic influenza to place extreme demands on healthcare resources (particularly ICU provision) has led to the development of detailed triage, admission and treatment guidelines by the Department of Health.

Patel M, Dennis A, Flutter C, Khan Z (2010). Br J Anaesth; 104: 128–42

Informed consent, *see Consent*

Infraorbital nerve block, *see Maxillary nerve blocks*

Infratrochlear nerve block, *see Ophthalmic nerve blocks*

Infusion regimens. Used to facilitate administration of potent iv drugs while minimising errors. Generally rely on adding a fixed amount of drug to a fixed volume of diluent to produce a set concentration, or varying one component (usually the amount of drug) according to the patient's weight to produce a concentration expressed in terms of amount of drug per kilogram. Other considerations relate to the kind of infusion device used and whether the dose is commonly expressed as drug per unit time (e.g. µg/h), volume per unit time (e.g. ml/h) or drug per kilogram per unit time (e.g. µg/kg/h). A common and useful method of preparing drugs (e.g. **inotropic drugs**) is to add (body weight × 3) mg of drug to diluent to make 50 ml solution; 1 ml/h is then equivalent to 1 µg/kg/h.

Inguinal hernia field block. May be used as the sole technique for surgery in high-risk patients, or as an adjunct to general anaesthesia to reduce the anaesthetic requirement and to provide **postoperative analgesia**.
- Anatomy (*see Fig. 69;* **Femoral triangle**):
  - the inguinal canal represents the path taken by the descending testicle, and contains the spermatic cord in the male (round ligament in the female). It runs downwards and medially, above and parallel to the inguinal ligament, which passes from the superior anterior iliac spine to the pubic tubercle.
  - anterior abdominal wall muscle layers, from within outwards: transversus abdominis, internal oblique, external oblique.
  - the canal emerges through the deep ring of the transversalis fascia and transversus abdominis above the midpoint of the inguinal ligament. The internal oblique lies in front laterally, but its conjoint tendon (formed with transversus abdominis) arches over the canal superiorly to lie behind it medially. The external oblique lies anteriorly along its length. The superficial ring is the defect in the external oblique aponeurosis just lateral and above the pubic tubercle.
  - nerve supply (branches from the **lumbar plexus**):
    - iliohypogastric (L1): anterior cutaneous branch is given off at the iliac crest; it passes between transversus abdominis and the internal oblique, piercing the latter 2 cm medial to the anterior superior iliac spine. It then runs deep to the aponeurosis of the external oblique, piercing it above the superficial ring to supply the skin above the pubis.
    - ilioinguinal (L1): passes just caudal to the iliohypogastric nerve, passing through the superficial ring to supply the skin of the groin and scrotum/labia majora.
    - genitofemoral (L1, 2): genital branch passes with the spermatic cord (in the male) through the deep ring, supplying the skin of the scrotum/labia majora.
- Technique of block:
  - iliohypogastric and ilioinguinal nerves: with the patient supine, a short, bevelled needle is introduced vertically downwards, 2 cm medial and caudal to the anterior superior iliac spine. A click is felt as the external oblique aponeurosis is penetrated. 10–20 ml **local anaesthetic agent** is injected, repeated with the needle directed medially and laterally. Subcutaneous infiltration from the pubis, 10 cm cranially, blocks fibres from the other side.
  - subcutaneous infiltration along the incision site.
  - genitofemoral nerve: injection of 20 ml solution at the deep ring, 1–2 cm above the midpoint of the inguinal ligament, deep to the external oblique aponeurosis as before. This may be left to the surgeon to reduce risk of vascular or peritoneal puncture.
  - the neck of the hernia sac may also be infiltrated by the surgeon.

Prilocaine 0.5% with adrenaline is suitable, and allows use of a large volume of solution. The maximal safe dose allowable is calculated and divided between the above injections. For an adjunct to general anaesthesia and postoperative analgesia, smaller volumes of **bupivacaine** with adrenaline may provide several hours' analgesia. Leg weakness has been reported due to unintentional **femoral nerve block**.

Inhalational anaesthetic agents. Since the discovery of anaesthesia, a variety of gases and volatile agents have been tried and discarded, including: **diethyl ether** (first used in 1842), **N_2O** (1844), **chloroform** (1847), **ethyl chloride** (1848), **ethylene** (1923), **cyclopropane** (1930), **divinyl ether** (1933), **trichloroethylene** (1935), **xenon** (1946), **halothane** and **fluroxene** (1956), **methoxyflurane** (1960), **enflurane** (1966), **isoflurane** (1971), **desflurane** (1994) and **sevoflurane** (1996). Some properties of inhalational agents are shown in Table 27.

Inhalational agents are popular because alveolar levels (and thus blood levels) are easily controllable by adjusting inspired concentration. However, side effects and **pollution** concerns have led to increased use of **iv anaesthetic agents**, i.e., **TIVA**.

Volatile anaesthetic agents are convenient to supply and store, but require special **vaporisers**. Many are ethers; **flammability** and risk of **explosion and fires** are reduced by addition of halogen atoms to the basic molecule.

Gases are supplied in **cylinders** or via pipelines. Cylinders are bulky to store. Administration of gases is controlled

Table 27 Properties of inhalational anaesthetic agents

Agent	Structure	Molecular weight	Boiling point (°C)	SVP at 20°C (kPa [mmHg])	MAC (% vol.) (young adults)	Partition coefficients at 37°C	
						Blood/gas	Oil/gas
Chloroform	$CHCl_3$	119	61	21 (160)	0.5	110	260
Cyclopropane	$(CH_2)_3$	42	−33	−9.2	0.45	11.5	
Desflurane	$CF_3\text{–}CHF\text{–}O\text{–}CF_2H$	168	23	88 (673)	5–10	0.42	19
Diethyl ether	$CH_3\text{–}CH_2\text{–}O\text{–}CH_2\text{–}CH_3$	74	35	59 (425)	1.9	12	65
Divinyl ether	$CH_2{=}CH\text{–}O\text{–}CH{=}CH_2$	70	28	74 (553)	3	2.8	60
Enflurane	$CHFCl\text{–}CF_2\text{–}O\text{–}CF_2H$	184.5	56	24 (175)	1.68	1.9	98
Ethyl chloride	$CH_3\text{–}CH_2Cl$	64.5	13	131 (988)	2	3	–
Ethylene	$CH_2{=}CH_2$	28	−104	–	65	0.4	1.3
Fluroxene	$CF_3\text{–}CH_2\text{–}O\text{–}CH{=}CH_2$	126	43	38 (286)	3.4	1.4	48
Halothane	$CF_3\text{–}CHClBr$	197.4	50	32 (243)	0.76	2.4	225
Isoflurane	$CF_3\text{–}CHCl\text{–}O\text{–}CF_2H$	184.5	49	33 (250)	1.28	1.4	97
Methoxyflurane	$CF\text{–}CHCl\text{–}O\text{–}CH_3$	165	105	3 (23)	0.2	13	14
Nitrous oxide	N_2O	44	−88	–	105	0.47	1.4
Sevoflurane	$(CF_3)_2CH\text{–}O\text{–}CH_2F$	200	58	21 (160)	2.5	0.69	53
Trichloroethylene	$CCl_2{=}CHCl$	131	87	8 (60)	0.17	9	960
Xenon	Xe	131	−108	–	71	0.14	1.9

using **flowmeters** alongside the O_2 flowmeter of an **anaesthetic machine**.

- Features of the ideal inhalational anaesthetic agent:
  - physical/chemical properties:
    - chemically stable, e.g. in the presence of heat, light, **soda lime**; long shelf-life. No additives (e.g. **thymol**) required and non-flammable.
    - non-irritant, with pleasant smell.
    - no corrosion of metal or adsorption on to rubber.
    - **SVP** should be high enough to enable production of clinically useful concentrations (depends on potency, **MAC**).
    - low blood/gas partition coefficient.
    - cheap.
  - pharmacology:
    - smooth, rapid induction with no breath holding, laryngospasm, coughing or increased secretions.
    - sufficiently potent to allow concurrent high F_IO_2.
    - analgesic, antiemetic and anticonvulsant properties, with skeletal muscle relaxation. No increase in **cerebral blood flow** or **ICP**.
    - no respiratory depression. Bronchodilatory action.
    - no cardiovascular depression or sensitisation of myocardium to **catecholamines**. No decrease in coronary, renal or hepatic perfusion.
    - minimal metabolism, with excretion via the lungs. No **fluoride ion** production.
    - no adverse renal, hepatic or haematological effects.
    - non-trigger for **MH**.
    - no effects on the **uterus**.
    - non-teratogenic/carcinogenic/neurotoxic.

No currently available agent fulfils all the above. All the volatile agents currently used have undesirable effects; in addition to those listed in Table 28, they all depress respiration, reduce uterine tone, and may trigger MH. All increase cerebral blood flow, although isoflurane and sevoflurane less so. N_2O is not potent enough for use as a sole agent and is losing popularity because of its emetic action, effects on **methionine** metabolism, cardiovascular and cerebral function, expansion of gas-containing cavities (e.g. **pneumothorax**) and its environmental effects. Trichloroethylene is analgesic and extremely cheap but is no longer produced due to costs associated with renewal of its product licence. Diethyl ether has been available on a named-patient basis. Cyclopropane, previously used mainly in paediatric anaesthesia, is now no longer available. Sevoflurane and desflurane are considered the agents of choice for **day-case surgery** because their low blood-gas solubility promotes rapid recovery.

The potency of anaesthetic agents depends on their **solubility** in the CNS, estimated by the oil/gas partition coefficient. Clinical effect depends on the partial pressure (rather than the total amount present) of the agent in the brain, which is related to arterial partial pressure, which is related to alveolar partial pressure. Thus steady-state brain concentration requires steady-state alveolar concentration. Drug is distributed from alveoli via bloodstream to:
  - vessel-rich tissues (e.g. brain, heart, kidney, liver; receive 70%–80% of cardiac output) until equilibrium is reached, then:
  - vessel-intermediate tissues (muscle, skin; 18% of cardiac output).
  - fat (6% of cardiac output) and other vessel-poor tissues, e.g. bone, ligaments.

In prolonged anaesthesia, the agent dissolves in fat, especially if it is very fat-soluble (i.e., potent). Thus it takes 80 min for the partial pressure of N_2O in fat to equal half that in arterial blood; halothane requires 32 h.

- Factors affecting uptake:
  - delivery to alveoli:
    - vaporisation: SVP, gas flow, temperature, vaporiser design, **pumping effect**.
    - **anaesthetic breathing system**: gas flow, volume of system and dilution of agent, adsorption on to rubber.
    - **alveolar ventilation**: increased alveolar ventilation shortens the time required for equilibration between inspired agent partial pressure and alveolar agent partial pressure. Hyperventilation thus hastens onset of anaesthesia.
    - **concentration effect** and **second gas effect**.
  - uptake from alveoli:
    - blood/gas partition coefficient (solubility in blood): if high, uptake and dissolution into blood are rapid;

Table 28 Undesirable features of the more modern volatile anaesthetic agents

Feature	*Halothane*	*Isoflurane*	*Enflurane*	*Desflurane*	*Sevoflurane*
Thymol required	+	–	–	–	–
Decomposed by light	+	–	–	–	–
Approximate cost/100 ml (£)	4–5	15–20	10–13	15–20	45–50
Irritant to breathe	–	+	+/–	++	–
Cardiac output	↓↓	↓	↓↓↓	↓	↓
SVR	(↓)	↓↓	↓	↓↓	↓↓
Heart rate	↓	↑	↑↑	↑	↑↓
Sensitivity to catecholamines	+++	+	++	–	–
Metabolised (%)	20	0.2	2	0.02	3–5
Others	Halothane hepatitis	Coronary steal	Epileptiform EEG	Direct metering vaporiser required	Decomposed by soda lime/baralyme

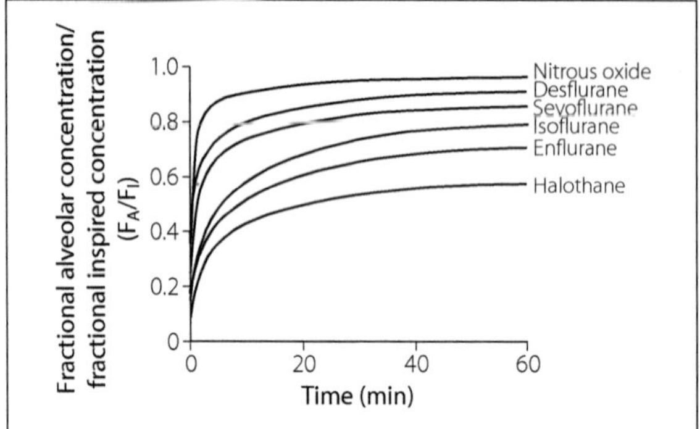

Fig. 88 'Wash-in' curves for some inhalational anaesthetic agents: equilibration between inspired and alveolar concentrations is faster for agents with lower solubility in blood

thus alveolar concentration falls rapidly until the next breath. Build-up of stable alveolar partial pressure and thus arterial partial pressure is therefore slow. If solubility is low, only a small proportion of agent dissolves in the blood, leaving a large reserve in the lungs. Thus alveolar and arterial partial pressures build up rapidly, with rapid clinical effects (Fig. 88). Changes in vaporiser settings are more rapidly reflected in arterial concentrations with insoluble agents than with soluble ones.

- cardiac output and pulmonary blood flow: uptake is more rapid if cardiac output is high, leading to slow build-up of alveolar concentration. If cardiac output is low, alveolar partial pressure builds up more quickly; in addition, a greater proportion of cardiac output goes to vital organs, e.g. brain and heart, increasing clinical effects. Thus overdose is more likely if cardiac output is low. The effect is more marked with soluble agents.
- concentration of agent in the pulmonary artery (i.e., mixed venous). As it approaches pulmonary venous concentration, alveolar and arterial levels approach equilibrium. Occurs as body tissues become saturated, or in severe low-output states when tissue perfusion is reduced.
- **$\dot{V}/\dot{Q}$ mismatch**: rarely significant unless large, e.g. accidental endobronchial intubation. Effects are greater for insoluble agents.
- impaired diffusion across alveolar wall is rarely significant.

Factors affecting recovery are similar to those described earlier. If body tissues are unsaturated, recovery is more rapid because the agent moves from arterial blood to both tissues and alveoli. If tissues are saturated after prolonged anaesthesia, recovery is slower, but is hastened by hyperventilation. However, drug movement from tissues into blood may cause reaccumulation of anaesthetic alveolar concentrations after initial wakening.

See also, Anaesthesia, mechanisms of; Coronary steal; Meyer–Overton rule

Injector techniques. Use of intermittent jets of driving gas, usually O_2, for IPPV by entraining room air. The jet is delivered to the proximal end of a bronchoscope by a metal cannula (Sanders injector), and entrains stationary gas within the bronchoscope by **jet mixing**. Room air is drawn in from the open end to replace the air delivered to the lungs. Expiration occurs by passive recoil of the lungs. A 14–16 G cannula is suitable for adults (delivers up to 30–50 cmH_2O pressure); 17–18 G for adolescents and small adults (up to 25 cmH_2O); 19 G for children (up to 15 cmH_2O). The Carden jetting device was described for attachment to a bronchoscope side-arm; higher inflation pressures and F_IO_2 are achieved with lower driving pressures.

The system usually consists of tubing and a connector for wall socket or gas cylinder, a pressure-reducing valve and gauge, a hand-operated trigger and attachment for the cannula. It may also be attached to commercially available **cricothyroidotomy** devices, or to iv cannulae used for emergency cricothyroidotomy. Similar principles are also used in high-frequency jet ventilation.

Commonly used for **bronchoscopy** and laryngoscopy because of its convenience.

- Disadvantages:
  - tidal volume and minute ventilation are difficult to assess.
  - trachea is unprotected during airway surgery.
  - possible interference with surgery from movement of vocal cords during ventilation.
  - **barotrauma** is possible if expiration is obstructed.
  - volatile anaesthetic agents cannot be delivered.

[Richard D Sanders (1906–1977) and Edward Carden, US anaesthetists]

See also, High-frequency ventilation

Injury severity score (ISS). **Trauma scale** used to grade severity of multiple injuries and based on the **abbreviated injury scale** (AIS). Mostly used for **audit** purposes, it takes the square of the AIS scores for the three worst affected anatomical regions, with scores ranging from 0 to 75 (any AIS score of 6 automatically converts the total to 75). A score under 24 indicates probable survival, 25–50 reflects progressive increase in mortality and >50 suggests very high mortality rates. Accounts only for anatomical injury, not other factors, and concentrates on only one injury per anatomical site.

The new injury severity score (NISS) differs by including all the most severe injuries rather than the most severe injury per body area. NISS performs better than ISS and is more accurate in distinguishing between survivors and non-survivors.

Baker SP, O'Neill B (1976). J Trauma; 16: 882–5

Inosine. Metabolite of **adenosine**, with some similar actions. Causes vasodilatation via a direct action on vascular smooth muscle. Also has a positive inotropic effect, but not via **β-adrenergic receptors**. Thought to improve cell survival following ischaemia and reperfusion (e.g. in cardiac and renal surgery), possibly by increasing intracellular levels of energy-rich phosphates and reducing **ATP** depletion. Has been used in proximal aortic and renal surgery; e.g. 30 mg/kg iv before clamping. Hypotension may occur.

Inotropic drugs. Drugs that increase myocardial contractility, increasing cardiac output.

- Drugs available include:
  - **catecholamines**: act via **G protein-coupled receptors** to increase intracellular **cAMP** levels via adenylate cyclase stimulation; cAMP increases intracellular **calcium** ion mobilisation and force of contraction.
    - **adrenaline**: a **β-adrenergic receptor agonist** mainly at low doses, **α-adrenergic receptor agonist** mainly at higher doses. Causes peripheral and renal vasoconstriction, especially at higher doses. Tachycardia and arrhythmias may occur, increasing myocardial O_2 demand.
    - **noradrenaline**: α-receptor agonist mainly, with some β-receptor agonist properties. Causes peripheral and renal vasoconstriction, with raised BP and compensatory bradycardia. Depending on the SVR, myocardial O_2 demand may be markedly increased.
    - **isoprenaline**: β-receptor agonist only. Increases cardiac output and rate, with peripheral and pulmonary vasodilatation. Arrhythmias are common, and myocardial O_2 demand is increased; ischaemia may occur due to lowered BP.
    - **dopamine**: β_1-receptor agonist at lower doses, with increased cardiac output and BP. α-Receptor-mediated vasoconstriction occurs at higher doses. Myocardial O_2 demand is increased, but ischaemia is less likely as BP also increases. Tachycardia is less common. **Dopamine receptor**-mediated renal and mesenteric vasodilatation may occur at low doses (so-called 'renal dose'), although accompanying diuresis may be simply due to improved cardiac output.
    - **dobutamine**: mainly a β_1-receptor agonist, with weak β_2- and weaker α-receptor agonist properties. Causes less tachycardia than other catecholamines for a given inotropic effect, possibly due to a smaller effect on the sinoatrial node, and activation of the **baroreceptor reflex** by increased BP. Coronary perfusion may increase as left ventricular end-diastolic pressure falls.
    - **dopexamine**: derived from dopamine; more active at β_2-receptors and less active at dopaminergic receptors. Causes peripheral and renal vasodilatation, with little tachycardia.
    - **pirbuterol**: mainly a β_1-receptor agonist. Causes some vasodilatation.
    - **salbutamol**: not a direct inotrope but has been used in circulatory failure. A β_2-receptor agonist, reducing SVR. Tachycardia is common.
  - phosphodiesterase inhibitors:
    - specific for cardiac phosphodiesterase: e.g. **amrinone, milrinone, enoximone.** Cause vasodilatation and increased cardiac output.
    - non-specific: e.g. **aminophylline.**
  - **calcium sensitisers**: e.g. **levosimendan**. Increase myocardial contractility without increasing myocardial energy/O_2 requirements. Also cause vasodilatation (by opening K^+ channels in vascular smooth muscle), thus reducing **afterload** and **preload.**
  - others:
    - calcium: effect lasts for about 5 min. Used as a temporary measure. Ventricular arrhythmias may occur.
    - **cardiac glycosides**: e.g. **digoxin**. Increase cardiac output and reduce heart rate; possibly also cause vasoconstriction. Thought to increase intracellular calcium ion activity via other ionic effects. Their use in **cardiac failure** is confined to those with severe functional limitation and ejection fractions <25%.
    - **glucagon**: mechanism is unclear; adrenergic receptors are not thought to be involved. May increase calcium flux into myocardial muscle by stimulating adenylate cyclase.

Choice of drug depends on clinical context. Dopamine is sometimes used in low dosage for its purported renal effect; dobutamine is commonly used for cardiac support. Adrenaline and noradrenaline are also used, the latter, for example, when vasodilatation is a particular problem, e.g. **septic shock. Milrinone** is often used where tachycardia is particularly undesirable, e.g. after **cardiac surgery**. Isoprenaline is indicated in bradycardia and raised pulmonary vascular resistance.

Often used in combination with **vasodilator drugs**, to reduce filling pressures while providing inotropic support. Milrinone and dopexamine especially fulfil both functions.

INPB, Intermittent negative pressure breathing, *see Intermittent negative pressure ventilation*

INPV, *see Intermittent negative pressure ventilation*

INR, International normalised ratio, *see Coagulation studies*

Insensible water loss. Volume of pure water (i.e., solute-free) lost per day through evaporation from the respiratory tract or **diffusion** through the skin (with subsequent evaporation). Normally up to 1200 ml at rest, increasing with body temperature (by up to 20% per °C above normal) and metabolic rate, and also in tachypnoea. Reduced as ambient humidity increases. During IPPV, exhaled losses may be reduced by **humidification** of inspired gases.

See also, Fluid balance

Inspiratory capacity. Maximal possible volume of air inspired from **FRC**. Composed of **tidal volume** and **inspiratory reserve volume**. Normally 3–4 l.
See also, Lung volumes

Inspiratory:expiratory ratio (I:E ratio). Ratio of inspiratory time to expiratory time. Usually 1:2, allowing recovery from the cardiovascular effects of **IPPV** during expiration. Adjustable on most **ventilators** between 1:1 and 1:4. If expiration is too short, air trapping may occur, with increasing intrathoracic volume and pressure, increasing adverse effects of IPPV. However, a reversed I:E ratio of up to 4:1 (**inverse ratio ventilation**) has been used to improve oxygenation in respiratory failure, especially combined with **PEEP**.

Inspiratory pressure support. Augmentation of spontaneous inspiration with supplementary gas flow. A more refined form of **assisted ventilation**, provided by modern ICU **ventilators**. Inspiratory flow rate is adjusted to produce a preset inspiratory airway pressure; when flow rate falls to a certain value, inspiration ends. Increases tidal volume, reducing work of breathing and respiratory rate during **weaning from ventilators**. However, negative pressure must be generated by the patient to trigger augmentation. Tidal volume may vary according to the patient's inspiratory flow pattern. During weaning, the amount of support supplied may be reduced either by lowering the preset airway pressure, or by increasing the negative pressure required to trigger the support.

A combination of pressure support and a decelerating inspiratory flow pattern and a guaranteed tidal volume, **inspiratory volume support**, has recently been developed, in which changes in lung properties during inspiration are continuously monitored.

Inspiratory reserve volume. **Inspiratory capacity** minus **tidal volume**. Normally about 3 l.
See also, Lung volumes

Inspiratory volume support. Spontaneous ventilator breathing mode combining the benefits of **inspiratory pressure support** with a decelerating inspiratory flow pattern and a guaranteed tidal volume. The ventilator automatically monitors the lung properties and modifies the inspiratory pressure support to deliver a predetermined volume. Maximum inspiratory pressure support permitted is just below the preset upper pressure limit and, if the tidal volume cannot be delivered with this degree of pressure support, the ventilator alarms, indicating that the breath has been pressure-limited. Useful mode when there is a large variation in lung/chest compliance during inspiration, e.g. atelectasis, bronchospasm. As the patient increases spontaneous ventilation, the inspiratory support from the ventilator decreases. If apnoea occurs, volume support also ensures a back-up of **pressure-regulated volume control ventilation**. The maximum pressure change between two breaths is preset by the ventilator (approximately 3 cmH_2O).

Insufflation techniques. Passage of 4–6 l/min fresh gas through a fine-bore catheter, passed through the larynx into the trachea; the tip usually lies near the carina (tracheal insufflation). With spontaneous ventilation, fresh gas and room air are inhaled into the lungs, with exhaled gas passing out around the catheter. May also be used to maintain oxygenation in apnoeic patients, although with build-up of CO_2 (**apnoeic oxygenation**). Used to maintain oxygenation during **brainstem death** testing.

First used in the early 1900s. **Magill** and **Rowbotham** later provided a separate tube for expired gases, both tubes subsequently replaced by a single wide-bore tracheal tube. Still used by some anaesthetists for **bronchoscopy** and **laryngoscopy**, especially in children. Fresh gas may also be delivered via the rigid endoscope.

Pharyngeal insufflation is also possible, using a pharyngeal catheter, or by attaching the fresh gas source to a gag or airway.

Barotrauma may occur if escape of gas is obstructed.

Insulin. Hormone secreted by B (β) cells of the pancreatic islets of Langerhans (A [α] cells secrete **glucagon**, and D [δ] cells **somatostatin**). Composed of two polypeptide chains specific to species, linked by disulfide bridges. Synthesised as a precursor molecule, subsequently split before secretion.

- Secretion is increased by:
  - **glucose**, mannose, fructose.
  - **amino acids**.
  - glucagon and other gut hormones.
  - **β-adrenergic receptor** stimulation.
  - vagal stimulation.
  - phosphodiesterase inhibition, e.g. due to drugs.
  - sulfonylureas.
- Secretion is decreased by:
  - hypoglycaemia.
  - somatostatin.
  - α-receptor stimulation.
  - insulin.
  - drugs:
    - diazoxide.
    - thiazide diuretics.
    - **β-adrenergic receptor antagonists**.
- Actions:
  - increases:
    - glucose uptake by muscle and fat.
    - **glycogen** and **protein** synthesis.
    - **fat** synthesis and deposition.
    - potassium uptake by cells.
  - decreases:
    - glycogen breakdown and gluconeogenesis.
    - fat and protein breakdown.
    - hepatic **ketone body** synthesis.

  Thus lowers blood glucose levels and increases glucose utilisation. Binds to the extracellular portion of the transmembrane insulin receptors (tyrosine kinase family), causing autophosphorylation of intracellular **enzymes**.

Insulins for therapeutic administration (e.g. in **diabetes mellitus**) are now most commonly produced by recombinant genetic engineering; older preparations were derived from bovine or porcine pancreatic extract. Substitution/deletion of amino acids at specific sites of the insulin molecule confers different properties with regard to onset and duration of action, mostly via altered absorption from the injection site. Changing from one type to another, especially from bovine to human, may result in hypoglycaemia.

Usually administered sc; may also be injected iv, im and intraperitoneally. Recently an inhaled form has been developed. Insulin pumps that deliver a continuous infusion sc with additional calculated boluses depending on blood glucose levels are increasingly used.

- Generally classified according to their onset and duration of action:

- short-acting:
  - insulin lispro: recombinant human insulin analogue with a lesser tendency to form hexamers in solution (responsible for slowing uptake). Acts within 15–30 min of sc injection with duration of action 1–3 h.
  - insulin aspart: recombinant human insulin analogue; rapidly dissociates into monomers and dimers after injection, resulting in rapid absorption. Acts within 10–20 min of sc injection with duration of action 3–5 h.
  - insulin glulisine: similar properties to insulin aspart.
  - soluble insulin. Acts within 30–60 min of sc injection, with effects lasting up to 8 h. **Half-life** is determined by rate of absorption from tissue: about 2–5 h after sc injection, but 5 min after iv injection (with the latter having effects lasting 30 min). Used for emergency treatment of **hyperglycaemia** and perioperatively; also to lower plasma potassium in **hyperkalaemia**. May be adsorbed on to the infusion set plastic.
- intermediate and long-acting:
  - isophane insulin (suspension with protamine) and amorphous insulin zinc suspension. Acts within 1–2 h, lasting up to 20 h.
  - insulin detemir and insulin glargine: recombinant human insulin analogues: exhibit slower absorption from injection sites via protein-binding and precipitation, respectively. Act within 1–2 h with duration of action up to 24 h.
  - crystalline insulin zinc suspension. Acts within 1–2 h, lasting up to 36 h.

The last group is mainly used for maintenance sc administration. Several insulin mixtures (biphasic) are also available. Available as 100 units/ml in the UK; dosage is adjusted for each patient.

[Paul Langerhans (1847–1888), German pathologist]

See also, Glycolysis

Intensive care, costs of, *see Costs of intensive care*

Intensive care follow-up. Programme of ward visits, outpatient clinics and support groups for patients discharged from ICUs. Results in improved communication between ICU and ward staff, and may prevent readmission of patients to ICU through early detection of complications. Clinic appointments allow better assessment of the patient's post-ICU quality of life and the early identification of **post-intensive care syndrome**.

Detting-Ihnenfeldt DS, De Graaff AE, Nollet F, et al (2015). Minerva Anestesiol; 81: 865–75

Intensive care, history of. Closely linked to the history of anaesthesia, **CPR**, pain relief and monitoring. Modern techniques originate from respiratory care units in 1940–1950 along with developments in **IPPV** and CPR. **Coronary care units** were the first specialised units, set up in the 1960s.

- Major developments relating to ICUs include:
  - various tank **ventilators** described and used: 1800s.
  - iv salt solutions first used to treat cholera: 1830s.
  - concept of keeping all patients requiring 'special' attention and nursing in one place pioneered by Florence Nightingale: 1852.
  - **curare** used in the treatment of **tetanus**: 1872.
  - **blood gas interpretation** performed: 1872.
  - venous pressures measured in humans: 1902.
  - **pulse oximetry** described: 1913.
  - modern **oxygen therapy** introduced by **Haldane**: 1917.
  - **haemodialysis** described: 1940s.
  - worldwide **poliomyelitis** epidemic in the 1950s. Early **tracheostomy**, chest **physiotherapy** and manual IPPV by medical students used in Copenhagen in 1952 resulted in the establishment of the first ICU by **Ibsen**: 1953.
  - first clinical description of **brainstem death**: 1959.
  - modern CPR developed: 1960s.
  - **ALI** described: 1967. **High-frequency ventilation** described and developed in the 1970s.
  - **Intensive Care Society** formed in the UK; **Society of Critical Care Medicine** formed in the USA: 1970.
  - critical care training programmes commenced in Canada and the USA: 1970s.
  - intermittent mandatory ventilation introduced: 1971.
  - bedside pulmonary artery catheterisation described; journal *Critical Care Medicine* first published: 1972.
  - ***Intensive Care Medicine*** first published: 1975.
  - first conference of UK Royal Colleges on diagnosis of brainstem death: 1976.
  - **haemofiltration** introduced: 1977.
  - **APACHE, SAPS** and **MPM** severity of illness scoring systems described: 1980s.
  - **European Society of Intensive Care Medicine** formed: 1982.
  - **Resuscitation Council (UK)** formed: 1982.
  - **etomidate** found to cause adrenal suppression in intensive care patients if used as an infusion: 1983.
  - **British Association of Critical Care** Nurses formed: 1984.
  - first **CEPOD** report: 1987 (*see National Confidential Enquiry into Patient Outcome and Death*).
  - **European Resuscitation Council** formed; **European Diploma in Intensive Care Medicine** held: 1989.
  - **International Liaison Committee on Resuscitation** formed: 1992.
  - **Intensive Care National Audit and Research Centre** established: 1994.
  - Intercollegiate Board for Training in Intensive Care Medicine formed; first running of UK Intensive Care Diploma examination: 1998.
  - intensive care medicine granted specialty status by Specialist Training Authority: 1999.
  - creation of **care bundles** summarising best practice: early 2000s.
  - first programmes towards Certificate of Completion of Specialist Training in Intensive Care Medicine commenced: 2002.
  - **Faculty of Intensive Care Medicine** established at the **Royal College of Anaesthetists**: 2010.

[Florence Nightingale (1820–1910), English nurse]

Kelly FE, Fong K, Hirsch NP, Nolan JP (2014). Clin Med: 14: 376–9

See also, Anaesthesia, history of; individual topics

Intensive Care Medicine. Official journal of the **European Society of Intensive Care Medicine** and **European Society of Paediatric Intensive Care**, originally published in 1975 as the *European Journal of Intensive Care*.

Intensive Care National Audit and Research Centre (ICNARC). Charitable company established in the UK in 1994 with funding from the Department of Health to develop and undertake comparative audit and evaluative research in intensive care. Its development results directly from the **Intensive Care Society**'s study of the **APACHE II** severity of illness system. Now a non-profit-making organisation, funded primarily by research grants and subscription of ICUs to ICNARC's Case Mix Programme. Has developed an ICU coding method generated from data from over 10000 patients admitted to 26 UK ICUs; the system describes over 700 conditions categorised by body system, anatomical site, physiological/pathological process and condition.

Harrison DA, Rowan KM (2008). Curr Opin Crit Care; 14: 506–12

Intensive care, outcome of. Survival from ICU admission is influenced by:

- patient factors: age, pre-existing morbidity, physiological reserve, genetic makeup.
- disease factors: type, site, severity.
- treatment factors: available therapies, appropriate usage, response to therapy.
- organisational factors: early referral/admission, resources, quality of ICU care.

Scoring systems (e.g. **APACHE**) are used to estimate the risk of hospital mortality for a group of patients. Mortality in ICU varies between ICUs and is dependent upon patient population and case mix factors. In the UK, unadjusted ICU mortality varies between about 11% and 30%; post-ICU in-hospital mortality varies between about 20% and 45%.

There is an increasing awareness that other outcome measures, such as post-ICU morbidity and quality of life, are also important.

See also, Intensive care follow-up; Mortality/survival prediction on intensive care unit

Intensive Care Society. British society founded in 1970, for the furtherance of intensive care medicine. Aims include the promotion of education and research, defining standards of intensive care and providing information on the availability, coding and costing of care to its members, the Department of Health and NHS Executive. Currently has over 3400 members, the majority of whom are anaesthetists.

Intensive care, training in. Previously a subspecialty of anaesthesia, intensive care medicine (ICM) has been recognised by the General Medical Council (GMC) as a specialty of its own since 2009.

Applicants wishing to train in ICM have to complete core medical training, core anaesthetic training or the acute care common stem; they must also have passed the corresponding postgraduate examination (e.g. membership of the Royal College of Physicians, membership of the College of Emergency Medicine or primary fellowship of the **Royal College of Anaesthetists**). Once given a national training number in ICM, the training consists of three stages:

- stage 1 (specialty training [ST] years 3 and 4): provides exposure to aspects of ICM not covered in core placements. By the end of stage 1, trainees will have spent one year in anaesthesia, ICM and medicine. The remaining year can be spent in any acute area.
- stage 2 (ST years 5 and 6): provides exposure to subspecialties. In ST5, at least 3 months are spent in cardiac, neurological and paediatric ICM units. Training in the remaining months depends on the local availability and the needs of the trainee. The Fellowship of the **Faculty of Intensive Care Medicine** examination must be completed by the end of ST6.
- stage 3 (ST year 7): clinical knowledge and skills are consolidated and leadership ability developed in readiness for consultancy.

Although stand-alone training in ICM was approved by the GMC in 2011, many opt for 'dual accreditation' with another acute specialty e.g. anaesthesia, emergency medicine, respiratory medicine, etc. A second national training number in that partner specialty must be obtained in a standard competitive application.

Intensive care unit (ICU). Modern techniques originate from postoperative recovery units and respiratory care units in 1940s–1950s along with developments in **IPPV** and **CPR. Coronary care units** were the first specialised units, set up in the 1960s. An ICU usually provides 1%–2% of total hospital beds, although factors affecting this proportion include the number of operating theatres, the type of surgery (e.g. surgery such as cardiac surgery and neurosurgery has greater requirements), location of the hospital (e.g. near major motorways), the overall provision of ICUs within the region and the presence of an accident and emergency department. In general, the unit should have the capacity to accept around 95% of all appropriately referred cases and bed occupancy should be 60%–70%. Units larger than 10 beds should be subdivided into specialised units; those smaller than four beds are felt to be uneconomic. Distinction is no longer made between ICU and **HDU** beds (most units now have a mix of beds), with defined levels of **critical care** provided according to the type of support required.

- Design considerations:
  - size of unit/bed space (approximately 20 m^2 suggested per patient). Adequate bed separation is important for **infection control**. Provision of cubicles (e.g. one per six open beds) is necessary for isolation of infectious/immunocompromised patients.
  - proximity to theatres, accident and emergency department, x-ray and laboratory facilities.
  - equipment: **ventilators, monitoring,** infusion pumps, cardiac arrest trolley, blood gas analyser. Adequate electrical points, gas pipelines and suction.
  - lighting and basins.
  - staff facilities, e.g. on-call room, kitchen.
  - security measures, e.g. single entrance, closed circuit television surveillance.
- Staffing requirements:
  - designated consultant with administrative responsibility for the unit. 85% of ICUs are run by anaesthetists in the UK, although intensive care medicine is rapidly becoming an independent specialty (*see Intensive care, training in*).
  - adequate consultant sessions (15 per week for a unit larger than four beds has been suggested, with more for larger units).
  - resident trainee medical staff with responsibility solely to the unit.
  - nursing staff (one nurse per patient required for 24 h/day).
- Patient selection criteria:
  - according to the requirements in the defined levels of critical care.
  - reasons for admission: the disease state should be potentially reversible.
  - premorbid general health, age and **mortality/survival prediction** scores (although severity of illness scoring systems cannot be used to predict outcome of intensive care in individual patients).

- response to treatment so far.
- anticipated quality of life and the wishes of the patient and relatives.
- availability of beds.
- Admission to ICU should be:
  - before the patient's condition reaches a point from which recovery is impossible.
  - according to clear criteria to identify at-risk patients.
  - undertaken at senior level using appropriate transfer equipment. Unless the referral area is close to the ICU, full stabilisation (e.g. intubation, IPPV and inotropic therapy) should be undertaken before transfer.
- Problems may be related to:
  - original condition.
  - multiple organ failure; may follow many disease processes (e.g. **renal failure** and **ALI** are common in critical illness of any cause). Prognosis worsens as more organ systems are involved.
  - infection and **sepsis**.
  - adequate **nutrition**, and fluid and electrolyte balance.
  - gastric ulceration (**stress ulcers**). Prophylaxis is as for **peptic ulcer disease**; **proton pump inhibitors** and **H_2 receptor antagonists** are most commonly used.
  - immobility: **DVT** and **decubitus ulcers** may occur. Prophylactic sc **heparin** is usually administered, and pressure area care and physiotherapy instituted.
  - **sedation**.

Other considerations relate to the **cost of intensive care**, **consent**, and the **ethics** and **audit** of ICU practice.
See also, Care of the critically ill surgical patient; Intensive care follow-up; Intensive care, history of; Medical emergency team; Postoperative care team; Safe transport and retrieval team; Selective decontamination of the digestive tract; Transportation of critically ill patients

Intensive care unit, transport to, *see Transportation of critically ill patients*

Intercollegiate Diploma in Intensive Care Medicine (IDICM), *see Diploma in Intensive Care Medicine*

Intercostal nerve block. Used for peri- and **postoperative analgesia**, and for analgesia in patients with fractured **ribs**.
- Technique:
  - may be performed with the patient sitting, with shoulders flexed to pull the scapulae forwards (e.g. with the forearms resting on pillows), or in the lateral position, with the side to be blocked uppermost.
  - identification of selected ribs: by counting down from the spinous process of T1 (the most prominent palpable at the base of the neck) or up from L4–5 (level with the iliac crests). The rib is palpated laterally to the angle, about 6–10 cm from the midline. Injection at the angle blocks the lateral cutaneous branch of the intercostal nerve, that may be missed if injection is performed in the mid- or posterior axillary line.
  - a needle (attached to a syringe of **local anaesthetic agent**) is introduced at the lower edge of the rib, directed cranially. It contacts bone, and is 'walked' inferiorly until it slips off the rib's inferior surface. It is then advanced 2–3 mm. The patient is asked to breath-hold to reduce lung movement and risk of **pneumothorax**.
  - stretching of the overlying skin cranially before needle insertion has been suggested: release of stretch following insertion aids angling of the needle tip into the subcostal groove.
  - following aspiration to exclude intravascular placement, 3–5 ml of local anaesthetic agent is injected while moving the needle inwards and outwards 1–2 mm. **Bupivacaine** 0.25%–0.5% with **adrenaline** may provide analgesia lasting up to 12 h; **lidocaine** 1% with adrenaline up to 2–4 h. A catheter may be inserted for continuous infusion or intermittent boluses.
  - studies with dyes have shown extensive overlap of injected solution to adjacent spaces (and even to the other side). Systemic absorption of solution is significant; maximal 'safe' doses should not be exceeded.
  - pneumothorax and puncture of intercostal blood vessels may occur. Intra- or epidural spread via a dural cuff surrounding the proximal nerve is also possible.

See also, Intercostal spaces; Interpleural analgesia

Intercostal spaces. Contain the intercostal nerves and blood vessels as they run around the width of the body (Fig. 89).

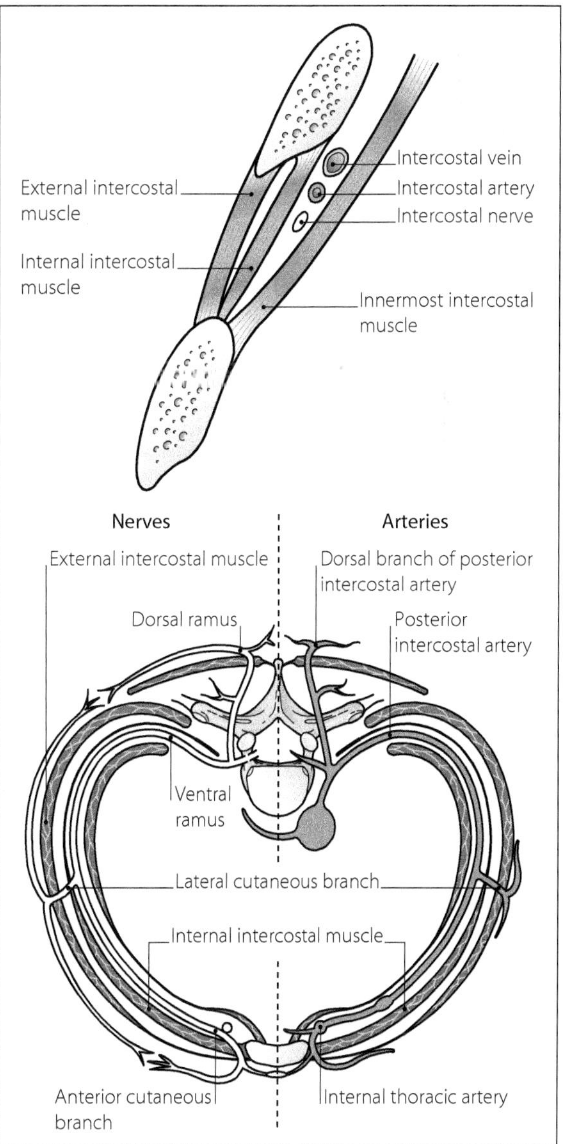

Fig. 89 Anatomy of intercostal spaces

- Muscle layers between **ribs**:
  - external intercostal muscle, passing down and forwards.
  - internal intercostal muscle, passing down and backwards. Becomes the internal intercostal membrane posterior to the rib angles.
  - innermost intercostal muscle, attached to the ribs' inner surfaces.
- Intercostal nerves:
  - ventral rami of **spinal nerves** T1–11. Each spinal nerve has dorsal and ventral roots, that join and then divide into dorsal and ventral rami. The dorsal rami supply the extensor muscles and skin of the back.
  - lie below the blood vessels in the intercostal space, running between the internal and innermost intercostal muscle layers.
  - each (except the first) gives off a lateral cutaneous branch anterior to the rib angles, and ends as the anterior cutaneous branch.
  - collateral branch arises at the angle, passing forward with main nerve.
- Intercostal arteries:
  - two anterior and one posterior supply each space except the lower two (posterior only).
  - anterior arteries arise from the internal thoracic artery or its terminal branch. They anastomose with the posterior artery and its collateral.
  - posterior arteries arise from the superior intercostal artery (first and second) or descending aorta. They each give off a collateral branch.

Venous drainage is via two anterior and one posterior intercostal veins, to internal thoracic and azygos veins.

Interferometer, *see Gas analysis*

Interferons, *see Cytokines*

Interleukins, *see Cytokines*

Intermittent-flow anaesthetic machines. To be distinguished from apparatus used for **draw-over techniques**, in which the patient's own inspiratory effort causes gas flow. Intermittent-flow machines provide gas flow usually on demand, i.e., when triggered by the patient's inspiration, but are more sophisticated than simple **demand valves**. Allow mixing of gases, usually **O_2** and **N_2O**, and addition of volatile agents using conventional **vaporisers**. Minnitt's machine (described in 1933) using an N_2O cylinder with indrawn air was used for analgesia in labour. Inspiration reduces pressure within the apparatus, moving a valve and allowing gas flow. In the **McKesson** machine, the force opposing fresh gas flow may be adjusted, so that continuous low flow may be provided if required, between breaths. Further adjustment provides continuous high flow, as with conventional **anaesthetic machines**.

Some machines feature **O_2 warning devices**, O_2 flushes and valves to cut off N_2O in case of potentially hypoxic gas mixtures.

Traditionally used for **dental surgery**, but less commonly used now because of unfamiliarity, inaccuracy of flow rates and gas composition, and relative lack of safety features.

[Robert J Minnitt (1889–1974), Liverpool anaesthetist]

Intermittent mandatory ventilation (IMV). Ventilatory mode used to assist **weaning from ventilators**. A mandatory minute volume is preset and delivered by the ventilator, but the patient is allowed to breathe spontaneously between ventilator breaths. As the patient weans, the proportion of minute volume delivered by the ventilator may be reduced, usually by reducing the ventilator rate.

IMV reduces average intrathoracic pressures and risk of **barotrauma**. The patient's progress may be monitored by counting the spontaneous respiratory rate.

Some ventilators will not deliver positive pressure breaths within a certain period of spontaneous breaths, to prevent over-distension of the patient's lungs and barotrauma (synchronised intermittent mandatory ventilation). Others simply incorporate a pressure-relief valve.

Although the weaning process is not shortened, IMV allows it to start earlier and be monitored more easily while requiring less **sedation**, and reducing risks of **IPPV**.

Intermittent negative pressure ventilation (INPV). Advocated in the 1800s as a means of controlled ventilation without the adverse effects of **IPPV**, although the latter were then overestimated. Tank **ventilators** ('iron lungs') were described first, then cuirass types; motor-driven devices were used in the 1930s.

Avoids the risk of **barotrauma** and other dangers of IPPV, while allowing the respiratory muscles to rest. Does not require tracheal intubation, although the risks of regurgitation and aspiration are still present. Indrawing of the soft tissues of the neck may result in upper airway obstruction. **Sedation** is not required. Continuous end-expiratory negative extrathoracic pressure has similar beneficial effects to **PEEP**, but without its adverse effects.

Largely superseded by IPPV, but still occasionally used for chronic ventilation, e.g. domiciliary night-time ventilation for neuromuscular disease; it has been used to aid **weaning** from prolonged IPPV.

The Hayek oscillator, first described in the late 1980s, consists of a clear plastic cuirass that fits over the chest and abdomen, connected to a power unit with wide-bore tubing. A wide range of frequencies (usually 30–300 Hz) and negative pressures may be generated. It has been used in **respiratory failure**, weaning, laryngeal surgery, and perioperatively in cases of failed intubation.

[Zamir Hayek (?–2005), Israeli-born English neonatologist]

Intermittent positive pressure ventilation (IPPV). Form of controlled ventilation. Performed by Vesalius in 1543 (via a tracheotomy in a pig) and Hooke in 1667 (used bellows via a tracheotomy in a dog). Used initially for **CPR**; later employed in animal experiments with **curare** by **Waterton** in the 1820s. Used in the late 1800s/early 1900s during anaesthesia, but wider acceptance accompanied the introduction of **neuromuscular blocking drugs** in the 1940s. Use in **respiratory failure** developed largely following the 1952 Danish **poliomyelitis** epidemic.

Modified forms (e.g. IMV, pressure control ventilation, pressure-regulated volume control ventilation) are mainly used in ICU during weaning from ventilators. **High-frequency ventilation** was developed from the early 1970s. **Non-invasive positive pressure ventilation** is available for patients with neuromuscular respiratory failure and **COPD**.

- Indications:
  - ICU:
    - respiratory failure.
    - **head injury**.
    - others, e.g. **coma**, post-CPR.
  - anaesthesia:
    - when neuromuscular blockade is required; often performed when tracheal intubation is indicated.
    - thoracic surgery.
    - when ventilation is inadequate.
    - to control arterial $P\text{CO}_2$.
    - to reduce requirement for inhalational agents, e.g. in cardiovascular disease.
    - to ensure adequate air entry, e.g. in respiratory disease.
- Technique:
  - usually via tracheal intubation, **tracheostomy** or **SAD**, but it may be performed via **facemask**.
  - manual ventilation was formerly used extensively; **ventilators** are now widespread. **Injector techniques** may also be used.
  - a tidal volume of 10–12 ml/kg, at a rate of 10–12 breaths/min, is commonly used, ideally adjusted to arterial (or end-tidal) $P\text{CO}_2$. **PEEP** is usually applied to reduce alveolar collapse and **atelectasis**. **Negative end-expiratory pressure** is no longer recommended.

    Mean intrathoracic pressure is lowest with accelerating gas flow, but ventilation is uneven. Ventilation is more uniform with decelerating flow, but mean pressure is highest. **Inspiratory:expiratory ratio** of 1:2 is usually employed but may be varied according to clinical requirements.
  - neuromuscular blockade is usually employed; deep anaesthesia using volatile agents may also be used, combined with **opioid analgesic drugs** and **hypocapnia** to suppress respiratory drive. Sedative/opioid infusions are commonly used in ICU (*see Sedation*).
  - **monitoring** is important to ensure adequate ventilation and gas exchange, and to detect disconnection.
- Physiological effects/hazards:
  - cardiovascular effects, due to increased intrathoracic pressure:
    - reduced **venous return** and **cardiac output**; may reduce BP, especially in **autonomic neuropathy** or **hypovolaemia**.
    - increased **pulmonary vascular resistance**, reducing right ventricular output.
    - reduced left ventricular **compliance** and filling, especially with **PEEP**. Bulging of the right ventricle and direct effects of lung expansion are thought to be responsible.
    - measured **CVP** is raised, and venous drainage from head and neck is reduced. **ICP** may increase.
  - respiratory effects:
    - **intrapleural pressure** is about –5 cmH_2O during expiration and up to +5 cmH_2O during inspiration, in contrast to spontaneous ventilation.
    - lung compliance and **FRC** fall. Atelectasis occurs in dependent lung tissue, increasing **alveolar–arterial O_2 difference** and **dead space**. Adding PEEP and increasing tidal volume may reduce these effects.
  - others:
    - renal: reduced arterial BP and increased venous pressure lower renal perfusion. Glomerular filtration is reduced, and the **renin/angiotensin system** stimulated. **Atrial natriuretic peptide** secretion is lowered and **vasopressin** secretion may be increased. The overall effect is reduced urine output (by up to 40%) and sodium retention.
    - **ileus** is common with prolonged IPPV; the cause is unclear but may involve changes in GIT neural activity and pressures. It may also be related to concurrent illness or drug therapy.
    - risks of tracheal intubation.
    - **barotrauma**, undetected disconnection.

[Andreas Vesalius (1514–1564), German anatomist; Robert Hooke (1635–1703), Curator of the Royal Society, England]

See also, Intermittent negative pressure ventilation; Intubation, tracheal; Ventilator-associated lung injury

Internal jugular venous cannulation. The internal **jugular vein** lies deep to the sternomastoid muscle, and follows a course from just anterior to the mastoid process to behind the sternoclavicular joint (Fig. 90). Cannulation may be performed at a number of sites; the most common are outlined below.

- Technique:
  - head-down position distends the vein and reduces the risk of **gas embolism**. The head is turned to the contralateral side. Aseptic techniques are used.
  - the distended vein may be palpable (or even visible) in thin subjects, lateral to the carotid pulsation.
  - a right-side approach is usually employed, because the right internal jugular vein, superior vena cava and right atrium are more directly aligned than on the left.
  - local anaesthetic is used if the patient is awake.

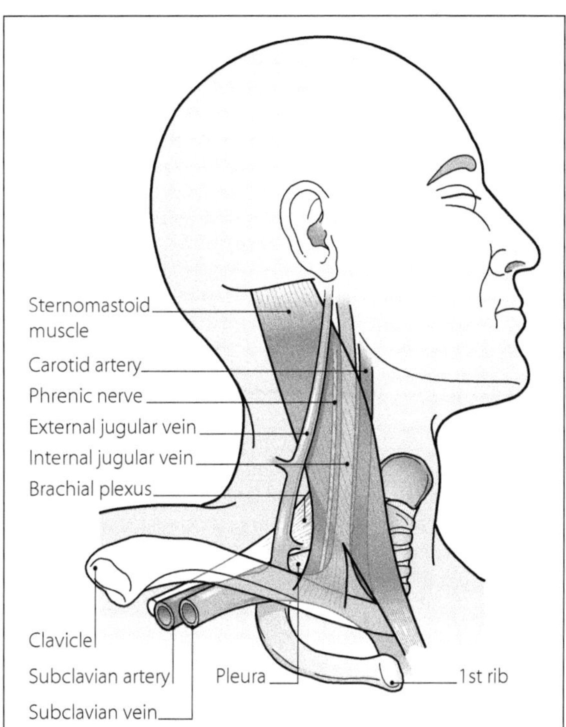

Fig. 90 Anatomy of right internal jugular vein

- high approach:
  - the carotid pulsation is located level with the cricoid cartilage (C6). With the fingers of one hand guarding the artery, the needle is introduced just laterally, angled at 30 degrees to the skin and directed towards the ipsilateral nipple. When blood is aspirated, the needle is lowered to align it more with the vein, and the cannula advanced or wire inserted (**Seldinger technique**). If no blood is aspirated, the needle may be redirected slightly medially. Some prefer to locate the vein with a small needle first before using the larger introducer needle.
  - alternatively, a slightly lower approach involves needle insertion at the apex of the triangle formed by the two heads of sternomastoid, a more reliable landmark when the carotid pulsation is weak or absent (e.g. cardiac arrest).
- low approach: the needle is introduced just above the sternoclavicular joint and directed caudally. A higher incidence of **pneumothorax** may result from this approach.

The routine use of ultrasound probes for location of the vein is now recommended by **NICE**.

See also, Central venous cannulation, for complications and comparisons with other techniques

International classification injury severity score (ICISS). **Trauma scale** based on the *International Classification of Diseases*, 9th edition (ICD-9). Has the advantage that most hospitals use the ICD for routine admission and discharge coding. Has been used for predicting survival, costing treatment and assessing outcome. Initial trials suggest it is superior in this respect to the **injury severity score** and **trauma revised injury severity score**.

Rutledge R, Osler T, Emery S, Kromhout-Schiro S (1998). J Trauma; 44: 41–9

International Liaison Committee on Resuscitation (ILCOR). Formed in 1992 to provide a forum for liaison between principal resuscitation organisations worldwide, producing its first advisory statements in 1997. Currently comprises the American Heart Association, the **European Resuscitation Council**, the Heart and Stroke Foundation of Canada, the Australian and New Zealand Resuscitation Council, the Resuscitation Councils of Southern Africa, the Inter American Heart Foundation and the Resuscitation Council of Asia. It aims to provide consensus opinions on all aspects of resuscitation, thereby producing consistent international guidelines.

International normalised ratio, *see Coagulation studies*

Interonium distance. Distance between quaternary ammonium groups in molecules of non-depolarising **neuromuscular blocking drugs**. Thought to relate to drug activity in blocking **acetylcholine receptor** sites at different locations; drugs with short interonium distances show a tendency for ganglion blockade, while those with longer distances favour neuromuscular junction blockade.

Lee C (2001). Br J Anaesth; 87: 755–69

Interpleural analgesia. Injection of **local anaesthetic agent** into the pleural cavity, performed for analgesia after thoracic and upper abdominal surgery and in **rib** fractures. Unilateral pain is the most suitable indication. An epidural catheter may be placed either under direct vision during thoracotomy, or via an epidural needle as follows:

- the midaxillary line or ~10 cm from the dorsal midline, in the 4th–8th interspace is usually employed.
- the pleural space is identified using a loss of resistance syringe, allowing the syringe plunger to be drawn in by the negative interpleural pressure, or a catheter is pushed through the needle as the latter is advanced; unobstructed passage of the catheter occurs when the parietal pleura is punctured. Alternatively, to avoid entrainment of air when the syringe is removed from the needle, a continuous infusion of saline attached via a three-way tap to the epidural needle allows demonstration of the negative pressure by free flow of saline; the catheter may be threaded though the needle without detaching the saline infusion. Utrasound has also been used.
- advancement of the needle is during the expiratory phase.
- 8–30 ml of 0.25%–0.5% **bupivacaine** with **adrenaline** produces up to 24 h analgesia. 0.1–0.5 ml/kg/h infusion may also be used. Gravity and positioning may be used to extend the block if inadequate. Solution may also be instilled through a pleural drain. Mechanism of analgesia is unclear, but is thought to involve blockade of **intercostal nerves.**

Complications are uncommon, but include **pneumothorax**, haemorrhage, local anaesthetic toxicity (maximal levels occur within 20 min of bolus injection), phrenic, recurrent laryngeal or sympathetic nerve blockade.

Dravid RM, Paul RE (2007). Anaesthesia; 62: 1039–49; 1143–53

Interstitial fibrosis, *see Pulmonary fibrosis*

Interstitial fluid. Fluid compartment comprising most of the **ECF**. Volume is approximately 9.5 l, about 14% of body weight of an average man; it is determined by subtracting **plasma** volume from ECF volume.

See also, Fluids, body, for composition.

Intestinal obstruction. Mechanical obstruction of transit of GIT contents, to be distinguished from **ileus**. May be caused by impaction within the lumen (e.g. faeces, foreign object), narrowing arising within the GIT wall (e.g. tumours, strictures) or compression from outside the GIT wall (e.g. strangulation, adhesions). In acute obstruction, gas and intestinal secretions accumulate, causing distension of the GIT proximal to the obstruction, resulting in pain, increased bowel activity and vomiting (especially in high obstruction). **Dehydration** and electrolyte disturbances may rapidly develop. If severe and unrelieved, obstruction may lead to **bowel ischaemia**, necrosis and perforation. Abdominal x-rays may reveal dilated loops of bowel with fluid levels. In high GI obstruction, anorexia and prolonged vomiting result in hypovolaemia, hypokalaemia, hypochloraemia and metabolic alkalosis. In low obstruction, bicarbonate loss through the bowel wall causes metabolic acidosis.

About 90% of cases will resolve spontaneously with nasogastric suction and iv fluid replacement; those that require surgery can usually wait until a routine list when appropriate staff are available. Preoperative management involves correction of circulating volume and electrolyte and acid–base imbalance. Anaesthetic and ICU considerations are those of **emergency surgery** in general, especially relating to dehydration, the risk of **aspiration of gastric** contents and sepsis if perforation occurs. Admission to a critical care area postoperatively markedly reduces mortality.

Chronic obstruction presents with distension and constipation; emergency surgery is less often indicated, although acute-on-chronic obstruction may occur. **Malnutrition** is more likely to be present than in acute obstruction.

Intra-abdominal pressure (IAP). Usually measured using a closed urinary drainage system, with the bladder acting as a transducer. Has also been measured using nasogastric or gastrostomy tubes. IAP is normally subatmospheric to zero relative to the symphysis pubis. In animals, IAP >10 mmHg has potentially deleterious effects on hepatic arterial flow, and >20 mmHg on mesenteric and bowel mucosal blood flow, portal venous flow and intestinal barrier function. In humans, there seems to be a strong relationship between IAP >20 mmHg and subsequent development of renal failure. There is consensus that abdominal decompression should occur at levels of IAP >20–25 mmHg.

Kirkpatrick A, Roberts DJ, De Waele J, et al (2013). Intensive Care Med; 39: 1190–206

See also, Abdominal compartment syndrome

Intra-abdominal sepsis. The leading cause of death in general surgical practice. May involve a wide variety of anaerobic and aerobic organisms; **bacterial translocation** has been implicated in many cases.

- Caused by:
  - spontaneous intra-abdominal disease (60%), e.g. perforated appendix, diverticulitis, primary liver abscess, perforated colonic cancer, **pancreatitis**.
  - **trauma** (10%).
  - complications of abdominal surgery (30%), especially colonic and biliary.
- Diagnosis:
  - clinical: fever, leucocytosis, localised tenderness.
  - ultrasound: fluid collection may be demonstrated.
  - radiological:
    - plain abdominal x-ray may reveal abnormal fluid and/or gas collections.
    - contrast studies may reveal filling defects, suggesting abscess.
    - radiolabelled leucocyte scan or gallium-67 imaging: may reveal collections.
    - abdominal/pelvic CT scan: in general, more sensitive than the above.

If sepsis is strongly suspected, exploratory laparotomy/laparoscopy should be performed, even in the absence of positive imaging tests.

- Management:
  - prevention: maintenance of careful asepsis during surgery; preoperative bowel preparation; prophylactic antibiotics.
  - treatment: general resuscitation; antibiotic therapy; drainage by open surgical procedure or percutaneously using CT/ultrasound guidance.

See also, Peritonitis

Intra-aortic counterpulsation balloon pump. Device used to support **cardiac output** by inflating a balloon within the descending aorta at the beginning of diastole, with deflation immediately before systole. Introduced percutaneously (e.g. via the femoral artery) and inflated with helium or CO_2. Triggered and timed according to the **ECG** and **arterial waveform**. Increases coronary and tissue blood flow, with reduced **afterload** and left ventricular work; i.e., increases myocardial O_2 supply while decreasing demand.

Used as a temporary measure, e.g. in left ventricular failure and **cardiogenic shock** pre-/post-**cardiac surgery** or after **MI**, although its efficacy has been questioned. Complications include: trauma and haemorrhage during insertion; **aortic dissection** and rupture; distal thrombus; embolism and ischaemia; and damage to platelets and red cells.

Ihdayhid AR, Chopra S, Rankin J (2014). Curr Opin Cardiol; 29: 285–92

Intra-arterial regional anaesthesia. Obsolete method of producing anaesthesia of the arm, described in 1908 by Goyanes, by injecting **local anaesthetic agent** into the brachial artery, a tourniquet having been inflated proximally to above systolic BP.

[J Goyanes (1876–1964), Spanish surgeon]

Intracellular fluid. Similar in composition between different cells; thus considered a single fluid compartment comprising about 28 l (40% of body weight) in an average man. Determined by subtracting **ECF** from total body water (measured using a **dilution technique** with deuterium oxide).

See also, Fluids, body, for composition, etc.

Intracranial haemorrhage, *see Extradural haemorrhage; Head injury; Stroke; Subarachnoid haemorrhage; Subdural haemorrhage; Traumatic brain injury*

Intracranial pressure (ICP). Pressure exerted by the **CSF** in the frontal horns of the lateral ventricles of the **brain**. Normally <15 mmHg (2 kPa) supine; it is a dynamic pressure that fluctuates with cardiac pulsations and the respiratory cycle as well as with changes in posture, **Valsalva manoeuvre**, etc. A sustained ICP >20 mmHg (e.g. following **TBI**) is considered pathological. Because the skull is rigid, and its contents incompressible, ICP depends on the volume of intracranial contents: brain volume 1300 cm^3 (85%); CSF 80 ml (10%); and blood 50 ml (5%) (*see Monro–Kellie doctrine*).

- Effects of increased intracranial volume:
  - movement of CSF into the spinal canal, increased absorption of CSF into the venous circulation, and venous sinus compression. Thus ICP is maintained at near-normal levels initially.
  - eventually, compensatory mechanisms are overwhelmed; small changes in volume are then accompanied by large increases in ICP (Fig. 91).

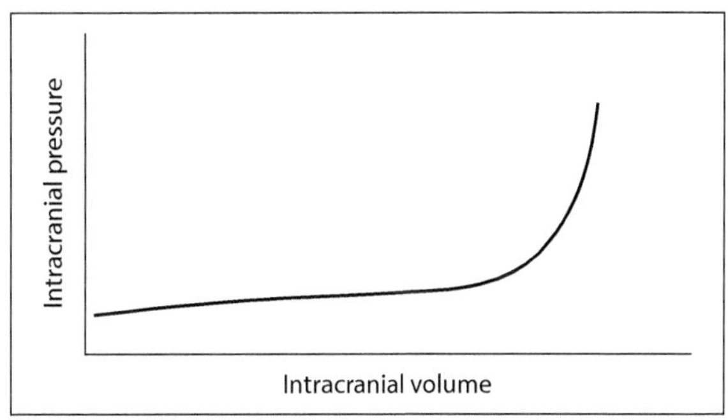

Fig. 91 Effects of increasing intracranial volume on intracranial pressure

- as ICP rises, **cerebral perfusion pressure** and **cerebral blood flow** are decreased. When venous blood vessels are obstructed, brain parenchymal swelling occurs. Regional ischaemia, structural distortion and **coning** may follow. During surgery, raised ICP is prevented by the open skull, but the brain may bulge and hinder surgery or closure.
- clinical features:
  - headache, nausea/vomiting, confusion. Headache is classically worse in the early morning and exacerbated by stooping or straining.
  - papilloedema (may take 24 h of raised ICP for it to occur), impaired consciousness, hypertension and bradycardia (**Cushing's reflex**) as ICP continues to rise.
  - hypotension, coma, irregular respiration or apnoea, fixed and dilated pupils.

- Raised ICP is caused by increased volume of the following compartments:
  - blood:
    - increased cerebral blood flow due to cerebral vasodilatation, e.g. due to hypercarbia, use of volatile anaesthetic agents.
    - impaired venous drainage, e.g. coughing, straining, obstructed jugular veins, head-down position.
  - brain:
    - tumour, abscess, haematoma.
    - **cerebral oedema.**
  - CSF: as for **hydrocephalus.**

Rarely, 'benign' (idiopathic) intracranial hypertension is associated with none of the above, especially in young obese women. It may cause permanent visual impairment due to optic nerve damage. Its management includes therapeutic lumbar puncture and CSF drainage, **corticosteroids**, **acetazolamide** and shunt insertion.

- Treatment of raised ICP involves reduction in volume of:
  - blood:
    - facilitation of venous drainage: head-up posture, adequate sedation/relaxation, avoiding jugular compression/kinking.
    - **hyperventilation** to arterial $P\text{CO}_2$ 3.5–4 kPa to produce cerebral vasoconstriction may be used as a temporary measure in life-threatening raised ICP. However, effectiveness is short-lived and it may result in **cerebral ischaemia** due to excessive cerebral vasoconstriction.
  - brain:
    - surgical decompression e.g. removal of cerebral tumour, decompressive craniectomy.
    - diuretics and corticosteroids in certain circumstances (*see Cerebral oedema*).
  - CSF: drainage, e.g. via the lateral ventricle. Long-term shunts as for hydrocephalus.
- Effects of anaesthetic agents on ICP:
  - iv agents: **barbiturates**, **etomidate**, **propofol**, **benzodiazepines**: reduce ICP. Opioids: no change or reduction, if normocapnia is maintained. **Ketamine** increases ICP.
  - inhalational agents: **halothane**, **enflurane**, **isoflurane**, **sevoflurane** and **desflurane**: cause a dose-dependent increase in ICP via increased cerebral blood flow and volume secondary to cerebral vasodilatation. At high concentrations cerebral vessel reactivity to CO_2 is lost and hyperventilation will not counteract the effect. **N_2O** also increases ICP via increased blood flow, or if air is contained in cavities within the skull, e.g. following surgery, head injury.
  - others: non-depolarising **neuromuscular blocking drugs** cause no change in ICP because they do not cross the **blood–brain barrier. Suxamethonium** may cause a transient increase (5–7 mmHg) during fasciculation, due to an increase in intrathoracic pressure. ICP is increased by laryngoscopy and tracheal intubation.
  - hypotensive drugs: ICP may increase following **sodium nitroprusside** and nitrates, due to vasodilatation and increased intracranial blood volume.

Anaesthesia for patients with raised ICP: as for **neurosurgery**.

See also, Cerebral protection/resuscitation

Intracranial pressure monitoring. Most commonly used for monitoring **intracranial pressure** following **TBI** although increasingly used in the management of **subarachnoid haemorrhage** and **stroke**. Two main types of monitor are available:

- intraventricular catheter pressure monitoring is the gold standard and measures global ICP; it also allows **CSF** drainage if necessary. Risks include brain trauma and haemorrhage (1%–7%) during insertion and ventriculitis on prolonged use. Insertion is contraindicated in patients with coagulopathy.
- microtransducer-tipped and fibreoptic devices placed either into brain parenchyma or into the subdural space; associated with fewer complications but may not reflect global ICP due to local pressure gradients around the device.

Monitoring of ICP following TBI allows treatment of raised ICP as well as goal-directed therapy aimed at maintaining a suitable **cerebral perfusion pressure**. However, the one randomised controlled trial available failed to show any benefit of ICP monitoring in TBI.

- Indications for ICP monitoring following TBI (Brain Trauma Foundation):
  - all patients with severe TBI and an abnormal CT scan.
  - patients with a normal scan with two or more of the following: age >40 years; unilateral motor posturing; systolic BP <90 mmHg.

The accepted threshold for treatment is an ICP >20–25 mmHg. Treatment consists of a stepwise approach of medical management (increase in sedation with or without neuromuscular blockade, use of hyperosmolar agents (e.g. **mannitol** or **hypertonic intravenous solutions**) and mild therapeutic **hypothermia** (*see Targeted temperature management*). **Barbiturates** are reserved for refractory raised ICP. Surgical therapy includes evacuation of mass lesions, drainage of CSF and decompressive craniectomy.

In addition to monitoring the level of ICP, variation of waveform (Lundberg waves) has also been described:

- A (plateau) waves: steep rises in ICP to 50–100 mmHg lasting 5–20 min. Always pathological, they represent severely reduced intracranial compliance with high risk of cerebral herniation.
- B waves: oscillations of ICP at frequency of 0.5–2 waves/min. Indicates unstable ICP and may be associated with cerebral vasospasm.
- C waves: amplitude <20 mmHg; occur at 4–8/min. Related to systemic vasomotor tone and BP. Seen in normal individuals.

[Nils Lundberg (1908–2002), Swedish neurosurgeon]

Kirkman MA, Smith M (2014). Br J Anaesth; 112: 35–46

Intractable pain, *see Pain; Pain management*

Intradural..., *see Spinal....*

Intramucosal pH, *see Gastric tonometry*

Intraocular pressure (IOP). Normally 1.3–2 kPa (10–15 mmHg), increased in **glaucoma**. Important during open **ophthalmic surgery** because of the risk of extrusion of intraocular contents and haemorrhage, with subsequent distortion of anatomy, scarring and loss of vision.

- Related to:
  - external pressure on the eye:
    - from facemask or leaning on the eye.
    - retrobulbar haematoma.
    - extrinsic muscles.
    - venous congestion of orbit.
  - scleral rigidity: increased in severe myopia and in the elderly.
  - intraocular contents:
    - choroidal blood volume:
      - increases with arterial $P\text{CO}_2$ and **hypoxaemia**, and vasodilatation.
      - increases transiently with acute rises in systolic BP; falls at systolic pressure of under 80–90 mmHg.
      - increases with **CVP**, e.g. due to straining, coughing, vomiting, head-down or prone position.
    - aqueous humour:
      - formed by the choroidal plexus of the posterior chamber, at about 0.08 ml/h. A small amount is formed in the anterior chamber.
      - passes through the pupil to the anterior chamber; drains from the angle between the iris and cornea via the canal of Schlemm into the venous circulation.
      - reduced by **acetazolamide**, although it also increases choroidal blood volume. Also reduced by oral glycerol and meiosis. Control is important in glaucoma, but less so during surgery.
    - vitreous humour: may be reduced by administration of **mannitol** 0.5–1.5 g/kg iv, 45 min preoperatively. Urinary catheterisation is usually required. Sucrose 50% 1 g/kg is shorter acting.
    - other structures, e.g. lens.
    - sulfur hexafluoride (SF_6) is sometimes injected into the vitreous in retinal surgery to splint the retina; $\mathbf{N_2O}$ markedly expands the SF_6 volume and increases IOP by diffusing into the bubble faster than SF_6 diffuses out (blood/gas **solubility** of N_2O is over 100 times that of SF_6). When N_2O is stopped at the end of surgery, IOP may decrease markedly. N_2O is therefore usually avoided. Atmospheric nitrogen diffuses into the bubble postoperatively, but its effect is smaller and slower because its blood/gas solubility is only 2–3 times that of SF_6.
- Effects of anaesthetic agents on IOP:
  - little effect, if any, of premedicant drugs.
  - no effect of **atropine**, unless administered topically to glaucomatous eyes (IOP may rise).
  - reduced by all iv induction agents except **ketamine**; **propofol** and **etomidate** cause a greater reduction than **thiopental**.
  - reduced slightly by **benzodiazepines** and **neuroleptanaesthesia**.
  - reduced by all volatile agents; the mechanism is unclear. Unaffected by N_2O.
  - increased by **suxamethonium**, possibly via choroidal vasodilatation and extrinsic eye muscle contraction, although the increase in IOP still occurs when the muscles are cut. The increase lasts only a few minutes. The use of suxamethonium in the presence of penetrating eye injury is controversial (*see Eye, penetrating injury*).
  - non-depolarising **neuromuscular blocking drugs** may lower IOP slightly.

Anaesthesia for open eye operations thus involves avoidance of factors that increase IOP and use of techniques and drugs that lower IOP, e.g. head-up tilt, hypocapnia, smooth anaesthesia.

IOP is estimated by measuring corneal indentation by a weighted plunger, or by measuring the force required to flatten an area of cornea.

[Friedrich Schlemm (1795–1858), German anatomist]

Intraosseous fluid administration. Infusion of fluids though a metal cannula into the bone marrow and thence, via a system of non-collapsible veins, into the general circulation. Used in emergencies when intravenous access is not readily available. Previously reserved for the resuscitation of infants and children; adult needles and insertion devices are now also routinely available. The upper tibia (anteromedial surface 1–3 cm below the tibial tuberosity) and proximal humerus are the most common sites chosen. A manual needle and trocar kit may be used to pierce the thin bony cortex, advancement continuing until a loss of resistance is felt. Alternatively, a battery-powered drill may be used. Easy injection of saline without obvious subcutaneous infiltration suggests correct placement. Aspiration of marrow is not always possible, but if successful, samples can be used for cross-matching. All standard drugs may be given by this route; they should be flushed through with 5–10 ml saline to ensure they reach the circulation. Fluids should be given under pressure to overcome venous resistance. Osteomyelitis is the major complication and can be minimised by sterile technique and by reverting to conventional venous cannulation following resuscitation. **Compartment syndrome** has been reported.

Intrapleural pressure. Pressure within the pleural cavity, perhaps better termed interpleural pressure. Measured indirectly using a balloon catheter placed within the lower third of the oesophagus (i.e., within the thorax but outside the lungs). Normally negative, due to the tendency of the thoracic cage to spring outwards, and the tendency of the lungs to collapse inwards. In the erect posture at normal resting lung volume, intrapleural pressure equals approximately −10 cm H_2O at the lung apex, −2.5 cm H_2O at the base.

Increases in magnitude as lung volume (and thus elastic recoil) increases. During spontaneous ventilation, it thus becomes more negative during inspiration. Normally changes by 3–4 cm H_2O, more if **airway resistance** is increased or breathing forceful. During expiration, it returns to its original value unless expiration is forced or resistance increased; it may then exceed zero.

During **IPPV**, pressure increases from the resting value, depending on the inflating pressure (usually by 10–20 cm H_2O). Thus it usually exceeds zero during inspiration. Increased by **CPAP** and **PEEP** (i.e., towards or beyond zero).

Intrathecal..., *see Spinal....*

Intravenous anaesthetic agents. Development of drugs and iv techniques occurred later than for **inhalational anaesthetic agents**, but iv **induction of anaesthesia** is usually preferred now because it is faster and smoother with less risk of laryngospasm. Popularised in the 1930s by **Weese**, **Lundy** and **Waters**, although **Oré** had used iv **chloral hydrate** in 1872. Subsequent agents include **hedonal** (1905), phenobarbital (1912), **paraldehyde** (1913), **bromethol** (1927), **hexobarbital** (1932; the first widely used iv **barbiturate**), **thiopental** (1932), **hydroxydione** (1955), **methohexital** (1957), **propanidid** (1956), **γ-hydroxybutyric acid** (1962), **ketamine** (1965), **Althesin** (1971), **etomidate** (1973) and **propofol** (1986). **Diethyl ether** has been injected iv.

Used for induction and maintenance of anaesthesia, including **TIVA**, and for **sedation**. Many iv agents have also been given im or rectally. **Benzodiazepines** (e.g. **midazolam**) are also used for induction, as are high doses of **opioid analgesic drugs**.

- May be classified thus:
  - rapid onset:
    - barbiturates: thiopental, methohexital.
    - imidazole compounds: etomidate.
    - alkyl phenol: propofol.
    - corticosteroids: Althesin, **minaxolone**, hydroxydione.
    - eugenols: propanidid.
  - slow onset:
    - ketamine.
    - benzodiazepines.
    - opioids.
- Features of the ideal iv anaesthetic agent:
  - physical/chemical properties:
    - chemically stable at room temperature and on exposure to light; long shelf-life.
    - water-soluble, not requiring reconstitution before use, nor any additives.
    - compatible with iv fluids and other drugs.
  - pharmacology:
    - painless on injection, without causing thrombophlebitis. Harmless if extravasated or injected intra-arterially.
    - low incidence of **adverse drug reactions**.
    - smooth onset of anaesthesia within one **arm–brain circulation time**, without unwanted movement, coughing or **hiccups**.
    - anticonvulsant, antiemetic and analgesic properties. No increase in **cerebral blood flow**, **ICP** or **intraocular pressure**. Reduces **CMRO$_2$**.
    - no respiratory depression. Bronchodilator.
    - no cardiovascular depression or stimulation, or arrhythmias.
    - predictable recovery, related to the dose injected.
    - rapid metabolism to non-active metabolites; i.e., non-cumulative.
    - no impairment of renal or hepatic function or corticosteroid synthesis.
    - no **emergence phenomena**.
    - no teratogenicity.

No currently available agent fulfils all of the above (Table 29).

Agents should be injected slowly, titrated to effect (except during **rapid sequence induction**), especially if the patient has reduced cardiac output. Overdose is easily produced by rapid injection of a large dose.

Following iv injection, brain levels depend on the amount of drug crossing the **blood–brain barrier**, related to:
- protein binding.
- ionisation; e.g. at pH of 7.4, 61% of thiopental and over 90% of propofol are unionised.
- cerebral blood flow: increased as a proportion of cardiac output in **hypovolaemia**.
- fat solubility: high for most anaesthetic agents; propofol and ketamine are particularly fat-soluble.
- distribution, metabolism and excretion.

Recovery from, for example, thiopental occurs by redistribution from vessel-rich tissues (brain, heart, liver, kidney; 70%–80% of cardiac output) to vessel-intermediate tissues (muscle, skin; 18% of cardiac output), thence to fat (6%) and vessel-poor tissues such as ligaments (Fig. 92). Thus significant amounts of thiopental remain in the body after recovery, compared with more rapidly metabolised agents, e.g. propofol.

See also, Anaesthesia, mechanisms of; Pharmacokinetics

Table 29 Properties of iv anaesthetic agents

Agent	*Thiopental*	*Methohexital*	*Ketamine*	*Etomidate*	*Propofol*	*Midazolam*
Additives	Sodium carbonate	Sodium carbonate	Benzethonium chloride	Propylene glycol	Soya-bean oil emulsion	–
Aqueous solution	+	+	+	–	–	+
Approximate cost/induction dose in UK (£)	3	Unavailable	2–4	1–2	2–4	2–4
Painful injection	–	+	–	+	+	–
Rapid onset	+	+	–	+	+	–
Unwanted movement	–	+	±	+	–	–
Respiratory/cardiovascular depression	+	+	–	±	+	±
Analgesic	–	–	+	–	–	–
Vomiting	–	–	+	+	–	–
Steroid inhibition	–	–	–	+	–	–
Rapid recovery	+	+	–	+	+	–
Emergence phenomena	–	–	+	–	–	–
pK_a	7.6	7.9	4.2	11	6.2	
Protein-binding (%)	85	85	12	75	98	98
Volume of distribution (l/kg)	1.5–2.5	1–2	2–3	2–5	3–5	1–2
Distribution half-life (min)	2–6	5–6	10–15	1–4	1–2	7–15
Elimination half-life (h)	5–10	2–4	2–3	1–5	1–5	2–5
Clearance (ml/kg/min)	2–4	10–12	18–20	18–25	25–30	6–11

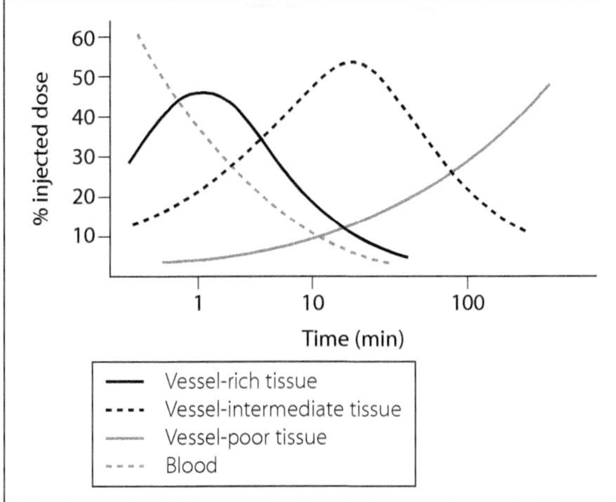

Fig. 92 Fate of thiopental after iv injection

Intravenous fluid administration. Described in the 1600s. **Saline solutions** were used sporadically in **dehydration** due to cholera, **diabetes mellitus** and **diarrhoea** in the 1800s. Infusions were widely used in World War I, including acacia solution as a **colloid**. Bacterial and chemical contamination and allergic reactions were common. Sterile fluids and administration sets became available in World War II; investigation into **fluid balance** since then has been prompted by subsequent wars, e.g. Korea, Vietnam. Balanced fluid therapy was developed in the 1950s–1960s.

- Practical considerations:
  - site of administration: usually forearm, because it is the least awkward for the patient. The arm or hand is preferred to the legs, because venous stasis is commoner in the latter. Placement near joints or known arteries is avoided when possible. **Central venous cannulation** is used for irritant or vasoactive drugs, if peripheral cannulation is unsuccessful or if long-term administration or CVP measurement is required.
  - cannulation: venous filling is increased by gentle slapping, squeezing of the hand or immersion of the limb in warm water. Intradermal injection of local anaesthetic or use of **EMLA** reduces the pain of insertion of large cannulae. Attempts are made to cannulate distal veins first, moving proximally if unsuccessful. Rarely, cut-down may be required:
    - an anatomically constant venous site is chosen, e.g. long saphenous vein (above and anterior to the medial malleolus).
    - the vein is exposed and two ties placed around it; only the distal one is tightened.
    - the cannula is introduced and secured with the proximal tie.
  - cannulae: plastic cannulae were developed in the 1970s. Their general design is similar but flow characteristics differ widely between different makes. More recent designs incorporate protective mechanisms to prevent needlestick injury, e.g. a metal clip or plastic cover that automatically shields the sharp point when the needle is withdrawn from the cannula. Since 2013, a European Union Directive has made the use of these safety needles mandatory whenever 'reasonably practicable'. British Standard for determining flow rate: a constant pressure of 10 kPa is maintained using a constant-level tank of distilled water at 22°C. It is connected via 110-cm tubing (internal diameter 4 mm) to the cannula, with the distal 4 cm and the cannula horizontal. The volume of water is collected over at least 30 s; an average of three readings is taken. Thus the flows are different from those achieved clinically, but the values are useful for comparison between differently sized cannulae:
    - 10 G: 550–600 ml/min.
    - 12 G: 400–500 ml/min.
    - 14 G: 250–360 ml/min.
    - 16 G: 130–220 ml/min.
    - 18 G: 75–120 ml/min.
    - 20 G: 40–80 ml/min.

    Gauge (G) numbers are equivalent to those used for **needles**. Colour-coding standard for iv cannulae:
    - 14 G: orange
    - 16 G: grey
    - 18 G: green
    - 20 G: pink
    - 22 G: blue
    - 24 G: yellow
    - 26 G: black
  - Blood giving sets: internal diameter is 4 mm, but increased turbulence and resistance arise from extra length, drip chambers and filter (170-µm pore size). Non-blood giving sets have no filter or float, and are narrower and cheaper.
  - syringe pumps, volumetric pumps, drip counters; high pressures may occur with the former two if obstruction to flow occurs. Some syringe pumps may empty rapidly if placed above the patient.
  - microfiltration: not routinely used, but 0.2-µm filters are claimed to reduce phlebitis, especially when repeated drug injections are given. They may also retain **endotoxin** and prevent **gas embolism**. The routine use of **blood filters** is controversial.
- Hazards:
  - during cannulation: haemorrhage, haematoma, trauma.
  - extravasation: especially harmful if the fluid is irritant, e.g. potassium or **bicarbonate** solutions, **thiopental**, antimitotic drugs. Flushing with saline, **hyaluronidase** or corticosteroids has been suggested as treatment.
  - thrombophlebitis: venous thrombosis accompanied by venous wall inflammation. Superficial thrombophlebitis does not lead to **DVT**. More common with small veins and concentrated or irritant infusates. Reduced if infusion sites are changed regularly, e.g. 24–48-hourly. Features include pain, redness of the overlying skin and hardening of the vein; there may be swelling and systemic features (e.g. pyrexia) if infection is involved. Infusion life may be prolonged with a **GTN** patch applied topically. Addition of heparin or hydrocortisone to the fluid bag has also been used. Heparinoid cream may be applied to existing phlebitis.
  - interactions between infused drugs or fluids, especially if multiple infusions are used through a single cannula.
  - gas embolism.
  - related to the iv fluid infused, e.g. hyponatraemia, pulmonary oedema.

- when one cannula is used for more than one infusion, temporary blockage of the cannula may lead to one infusion (e.g. of a drug) retrogradely filling the tubing of the second infusion (e.g. a saline infusion), especially if the former is driven by a pump. When the obstruction is relieved, a bolus of drug may be delivered instead of a saline flush; therefore a non-return valve/connector should be used.

Fluids may also be delivered into the circulation by **intraosseous fluid administration**; other routes, e.g. rectal, im or sc administration (the latter two aided by hyaluronidase), are rarely used now.
See also, Venous drainage of arm

Intravenous fluids. May be divided into **colloids** and **crystalloids** (Table 30).

- Simplistic effects of infused fluid on body fluid compartments:
  - initial expansion of the vascular compartment. Extent and duration depend on whether it can freely cross the vascular endothelium; i.e., crystalloids do, colloids do so only slowly, e.g. **gelatin solutions** after a few hours. Colloids may draw water into the vascular space by **osmosis** in addition to the volume infused (hence **plasma expanders**).
  - expansion of the **interstitial fluid** compartment as fluids pass into it from the vascular compartment. Fluids distribute within the **ECF** thus: three-quarters in interstitial fluid, one-quarter in **plasma**.
  - expansion of the intracellular space. Water moves across cell membranes by osmosis only if **osmolality** on one side of the membrane changes. Thus, if **saline** 0.9% is added to ECF, osmolality is unchanged, and no movement of water occurs; i.e., saline is confined to ECF. The dextrose in **dextrose solutions** is rapidly metabolised after administration; the resultant free water then redistributes to both intracellular and extracellular compartments.
- Summary:
  - colloids cause greater expansion of the vascular compartment for the volume infused, and were widely used to replace plasma/blood losses.
  - saline 0.9% and **Hartmann's solution** expand ECF (three-quarters interstitial, one-quarter plasma) and are ideally suited to replace ECF losses.
  - dextrose 5% expands total body water (one-third ECF, two-thirds interstitial). Thus only 1/12 infused volume of dextrose 5% remains in the vascular compartment. The main use of dextrose is to replenish a water deficit; infusing pure water would cause haemolysis.

See also, Bicarbonate; Colloid/crystalloid controversy; Dextrans; Haemorrhage; Hypertonic intravenous solutions; Intravenous fluid administration

Intravenous oxygenator (IVOX). Intravascular gas exchange device, consisting of a 30–40-cm long bundle of hollow gas-permeable polypropylene fibres (internal diameter 200 μm), introduced into the superior and inferior venae cavae via the right internal jugular or femoral veins. Was used in the 1990s for acute **respiratory failure** but its use was hampered by technical problems, e.g. obstruction of venous return, bleeding. No longer available.

Table 30 Compositions of commonly used iv fluids (in mmol/l unless otherwise stated)

Fluid	*Na^+*	*K^+*	*Ca^{2+}*	*Cl^-*	*Other*	*pH*
Crystalloids[a]						
Saline 0.9% ('normal')	154	–	–	154	–	5.0
Dextrose 4%–saline 0.18%	30	–	–	30	Dextrose 40 g	4–5
Dextrose 5%	–	–	–	–	Dextrose 50 g	4.0
Hartmann's solution	131	5	2	111	Lactate 29	6.5
Bicarbonate						
8.4%	1000	–	–	–	HCO_3^- 1000	8.0
1.26%	150	–	–	–	HCO_3^- 150	7.0
Colloids[b]						
Haemaccel	145	5.1	6.25	145	Gelatin 35 g	7.4
Gelofusine	154	–	–	120	Gelatin 40 g Mg^{2+} <0.4	7.4
Hetastarch/pentastarch/ tetrastarch 6%/10%						
In 0.9% saline	154	–	–	154	Starch 60 g/100 g	5.0–5.5
In balanced solution	137–140	4	0–2.5	110–118	Mg^{2+} 1–1.5; acetate 0–34; malate 0–5	
Albumin 4.5%	<160	<2	–	136	Albumin 40–50 g Citrate <15	7.4
Dextran						
In saline 0.9% (as above)	60 g dextran 70 or					4.5–5
In dextrose 5% (as above)	100 g dextran 40					5–6

[a]All have an osmolality of 280–300 mosmol/kg, except for bicarbonate 8.4% (200 mosmol/kg)
[b]Osmolality ranges between approximately 280 and 320 mosmol/kg

Intravenous regional anaesthesia (IVRA; Bier block). First described in 1908 by **Bier**, who injected **procaine** iv into an exsanguinated portion of the arm between two inflated tourniquets, to provide distal analgesia.
- Modern technique (described in the 1960s):
  - an iv cannula is placed in each hand.
  - the limb is exsanguinated by raising it with the brachial artery compressed, or by using a rubber bandage.
  - a **tourniquet** is inflated around the upper arm to a value higher than systolic BP (twice systolic BP is usually quoted).
  - local anaesthetic agent is injected slowly.
  - a more distal tourniquet may be inflated after 5–10 min and the original deflated, to reduce discomfort.
  - motor and sensory block occurs within 5–10 min.
  - for prolonged surgery, the cannula is left in situ. The cuff may be deflated after 60–90 min for 5 min, the arm re-emptied of blood and the tourniquet re-inflated. Half the initial dose is then injected. Thus safe tourniquet time is not exceeded.
- Solutions:
  - **prilocaine** is safest but **lidocaine** may also be used; 3 mg/kg (0.6 ml/kg) 0.5% solution is suitable, without adrenaline. Preservative-free prilocaine is no longer available for IVRA, but solution containing preservative has been safely used for many years.
  - **bupivacaine** is contraindicated because of its cardiotoxicity.
- Mechanism of action is unclear, but may include:
  - compression by the tourniquet.
  - ischaemia.
  - drug action on nerve trunks.
  - drug action on nerve endings.
- IVRA is a potentially dangerous technique, involving direct iv injection of local anaesthetic; therefore the following must apply:
  - all equipment is checked for leaks and other defects.
  - the patient is prepared and starved as for any anaesthetic procedure, with resuscitative drugs and equipment available.
  - full **monitoring** is applied throughout.
  - rapid injection is avoided (may force solution past the tourniquet).
  - injection near the antecubital fossa is avoided (solution may be forced into the systemic circulation).
  - the technique is used with caution in patients with severe arteriosclerosis and **hypertension**, because the tourniquet may not completely compress their arteries. Similar caution has been suggested in **obesity**.
  - contraindication has been suggested in prepubertal children, because intraosseous vessels may allow local anaesthetic to bypass the tourniquet.
  - the tourniquet is not deflated for at least 20 min. Intermittent deflation/reinflation has been suggested to reduce blood drug levels, e.g. deflation for 5–10 s, inflation for 1 s.
  - not to be used in patients with **sickle cell anaemia** or trait.

May be used for the leg, although larger volumes are required, e.g. 1.0 ml/kg. The block may be less effective than in the arm.

Has also been used for **sympathetic nerve block**, e.g. using **guanethidine** 10–25 mg in 20 ml saline for the arm (30–40 mg in 40 ml for the leg); lidocaine or prilocaine is often added. The tourniquet is deflated after 10–20 min. Hypotension may occur up to several hours later. It may be repeated for several weeks, e.g. on alternate days.

Intrinsic activity. Ability of a substance (e.g. drug) to produce a response by interacting with a surface receptor. Refers to the amount of response produced, i.e., **efficacy**. *See also, Affinity*

Intrinsic sympathomimetic activity (ISA). Ability of **β-adrenergic receptor antagonists** to stimulate **β-adrenergic receptors** as well as block them. Oxprenolol, **labetalol**, pindolol, celiprolol and acebutolol have ISA and are therefore partial **agonists**; they may cause less bradycardia than other β-receptor antagonists, although the importance of this is unclear.

Intubation aids. Used in difficult tracheal intubation.
- Designed for:
  - avoiding obstruction of the **laryngoscope** handle on the chest during insertion of the blade into the mouth:
    - laryngoscopes with adjustable handles or an increased angle between the blade and handle (e.g. polio **laryngoscope blade**).
    - adaptor to swing the handle to one side during insertion (Yentis adaptor).
    - short-handled laryngoscope.
  - improving the view of the glottis:
    - specialised laryngoscope blades (e.g. McCoy).
    - **fibreoptic instruments**: may be flexible, rigid or malleable; extendable forceps and stylets may be attached.
    - Optical/video devices and mirrors attached to or incorporated in the laryngoscope (*see Videolaryngoscope*). The Huffman prism clips to a standard laryngoscope blade, allowing a view of the larynx by refracting light 30 degrees from its original path. It must be warmed before use to prevent misting.
  - enabling intubation despite poor view:
    - long flexible introducer (often called a 'bougie', although this term refers to devices used for serial dilatation of strictures. Traditionally these were made of gum elastic). Usually bears an angled tip that assists placement through the larynx; may be inserted through the tracheal tube before intubation or placed first and the **tracheal tube** passed over it, with gentle rotation if required. It may be placed blindly; correct placement is suggested by feeling the tracheal rings during insertion, and feeling the distal end reach the carina. Directional bougies, controllable from their proximal end, are also available. **Airway exchange catheters** allow insufflation of O_2 during attempted intubation.
    - malleable stylet, inserted through the tube before intubation. Plastic-coated ones are less traumatic than those of bare metal; trauma is also reduced by avoiding protrusion of the stylet from the distal end of the tube.
    - **forceps** to guide the tube.
    - some tracheal tubes are able to be flexed by pulling a cord within their walls, aiding direction during placement.
    - laryngoscope blades have been described that incorporate forceps, allowing manipulation of the tracheal tube.
    - hooks introduced orally for pulling the tube anteriorly.

- allowing intubation without laryngoscopy:
  - malleable stylet with a bulb at its distal end (**lightwand**): passed through the tube and introduced through the mouth, with observation of the anterior neck. The light may be followed down the anterior larynx into the trachea; it disappears if intra-oesophageal.
  - **SAD**: either a blind technique using a specific 'intubating' SAD, e.g. **LM** or using a fibreoptic laryngoscope, which may be passed through a standard SAD.
  - retrograde epidural catheter technique: the catheter is introduced through the cricothyroid membrane via an epidural needle and passed upwards through the larynx and out of the mouth. The tracheal tube is advanced over it from the mouth into the trachea as the catheter is held from above. For nasal intubation, the catheter is tied with thread to a suction catheter passed through the nose and out through the mouth, then both are pulled out of the nose. Central venous cannulae and threads have also been used.
- detecting oesophageal intubation.

[John P Huffman (1933–2014), US nurse-anaesthetist; Eamon P McCoy, Belfast anaesthetist; SM Yentis, London anaesthetist]

See also, Intubation, difficult; Intubation, fibreoptic; Intubation, oesophageal; Intubation, tracheal

Intubation, awake.

- Indications:
  - known or suspected difficult airway or intubation, including an unstable cervical spine.
  - to isolate a leak and/or protect lung segments before applying IPPV, e.g. **bronchopleural fistula**, **tracheo-oesophageal fistula.**
  - in **neonates**: controversial; it is felt to be safer by many but with the possibility of causing undue stress and raised ICP.
- Requires anaesthesia of the **pharynx**, **larynx** and trachea, and **tongue** or nasal passages:
  - **nose**: **cocaine** spray 4%–10% to provide anaesthesia and vasoconstriction (3 mg/kg maximum). Alternatively, **xylometazoline** 0.1% and **lidocaine** 1%–4% may be used.
  - tongue and oropharynx: benzocaine lozenge 100 mg, sucked 30 min beforehand.
  - pharynx and larynx above the vocal cords: lidocaine or **prilocaine** 1%–4% via metered spray or swabs at increasing depths into the mouth. Maximum 'safe doses' should be observed. **Glossopharyngeal nerve block** has been used, but topical anaesthesia is easier to perform. Superior **laryngeal nerve** block provides anaesthesia of the epiglottis, base of tongue and mucosa down to the cords, and is performed either by holding a lidocaine-soaked pledget for 2–3 min in the piriform fossa on each side (e.g. using Krause's **forceps**) or by injecting 2–3 ml 1% lidocaine from the front of the neck just below the greater cornu of the hyoid bone on each side, with the bone displaced towards the side to be blocked with the operator's other hand. A click may be felt as the thyrohyoid membrane is pierced.
  - trachea and larynx below the cords: rapid transtracheal injection of 3–5 ml 1% lidocaine through the cricothyroid membrane, following aspiration of air to confirm correct placement. The patient is asked to breathe out fully before injection; the resultant inspiration and coughing aid spread of solution within the upper **tracheobronchial tree.** To reduce the risk of breakage and trauma during coughing, the needle is withdrawn immediately following injection, or an iv cannula used instead.
  - nebulised 4% lidocaine may be used as the sole local anaesthetic.

Alternatively, awake intubation can be performed solely using a remifentanil infusion at low dose.

Tracheal intubation then proceeds as usual, using laryngoscopy or a blind nasal technique. The upper airways are rendered insensitive to aspirated material, and the patient should be given nil by mouth for 4 h. Patients already at risk of regurgitation and aspiration are placed at further risk.

A similar technique may be used for awake fibreoptic **bronchoscopy**. **Fibreoptic instruments** for bronchoscopy/intubation have injection ports through which local anaesthetic may be sprayed as the bronchoscope is advanced. Awake intubation via a **SAD** or using a **videolaryngoscope** has also been described; it has been suggested that the latter should replace fibreoptic techniques because of greater familiarity.

See also, Intubation, blind nasal; Intubation, fibreoptic; Intubation, tracheal

Intubation, blind nasal. Technique of tracheal intubation without using laryngoscopes or other instruments; developed by **Magill** and **Rowbotham** as their first method of tracheal intubation (without use of neuromuscular blocking drugs). Of particular use in difficult intubation, because obtaining a view of the larynx is not required. Also used in awake intubation.

Originally described in spontaneously breathing patients, with use of 5%–10% inspired CO_2 to increase ventilation. May also be performed in paralysed patients, although induction of neuromuscular blockade may be hazardous in difficult intubation. Use of CO_2 is now generally considered dangerous.

- Technique:
  - the patient's head is positioned in the 'sniffing position'.
  - a lubricated tracheal tube is inserted into a nostril (usually the right, because most bevels face left). Uncuffed rubber tubes were originally used; cuffed tubes are also suitable. **Epistaxis** may occur; it is reduced if a soft tube, little force and **cocaine** paste or spray are used. Trauma to the nasopharynx may also occur, and the incidence of bacteraemia is higher than with oral intubation.
  - the tube is passed into the pharynx, keeping the head extended and mandible elevated. The head is rotated slightly towards the side of the nostril used.
  - in spontaneous ventilation, the opposite nostril is occluded. Audible breath sounds from the tube are used as a guide to the position of the tube's tip; i.e., if they disappear, the tube is withdrawn slightly and redirected.
  - the tube is gently inserted further; it may:
    - enter the trachea in approximately a third of cases.
    - enter the oesophagus; the tube is partially withdrawn and reinserted with the head extended further. Posterior external pressure on the larynx may help.
    - meet obstruction level with the larynx; the tube's tip may be:

- lateral to the glottis, e.g. in a piriform fossa, or against a false cord or arytenoid cartilage. A bulge may be visible at one side of the larynx at the front of the neck. The tube is partially withdrawn, rotated and reinserted. Head rotation or lateral external pressure on the larynx may help.
- against the anterior part of the cricoid or in the vallecula; tube rotation or head flexion may help.

Practice is required to achieve proficiency. Differently curved tubes may be required. Partial inflation of the tracheal tube cuff when the tube's tip is in the oropharynx may help to centre it and aid insertion into the larynx.

See also, Intubation, awake; Intubation, difficult; Intubation, oesophageal; Intubation, tracheal

Intubation, complications of. Complications may occur at the time of tracheal intubation or afterwards.

- During intubation:
  - trauma:
    - caused by leaning on the eyes.
    - to the neck or jaw.
    - to the **teeth**, lips, nasal mucosa, mouth, **tongue**, **pharynx**, **larynx**, **laryngeal nerves** and trachea. Infection, surgical emphysema and bleeding may result. Rigid introducers and bougies are particularly traumatic. Nasal polyps may be carried into the trachea during nasal intubation.
  - hypertensive response:
    - associated with sympathetic activity and tachycardia.
    - may increase **ICP** and **intraocular pressure**.
    - particularly undesirable in patients with **hypertension** and **ischaemic heart disease**.
    - caused by **laryngoscopy** alone; thus not obtunded by **lidocaine** spray.
    - methods to reduce the response:
      - **antihypertensive drugs**, e.g. **β-adrenergic receptor antagonists**, **hydralazine**, **nitroglycerine**, **sodium nitroprusside**. Some may be effective given orally, preoperatively (e.g. β-receptor antagonists) but bradycardia may occur.
      - **benzodiazepines**.
      - deep inhalational anaesthesia.
      - iv lidocaine 1–2 mg/kg.
      - **fentanyl** 6–8 μg/kg, **alfentanil** 30–50 μg/kg or **sufentanil** 0.5–1.0 μg/kg obtund the response if given 1–2 min before intubation.
  - **arrhythmias**, particularly if **hypoxaemia** and **hypercapnia** are present.
  - **laryngospasm**, **bronchospasm**, breath-holding, if intubation is attempted too early.
  - **aspiration of gastric contents**.
  - misplaced tube, e.g. oesophageal or endobronchial. Auscultation over both lungs and axillae and the stomach should be performed following intubation and positioning (*See Intubation, oesophageal*).
  - difficult/failed intubation: risk of misplacement of the tube. Hypoxaemia, hypercapnia, **awareness**, trauma and aspiration may occur during repeated attempts at intubation.
  - bacteraemia has been reported but the clinical significance is unclear. More likely with nasal intubation.
- Once the trachea is intubated:
  - displacement of the tube:
    - extubation.
    - endobronchial intubation. Suggested by:
      - lightening anaesthesia.
      - increased **airway pressures**.
      - hypoxaemia and/or reduced end-tidal CO_2 levels.
      - unequal lung expansion.

    Usually occurs on the right side. It may cause collapse of the unventilated lung (± right upper lobe) and postoperative infection. On the **CXR**, the tube's tip should be at T1–3 (carina lies at T4–5). The tube may move up to 2 cm with neck movement (caudad with flexion, cephalad with extension).
  - disconnection from the fresh gas supply.
  - **airway obstruction**:
  - blockage by sputum, blood or foreign object.
  - compression by mouth gag, surgeon or kinking.
  - related to the **cuff**.
  - tube ignition by **laser**.
  - complications of **extubation**.
- Late complications:
  - cord ulceration and granuloma: uncommon; typically occur at the junction of the posterior and middle thirds of the cord.
  - damage to the recurrent/superior laryngeal nerves. Stretching and compression are thought to be the most likely causes. Slow recovery usually occurs.
  - tracheal stenosis following prolonged intubation.
  - nasal/oral ulceration.
  - **sinusitis** may occur in prolonged nasotracheal intubation.

Tracheostomy is performed to avoid late complications.

See also, Anaesthetic morbidity and mortality; Intubation, difficult; Intubation, failed; Intubation, tracheal

Intubation, difficult. Incidence is thought to be about 1% in the general population, although definitions vary.

- Widely accepted classification (of Cormack and Lehane) according to the best view possible at direct laryngoscopy (Fig. 93a):
  - grade 1: complete glottis visible.
  - grade 2: anterior glottis not seen.
  - grade 3: epiglottis seen but not glottis.
  - grade 4: epiglottis not seen.

Grades 3 and 4 together are often termed 'difficult'. The grading system has been criticised for being too insensitive, especially for laryngoscopies between grades 2 and 3 (grades 2a [cords visible] and 2b [only corniculate/cuneiform cartilages or posterior glottis visible] have been

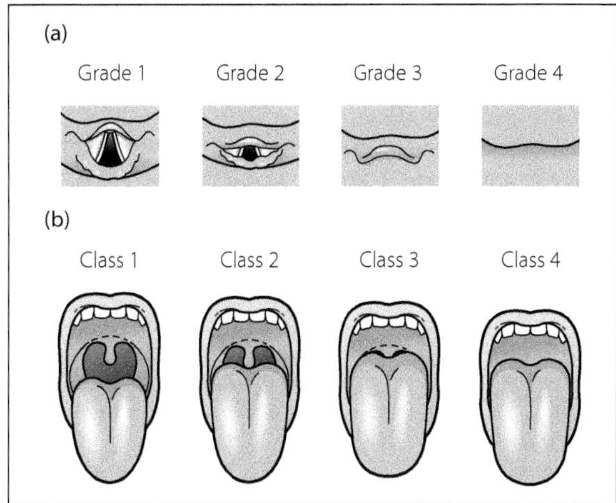

Fig. 93 (a) Cormack and Lehane classification of laryngoscopic views. (b) Modified Mallampati classification of pharyngeal appearance

suggested). The system has been applied to intubation using a **videolaryngoscope**; such use has been criticised because difficulty using these devices may be encountered despite having a good view of the glottis.

- Caused by:
  - inexperienced practitioner.
  - difficulty inserting the laryngoscope into the mouth, e.g. because its handle is obstructed by the patient's chest or by the hand applying **cricoid pressure** (e.g. **obesity**, **caesarean section**, barrel chest). This may also occur with reduced mouth opening and neck mobility.
  - reduced neck mobility, e.g. caused by osteoarthrosis, **rheumatoid arthritis**, **ankylosing spondylitis**, surgical fixation/traction.
  - reduced mouth opening, e.g. reduced **temporomandibular joint** (TMJ) mobility, **trismus**, scarring, fibrosis, local lesions/swelling.
  - lesions/swelling/fibrosis of **larynx**, **pharynx**, **tongue**.
  - congenital conditions, often associated with the above, e.g. **facial deformities**, **achondroplasia**, **Marfan's syndrome**, **cystic hygroma**.
  - anatomical variants of normal; they may be associated with the above but difficult intubation may occur in otherwise unremarkable patients.

Studies investigating difficult intubation have described many associated features; the large number of contributing factors may hinder reliable prediction of difficulty. Also, although many difficult cases share common features, many patients with these features present no difficulty; i.e., the **specificity** of most tests is poor.

- Difficulty may be suggested by:
  - previous difficulty recorded in the medical notes.
  - obesity, with short neck and reduced movement at the **cervical spine**, especially the atlanto-occipito-axial complex. The latter is tested by asking for full neck flexion, then asking the patient to look up with the examiner's hand at the back of the neck, holding it flexed. Normal movement exceeds 15 degrees.
  - reduced TMJ movement: anterior/posterior sliding of lower jaw (inability to protrude the lower teeth beyond the upper) or mouth opening (<3 cm).
  - protruding teeth, small mouth, high, narrow arched palate, receding mandible.
  - poor view of the pharyngeal structures with open mouth and tongue protruded maximally, with the observer level with the seated patient. The modified Mallampati classification is commonly used (Fig. 93b): soft palate, uvula, fauces and pillars visible (class 1); soft palate, fauces and uvula visible (class 2); only soft palate visible (class 3); and soft palate not visible (class 4). A 'class 0' has been suggested in which the tip of the epiglottis itself is visible. The test is also valid if performed with the patient supine but there may be significant interobserver differences in any position. Phonation during testing misleadingly improves the rating.
  - thyromental distance, with neck extended, of <6.5 cm.
  - x-ray assessment: formal measurement of jaw dimensions is rarely done. Movement of the neck in extension/flexion, especially middle/upper vertebrae, may be useful. There should be a gap between the occiput and posterior arch of the atlas. The gap should increase on neck flexion. An absent gap or little change on flexion suggests limited movement at the top of the spine. Not performed routinely, unless neck disease is suspected.

Grouping of several tests in various combinations has been proposed to improve the predictive power, although because the incidence of difficulty (and especially failure) is low, even the best tests have poor **positive predictive value**.

- Management:
  - known or anticipated difficulty:
    - consideration of alternatives to intubation:
      - **regional anaesthesia**.
      - **facemask** ± **airway**.
      - **SAD**.
      - **tracheostomy/cricothyroidotomy**.
    - if oro/nasal intubation is deemed necessary, it may be performed with the patient awake or anaesthetised. In the latter, inhalational induction (e.g. with **sevoflurane**) with maintenance of spontaneous ventilation during intubation is classically advocated.
    - iv induction may be performed if ventilation by facemask or SAD is unlikely to be difficult, although this approach should be undertaken with extreme caution as it may precipitate a 'can't intubate, can't oxygenate' scenario.
    - techniques of intubation:
      - the position of the head should be optimised. **Cricoid pressure** (especially backward, upward and to the patient's right [BURP]) may help if the larynx is anteriorly placed.
      - blind nasal intubation.
      - use of **intubation aids**, e.g. bougies, **forceps**, **fibreoptic instruments**, specialised **laryngoscopes** (e.g. videolaryngoscope) and **tracheal tubes**, retrograde catheter technique.

    Preoxygenation should precede all attempts at intubation. **Neuromuscular blocking drugs** are avoided by some until the airway is secure; others advocate their use in order to provide optimum intubating conditions. Experienced help and facilities for tracheostomy or **cricothyroidotomy** should be available. Special considerations apply if **airway obstruction** is present.

    In patients at risk of regurgitation, risk of aspiration is increased if laryngeal protective reflexes are obtunded by local anaesthetic during awake intubation. If inhalational induction is chosen, the left lateral head-down position is traditionally advocated, but reduced familiarity with the position may exacerbate difficulty in intubation.

    Emphasis should be on a plan A, plan B, plan C, with clear communication of the strategy chosen throughout the team.
  - unanticipated difficulty:
    - maintenance of oxygenation.
    - remove cricoid pressure if applied.
    - consideration of alternative strategies:
      - allowing the patient to wake, with subsequent management as above.
      - continuing inhalational anaesthesia without intubation.
      - persisting in intubation attempts as above. Increases the risk of trauma, **awareness** and oesophageal intubation.
      - a failed intubation drill should be instituted early, especially if at risk of regurgitation.
  - airway obstruction may follow tracheal **extubation** unless measures are taken to protect the airway; options include tracheostomy/cricothyroidotomy, use of an **airway exchange catheter** or delaying extubation

until further equipment and/or personnel are available or until airway oedema has subsided.
- anaesthetic records and notes should be clearly marked to warn other anaesthetists. The patient should be visited postoperatively, to discuss the events and implications.

The routine availability of a 'difficult airway trolley', containing all the equipment required, is considered essential.
[Ronald S Cormack, London anaesthetist; John R Lehane, Oxford anaesthetist; Seshagiri R Mallampati, Indian-born Boston anaesthetist]
Frerk C, Mitchell VS, McNarry AF, et al (2015). Br J Anaesth; 115: 827–48
See also, Intubation, awake; Intubation, blind nasal; Intubation, complications of; Intubation, failed; Intubation, fibreoptic; Intubation, oesophageal; Intubation, tracheal

Intubation, endobronchial, *see Differential lung ventilation; Endobronchial tubes and blockers; Intubation, complications of*

Intubation, failed. Incidence is approximately 1:2500–3000 in general patients, and 1:300–500 in obstetrics. If it occurs, the priority is maintenance of oxygenation.
- Management:
  - early acceptance of failure is important; a maximum of three attempts at intubation is recommended, during which conditions should be optimised (e.g. head-up/'ramped' positioning, full neuromuscular blockade, removal of **cricoid pressure**) and oxygenation maintained with facemask ventilation. Anaesthesia should be maintained with either inhalational or intravenous agents.
  - help should be summoned whatever the level of experience of the anaesthetist.
  - attempt to place a second-generation **SAD**. A maximum of three attempts at placement is recommended. If successful, decide whether to wake the patient, intubate the trachea via the SAD, proceed without intubation or perform a **cricothyroidotomy** or **tracheostomy**.
  - if placing a SAD fails, and facemask ventilation is unsuccessful, ensure the patient has received an adequate dose of a **neuromuscular blocking drug** and reattempt facemask ventilation. If successful, wake the patient. If not, declare a 'can't intubate-can't oxygenate' (CICO) situation and proceed to cricothyroidotomy.

Frerk C, Mitchell VS, McNarry AF, et al (2015). Br J Anaesth; 115: 827–48
See also, Intubation, awake; Intubation, difficult

Intubation, fibreoptic. Usually refers to use of flexible **fibreoptic instruments**, although there are also rigid fibreoptic **laryngoscopes** available. May be used for awake intubation or as an alternative to direct laryngoscopy in the anaesthetised patient, in both routine and difficult cases. Oral intubation may be assisted by passage of the laryngoscope via a specialised oral airway (*see Airways*) or **SAD**. Causes less trauma and cardiovascular response than direct laryngoscopy and intubation.
Collins SR, Blank RS (2014). Resp Care; 59: 865–80
See also, Intubation, awake; Intubation, tracheal

Intubation, oesophageal. A potential complication of attempted tracheal intubation. If undetected, it may lead to severe **hypoxaemia**, resulting in death or brain injury. Particularly likely if intubation is difficult or the practitioner unskilled. Detection is often difficult, because observation of chest movement and auscultation over the chest and stomach may wrongly suggest successful tracheal intubation. The belching noise on manual inflation that usually accompanies oesophageal intubation may be absent. The reservoir bag may move convincingly during spontaneous ventilation. Condensation of water vapour within the tube may occur in both oesophageal and tracheal intubation. **Preoxygenation** may delay subsequent hypoxaemia and cyanosis.
- Methods of detection:
  - **capnography**: the gold standard; although CO_2 may be present in the stomach, sustained levels in repeated expirations indicate tracheal intubation. Disposable detectors may be attached to the tube, giving breath-by-breath colour changes in response to exhaled CO_2.
  - fibreoptic endoscopy through the tube.
  - injection and withdrawal of air through the tube, using a large syringe or rubber bulb (oesophageal intubation detector device; Wee detector). Oesophageal intubation is suggested by a belch on inflation, followed by absent or obstructed withdrawal of air. Both components are silent and unobstructed if intubation is tracheal.
  - passage of an illuminated stylet down the tube; tracheal placement is suggested by visible light at the front of the neck.
  - use of sound: a simple stethoscope attachment at the proximal end of the tracheal tube has been used to distinguish tracheal and oesophageal tube placement. A hand-held device (SCOTI; Sonomatic Confirmation of Tracheal Intubation) that emits sound waves along the tracheal tube and analyses the reflected waves has also been used but is no longer manufactured because of poor performance.

Removal of the tube has been advocated if there is any doubt as to its position. Alternatively, disconnecting the tube but leaving it in place may allow manual ventilation using a facemask placed over it.
[Michael Wee, UK anaesthetist]

Intubation, tracheal. Oro/nasal intubation was initially described for resuscitation (e.g. by **Kite** in 1788) and for laryngeal obstruction, although tracheal insufflation in animals had been described earlier. **Macewen** was the first to advocate tracheal intubation instead of **tracheostomy** for anaesthesia for head and neck surgery, in 1880. An intubating tube was described by **O'Dwyer** in 1885. **Laryngoscopy** was pioneered by **Kirstein**, **Killian** and **Jackson** between 1895 and 1915. Modern endotracheal anaesthesia and blind nasal intubation were developed by **Magill** and **Rowbotham** after World War I. **Tracheal tubes** and **laryngoscopes** are continually being developed and adapted.
- Indications for intubation:
  - anaesthetic:
    - restricted access to the patient, e.g. head and neck surgery, prone position.
    - to protect against tracheal soiling by gastric contents and blood, e.g. **dental**, **ENT** and **emergency surgery**.
    - to secure the airway, e.g. in **airway obstruction**.
    - when muscle relaxation is required, e.g. abdominal surgery.
    - when **IPPV** is required, e.g. respiratory disease, **thoracic** or **cardiac surgery**, **neurosurgery**, prolonged surgery.

- non-anaesthetic:
  - CPR.
  - when IPPV is required, e.g. respiratory failure.
  - to secure/protect the airway, e.g. in airway obstruction, unconscious patients, impaired protective laryngeal reflexes.
  - to allow suctioning/clearance of sputum/secretions.
- Technique:
  - at least two laryngoscopes, a selection of tubes, syringe for **cuff** inflation, **suction equipment**, **intubation aids**, emergency equipment and drugs should always be available and checked before use.
  - oral:
    - the patient is positioned with the neck flexed about 35 degrees and head extended about 15 degrees ('sniffing the morning air'). A pillow is required.
    - with the lungs oxygenated and the patient either paralysed or adequately anaesthetised if breathing spontaneously, the mouth is opened with the right hand and the laryngoscope introduced at the right side, using the left hand. The blade's tip is passed back along the upper surface of the tongue until the epiglottis is visible.
    - if a curved blade (e.g. **Macintosh**'s) is used, the tip is placed between the epiglottis and the base of the tongue, and the laryngoscope lifted in the direction of the handle, avoiding pivoting or pressure on the upper teeth. The glottis is visible under the epiglottis as the latter is lifted forward (Fig. 94a). This method is thought to be less stimulating than with a straight blade, because the dorsal surface of the epiglottis (innervated by the superior laryngeal branch of the vagus) is not touched.
    - if a straight blade (e.g. Magill's) is used, the tip is placed posterior to the epiglottis and lifted as above. The glottis is visible beyond the tip (Fig. 94b). Alternatively, the tip is passed into the oesophagus and slowly withdrawn until the glottis appears. Epiglottic bruising is more likely with this technique. In the paraglossal technique, the straight blade is introduced to the (right) side of the tongue and angled so that the blade's tip lifts the epiglottis in the midline (a similar technique is also possible using a curved blade).
    - **lidocaine** spray 4% is sometimes applied to the larynx, to reduce stimulation by the tube. Lidocaine gel is also available.
    - size 8–9 mm tubes are often used for men, 7–8 mm for women (smaller tubes are associated with a lower incidence of sore throat and hoarseness); average suitable length is 20–21 cm in women and 22–23 cm in men. The tube is inserted under direct vision if possible, from the right side of the mouth with conventional laryngoscopes. The view may be improved by backward, upward and rightward pressure on the larynx (BURP) from the front of the neck. If the view is incomplete or insertion difficult, intubation aids (e.g. stylet, bougie) may help. If the glottis is not seen, the bougie or tube may be placed blindly, by careful advancement posterior to the epiglottis or laryngoscope tip. Tracheal rings may be felt if placement is successful; oesophageal intubation must be excluded.
    - the tube cuff is inflated slowly until the audible leak stops. Low-pressure inflators are available.
    - observation of the chest and auscultation of both lungs (e.g. high in the axilla) are required to exclude accidental intubation of the right main bronchus. Auscultation over the stomach and in the suprasternal notch has also been suggested to help indicate gastric inflation and tracheal leak, respectively.
    - the tube is tied or taped in position.
    - other techniques include awake intubation, fibreoptic intubation, use of **SADs** (especially those specifically designed for intubation) and retrograde catheters. Intubation may also be performed without instruments, by hooking the fingers or thumb of one hand over the back of the tongue, and guiding the tube by touch.

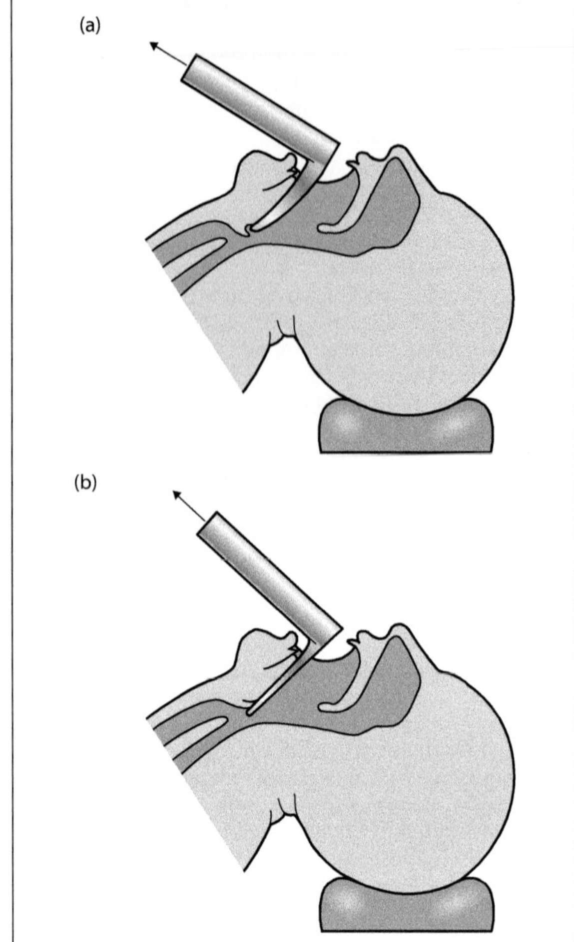

Fig. 94 Tracheal intubation using (a) curved and (b) straight laryngoscope blades

  - nasal:
    - **cocaine** paste/spray 10%, or **xylometazoline** 0.1% is used to reduce epistaxis, which may be severe.
    - tubes of diameter 1 mm less than for oral intubation are usually employed; average suitable length is 25–28 cm. The lubricated tube is gently inserted directly backwards, twisting to ease its passage. Intubation is achieved blindly, with **fibreoptic instruments** or with laryngoscopy as above, using **forceps** to position the tube if required.
    - checking/securing as above.

Special considerations apply for **paediatric anaesthesia**, or when risk of aspiration is present (*see Induction, rapid sequence*).

In ICU, nasal intubation was previously preferred because of increased patient comfort, easier securing of the tube and mouth care. However, narrower, longer tubes are required, and thus suction is more difficult and occlusion more likely. The incidence of nasal **sinusitis** is also increased. Early tracheostomy is now preferred.
See also, Intubation, awake; Intubation, blind nasal; Intubation, complications of; Intubation, difficult; Intubation, oesophageal

Inverse ratio ventilation (IRV). Ventilatory mode used in neonatal **IPPV** and **ALI**. Consists of a prolonged inspiratory phase of up to four times the duration of the expiratory phase. Increases mean **airway pressure** and is thought to improve oxygenation by keeping collapsible alveoli open for longer periods and by keeping alveoli distended through 'intrinsic **PEEP**' associated with shortened expiratory time. May require a few hours for alveolar recruitment to become apparent. Risk of **barotrauma** may be increased, and air trapping may occur if the expiratory phase is too short. It is therefore contraindicated in obstructive lung disease when hyperventilation may occur. Spontaneous ventilation is prevented by most ventilators during the long inspiratory phase; thus it is unsuitable for **weaning from ventilators**. Usually requires neuromuscular blockade and **sedation**.

Investigations, preoperative. Aid clinical **preoperative assessment** of patients' fitness for surgery and whether optimisation is possible, providing a baseline for subsequent testing. Indications and requirements vary and are sometimes controversial; history and examination are generally considered more useful in routine preoperative screening for disease. Unnecessary testing is expensive, time-consuming and may be worrying for the patient; it may be performed because of ignorance, supposed medicolegal security and to avoid postponement of surgery if a test result is required later. Conversely, anaesthetists are often pressed to proceed with anaesthesia despite inadequate investigation.

- Guidelines for investigation are related to:
  - cost and availability.
  - **sensitivity** and **specificity** of the test.
  - incidence of abnormality in the population concerned.
  - clinical significance of the result if abnormal.
  - extent of planned surgery.
- In 2016 **NICE** published updated guidelines for routine preoperative tests for elective surgery, taking into account the patient's **ASA physical status** and grade of surgery:
  - **ECG**: indicated for ASA 3–4 patients and all those undergoing major surgery; consider for age >65 years, those with cardiovascular, renal or diabetic co-morbidity.
  - **echocardiography**: consider if heart murmur and any cardiac symptoms are present, or if there are signs of heart failure.
  - full blood count: indicated in all those undergoing major/complex surgery, or those with significant cardiovascular or renal disease. Routine testing in all women and in all patients has been suggested, but is not supported by best evidence.
  - **coagulation studies**: should not be routinely performed; consider in those with chronic liver disease having intermediate or major/complex surgery. Those taking **anticoagulant drugs** requiring alteration of their regimen should have a personalised plan according to local guidance.
  - biochemistry: indicated in all those undergoing major/complex surgery or those at risk of perioperative **AKI**. Consider for metabolic diseases, **dehydration**, drug therapy known to alter biochemistry (e.g. **diuretics**) or whose actions are affected by abnormalities, e.g. **digoxin**. **Creatinine** has been suggested as a better routine test than **urea**.
  - pregnancy testing: all women of childbearing potential should be asked if there is any possibility of pregnancy and tested according to local guidance if there is any doubt.
  - other investigations if suggested by history/examination/proposed surgery include testing for **sickle cell anaemia, liver function tests, lung function tests, cardiopulmonary exercise testing, arterial blood gas interpretation, cervical spine** x-rays.

CXR is no longer recommended as a routine preoperative investigation in elective surgery.

O'Neill F, Carter E, Pink N, Smith I (2016). Br Med J, 354: i3590

Ionisation of drugs. Important determinant of a drug's passage through **membranes**, because charged (ionised) particles are relatively lipid-insoluble and therefore do not cross easily. Once a drug has dissociated, passage across the membrane depends on the concentration of the unionised form. Weak **acids** dissociate in alkaline environments; thus passage across membranes is favoured by acid environments. The opposite applies for weak bases.

Degree of ionisation is derived from the **Henderson–Hasselbalch equation**:

$$\text{acidic drug: pH} - \text{p}K_a = \log\frac{[\text{ionised drug}]}{[\text{unionised drug}]}$$

$$\text{basic drug: pH} - \text{p}K_a = \log\frac{[\text{unionised drug}]}{[\text{ionised drug}]}$$

At 50% ionisation, pH = pK_a.

- Examples of acidic drugs:
  - **phenytoin**.
  - **barbiturates**, e.g. **thiopental** (pK_a 7.6).
  - **salicylates**.
  - **penicillins**.
- Examples of basic drugs:
  - **diazepam** (pK_a 3.3).
  - **local anaesthetic agents**, e.g. **lidocaine** (pK_a 7.9), **bupivacaine** (pK_a 8.1).
  - **opioid analgesic drugs**, e.g. **morphine** (pK_a 7.9), **pethidine** (pK_a 8.5).
  - non-depolarising **neuromuscular blocking drugs**.
- Examples of anaesthetic relevance:
  - in **acidosis**, dissociation of thiopental is decreased; thus the concentration of unionised portion increases. The amount of drug entering the brain therefore increases; thus the effect per mg increases.
  - conversely, in infected tissues with a relatively acidic pH, the dissociation of local anaesthetic agents is increased, rendering them less effective.
  - 'trapping' of drugs in the ionised form in urine, by manipulating urinary pH to aid excretion (**forced diuresis**).

See also, Pharmacokinetics

Iontophoresis. Use of electric current to aid penetration of drug into the tissues. Suitable for drugs of low mw and high lipid solubility and potency, e.g. **GTN**, **fentanyl**. The drug is applied to the skin in the ionised form using an electrode of the same charge as the drug; current is applied using a nearby reference electrode to complete the circuit. Drug is repelled from the electrode and passes into the skin and subcutaneous tissues.

Ipecacuanha. **Emetic drug**, a mixture of plant alkaloids, formerly used in the treatment of **poisoning and overdoses**. Activates peripheral GIT sensory receptors and stimulates the **chemoreceptor trigger zone**. Produces vomiting within 20–30 min, with effects lasting up to 2 h. Its use is no longer advocated as there is no evidence that it reduces absorption of poisons and it may increase the risk of **aspiration of gastric contents**.

IPPV, *see Intermittent positive pressure ventilation*

Ipratropium bromide. Quaternary amine **anticholinergic drug**, used to treat **asthma** and chronic bronchitis. Of slower onset than **salbutamol** and similar drugs; there may be synergy between them. Oxitropium (taken 8–12-hourly) and tiotropium (taken once daily) are similar drugs; the latter has been associated with fewer exacerbations of **COPD** (but more dry mouth) than ipratropium.

- Dosage:
  - 1–2 puffs aerosol (20–40 μg) tds/qds.
  - 0.1–0.5 mg nebuliser solution (0.4–2.0 ml 0.025% solution) tds/qds. Paradoxical bronchospasm in earlier preparations was caused by preservatives.
- Systemic anticholinergic effects are rare, although **glaucoma** has occurred in susceptible patients following delivery of nebulised ipratropium through poorly fitting masks.

IPSP, Inhibitory postsynaptic potential, *see Synaptic transmission*

Iron lung, *see Intermittent negative pressure ventilation*

Iron poisoning. Occurs almost exclusively in children who accidentally consume iron tablets. Doses exceeding 40–60 mg/kg of elemental iron, or serum concentrations exceeding 90 μmol/l in children or 140 μmol/l in adults represent severe poisoning. Early symptoms (within an hour) include nausea, vomiting, upper abdominal pain and GIT bleeding (caused by the corrosive action of iron on the gastric mucosa); later symptoms include hypotension, hypoglycaemia, convulsions, **acute kidney injury** and coma. Hepatic failure and pyloric stenosis may occur. With intensive treatment, mortality is about 1%.

- Management:
  - general measures as for **poisoning and overdose**, e.g. O_2 therapy, iv fluids.
  - in severe cases, **desferrioxamine** iv up to 15 mg/kg/h to a maximum of 80 mg/kg in 24 h. With features of severe toxicity, treatment should be started without waiting for the serum iron level. Instillation of 5 g into the stomach has also been suggested to reduce absorption. **Gastric lavage** is not routinely recommended, though may be considered if a child presents within minutes of ingesting a life-threatening dose. Whole bowel irrigation has been performed after ingestion of enteric-coated preparations, although evidence of benefit is unclear. Exchange transfusion and plasmapheresis have also been used successfully in refractory cases.
  - treatment should be monitored by serial serum iron measurements.

Chang TP, Rangan C (2011). Pediatr Emer Care; 27: 978–85

IRV, *see Inverse ratio ventilation*

ISA, *see Intrinsic sympathomimetic activity*

Ischaemic heart disease. Most common cause of death in the developed world (20%–30%); its incidence is now declining in many countries including the UK, due to improvements in treatment, secondary prevention and the reduction of preventable risk factors.

- Risk factors include:
  - increasing age, male gender, postmenopausal women.
  - family history: incidence is increased if a person has a first-degree relative with angina or previous **MI** aged <55 years.
  - **smoking**.
  - hypercholesterolaemia associated with high plasma levels of low-density lipoproteins and low levels of high-density lipoproteins. Mortality and morbidity are reduced by treating hypercholesterolaemia.
  - **hypertension**, **diabetes mellitus**.
  - **obesity**, lack of exercise, poverty, stress and alcohol have been implicated in some studies.
- Main pathophysiological feature: reduction in coronary artery patency by lipid atheromatous plaques, which may be exacerbated by coronary spasm. This may lead to:
  - myocardial ischaemia when O_2 demand exceeds supply.
  - fissuring of plaques with thrombus formation; may lead to **acute coronary syndromes** or sudden death.
- Clinical features:
  - angina (*see Myocardial ischaemia*).
  - **dyspnoea**, related to ischaemia, **cardiac failure** or smoking-related respiratory disease.
  - palpitations, syncope due to **arrhythmias** (including **heart block**).
  - hypertension, cardiomegaly, peripheral or **pulmonary oedema**.
  - fatty deposits due to hyperlipidaemia, e.g. around the eyes, arcus senilis in the cornea.
  - sudden death.
- Investigations:
  - resting **ECG** and exercise testing.
  - **echocardiography**.
  - **nuclear cardiology** ± gated scanning.
  - **cardiac catheterisation**.
  - **CT scanning** and **MRI**.
  - digital subtraction angiography: computerised subtraction of background signals in order to enhance vessel images. Allows iv contrast injection instead of cardiac catheterisation.
- Management (*see Acute coronary syndromes for treatment of unstable disease*):
  - general measures: stopping smoking; treatment of hypertension and hypercholesterolaemia (e.g. with **statins**).
  - first-line specific treatment is with nitrates (e.g. **GTN**, **isosorbide**), **antiplatelet drugs**, **β-adrenergic receptor antagonists** and **calcium channel blocking drugs**. Oral/sublingual therapy is started first.

- percutaneous coronary intervention is increasingly used to avoid surgery.
- **coronary artery bypass graft.**
- Anaesthetic management: the main aim is to prevent perioperative myocardial ischaemia and infarction (reinfarction rate is up to 6%, usually on the third day; infarction rate if none previously is about 0.1%–0.2%):
  - preoperatively:
    - **preoperative assessment** of risk factors and severity of disease. **Cardiac risk index** is sometimes used. Conditions are optimised before surgery if possible; e.g. treatment of cardiac failure, arrhythmias.
    - continuation of antianginal therapy up to and including the morning of surgery.
    - addition of further therapy if required; e.g. GTN skin patch.
    - sedative **premedication** is often prescribed, to reduce anxiety and endogenous **catecholamine** secretion.
  - perioperatively:
    - the main principle is the optimisation of myocardial oxygen delivery while minimising demand. The combination of tachycardia and hypotension is particularly hazardous and should be avoided. In general, drugs with minimal cardiovascular effects are chosen, e.g. **vecuronium, atracurium, fentanyl. Pancuronium** has traditionally been preferred because hypotension is less likely. Previous concerns over isoflurane-induced **coronary steal** have been refuted.
    - direct **arterial BP measurement** is useful if disease is severe or surgery extensive. **Pulmonary artery catheterisation** is rarely indicated.
    - smooth **induction of anaesthesia**, using a minimal dose of **iv anaesthetic agent** given slowly, as the **arm–brain circulation** time may be prolonged. **Etomidate** causes less myocardial depression than other drugs, but others are often used. **Ketamine** may increase cardiac work and is usually avoided.
    - **spinal** and **epidural anaesthesia** risk hypotension and worsening of myocardial ischaemia, although they may reduce myocardial work by reducing **preload** and **afterload**.
    - hypertensive response to intubation increases myocardial O_2 demand with risk of myocardial ischaemia (*see Intubation, complications of*).
    - routine preoperative treatment with β-blockers is no longer advocated as it has been shown to increase the incidence of **stroke** and death.
    - myocardial ischaemia may be demonstrated by ECG or assessed by **rate–pressure product**.
  - postoperatively:
    - admission to HDU/ICU if severe.
    - **postoperative analgesia** is particularly important, to reduce sympathetic overactivity.

See also, Atherosclerosis

Ischaemic preconditioning. Protective effect of short non-lethal ischaemic periods on subsequent infarct size, originally described in animal experiments and relating to **myocardial ischaemia** (although has also been applied to the brain and other tissue). Thought to be due to release of autocoids by ischaemic myocytes; the precise mechanism is unknown but involves multiple **second messenger** systems resulting in inhibition of apoptosis and improved mitochondrial function. The effect is transient, although some protective effect has been described up to 72 h later; improved ventricular function may also follow. Also seen when ischaemia is applied to tissue away from the organ being 'preconditioned' (e.g. with a tourniquet applied to the upper limb), termed remote ischaemic preconditioning. Its importance in humans is uncertain but has been suggested by in vitro work, and several initial clinical trials have yielded promising results.

Sivaraman V, Pickard JM, Hausenloy DJ (2015). Anaesthesia; 70: 732–48 and Kunst G, Klein AA (2015). Anaesthesia; 70: 467–82

Isosbestic point. A wavelength of light that is absorbed by two substances to the same extent. In **oximetry**, the different absorption profiles of oxyhaemoglobin and deoxyhaemoglobin are utilised to quantify the percentage saturation of **haemoglobin**. Isosbestic points occur at 590 and 805 nm; these may be used as reference points where light absorption is independent of degree of saturation (*see Fig. 127;* **Oximetry**).

Isoflurane. 1-Chloro-2,2,2-trifluoroethyl difluoromethyl ether (Fig. 95). **Inhalational anaesthetic agent**, first synthesised in 1965 with its isomer **enflurane**, but not introduced until 1980 because of earlier (erroneous) reports of hepatic carcinogenicity in mice.

- Properties:
  - colourless liquid; pungent vapour, 7.5 times denser than air.
  - mw 184.5.
  - boiling point 49°C.
  - **SVP** at 20°C 33 kPa (250 mmHg).
  - **partition coefficients**:
    - blood/gas 1.4.
    - oil/gas 97.
  - **MAC** 1.05% (>60 years) to 1.28% (young adults); 1.6%–1.8% in children.
  - non-flammable, non-corrosive. Dissolves certain plastics, e.g. some makes of syringe.
  - supplied in liquid form with no additive.
- Effects:
  - CNS:
    - smooth, rapid induction, but speed of uptake is limited by respiratory irritation. Recovery is slower than with **sevoflurane** and **desflurane.**
    - anticonvulsant properties, unlike enflurane. Causes more reduction of EEG activity than other agents, producing an isoelectric EEG at greater than 2 MAC.
    - reduces $CMRO_2$.
    - increases **cerebral blood flow** and **ICP**.
    - decreases **intraocular pressure**.
    - has poor analgesic properties.
  - RS:
    - irritant; more likely to cause coughing and laryngospasm than sevoflurane.

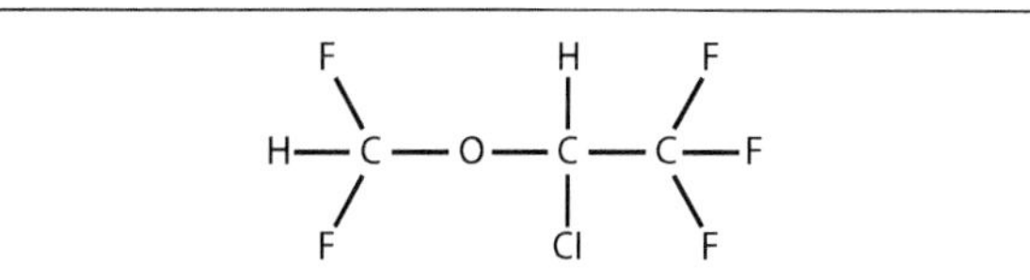

Fig. 95 Structure of isoflurane

- respiratory depressant, with increased rate and decreased tidal volume.
- causes bronchodilatation.

- CVS:
  - myocardial depression is less than with **halothane**, enflurane and sevoflurane, but vasodilatation and hypotension commonly occur. Compensatory tachycardia is common, especially in young patients.
  - myocardial O_2 demand decreases, but tachycardia may reduce myocardial O_2 supply.
  - **coronary steal** is not thought to occur in humans.
  - arrhythmias are less common than with other agents. Little myocardial sensitisation to **catecholamines**.
- other:
  - dose-dependent uterine relaxation.
  - nausea/vomiting is uncommon.
  - skeletal muscle relaxation; **non-depolarising neuromuscular blockade** may be potentiated.
  - may precipitate **MH**.

Less than 0.2% metabolised, the rest being excreted by the lungs. Widely used in **neurosurgery**, for the above properties. **Fluoride ion** production is minimal, even after prolonged surgery; higher levels have been reported after several days' use on ICU.

1%–2.5% is usually adequate for maintenance of anaesthesia, with higher concentrations at induction. Tracheal intubation may be performed easily with spontaneous respiration, once the patient is adequately anaesthetised.

See also, Vaporisers

Isolated forearm technique. Method for detecting **awareness** during anaesthesia. A tourniquet is inflated on the upper arm to above systolic BP, before systemic injection of **neuromuscular blocking drug**. Arm movement, both spontaneous and in response to verbal command, can be observed during anaesthesia but responses may be open to interpretation. Patients may respond to command without postoperative recall (wakefulness).

Pandit JJ, Russell IF, Wang M (2015). Br J Anaesth; 115 Suppl 1:i32–45

Isomerism. Existence of two or more ions or compounds that have the same atomic composition but different structural arrangement, often with different properties.

- Two types exist:
  - structural: compounds have the same molecular formula but different chemical structures, that is, their atoms are arranged differently. Structural isomers may have similar actions (e.g. **isoflurane** [$CF_3CHClOCHF_2$] and **enflurane** [$CHClFCF_2OCHF_2$]) or different actions (e.g. promazine and **promethazine**). Tautomerism (or dynamic isomerism) refers to two structural isomers existing in equilibrium. Following iv administration, pH changes convert one isomer into the other: e.g. **thiopental**, ionised and water-soluble in the syringe but rapidly converted to the largely unionised, water-insoluble form after injection. **Midazolam** undergoes similar changes in lipid solubility after injection.
  - stereoisomerism: compounds have the same molecular formulae and chemical structure but have different spatial orientation. Two types exist:
    - enantiomers: (optical isomers; chiral substances): the compounds are mirror images of each other, and have the ability to rotate the plane of polarisation of polarised light to the right (+, dextro, *d* or D) or left (–, laevo/levo, *l* or L). This classification has been largely superseded by the R/S system (standing for rectus and sinister, the Latin for right and left, respectively), that describes the configuration of the atoms around the chiral atom (around which the other components differ between the isomers) according to set rules involving the mw of the other atoms. An R(–) enantiomer thus has its atoms arranged in a clockwise manner; an R(+) enantiomer also rotates light to the right. Each enantiomer typically has very different effects to those of its mirror image. That such closely related isomers may have different effects is one piece of evidence supporting **receptor theory**. A racemic mixture is one containing equal amounts of the two enantiomers and has no optical activity.
    - diastereomers: the compounds are not mirror images but have identical molecular formulae and chemical structure. They generally have more than one chiral centre.
    - different profiles of drug activity have been identified as resulting from specific isomers, e.g. S(+) **ketamine** has greater anaesthetic and amnesic potency than the R(–) isomer, with fewer **emergence phenomena** and faster recovery. Similarly, levobupivacaine is less cardiotoxic than the racemic **bupivacaine** preparation. Future drug development will be directed at production of single stereoisomers. Currently available drugs in single stereoisomer form include l-**hyoscine**, **etomidate**, **cisatracurium** and **ropivacaine**. Drugs administered as a mixture of two isomers include ketamine, bupivacaine, **atropine**, **adrenaline**, **halothane** and isoflurane. **Mivacurium** and **atracurium** are presented as a mixture of more than two stereoisomers.

Cis-trans isomerism refers to the arrangements of paired atoms or groups around a double bond; *cis* refers to both substituents being on the same side of the double bond, while *trans* refers to one on each side.

Nau C, Strichartz GR (2002). Anesthesiology; 97: 497–503

Isoniazid. **Antituberculous drug**, usually included in all anti-**TB** regimens.

- Dosage: 300 mg/day iv, im or orally in adults; 10 mg/kg/day up to 300 mg/day in children.
- Side effects: peripheral neuropathy (especially in diabetes, alcoholism, malnutrition or chronic renal failure, when concurrent treatment with pyridoxine 10 mg/day should be given); nausea, hepatitis, agranulocytosis, psychosis, convulsions, lupus-like syndrome and erythema multiforme are rare.

Isoprenaline hydrochloride/sulfate. Synthetic **catecholamine** and **inotropic drug**. A non-selective **β-adrenergic receptor agonist**, used for its effects on heart rate, vasomotor tone and bronchial muscle. Only available in the UK on 'special order'.

- Actions:
  - increased heart rate and force of myocardial contraction (via β_1 receptors).
  - peripheral and pulmonary vasodilatation (via β_2 receptors).
  - systolic BP may therefore rise or fall; diastolic BP usually falls.
  - bronchodilatation (via β_2 receptors).

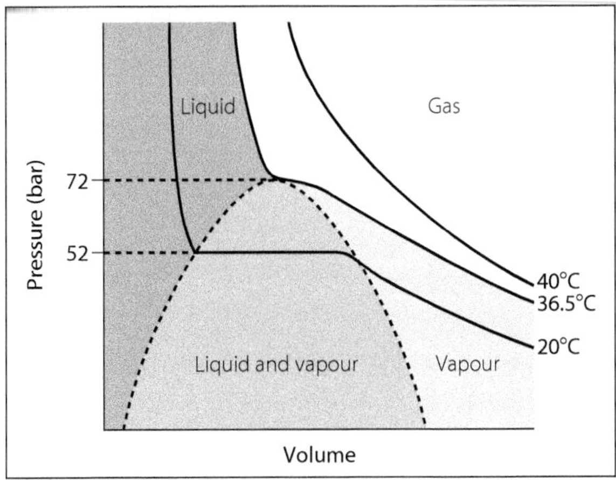

Fig. 96 Isotherms for N_2O

- Dosage:
  - 0.02–0.2 µg/kg/min iv for complete **heart block** or severe bradycardia. A bolus of 5–20 µg may also be given.
  - may also be given orally, rectally or sublingually: 10–30 mg tds; absorption may be unreliable.

May cause tachycardia, tremor and ventricular arrhythmias. May worsen coronary perfusion in **ischaemic heart disease**.

Isoprostanes. Substances related to **prostaglandins**, formed by peroxidation of **arachidonic acid** by a reaction catalysed by **free radicals** (not involving **cyclo-oxygenase**). Have been studied as markers of oxidative stress, e.g. occurring during **reperfusion injury**. Isoprostanes themselves disrupt cell membranes and cause vasoconstriction.

Isoproterenol, *see Isoprenaline*

Isosorbide di- and mononitrate. Vasodilator drugs, with similar actions to **GTN** but of longer duration (up to 12 h with sustained release preparations). IV infusion of the dinitrate has been suggested in preference to infusion of GTN preparations because the latter contains additives (e.g. propylene glycol). The mononitrate is a metabolite of the dinitrate. Used in **ischaemic heart disease**, **cardiac failure** and as an **antihypertensive drug** perioperatively.
- Dosage:
  - dinitrate:
    - 5–10 mg sublingually.
    - up to 240 mg/day orally; given 1–4 times daily.
    - 2–10 mg/h iv (0.5–2 µg/kg/min).
  - mononitrate: 20–120 mg/day orally in divided doses.
- Side effects: as for GTN.

Isothermal change. Alteration in the state of a **gas** while **temperature** remains constant, e.g. by removal of heat produced during compression. Thus **Boyle's law** applies.
See also, Adiabatic change

Isotherms. Lines on a chart or graph denoting changes in volume or **pressure** with **temperature** remaining constant. The graph for an ideal gas would consist of rectangular hyperbolas according to the gas laws. In fact, for $\mathbf{N_2O}$ (Fig. 96), the isotherms approach those of an ideal gas at temperatures above its **critical temperature** (36.5°C). Compression of the N_2O below its critical temperature causes liquefaction, thus resisting an increase in pressure. Once all the N_2O is liquid, further compression causes a large increase in pressure, because liquids are less compressible than gases.

Isoxane. Trade name for premixed **Entonox** with 0.25% **isoflurane**. Has been used to provide analgesia during labour and minor surgery in a similar way to Entonox.
See also, Obstetric analgesia and anaesthesia

ISS, *see Injury severity score*

Itraconazole. Triazole **antifungal drug**, related to fluconazole.
- Dosage: 100–400 mg orally/iv daily.
- Side effects: as for fluconazole, though hepatic impairment is more common. Heart failure has been reported.

ITU, Intensive therapy unit, *see Intensive care unit*

Ivabridine hydrochloride. Antianginal drug, licensed for patients in normal sinus rhythm and heart rate >70/min, in whom **β-adrenergic receptor antagonists** are contraindicated or not tolerated. Acts purely on the sinoatrial node, lowering heart rate by selectively inhibiting the cardiac pacemaker I_f ('funny') current—a mixed sodium/potassium inward current that controls diastolic depolarisation. Also used for chronic **cardiac failure**.
- Dosage: 2.5–7.5 mg orally bd.
- Side effects: bradycardia, first-degree heart block, ventricular ectopics, headache, dizziness, visual disturbances; less commonly, GIT upset, supraventricular ectopics.

IVOX, *see Intravenous oxygenator*

IVRA, *see Intravenous regional anaesthesia*

J receptors, *see Juxtapulmonary capillary receptors*

J wave, *see Hypothermia*

Jackson, Charles T (1805–1880). US chemist, present at **Wells'** unsuccessful demonstration of N_2O in 1846; suggested **diethyl ether** to **Morton** for dental topical anaesthesia instead. Applied for the patent rights to ether jointly with Morton, the latter subsequently taking over 90% of Jackson's share. Jackson later claimed sole credit for the discovery of anaesthesia.
Martin RF, Desai SP (2015). J Anesth Hist; 1: 38–43

Jackson, Chevalier (1865–1958). Renowned US laryngologist. Perfected a direct-vision **laryngoscope** in the early 1900s, and wrote extensively on laryngoscopy and tracheal insufflation.
Boyd AD (1994). Ann Thorac Surg; 57: 502–5

Jaundice. Yellow discoloration of the skin caused by high plasma bilirubin concentration. Clinically detectable at total bilirubin > 50 µmol/l (normally < 17 µmol/l).

- Normal formation and metabolism of bilirubin:
  - **haemoglobin** is broken down to amino acids and haem in the reticuloendothelial system. Haem is further metabolised to lipid-soluble unconjugated bilirubin that is transported (bound to **albumin**) to the liver.
  - in the liver, unconjugated bilirubin is conjugated with glucuronic acid, rendering it water-soluble.
  - conjugated bilirubin is stored in the gallbladder with bile salts and acids, passing into the small bowel.
  - bilirubin is converted to urobilinogen and thence urobilin by gut bacteria. Reabsorbed from the gut, with some urobilinogen passing back to the liver to be re-excreted; a small amount is extracted by the kidneys.
- Causes of jaundice:
  - increased bilirubin production, e.g. **haemolysis**. Usually mild. Unconjugated and conjugated bilirubin levels are raised, with increased urinary urobilinogen.
  - impaired conjugation of bilirubin, e.g. **hepatitis**, cirrhosis, drug-induced (e.g. **α-methyldopa, paracetamol**), **hepatic failure**. Unconjugated bilirubin is raised; urinary urobilinogen may be raised because the liver is unable to re-excrete it.
  - congenital abnormalities of bilirubin transport are rare, except for Gilbert's syndrome (hepatic glucuronyltransferase deficiency causing mild unconjugated bilirubinaemia with otherwise normal **liver function tests** and no urinary bilirubin).
  - obstruction of bile drainage, e.g. gallstones, pancreatic carcinoma, **cholangitis, cholecystitis** (extrahepatic), primary biliary cirrhosis, drug-induced, e.g. **contraceptives**. Conjugated bilirubin is raised, often markedly, and is excreted in the urine, which is dark (but with reduced urobilinogen). Faeces are pale and fatty. Itching is common.

The latter two types are frequently mixed and difficult to distinguish.

Assessment should include questioning for a history of tattoos, drug abuse, sexual contacts, contacts with jaundiced people, travel abroad, drugs, blood transfusions, alcohol, acupuncture, abdominal symptoms and recent anaesthetics.

Jaundice in ICU patients is often part of the presenting problem (e.g. in hepatic failure, biliary obstruction, **sepsis**) or may result from drug therapy, the development of acalculous cholecystitis, haemolysis of intra-abdominal haematoma, ischaemic hepatitis (in shocked patients) or the administration of **TPN**. It may also be part of **multiple organ dysfunction syndrome**.

- ICU management:
  - support of other organs, e.g. circulation, respiration.
  - treatment of cause, e.g. endoscopic retrograde cholangiopancreatography/surgery for obstructive causes, cessation of drugs likely to cause jaundice.
  - treatment of associated clotting abnormalities, e.g. with clotting factors, **vitamin K**.
  - early treatment of infection.
- Anaesthetic management:
  - preoperative assessment as above, and for hepatic failure, depending on severity and cause.
  - risk of perioperative **acute kidney injury** due to acute tubular necrosis or **hepatorenal syndrome**:
    - especially common with obstructive jaundice, because bilirubin levels are often highest.
    - more likely if dehydration or biliary sepsis is present.
    - plasma urea/creatinine is monitored preoperatively.
    - preoperative iv hydration is instituted to maintain urine flow above 1 ml/kg/h.
    - **mannitol** may be given if bilirubin is very high or urine output inadequate despite hydration. **Furosemide** has also been used.
  - antibacterial therapy.
  - anaesthetic drugs/techniques as for hepatic failure.
- Postoperative jaundice may be due to:
  - Gilbert's syndrome.
  - underlying medical/surgical conditions.
  - drugs.
  - haemolysis, e.g. due to **blood transfusion** reaction, or following extensive bruising and haematoma.
  - infection, e.g. transmitted via transfused blood/needles, sepsis, pre-existing subclinical hepatitis becoming apparent postoperatively.
  - hepatic injury due to severe hypoxia/hypotension.
  - surgical iatrogenic biliary obstruction.

Jaundice is particularly hazardous in **neonates**; the immature blood–brain barrier allows penetration of bilirubin into the basal ganglia of the brain, causing kernicterus (convulsions may occur, leading to brain damage).

[Nicolas Gilbert (1858–1927), French physician]

See also, Biliary tract

Jaw, fractured, *see Facial trauma*

Jaw, nerve blocks, *see Gasserian ganglion block; Mandibular nerve blocks; Maxillary nerve blocks*

Jehovah's Witnesses. Religious group founded in the USA in the 1870s. Believe that they alone will survive the imminent destruction of the world, with a small proportion passing into Heaven to rule over the remainder of worthy individuals who will reside in an earthly paradise. Since 1945, also believe that to receive **blood products** is against God's will, thus causing potential difficulties perioperatively. Special **consent** forms are usually employed. For paediatric surgery, a court order is required to overrule parents' wishes. Although blood, plasma and autologous predonation are unacceptable, **cell salvage**, **cardiopulmonary bypass** and recombinant **erythropoietin** and factor VIIa are usually permitted. Autologous **blood transfusion** is usually permitted only if contact of blood with the body is not broken. Other factors such as platelets, clotting factors, albumin and intravenous immunoglobulin are 'matters of conscience' for individual Witnesses. Special measures to reduce **blood loss** may be required, e.g. **hypotensive anaesthesia**, recombinant factor VIIa.
[Jehovah (Old Testament); divine being]
Lawson T, Ralph C (2015). Br J Anaesth; 115: 676–87
See also, Medicolegal aspects of anaesthesia

Jet mixing. Effect of a jet of **gas** (e.g. O_2) delivered from a nozzle into ambient gas, e.g. air. Energy is transferred from O_2 molecules to adjacent air molecules; the latter are entrained into the jet due to viscous shearing between the gas layers. Employed in **injector techniques** for IPPV, and in fixed performance O_2 masks. In the latter, air is entrained to a fixed degree depending on O_2 flow rate and the size of side ports in the entrainment device.
See also, Oxygen therapy; Venturi principle

Jet ventilators, *see High-frequency ventilation; Injector techniques; Ventilators*

JG cells, *see Juxtaglomerular cells*

Joule. SI **unit** of **energy**. 1 **joule** = **work** done when the point of application of a **force** of 1 **newton** moves 1 **metre** in the direction of the force (1 J = 1 N × 1 m).
[James Joule (1818–1889), English physicist]

Joule–Thomson effect (Joule–Kelvin effect). Lowering of temperature when a gas expands, e.g. passing from a **cylinder** under pressure to a large space. The principle is employed in the **cryoprobe**. Conversely, temperature rises if gas within a small space is compressed.
See also, Adiabatic change

Jugular bulb catheterisation. Performed to allow access to the blood draining the brain, and used to estimate the balance between cerebral oxygen delivery and utilisation. The jugular bulb is a dilatation of the internal **jugular vein** just below the base of the skull and may be catheterised using a **Seldinger technique** with the needle inserted lateral to the carotid pulsation at the level of the thyroid cartilage and directed cranially towards the external auditory meatus.

Cerebral oxygenation can only be accurately monitored if the dominant jugular bulb is used. The right side is often chosen as it is usually dominant; more accurate identification of dominance can be made by ultrasound examination of the internal jugular veins or by identifying the larger increase in **intracranial pressure** that occurs during manual compression of each internal jugular vein.

Blood may be sampled for PO_2 and O_2 saturation (S_jO_2), giving an indication of **cerebral blood flow** (lower values reflecting greater uptake by the brain and therefore less blood flow, assuming O_2 consumption remains constant), and concentrations of **lactate** and other substances. Indwelling fibreoptic sensors may also be placed to give a continuous reading of global cerebral O_2 saturation; this has been used particularly during **cardiopulmonary bypass**, in **neurosurgery** and after **TBI**. Desaturation ($S_jO_2 < 55\%$) indicates impending cerebral ischaemia, e.g. caused by hypotension, hypoxaemia, high intracranial pressure, (e.g. due to **cerebral oedema**), high temperature and seizures.

Although supported by many enthusiasts, monitoring of jugular bulb O_2 saturation gives information only about global cerebral function, not regional differences. In addition, if cerebral blood flow and O_2 consumption both decrease, e.g. in severe brain injury, S_jO_2 may be unchanged. There is no evidence that clinical management based on jugular bulb oximetry influences outcome in TBI.
Kirkman MA, Smith M (2016). Anesthesiol Clin; 34: 537–56

Jugular veins. Include the internal, external and anterior jugular veins (Fig. 97; *see also Fig. 115;* **Neck, cross-sectional anatomy**).
- Internal jugular vein:
  - passes through the jugular foramen at the base of the **skull**, draining the intracranial structures via the sigmoid sinus.
  - lies at first posterior, then lateral, to the internal **carotid artery**. Contained within the carotid sheath with the carotid artery and **vagus nerve**; the cervical sympathetic chain lies behind the sheath.
  - receives tributaries from the pharynx, face, scalp, tongue and thyroid gland. Receives the thoracic duct on the left and right lymph duct on the right.
  - has a dilatation at each end (jugular bulb), with valves above the lower bulb.

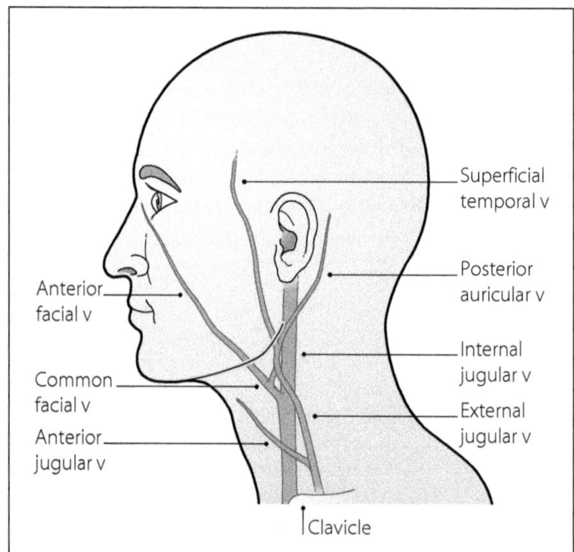

Fig. 97 Venous drainage of head and neck

- terminates behind the sternoclavicular joint by joining with the subclavian vein to form the brachiocephalic vein.
- External jugular vein:
  - drains the lateral parts of the head; passes over the sternomastoid muscle to join the subclavian vein behind the clavicle at its midpoint.
  - receives the anterior jugular vein (passing down from in front of the hyoid bone) behind the clavicle.

See also, Cerebral circulation; External jugular venous cannulation; Internal jugular venous cannulation; Jugular bulb catheterisation

Jugular venous pressure (JVP). Assessed by observing the height (in cm) of visible pulsation in the **jugular veins** above the sternal angle, with the patient reclining at 45 degrees. The normal value is zero, i.e., the venous pulsations are not normally visible. The JVP falls during inspiration, and rises during expiration and when pressure is applied to the abdomen (Q sign). Pulsations are usually non-palpable. The **venous waveform** may be apparent. JVP may be difficult to identify in obese patients.

Used as a clinical guide to right atrial pressure; raised in right-sided **cardiac failure**, hypervolaemia and mechanical obstruction, e.g. tricuspid stenosis or **superior vena caval obstruction**.

See also, Central venous pressure

Junctional arrhythmias (Nodal arrhythmias). **Arrhythmias** arising from the atrioventricular node. Common during anaesthesia, especially deep inhalational anaesthesia.

- May consist of:
  - ectopic beats.
  - bradycardia.
  - tachycardia.

On the **ECG**, inverted **P waves** may precede, follow or be hidden by the (normal) **QRS complexes**. Often of little clinical significance, although cardiac output may be reduced. Cannon waves may be visible in the jugular **venous waveform**.

Atropine and **ephedrine** have been used to restore sinus rhythm in bradycardia; junctional tachycardias may respond to **lidocaine** or **amiodarone**.

See also, Heart, conducting system

Juxtaglomerular apparatus. System adjacent to renal glomeruli, composed of:

- juxtaglomerular cells; epithelioid cells within the media of afferent arterioles entering the glomeruli. Contain renin in granules.
- macula densa; specialised tubular epithelial cells, just before the start of the distal convoluted tubule. Thought to be involved in the control of renin secretion.
- granular cells within surrounding connective tissue; contain some renin granules.

Responds to reductions in renal perfusion pressure by secreting renin, although the exact mechanism is unclear. Possibly renal vasodilatation is involved, since **β-adrenergic receptor agonists**, **prostacyclin**, **bradykinin**, **dopamine**, **furosemide** and **vasodilator drugs** all increase renin secretion. Conversely, **α-adrenergic receptor agonists**, **vasopressin**, and angiotensin reduce renin secretion.

Richly innervated with adrenergic nerve fibres; β-adrenergic activity increases secretion, and antagonism reduces it, independently of vasodilatation.

See also, Nephron; Renin/angiotensin system

Juxtapulmonary capillary receptors (J receptors). Receptors present in alveolar walls near the pulmonary capillaries. Thought to be responsible for the tachypnoea seen in **pulmonary oedema** and interstitial lung disease, via vagal afferent fibres. Their role in normal lungs is unknown.

Kallikreins. Serine protease **enzymes** in tissue and plasma, performing diverse physiological functions. Produce **kinins** from kininogens and may also catalyse formation of renin from prorenin. Plasma kallikrein is produced from prekallikrein by various activating substances, including part of activated **coagulation** factor XII. Plasmin, a fibrinolytic enzyme, catalyses the reaction, as does kallikrein itself. Inhibited by **aprotinin**. Prostate-specific antigen (PSA) is a kallikrein used as a biomarker for prostatic cancer.

Katharometer. Device used for **gas analysis**, following separation, e.g. by **gas chromatography**. A heated wire is placed in the gas flow; different gases have different thermal conductive properties and therefore produce different changes in electrical resistance of the wire. Particularly useful in detecting inorganic gases, e.g. helium, CO_2, N_2O and O_2. Used to quantify the amount of a known gas, not to identify unknown ones.

Kawasaki disease (Musculocutaneous lymph node syndrome). Autoimmune systemic vasculitis of unknown aetiology, usually affecting children <5 years old. Incidence is 3.4 per 100 000 in the UK; 3 and 30 times more common in the USA and Japan, respectively. Important because arteritis can lead to formation of coronary artery aneurysms in 15% of cases if untreated, with mortality of up to 4%. May present with fever (typically for more than 5 days), conjunctivitis, reddened lips, mouth and tongue, desquamating rash, peripheral oedema and cervical lymphadenopathy. Diagnosis may be difficult because not all these features may be present at once, other non-specific symptoms may be present (e.g. cough, abdominal pain, vomiting, arthralgia) and there is no diagnostic test. Treatment is with iv **immunoglobulin** 2 g/kg over 10 h and **aspirin** 30 mg/kg/day in 3–4 divided doses.

[Tomisaku Kawasaki, Japanese paediatrician]

Rashid AK, Kamal SM, Ashrafuzzaman M, Mustafa KG (2014). Curr Rheumatol Rev; 10: 109–16

See also, Vasculitides

KCT, Kaolin cephalin time, *see Coagulation studies*

Kelvin. SI **unit** of **temperature**. One kelvin (K) = 1/273.16 of the thermodynamic scale temperature of the **triple point** of water (point at which solid, liquid and gaseous water are at equilibrium). nK = (n – 273.16)°C.

[William Thomson (1824–1907), Irish-born Scottish physicist; became Lord Kelvin in 1892]

Kerley's lines. Opaque markings seen on the **CXR**:
- type A: thin 2–6-cm unbranched lines, radiating from the hila. Probably represent anastomoses between central and peripheral lymphatic vessels.
- type B: transverse lines, under 3 cm long, seen at the lung bases, especially costophrenic angles. Represent thickened interlobular septa, e.g. due to fluid (e.g. **pulmonary oedema**), fibrosis or tumour.
- type C: short reticular fine lines. Not commonly seen.

[Peter Kerley (1900–1978), Irish radiologist]

Ketamine hydrochloride. Phencyclidine derivative (Fig. 98), first used as an **iv anaesthetic agent** in 1965. An antagonist at **NMDA** receptors, inhibiting the **ascending reticular activating system** at thalamic level and the cortical part of the **limbic system**; also interacts with opioid, monoamine and cholinergic receptors. Recently described anti-inflammatory effects may be via reduced expression of **cytokines** (e.g. interleukin-6) by activated macrophages.
- Uses include:
  - **induction of anaesthesia**, traditionally in shocked patients. Produces a state of 'dissociative anaesthesia': intense analgesia with light sleep. Increased thalamic and limbic activity occurs, with dissociation from higher centres.
  - maintenance of anaesthesia as the sole agent, especially in **burns** and **trauma**, or short procedures (e.g. **radiotherapy** and radiological investigations). Widely used in battlefield and prehospital anaesthesia due to its relative preservation of upper airway reflexes. Its routine use at anaesthetic doses in adults is limited by psychomimetic **emergence phenomena** (*see later*).
  - **postoperative analgesia**: when given perioperatively, has a potent opioid-sparing effect, with reduced **PONV** and minimal side effects.
  - treatment of acute (e.g. post-amputation) and chronic neuropathic pain.
  - adjunct in **regional anaesthesia**: has local anaesthetic properties, and has been used for **spinal** and **epidural anaesthesia** within clinical trials; concerns over direct neurotoxicity have restricted its use beyond the trial setting.
  - **sedation** in the ICU.
  - possible neuroprotective effects via its NMDA receptor antagonism.

Also a drug of abuse ('K', 'Special K'), leading to its classification as a Class C drug under the **Misuse of Drugs Act** in 2006.

Commercially available as a racemic mixture of two isomers or as the pure S(+) enantiomer. The latter is 2–4 times as potent as the R(–) enantiomer and less

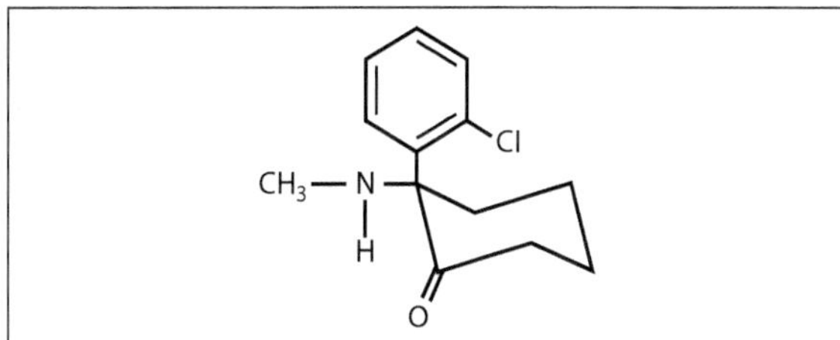

Fig. 98 Structure of ketamine

psychoactive, with a higher **clearance** and thus more rapid recovery.

Presented in 10, 50 and 100 mg/ml solutions, containing benzethonium chloride (the 10 mg/ml solution since 1997). pH is 3.5–5.5; pK_a 7.5. 12% bound to plasma albumin. Elimination **half-life** is about 3 h. Metabolised in the liver to norketamine, which is weakly active; excreted in urine.

- Effects:
  - iv induction: smooth, but slower than **thiopental** (about 30 s).
  - CVS/RS:
    - BP and heart rate usually increase; cardiac output is maintained. Changes are probably via direct myocardial and central sympathetic stimulation, and blockade of noradrenaline uptake by sympathetic nerve endings. Contraindicated in severe **ischaemic heart disease** and **hypertension.**
    - respiratory depression after rapid iv injection, but less than with other agents.
    - relative preservation of laryngeal and pharyngeal reflexes, although increased salivation is common. Airway obstruction, laryngospasm and aspiration may still occur.
    - bronchodilatation via a direct action and sympathomimetic effects.
  - CNS:
    - analgesia at subanaesthetic doses.
    - increased muscle tone, twitching, blinking and nystagmus.
    - increased **cerebral blood flow** and **ICP**; contraindicated in **pre-eclampsia** and severe intracranial pathology.
    - anterograde amnesia in some cases.
    - at anaesthetic doses may cause vivid dreams and **emergence phenomena**, e.g. unpleasant hallucinations. Usually less distressing in patients <15 or >65 years. Hallucinations may be reduced by **benzodiazepines**, and delirium by **butyrophenones. Physostigmine** has also been used. Preoperative counselling, opioid/hyoscine premedication and recovery in a quiet, darkened room may also reduce their incidence.
    - there are concerns that the NMDA-blocking activity of ketamine may induce neurodegeneration in the developing brain of infants and children; trials are ongoing.
  - other:
    - may cause nausea and vomiting. Salivation is increased.
    - may increase uterine tone.
    - increases **intraocular pressure**; contraindicated in open eye operations.
    - does not cause **histamine** release.
- Dosage (for racemic ketamine; dosages for S-ketamine are approximately 50% lower):
  - iv induction: 1–2 mg/kg. Effects last for 5–10 min. Supplementary doses 0.5 mg/kg.
  - im induction; 10 mg/kg. Acts in 3–5 min, lasting 20–30 min.
  - **sedation** (e.g. while performing regional techniques or on ICU): 2 mg/kg im, 10-mg increments iv, or 1–2 mg/kg/h infusion.
  - as an adjunct to general anaesthesia and postoperative opioid analgesia: 0.5 mg/kg slow iv bolus before skin incision, followed by 0.125–0.25 mg/kg iv boluses at 30-min intervals (in operations lasting >2 h, the last dose is given at least 60 min before the end of surgery, to prevent prolonged recovery).
  - to treat severe **asthma**: 0.5–2.5 mg/kg/h infusion.

Himmelseher S, Durieux ME (2005). Anesthesiology; 102: 211–20

See also, Isomerism

Ketanserin. **5-HT** antagonist, and weak **α_1-adrenergic receptor antagonist**. Also has class III antiarrhythmic properties. Has been used to prevent vasoconstriction and bronchospasm in **carcinoid syndrome**, and also to provide vasodilatation and hypotension in **cardiac surgery**.

Ketoacidosis. Metabolic **acidosis** due to accumulation of **ketone bodies** in plasma. Occurs when there is reduced availability of glucose (e.g. starvation, commonly seen in chronic **alcoholism**) or reduced ability to utilise glucose (e.g. diabetic ketoacidosis). The latter is associated with **hyperglycaemia**; the former is not.

- Features:
  - of acidosis, including hyperventilation and **hyperkalaemia**.
  - characteristic sweet smell on the patient's breath due to ketosis.
  - nausea and vomiting, **dehydration**.

Treatment includes rehydration, correction of electrolyte imbalance and **hypoglycaemia** if present. Diabetic ketoacidosis is treated with **insulin**.

See also, Diabetic coma

Ketobemidone hydrochloride. **Opioid analgesic drug**, with similar potency and properties to **morphine**. Mainly used in Scandinavia.

Ketoconazole. Imidazole **antifungal drug**, active against a wide range of fungi, including yeasts. No longer licensed for systemic treatment of fungal infections because of the risk of fatal hepatotoxicity. Suppresses synthesis of **glucocorticoids** and thus continues to be used for treatment of **Cushing's disease**.

- Dosage: 400–600 mg daily in divided doses.
- Side effects include hepatic impairment (occurs commonly; liver function must be monitored), GIT disturbances, gynaecomastia, rashes.

Ketone bodies. Acetone, acetoacetic acid and hydroxybutyric acid; formed from hepatic metabolism of free fatty acids released from adipose tissue. Normally utilised by brain, heart and other tissues as an energy source, keeping blood levels low. Levels increase when **fat** metabolism increases, especially when intracellular **glucose** is deficient, e.g. in **diabetes mellitus**, chronic **alcoholism**, starvation, and high fat/low **carbohydrate** diet. Increased levels may lead to **ketoacidosis**.

Ketoprofen **NSAID**, similar to **ibuprofen** but with greater incidence of GIT side effects.

- Dosage: 50–100 mg bd–qds up to 200 mg/day; may be given orally, pr or by deep gluteal im injection (the latter for up to 3 days). A modified release preparation (100–200 mg orally od) and a topical gel are also available.

Ketorolac trometamol/tromethamine. **NSAID**, licensed for short-term **postoperative analgesia**. Has a marked analgesic effect with little anti-inflammatory effect. Maximal plasma levels occur within 60 min of im injection and

5 min of iv injection, with **half-life** of 5–6 h. Pain relief may not occur until 30 min after injection. Over 99% protein-bound, with hepatic metabolism (reduced in the elderly). Over 95% of metabolites are excreted in urine, with ~6% in the faeces. Recommended parenteral doses have been reduced from those originally proposed, following adverse events, including death from GIT perforation/haemorrhage, asthma, anaphylaxis and renal failure. The datasheet specifies intraoperative and prophylactic use before surgery as contraindications because of the increased risk of bleeding.

- Dosage: 10 mg im/iv (the latter over at least 15 s) 4–6-hourly, up to 90 mg/day (60 mg in elderly or patients <50 kg) for up to 2 days. May also be given orally: 10 mg 4–6-hourly, up to 40 mg/day for up to 7 days.
- Side effects: as for NSAIDs. CNS effects, including drowsiness, dizziness, psychological changes and convulsions. Contraindications include peptic ulcer disease, coagulation abnormalities/anticoagulant drugs (including low-dose **heparin**), asthma, concurrent treatment with or allergy to any other NSAID, renal impairment, hypovolaemia, stroke, pregnancy and lactation.

Kety–Schmidt technique. Method of measuring **cerebral blood flow** using the **Fick principle**, using N_2O. 10% N_2O is inhaled for 10–15 min, and the jugular venous concentration is assumed to be equal to the brain concentration. Cerebral N_2O uptake is therefore calculated.
[Seymour S Kety (1915–2000) and Carl F Schmidt (1893–1988), US neuroscientists]

Key filling system. System for filling modern **vaporisers** with volatile anaesthetic agent, preventing filling with incorrect agent and supposedly reducing spillage and pollution by using closely fitting interlocking components.

- Composed of:
  - filler tube: a base at one end screws on to the bottle; the other end bears a plastic block that only fits into the correct vaporiser filling port.
  - collar around the neck of the bottle of volatile agent; protruding pegs slot into corresponding slots in the filler-tube base. Position of pegs and slots is specific for each agent.

Collar, filler-tube base and block are colour-coded for the particular agent (**halothane**, red; **enflurane**, orange; **isoflurane**, purple; **trichloroethylene**, blue; **methoxyflurane**, green) and the name of the agent is written on the filler-tube base.

Vaporisers for **desflurane** and **sevoflurane** do not utilise the key filling system, their bottles fitting to the vaporiser by an agent-specific attachment already on the bottle (desflurane) or fitted to it (sevoflurane).

See also, COSHH regulations; Environmental safety of anaesthetists

Kidney. Situated on the posterior abdominal wall, with the diaphragm and 11th and 12th ribs posteriorly. The renal hila are approximately level with the pylorus. Each kidney is about 10 cm long, 5 cm wide and 3 cm thick. Nerve supply is via the coeliac ganglion from T12 and L1. Blood supply is from the renal arteries that arise from the descending aorta, and venous drainage is via the renal veins into the inferior vena cava. **Renal blood flow** is 1200 ml/min (22% of cardiac output), about 400 ml/100 g/min. O_2 consumption is 20 ml/min, or 6 ml/100 g/min.

Composed of outer cortex and inner medulla, forming pyramids. Functional unit is the **nephron**, with accompanying arterioles and capillaries.

- Functions:
  - filtration of plasma and excretion of waste products of **metabolism**, while maintaining water, **osmolality**, electrolyte and acid–base homeostasis.
  - secretion of renin.
  - secretion of **erythropoietin**.
  - formation of 1,25-dihydroxycholecalciferol (important in **calcium** homeostasis).
  - metabolism and excretion of drugs.
- May be affected by anaesthesia/surgery:
  - drug effects, e.g. **methoxyflurane**, **diuretics**.
  - alteration of renal blood flow, e.g. **hypotension**, **aortic aneurysm** repair.
  - renal impairment following incompatible **blood transfusion**, severe **jaundice**, **sepsis**, obstetric emergencies or **crush syndrome**.

See also, Acid–base balance; Acute kidney injury; Fluid balance; Renal failure; Renal transplantation; Renin/angiotensin system

Killian, Gustav (1860–1921). German laryngologist; published extensively on the structure and function of the **larynx**. A former student of **Kirstein**, he helped popularise direct **laryngoscopy**. Also performed the first translaryngeal removal of a foreign body from the right main bronchus in 1897, using a rigid oesophagoscope and **cocaine** local anaesthesia, thus pioneering **bronchoscopy**.

Kilogram. SI **unit** of **mass**. The standard kilogram is the mass of a cylindrical piece of platinum–iridium alloy kept at Sèvres, France.

Kilogram weight. Weight of a **mass** of 1 **kilogram** subjected to standard Earth gravity. Also called kilogram force.

$$\begin{aligned} 1\ \text{kg wt (or kgf) due to gravity} &= 1\ \text{kg} \times 9.81\ \text{m/s}^2 \\ &= 9.81\ \textbf{newton} \end{aligned}$$

Kinins. Vasodilator peptides derived from precursor molecules (kininogens) by the action of **kallikreins**. Involved in many inflammatory and immune reactions, and possibly in **shock**. Also thought to be involved in **carcinoid syndrome**. Bradykinin is the main plasma kinin, causing vasodilatation and increased vascular permeability. **Glucocorticoids** inhibit their release. Broken down by angiotensin converting enzyme, mainly in the lung. Elimination **half-life** is less than 15 s.

Kirstein, Alfred (1863–1922). German laryngologist; described the first direct **laryngoscopy** in 1895. His **laryngoscopes** could be placed anterior or posterior to the epiglottis. Stressed the importance of the 'sniffing the morning air position' for laryngoscopy. Also suggested translaryngeal removal of bronchial foreign bodies as being easier than via tracheostomy.
Hirsch NP, Smith GB, Hirsch PO (1986). Anaesthesia; 41: 42–5

Kite, Charles (1768–1811). English doctor, practising in Gravesend, Kent. Awarded the silver medal by the Humane Society (now Royal Humane Society) in 1787 for his *Essay on the Recovery of the Apparently Dead*, later published as a book. Described oro- and nasotracheal catheterisation for lung inflation, and suggested laryngospasm as a cause for hypoxia in drowning. Also described successful resuscitation of a young girl by passing an electric current across her thorax.

Klippel–Feil syndrome. Inherited condition characterised by congenitally fused cervical vertebrae; subdivided according to the extent of vertebral involvement:
- type I: several vertebrae (cervical and upper thoracic) form a single unit.
- type II: one or two cervical vertebrae affected only.
- type III: types I or II with thoracic or lumbar abnormalities too.

Most commonly restricted to C2–3 and C5–6. Associated with scoliosis, other skeletal malformations, cardiac and genitourinary abnormalities. Typically, the patient has a short neck with limited movement and a low posterior hairline. Both autosomal dominant and recessive inheritance has been suggested for different subtypes.
- Anaesthetic considerations:
  - cervical instability.
  - difficult intubation.
  - **epidural** and **spinal anaesthesia** may be technically difficult.
  - related to abnormalities of other systems.

[Maurice Klippel (1858–1942) and Andre Feil (1884–1955), French neurologists]

Naguib M, Farag H, Ibrahim AEW (1986). Can Anesth Soc J; 33: 66–70

Knee, nerve blocks. Blockade of nerves at or near the knee joint, performed for surgery to the lower leg and foot. Blocks may be performed using **ultrasound** guidance or **nerve stimulator** techniques.
- Nerves that may be blocked (*see Fig. 69;* **Femoral nerve block**):
  - tibial nerve (L4–S3): terminal branch of the sciatic nerve; supplies the anteromedial part of the sole of the foot via plantar branches. In the **popliteal fossa**, the nerve lies superficial and lateral to the popliteal vessels, with vein medially and artery most medial.

    With the patient prone and knee extended, a needle is inserted in the midline of the popliteal fossa, level with the femoral condyles. 5–10 ml **local anaesthetic agent** is injected at a depth of 2–3 cm.
  - common peroneal (L4–S2): terminal branch of the sciatic nerve; supplies the dorsum of the foot via its superficial peroneal branch, and the area between the first and second toes via the deep peroneal branch. The region posterior to the head of the fibula is infiltrated with 5 ml solution.
  - sciatic (L4–S3): may be blocked before it divides into tibial and common peroneal nerves above the popliteal fossa, at a point 7 cm cranial to the skin crease behind the knee, and 1 cm lateral to the midline. 5–10 ml solution is injected at a depth of 3–5 cm.
  - saphenous (L4–5): a continuation of the femoral nerve; supplies the medial part of the lower leg, ankle and foot. May be blocked by infiltration from the medial border of the tibial tuberosity to the posterior edge of the tibia (taking care to avoid the saphenous vein).

See also, Adductor canal block

Koller, Carl (1857–1944). Austrian ophthalmologist; first described the use of **local anaesthetic agent** (**cocaine**) for a surgical operation (for glaucoma) in Vienna in 1884, having previously investigated the drug with **Freud**. This was reported by a colleague at an ophthalmological congress in Heidelberg on the following day. Disappointed with his subsequent career progress, he emigrated to New York in 1888.

Goerig M, Bacon D, Zundert A (2012). Reg Anesth Pain Med; 37: 318–24

Korotkoff sounds. Sounds heard during auscultation over the brachial artery, while a proximal cuff is slowly deflated from above systolic pressure. Thought to result from turbulent flow within the artery, causing vessel wall vibration and resonance. Used in **arterial BP measurement.** Three phases were originally described by Korotkoff; these were subsequently increased to five:
- phase I: intermittent tapping sound, corresponding to the heartbeat. Represents systolic pressure.
- phase II: sounds quieten or even disappear (auscultatory gap). The significance is unknown, but it emphasises the importance of palpating the artery before auscultation, in order to ensure that the absence of sounds is because the pressure is above systolic, and not within this 'silent' gap
- phase III: sounds become louder again.
- phase IV: sounds suddenly become muffled.
- phase V: sounds disappear.

Argument over whether diastolic pressure is best recorded at phase IV or V continues (the latter being more reproducible); traditionally phase IV is used in the UK, phase V in the USA. Recording of both has been suggested, e.g. 120/80/75.

[Nicolai Korotkoff (1874–1920), Russian physician]

Krebs cycle, *see Tricarboxylic acid cycle*

Kuhn, Franz (1866–1929). German physician; wrote extensively on **tracheal intubation** for anaesthesia. Described tracheal insufflation in 1900 and nasotracheal intubation in 1902.

Thierbach A (2001). Resuscitation; 48: 193–7

Kussmaul breathing (Air hunger). **Hyperventilation** originally described in diabetic hyperglycaemic **ketoacidosis.** Caused by stimulation of central **chemoreceptors** by hydrogen ions. Occurs in severe metabolic **acidosis** from any cause.

[Adolf Kussmaul (1822–1909), German physician]

Kussmaul's sign, *see Cardiac tamponade*

Kyphoscoliosis
- Definitions:
  - kyphosis: posterior curvature of spine.
  - scoliosis: lateral curvature.

There may also be rotational deformity.

May be associated with congenital skeletal, muscular or neurological abnormalities. Idiopathic scoliosis develops in childhood and is the most common form. The angle of curvature is measured from x-rays of the spine (Fig. 99) and an angle >10 degrees is abnormal. There may be rotation of the vertebrae, with the spinous processes turned inward towards the concavity of the curve. Thoracic, rib and chest wall deformity may cause restriction of ventilation, especially if the curve exceeds 65 degrees. Surgical fixation is increasingly performed early using metal Harrington rods, which allow progressive distraction of the vertebrae as the child grows.

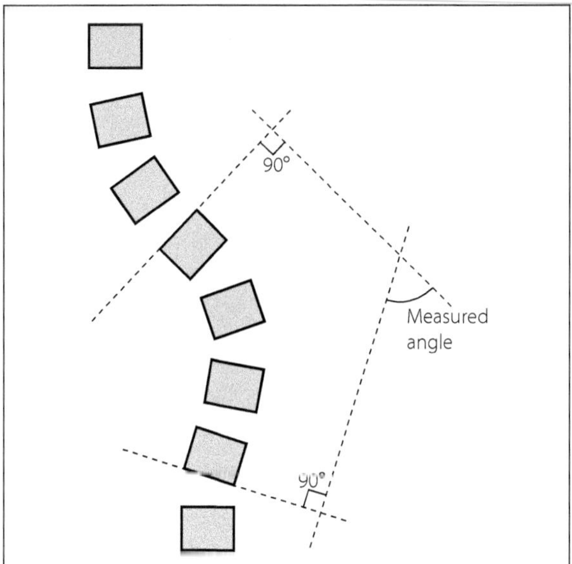

Fig. 99 Measurement of the angle of curvature in scoliosis

- Anaesthetic management:
  - preoperatively:
    - assessment for associated disease.
    - **MH** may be commoner in this group.
    - assessment of RS: lung volumes and **compliance** are reduced; the main defect is restrictive. **$\dot{V}/\dot{Q}$ mismatch** may be present. Repeated aspiration may occur in neuromuscular disease. **CXR, lung function tests** and arterial **blood gas interpretation** may be useful.
    - chronic **hypoxaemia** may lead to **pulmonary hypertension** and **cor pulmonale**.
    - preoperative **physiotherapy** and antibiotics may be required.
  - perioperatively:
    - tracheal intubation may be difficult, especially if the patient is unable to lie flat.
    - surgery may be prolonged, with risk of major blood loss and hypothermia.
    - transthoracic surgery may involve anterior or posterior approaches.
    - **hypotensive anaesthesia** is advocated by some, to reduce blood loss and ease surgery. Others argue that the risk of spinal cord ischaemia precludes this. Careful positioning of the patient is required to prevent pressure on the abdominal inferior vena cava.
    - risk of cord damage during distraction of **vertebrae** may be assessed by the **wake-up test** or monitoring of **evoked potentials**.
    - access to the patient may be restricted.
  - postoperatively: ventilatory failure is possible; close monitoring is required. CXR is usual to exclude **pneumothorax**. An epidural catheter may be placed by the surgeon for postoperative analgesia.

Central neural blockade (e.g. for labour) may be difficult in scoliotic patients. The incidence of accidental dural puncture during epidural anaesthesia may be increased, and its efficacy may be reduced following prior surgery.

[Paul R Harrington (1911–1980), Texas surgeon]

Soundararajan N, Cunliffe M (2007). Br J Anaesth; 99: 86–94

L

Labat, Gaston (1877–1934). Anaesthetist, born in the Seychelles; worked in Paris and at the Mayo Clinic and New York University, USA. Pioneer of regional anaesthesia, writing a classic text on the subject in 1922. Founded the American Society of Regional Anaesthesia in 1923.
Brown DL, Winnie AP (1992). Reg Anesth; 17: 249–62

Labetalol hydrochloride. Combined β- and **α-adrenergic receptor antagonist**, with ratio of activities usually quoted between 2:1 and 5:1, respectively. Selective for α_1-receptors, but non-selective at β-receptors, with some **intrinsic sympathomimetic activity**. Used to treat severe **hypertension** and **pre-eclampsia**, and in **hypotensive anaesthesia**. 90% protein-bound. **Half-life** is 4 h. Metabolised in the liver and excreted in urine and faeces. Undergoes extensive **first-pass metabolism** when given orally.

- Dosage:
  - 5–50 mg iv by slow injection, up to 200 mg. Effects occur usually within 5 min, lasting 6–18 h.
  - 10–200 mg/h infusion.
  - 50–100 mg orally bd; increased up to a maximum 2.4 g/24 h.
- Side effects:
  - as for β-adrenergic receptor antagonists. Liver damage and **jaundice** may occur rarely.

Labour, active management of. Term referring to a collection of medical interventions and management, including strict diagnostic criteria for the onset and course of labour, artificial rupture of membranes, early use of **oxytocic drugs** and continuous obstetric input so that the duration of labour is limited. Despite claims of improved outcome, evidence is at best conflicting.

Medical intervention depends on the plot of cervical dilatation and descent of the fetal head against time, usually starting from presentation in labour. The curve obtained is compared with curves derived from studies of normal labours, primiparous or multiparous as appropriate (partograms). The normal curve is composed of latent (up to 3–4 cm cervical dilatation) and active (until 10 cm dilatation) phases. Delay in progress is represented by a lag of more than 2 h to the right of the expected curve.

- Different patterns of delay may occur:
  - prolonged latent phase: its relevance is disputed by some obstetricians, because the onset of labour is variable and difficult to define. Others claim up to 30% instrumental rate and up to 15% caesarean section (CS) rate. More common in primiparous women.
  - primary delay: i.e., slow progress of the active phase, e.g. due to ineffective uterine contraction. Instrumental rate is 7%–8%, CS rate 4%–5%. More common in primiparous women.
  - secondary arrest: normal progress to 7–8 cm, then delay. Commonly due to malposition. Instrumental rate is 2%–3%, CS rate 1%–2%.

Cephalopelvic disproportion may cause delay at any stage, but especially secondary arrest. Most other causes are treated successfully with oxytocic drugs (with continuous **fetal monitoring**).

Epidural blockade is often instituted to provide analgesia for augmented contractions, possibly to restore co-ordinated uterine activity, and in case of operative delivery.

Lack breathing system, *see Coaxial anaesthetic breathing systems*

Lacosamide. Functionalised amino acid anticonvulsant drug, introduced in 2008. Used as adjunctive therapy to treat partial epilepsy with or without secondary generalised seizures. Has also been used to treat convulsive, non-convulsive and refractory **status epilepticus** and pain due to diabetic neuropathy. Acts by slow inactivation of neuronal voltage-gated sodium channels.

- Dosage:
  - initially 100 mg orally/iv bd, followed by weekly increases of 50 mg bd up to 150–200 mg bd.
  - for status epilepticus: 200–400 mg iv bolus over 3–5 min.
- Side effects: visual disturbance, dizziness, drowsiness, nausea and vomiting, confusion, worsening of cardiac conduction abnormalities.

β-Lactams. Group of substances containing the 4 atom β-lactam ring (Fig. 100). Include the **penicillins**, **cephalosporins**, the monobactam **aztreonam** and the **carbapenems**. The β-lactam ring is a site of breakdown by bacterial β-lactamase, leading to **bacterial resistance**.

Lactate ($CH_3CH(OH)CO_2^-$). Byproduct of anaerobic metabolism of the products of **glycolysis**. **Hypoxia** prevents aerobic metabolism of pyruvate to CO_2 and water (via the **tricarboxylic acid cycle**); instead lactic acid is formed, dissociating to lactate and H^+ with consequent increases in plasma lactate/pyruvate ratio (normally 10) and plasma lactate (normally 0.3–1.3 mmol/l). The liver metabolises 70% of lactate and the rest is converted to pyruvate by mitochondria-rich skeletal and cardiac muscle.
See also, Lactic acidosis

Lactic acidosis. Metabolic **acidosis** accompanied by raised plasma **lactate** levels.

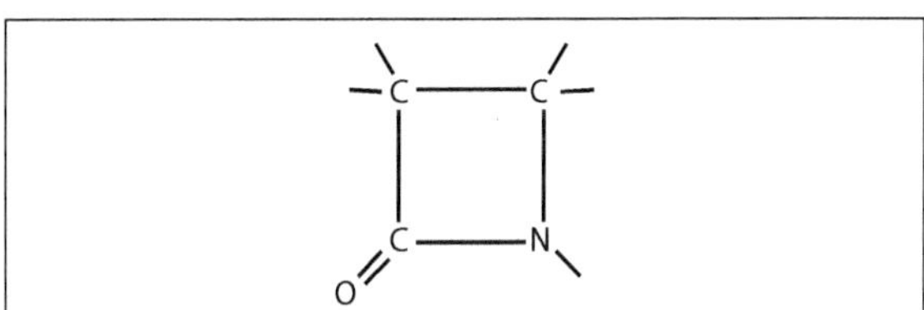

Fig. 100 Structure of β-lactam ring

- Causes are divided into:
  - those with overt tissue hypoxia and anaerobic respiration (type A):
    - severe **hypoxaemia**.
    - severe **anaemia**.
    - **shock/haemorrhage/hypotension**.
    - **cardiac failure**.
    - severe **exercise**.
    - **carbon monoxide poisoning**.
    - mesenteric ischaemia.
  - those without apparent initial tissue hypoxia (type B), further subdivided into:
    - **hepatic failure/renal failure** (delayed clearance of lactate).
    - severe infection and **sepsis** (where lactate levels are useful for diagnosis, assessing efficacy of treatment to reverse tissue hypoperfusion and prognosis).
    - thiamine deficiency, alcoholic and diabetic **ketoacidosis** (pyruvate dehydrogenase dysfunction).
    - **cyanide poisoning**, **biguanides**, **salicylates**, **sodium valproate** (uncoupling of oxidative phosphorylation).
    - exercise, severe infection, seizures, **β-adrenergic receptor agonists**, fructose and sorbitol in **TPN**, malignancies (increased glycolysis such that the aerobic pathway is overwhelmed).
    - **glycogen storage disorders**, **inborn errors of metabolism**.

In critical illness, type A and B causes frequently coexist (e.g. hypoxaemia with severe infection and increased glycolysis).
- Treatment:
  - directed at the underlying cause (with supportive therapy).
  - minimisation of drugs that may exacerbate the problem (e.g. **adrenaline**).
  - cautious use of **bicarbonate** (increased lactate levels have followed its use).
  - amine buffers, insulin and glucose infusions, and stimulation of pyruvate dehydrogenase with sodium dichloroacetate have also been tried.

Kraut JA, Madias NE (2014). N Engl J Med; 371: 2309–19

Laevobupivacaine, *see Bupivacaine*

Lambert–Beer law, *see Beer–Lambert law*

Lamotrigine. Anticonvulsant drug, blocks voltage-gated sodium channels and thus inhibits the presynaptic release of **glutamate** and other excitatory **neurotransmitters**. Used for partial or secondary generalised seizures, either alone or in combination with other anticonvulsants. Has also been used for the treatment of bipolar disorders and in chronic **pain management**. Rapidly absorbed after oral administration with peak plasma concentrations at 2.5 h; **half-life** is 24–36 h. Plasma concentration is increased by **sodium valproate** but decreased by drugs causing **enzyme induction** (e.g. other anticonvulsants). It also induces its own metabolism.
- Dosage: depends on the drug combination used; generally starts at 25 mg/day, increased as necessary up to 500 mg/day, orally.
- Side effects: rash and serious skin reactions, fever, malaise, blood dyscrasias, hepatic impairment, visual disturbances, GIT upset.

Lanreotide. Long-acting **somatostatin** analogue; actions and effects are similar to those of **octreotide**. Used in the management of **acromegaly** and **carcinoid syndrome**.

Lansoprazole. Proton pump inhibitor; actions and effects are similar to those of **omeprazole**.
- Dosage: 15–30 mg orally od.
- Side effects: as for omeprazole.

LAP, *see Left atrial pressure*

Laparoscopy. Minimally invasive surgery in which an endoscope (laparoscope) is inserted into the abdominal cavity via a small incision, allowing the abdominal and pelvic organs to be seen. Originally used for diagnostic gynaecological procedures, now commonly performed for more extensive procedures (e.g. hysterectomy) and other types of surgery, e.g. cholecystectomy, gastric banding. Although benefits include faster recovery, reduced morbidity and postoperative pain and wound infection, patients may be exposed to prolonged operating times. Requires induction of a pneumoperitoneum, usually with CO_2. Specific complications are related to:
  - gas insufflation:
    - trauma to abdominal viscera (including stomach if previously distended with gas during **IPPV** via facemask) and great vessels when the trocar is introduced or gas insufflated.
    - intravascular insufflation resulting in gas emboli. CO_2 is rapidly absorbed from the blood, reducing the size of emboli.
    - subcutaneous/mediastinal emphysema and **pneumothorax**.
    - bradycardia or asystole due to vagal stimulation.
    - caval compression reducing venous return if intraperitoneal pressure exceeds 3–4 kPa. Higher pressures may compress the aorta.
    - gas may splint the diaphragm and reduce lung expansion.
    - raised intra-abdominal pressure may increase risk of regurgitation and **aspiration of gastric contents**. High incidence of **PONV**.
    - **ICP** is increased.
    - CO_2 may be extensively absorbed across the peritoneum, requiring increased alveolar ventilation to maintain normocapnia.
    - postoperative pain or discomfort, typically referred to the shoulder tip, due to presence of subdiaphragmatic gas; incidence reduced if gas is xpelled from abdominal cavity at the end of the procedure.
    - explosion through ignition of intestinal methane by diathermy has been reported.
  - patient's position: for upper GIT procedures patients are positioned head-up, which may encourage venous pooling in the legs and further hinder venous return. For gynaecological procedures the semi-lithotomy position is used, which may be associated with:
    - reduced **FRC** and diaphragmatic splinting, with risk of atelectasis, **hypoxaemia** and **hypoventilation**.
    - increased risk of regurgitation.
    - increased venous return when the legs are raised. Pooling of blood in the legs may occur when they are lowered afterwards, with resultant hypotension.
  - surgical procedure:
    - bleeding may go unnoticed if not in the immediate area being worked on.

- large amounts of irrigating fluid may be used, with the risk of **hypothermia** if not warmed.
- sudden coughing during upper GIT surgery may risk damage to vital structures (e.g. bile ducts, vessels).
- may involve **laser surgery**.

Other considerations include patient co-morbidity; e.g. **obesity** in patients for gastric banding. The above complications lead many anaesthetists to choose tracheal intubation and IPPV as the technique of choice, although a **SAD** may also be used for short gynaecological procedures in suitable patients.

- Recommended maximal safe limits for insufflation:
  - 4 L/min.
  - 3–5 L total gas volume.
  - 3 kPa maximal intraperitoneal pressure.

Gynaecological laparoscopy may also be performed using local anaesthesia, with infiltration of the abdominal puncture site. Discomfort may result from peritoneal stretching and pneumoperitoneum. Use of epidural/spinal anaesthesia has been described but is rarely attempted because of the above considerations.

Oti C, Mahendran M, Sabir N (2016). Br J Hosp Med; 77: 24–8

Laplace's law. For a hollow distensible structure:

$$P = \frac{T}{R_1} + \frac{T}{R_2}$$

where P = transmural pressure
T = tension in the wall
R_1 = radius of curvature in one direction
R_2 = radius of curvature in the other direction

For a cylinder, one radius = infinity; therefore $P = \frac{T}{R}$

For a sphere, both radii are equal; therefore $P = 2\frac{T}{R}$

- Physiological/clinical importance:
  - cylinders:
    - arteriolar smooth muscle response to fluctuating intraluminal pressure: wall tension varies in order to maintain constant radius and blood flow (one theory of the mechanism of **autoregulation**).
    - as intraluminal pressure in arterioles or airways falls, or external pressure rises, there is a critical closing pressure across the wall at which collapse may occur. In the lungs, this may occur during **forced expiration**, limiting expiratory air flow.
  - spheres:
    - ventricular cardiac muscle must generate greater tension when the heart is dilated than when of normal size, in order to produce the same intraventricular pressure. Thus an enlarged failing heart must contract more forcibly to sustain BP; hence the benefit of reducing **preload**.
    - in the lungs, alveoli would tend to collapse as they became smaller, were it not for **surfactant**, which reduces surface tension.
    - if the outlet of an **anaesthetic breathing system** is obstructed, the **reservoir bag** distends, thus limiting the dangerous build-up of pressure that would occur within a non-distensible bag.

[Pierre-Simon Laplace (1749–1827), French scientist]

Larrey, Baron Dominique Jean (1766–1842). French surgeon-in-chief to Napoleon. Employed **refrigeration anaesthesia** in 1807, and again in 1812 during the Russian campaign to allow painless amputations in half-frozen soldiers. Also employed **triage** and horse-drawn 'flying ambulances' to transport the injured to field hospitals outside the battle zone. Supported **Hickman** when the latter presented his experiments on 'suspended animation' to the French Academy in 1828.

[Napoleon Bonaparte (1769–1821), French Emperor]

Baker D, Cazalaà JB, Carli P (2005). Resuscitation; 66: 259–62

Laryngeal mask (LM). Generic term for **SADs** that are based on the original laryngeal mask airway (LMA), invented by Brain and introduced in 1988 for supporting and maintaining the airway without tracheal intubation (Fig. 101a) (*see Supraglottic airway device* for indications and insertion technique). The LMA revolutionised general anaesthesia by enabling a third option between holding a facemask and intubating the trachea, the concept subsequently developed by Brain himself and other manufacturers/designers into a wide range of devices, all consisting of the same basic components (supraglottic inflatable cuff attached to wide-bore breathing tube). Does not protect against **aspiration of gastric contents**. May be removed before the patient wakes, or left in position. A bite block is required to prevent obstruction or damage by/to the teeth.

Available in several sizes from 1 (neonates <5 kg) to 6 (adults >100 kg), each with its own maximum recommended volume for cuff inflation, although a maximum cuff pressure of 60 cmH_2O has been suggested as more logical than maximal volumes.

Also available with reinforced tubes to prevent kinking. Other developments of the original LMA (LMA Classic) include: the LMA ProSeal, which features a larger cuff (providing a better seal), and a gastric drainage port that opens at the tip of the cuff (Fig. 101b); the LMA Supreme, similar to the ProSeal but disposable and incorporating a bite block (Fig. 101c); and the LMA Fastrach (previously called intubating LMA), in which the tube is shorter and rigid, with a sharp angle. In the latter, the bars covering the laryngeal aperture are replaced by a single flap that lifts the epiglottis when a tracheal tube (a soft silicone one specifically provided for the purpose) is passed blindly through it (Fig. 101d). The LMA CTrach incorporates a small display screen mounted at the proximal end of the airway so that intubation can be observed in real time. The LMA Gastro is designed to allow endoscopy.

Previously washed and autoclaved between uses; disposable, single-use LMs are now widely used. (N.B. 'LMA' refers to one manufacturer's products [The Laryngeal Mask Company Ltd]; similar devices are made by other manufacturers but strictly should be referred to as 'laryngeal masks', not LMAs).

[Archie Brain, British anaesthetist]

Laryngeal nerve blocks, *see Intubation, awake*

Laryngeal nerves. Derived from the **vagus nerves**:

- superior laryngeal nerve:
  - arises at the base of the **skull** and passes deep to the **carotid arteries**.
  - divides into internal and external branches below and anterior to the greater cornua of the hyoid bone.

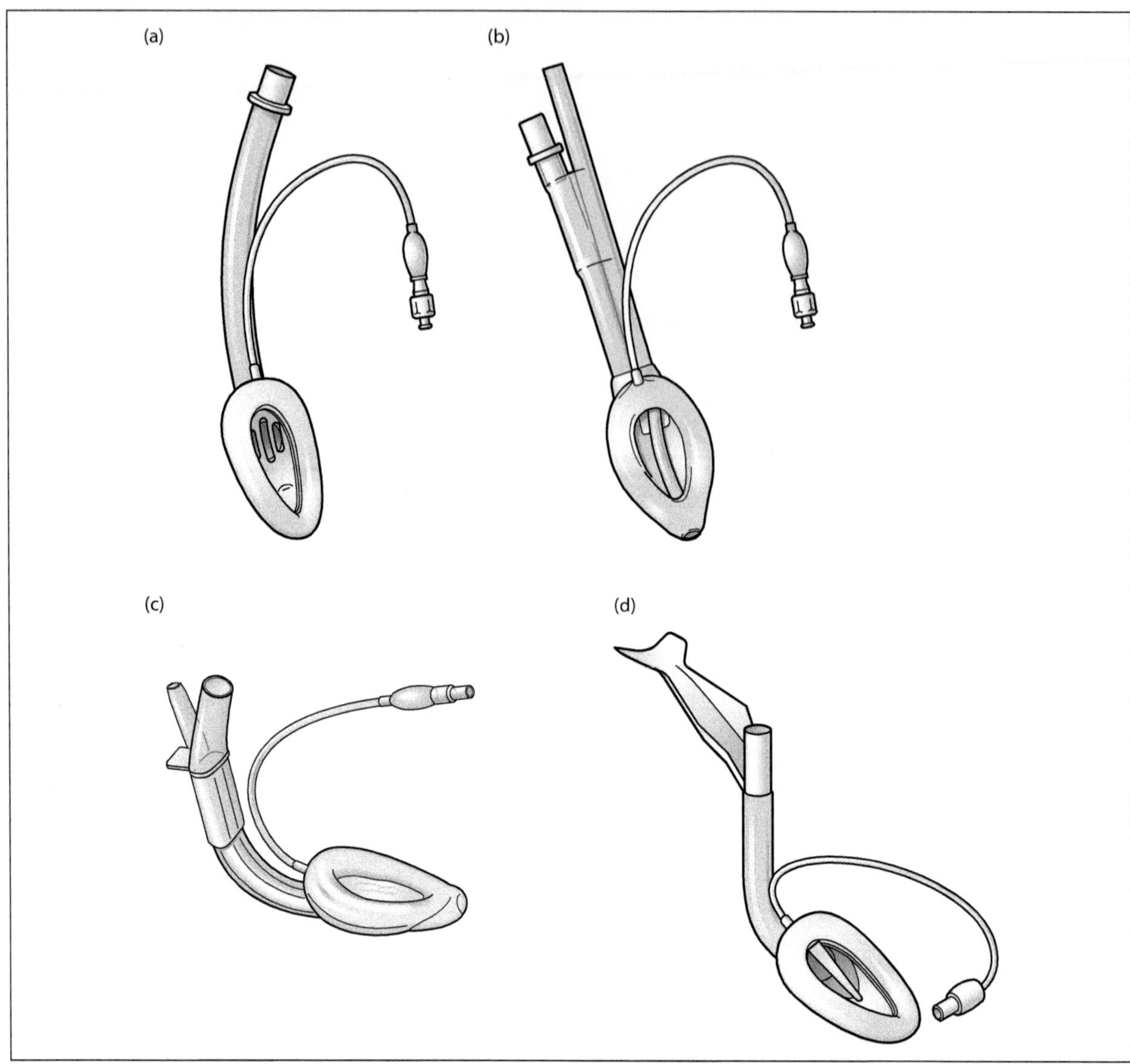

Fig. 101 Types of LMA: (a) Classic; (b) ProSeal; (c) Supreme; (d) Fastrach

   - the internal laryngeal nerve pierces the thyrohyoid membrane with the superior laryngeal vessels, supplying the mucous membrane of the **larynx** down to the vocal cords. Special sensory afferent fibres (taste) from the vallecula run with the internal laryngeal nerve.
   - the external laryngeal nerve passes deep to the superior thyroid artery, supplying cricothyroid muscle and the inferior constrictor muscle of the pharynx.
- recurrent laryngeal nerve:
   - on the left, arises anterior to the ligamentum arteriosus, passes below and behind it and the aorta and ascends in the neck (*see Fig. 116;* **Neck, cross-sectional anatomy**).
   - on the right, given off at the right subclavian artery, passing below and behind it and ascending in the neck.
   - in the neck, ascends in the groove between the **oesophagus** posteriorly and trachea anteriorly.
   - enters the larynx posterior to the thyrocricoid joints, deep to the inferior constrictor. Supplies all the intrinsic laryngeal muscles except cricothyroid, and the mucous membrane of the larynx below the vocal cords.

Sympathetic branches pass with the arterial supply.

- Effects of nerve damage:
   - superior laryngeal: slack cord and weak voice.
   - recurrent laryngeal (partial): cord held in the midline because the abductors are affected more than the adductors (Semon's law). The voice is hoarse. If bilateral, severe airway obstruction may occur.
   - recurrent laryngeal (complete): cord held midway between the midline and abducted position. If bilateral, the cords may be snapped shut during inspiration, causing stridor. The voice is lost.
   - if one side only is affected, the contralateral cord may move across and restore the voice.

Branches may be damaged during surgery (e.g. thyroidectomy) and tracheal intubation, especially if undue force is used or the **cuff** is inflated within the larynx. The recurrent laryngeal nerve may be involved by lesions in the neck, thorax or mediastinum (on the left).

The superior laryngeal nerve may be blocked to allow awake tracheal intubation.
[Sir Felix Semon (1849–1921), German-born English laryngologist]
See also, Intubation, awake

Laryngeal reflex. **Laryngospasm** in response to stimulation of the laryngeal/hypopharyngeal mucosa. Afferent pathway is via the **laryngeal nerves, vagus** and **brainstem.**

Laryngeal tube, *see Airways*

Laryngoscope. Instrument used to perform **laryngoscopy**. The first direct-vision laryngoscope was invented by **Kirstein** and later developed by **Jackson**; the principle was later modified by **Magill**, **Macintosh** and others.

- Most consist of:
  - handle:
    - contains a battery power source.
    - fibreoptic laryngoscopes have batteries and bulb in the handle, with transmission of light along a fibreoptic bundle set in the blade.
    - short or adjustable handles are available; smaller, lighter handles are usually used for **paediatric anaesthesia.**
  - blade:
    - usually set at right angles to the handle.
    - many different **laryngoscope blades** have been described, most of them interchangeable when standard attachments are used.
    - older type of attachment: secured by screwing a pin through the handle and blade seatings (Longworth fitting). Newer forms employ a 'hook-on' attachment at the base of the blade, locked on to the handle by a spring-loaded ball-bearing.

Devices incorporating viewing channels or with video cameras in the blade (**videolaryngoscopes**) allow either placement of the device in the trachea under visual control, with advancement of the tracheal tube over it, or identification of the glottis and observation of the tube's passage through the vocal cords. The image may be viewed by looking through an eyepiece, attachment to a camera/video system or via a screen incorporated into the device itself. Flexible **fibreoptic instruments** are also available.

Surgical (suspension) laryngoscopes resemble Jackson's more closely; they are composed of a viewing tube with a right-angled handle, the two components together forming three sides of a rectangle. They are illuminated by an external light source attached to the proximal end of the tube.

Concerns over cross-infection, especially transmission of variant **Creutzfeldt–Jakob disease**, have led to the widespread use of disposable laryngoscope blades, laryngoscopes or blade covers/sheaths.
[Longworth Scientific Instrument Co. Ltd, original name for Penlon Ltd].

Laryngoscope blades. Parts of **laryngoscopes** inserted into the mouth.

- Consist of:
  - base for attachment to handle.
  - tongue: straight or curved; the former is designed for placement posterior to the epiglottis, the latter for anterior placement. The tip is usually blunt and thickened to reduce trauma.
  - web: forms a shelf along one edge of the tongue, connecting the latter to the flange. Incorporates electric connections and bulb (or fibreoptic bundle). Connection channels are completely removable in older models, and fixed to the web in newer ones.
  - flange: parallel to the tongue; usually only present for the proximal one- to two-thirds of the blade.

Most are designed for use with the laryngoscope handle held in the left hand; i.e., the tongue is pushed to the left side of the patient's mouth by the flange and web.

- Common varieties (Fig. 102a):
  - **Macintosh** (1943): tongue, web and flange form a reverse Z shape in cross-section. The most commonly used blade in the UK; also popular in the USA. Available in large adult, adult, child and baby sizes; the latter size was not designed by Macintosh and was criticised by him as being anatomically incorrect. A 'left-handed' version is available, for use when anatomical features of the airway require insertion of the tracheal tube from the left side of the mouth instead of the right. The McCoy blade (1993) is hinged at the tip, and is controlled by a lever on the laryngoscope handle. It allows elevation of the epiglottis while reducing the amount of force required during laryngoscopy. Although it may make a difficult laryngoscopy easier, it may also make an easy one more difficult.
  - polio Macintosh (1950s): mounted at 135 degrees to the handle, to allow intubation in patients confined to iron lung ventilators (e.g. in the Scandinavian polio epidemics of the 1950s). Useful when insertion of the blade into the mouth is hindered, e.g. by barrel chest, enlarged breasts, especially in obstetrics.
  - **Magill** (1926): U-shaped in cross-section.
  - Miller (1941): similar to Magill's, but with a curved tip and flatter flange and web, requiring less mouth opening for insertion. Available in six sizes from premature baby to large adult. Popular in the USA.
  - Wisconsin (1941): bigger than Magill's, with the bulb nearer the tip. Available in similar sizes to Miller's blade. Popular in the USA.
  - Soper (1947): straight version of the Macintosh blade. The small transverse slot near the tip was designed to prevent the epiglottis slipping off the blade. Available in adult, child and baby sizes.
  - Bellhouse (1988): angled along its length to give the advantage of a straight blade, while the end nearest the anaesthetist is brought anteriorly to avoid obstruction of the anaesthetist's view. May be fitted with an optical prism to enable an indirect view of the glottis when a direct view is impossible.
- Specific paediatric blades (Fig. 102b):
  - Robertshaw (1962): straight tongue with gently curving tip; the flange is folded inwards over the tongue. Available in infant and neonatal sizes.
  - Seward (1957): similar to Robertshaw's but with the flange folded outwards. Available in child and baby sizes.
  - Oxford infant (1952): straight tongue with slightly curved tip. Available in one size. Useful for intubation in children with cleft palate.
- Others:
  - **Guedel** and Flagg (1928): similar to Magill's, but with the bulb at the tip. Guedel's is set at an acute angle to the handle.
  - Bowen–Jackson (1952): similar to Macintosh's but with a cleft tip, designed to straddle the glossoepiglottic fold.
  - Siker (1956): angled blade incorporating a mirror at the angle.

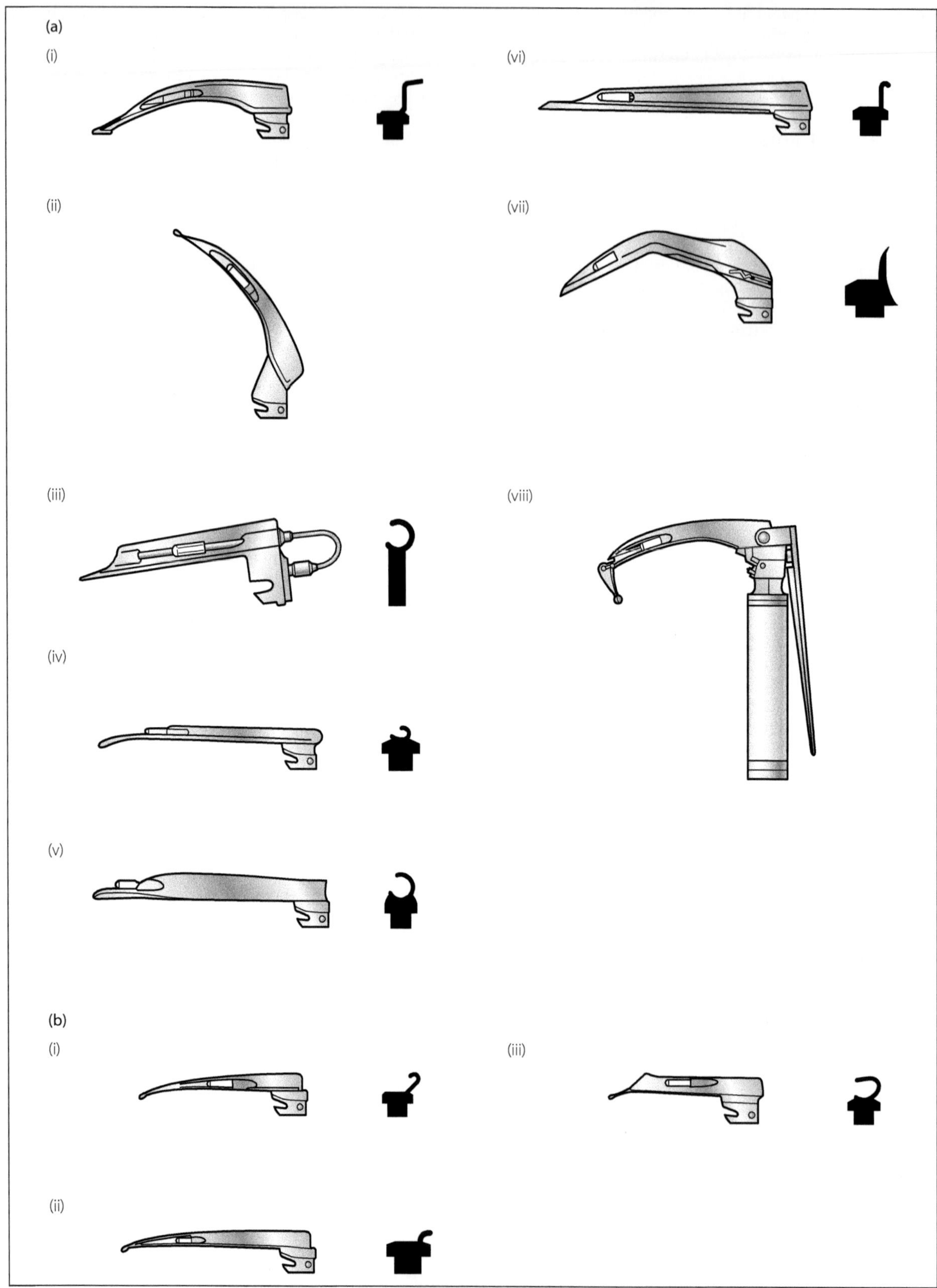

Fig. 102 Laryngoscope blades (not to scale). (a) Adult/paediatric: (i) Macintosh; (ii) polio Macintosh; (iii) Magill; (iv) Miller; (v) Wisconsin; (vi) Soper; (vii) Bellhouse; (viii) McCoy. (b) paediatric only: (i) Robertshaw; (ii) Seward; (iii) Oxford infant

- Bizzarri–Giuffrida (1958): similar to Macintosh's but with virtually no web and a very small flange; designed for patients with little mouth opening.

Disposable blade covers are available but increasingly, disposable blades are used in order to reduce the risk of cross-contamination and reduce the risk of transmission of **Creutzfeldt–Jakob disease. Videolaryngoscope** blades have similar shapes/designs to those used for direct laryngoscopy, but can be more curved because a direct view along the blade is no longer required. They may also incorporate a video camera.

[Robert L Soper (1908–1973), RAF anaesthetist; Eamon P McCoy, Belfast anaesthetist; Paul Bellhouse, Australian anaesthetist; Frank L Robertshaw (1918–1991), Manchester anaesthetist; Edgar H Seward (1917–1995), Oxford anaesthetist; Ronald A Bowen (1913–1999) and Ian Jackson, London anaesthetists; Paluel Flagg (1886–1970), Robert A Miller (1906–1976), Ephraim S Siker, Dante V Bizzarri (1914–1994) and Joseph G Giuffrida (?–1993), US anaesthetists]

See also, Intubation aids; Intubation, tracheal

Laryngoscopy. Act of viewing the **larynx**. Indirect laryngoscopy was first described in 1855 in London by Garcia using a mirror. Direct laryngoscopy was pioneered by **Kirstein, Killian** and **Jackson** in the late 1800s/early 1900s, and is now the technique most commonly used for tracheal intubation. The view of the larynx during direct laryngoscopy is shown in Fig. 103.

Anaesthesia for diagnostic or therapeutic laryngoscopy must provide relaxation of the jaw and vocal cords, with rapid recovery of laryngeal reflexes without **laryngospasm**. Problems include sharing of the airway, the hypertensive response to laryngoscopy and contamination of the airway with blood and debris. Usually performed under general anaesthesia, with IPPV through a special 5–6-mm 'microlaryngoscopy' cuffed tracheal tube (resistance is too high for spontaneous ventilation). Other methods include **injector** and **insufflation techniques** as for **bronchoscopy**. Spraying the cords with **lidocaine** reduces intraoperative laryngospasm but at the expense of diminished laryngeal reflexes postoperatively.

[Manuel Garcia (1805–1906), Spanish singing teacher]

See also, Intubation, complications of; Intubation, difficult; Intubation, tracheal

Laryngospasm. Sustained closure of the glottis by adduction of the vocal cords resulting in partial or complete **airway obstruction**. Although a protective reflex against aspiration, it may persist after cessation of its stimulus. The precise mechanism is controversial; the lateral cricoarytenoid muscles are thought to be most important in adducting the cords whereas cricothyroid tenses them. The extrinsic muscles of the **larynx** may also have a role.

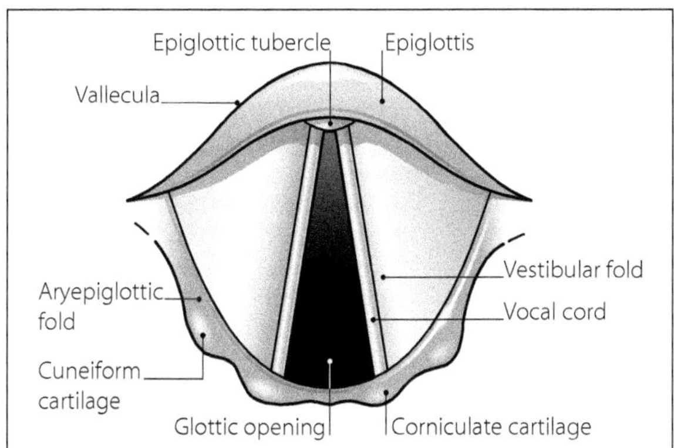

Fig. 103 View obtained during direct laryngoscopy

- Risk factors:
  - inadequate depth of anaesthesia—reflex is abolished in planes 2–4 of anaesthesia.
  - local stimulation of the larynx by saliva, blood, vomitus or foreign body (including laryngoscope, airway or tracheal tube).
  - patient factors: airway hypersensitivity (e.g. asthma, smoking), **gastro-oesophageal reflux, obstructive sleep apnoea.**
  - response to other stimulation, e.g. surgery, movement, stimulation of anus, cervix (**Brewer–Luckhardt reflex**).

Occurs in about 1% of the general population during general anaesthesia and up to 3% in infants. Incidence following tonsillectomy may reach 25%.

May cause complete or partial airway obstruction, the latter often presenting as inspiratory stridor. Causes **hypoxaemia** and **hypoventilation**; **pulmonary oedema** has been reported.

- Management:
  - cessation of stimulus.
  - application of **CPAP** with administration of 100% O_2.
  - increased jaw thrust and introduction of an airway device (e.g. Guedel).
  - increasing depth of anaesthesia, either with intravenous or inhalational agent.
  - if the above measures fail, laryngeal muscle relaxation may be achieved with **suxamethonium** (as little as 8–10 mg may suffice), followed by ventilation with O_2 and tracheal intubation if necessary.
- Prevented by:
  - achieving adequate depth of anaesthesia before attempting laryngoscopy, insertion of airway, surgery, etc.
  - local anaesthetic spray to the larynx and laryngeal nerve blocks.
  - use of neuromuscular blocking drugs and tracheal intubation.

Gavel G, Walker RWM (2014). Cont Edu Anaesth Crit Care Pain; 14: 47–51

Larynx.
- Functions:
  - protects the **tracheobronchial tree** and lungs, e.g. during swallowing.
  - allows coughing.
  - allows speech.
  - allows straining, e.g. during defecation.

Extends from the root of the **tongue** to the cricoid cartilage, i.e., level with C3–6 (at higher level in children).
- Dimensions:
  - length: 45 mm (men); 35 mm (women).
  - anteroposterior: 35 mm (men); 25 mm (women).
  - transverse: 45 mm (men); 40 mm (women).
- Composed of hyoid bone, and epiglottic, thyroid, cricoid, arytenoid, corniculate and cuneiform cartilages, joined by several muscles and ligaments (Fig. 104):
  - hyoid bone:
    - level with C3.
    - U-shaped, with horizontal body and bilateral greater and lesser horns, which pass backwards and upwards, respectively.
    - attached superiorly to the mandible and tongue (by hyoglossus, mylohyoid, geniohyoid and digastric

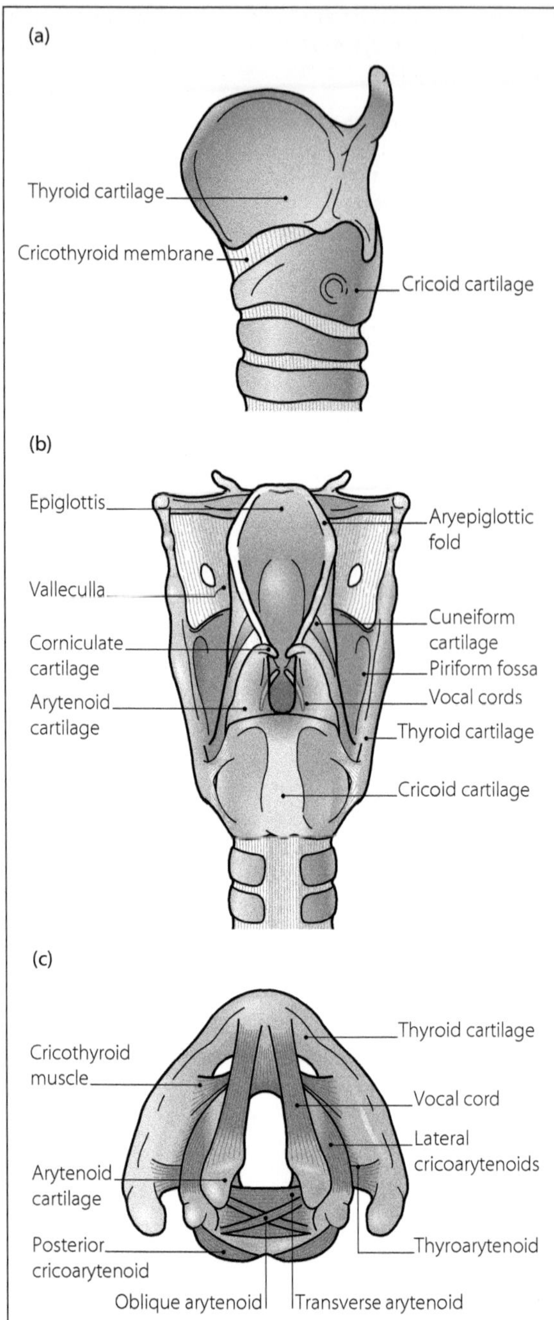

Fig. 104 Anatomy of the larynx: (a) lateral view; (b) posterior view; (c) superior view with intrinsic muscles

muscles) and styloid process (by stylohyoid ligament and muscle).
  - attached inferiorly to the thyroid cartilage (by thyrohyoid membrane and muscle), sternum (by sternohyoid muscle) and clavicle (by omohyoid muscle).
  - attached posteriorly to the **pharynx** by the middle constrictor muscle.
- epiglottis:
  - leaf-shaped, attached anteriorly to the base of the tongue, body of the hyoid and back of the thyroid cartilage above the vocal cords. The depression on either side of the midline glossoepiglottic fold is the vallecula, with the pharyngoepiglottic folds laterally.
  - attached to the arytenoid laterally by the aryepiglottic membrane.
- thyroid cartilage:
  - formed from two quadrilateral halves, meeting anteriorly to form the thyroid notch level with C4. The posterior edge forms superior and inferior horns on each side, the latter articulating with the cricoid cartilage.
  - attached superiorly to the hyoid bone by the thyrohyoid membrane and muscle.
  - attached posteriorly to the pharynx (by inferior constrictor muscle, palatopharyngeus and salpingopharyngeus muscles) and styloid process (by stylothyroid muscle).
  - attached inferiorly to the cricoid (by cricothyroid membrane and muscle) and sternum (by sternothyroid muscle).
  - attached inferomedially to the arytenoids by thyroarytenoid muscle; part of it attaches to the free border of cricothyroid, forming vocalis muscle, and part attaches to the lateral epiglottis, forming thyroepiglottic muscle.
- cricoid cartilage:
  - signet ring–shaped, broadest posteriorly. Level with C6. The lateral surface articulates with the inferior horn of the thyroid cartilage; its upper surface posteriorly articulates with the arytenoids.
  - attached via its superior surface to the thyroid cartilage by the cricothyroid membrane.
  - attached via its lateral surface to the thyroid cartilage (by cricothyroid muscle) and arytenoids (by lateral cricoarytenoid muscles).
  - attached via its posterior surface to the arytenoids by the posterior cricoarytenoid muscles.
  - attached inferiorly to the trachea by the cricotracheal membrane.
- arytenoid cartilages:
  - pyramid-shaped, the bases articulating with the back of the cricoid.
  - also attached to the cricoid by posterior and lateral cricoarytenoid muscles.
  - the vocal cords pass from the vocal processes anteriorly to the back of the thyroid cartilage.
  - attached to the epiglottis superomedially via the aryepiglottic folds and muscles.
  - attached anterolaterally to the back of the thyroid cartilages by the thyroarytenoid muscles.
  - attached to each other by the transverse arytenoid muscle.
- corniculate cartilages: form tubercles in the posterior aryepiglottic folds, at the apex of the arytenoids.
- cuneiform cartilages: lie anterior to the corniculate cartilages, in the aryepiglottic folds.

- Membranes and areas of the larynx:
  - aryepiglottic membrane:
    - passes from the anterior arytenoid to lateral epiglottis.
    - forms the vestibular fold at the lower border. The area between vestibular folds is termed the rima vestibuli; that between the aryepiglottic fold and vestibular fold is the vestibule; the recess between the vocal and vestibular cords is the laryngeal sinus (saccule).
  - cricothyroid membrane: free upper border forms the vocal cord (level with C5) between the back of

the thyroid cartilage and vocal process of the arytenoid; it contains the vocal ligament beneath its mucosa. The area between vocal cords is the rima glottidis (glottis).
  - thyrohyoid membrane: lateral borders are thickened to form the lateral thyrohyoid ligaments.

The entrance to the larynx slopes downwards and backwards, bounded anteriorly by the epiglottis, laterally by the aryepiglottic folds and posteriorly by the arytenoid cartilages. The piriform fossa is the recess on each side, between the aryepiglottic folds medially and thyroid cartilage and thyrohyoid membrane laterally. The rima glottidis is the narrowest part of the airway in adults; the cricoid is the narrowest in children.
- Epithelium: squamous above the cords, columnar below. Mucosa of the cords is closely adherent.
- Muscle actions (Fig. 104c):
  - the cords are tensed by cricothyroid and relaxed by thyroarytenoid and vocalis muscles.
  - the cords are abducted by the posterior cricoarytenoids, causing outward rotation and movement of the arytenoids.
  - the cords are adducted by the lateral cricoarytenoids (causing inward rotation of the arytenoids) and transverse arytenoid muscle (causing the arytenoids to move together).
  - the inlet is opened by the thyroepiglottic muscle and closed by the aryepiglottic muscle.
  - the larynx is elevated by muscles from the pharynx and those above the hyoid, and depressed by sternothyroid.
- Nerve supply:
  - recurrent **laryngeal nerve**: all muscles except cricothyroid, and sensation below vocal cords.
  - superior laryngeal nerve: cricothyroid muscle, and sensation above vocal cords.
- Blood supply: branches of superior and inferior thyroid arteries and accompanying veins.
- Lymphatic drainage:
  - above cords: to upper deep cervical nodes.
  - below cords: to lower deep cervical nodes.

See also, Laryngoscopy

Laser surgery. Use of laser (light amplification by stimulated emission of radiation) radiation to cause tissue destruction by producing intense local heat. Involves stimulation of atoms, ions or molecules within a tube using high voltage. Energy is absorbed and emitted by the particles; the emitted energy is amplified and allowed to escape as a parallel beam of coherent light, of precise wavelength and in phase.
- Effects of the laser beam on tissues depend on its wavelength:
  - CO_2 laser (wavelength 10600 nm): used for precise surgical cutting and coagulation, e.g. in **ENT surgery**, **neurosurgery**, general and gynaecological surgery and dermatology.
  - neodymium yttrium–aluminium–garnet (Nd:YAG) laser (1060 nm): used for photocoagulation and debulking of tumours, e.g. bronchial carcinoma.
  - argon or krypton (400–700 nm): used for photocoagulation in ophthalmology and dermatology.
- Risks to patient and operating staff:
  - ocular (corneal and retinal) damage: prevented by containment of the laser beam, and by wearing protective glasses. Most glasses will absorb energy from the CO_2 laser; specifically tinted goggles are required for the other types.
  - skin damage: prevented by appropriate draping of the patient.
  - **explosions and fires**: particularly problematic during upper airway surgery, when the high-energy beams may cause ignition of anaesthetic vapours, rubber, PVC or silicone tracheal tubes or drapes. The following precautions are available:
    - flexible metal tracheal tubes without cuffs.
    - metallic-coated tubes: expensive, and may still be susceptible to damage. Cuff inflation is with saline instead of air.
    - protection of the tube by wrapping in metallic tape: no longer recommended now that coated or metal tubes are available.
    - avoidance of tracheal intubation, e.g. use of **insufflation** or **injector techniques**, including **high-frequency ventilation**.
    - use of non-explosive mixtures of gases, e.g. <30% O_2 in nitrogen or helium. Intermittent flushing with 100% nitrogen or helium has been used
    - limitation of laser power and duration of bursts.

    Vigilance should be high. If ignition occurs, the O_2 source should be disconnected and the operative site doused with water.
  - gas embolism if the probe's tip is gas-cooled.
  - production of noxious/potentially infective fumes: adequate suction is required.

Latent heat. Energy released or absorbed when a substance undergoes a change of state, without a change in its temperature, e.g.:
  - liquid to gas or vice versa (latent heat of vaporisation).
  - solid to liquid or vice versa (latent heat of fusion).

Heat is required to change liquid to a gas, in order to overcome the attraction between molecules and expand the substance; heat is given out when the reverse occurs, e.g. when steam condenses.

Specific latent heat is the energy required to alter the state of unit mass of substance at specified temperature; e.g. specific latent heat of vaporisation of water = 2.26 MJ/kg at 100°C. It is greater at lower temperatures, and falls at higher temperatures until it reaches zero at the **critical temperature**.

Lateral cutaneous nerve of the forearm, block, *see Elbow, nerve blocks*

Lateral cutaneous nerve of the thigh, block. Provides analgesia of the lateral thigh (e.g. in **fractured neck of femur** and total hip replacement), following skin harvesting, and to reduce leg tourniquet pain. Has also been used in pain states and to diagnose entrapment neuropathy of the nerve caused by the latter's piercing the inguinal ligament instead of passing under it (meralgia paraesthetica), before surgical treatment.

The nerve (L2–3) arises from the **lumbar plexus** (may arise from the femoral nerve), passing under the inguinal ligament just medial to the anterior superior iliac spine to supply the skin of the lateral side of the thigh (*see Fig. 69*; **Femoral triangle**). A needle is inserted 2 cm medial and inferior to the iliac spine, at right angles to the skin. A click is felt as the fascia lata is pierced. 10–15 ml **local anaesthetic agent** is injected fanwise, mediolaterally.

May also be blocked via **femoral nerve block** (three-in-one block). Usually blocked during **fascia iliaca block**.

Latex allergy. Typically occurs in individuals repeatedly exposed to latex, e.g. healthcare workers and patients undergoing repeated urinary catheterisation (e.g. those with spina bifida) or surgery. Thought to be true **anaphylaxis** to various soluble proteins in latex. Accounts for 20% of anaphylactic reactions during the perioperative period, although its incidence is decreasing with better awareness.

May present as cardiovascular collapse during surgery, when the cause may not be easily identifiable. A history of allergy to rubber (e.g. rubber gloves, condoms) may be obtained. Typically associated with allergy to bananas, avocados and chestnuts.

Evaluation includes skin testing, in vitro leucocyte studies and testing for anti-latex IgE antibodies. Perioperative management includes avoidance of all latex-containing equipment including **facemasks**, gloves, airways/tubes, rebreathing bags/bellows, bungs, drains and catheters. Drug vials with rubber tops and iv tubing with rubber injection ports should be avoided. Protection of the arm with gauze before application of a rubber BP cuff has been suggested, although cuffs and other equipment are increasingly manufactured without latex. Pretreatment with **antihistamine drugs, H_2 antagonist drugs** and **corticosteroids** has been used but may not be necessary if proper precautions have been taken. Because airborne latex particles have triggered allergic reactions, no latex-containing equipment should be used in the operating room before a known case; scheduling surgery for the beginning of the operating list has been advocated. A high index of suspicion and availability of resuscitation drugs are important; management of a reaction should follow standard lines as for **adverse drug reactions.**

Hepner DL, Castells MC (2003). Anesth Analg; 96: 1219–29

Laudanosine. Tertiary amine, a product of **atracurium** metabolism via **Hofmann degradation. Half-life** is about 2–3 h, i.e., considerably longer than for atracurium; approximately doubled in renal failure. In anaesthetised dogs, causes epileptiform EEG changes at blood levels over 17 µg/ml. Blood levels in humans, even after several days' infusion of atracurium in patients with renal and hepatic failure, rarely rise above 5 µg/ml, although fears have been expressed about central stimulation in patients at risk, e.g. those with an impaired **blood–brain barrier. Cisatracurium** at equipotent doses produces one-fifth of the level of laudanosine. Has recently been found to have analgesic effects in animals, and to interact with central GABA, opioid and acetylcholine receptors.

Fodale V, Santamaria LB (2002). Eur J Anaesthesiol; 19: 466–73

Lavoisier, Antoine Laurent (1742–1794). French chemist. Disproved the **phlogiston** theory, showing that the gain in weight of sulfur or phosphorus on combustion was due to combination with air. Concluded that air consists of two elastic fluids: one necessary for combustion and respiration, and one that would support neither. Renamed the former (previously called dephlogisticated air) *oxygène*, estimating its concentration in air to be about 25%.

Lawen, Arthur (1876–1958). German surgeon, the first to perform **caudal analgesia** for abdominal surgery, using large volumes of **procaine.** Also described **paravertebral block,** and helped popularise regional anaesthesia. Described the use of **curare** to produce relaxation during surgery in 1912.

Laxatives.

- Perioperative/ICU usage:
  - to prepare the lower GIT before surgery.
  - to reduce pain following rectal or anal surgery.
  - to treat **constipation**, e.g. on ICU or postoperatively.
  - to treat **poisoning and overdoses**, e.g. **whole bowel irrigation**, especially in children.
- Divided into:
  - bulk-forming laxatives: increase faecal mass and stimulate peristalsis. Useful in patients with enterostomies and colonic disease. Include bran, methylcellulose, ispaghula and sterculia.
  - stimulants: increase GIT motility. Include senna, bisacodyl, dantron, docusate sodium, glycerol (also acts as an osmotic laxative and faecal softener) and sodium picosulfate.
  - faecal softeners: liquid paraffin is rarely used because, if aspirated, may cause severe pneumonitis. Arachis oil enemas may be useful for impacted faeces.
  - osmotic laxatives: cause retention of water within the bowel. Include lactulose (broken down by gut bacteria to osmotically active compounds; also reduce ammonia production; hence its use in **hepatic failure**), polyethylene glycols and rectal citrate or phosphates (caution in renal impairment because **hyperphosphataemia** may result). Magnesium salts act within 2–4 h but should not be used in renal impairment because of systemic absorption.
  - bowel cleansers: usually mixtures of agents; should not be used in constipation. In frail patients, preoperative use may result in significant **dehydration.** Used in whole bowel irrigation.

Dosage depends on the particular preparation used. Complications include dehydration and electrolyte disturbances. Stimulants may cause abdominal cramps; osmotic laxatives may cause bloating. Laxatives (especially stimulants) are contraindicated in **intestinal obstruction.**

LBBB, Left bundle branch block, *see Bundle branch block*

LD_{50}, *see Therapeutic ratio/index*

Le Fort classification, *see Facial trauma*

Left atrial pressure (LAP). Mean pressure approximates to **left ventricular end-diastolic pressure,** unless the mitral valve is abnormal. Pressure wave abnormalities are similar to the **venous waveform,** but with reference to mitral and aortic valves and systemic circulation, instead of tricuspid and pulmonary valves and pulmonary circulation.

May be measured via a catheter inserted directly into the left atrium, or indirectly via **pulmonary artery catheterisation,** which measures **pulmonary capillary wedge pressure.** Usually measured from mid-axilla or sternal angle. Normal value is 2–10 mmHg.

See also, Cardiac cycle

Left ventricular ejection time, *see Systolic time intervals*

Left ventricular end-diastolic pressure (LVEDP). Reflects the **preload** of the left ventricle. Provided ventricular compliance is constant, a constant relationship (exponential rather than linear) exists between LVEDP and **left ventricular end-diastolic volume**. Normal LVEDP does not ensure normal ventricular function, and abnormal LVEDP may not indicate degree of dysfunction. Elevations of LVEDP (normally under 12 mmHg) may reflect increased blood volume, reduced **myocardial contractility**, reduced ventricular compliance and increased **venous return**. Coronary perfusion pressure is the difference between aortic diastolic pressure and LVEDP; thus, raised LVEDP may compromise **coronary blood flow**, leading to a vicious cycle of **myocardial ischaemia**, LV failure/dilatation and increasing LVEDP. May be measured directly via a ventricular cannula or arterial cannulation, or inferred from **left atrial pressure** measurements.

Left ventricular end-diastolic volume. Nearest physiological variable to left ventricular **preload**, as described by **Starling's law**. May be assessed using **echocardiography** or radiology, but indicators of **left ventricular end-diastolic pressure** are easier to measure. Normally 70–95 ml/m^2.

Left ventricular failure, *see Cardiac failure*

Left ventricular fractional shortening. Indicator of left ventricular function derived from M-mode **echocardiography**.

Equals:

$$\frac{\left(\begin{array}{c}\text{end-diastolic}\\ \text{internal dimension}\end{array}\right)-\left(\begin{array}{c}\text{end-systolic}\\ \text{internal dimension}\end{array}\right)}{\text{end-diastolic internal dimension}}$$

Normally 34%–44%; often easier to estimate during echocardiography than doing a formal evaluation of **ejection fraction**.

Left ventricular stroke work, *see Stroke work*

Legionnaires' disease. Atypical pneumonia caused by *Legionella pneumophila*, a gram-negative aerobic **bacterium**. First came to prominence when it killed 29 delegates at an American Legion convention in 1976. Accounts for 2%–9% of community-acquired pneumonia. More likely to affect elderly patients. Acquired by inhaling contaminated water particles, especially derived from cooling towers; typically occurs in epidemics involving a single building. Presents as an acute febrile **chest infection**, typically with myalgia, fatigue and GIT upset before respiratory symptoms develop. Pleuritic chest pain and confusion may occur. Widespread infiltrates may be present on **CXR**. Diagnosis is via sputum culture ± serological testing. Treatment is with **erythromycin** or **clarithromycin**; **4-quinolones** are also used. The disease lasts for 7–10 days. Mortality rates of 10%–30% have been reported.

Cunha BA, Burillo A, Bouza E (2016). Lancet; 387: 376–85

Lenograstim, *see Granulocyte colony-stimulating factor*

Lepirudin. Recombinant **hirudin**, used as an alternative to **heparin** if the latter induces **heparin-induced thrombocytopenia**.

- Dosage: 400 µg/kg slowly iv followed by 150 µg/kg/h up to 16.5 mg/h, adjusted according to **coagulation studies**.
- Side effects: bleeding; hypersensitivity.

Leptospirosis (Weil's disease). Caused by species of leptospira, gram-negative aerobic **bacteria**. Passed from asymptomatic animals (dogs, rodents, livestock and wild animals) via their urine to water, where it may survive for many months. Typically affects sewage workers. Acquired via mucous membranes and broken skin; it causes widespread vasculitis affecting the kidney, liver, lungs and heart. Clinical features include fever, myalgia, headache/neck stiffness, cough, chest pain, confusion, rash and occasionally renal and hepatic failure. Diagnosed retrospectively by increases in antibody titre. Treatment is with **benzylpenicillin**, **erythromycin** or **tetracyclines**. Normal organ function returns usually within 1–2 months. Mortality is up to 11% if hepatic failure occurs.

[H Adolph Weil (1848–1916), German physician]

Haake DA, Levett PN (2015). Curr Top Microbiol Immunol; 387: 65–97

LES, *see Lower oesophageal sphincter*

Letheon. Name given to **diethyl ether** by **Morton** in 1846 when he patented his discovery. Despite this patent, ether was widely used without acknowledgement of Morton's claim. His attempts to enforce the patent and payments of royalties included approaching the governments of the USA and France, but were unsuccessful.

[Lethe (Greek mythology), river in Hades whose waters induced forgetfulness in those who drank them]

Leucocytes. White blood cells; normal total count in peripheral **blood** is 4–10 × 10^9/l.

- Exist as three morphologically different types:
  - granulocytes: derived from common bone marrow precursor stem cells:
    - neutrophils (60%–70%; 2.5–7 × 10^9/l): phagocytic with high enzyme content.
    - eosinophils (1%–4%; 0.01–0.4 × 10^9/l): contain **histamine** and are involved in cell-mediated hypersensitivity reactions.
    - basophils (0%–1%; 0–0.2 × 10^9/l): contain histamine and **heparin**; non-phagocytic.
  - lymphocytes (23%–35%: 1–3.5 × 10^9/l): derived from lymphoid stem cells throughout the body, including bone marrow. Mainly concerned with immune mechanisms: B (bursa) cells with **immunoglobulin** production and T (thymus) cells with immune system regulation and killing of infected cells.
  - monocytes (4%–8%; 0.2–0.8 × 10^9/l): formed in spleen, lymphoid tissue and marrow. Differentiate into phagocytic tissue macrophages.

Leucocytosis may be caused by almost any acute illness as part of the inflammatory response. Other causes include strenuous exercise, **trauma**, surgery, **burns**, and glucocorticoid therapy. Leucopenia may be caused by reduced production (e.g. drugs, radiation, inflammation, infection, infiltration of bone marrow by malignancy, fibrosis) or increased utilisation (e.g. sequestration into the tissues). Thus in severe illness white cell count may be increased or decreased. A low count appears to be prognostic of increased mortality in ICU patients.

Bellingan G (2000). Intensive Care Med; 26: S111–18

See also, Erythrocytes; Platelets

Leukotriene pathway inhibitors. Group of drugs that block the synthesis of all **leukotrienes**; have been used in **asthma** along with the **leukotriene receptor antagonists**. Zileuton is an example, and inhibits the action of 5-lipoxygenase.

Leukotriene receptor antagonists. Group of drugs that block the action of cysteinyl **leukotrienes** at their receptors, especially on bronchial smooth muscle. Have been used orally in mild/moderate **asthma** but not indicated for treatment of acute attacks. Churg–Strauss syndrome (eosinophilia, systemic vasculitis and worsening pulmonary symptoms) has been reported following their use. Examples include montelukast, zafirlukast and pranlukast.
[Jacob Churg (1910–2005; Polish-born) and Lotte Strauss (1913–1985; German-born), US pathologists]

Leukotrienes. Inflammatory mediators derived from **arachidonic acid** by the action of lipoxygenases. Released from **mast cells**, **platelets** and some **leucocytes** following various stimuli (e.g. mechanical, thermal, infective and immunological). Actions include bronchoconstriction, vasoconstriction, increased vascular permeability and chemotaxis of other inflammatory cells.

They have been implicated in the pathophysiology of **sepsis**, **ALI** and **asthma. Leukotriene pathway inhibitors** and **leukotriene receptor antagonists** have been developed for use in asthma.

Peters-Golden M, Henderson WR (2007). N Engl J Med; 357: 1841–54

Levallorphan tartrate. Opioid receptor antagonist with partial agonist properties, the *n*-allyl derivative of **levorphanol.** Synthesised in 1950. 1.25 mg levallorphan has been combined with 100 mg **pethidine** as pethilorphan, but hopes of analgesia without respiratory depression were not realised. Its use has been superseded by **naloxone.**

Levetiracetam. Anticonvulsant drug used as monotherapy or as an adjunct in the treatment of partial or generalised **epilepsy**; it is the first-line therapy for myoclonic seizures. Mechanism of action is unknown. Oral **bioavailability** is close to 100%. Minimally metabolised, with 95% excreted unchanged in the urine; dose adjustment in renal failure and the elderly is therefore required.
- Dosage: 250 mg–1.5 g bd orally or iv, titrated to response.
- Side effects: GIT upset, cough, ataxia, visual disturbance, thrombocytopenia.

Levobupivacaine, *see Bupivacaine*

Levofloxacin. Antibacterial drug, one of the **4-quinolones** related to **ciprofloxacin** but more active against pneumococci.
- Dosage: 250–500 mg od/bd orally or iv.
- Side effects: as for ciprofloxacin. Hypotension and thrombophlebitis may occur on iv administration.

Levorphanol tartrate. Synthetic **opioid analgesic drug**, synthesised in 1949. Similar to **morphine** but less sedating. Onset of action is under 30 min, lasting for up to 8 h. No longer available in the UK.

Levosimendan. Calcium sensitiser, used as an **inotropic drug** in the treatment of decompensated congestive **cardiac failure.** Shown to improve survival and cardiac function compared with placebo and **dobutamine**; unlike the latter, levosimendan has no pro-arrhythmic side effects.

Acts by binding to cardiac troponin C, increasing its sensitivity to **calcium**; thus increases **myocardial contractility** without increasing myocardial O_2 consumption. Also causes vasodilatation by opening ATP-sensitive K^+ channels in smooth muscle; hence sometimes referred to as an 'ino-dilator'. Reductions in arterial (systemic and pulmonary) and venous tone decrease **afterload** (both right and left ventricular) and **preload**, respectively.

Haemodynamic effects are seen within 5 min of loading dose administration; peak effect is at 10–30 min. 98% protein-bound with an elimination half-life of 1 h.
- Dosage: 6–12 μg/kg iv loading dose over 10 min, followed by infusion of 0.05–0.2 μg/kg/min titrated to effect.
- Side effects: related to vasodilatation (e.g. hypotension, headache).

Lidocaine hydrochloride (Lignocaine). Amide **local anaesthetic agent**, introduced in 1947 (revolutionising regional anaesthesia because of its superior safety to previous agents). The standard drug against which other local anaesthetics are compared. pK_a is 7.9. 65% protein-bound; 95% of an injected dose undergoes hepatic metabolism and renal excretion. Onset is rapid by all routes; usual duration of action for 1% solution is about 1 h, increased to 1.5–2 h if **adrenaline** is added.
- Uses:
  - local anaesthesia. Often combined with adrenaline, because lidocaine tends to produce local vasodilatation; 1:200000 and 1:80000 solutions are commonly available, the latter usually restricted to dental use.
  - iv administration:
    - depression of laryngeal and tracheal reflexes (e.g. during tracheal intubation/extubation). Commonly used to reduce the increase in **ICP** caused by laryngoscopy. Possibly reduces muscle pains and potassium increase after **suxamethonium.** It has been used to produce analgesia and general anaesthesia (although its **therapeutic ratio** is low). 4%–10% lidocaine has been used instead of air to inflate the tracheal tube cuff, thereby reducing postoperative sore throat and hoarseness.
    - class I **antiarrhythmic drug** in ventricular tachyarrhythmias.
    - may be useful in treatment of neuropathic pain.
- Many preparations are available, including:
  - 0.25%–0.5% solutions for **infiltration anaesthesia** and **IVRA.**
  - 1%–2% solutions for nerve blocks and **epidural anaesthesia.**
  - 4% solution for **topical anaesthesia** of the mucous membranes of the mouth, pharynx and respiratory tract.
  - 10% spray for topical anaesthesia as above. Available in metered dose delivery systems (10 mg/spray).
  - also available in 1%–2% gel for urethral instillation, and 5% ointment for skin, rectum and other mucous membranes. A constituent of **EMLA cream**; it is also available as a cream containing lidocaine 7% and tetracaine 7%, used for minor dermatological procedures and venepuncture (a 1-mm layer is applied 30 min before, then peeled off immediately before, the procedure, up to 400 cm² total area). In other countries (especially the USA), 5% hyperbaric solution has been used in **spinal anaesthesia** (*but see later*).
- Dosage:
  - depends on the block.
  - 1–2 mg/kg iv 2–5 min before intubation/extubation.
  - for ventricular arrhythmias: 1 mg/kg iv initially, then 4 mg/kg/min for 30 min, 2 mg/kg/min for 2 h and 1 mg/kg/min thereafter.

Adverse effects are as for local anaesthetic agents. Lidocaine is thought to be more directly neurotoxic than other local anaesthetics; hence the increased incidence of **transient radicular irritation syndrome** following spinal injection compared with other drugs (hyperbaricity of the solution and use of very thin needles/catheters are also thought to contribute by encouraging pooling of drug around spinal nerves). This has led to revision of the drug's data sheet to specify dilution to 2.5% before administration (even this concentration has been implicated in causing transient symptoms). Maximal recommended dose: 3 mg/kg without adrenaline, 7 mg/kg with adrenaline. Toxic plasma levels: >10 μg/ml.

Life support, *see Cardiopulmonary resuscitation*

Lightwand. Device used to place a tracheal tube without requiring **laryngoscopy**. Consists of a flexible malleable stylet incorporating a light bulb at the distal end, with the battery and handle at the proximal end. Placed inside a tracheal tube with the bulb at the tube's tip, the tube/lightwand combination is bent into a J shape and manoeuvred into the larynx, with successful placement indicated by a glow at the anterior neck below the thyroid prominence. The tracheal tube is then passed into the trachea and the lightwand removed. Oesophageal placement is suggested by a more diffuse glow above the prominence.

Several different types exist. The technique has been used for both routine and difficult intubations.

Agro F, Hung OR, Cataldo R, et al (2001). Can J Anesth; 48: 592–9

Lignocaine, *see Lidocaine*

Likelihood ratio. Method of quantifying the relative probabilities of two complementary hypotheses. For a predictive test, it equals the probability that a person with the condition has a positive test, over the probability that a person without the condition has a positive test. Also equals **sensitivity** ÷ (1 – **specificity**).

Limbic system. Part of the **brain**, formerly termed the rhinencephalon. Composed of left and right lobes, each consisting of:

- rim of cortical tissue around the hilum of the cerebral hemisphere.
- associated deep structures: hippocampus and gyrus, uncus, amygdala, cingulate gyrus, part of insula, septal area, isthmus, Broca's olfactory area and orbital surface of the frontal lobe. Also includes the hippocampal formation and thus associated with memory.

Responsible for olfaction, feeding behaviour, motivation, sexual behaviour and generation of emotions. Damage to the amygdala is associated with rage reactions, hyperphagia and increased sexual activity; lesions in the uncus with olfactory and gustatory hallucinations.

Thought to be one site of action of **benzodiazepines**, **ketamine** and possibly other anaesthetic drugs.

[Pierre P Broca (1824–1880), French surgeon]

LiMON. Commercial non-invasive monitor of liver function and blood volume. Requires peripheral or central venous access and uses a four-wavelength near infrared finger sensor. Measures the plasma disappearance rate and the 15-min retention rate of an intravenous marker, **indocyanine green**. Knowledge of the **cardiac output** permits estimation of circulating blood volume and indocyanine green **clearance** within minutes. As the elimination of indocyanine green is dependent on both liver blood flow and hepatocellular function, the system cannot differentiate the cause of a reduced clearance of indocyanine green. However, any sudden reduction in clearance will reflect a fall in liver blood flow. Up to 10 measurements are possible in any 24-h period.

See also, Liver function tests

Linear analogue scale (Visual analogue scale). Method of evaluating **pain**, nausea, anxiety and other symptoms, e.g. for statistical analysis. For example, for **pain evaluation**, a horizontal 10 cm line is drawn on plain paper, with 'no pain' written at the left-hand end, and 'worst possible pain' at the right-hand end. The patient marks his or her position on the line. Thought to be more reliable than assessments where patients choose the most appropriate number or word from a list, which may be influenced by personal preference for certain words or numbers and limited by the number of choices offered. Thought to be consistent for any individual; however, because patients may interpret the analogue scale differently, comparison between patients may be unreliable. Also, patients tend to avoid the extremes of the scale, clustering their scores around the middle; the scale is thus not truly linear.

Linezolid. Oxazolidinone **antibacterial** drug active against gram-positive bacteria, including multiresistant staphylococci and enterococci, but poorly active against gram-negative organisms.

- Dosage: 600 mg bd orally or iv over 30–120 min, for a maximum of 28 days.
- Side effects: GIT disturbance, headache, dry mouth, blood dyscrasias (full blood count must be monitored weekly). Has weak **MAOI** properties.

Lingual nerve block, *see Mandibular nerve blocks*

Lipid emulsion. Fat emulsion for iv administration composed of soya bean oil, glycerol and egg phospholipids. Available in 10%, 20% and 30% concentration (of soya oil) for parenteral **nutrition**. 20% emulsion is the recommended treatment for circulatory arrest due to **local anaesthetic agents** (and should also be considered for severe toxicity without loss of circulation [*for mechanism, see Local anaesthetic agents*]). Animal studies and case reports also support its use in the treatment of poisoning with other lipophilic drugs, including: **β-adrenergic receptor antagonists**; **calcium channel blocking drugs**; **tricyclic antidepressant drugs**; and neuroleptic drugs (e.g. **haloperidol**). Few adverse effects have been associated with its use in acute poisoning, although **pancreatitis** may occur with acute hyperlipidaemia.

- Dosage: for local anaesthetic toxicity: 1.5 ml/kg of 20% emulsion over 60 s, followed by an infusion of 15 ml/kg/h; maximum of two repeat boluses every 5 min if circulation not restored (infusion rate should also be doubled), up to a maximum of 12 ml/kg total dose. Similar regimens have been used for poisoning with other agents.

Picard J, Meek T (2016). Anaesthesia; 71: 879–82

Lipopolysaccharide, *see Endotoxins*

Liquid ventilation. Technique of partially or totally filling the lungs with **perfluorocarbons** (especially perfluorooctylbromide) and ventilating with this liquid instead of

O_2-enriched air. First done experimentally in animals in the early 1960s, using pressurised crystalloid solutions. Has been used in neonatal **respiratory distress syndrome** and **ALI**, mostly in animal models, but human studies have been and are currently being performed.

In total liquid ventilation, the entire lung volume and ventilator circuit are filled, requiring a specialised ventilator. The liquid is oxygenated to a P_{O_2} of 50–90 kPa (350–675 mmHg) by either bubbling O_2 through it or by using a standard extracorporeal device. Tidal volumes of 15–20 ml/kg are given at a rate of about 5 breaths/min. In partial liquid ventilation (perfluorocarbon-associated gas exchange; PAGE) a volume approximating to **FRC** is instilled and standard **IPPV** continued. Results in improved oxygenation and increased **compliance**, thought to be via increased recruitment of non-aerated alveoli and redistribution of perfusion. A protective effect against further lung injury has been suggested.

Kaisers U, Kelly KP, Busch T (2003). Br J Anaesth; 91: 143–51

Lissive anaesthesia. Obsolete technique of anaesthesia in which small doses of non-depolarising neuromuscular blocking drugs (originally **tubocurarine**) were used to produce muscle relaxation without causing complete paralysis, allowing spontaneous respiration ('diaphragmatic sparing').

Liston, Robert (1794–1847). Scottish-born surgeon; performed the first operation under **diethyl ether** anaesthesia in England on 21 December 1846, at University College Hospital, London, having been told about ether by **Boott**. William Squire administered the anaesthetic from a glass inhaler made by his uncle, Peter, while Frederick Churchill had an above-knee amputation. The operation allegedly lasted 25 s.

[William Squire (1825–1899), London medical student, later physician; Peter Squire (1798–1884), London chemist; Frederick Churchill (1810–?), Harley Street butler]

Lithium carbonate/citrate. Salts used for treatment of mania in bipolar disease. Lithium mimics sodium in the body, entering excitable cells during depolarisation. It decreases release of central and peripheral **neurotransmitters** and may prolong **depolarising** and **non-depolarising neuromuscular blockade** and decrease requirements for anaesthetic agents. Shown to have **cerebral protection** properties. Termination 24 h before anaesthesia has been suggested but this is disputed. Has low **therapeutic ratio**, with optimal plasma concentration of 0.4–1.0 mmol/l and toxicity occurring at >1.5 mmol/l. Distributed slowly within the tissues (24–36 h with slow-release preparations). Almost entirely excreted by the kidneys, with **half-life** 6–12 h initially but >24 h if the tissue compartment contains significant amounts of drug. **Lithium poisoning** may occur acutely and deliberately, or insidiously during chronic treatment as a result of dehydration, impaired renal function, infection and use of drugs, e.g. **NSAIDs**, **diuretics**.

- Dosage: 200 mg–2.0 g/day depending on the preparation, indication, plasma level and clinical response.
- Side effects: as for lithium poisoning.

Lithium poisoning. Toxic effects of **lithium** may be seen at plasma concentrations of <1.0 mmol/l but are common at >1.5 mmol/l; severe toxicity is usual at levels >2.0 mmol/l, although acute poisoning may produce high concentrations before the onset of symptoms. Features include lethargy or restlessness initially; then tremor, ataxia, GIT upset, weakness and muscle twitching; finally, **hypokalaemia**, **arrhythmias**, **renal failure**, **convulsions** and **coma**.

Management consists of increasing urine output if symptoms have not yet developed; general treatment is supportive with control of electrolyte imbalance and convulsions, and **haemodialysis** (which may need repeating as lithium redistributes from the tissues to the circulation) if neurological symptoms are present or if plasma concentration is >7.5 mmol/l after acute overdose (or >4 mmol/l in chronic overdose). The possibility of prolonged absorption of lithium from slow-release preparations should be remembered. Activated **charcoal** is relatively ineffective at preventing further absorption; **whole bowel irrigation** has been used but is not standard therapy.

Litre. SI **unit** of volume. Originally defined as the volume of 1 kg pure water at 4°C, but redefined as equal to 1000 cm^3 in 1964, because of an error in the standard **kilogram** constructed in 1889.

Liver. Largest body organ, weighing about 1200–1500 g, lying in the right upper abdominal quadrant. Two major lobes, right and left, are divided into lobules based on a central vein connected by a network of sinusoids to peripheral portal tracts. Central veins are tributaries of hepatic veins; portal tracts contain branches of the hepatic artery, portal vein, lymphatics and bile ducts. Blood from the hepatic arterial and portal venous systems is conveyed to the central veins via the sinusoids, lined with endothelial and phagocytic (Kupffer) cells and separated by hepatocytes. Bile canaliculi form networks between the hepatocytes, conveying bile towards the **biliary tract**.

Blood flow is about 20%–30% of cardiac output (80% via the portal vein, 20% via the hepatic artery).

- Functions:
  - **carbohydrate** and **lactate** metabolism; **glycogen** storage and breakdown.
  - **protein** metabolism: synthesises many, including **albumin**, globulins, **coagulation** factors (all except factor VIII), **complement** proteins, transferrin, haptoglobulins, caeruloplasmin, plasma **cholinesterase** and α_1-antitrypsin. Important site of **amino acid** deamination before interconversion and oxidation. **Ammonia** produced by deamination is converted to **urea**.
  - **fat** metabolism: breakdown of dietary triglycerides and fatty acids, and synthesis of triglycerides, phospholipid and cholesterol, released into the bloodstream as lipoproteins. Cholesterol is also used to make bile acids.
  - bilirubin metabolism: unconjugated fat-soluble bilirubin is transported to the liver bound to albumin; it is conjugated with glucuronide to the water-soluble form (*see Jaundice*).
  - formation of bile acids: cholic and chenodeoxycholic acids are produced from cholesterol and secreted in the bile. Reabsorbed via enterohepatic circulation.
  - **vitamin** storage: A, D, K, B_{12} and folate.
  - hormone metabolism and inactivation: include cortisol, oestrogens, **aldosterone**, **vasopressin** and thyroxine.
  - haematological role: site of haemopoiesis during fetal and early neonatal life. Also acts as a reservoir for blood that can be redistributed to the body by stimulation of the liver's autonomic innervation.

Kupffer cells phagocytose antigens and bacteria absorbed from the GIT, and destroy old red cells.
 - drug metabolism: achieved by transforming lipid-soluble compounds into water-soluble ones via **enzymes** located in the hepatocyte microsomes. Several processes are involved, including oxidation, conjugation, reduction, hydrolysis, methylation and acetylation. Most drugs are metabolised by a combination of oxidation by cytochromes and conjugation (*see Pharmacokinetics*).
- Effects of anaesthetic agents:
 - both hepatic artery and portal vein blood flow are reduced by most agents, probably as a consequence of reduced cardiac output. The effect is opposed by hypercapnia and exacerbated by hypocapnia and IPPV, although this is rarely significant.
 - drug metabolism may be reduced in the presence of volatile agents, although whether due to alterations in hepatic blood flow or a direct inhibitory effect is unclear.
 - **enzyme induction** by volatile agents has been reported but is controversial.
 - toxic effects: e.g. halothane **hepatitis**.

[Karl W von Kupffer (1829–1902), German anatomist]

Liver dialysis. Term used to describe various techniques for extracorporeal detoxification of blood in acute-on-chronic **hepatic failure**. Includes the molecular adsorbents recirculation system (MARS) in which a **dialysis** circuit, containing albumin, is separated from the patient's blood by a semi-permeable membrane, the albumin filtered in a second circuit before being reused. Single-pass albumin dialysis (SPAD) uses a single disposable circuit containing albumin. Continuous venovenous **haemodiafiltration** and other variants of **haemoperfusion** and **haemodialysis** have also been investigated. Few are in routine use, although MARS was approved in the USA in 2005 for patients awaiting **liver transplantation**.

Liver failure, *see Hepatic failure*

Liver function tests. Most commonly measured:
 - bilirubin (*see Jaundice*).
 - liver enzymes:
   - aspartate aminotransferase (AST) and alanine aminotransferase (ALT): released by damaged hepatocytes. Very high levels suggest **hepatitis**. Normally 5–40 IU/l.
   - alkaline phosphatase (ALP): highly raised in cholestasis, both intra- and extrahepatic. Isoenzyme analysis differentiates between hepatic and other sources, e.g. bone. Normally 40–110 IU/l.
   - γ-glutamyl transferase (γGT): non-specific, but often raised following drug ingestion, e.g. alcohol. Normally 10–50 IU/l.
 - plasma proteins:
   - albumin: reduced in chronic liver disease after a few weeks. Normally 35–55 g/l.
   - globulins: increased to varying extents, depending on the underlying cause. Normally 25–35 g/l.
 - **coagulation studies**.
 - others, including:
   - rate of **clearance** of indocyanine green following a bolus iv injection allows assessment of hepatic excretory function; improvement in clearance has been associated with better outcome in ICU patients.
   - α_1-fetoprotein, increased in hepatoma.
   - **cholinesterase**.
   - 5′ nucleotidase, increased in biliary obstruction.

Agrawal S, Dhiman RK, Limdi JK (2016). Postgrad Med J; 92: 223–34

Liver transplantation. First performed in 1963. Indicated for end-stage **hepatic failure**, e.g. due to inherited disease, chronic **hepatitis**, acute toxic hepatitis, primary biliary cirrhosis and some cases of liver tumour. Scoring systems are commonly used to prioritise potential recipients, based on the likelihood of death while waiting for transplantation. Surgery involves vascular and biliary isolation of the diseased organ (pre-anhepatic and anhepatic phases) with re-anastomosis of a donor cadaveric organ (reperfusion phase); partial donation by live donors is also performed. The recipient's liver is dissected to its vascular pedicle, the portal vein, hepatic artery and inferior vena cava above and below the liver are clamped, and the diseased organ is removed. Venovenous bypass is often employed from the portal and femoral veins to the axillary or internal jugular veins, although practice varies between centres. Donor liver viability is up to 8 h from harvesting. It is flushed with crystalloid solution via the portal vein to remove the transport infusate and air bubbles. Anastomosis of the portal vein and hepatic artery is followed by release of vascular clamps, incorporating the donor liver into the recipient's circulation.
- Anaesthesia:
 - as for hepatic failure. Preoperative assessment includes evaluation of cardiovascular status and other co-morbidity. Those with encephalopathic fulminant liver failure are at risk of raised **ICP** (and higher mortality), and neuroprotective measures as for **neurosurgery** are routinely employed. Opioid, volatile agent, neuromuscular blockade and IPPV are usual; N_2O is avoided to reduce bowel distension and risk of **gas embolism** during reanastomosis. Aseptic techniques are used to reduce infection. **Ciclosporin** and **corticosteroids** are given.
 - monitoring and vascular lines include direct BP and CVP measurement, **pulmonary artery catheterisation** (or a non-invasive method of **cardiac output measurement**), **transoesophageal echocardiography**, several large iv cannulae, temperature probes and urinary catheter.
 - frequent measurement of plasma electrolytes, glucose, haemoglobin, platelets, arterial blood gases and **coagulation studies** is required. **Thromboelastography** is useful.
 - blood loss is usually 8–10 units but may be up to 200 units. **Cell salvage** is often used. Rapid **blood transfusion** devices are required to keep up with losses; they include a reservoir of several units of blood, driven by a pump. Venous return may also be reduced by surgical manipulation.
 - SVR and cardiac rhythm/output may change frequently. Myocardial depression may be caused by **hypocalcaemia**, **hypothermia** and **acidosis**. Acidosis is common but treated cautiously, as postoperative metabolic alkalosis is also common, due to metabolism of lactate and citrate. **Inotropic drugs** are often required.
 - **hypoglycaemia** and **hyperglycaemia** may occur, especially during the anhepatic phase.
 - potassium levels fluctuate due to acid–base changes, flushing out of liver perfusate and uptake by the transplanted liver.

- surgery usually lasts 8–10 h but may be up to 24 h, with major biochemical, haematological and temperature disturbances that may persist postoperatively. IPPV is usually maintained for 24–48 h. Postoperative problems include infection, atelectasis and **pleural effusion**, graft failure, hepatic artery thrombosis, biliary leaks or obstruction, neurological impairment and renal failure.

Dalal A (2016). Transplant Rev; 30: 51–60

See also, Liver dialysis; Organ donation; Transplantation

Living will, *see Advance decision*

Local anaesthesia, *see Infiltration anaesthesia; Local anaesthetic agents; Regional anaesthesia; Topical anaesthesia; specific blocks*

Local anaesthetic agents. **Cocaine** was introduced in 1884 by **Freud** and **Koller**; less toxic agents subsequently introduced include **procaine** and **stovaine** (1904), **cinchocaine** (1925), **tetracaine** (amethocaine) (1931) and **lidocaine** (lignocaine) (1947). Lidocaine is particularly non-toxic. Later drugs include **chloroprocaine** (1952), **mepivacaine** (1956), **prilocaine** (1959), **bupivacaine** (1963), **etidocaine** (1972), **articaine** (1974), **ropivacaine** and levobupivacaine (both 1997). Others are used only for **topical anaesthesia**, e.g. benzocaine.

- General properties (Table 31):
  - poorly water-soluble weak bases with pK_a >7.4.
  - composed of hydrophilic and hydrophobic portions separated by an alkyl chain. The hydrophilic part is usually a tertiary amine; the lipophilic part (essential for local anaesthetic action) is usually an unsaturated aromatic ring, e.g. *para*-aminobenzoic acid.
  - modification of chemical structure (lengthening the alkyl chain or increasing the number of carbon atoms in the aromatic ring or tertiary amine) may alter lipid solubility, potency, rate of metabolism and duration of action.
  - classified according to the nature of linkage between the amine and aromatic parts into ester or amide drugs:
    - esters:
      - allergic reactions are common.
      - rapidly metabolised by plasma and liver **cholinesterase**. One metabolite, *para*-aminobenzoic acid, is thought to be responsible for allergic reactions. Metabolism may be prolonged when plasma cholinesterase level is low, e.g. liver disease, **pregnancy** or atypical enzymes.
    - amides:
      - allergic reactions are rare; they may be associated with the preservative vehicle.
      - metabolised by liver microsomal enzymes, initially to aminocarboxylic acid and a cyclic aniline derivative, subsequently via *N*-dealkylation and hydroxylation, respectively. Dependent on liver blood flow and function.
  - presented in solution as acidic hydrochloride salts.
- Mechanism of action:
  - produce reversible blockade of peripheral and central neural transmission in autonomic, sensory and motor nerve fibres, depending on the concentration of drug applied.
  - bind to fast **sodium** channels in the axon membrane from within, preventing sodium entry during depolarisation. The threshold potential is thus not reached and the **action potential** of the nerve not propagated (membrane-stabilising effect).
  - fate of injected drug:
    - diffuses to axons; thus more effective if deposited close to the nerve (*see Minimal blocking concentration*).
    - crosses the membrane in the unionised form; thus activity depends on extracellular pH, because the degree of ionisation and thus lipid insolubility are increased by acidosis. The pH of infected tissue is lower than normal; hence the effectiveness of local anaesthetics is reduced.
    - dissociates within the axon to the ionised form; thus dependent on intracellular pH.
    - binds to sodium channels in their open state.
    - smallest **nerve fibres** are blocked first.
- Features of block are affected by:
  - patient variables, e.g. tissue pH, pregnancy.
  - drug characteristics.
  - concentration and dose used: e.g. higher concentrations and doses reduce onset time, and increase density and duration of block.
  - site of injection, e.g. rapid onset of **spinal anaesthesia** but slow onset of **brachial plexus block.**
  - additives:
    - vasoconstrictors, e.g. **adrenaline**, **felypressin**, **phenylephrine**: reduce systemic absorption and prolong the block. Intensity and onset may be improved. Effects are greatest with local anaesthetics that cause vasodilatation (e.g. lidocaine) and less with prilocaine and bupivacaine. Cocaine itself causes vasoconstriction.
    - CO_2 dissolved under pressure (carbonated solutions): passes into axons, lowering pH; intracellular dissociation is thus favoured, with faster block.
    - sodium hydroxide: remains extracellular, raising pH and increasing the unionised fraction of drug; uptake into the axon is thus favoured.
    - potassium: has been shown to increase duration of block.
    - **dextrans**: used to prolong blocks, perhaps by combining with local anaesthetic and trapping it within the tissues. Results are inconsistent.

Table 31 Properties of local anaesthetic agents

Agent	pK_a	% Protein binding	Equivalent concentration (%)	Recommended maximal safe dose (mg/kg)
Esters				
Amethocaine	8.5	76	0.25	1.5
Chloroprocaine	8.7	–	1	15
Cocaine	8.7	–	1	3
Procaine	8.9	6	2	12
Amides				
Bupivacaine	8.1	96	0.25	2
Cinchocaine	7.9	–	0.25	2
Etidocaine	7.7	94	0.5	2
Lidocaine	7.9	64	1	3–7
Mepivacaine	7.6	78	1	5
Prilocaine	7.9	55	1	5–8
Ropivacaine	8.1	94	1	3.5

- **hyaluronidase**: formerly used to increase spread by breaking down tissue stroma. Benefits are doubtful; thus rarely used now except in eye blocks.
- dextrose to increase baricity for spinal anaesthesia: affects spread.

- Toxicity:
  - may follow accidental iv injection, or systemic absorption, the latter affected by:
    - total dose administered. Recommended maximal 'safe' doses are useful as a guide but are rough estimations only, because other factors are involved (*Table 31*).
    - site of injection: e.g. absorption is large after topical anaesthesia and **intercostal block** and slow after brachial plexus block and **infiltration anaesthesia**. Affected by blood flow and tissue vascularity.
    - vasoconstrictor additives.
    - individual drug: e.g. lidocaine causes vasodilatation; bupivacaine binds extensively to tissues. Ropivacaine and levobupivacaine are less toxic than bupivacaine.
  - due to membrane-stabilising effects on other cells, especially heart and CNS. Features:
    - tingling, typically around the mouth and tongue.
    - lightheadedness, agitation and tremor.
    - unconsciousness and/or convulsions.
    - hypotension may be caused by hypoxaemia following central apnoea, direct myocardial depression or vasodilatation. Arrhythmias and cardiac arrest may occur; resistant ventricular arrhythmias are particularly likely with bupivacaine.
  - treatment:
    - supportive, with oxygenation/cardiovascular support as for **CPR**.
    - **lipid emulsion** 20%: 1.5 ml/kg bolus over 1 min, repeated up to two times, followed by 15 ml/kg/h increased to 30 ml/kg/h if the CVS is stable. Originally thought to act via either sequestration of local anaesthetic within circulating lipid ('lipid sink'), or enhanced metabolism of drug in cardiac muscle. More recent evidence suggests that lipid traps local anaesthetic in the blood to reduce the amount reaching the brain/heart, and carries it to lesser perfused parts of the body, thus accelerating initial clearance of the drug. There may be a beneficial secondary action on the heart as local anaesthetic levels fall, boosting cardiac output.

      Propofol is not a viable alternative because of the drug's haemodynamic effects and low concentration of intralipid.
    - **thiopental** or **diazepam/midazolam** may be used for convulsions, although hypotension may be exacerbated.
  - other complications may be related to:
    - vasoconstrictors, e.g. tachycardia, arrhythmias, pallor, agitation, caused by adrenaline.
    - regional technique, e.g. intraneural injection, hypotension following spinal anaesthesia.
    - preservatives, e.g. allergic reactions (e.g. to methylparaben), neurological damage and **arachnoiditis**.

See also, Ionisation of drugs; Regional anaesthesia; specific blocks

Locked-in syndrome. Syndrome of complete paralysis with preservation of vertical eye movements only. May mimic **brainstem death** except that the patient is conscious and aware of the environment but is only able to communicate via eye movements, which are often slow. 'Automatic' breathing continues but the patient is unable to control the rate or depth of breathing because of disruption to the corticospinal tract. Caused by damage to the ventral pons of the **brainstem**, usually following occlusion of the vertebrobasilar artery. May also follow **central pontine myelinolysis**. Prognosis is very poor, with death usually due to respiratory complications.

Smith E, Delargy M (2005). Br Med J; 330: 406–9

LODS, *see Logistic organ dysfunction system*

Lofentanil *cis*-oxalate. Opioid analgesic drug derived from **fentanyl**; developed in 1975. 20 times as potent as fentanyl and 6000 times as potent as **morphine** in animal studies. Of similar pK_a to fentanyl, highly lipophilic and with a particularly long duration of action due to persistent binding to **opioid receptors** (about 10 h). Has been used via the epidural route to provide long-lasting analgesia, but not generally available.

Logistic organ dysfunction system (LODS). Scoring system developed to predict hospital mortality from 11 variables measured on the first day of admission to ICU (**Glasgow coma scale**, heart rate, systolic BP, urea, creatinine, urine output, P_aO_2/F_IO_2 ratio, white cell count, platelets, bilirubin and international normalised ratio). The total score ranges from zero (normal) to 22. The difference between LODS score on day 3 and day 1 is highly predictive of hospital outcome.

Has been modified by adding infection as a 12th item (organ dysfunction and/or infection; ODIN).

Keegan MT, Gajic O, Afessa B (2011). Crit Care Med; 39: 163–9

See also, Mortality/survival prediction on intensive care unit

Long, Crawford Williamson (1815–1878). US general practitioner; administered **diethyl ether** several times for minor surgery from 1842 in Georgia, but did not report it until after **Morton**'s demonstration.

Hammonds WD, Steinhaus JE (1993). J Clin Anesth; 5: 163–7

Long Q–T syndromes, *see Prolonged Q–T syndromes*

Lorazepam. Benzodiazepine, used for insomnia, **epilepsy**, **sedation** and **premedication**. It is the first-line drug of choice in **status epilepticus. Half-life** is approximately 12 h with prolonged duration of action. Said to produce more amnesia than other benzodiazepines. Similar rates of absorption follow im and oral administration.

Metabolised to an inactive metabolite.

- Dosage:
  - 1–4 mg orally. If given the night before surgery, a further 1–2 mg may be given 1–2 h preoperatively.
  - 25–30 µg/kg iv (50–100 µg/kg in status epilepticus).

LOS, *see Lower oesophageal sphincter*

Lower oesophageal sphincter. 2–5 cm portion of **oesophagus** of increased intraluminal pressure, extending above and below the diaphragm. Opens reflexively during swallowing, and helps to prevent retrograde passage of gastric contents into the oesophagus via:
  - increased muscle tone: muscle of the sphincter zone, especially the inner circular layer, has higher resting

tone than other oesophageal muscle, possibly via increased **calcium** ion uptake and utilisation.
- neural input:
  - vagal: muscle tone reflexively increases as gastric pressure increases, thus maintaining barrier pressure (normally about 20 cmH_2O). The reflex is abolished by **atropine**.
  - sympathetic: tone is increased by α-stimulation and β-blockade, and decreased by β-stimulation and α-blockade.
- mechanical factors:
  - oesophageal compression by the diaphragm.
  - acute angle of entry of the oesophagus into the stomach.
  - mucosal flap or rosette at the oesophageal opening.
- Muscle tone is decreased by:
  - **anticholinergic drugs** given iv; possibly less with **glycopyrronium**. Atropine im does not affect sphincter pressure, but inhibits the action of **metoclopramide**.
  - gut hormones, e.g. **vasoactive intestinal hormone**, **glucagon** and gastric inhibitory peptide. Gastrin may increase tone at very high levels.
  - progesterone.
  - **opioid analgesic drugs**, volatile anaesthetic agents and most iv anaesthetic agents.
  - **ganglion blocking drugs**.
- Tone is increased by:
  - metoclopramide, **domperidone** and **prochlorperazine**.
  - **neostigmine**.
  - **pancuronium**.

No change is found with **H_2 receptor antagonists**. Although **suxamethonium** may increase intragastric pressure, the corresponding increase in lower oesophageal sphincter tone maintains barrier pressure.

Sphincter incompetence may result in **gastro-oesophageal reflux**. It becomes less competent in **hiatus hernia**, particularly if intra-abdominal pressure increases, e.g. in the head-down position.

Cotton BR, Smith G (1984). Br J Anaesth; 56: 37–46

Lown–Ganong–Levine syndrome. Tendency to **SVT** caused by an accessory conducting pathway bypassing the atrioventricular node. Impulses may pass directly from the atria to the distal **heart conducting system**, without the usual delay at the node.

Characterised by a normal **P wave**, short **P–R interval** and normal **QRS complex** on the **ECG**. Anaesthetic management is as for **Wolff–Parkinson–White syndrome**.

[Samuel A Levine (1891–1966) and Bernard Lown, US cardiologists; William F Ganong (1924–2007), US physiologist]

LPS, Lipopolysaccharide, *see Endotoxins*

Lucid interval. Period of apparently normal function and behaviour following **TBI**, during which blood is accumulating inside the skull from a slowly bleeding vessel. Classically occurring with **extradural haemorrhage**, features only become apparent when the collection causes compression of intracranial structures; because this may occur up to several hours after injury, diagnosis may be delayed and significant morbidity may result.

Ludwig's angina. Cellulitis of the floor of the mouth and submandibular region, with massive swelling. Often due to anaerobic infection. May progress to laryngeal obstruction and death unless treated with antibiotics initially, or by deep incision of the tissues under the mandible.

Anaesthetic management is as for **airway obstruction**; antibiotic therapy may reduce the swelling and improve obstruction preoperatively. Local anaesthesia may be preferable in extreme cases.

[Wilhelm von Ludwig (1790–1865), German surgeon]

Luer connectors. Worldwide system of standard fittings designed to provide leak-free (for air and fluid) connections between **syringes**, hypodermic **needles** and three-way taps. Two standard types exist:
- Luer-Lok (Lock): ends joined securely via a screw thread and matching hub on the male and female connections, respectively.
- Luer-Slip: tapered male and female connections held in place by friction.

Although originally designed for iv equipment, Luer connections are now present on many others, e.g. nasogastric tubes, airway monitoring tubing, and equipment for **spinal** and **epidural anaesthesia**. Fatal wrong-route errors have involved the latter (e.g. iv administration of **local anaesthetic agents** or intrathecal/epidural administration of iv **cytotoxic drugs**). Work on the new ISO 80369 standard for small-bore connectors began in 2007, with ISO 80369-1 (general requirements including testing methods and non-interchangeability) published in 2011. Other standards include:
- ISO 80369-2: breathing systems and driving gases.
- ISO 80369-3: enteral and gastric.
- ISO 80369-4: urethral and urinary.
- ISO 80369-5: limb cuff inflation (e.g. BP measurement).
- ISO 80369-6: neuraxial devices. The trademarked description for this category is the 'NRFit' connector, which is similar but ~20% smaller than the standard Luer; it has slip and lock forms, with the male half having a non-screw collar and screw collar, respectively. Introduced into practice in 2017.
- ISO 80369-7: intravascular/hypodermic (Luer + additional specifications).

[Hermann W. Luer (1836–1910), German medical instrument maker]

Cook TM (2012). Anaesthesia; 67; 7: 784–92

Lumbar epidural anaesthesia, *see Epidural anaesthesia*

Lumbar plexus. Formed in front of the transverse processes of the lumbar vertebrae from the anterior primary rami of the first four lumbar nerves, occasionally with a contribution from T12 (Fig. 105).

May be blocked via **paravertebral**, **psoas compartment**, **fascia iliaca compartment** and 'three-in-one' **femoral nerve blocks**. Individual nerves may also be blocked. Block is useful for hip surgery and operations on the thigh and anterior gluteal region, together with adjacent perineal and suprapubic areas.

See also, Inguinal hernia field block

Lumbar puncture. Procedure for removing **CSF** either for diagnostic purposes (e.g. **meningitis**) or treatment (e.g. benign intracranial hypertension, intrathecal injection of chemotherapy, **CSF filtration**). First performed by **Quincke** for the treatment of **hydrocephalus**. Forms part of the procedure of **spinal anaesthesia**. May be required in the

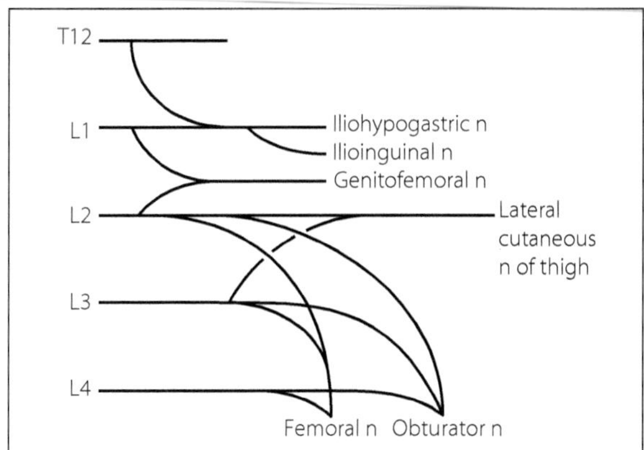

Fig. 105 Plan of the lumbar plexus

ICU for diagnosis of neurological conditions. Technique, contraindications and complications are as for spinal anaesthesia but without the drug effects; CSF 'opening pressure' may also be measured, using a simple manometer. Neurologists, general physicians and radiologists are more likely to use larger needles with cutting points than anaesthetists; whether subsequent **post-dural puncture headache** (PDPH) is masked by the presenting symptoms is uncertain. The incidence of PDPH may be decreased if the stylet is reinserted after aspiration before removal of the needle, presumably by preventing avulsion of dural strands sucked into the needle's shaft during removal of CSF.

Costerus JM, Brouwer MC, van de Beek D (2018). Lancet Neurol; 17: 268–78

Lumbar sympathetic block. Performed for peripheral vascular disease, including incipient **gangrene**, and in chronic **pain management** (e.g. post-traumatic dystrophies).

The lumbar sympathetic chain lies on the anterolateral aspect of the lumbar vertebral bodies within a fascial compartment formed by the vertebral column, psoas sheath and posterior peritoneum.

With the patient in the lateral position and with a soft pillow between the iliac crest and costal margin to curve the spine laterally, skin wheals are raised 5–8 cm lateral to the upper borders of the spinous processes of L2–4. A 12–18-cm long needle is directed medially, to strike the transverse process at about 3–5 cm. The lateral aspect of the vertebral body is contacted usually 4–6 cm deeper, and the needle advanced a further 1–2 cm. Correct positioning is confirmed by negative aspiration for CSF or blood, and radiographic imaging: the needles should barely reach the anterior borders of the vertebral bodies in the lateral view, and should overlie their lateral edge in the anteroposterior view. Further confirmation of positioning is made by injecting contrast medium. 25–30 ml local anaesthetic solution (e.g. 0.5% **lidocaine** or **prilocaine**) is injected at L2, or 15 ml at L2 and L4. Catheters may be inserted for repeated injection. **Phenol** or absolute alcohol is used for chemical sympatholysis, 3 ml at each of L1, L2 and L3. The block may also be performed with the patient prone.

Complications include hypotension, genitofemoral neuritis, bleeding into psoas and accidental epidural, subarachnoid or iv injection.

Similar blocks have been performed in the thoracic region but with risk of pneumothorax.

Lundberg waves, *see Intracranial pressure monitoring*

Lundy, John Silus (1894–1973). US anaesthetist; he became head of department at the Mayo Clinic in 1924. Co-founder of the **American Board of Anesthesiology**. An advocate and developer of regional techniques, **balanced anaesthesia**, **thiopental** and post-anaesthetic **recovery rooms**. Established the first blood bank in the USA.

Ellis TA 2nd, Narr BJ, Bacon DR (2004). J Clin Anesth; 16: 226–9

Lung. Organ of respiration. Continues to develop after birth, with alveolar proliferation complete at about 8 years.

- Anatomy:
  - cone-shaped, with bases applied to the **diaphragm**.
  - enveloped in **pleura**, attached to the **mediastinum** at the hila.
  - the right lung is larger than the left and divided into three lobes separated by the oblique and transverse fissures.
  - the left lung is divided into two lobes by the oblique fissure. The lingula is the anteroinferior portion of the upper lobe.
  - lobes are divided into segments (*see Tracheobronchial tree*).
  - surface anatomy:
    - as for pleura, except for the lower border, which lies two ribs cranial to the caudal pleural limit.
    - on the left side, the medial anterior border lies 2–3 cm lateral to the sternum at the fifth and sixth costal cartilages (cardiac notch).
    - the oblique fissure follows a line from the spine of T4 downwards and outwards to the sixth costal cartilage.
    - the transverse fissure follows a horizontal line from the fourth costal cartilage until it hits the previous line.
- Blood supply: via bronchial and pulmonary arteries (*see Pulmonary circulation*).
- Nerve supply: sympathetic and vagal plexuses; sensory pathways are mainly via the latter.
- Lymph drainage: via bronchopulmonary, tracheobronchial and paratracheal nodes to mediastinal lymph trunks and thence brachiocephalic veins.
- Functions:
  - gas exchange.
  - filtering of inhaled particles.
  - synthesis of associated phospholipids, e.g. **surfactant**, carbohydrates (e.g. mucopolysaccharides) and proteins (e.g. collagen).
  - metabolism and deactivation of certain compounds, e.g. angiotensin, bradykinin and **5-HT**. Takes up amide **local anaesthetic agents**.
  - synthesis and release of compounds, e.g. **prostaglandins** and **histamine**.
  - involvement in the immune system, with pulmonary alveolar macrophages especially effective against bacteria.
  - coagulation effects: pulmonary endothelial fibrinolysin and presence of high levels of heparin within the lung help prevent **PE** and possibly contribute to overall systemic coagulability.
  - acts as a reservoir for blood; the pulmonary circulation contains 500–900 ml blood. Moving from the supine to erect position results in the transfer of ~400 ml into the systemic circulation.

See also, Alveolus; Lung…; Pulmonary…

Lung function tests. Used to determine the nature and extent of pulmonary disorders. Clinical assessment, e.g. ability to walk up stairs, breath-hold for >30 s, or blow out a lighted match held 15 cm (6 inches) away, are imprecise and non-specific indicators.

- Include tests of:
  - ventilation mechanics:
    - measurement of static **lung volumes**: cumbersome apparatus is required. **Dead space** and **closing capacity** may be measured.
    - assessment of **forced expiration** and derived variables (e.g. **FEV_1, FVC, forced expiratory flow rate**), e.g. using a spirometer. The FEV_1/FVC ratio typically is reduced in obstructive lung disease, and is normal or high in restrictive disease. **Peak expiratory flow rate** is another simple bedside test for obstructive disease. Reversibility of obstructive disease is assessed using inhaled **bronchodilator drugs**. Airway reactivity is assessed by challenging with histamine or methacholine while measuring FEV_1.
    - **flow–volume loops** require more sophisticated apparatus, with instantaneous flow rate measurement.
    - **airway resistance** and lung **compliance** may be measured.
    - **maximal voluntary ventilation** is non-specific and related to effort as well as pulmonary function.
    - **respiratory muscle** function may be assessed, e.g. maximal mouth or nasal sniff pressures when breathing against a closed valve. Work of breathing and O_2 consumption may also be measured.
  - gas exchange:
    - **blood gas interpretation** and pulse **oximetry**.
    - **diffusing capacity** for carbon monoxide (transfer factor); now thought to be related more to $\dot{V}/\dot{Q}$ **mismatch** than to diffusion impairment.
    - distribution of ventilation and perfusion as for $\dot{V}/\dot{Q}$ mismatch.
  - pulmonary circulation: assessment is difficult. **Radioisotope scanning** may be used as for $\dot{V}/\dot{Q}$ mismatch.
  - control of breathing: CO_2 response curve or response to hypoxia may be used.
  - response to exercise, using the above tests.

ERS Guidelines (2005). Eur Resp J; 26: 319–38, 511–22 and 720–35

See also, Body plethysmograph; Breathing, control of; Nitrogen washout

Lung protection strategies. Principles of mechanical ventilation demonstrated to improve outcomes in **ALI**. Components include:

- avoidance of overdistension of alveoli.
- **permissive hypercapnia.**
- maintenance of alveolar volume.
- prevention of radial stress associated with cyclical end-expiratory collapse and re-expansion at low lung volumes.

Inspiratory plateau pressure is usually limited to <35 cmH_2O. Pressure–volume curves may be used to identify an upper inflection point (UIP), thought to represent the point of alveolar overdistension, and a lower inflection point (LIP), thought to represent the point of alveolar recruitment during inflation. **PEEP** levels are set at or above LIP; maximum inspiratory plateau pressure is set below UIP. **Extracorporeal CO_2 removal** has also been used to reduce the minute ventilation requirement.

Yilmaz M, Gajic O (2008). Eur J Anaesthesiol; 25: 89–96

Lung transplantation. First performed in 1963; includes transplantation of a single lung, both lungs, or sequential single lungs during the same operation. Most commonly performed for **COPD** and idiopathic **pulmonary fibrosis**, but also for **cystic fibrosis** and other causes of end-stage lung disease. Similar considerations apply as to **heart–lung transplantation**:

- Donor:
  - as for heart–lung transplantation; those with significant respiratory disease are excluded. HLA mismatching is not associated with reduced long-term rejection, although matching of size is important.
  - up to 9 h is thought to be acceptable before transplantation, although up to 3 h is best. Preservative techniques may include iv **heparin** and **prostacyclin** (the latter into the pulmonary artery) before removal from the donor. A left atrial cuff, pulmonary veins, main bronchi and pulmonary artery are taken in addition to the lungs.
- Recipient:
  - immunosuppression and antibiotic therapy as for heart–lung transplantation.
  - a double-lumen endobronchial tube or single-lumen tube with bronchial blocker is used. Initial problems are those of **thoracic surgery** in general, especially **one-lung ventilation.**
  - monitoring may include **pulmonary artery catheterisation** (the catheter usually flows to the better perfused lung; it may require withdrawal before the lung is removed).
  - control of **pulmonary vascular resistance** may be difficult; options include **milrinone** and inhaled **nitric oxide** or **prostacyclin.** If the patient remains markedly unstable, **cardiopulmonary bypass** may be used.
  - postoperative problems include non-cardiogenic pulmonary oedema (pulmonary reimplantation response), hypoxaemia, disrupted anastomosis, infection and rejection. Obliterative bronchiolitis may occur.

Anaesthetic management of patients with transplanted lungs is as standard, remembering the risks of infection and graft rejection, **pulmonary hypertension** and impaired lung function (**lung protection strategies** are employed).

Castillo M (2011). Curr Opin Anesthesiol; 24: 32–6

Lung volumes. Functional, not anatomical, volumes of the lungs, usually expressed as if both lungs compose one unit. May be derived from a **spirometer** tracing of inhaled/exhaled volumes, with maximal inspiration and expiration following normal tidal breathing (Fig. 106).

- Approximate normal values for a 70-kg man:
  - **tidal volume**: 0.5 l
  - **inspiratory reserve volume**: 2.5 l
  - **inspiratory capacity**: 3.0 l
  - **vital capacity**: 4.5 l
  - **expiratory reserve volume**: 1.5 l
  - **residual volume**: 1.5 l
  - **FRC**: 3.0 l
  - **total lung capacity**: 6.0 l.

Capacities are sums of volumes.

Tidal volume, inspiratory reserve volume, expiratory reserve volume and capacities derived from them may

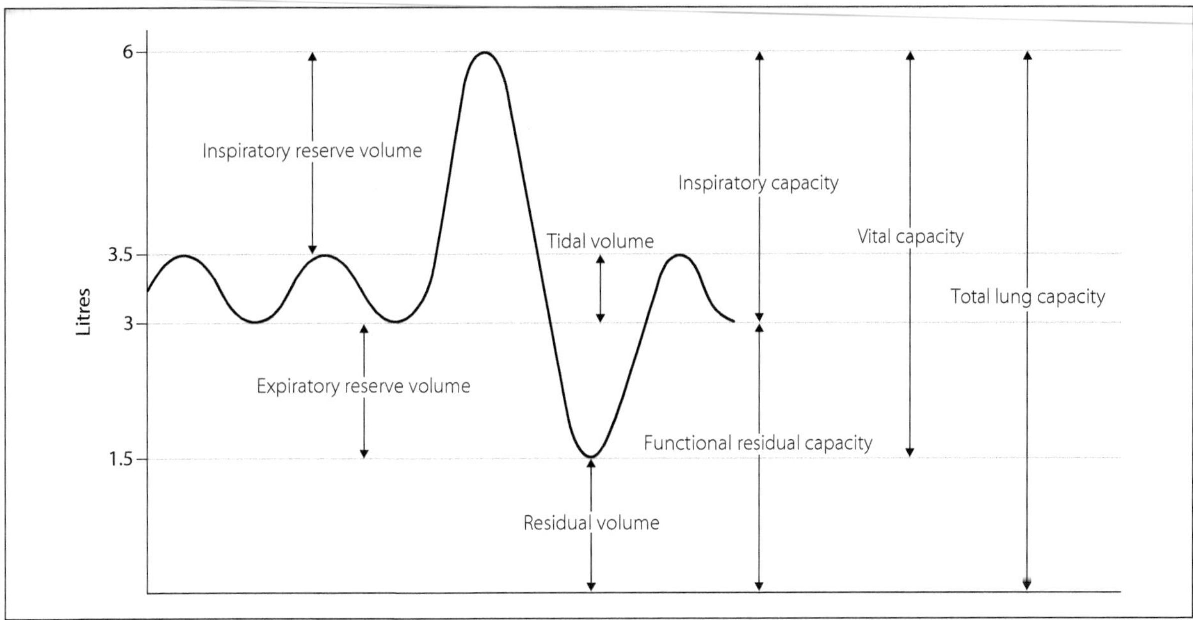

Fig. 106 Lung volumes

be measured using a wet spirometer. Residual volume may be measured using helium dilution or the **body plethysmograph**.

Other lung volumes measured include **dead space** and **closing capacity**. Differential spirometry is used to examine function of single lungs.

See also, Lung function tests

LVEDP, *see Left ventricular end-diastolic pressure*

LVEDV, *see Left ventricular end-diastolic volume*

LVET, Left ventricular ejection time, *see Systolic time intervals*

LVF, Left ventricular failure, *see Cardiac failure*

LVH, Left ventricular hypertrophy, *see Cardiac failure*

Lyme disease. Tick-borne disease caused by the spirochaete *Borrelia burgdorferi*. First recognised as a cause of paediatric arthropathy in Lyme, Connecticut, USA, in 1975. Widespread in the USA and parts of Europe and Asia, becoming more common in the UK. Causes characteristic expanding skin lesions (erythema migrans) at the site of the tick's bite, associated with systemic flu-like symptoms. Weeks to months later, neurological features (**meningitis, encephalitis**, cranial neuritis) lasting for months occur in 15% of cases whereas 8% develop cardiac features (**heart block, myocarditis**) lasting a few days. Arthritis occurs up to 2 years later in 60% of cases. Diagnosis is on clinical grounds, aided by serological testing. Treatment is with **penicillins, tetracyclines, cephalosporins** or **macrolides** depending on the presentation and stage of illness. Outcome is usually favourable, although late neurological complications may persist.

[Willy A Burgdorfer (1925–2014), Swiss-born US entomologist]

Shapiro ED (2014). N Engl J Med; 370: 1724–30

Lypressin, *see Vasopressin*

Lytic cocktail. Obsolete mixture of **chlorpromazine**, **promethazine** and **pethidine**, described in the 1940s as a means of **sedation**, e.g. for premedication and labour. Produced a state of drowsiness and apathy ('artificial hibernation') but effects were long lasting and accompanied by hypotension.

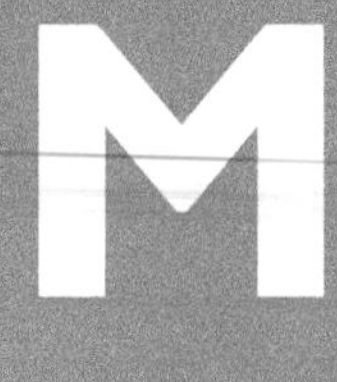

MAC, *see Minimal alveolar concentration*

Macewen, William (1847–1924). Eminent Scottish surgeon; Professor at Glasgow University, knighted in 1902. Advocated and practised tracheal intubation, usually oral, for laryngeal obstruction, e.g. due to **diphtheria**; he performed this by touch without anaesthetic. Was the first to advocate tracheal intubation instead of tracheotomy for head and neck surgery, in 1880. The tube was inserted before introduction of **chloroform**, and the patient allowed to breathe spontaneously. Packing around the tube achieved a seal.
James CDT (1974). Anaesthesia; 29: 743–53

Macintosh, Robert Reynolds (1897–1989). New Zealand–born anaesthetist, he became the first British Professor of Anaesthetics in Oxford in 1937. Lord Nuffield, a friend of Macintosh, had insisted that such a chair be set up as a precondition for endowing further chairs in Medicine, Surgery and Obstetrics and Gynaecology. Established Oxford as a centre for anaesthesia, and helped to establish anaesthesia as a medical specialty. Wrote books and articles about many aspects of local and general anaesthesia, and designed many pieces of equipment, including his **laryngoscope**, **spray**, **endobronchial tube**, **vaporisers** and devices for locating the epidural space. Also helped research the hazards of aviation and seafaring. Knighted in 1955, and received many other medals and awards.
[William Morris (1877–1963), English automobile industrialist and philanthropist—became Lord Nuffield in 1934]
Mushin WW (1989). Anaesthesia; 44: 950–2

Macitentan, *see Endothelin receptor antagonists*

McKesson, Elmer Isaac (1881–1935). US anaesthetist, founder and member of many US and international anaesthetic bodies. Also invented and manufactured expiratory valves, **pressure regulators**, **flowmeters**, **suction equipment**, **vaporisers** and **intermittent flow anaesthetic machines**. A major proponent of the use of N_2O in modern anaesthesia.

McMechan, Francis Hoeffer (1879–1939). US anaesthetist, practising in Cincinnati. A pioneer of the development of anaesthesia in the USA. Founded the American Association of Anesthetists in 1912, and instrumental in founding the National Anesthetic Research Society (subsequently the International Anesthesia Research Society) whose publication (which became ***Anesthesia and Analgesia***) he edited.

Macrolides. Group of **antibacterial drugs** containing a lactam ring but distinct from β-lactams. Interfere with RNA-dependent protein synthesis. Includes **erythromycin**, **azithromycin**, **clarithromycin** and telithromycin. All have similar antibacterial activities (gram-positive and some gram-negative bacteria, mycoplasma, rickettsia and toxoplasma) but varying properties otherwise; the latter three drugs have longer durations of action than erythromycin and cause less nausea and vomiting.

Macrophage colony-stimulating factor, *see Granulocyte colony-stimulating factor*

Magill breathing system, *see Anaesthetic breathing systems*

Magill, Ivan Whiteside (1888–1986). Irish-born anaesthetist, responsible for much of the innovation in, and development of, modern anaesthesia. With **Rowbotham** in Sidcup after World War I, he developed endotracheal anaesthesia as an alternative to **insufflation techniques**, originally for facial plastic surgery. Introduced his own **anaesthetic breathing system**, **forceps**, **laryngoscope** and **connectors**, and developed blind nasal intubation. A pioneer of anaesthesia for thoracic surgery, he developed **one-lung anaesthesia**, **endobronchial tubes** and **bronchial blockers**. Also introduced bobbin **flowmeters**, portable anaesthetic apparatus and other equipment.

Co-founder of the **Association of Anaesthetists of Great Britain and Ireland**, he also helped establish the **DA examination**, the **Faculty of Anaesthetists** and the **FFARCS examination**. Worked at the Westminster and Brompton Hospitals, London. Knighted in 1960, and received many other medals and awards.
Edridge AW (1987). Anaesthesia; 42: 231–3

Magnesium. Largely intracellular ion, present mainly in bone (over 50%) and skeletal muscle (20%); the remainder is found in the heart, liver and other organs. 1% is in the **ECF**. Normal plasma levels: 0.75–1.05 mmol/l (although the value of measurement has been questioned, because most magnesium is intracellular). Deficiency is common in critical illness and is associated with increased mortality. Causes include decreased intake (due to reduced GI activity, malnutrition), increased renal excretion (due to diuretic therapy, **digoxin**), **diabetes mellitus**, **hypokalaemia** and **hypocalcaemia**. Required for protein and nucleic acid synthesis, regulation of intracellular **calcium** and **potassium**, and many enzymatic reactions, including all those involving **ATP** synthesis/hydrolysis. Inhibits voltage-gated calcium channels, acting as a physiological antagonist; also an antagonist at **NMDA receptors**.
Herroeder S, Schonnher ME, De Hert SG, Hollman MW (2011). Anesthesiology; 114: 971–93
See also, Hypermagnesaemia; Hypomagnesaemia

Magnesium sulfate. Drug with varied clinical indications, reflecting its numerous sites of action, e.g. non-competitive inhibition of phospholipase C-mediated **calcium** release; antagonism of **NMDA receptors**; inhibition of voltage-gated calcium channels and **sodium/potassium pumps**; and attenuation of catecholamine release from the **adrenal glands**. Its actions thus include neuronal/myocardial membrane stabilisation and bronchial and vascular smooth muscle relaxation. Magnesium chloride is also used.

- Clinical indications:
  - as the **anticonvulsant drug** of choice in **pre-eclampsia** and **eclampsia**. Thought to act by reducing cerebral vasospasm seen in the condition. Also causes systemic vasodilatation, helping to lower BP. Superior to **diazepam** and **phenytoin** in preventing primary eclampsia, as well as preventing recurrence of seizures.
  - increasingly used before surgery to promote **pre-emptive analgesia** and perioperatively to reduce opioid requirements postoperatively (30–50 mg/kg and/or infusion of 1–15 mg/kg/h).
  - as a **tocolytic drug**.
  - severe **asthma** resistant to conventional bronchodilator therapy.
  - perioperative management of **phaeochromocytoma**.
  - cardiac **arrhythmias** (e.g. **torsade de pointes**), especially those caused by **hypokalaemia**.
  - has also been used in **migraine** and depression.
- Dosage: 2–4 g (8–16 mmol) iv over 5–15 min, followed by 1–2 g/h.
- Side effects:
  - cardiac conduction defects, drowsiness, reduced tendon reflexes, muscle weakness, hypoventilation and cardiac arrest may occur with increasing **hypermagnesaemia**.
  - augments non-depolarising and depolarising neuromuscular blockade. Neonatal hypotonia may also occur.

Overdosage may be treated with iv **calcium**.

- Therapeutic plasma levels: 2.0–3.5 mmol/l; side effects may occur above 4–5 mmol/l, with cardiac arrest above 12 mmol/l. Loss of deep tendon reflexes (e.g. knee jerk) may indicate impending toxicity.

Herroeder S, Schonnher ME, De Hert SG, Hollman MW (2011). Anesthesiology; 114: 971–93

Magnesium trisilicate. Particulate **antacid**, used in dyspepsia. Has been used to increase gastric pH preoperatively in patients at risk from **aspiration of gastric contents**, but may itself cause pneumonitis if inhaled. Has also been used to reduce risk of peptic ulceration on **ICU**, e.g. by hourly nasogastric administration to keep pH above 3–4.

Magnetic resonance imaging (MRI; Nuclear magnetic resonance, NMR). Imaging technique, particularly useful for investigating CNS, pelvic and musculoskeletal pathology, where tissue movement is minimal. By using gating techniques it can also be used in other parts of the body, including the chest and heart.

Involves placement of the patient within a powerful magnetic field, causing alignment of atoms with an odd number of protons or neutrons, e.g. hydrogen. Radiofrequency pulses are then applied, causing deflection of the atoms with absorption of energy. When each pulse stops, the atoms return to their aligned position, emitting energy as radiofrequency waves. Computer analysis of the emitted waves provides information about the chemical make-up of the tissue studied. MRI can provide graphic tissue slices in any plane, or may be used to analyse metabolic processes, e.g. distribution and alterations of intracellular phosphate (spectroscopy). So-called functional MRI (fMRI) techniques demonstrate regional differences in tissue oxygenation and **cerebral blood flow**. Interventional MRI involves surgery within the MRI suite to allow scanning during operative procedures.

- Problems and anaesthetic considerations:
  - magnets used are very powerful but not considered directly harmful; however, the maximal 'safe' level for occupational exposure to static magnetic fields is set at 200 mT over a single 8-h period. Indirect problems:
    - metal objects may become dangerous projectiles if they are placed near the magnet. All ferromagnetic metal equipment, including cylinders, needles and laryngoscope batteries, must be kept away from the machine. Intracranial clips, pacemakers and heart valves may also be affected. Non-ferromagnetic anaesthetic equipment is increasingly available.
    - monitoring may be difficult because of poor access to the patient and the need for special equipment. Remote monitoring from outside the scanning room requires a window and protective brass tubes (waveguides) for cables passing between the scanning and observation rooms, with the ability to communicate with the patient. Audible alarms may not be heard because of the background noise of the scanner and the need for ear protection. Automatic BP devices using plastic connectors, capnography, oesophageal stethoscopes and non-magnetic oximeters using fibreoptic cabling are used. ECG artefacts (especially in the S–T region) may be caused by currents induced by aortic blood flow within the magnetic field. The length of capnography tubing (in side-stream analysers) introduces a long delay before the CO_2 signal is obtained.
    - some magnets may be switched off in emergencies, but may require lengthy and expensive restarting procedures. Rapid, sudden shutdown may result in the liquid coolant of the magnet (cryogen; usually helium in modern devices) boiling off and flooding the immediate area if not properly vented (quenching). This may cause a dangerous reduction in available O_2 with the risk of asphyxia; proper procedures and O_2 sensors are therefore required.
  - radiofrequency pulses may cause heating effects, thought to be relatively insignificant. These effects may be increased with metal prostheses.
  - sedation/anaesthesia may be required, especially in children or nervous adults, because the subject has to lie within a very small space and the scans are accompanied by loud knocking noises. Problems include those of **radiology** in general, in addition to the above. Scans originally took up to 2–3 h but are shorter with newer machines.

Malaria. Tropical disease caused by the protozoan plasmodium (*Plasmodium vivax, P. malariae, P. ovale* or *P. falciparum*), and spread by the anopheles mosquito, which carries infected blood between individuals. Although not endemic in Europe, about 5000–7000 cases are reported each year because of widespread air travel. All febrile or ill patients who have travelled to endemic areas within 6 months should be screened for the disease.

Severe illness and death are almost exclusively due to infection with *P. falciparum*, particularly common in tropical Africa and Southeast Asia. Incubation period is 12–14 days. Many features result from microvascular obstruction by damaged infected red blood cells, resulting in organ ischaemia and **lactic acidosis**.

- Features are non-specific but include:
  - fever/sweats/chills, malaise, myalgia, vomiting, headache.
  - diarrhoea, cough.
  - confusion, **coma, seizures** (cerebral malaria).
- World Health Organization criteria for severe malaria include:
  - cerebral malaria—accounts for 80% of deaths.
  - **ALI, pulmonary oedema**, hypotension.
  - spontaneous bleeding, **DIC**, intravascular **haemolysis, thrombocyctopaenia, jaundice**.
  - **hypoglycaemia** (<2.2 mmol/l): may be due to a failure of hepatic gluconeogenesis; it may also result from **quinine** therapy, which increases **insulin** secretion.
  - lactate >5 mmol/l, pH <7.35.
  - anaemia (Hb <50 g/l).
  - **acute kidney injury**.

Diagnosis is made by examining thick and thin blood films (or rarely, bone marrow) for parasites. Rapid diagnostic tests that detect parasite-associated proteins and enzymes are helpful but do not allow separation of malaria types.

- Prevention:
  - use of insect repellents, mosquito nets over beds, etc.
  - drug prophylaxis, e.g. mefloquine, doxycycline or malarone.
  - vaccination: a vaccine has been developed that can halve the infection rate.
- Treatment regimens vary according to drug availability and local resistance, but include the following drugs:
  - **chloroquine** and primaquine for mild infections.
  - artemisinin derivatives (artemether and artesunate): drugs of choice in severe falciparum infection. If not available, iv quinine is used.
- Severe malaria requires admission to an HDU or ICU. Management includes:
  - expert advice from a tropical diseases unit.
  - respiratory support as necessary.
  - fluid balance to maintain normovolaemia; fluid overload must be avoided as patients are susceptible to pulmonary oedema.
  - regular monitoring of blood glucose to detect hypoglycaemia. Enteral feeding should be started as soon as feasible.
  - regular Hb, electrolyte, liver function, coagulation and parasite count testing.
  - treatment for gram-negative sepsis if the patient is shocked.

Malaria may be transmitted by **blood transfusion**; those with known infection or recent travel to an endemic area are therefore excluded from being donors.

Marks M, Gupta-Wright A, Doherty JF, et al (2014). Br J Anaesth; 113: 910–21

Malignancy. Now the commonest cause of death in the UK (previously this was cardiovascular disease). Patients may present to anaesthetists for investigative, therapeutic or unrelated procedures. ICU management may be required after major surgery related to the malignancy or for incidental conditions. Considerable ethical issues surround ICU provision for patients with terminal disease.

- General anaesthetic considerations:
  - effects of malignancy itself:
    - primary:
      - local, e.g. pressure effects, ulceration, haemorrhage.
      - systemic, e.g. **anaemia**, cachexia, susceptibility to infection, electrolyte disturbances (e.g. **hypercalcaemia**), endocrine effects (e.g. **Cushing's syndrome** caused by **bronchial carcinoma, carcinoid syndrome, myasthenic syndrome**).
    - metastatic, e.g. lung, liver, bone.
  - effects of previous treatment:
    - surgery/**radiotherapy**, e.g. scarring, deformities.
    - **cytotoxic drugs, corticosteroids, opioid analgesic drugs** and **antidepressant drugs**.
  - possible effects of anaesthesia on outcome: animal studies and retrospective human ones suggest that surgery for cancer under inhalational anaesthesia may be associated with poorer outcomes than **TIVA**, possibly related to:
    - increased growth factors associated with angiogenesis and spread of cancer cells.
    - impaired **immune system** function, favouring survival of cancer cells.

    Other factors that may also have an effect include regional anaesthesia and use of COX-2 inhibitors (protective), and administration of blood during bowel cancer resection (may decrease survival, possibly via immunosuppression).
  - anxiety, depression.
  - **pain management**.

Arain MR, Buggy DJ (2007). Curr Opin Anaesthesiol; 20: 247–53

Malignant hyperthermia (MH). Condition first described by Denborough in 1961, consisting of increased temperature and rigidity during anaesthesia. Reported incidence is between 1:5000 and 1:200 000. Results from abnormal skeletal **muscle contraction** and increased metabolism affecting muscle and other tissues. Exhibits autosomal dominant inheritance; in 50%–70% of affected families the predisposing genetic loci are found on the long arm of chromosome 19, coding for the ryanodine/dihydropyridine receptor complex at the T-tubule/sarcoplasmic reticulum complex of striated muscle. This receptor regulates **calcium** flux in and out of the sarcoplasmic reticulum; this control is lost in MH, resulting in a massive influx of calcium leading to uncontrolled muscle contraction. MH susceptibility is also genetically related to central core disease, a rare **muscular dystrophy**. Several other gene mutations have been implicated, thus reducing the sensitivity of genetic analysis as a test for MH.

MH follows exposure to triggering agents, particularly the volatile anaesthetic agents and **suxamethonium**, although it is thought that a single dose of the latter by itself will not cause the syndrome. It may occur in patients who have had previously uneventful anaesthetics. MH may also be triggered by stress and strenuous exercise. Thus patients' sensitivity to triggering agents may vary at different times. Reactions have been reported up to 11 h postoperatively.

Most common in young patients undergoing musculoskeletal surgery, including trauma surgery. Whether this reflects an underlying abnormality of muscle predisposing to trauma is unknown. Operations in the young are commonly for squints and orthopaedic problems, and increased incidence in this group may simply represent the first exposure to anaesthesia in susceptible patients.

All patients should be questioned for family history of anaesthetic problems, because many susceptible patients give a positive family history. Susceptible patients should wear MedicAlert bracelets.

- Features are related to muscle abnormality and hypermetabolism, but not all may be present:
  - sustained muscle contraction; results from breakage of the normal impulse/contraction sequence (excitation/contraction uncoupling) relating to abnormal calcium ion mobilisation, and is unrelieved by neuromuscular blocking drugs. **Masseter spasm** may be an early sign.
  - muscle breakdown with release of potassium, myoglobin and muscle enzymes, e.g. creatine kinase. **Hyperkalaemia** may cause cardiac **arrhythmias**.
  - increased O_2 consumption, leading to **cyanosis**.
  - increased CO_2 production and **hypercapnia**. Hyperventilation may occur in the spontaneously breathing patient.
  - rapidly increasing body temperature (e.g. >0.5°C every 10 min) and sweating.
  - tachycardia and unstable BP.
  - metabolic **acidosis**.
- Management:
  - discontinuation of the triggering agent, and abandonment of surgery if feasible. Changing the anaesthetic machine, tubing and soda lime has been suggested if possible. If not, because the modern volatile agents are hardly adsorbed on to modern plastic breathing tubing, simply removing the vaporisers and emptying the reservoir bag (or flushing the ventilator bellows) may be sufficient.
  - **dantrolene** is the only available specific treatment. 1 mg/kg is given iv, repeated as required up to 10 mg/kg.
  - supportive treatment:
    - hyperventilation with 100% O_2. Anaesthesia is maintained with **TIVA**.
    - correction of acidosis with **bicarbonate**, according to the results of **blood gas interpretation**.
    - cooling with cold iv fluids, fans, sponging and irrigation of body cavities. Other causes of **hyperthermia** should be considered.
    - treatment of hyperkalaemia if severe.
    - **diuretic** therapy (**mannitol** or **furosemide**) and urinary alkalinisation to reduce renal damage caused by myoglobin.
    - treatment of any arrhythmias as they occur.
    - **corticosteroids** (e.g. **dexamethasone** 4 mg) have been advocated.
    - close **monitoring** in an ICU for 36–48 h postoperatively. Creatine kinase levels should be measured 12-hourly for 36–48 h, and the urine analysed for myoglobin.
    - **acute kidney injury** and **DIC** are treated as necessary.

Treatment with dantrolene should be instituted as soon as the diagnosis is suspected. Arterial blood gas analysis and measurement of plasma potassium should be performed early to detect acidosis and hyperkalaemia.

Prognosis is good if treated appropriately and early; mortality was 80% before dantrolene became available but is <5% with modern management.

- Investigation:
  - serum creatine kinase elevation and **myoglobinuria** are suggestive, but not diagnostic. The former is not reliable as a screening test. Creatine kinase and myoglobin may both increase after suxamethonium administration in normal patients.
  - muscle biopsy may appear normal histologically.
  - caffeine and halothane contracture testing is the investigation of choice. Biopsied muscle is exposed to caffeine and halothane, and tension in the muscle measured. Contractures are induced in susceptible muscle. Results are divided into positive, negative or equivocal. False-positive results may occur. All suspected cases and immediate relatives should be tested for susceptibility.
  - genetic testing for the RYR1 variants associated with MH can aid investigation of susceptibility.
- Management of known cases:
  - pretreatment with oral dantrolene is no longer recommended.
  - sedative **premedication** is sometimes given to reduce 'stress', but this is controversial.
  - avoidance of known triggering agents: volatile agents and suxamethonium. **N_2O** is considered safe. Many other drugs have been implicated at some time, but the above are the only definite triggers. TIVA is a useful technique. Local anaesthetic techniques may be used, but MH may still occur. All local anaesthetic agents are considered as safe as each other. Some would avoid **phenothiazines** and **butyrophenones** because of the **neuroleptic malignant syndrome**, but there is no evidence that the two conditions are related.
  - formerly, use of an anaesthetic machine not previously exposed to volatile agents was considered mandatory, but a new breathing system, flushed with fresh gas for 10–20 min, has been suggested as being adequate.
  - routine monitoring should include core temperature. Some would consider arterial cannulation mandatory. Close monitoring should continue postoperatively.
  - dantrolene and supportive treatments should be readily available.
  - reactions have been reported following apparently 'trigger-free' anaesthetics, but these have not been severe.

[Michael Denborough (1929–2014), Australian physician]

Wappler F (2010). Curr Opin Anesthesiol; 23: 417–22

Mallampati score, *see Intubation, difficult*

Malnutrition. Nutrient deficiency, usually of several dietary components. **Protein** depletion with near-normal **energy** supply may lead to kwashiorkor, with **hypoproteinaemia** and **oedema**. Protein and energy depletion may lead to marasmus, with normal plasma protein concentration.

- Body reserves during total starvation under basal conditions:
  - **carbohydrate**: about 0.5 kg, mainly as liver and muscle glycogen; lasts <1 day.
  - protein: 4–6 kg, mainly as muscle; lasts 10–12 days.
  - **fat**: 12–15 kg, as adipose tissue; lasts 20–25 days.

Protein breakdown is reduced by even small amounts of **glucose**, possibly via resultant **insulin** secretion, inhibiting protein **catabolism**.

- Malnutrition is common to some degree in hospital patients. It may be associated with:
  - decreased intake, e.g. **vomiting**, malabsorption, anorexia, poor diet, nil-by-mouth orders.
  - decreased utilisation, e.g. **renal failure**.
  - increased **basal metabolic rate**, e.g. **trauma**, **burns**, severe illness, pyrexia.

Thus common perioperatively, especially in severe chronic illness, GIT disease/surgery, alcoholics, the elderly and the mentally ill. May result in impaired wound healing, pressure sores, increased susceptibility to infection, weakness, **anaemia**, hypoproteinaemia, electrolyte disturbances and **dehydration**, **vitamin deficiency** disorders and predisposition to **hypothermia**. Respiratory muscle weakness may predispose to respiratory complications including difficulty **weaning from ventilators**.

Long-term **nutrition**, via enteral or parenteral routes, is thought to be beneficial preoperatively (at least 14 days). The place of short-term feeding is less certain. Progress may be monitored by weight or skin thickness measurements.

Casaer MP, Van den Berghe G (2014). N Engl J Med; 370: 1227–36

Managing Obstetric Emergencies and Trauma course (MOET course). Training programme, devised in 1998, designed for medical staff working within obstetrics, obstetric anaesthesia, and accident and emergency medicine. Similar to other acute life support courses in its systematic approach and structure.

Mandatory minute ventilation (MMV). Ventilatory mode used to assist **weaning from ventilators**. The required mandatory minute ventilation is preset, and the patient allowed to breathe spontaneously, with the ventilator making up any shortfall in minute volume. Thus with the patient breathing adequately, the ventilator is not required. However, a minute ventilation made up of rapid, shallow breaths will also 'satisfy' the ventilator, despite **alveolar ventilation** being inadequate. In addition, not all ventilators allow spontaneous minute ventilation to exceed the preset one (extended mandatory minute ventilation; EMMV). Thus MMV is less popular than **IMV**.

Mandibular nerve blocks. Performed for facial and intraoral procedures.

- Anatomy: the mandibular division (V_3) of the trigeminal nerve passes from the **Gasserian ganglion** through the foramen ovale.
- Divisions:
  - motor nerves to the muscles of mastication and tensor muscles of the palate and tympanic membrane.
  - sensory nerves (*see Fig. 79*; **Gasserian ganglion block**):
    - meningeal branch: passes through the foramen spinosum and supplies the adjacent dura.
    - buccal nerve: supplies the skin and mucosa of the cheek.
    - auriculotemporal nerve; supplies the anterior eardrum, ear canal, **temporomandibular joint**, cheek, temple, temporal scalp and parotid gland.
    - inferior alveolar nerve: enters the mandible at its ramus, supplying the lower teeth and gums; the central incisors are innervated bilaterally. Emerges through the mental foramen to supply the mucosa and skin of the lower lip, chin and gum.
    - lingual nerve: passes alongside the **tongue** to supply its anterior two-thirds, the floor of the mouth and lingual gum.

The supraorbital foramen, pupil, infraorbital notch, infraorbital foramen, buccal surface of the second premolar and mental foramen all lie along a straight line.

- Blocks:
  - mandibular: a needle is inserted at right angles to the skin between the coronoid and condylar processes, just above the bone. After contacting the pterygoid plate, it is redirected posteriorly until paraesthesiae are obtained, and 5 ml **local anaesthetic agent** injected (N.B. the pharynx lies 5 mm internally).
  - inferior alveolar/lingual: with the mouth wide open, a needle is inserted parallel to the teeth and 1 cm above their occlusal surface, medial to the oblique line of the mandibular ramus. It is advanced 1.5–2.0 cm and the syringe barrel swung across to the opposite side. 1–1.5 ml solution is injected with a further 0.5 ml on withdrawal (to block the lingual nerve).

    May also be performed extraorally, by injecting 1.5–2.0 ml between the mandibular ramus and maxilla, level with the upper teeth gingival margins; the needle is inserted from the front with the mouth shut.

    Buccal infiltration is required for surgery to the molar teeth; 0.5–1.0 ml is injected into the cheek mucosa opposite the third molar. The incisors receive bilateral innervation.
  - mental/incisive branches of the inferior alveolar nerve (supplying from the incisors to the first premolar): 0.5–1.0 ml is injected at the mental foramen from behind the second molar intraorally, or extraorally.
  - buccal nerve: 0.5–1.0 ml is injected lateral and posterior to the last molar, by the anterior border of the mandibular ramus.
  - submucous infiltration on both sides of individual teeth, directed along its long axis, may also be used.
  - auriculotemporal nerve: 1.5–2.0 ml is injected in the anterior wall of the ear canal, at the junction of its bony and cartilaginous parts. Allows myringotomy to be performed.

1%–2% **lidocaine** or **prilocaine** with **adrenaline** is most commonly used. Systemic absorption of adrenaline may cause symptoms, especially if high concentrations are used, e.g. 1:80 000. Immediate collapse following dental nerve blocks is thought to result from retrograde flow of solution via branches of the external carotid artery, reaching the internal carotid; perineural spread to the medulla has also been suggested.

See also, Gasserian ganglion block; Maxillary nerve blocks; Nose; Ophthalmic nerve blocks

Mandragora (Mandrake). Plant, supposedly human-shaped, thought to hold magic powers, including the ability to induce sleep and relieve pain. Contains **hyoscine** and similar alkaloids. According to legend, its scream on uprooting killed all who heard it; hence the supposedly 'safe' method of collection: a dog is tied to the plant at midnight, while its owner retreats to a safe distance with ears stopped with wax. The dog is enticed to run after food, pulling out the mandrake and dying in the process.

Carter AJ (2003). J R Soc Med; 96: 144–7

Mannitol. Plant-derived alcohol with molecular weight of 182. An osmotic **diuretic**; it draws water from the extracellular and intracellular spaces into the vascular compartment, expanding the latter transiently. Not reabsorbed once filtered in the kidneys, it continues to be osmotically active in the urine, causing diuresis. Used mainly to reduce the risk of perioperative **renal failure** (e.g. during vascular surgery, surgery in obstructive **jaundice**) and to treat **cerebral oedema**. Efficacy in the latter depends on integrity of the **blood–brain barrier** that may be altered in neurological disease, although some benefit is derived from the systemic dehydration produced. Has also been used to lower **intraocular pressure**. It may also act as a **free radical** scavenger. Oral mannitol has been used (together with activated **charcoal**) as an osmotic agent to increase intestinal removal of poisons.

Temporarily increases **cerebral blood flow**; **ICP** may rise slightly before falling, especially after rapid injection. Excessive brain shrinkage in the elderly may rupture fragile subdural veins. A rebound increase in ICP may occur if treatment is prolonged, due to eventual passage of mannitol into cerebral cells; the effect is small after a single dose. A transient increase in vascular volume and CVP may cause **cardiac failure** in susceptible patients. Other complications include **hypernatraemia**, **metabolic acidosis**, thrombophlebitis, skin necrosis if extravasation occurs and allergic reactions including **anaphylaxis**.

- Dosage: 0.25–2 g/kg by iv infusion of 10%–20% solution over 20–30 min. Effects occur within 30 min, lasting 6 h. 0.25–0.5 g/kg may follow 6-hourly for 24 h, unless diuresis has not occurred, cardiovascular instability ensues or plasma **osmolality** exceeds 315 mosmol/kg.

Available as 10% and 20% solutions with osmolality 550 and 1100 mosmol/kg, respectively.

Shawkat H, Westwood M-M, Mortimer A (2012). Cont Educ Anaesth Crit Care Pain; 12: 82–5

Mann–Whitney rank sum test, *see Statistical tests*

Manslaughter. Unlawful killing of another person; a criminal charge (as opposed to the civil charge of **negligence**) that has been applied to anaesthetists in cases where the care provided was so poor as to constitute a reckless or grossly negligent act or omission. Examples have included fatal cardiac arrest following disconnection of the breathing system and inadequate immediate postoperative care. Requires a 'burden of proof' of 'beyond reasonable doubt', unlike negligence and other civil claims in which the burden is the 'balance of probabilities'.

The charge of corporate manslaughter exists in common law but actions against large organisations have often been unsuccessful because of difficulties identifying the person(s) responsible for the decisions that led to death. The Corporate Manslaughter and Corporate Homicide Act 2007 raises the possibility of senior managers, including clinicians (i.e., not just directors and executives), facing charges if they are implicated in playing 'a significant role' that leads to a 'breach in decision making related to operational processes within the organisation that subsequently results in the death of a person'.

Ferner RE, McDowell SE (2006). J R Soc Med; 99: 309–14

See also, Medicolegal aspects of anaesthesia

MAO, *see Monoamine oxidase*

MAOIs, *see Monoamine oxidase inhibitors*

MAP, *see Mean arterial pressure*

Mapleson classification of breathing systems, *see Anaesthetic breathing systems*

Marey's law. Increased pressure in the aortic arch and **carotid sinus** causes bradycardia; decreased pressure causes tachycardia.

[Etienne Jules Marey (1830–1904), French physiologist]

See also, Baroreceptor reflex

Marfan's syndrome. **Connective tissue disease**, inherited as an autosomal dominant gene. Prevalence is 1:20000.

- Features:
  - tall stature, with long, thin extremities. Joint dislocations, **kyphoscoliosis**, pes excavatum, inguinal and diaphragmatic herniae are common.
  - cataracts and subluxation of the ocular lens (50%).
  - cardiovascular:
    - **aortic regurgitation** (<90%).
    - ascending **aortic aneurysm**.
    - **mitral valve prolapse**.
    - conduction defects.
  - respiratory:
    - kyphoscoliosis.
    - emphysema.
    - **pneumothorax**.
    - tracheal intubation may be difficult (high arched palate).
  - neurological: **subarachnoid haemorrhage**.

Death usually results from aortic dilatation and its complications. Careful **preoperative assessment** for **congenital heart disease** and its sequelae is required.

[Bernard J Marfan (1858–1942), French paediatrician]

von Kodolitsch Y, Robinson PN (2007). Heart; 93: 755–60

MARS, Molecular adsorbents recirculation system, *see Liver dialysis*

Masks, *see Facemasks; Oxygen therapy*

Mass. Precise definitions vary, but include the inertial resistance to movement of a body, and the amount of matter contained in a body. Under conditions of differing gravity, mass remains constant, whereas **weight** varies. SI **unit** is the **kilogram**.

Mass spectrometer. Device used to analyse mixtures of substances according to mw. The sample passes through an ionising chamber, and becomes charged by electrons arising from a cathode. The charged sample particles are then accelerated by an electric field that imparts a certain velocity. When they subsequently pass through a strong magnetic field, the particles are deflected to varying degrees depending on their mass and velocity. The electrical charge arriving at certain distances from the accelerating chamber is measured, and corresponds to the amount of differently sized particles present in the original sample. Different ranges of particle size may be analysed by altering accelerator characteristics. Compounds of identical mw may be distinguished by identifying breakdown products.

Alternatively, in the quadrupole mass spectrometer, the accelerated beam passes longitudinally between four rods, of variable potential. Particles are removed from the beam unless of a certain mass, depending on the rods' potential.

Mass spectrometers may be used for on-line **gas analysis** during anaesthesia.

Masseter spasm. Increase in jaw tone occurring after **suxamethonium**. More common in children and after **halothane** induction, although the incidence is hard to determine because of diagnostic variability. A 1:100–1:3000 incidence has been reported, but is controversial. A protective effect of **thiopental** has been suggested. Spasm may represent a normal dose-related response to suxamethonium, but has been associated with **MH** susceptibility, especially if spasm is severe and prolonged, and associated with markedly raised serum creatine kinase and **myoglobinuria**. May also be seen in **dystrophia myotonica** following suxamethonium and acetylcholinesterase inhibitors.

Management of spasm is controversial: termination of anaesthesia and referral for muscle biopsy, treatment with **dantrolene**, and proceeding with caution have all been recommended.

MAST, Military antishock trousers, *see Antigravity suit*

Mast cells. Basophilic cells in connective and subcutaneous tissues, involved in inflammatory reactions and immune responses. Storage granules contain lytic **enzymes** (e.g. tryptase) and inflammatory mediators, e.g. **histamine, kinins, heparin, 5-HT, hyaluronidase, leukotrienes, platelet** aggregating and leucocyte chemotactic factors. Release is caused by: tissue injury; **complement** activation; drugs (e.g. **atracurium**); and cross-linkage of surface IgE molecules by antigen (i.e., **anaphylaxis**). Also involved in presentation of antigen to lymphocytes. Occur in excess in mastocytosis, either in the circulation or as tissue infiltrates.

Maternal mortality, *see Confidential Enquiries into Maternal Deaths*

Maxillary nerve blocks. Performed for facial and intraoral procedures.

- Anatomy: the maxillary division (V_2) of the trigeminal nerve passes from the **Gasserian ganglion** through the foramen rotundum into the pterygopalatine fossa, dividing into sensory branches and continuing as the infraorbital nerve (*see Fig. 79;* **Gasserian ganglion block**). Branches:
  - via the pterygopalatine ganglion to the **nose**, nasopharynx and palate via nasal, nasopalatine, greater and lesser palatine and pharyngeal nerves.
  - nasopalatine nerve: supplies the anterior third of the hard palate and palatal gingiva of the upper incisors.
  - greater palatine: supplies the posterior hard palate and palatal gingiva of adjacent teeth.
  - zygomatic nerve: supplies the temple, cheek and lateral eye.
  - posterior superior alveolar nerve: supplies the molar/premolar teeth.
  - infraorbital nerve: supplies the lower eyelid, conjunctiva, side of the nose, upper lip, cheek, and via its anterior superior alveolar branch, the upper canines and incisors, maxillary sinus and cheek mucosa.

The supraorbital foramen, pupil, infraorbital notch, infraorbital foramen, buccal surface of the second premolar and mental foramen all lie along a straight line.

- Blocks:
  - maxillary nerve: a needle is inserted extraorally 0.5 cm below the midpoint of the zygoma and directed medially until bone is contacted. It is redirected anteriorly and advanced a further 1 cm, anterior to the lateral pterygoid plate. 3–4 ml **local anaesthetic agent** is injected. May also be blocked via the intraoral route: the needle is inserted behind the posterior border of the zygoma and directed upwards, medially and posteriorly 3 cm. Up to 5 ml solution is injected within the pterygopalatine fossa.
  - nasopalatine nerve: 0.5–1.0 ml is injected at the incisive foramen, 0.5–1.0 cm posterior to the upper incisors in the midline.
  - greater palatine nerve: 0.5–1.0 ml is injected at the greater palatine foramen, marked by a depression in the palate opposite the second/third molar 1 cm above the gingival margin.
  - infraorbital nerve: 1–2 ml is injected at the infraorbital foramen, 0.5–1.0 cm below the infraorbital notch. Injection may be performed intraorally or extraorally.
  - superior alveolar nerve branches to individual teeth may be blocked by submucous infiltration above each tooth.
  - for the Cadwell–Luc approach, the mucosa and periosteum above the upper premolars may be infiltrated with 5–10 ml solution, to block branches of the anterior superior alveolar nerve. Topical application of, e.g. **lidocaine** may assist the block. Further solution may be injected into the mucosa of the maxillary sinus once opened. Alternatively, maxillary or infraorbital nerve blocks may be performed.

1%–2% lidocaine or **prilocaine** with **adrenaline** is most commonly used. Systemic absorption of adrenaline may cause symptoms, especially if high concentrations are used, e.g. 1:80 000.

Immediate collapse following dental nerve blocks is thought to result from retrograde flow of solution via branches of the external carotid artery, reaching the internal carotid; perineural spread to the medulla has also been suggested.

[George Caldwell (1834–1918), US ENT surgeon; Henri Luc (1855–1925), French ENT surgeon]

See also, Mandibular nerve blocks; Ophthalmic nerve blocks

Maxillofacial surgery. Anaesthesia may be required for elective surgery (e.g. for **facial deformities**, tumours) or because of **facial trauma**, infection or **airway obstruction**. General considerations are as for **ENT**, **plastic** and **dental surgery**, particularly problems of access, protection of the airway and the potential for long and bloody surgery. Bradycardia may occur during procedures around the face (*see Oculocardiac reflex*).

Maximal breathing capacity, *see Maximal voluntary ventilation*

Maximal voluntary ventilation (Maximal breathing capacity). Maximal minute volume of air able to be breathed, measured over 15 s. Normally about 120–150 l/min. Equals approximately 35 × **FEV**$_1$. Rarely used, because very tiring to perform.

See also, Lung function tests

MCH/MCHC/MCV, Mean cell haemoglobin/Mean cell haemoglobin concentration/Mean cell volume, *see Erythrocytes*

MDEA, Methylenedioxyethylamfetamine, *see Methylenedioxymethylamfetamine*

MDMA, *see Methylenedioxymethylamfetamine*

MEA syndrome, *see Multiple endocrine adenomatosis*

Mean (Average). Expression of the central tendency of a set of observations or measurements. Equals the sum of all the observations divided by the number of observations (n), i.e.,

$$\bar{x} = \frac{\sum x}{n}$$

Population mean is denoted by μ; sample mean by $\bar{x}$.

Means of more than one sample group may be compared using **statistical tests**.

See also, Median; Mode; Standard error of mean; Statistical frequency distributions; Statistics

Mean arterial pressure (MAP). Average **arterial BP** throughout the **cardiac cycle**. The area contained within the **arterial waveform** pressure trace above MAP equals the area below it.

$$\text{equals approximately } \frac{(2 \times \text{diastolic}) + \text{systolic}}{3}$$

$$\text{or diastolic} + \frac{(\text{systolic} - \text{diastolic})}{3}$$

Preferred by some clinicians to measures of systolic or diastolic pressures, because it is less liable to errors or differences due to measuring techniques. Also represents the mean pressure available for perfusion of tissues.

Mechanocardiography. Recording of the mechanical pulsations of the CVS; includes tracings of the **JVP** and **venous waveform, arterial waveform** and recordings at the apex using an externally applied transducer. Has been used to investigate cardiovascular disease, especially valvular disease, and to determine **systolic time intervals**.

Median. Expression of the central tendency of a set of measurements or observations.

$$\text{equals the } \frac{(n+1)\text{th}}{2} \text{ measurement.}$$

Half the population or sample above it, half below. Equals the **mean** for a **normal distribution**.

See also, Statistical frequency distributions; Statistics

Median nerve (C6–T1). Arises from the medial and lateral cords of the **brachial plexus** in the lower axilla, lateral to the axillary artery. Passes down the front of the arm to the **antecubital fossa**, first lateral to the **brachial artery**, then crossing it anteriorly at mid/upper arm to lie medially. Entering the forearm, it crosses the **ulnar artery** anteriorly, passing between the two heads of pronator teres. Passes between flexor digitorum superficialis and profundus; at the wrist it lies between the tendons of palmaris longus (medially) and flexor carpi radialis (laterally).

- Apart from branches to the joints of the wrist and hand, it supplies:
  - superficial flexor muscles (except flexor carpi ulnaris), abductor pollicis brevis, flexor pollicis brevis and opponens pollicis.
  - radial side of the palm and the palmar surface of the radial 3½ digits, extending to their dorsal surface at their tips.
  - via the anterior interosseus branch arising at the distal antecubital fossa: flexor pollicis longus, radial part of flexor digitorum profundus and pronator quadratus.

May be blocked at the brachial plexus, elbow, forearm and wrist.

See also, Brachial plexus block; Elbow, nerve blocks; Wrist, nerve blocks

Mediastinum. Region of the thorax between the two pleural sacs. It is in contact with the **diaphragm** inferiorly, and continuous with the tissues of the neck superiorly. Lies between the vertebral column posteriorly and sternum anteriorly. Contains the **heart**, great vessels, **trachea**, **oesophagus**, thoracic duct, vagi, **phrenic** and recurrent **laryngeal nerves**, sympathetic trunk, thymus and lymph nodes (Fig. 107).

- Divided into:
  - superior mediastinum: above a horizontal line level with T4/5 and the angle of Louis.
  - inferior mediastinum: below this line. Composed of anterior (between heart and sternum), middle (containing **pericardium** and contents) and posterior (between heart and **vertebrae**) portions.

  Thus mediastinal enlargement may be caused by:
  - enlargement of any of the above constituent structures (central).
  - spinal and vertebral masses (posterior).
  - thymic, thyroid, teratoma and dermoid tumours (anterior). Tumours (e.g. **bronchial carcinoma**) may involve local structures within the mediastinum, e.g. recurrent laryngeal or phrenic nerves, pericardium. Bleeding from the aorta following **chest trauma** or dissection may cause widening of the superior mediastinum.

Patients with mediastinal enlargement may present for biopsy (e.g. via mediastinoscopy through a suprasternal incision) or resection.

- Main anaesthetic considerations:
  - preoperative state, e.g. related to the primary **malignancy**. Tracheal compression and **airway obstruction, superior vena caval obstruction**, phrenic and recurrent laryngeal nerve involvement and drug/radiotherapy effects may be present.
  - classically, **induction of anaesthesia** is inhalational, but some advocate iv induction. Reinforced tracheal/bronchial tubes are often preferable.
  - severe haemorrhage may occur. Fluid replacement via the femoral vein may be required if the superior vena cava and its tributaries are involved.
  - **one-lung anaesthesia** and even **extracorporeal circulation** may be required during resection.

[Antoine Louis (1723–1792), French surgeon]

See also, Chest x-ray

Medical emergency team (MET). Team consisting of medical and nursing staff skilled in resuscitation (in its broadest sense) responding to standardised calling criteria, including abnormal physiological variables (e.g. systolic BP <90 mmHg), specific conditions or 'any time urgent medical assistance is required'. May replace existing **cardiac arrest** teams on the basis that prevention of cardiac arrest or severe physiological deterioration is likely to have a better outcome than treatment applied after cardiac arrest. Its effect on preventing cardiac arrest, decreasing ICU admission and improving mortality has not been proven.

Lee A, Bishop G, Hillman KM, Daffurn K (1995). Anaesth Intens Care; 23: 183–6

See also, Acute life-threatening events—recognition and treatment; Outreach team; Postoperative care team

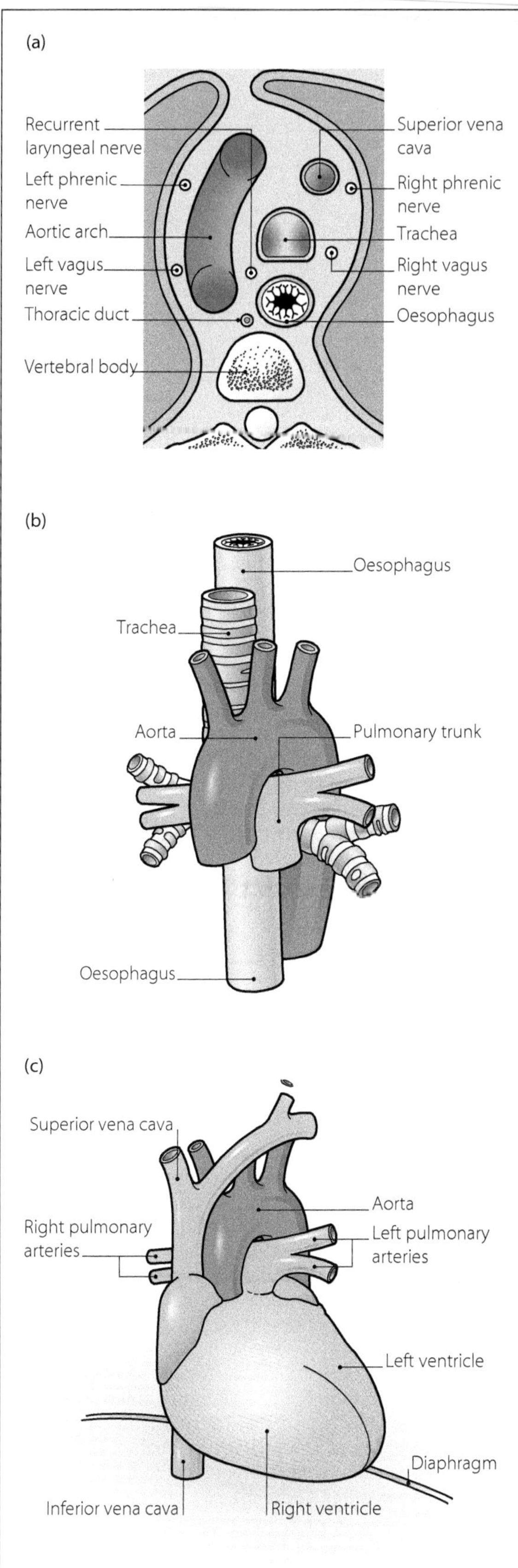

Fig. 107 Anatomy of the mediastinum: (a) transverse section through T4; (b) trachea and relations; (c) heart and great vessels

Medicines and Healthcare products Regulatory Agency (MHRA). UK government agency formed in 2003 from the Medicines Control Agency and Medical Devices Agency. Responsible for regulating medicines, medical devices and blood components for transfusion and ensuring their safety, via approval/regulation/monitoring of **clinical trials**, reporting/investigating **adverse drug reactions** and licensing/testing medicinal products and devices.

Medicolegal aspects of anaesthesia. In the UK, these usually concern matters of civil law (e.g. **negligence**) breach of contract or battery; proof must be according to 'balance of probabilities'. Criminal law is involved less commonly, e.g. involving murder or **manslaughter** due to criminal neglect or reckless disregard of clinical duties; proof must be 'beyond reasonable doubt'.

- Usually related to:
  - negligence: harm resulting from a failure in the duty of care. In the National Health Service (NHS), employing Trusts are legally liable for the negligent acts/omissions of their employees during their employment (the principle of vicarious liability), providing indemnity for NHS work since 1990.

    Anaesthesia is considered a high-risk specialty because of common minor claims (e.g. damage to **teeth**) and very expensive major claims.
  - perioperative deaths: those occurring within 24 h of anaesthesia are reported to the **coroner**, who may order an inquiry or inquest, although the time interval is not specified by law. Once reported, organs may not be harvested for transplantation without the coroner's permission.
  - **Misuse of Drugs Act**.
  - fitness to practise: investigated by a committee of the **General Medical Council** (GMC) that regulates licensing to practise medicine in the UK; although not a civil court, the process may be broadly similar.

More than one process may follow a single incident; thus a serious error that results in a patient's death may result in an inquest, a claim of negligence, a charge of manslaughter and/or a referral to the GMC.

Similar considerations apply to ICU, although claims arising from ICU itself are less common; however, ICU may be required for critical illness arising from negligent practice. Specific ICU issues with medicolegal implications include competence (whether the patients are able to make their own decisions), non-provision of life-sustaining treatment or **withdrawal of treatment** (justified if it is in the patient's best interests to be allowed to die) and **brainstem death**. The need for attention to detail and proper record-keeping is as important as in general anaesthetic practice.

In general, risks are reduced by: **checking of anaesthetic equipment**; use of the **WHO Surgical Safety Checklist**; adequate **preoperative assessment** and preparation (including warning patients of risks); consultation with senior colleagues when appropriate; adherence to generally accepted techniques, including adequate **monitoring**; careful writing of clinical notes and anaesthetic **record-keeping**, with copies kept for later use; and full and honest explanation with patients and/or relatives when anything goes wrong.

See also, Abuse of anaesthetic agents; Anaesthetic morbidity and mortality; Ethics; Sick doctor scheme

Meglitinides. Oral **hypoglycaemic drugs** used in the management of diabetes mellitus. Stimulate **insulin** release from the functioning β cells of the pancreas. Taken just before meals. Two available agents are nateglinide and repaglinide; the former is only licensed for use in combination with metformin. Common side effects include headache and upper respiratory tract infections.

Melatonin. Hormone synthesised and released by the pineal gland. Formed from the amino acid tryptophan, its formation is promoted by darkness and inhibited by light. Actions include control of circadian rhythms, modulation of seasonal changes in physiology, timing of puberty and thermoregulation. Also has analgesic, anti-inflammatory and antioxidative properties. Its function of regulating **sleep** has resulted in its use in combating sleep deprivation in ICU patients.
Andersen LP, Werner MU, Rosenberg J, Gögenur I (2014). Anaesthesia; 69: 1163–71

Membrane potential. Electrical potential difference across a cell membrane, present in almost all living eukaryotic cells. Results from the differential distribution of charged particles across cell **membranes**. The distribution of each particle is determined by its permeability across the membrane, the distribution of other particles (e.g. **Donnan effect**) and **active transport** systems, e.g. **sodium/potassium pump**. Membranes are impermeable to proteins (negatively charged), which thus remain intracellular; membranes are poorly permeable to **sodium** ions and moderately permeable to chloride and **potassium** ions.

Electrochemical gradients exist across the cell membrane for each ion; the membrane potential at equilibrium for each is calculated by the **Nernst equation**. Membrane potentials at given intracellular/extracellular concentrations of sodium, chloride and potassium ions together are calculated by the **Goldman constant-field equation**.

Potential is conventionally written as negative; i.e., the inside is negative relative to the outside. The potential's magnitude varies between tissues, e.g. −70 mV for nerves and −90 mV for muscle.

Changes in membrane permeability may alter, or be altered by, membrane potential, e.g. during **action potentials**.

Membranes. Biological membranes share certain features:

- phospholipid bilayer; the hydrophilic end of each phospholipid molecule faces the membrane surface and the hydrophobic end lies within the membrane substance.
- protein molecules at intervals within the membrane; they may traverse it or project on one side only, according to the water/lipid solubility of the protein subunits. Proteins are able to 'float' within the lipid molecules.
- proteins may function as enzymes, receptors, pumps or channels for ions. They also have antigenic properties.
- resting **membrane potential** is created by differential permeability for certain ions, together with **active transport** pumps. Most membranes are relatively permeable to chloride and **potassium** ions, less so to **sodium** ions, and relatively impermeable to proteins and anions. Non-charged substances (e.g. CO_2 and non-ionised drugs) are able to cross freely, as is water.
- function of cells is dependent on the features of their membrane proteins, which may be altered by electrical signals or chemicals, e.g. drugs, hormones, **neurotransmitters**. The action of anaesthetic agents is thought to involve alteration of membrane configuration within the nervous system.

See also, Action potential; Anaesthesia, mechanisms of

Memory. Classically divided into explicit and implicit memory; the latter not requiring conscious retrieval (e.g. driving a car), the former subdivided into episodic (information regarding specific events, places and times) and semantic (concepts about the world and linguistic meaning). The hippocampus, amygdala, frontal lobes, and thalamic and hypothalamic nuclei are thought to be concerned with memory storage and retrieval.

Anaesthetic agents are thought mainly to impair acquisition of short-term memory, although transfer into intermediate and long-term memory may also be affected.
Wang DS, Orser BA (2011). Can J Anesth; 58: 167–77
See also, Amnesia; Postoperative cognitive dysfunction

Mendelson's syndrome, *see Aspiration pneumonitis*

Meninges. Tissue layers surrounding the **brain** and **spinal cord**, composed of:

- pia mater: delicate vascular layer, closely adherent to the brain and cord, following their surfaces into clefts, sulci, etc. Surrounded by **CSF** within the arachnoid. Thin projections of the latter cross the subarachnoid space to the pia. Blood vessels lie within the space.

  Within the **vertebral canal**, the denticulate ligament passes laterally from the pia along its length and attaches at intervals to the dura. The subarachnoid septum lies posteriorly, attaching to the arachnoid intermittently. The pia terminates as the filum terminale, which passes through the caudal end of the dural sac and attaches to the coccyx.
- arachnoid mater: delicate membrane, containing CSF internally. Does not project into clefts and sulci, apart from the longitudinal fissure. Applied to the dura externally; the potential subdural space lies between them, containing vessels. Fuses with the dura at S2. Arachnoid granulations project into the venous sinuses, for drainage of CSF.
- dura mater: composed of two fibrous layers: the outer is adherent to the periosteal lining of the **skull**; the inner attaches to the outer but is separated by venous sinuses. The inner layer forms sheets within the skull:
  - vertical: falx cerebri and falx cerebelli between the cerebral and cerebellar hemispheres, respectively.
  - horizontal: tentorium cerebelli above the cerebellum and the diaphragma sellae above the pituitary gland.

  The dura also forms two layers within the vertebral canal: the external adherent to the inner periostium of the **vertebrae** and the internal lying against the outer surface of the arachnoid. The space between the two dura layers is the epidural space. Projections and fibrous bands are present within the epidural space, especially in the midline. Dura projects intermittently to the posterior longitudinal ligament of the vertebrae, especially lumbar. Dura ends at about S2.

All layers donate a thin covering 'sleeve' to **cranial nerves** and **spinal nerves** as they leave the CNS. These dural cuffs, which contain CSF, may accompany spinal nerves through the intravertebral foramina.

- Blood supply:
  - intracranial:
    - from ascending pharyngeal, occipital and maxillary branches of the external **carotid artery**. The maxillary artery gives rise to the middle meningeal artery, which enters the skull through the foramen spinosum.
    - from branches of the internal carotid and vertebral arteries.
  - spinal: as for the spinal cord.

See also, Meningitis; Vertebral ligaments

Meningitis. Inflammation of the **meninges**. Usually infective:

- viral: most commonly coxsackie, echo and herpes viruses. Mumps and measles viruses are less common since the introduction of the MMR vaccine. Meningitis can occur early in the course of **HIV** infection. Usually has good prognosis, unless associated with generalised **encephalitis**.
- bacterial:
  - incidence in Europe of 1–2 per 100 000 population per year. Incidence has decreased markedly (especially in children) with the introduction of conjugate vaccines.
  - *Streptococcus pneumoniae* (pneumococcal meningitis) is the most common cause followed by *Neisseria meningitidis* (meningococcal meningitis). *Haemophilus influenza* type b was a significant cause but, like meningococcal meningitis, has virtually disappeared in areas where vaccination has been carried out.
  - rarer causes include **TB**, listeria, fungi.

Organisms initially colonise membranes of the upper respiratory tract adhering to the mucosa with pili attaching to receptors; they then enter the bloodstream by passing through or between cells and then into the subarachnoid space. Direct spread may occur from nasal sinuses. People with **complement** deficiency are more susceptible.

Aseptic meningitis may also occur; it may be caused by malignant infiltration, chemical irritation (e.g. alcoholic solutions used to clean the skin before lumbar puncture) and occasionally drugs (e.g. **NSAIDs**, **H_2 receptor antagonists**).

- Features:
  - fever, nausea, vomiting, headache, photophobia, convulsions, coma.
  - neck stiffness, with muscle resistance to passive knee extension from the flexed position with the thigh flexed (caused by stretching of inflamed sciatic nerve roots [Kernig's sign]).
  - cranial nerve lesions or signs of **cerebral oedema** may be present.
  - may be associated with systemic involvement, e.g. effects of severe **sepsis** in **meningococcal disease**.
  - CT scan is usually required to exclude space-occupying lesions and raised **ICP** before **lumbar puncture**.
  - **CSF**: Typical findings include:
    - viral: increased lymphocytes, slightly raised protein and normal glucose.
    - bacterial: increased polymorphs and protein, and reduced glucose. Bacteria may be visible on staining. A high lactate before starting antibacterial therapy has a high sensitivity and specificity in differentiating bacterial from viral meningitis. PCR analysis is useful for detecting *S. pneumoniae* and *N. meningitidis*.
    - aseptic: increased polymorphs and protein, and normal glucose. The CSF may appear cloudy but no organisms are seen or grown.

Recovery may be complete or there may be neurological deficit, particularly in bacterial meningitis and especially if treatment with antibacterial agents and corticosteroids is delayed. Factors associated with poor prognosis include older age, reduced conscious level at presentation, a low CSF leucocyte count and reduced blood platelet count. Aseptic chemical meningitis is characterised by its short and benign course.

Treatment is directed at the underlying organism. Recent UK guidelines suggest **cefotaxime** or **ceftriaxone** (both 2 g iv) as soon as possible (i.e., before definitive microbiological diagnosis). **Ampicillin** 2 g is added if >55 years, to cover listeria or **vancomycin** ± **rifampicin** if penicillin-resistant pneumococcus is suspected. **Dexamethasone** (e.g. 10 mg iv qds for 4 days) reduces mortality and neurological morbidity.

[Vladimir M Kernig (1840–1917), Russian neurologist]

McGill F, Heyderman RS, Panagiotou S, et al (2016). Lancet; 388: 3036–47

Meningococcal disease. Strictly, refers to any illness caused by *Neisseria meningitidis*, although the term is often used to describe the severe systemic illness that often results in admission to an ICU. Most infections in the UK are caused by the B serotype, although the C serotype more frequently causes outbreaks. The A serotype may also cause clinical infection.

Important because of its innocuous early course, rapid progression and potentially disastrous outcome; the latter is thought to be related to the extremely toxic **endotoxin** present in the outer wall of the organism. An important cause of morbidity and mortality in children and young adults; epidemics (e.g. in schools/colleges) occur periodically. Asplenia and **complement** deficiency are specific risk factors. Shows seasonal variation (approximately 40% of cases occurring between January and March). The organism is present in the nasopharynx of about 5% of otherwise healthy subjects, increasing to about 30% during epidemics. Case mortality is 10%–12% in the UK.

- Features:
  - non-specific (especially initially), e.g. cough, sore throat, fever, vomiting, headache.
  - signs and symptoms of **meningitis**: may develop in about 85% of cases but bacteraemia and severe **SIRS** may occur without overt meningitis being present, and has a higher mortality.
  - petechial rash: present in up to 80% of patients, although sometimes limited to the mucous membranes. May become maculopapular. **DIC** is common. Vasculitic lesions or extensive skin digit or limb necrosis (purpura fulminans) may also occur.
  - **MODS** and **septic shock** may occur.
  - **adrenocortical insufficiency** due to sepsis or adrenal haemorrhage.

Diagnosis is often suggested by the history and clinical examination, although similar rashes can occur with staphylococcal, streptococcal or *Haemophilus influenzae* infections. **Blood cultures** reveal the meningococcus in up to 80% of untreated cases. The organism may also be isolated from the skin lesions or CSF. Polymerase chain reaction (PCR) is increasingly used to identify the organism.

- Treatment:
  - iv antibiotic therapy as for meningitis.
  - supportive: includes management of meningitis (depressed consciousness, etc.), coagulopathy and septic shock.
  - limb fasciotomies or amputation may be necessary.
  - others: specific **anti-endotoxin antibodies** and anti-**cytokine** therapies, **corticosteroids** and other treatments of severe sepsis have been studied but their place is uncertain.

If exposed before the patient has received appropriate antibiotics, close contacts (including ICU staff) should receive prophylaxis, e.g. with **rifampicin** or **ciprofloxacin.** At-risk subjects may be protected by immunisation with a polysaccharide vaccine against types A and C meningococci; the B serogroup has a number of subtypes and an effective vaccine against it has not yet been developed. Public health officials should be contacted (it is a **notifiable disease**) to organise contact tracing and prophylaxis.

Other forms of meningococcal disease are often trivial (e.g. conjunctivitis, pharyngitis, otitis media) but some may be severe (e.g. pericarditis, endocarditis, myocarditis, septic arthritis).

Campsall PA, Laupland KB, Niven DJ (2013). Crit Care Clin; 29: 393–409

Mental Capacity Act 2005. Act providing a framework for decision making on behalf of adults without capacity; came into force in England and Wales in April 2007. Largely building on pre-existing common law, the Act confers formal statutory status on advance directives (termed **advance decisions**) and creates new 'lasting powers of attorney' and 'court-appointed deputies' with the ability to make medical decisions on behalf of adults >16 years who lack capacity.

Based on the following principles:

- capacity must be presumed unless proven otherwise.
- everything practicable must be done to support individuals to make their own decisions, before deciding they lack capacity.
- individuals may make unwise or irrational decisions and doing so is not evidence of incapacity.
- any decision made on behalf of another person must be in their best interests (not necessarily their best *medical* interests).
- if a decision is made on another's behalf, it should be the least restrictive option; i.e., the one that interferes least with the individual's freedoms in order to achieve the required aim.

Requires providers of healthcare to consider advance decisions and to assess capacity before initiating, withholding or withdrawing treatment. The new Court of Protection, created by the Act, has ultimate responsibility for the Act's proper functioning, including deciding on individual cases.

The Adults with Incapacity (Scotland) Act 2000 and the Mental Capacity Act (Northern Ireland) 2016 cover similar ground.

White SM, Baldwin TJ (2006). Anaesthesia; 61: 381–9

MEOWS, *see Modified Early Obstetric Warning Score*

Meperidine, *see Pethidine*

Mepivacaine hydrochloride. Amide **local anaesthetic agent**, first used in 1956. Similar to **lidocaine**, but more protein-bound. Does not cause vasodilatation. Not available in the UK. Used in 1%–2% solutions for **epidural anaesthesia** and 4% solution for **spinal anaesthesia**, in the same doses as lidocaine. Maximal safe dose is 5 mg/kg; toxic plasma level is about 6 μg/ml. Rarely used in obstetrics because of greater fetal protein-binding and longer fetal **half-life** than alternative drugs.

MEPP, Miniature end-plate potential, *see End-plate potentials*

Meptazinol hydrochloride. Synthetic **opioid analgesic drug**, first investigated in 1971. Has partial agonist properties, and therefore antagonises respiratory depression caused by morphine. Causes less respiratory depression or sedation than morphine. Analgesic effects are almost completely reversed by **naloxone.** 100 mg is equivalent to 10 mg morphine or 100 mg **pethidine.**

- Dosage: 50–100 mg iv/im 2–4-hourly as required; 200 mg orally, 3–6-hourly.

Meropenem. Broad-spectrum **carbapenem** and **antibacterial drug**, similar to **imipenem** but not broken down by renal enzymatic action. Less likely to cause convulsions than imipenem; thus more useful for CNS infections.

- Dosage: 500 mg–1 g iv over 5 min tds (2 g in **meningitis** or infection in **cystic fibrosis**).
- Side effects: as for imipenem.

MERS, *see Middle East respiratory syndrome*

Mesmerism. Treatment of various maladies (including postoperative pain relief) by 'animal magnetism', the transmission between individuals of healing force derived from the ubiquitous magnetic fluid that pervaded the universe. Named after Mesmer, who originally passed magnets over his patients' bodies to treat them. He later used only his touch, and then speech, to achieve the same effects. Investigated in Paris by a French Royal Commission in 1784, which included Benjamin Franklin and **Lavoisier**; mesmerism was declared to have no scientific foundation, relying on suggestion alone. It continued to be popular until the 1840s, when the importance of psychological suggestion by the therapist was emphasised, leading to the concept of hypnotism.

[Franz A Mesmer (1734–1815), Swiss-born French physician; Benjamin Franklin (1706–1790), US statesman and scientist]

See also, Hypnosis

MET, *see Medical emergency team*

Meta-analysis (Systematic review). Technique for determining the efficacy of a treatment by combining trials that may individually have been too small to show a statistically significant difference. Requires careful inclusion of all randomised controlled trials (RCTs) of the particular treatment, some of which may not have been published. The RCTs are then scored according to their methodology, excluding any that are inadequately randomised or blinded. The results of the remaining RCTs are then pooled to increase the overall number of subjects and **power**; the outcome of each RCT is expressed in a standard format (e.g. **odds ratio, number needed to treat, absolute** or **relative risk reduction**) and the value for the

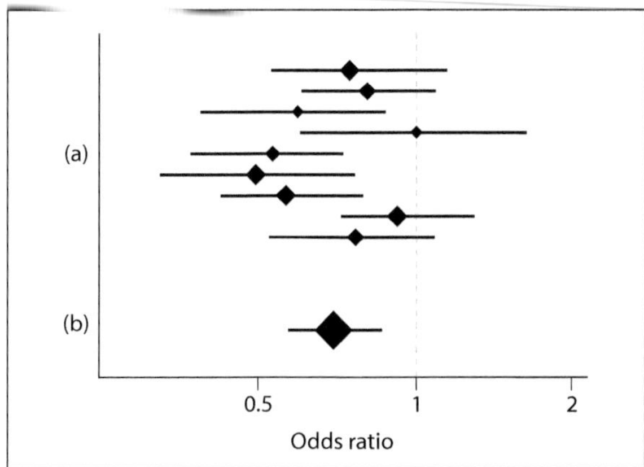

Fig. 108 Meta-analysis (forest plot): nine small trials (a) are pooled to give a combined result (b)

combined data given. Typically, each separate RCT's result is shown on a graph, with horizontal lines representing **confidence intervals**; the size of the central mark represents the sample size (forest plot; Fig. 108). The combined result therefore has smaller confidence intervals and larger central mark than the constituent RCTs, representing the greater certainty of the combined result and the larger number of subjects. Those trials whose confidence intervals cross the line of equivalence (for odds ratio, a value of one) are statistically 'non-significant' whereas those that do not are 'significant'. In the example given, the overall conclusion is that there is a statistically significant difference, as demonstrated by the combined confidence intervals' not crossing the line.

Although meta-analysis has the ability to demonstrate true treatment effects and thus represents the best evidence on which to base clinical practice, the technique may not always be valid because of:

- bias in the identification of RCTs included (e.g. 'positive' studies have traditionally been more likely to be published than 'negative' ones).
- differing definitions of selection criteria for RCTs.
- use of different outcomes in the component studies.
- the ability for single RCTs to influence unduly the overall result in certain circumstances.
- uncertainty in applying the result to a particular patient (e.g. man aged 45 years) when the RCTs included all refer to a specific patient population (e.g. men aged 60–70 years).

Thus there have been some famous examples of treatment effects apparently demonstrated by meta-analysis that have not been supported by subsequent huge RCTs, e.g. the 'beneficial' effect of **magnesium sulfate** following **MI**. However, meta-analysis has had notable successes too, e.g. by demonstrating clearly the reduction in mortality when **β-adrenergic receptor antagonists** are given following MI despite conflicting results of the many small RCTs that previously existed.

Møller AM, Myles PS (2016). Br J Anaesth; 117: 428–30

Metabolic syndrome. Term used to describe the association of: **insulin** resistance; dyslipidaemia; **hypertension**; and **obesity** (central in particular). Also variously termed 'syndrome X', 'insulin resistance syndrome' and 'visceral obesity syndrome'. Likely to be caused by a combination of genetic predisposition and chronic caloric excess. Previously the subject of much research, but recently criticised as an overly simplistic concept and no longer considered useful for diagnosis or management.

Ball J (2014). Anaesthesia; 69: 203–7

Metabolism. Physical and chemical reactions occurring in an organism in order to sustain life. Involves anabolism (building up; i.e., incorporation of substrate into living cells) and **catabolism** (breaking down; usually concerned with **energy** liberation). Metabolic pathways are mediated by **enzymes**, subject to various control mechanisms (e.g. hormonal). Basic pathways may be discussed in terms of dietary substrate:

- **carbohydrates**: digested to monosaccharides, absorbed and passed to **liver** and **muscle**. **Glucose** is converted to **glycogen** for storage or broken down via **glycolysis**, **tricarboxylic acid cycle** and **cytochrome oxidase system** to CO_2 and water with liberation of energy that is stored in **ATP** and other compounds.
- **fats**: digested to fatty acids and glycerol, which pass to the liver. Stored as adipose tissue or oxidised to CO_2, water and energy.
- **proteins**: digested to **amino acids**; form new proteins, e.g. enzymes, secretions, cellular components such as **muscle**. Subsequently broken down to **urea**.

Carbohydrate, fat and protein subunits are interchangeable via many pathways, and are interlinked with other substances, e.g. purines, nucleic acids.

See also, Basal metabolic rate; Inborn errors of metabolism

Metaraminol tartrate/bitartrate. **Vasopressor drug**, acting directly via **α-adrenergic receptors**, and indirectly via **adrenaline** and **noradrenaline** release. Increases **cardiac output** and **SVR**, and thus **arterial BP**. Used to raise BP following **epidural/spinal anaesthesia** and cardiogenic shock. May cause excessive hypertension in **hyperthyroidism** and **monoamine oxidase inhibitor** therapy, and **myocardial ischaemia** in **ischaemic heart disease**.

- Dosage:
  - 2–10 mg sc or im; acts within 10 min and lasts 1–1.5 h.
  - in severe hypotension or **shock**: 0.5–5 mg iv, titrated to effect; acts within 1–2 min, lasting for 20–30 min.

Methadone hydrochloride. Synthetic **opioid analgesic drug**, formulated in 1947. Due to its long duration of action (up to 24 h), used for chronic **pain management**, maintenance in opioid addicts and cough suppression in palliative care. Has similar actions and side effects to morphine, but is generally milder with less sedation. Elimination **half-life** exceeds 18 h. Accumulation may be problematic.

- Dosage: 5–10 mg orally/im/sc, tds/qds (bd in chronic use).

See also, Spinal opioids

Methaemoglobinaemia. Increased circulating **haemoglobin** in which the iron atom of haem is in the ferric (Fe^{3+}) state (normally <1%). Levels determined by co-oximetry.

- May be:
  - congenital:
    - deficiency of reducing **enzymes** (especially cytochrome b5 oxidase), which normally convert endogenously formed methaemoglobin to haemoglobin. Usually autosomal recessive inheritance; heterozygotes may be at risk of acute acquired methaemoglobinaemia.

- abnormal haemoglobin chains, with fixation of iron in Fe^{3+} state; autosomal dominant inheritance.
- **glucose-6-phosphate dehydrogenase deficiency**.
  - acquired: drugs and chemicals, e.g. **prilocaine, sodium nitroprusside**, chlorate, quinones, nitrites, phenacetin, sulfonamides, aniline dyes.
- Effects:
  - because methaemoglobin is dark (brownish), patients appear to have **cyanosis** when levels exceed 8%–12% (at normal haemoglobin concentrations). Inaccurate readings of haemoglobin saturation may occur with pulse **oximetry** (as the level of methaemoglobin increases, measured arterial O_2 saturation tends towards 85% because both oxygenated and deoxygenated forms absorb light equally at 660 nm and 940 nm).
  - the **oxyhaemoglobin dissociation curve** of the unaffected haem is shifted to the left, reducing O_2 delivery to tissues. Patients already anaemic are more at risk. Most patients are symptomatic at levels >8%, with dyspnoea and headache common at >20% methaemoglobin, although rate of formation is also important.
- Treatment: discontinuing the causative agent may be all that is required. Reducing agents (e.g. iv methylthioninium chloride [methylene blue]) if acute and severe: 1–2 mg/kg over 5 min, repeated as necessary. Oral therapy with methylthioninium chloride or ascorbic acid may suffice in chronic methaemoglobinaemia. In life-threatening cases, blood or exchange transfusion may be required.

Cortazzo JA, Lichtman AD (2014). J Cardiothorac Vasc Anaesth; 28: 1043–7

See also, Sulfhaemoglobinaemia

Methanol poisoning, *see Alcohol poisoning*

Methionine and methionine synthase. Methionine (an **amino acid**) is the main source of methyl groups in the body, and is involved in many biochemical reactions, including myelination. It is also the precursor of glutathione, depleted in the liver by toxins, e.g. **paracetamol poisoning**; hence its use in the latter. Formation from homocysteine by methionine synthase is involved in folate metabolism, and thymidine and DNA synthesis.

Methionine synthase containing **vitamin B_{12}** as a cofactor is inhibited by **N_2O**, which interacts directly with the vitamin. Prolonged exposure to N_2O may result in features of folate/vitamin B_{12} deficiency, e.g. subacute combined degeneration of the cord and megaloblastic **anaemia**. Myelination may also be affected. Significant effects are thought to be minimal up to 8 h normal anaesthetic use, but biochemical changes have been found after a few hours. Megaloblastic changes have been found in dentists who use N_2O. Effects on DNA synthesis may mediate teratogenesis after prolonged exposure in animal models, but teratogenicity in humans during routine anaesthesia is considered negligible.

Methohexital sodium (Methohexitone). **Intravenous anaesthetic drug**, first used in 1957 and discontinued in the UK in 2000. A methyl **barbiturate**, presented as a white powder with 6% anhydrous sodium carbonate. pH of 1% solution: 10–11. pK_a is 7.9; thus a greater proportion remains unionised in plasma than with **thiopental**. Used mainly for **day-case surgery** and short procedures, including **electroconvulsive therapy** (because of its pro-convulsant properties).

Properties are similar to those of thiopental but pain on injection, involuntary movement, hiccup and laryngospasm are more likely. Adverse effects of intra-arterial injection are less than with thiopental, due to the more dilute solution. Recovery is within 3–4 min of a single dose of 1.0–1.5 mg/kg, with **half-life** 2–4 h.

Methotrexate. Antimetabolite **cytotoxic drug**; inhibits dihydrofolate reductase, thus blocking purine and pyrimidine synthesis and preventing cell division. Used in the treatment of various malignancies, including acute lymphoblastic leukaemia; also used in severe psoriasis and **rheumatoid arthritis**. May accumulate in pleural or ascitic fluid, producing systemic toxicity subsequently. Excreted renally; thus **NSAIDs** are contraindicated because reduced renal function may increase toxicity.
- Dosage varies widely according to the condition and route; usual range is 7.5–100 mg every 2–7 days. May be given orally, iv, im or intrathecally.
- Side effects: myelosuppression, mucositis, pneumonitis (especially likely in rheumatoid arthritis), GIT disturbance, hepatic impairment.

Methoxamine hydrochloride. **Vasopressor drug**, acting via selective **α_1-adrenergic receptor** stimulation. Used (1–2 mg iv) to raise BP (e.g. during **epidural** or **spinal anaesthesia**) and to treat **SVT**. Causes a reflex bradycardia via the **baroreceptor reflex**. Discontinued in 2001 because of falling global demand.

Methoxyflurane. $CHCl_2CF_2OCH_3$. **Inhalational anaesthetic agent**, first used in 1960. Cheap and non-explosive, but withdrawn from UK practice in 1980 because of high-output **renal failure** caused by **fluoride ion** and dichloroacetic acid production. Has high boiling point (105°C) and therefore difficult to vaporise. Very soluble in blood (blood/gas **partition coefficient** of 13); induction and recovery are therefore slow. Extremely potent (**MAC** 0.2) and a powerful analgesic. Formerly used for general anaesthesia and draw-over analgesia, e.g. during labour, using the Cardiff fixed output (0.35%) inhaler.

Remained in use in Australia and New Zealand for prehospital analgesia, and reintroduced in the UK in 2016 for self-administered inhalational analgesia via a hand-held inhaler containing 3 ml volatile agent. Analgesia occurs within 6–10 inhalations, lasting 25–30 min with continuous inhalation.

N-Methyl-D-aspartate receptors (NMDA receptors). Heterotetrameric ligand-gated ion channels; activated by **glutamate** (but requiring **glycine** as a co-agonist) and to a lesser extent aspartate, resulting in influx of Na^+ and Ca^{2+} ions into neurones. At resting **membrane potential**, the ion channel is largely 'blocked' by extracellular **magnesium**; maximal ion flux therefore requires membrane depolarisation as well as presynaptic glutamate release. Involved in the plasticity of the CNS to afferent impulses, especially **pain**.

Activation by repeated C-fibre stimulation leads to increased intracellular **calcium**, which in turn activates various intracellular second messenger systems, leading to an increased response to glutamate (a positive feedback mechanism). Thus input via NMDA receptors is thought to lead to a hyperexcitable state (**'wind-up'**) whereby repeated stimuli cause increasing degrees of pain sensation and expansion of the receptive field of individual sensory neurones involved in **pain pathways**. NMDA receptor antagonists (e.g. **ketamine**) are thought to prevent these phenomena and may thus have a role in **pre-emptive analgesia**.

Also involved in long-term neuronal potentiation (required for memory and learning) and activity-dependent neuronal survival; interference with the latter in the developing brain has been suggested as a mechanism for anaesthetic-induced neurotoxicity seen in vitro and in some animal studies.

NMDA receptor-mediated calcium influx is also thought to contribute to neuronal cell death in **cerebral hypoxic ischaemic injury** and in neurodegenerative disorders. An autoimmune **encephalitis** due to antibodies directed at NMDA receptors is increasingly recognised.

Vyklicky V, Korinel M, Smejkulova T, et al (2014). Physiol Rev; 63: S191–203

α-Methyldopa. **Antihypertensive drug**, originally thought to act via uptake into **catecholamine** synthetic pathways and formation of a 'false transmitter', α-methylnoradrenaline. The latter is now thought to have a direct antihypertensive action of its own, possibly via stimulation of central inhibitory **α-adrenergic receptors**, or reduction of plasma renin activity. Superseded by newer drugs, but it is still occasionally used, e.g. in **pre-eclampsia** (shown to be non-teratogenic).

- Dosage:
  - 250 mg orally bd/tds, titrated to response (maximum 3 g/day).
  - 250–500 mg iv over 30–60 min (as methyldopate hydrochloride). Onset of action is 4–6 h, lasting up to 16 h.
- Side effects:
  - leucopenia, hepatitis, haemolytic anaemia. 10%–20% of patients have a positive direct Coombs' test that may interfere with **blood compatibility testing** (*see Haemolysis*). An **SLE**-like syndrome has been reported.
  - sedation, confusion.
  - bradycardia, hypotension, oedema.
  - GIT disturbances.
  - paradoxical hypertension has occurred after iv use.

[Robin RA Coombs (1921–2006), Cambridge immunologist]

Methylenedioxyethylamfetamine, *see Methylenedioxymethylamfetamine*

Methylenedioxymethylamfetamine (MDMA; 'Ecstasy'). Synthetic **amfetamine**-like stimulant drug, abused recreationally, especially in association with prolonged dancing. Psychological effects include feelings of euphoria and increased intimacy with others. Toxicity has been associated with collapse and sudden death, particularly when combined with extreme physical exertion and dehydration. Has been associated with **hyperthermia** (thought to involve central **5-HT** pathways and not peripheral mechanisms as in **MH**), **arrhythmias** and **hepatic failure**. With increasing awareness that concurrent dehydration may be harmful, cases of **hyponatraemia** caused by excessive water intake have been reported. Degeneration of central neurones has also been reported after prolonged exposure. Most cases of acute critical illness involve hyperthermia that may be associated with severe acidosis, **DIC** and **rhabdomyolysis**.

Management of acute toxicity is mainly supportive. Hyperthermia is treated with active cooling; **dantrolene** has been used.

Similar concerns exist for the related drug methylenedioxyethylamfetamine ('Eve'), which is less commonly used.

White CM (2014). J Clin Pharmacol; 54: 245–52

Methylmethacrylate, *see Bone cement implantation syndrome*

Methylnaltrexone bromide. Peripherally acting mu **opioid receptor antagonist** licensed as a treatment for opioid-induced constipation in patients receiving palliative care. Has been investigated for preventing/treating postoperative **ileus**. Does not cross the **blood–brain barrier**; thus devoid of central effects.

- Dosage: 8–12 mg sc on alternate days.
- Side effects include abdominal pain, diarrhoea, nausea.

Methylprednisolone, *see Corticosteroids*

α-Methyl-*p*-tyrosine (Metirosine). **Antihypertensive drug**; inhibits conversion of tyrosine to dopa, thus blocking **catecholamine** synthesis. Available on a named patient basis in the UK. Has been used to reduce the incidence and severity of hypertensive episodes in **phaeochromocytoma**, e.g. before or instead of surgery. Should not be used in essential hypertension.

- Dosage: 2–4 g/day orally.
- Side effects include sedation, extrapyramidal movements, renal stones and diarrhoea.

Meticillin-resistant *Staphylococcus aureus*, *see Infection control; Staphylococcal infections*

Metoclopramide hydrochloride. **Antiemetic drug**, used in migraine, chemo-/radiotherapy-induced nausea and vomiting, and for prevention of **PONV**. Acts via **dopamine receptor** antagonism at the **chemoreceptor trigger zone**. Also a **prokinetic drug**, increasing **gastric emptying** and **lower oesophageal sphincter** pressure via a peripheral cholinergic action, but will not reverse the effects of **opioid analgesic drugs** in this respect unless given iv. It also decreases the sensitivity of visceral afferent nerves to local emetics and irritants. **Half-life** is about 4–6 h.

- Dosage:
  - 10 mg iv, im or orally tds as required.
  - has been used in very high doses (up to 5 mg/kg iv) to treat **vomiting** caused by cytotoxic therapy; thought to antagonise central **5-HT$_3$** receptors.
- Side effects: extrapyramidal effects and **dystonic reactions** (particularly affecting the face), especially following iv administration in children or young adults. Hypotension and tachy- or bradycardia may occur after rapid injection. Has been associated with **methaemoglobinaemia** and **sulfhaemoglobinaemia** if taken chronically or in high dosage.

Metocurine, *see Dimethyl tubocurarine chloride/bromide*

Metoprolol tartrate. **β-Adrenergic receptor antagonist**, available for oral and iv administration. Relatively selective for β$_1$-receptors. Uses and side effects are as for β-adrenergic receptor antagonists in general.

- Dosage:
  - hypertension, migraine: 100–200 mg orally od/bd; arrhythmias, angina: 50–100 mg bd/tds; thyrotoxicosis: 50 mg qds.
  - acute administration: 2–4 mg slowly iv, repeated up to 10 mg.
  - **acute coronary syndromes**: 5 mg iv every 2 min up to 15 mg if haemodynamically tolerated; then 15 min later 50 mg orally qds for 48 h.

Metre. SI **unit** of length. Originally defined according to the length of a platinum–iridium bar kept at Sèvres, France, but redefined in 1960 according to the speed of light in a vacuum, following doubts as to the bar's constant length over time: 1 metre = the distance occupied by 1 650 763.73 wavelengths of a specified orange-red light from gaseous krypton-86.

Metronidazole. **Antibacterial drug**, active against a wide range of anaerobic bacteria and protozoa. Used in many infections, especially gastrointestinal and gynaecological. Undergoes hepatic metabolism and renal excretion, with a **half-life** of 8.5 h. Tinidazole has similar actions but a longer duration of action and is given once daily.

- Dosage:
  - 200–800 mg orally/iv tds.
  - 1 g pr tds for 3 days, then bd.
- Side effects: **disulfiram**-like reaction, nausea, vomiting, urticaria; rarely drowsiness, ataxia; on prolonged dosage peripheral neuropathy, convulsions, leucopenia, urine discoloration.

MEWS, *see Modified early warning score*

MEOWS, Modified early obstetric warning score, *see Modified early warning score*

Mexiletine hydrochloride. Class Ib **antiarrhythmic drug**; reduces fast sodium entry and shortens the refractory period. Chemically related to **lidocaine**, but active orally. **Half-life** is 10 h. Used to treat ventricular **arrhythmias**.

- Dosage:
  - 400 mg orally, followed by 200–250 mg tds/qds.
  - 100–250 mg iv over 10 min, followed by 250 mg over 1 h, then 250 mg over 2 h, then 30 mg/h thereafter.
- Side effects:
  - hypotension, bradycardia.
  - confusion, ataxia, nystagmus, tremor, convulsions.
  - hepatitis, jaundice, GIT disturbances.

Meyer–Overton rule. Describes the positive correlation between anaesthetic potency of **inhalational anaesthetic agents** and lipid solubility. Can be seen if **MAC** is plotted against oil/gas **partition coefficients** at 37°C for various agents, using logarithmic scales (Fig. 109).

[Hans Meyer (1853–1939), German pharmacologist; Charles Ernest Overton (1865–1933), English-born German pharmacologist]

Perouansky A (2015). Br J Anaesth; 114: 537–41

See also, Anaesthesia, mechanism of

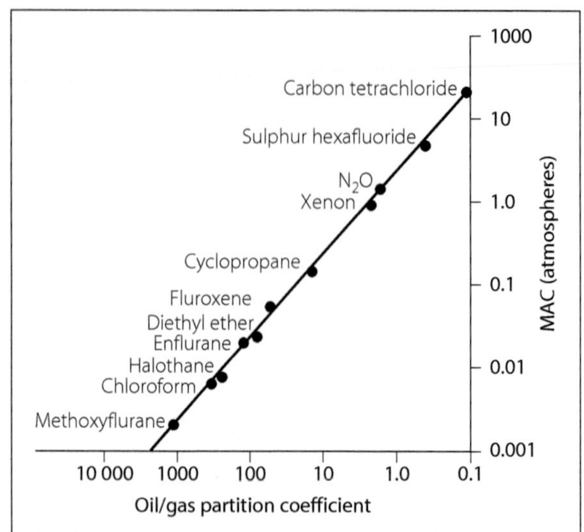

Fig. 109 Meyer–Overton rule

MH, *see Malignant hyperthermia*

MHRA, *see Medicines and Healthcare products Regulatory Agency*

MI, *see Myocardial infarction*

Michaelis–Menten kinetics. Refers to the reaction between a single substrate S and an **enzyme** E, via an intermediate complex ES to give a single product P:

$$S + E \rightleftharpoons ES \rightleftharpoons P$$

As the concentration of S ([S]) increases from zero, rate of reaction increases, until the enzyme binding sites become

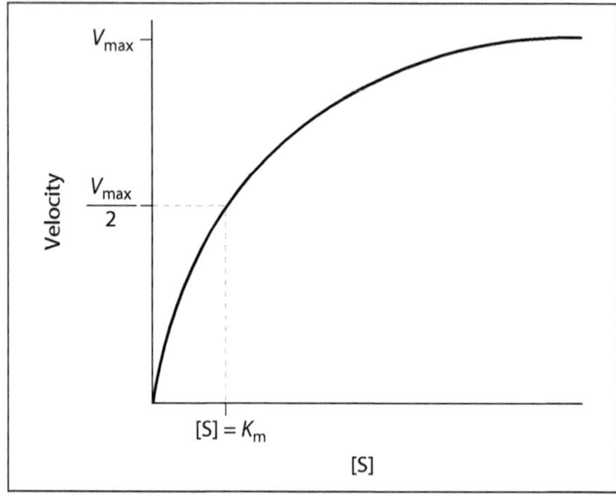

Fig. 110 Michaelis–Menten kinetics

saturated, and maximal rate of reaction is reached. Thus, initially, velocity of reaction (V) is proportional to [S]; i.e., first-order kinetics apply. Eventually, V does not increase as [S] increases; i.e., zero-order kinetics apply (Fig. 110).

$$\text{Michaelis-Menten equation } V = \frac{V_{max}[S]}{K_m + [S]}$$

where V_{max} = maximal reaction velocity

K_m = Michaelis constant, the concentration of S at which $V = \frac{1}{2} V_{max}$

V_{max} and K_m are found by plotting $1/V$ against $1/[S]$ to obtain a straight line; the x-intercept is $-1/K_m$, the y-intercept is $1/V_{max}$ and the slope is K_m/V_{max}.

May also be applied to pharmacology, to describe absorption, distribution and elimination of drugs.

[Leonor Michaelis (1875–1945), German-born US chemist; Maud Menten (1879–1960), US physician]

See also, Pharmacokinetics

Miconazole. Imidazole **antifungal drug**, active against a wide range of fungi and yeasts. Used for local treatment, or by mouth (as tablets or oral gel) for intestinal infection.

- Dosage: tablets: 250 mg qds for 10 days; gel: 2.5 ml qds.
- Side effects include GIT disturbances and rash. Should be avoided in **porphyria**.

Microshock, *see Electrocution and electrical burns*

Midazolam hydrochloride. **Benzodiazepine**, used for **sedation**, **premedication** and **induction of anaesthesia**. Also used for **status epilepticus**. Water-soluble at pH <4 due to its open imidazole ring (five-membered ring containing carbon and nitrogen atoms); it becomes highly lipid-soluble at body pH due to ring closure (an example of structural **isomerism**), resulting in rapid onset of action following iv administration. Also rapidly absorbed after im injection. Elimination **half-life** is 1.5–2.5 h. Undergoes hepatic metabolism to an active compound (alpha-hydroxymidazolam), which is excreted renally. Anterograde **amnesia** is marked.
Has relatively slow onset when used for induction, with prolonged recovery. Effects are antagonised by **flumazenil**.

- Dosage:
  - premedication: 0.07–0.1 mg/kg im, 30–60 min preoperatively. Paediatric oral dosage: 0.5–0.75 mg/kg 30 min preoperatively.
  - sedation: 0.5–2 mg increments iv. By infusion: 0.05–0.2 mg/kg/h.
  - induction: up to 0.3 mg/kg.

Respiratory and cardiovascular depression may occur, especially in elderly and sick patients, in whom reduced dosage is required.
See also, Intravenous anaesthetic agents

MID-CM, *see Minimally invasive direct cardiac massage*

Middle East respiratory syndrome (MERS). Coronavirus infection first described in 2012, originating in the Arabian Peninsula, with sporadic cases elsewhere thought to result from air travel. An outbreak occurred in South Korea in 2015, affecting 186 people, with 36 deaths. Approximately 1900 cases have been confirmed worldwide. More common in males. Incubation period is thought to be 2–15 days. Transmission via camels has been implicated, though person-to-person transmission has also been reported. Typically presents with fever, cough, breathlessness, myalgia and GIT symptoms. Mortality is ~40%. No specific treatment is available.

Arabi YM, Balkhy HH, Hayden FG, et al (2017). N Engl J Med; 376: 584–94

Midwives, prescription of drugs by. Approved hospital midwives in the UK are usually permitted to administer certain drugs on the labour ward without individual prescription by doctors, according to agreement with the local health authority and obstetricians. Specified drugs thus vary between hospitals, but usually include:

- **opioid analgesic drugs**, usually **pethidine** 100–150 mg im, repeated once.
- **Entonox** and O_2.
- oxytocics, e.g. **oxytocin** and **ergometrine** separately or combined.
- **antiemetic drugs/H_2 receptor antagonists**, e.g. **metoclopramide/ranitidine**.
- **lidocaine** 0.5% 10–20 ml for local perineal infiltration.
- **vitamin K** and **naloxone** for the **neonate**.

Others include hypnotics, traditionally **chloral hydrate** or **triclofos**. **Temazepam** and alternative opioids (e.g. **pentazocine**) are sometimes given. Community midwives usually have freedom to prescribe iron, **antacids**, etc., in addition.

Midwives may give epidural solutions (but not the first injection) according to written instructions; responsibility for administration lies with the prescribing doctor. They may also administer **TENS**.
See also, Nurses, prescription of drugs by

Migraine. Episodic form of primary headache; classified into migraine without aura (75% of cases; headache is typically unilateral and throbbing; there may be nausea and photophobia) and migraine with aura (25% of cases; headache is preceded by visual disturbances, tinnitus, numbness, etc.). May be difficult to distinguish from tension headaches (caused by muscular contraction), headache caused by cervical spondylosis, temporal arteritis, **trigeminal neuralgia**/other facial pain syndromes and headache caused by drugs. **Subarachnoid haemorrhage**, **meningitis** and **post-dural puncture headache** may also pose diagnostic difficulties. Neurological features may occasionally be severe and mimic **stroke**. Typically provoked by triggers such as emotional stress (80%), hormonal changes (65%), sleep disturbances (50%), alcohol (40%) and certain foods (30%). The pathophysiology is thought to involve activation of neurones originating from the trigeminal ganglion and upper cervical spinal cord that supply large cerebral blood vessels and the meninges. Activation releases neurotransmitters (**5-HT**, **substance P**, **glutamate**) that cause sensitisation with increased responsiveness to painful stimuli. This, in turn, results in sensitisation of thalamic and hypothalamic neurone networks.

- Management is divided into:
  - prophylactic: includes **β-adrenergic receptor antagonists** (**metoprolol**, **propranolol** or bisoprolol), **anticonvulsant drugs** (**sodium valproate**, **topiramate**) and **amitriptyline**.
  - therapeutic: includes simple analgesic/antiemetic combinations and **triptans**. 2%–3% of patients have chronic migraine (15 days of headache/month for 3 months); in addition to drug treatment, they may benefit from greater occipital nerve block or stimulation and **botulinum toxin** injection.

Anaesthetic management of a migraine sufferer is along standard lines. Management in the presence of an actual migraine attack is uncertain; if severe it may be wiser to postpone surgery, although there is no evidence to support this. Recent registry analysis data from the USA suggests that patients with migraine (especially with aura) have an increased risk of perioperative ischaemic stroke.

Poply K, Bahra A, Mehta V (2016). BJA Educ; 16: 357–61

Military antishock trousers, *see Antigravity suit*

Milrinone lactate. **Phosphodiesterase inhibitor**, used as an **inotropic drug** in low **cardiac output** states (e.g. after **cardiac surgery** or severe congestive **cardiac failure**). Increases **cardiac output** and reduces **SVR** without increasing **heart rate** or myocardial O_2 demand, although rate of atrioventricular conduction may increase slightly. BP may fall due to peripheral vasodilatation, despite increased cardiac output. Elimination **half-life** is about 2–2.5 h. Excreted mainly via urine.

- Dosage: 50 μg/kg over 10 min iv, followed by 0.3–0.75 μg/kg/min up to 1.1 mg/kg/day; accumulation may occur in renal impairment.
- Side effects: hypotension, ventricular and supraventricular arrhythmias, angina, headache.

Minaxolone. Water-soluble corticosteroid **iv anaesthetic agent** derived from **Althesin**, investigated in the late 1970s/early 1980s. Causes rapid induction with involuntary muscle movement, anaesthesia lasting up to 20 min. Development was terminated because of reported toxicity in rats.

Mineralocorticoids. Group of **corticosteroids**; typically comprise **aldosterone** physiologically and **fludrocortisone** therapeutically. Chief function is to regulate the transport of sodium and potassium ions in the kidney and other organs; hence they cause renal sodium reabsorption and loss of potassium. **Hydrocortisone** and other corticosteroids have some mineralocorticoid effects but these are generally too weak to make hydrocortisone a useful therapeutic mineralocorticoid (although they may limit its usefulness as a long-term **glucocorticoid** when used for disease suppression).

Miniature end-plate potential, *see End-plate potentials*

Minimal alveolar concentration (MAC). Minimal alveolar concentration of **inhalational anaesthetic agent** that prevents movement in response to a standard skin incision in 50% of subjects studied, when breathed in oxygen in the absence of any other analgesic or anaesthetic/depressant drugs. Thus inversely related to anaesthetic potency. Useful as a means of comparing different agents, and may be used to guide clinical dosage if end-tidal concentration of agent is monitored. Defined in terms of percentage of one atmosphere; therefore influenced by altitude, e.g. when barometric pressure is low (at high altitude), the MAC is increased because it is the partial pressure of inhalational agent that determines level of anaesthesia, not concentration, and a greater alveolar concentration is required to achieve the same partial pressure as at sea level. Minimal alveolar partial pressure (MAPP) has therefore been suggested as a more logical and practically useful measurement than MAC.

- MAC is reduced by:
  - other depressant drugs (e.g. opioids, sedatives, other inhalational agents).
  - CNS depletion of catecholamines, e.g. by **α-methyldopa**, **reserpine**.
  - **hypothermia**.
  - **hypoxaemia**, hypotension, **hyponatraemia**, **metabolic acidosis**.
  - **pregnancy**, possibly due to increased progesterone levels.
  - extremes of age.
- MAC is increased in:
  - children.
  - **hyperthermia**.
  - **hyperthyroidism**.
  - chronic **alcoholism**.
  - use of **cocaine**, **amfetamines**, **ephedrine**.

It is unaffected by duration of anaesthesia, sex, acidaemia/alkalaemia, hypercapnia or hypocapnia. Its limitations are that it is not a reliable indicator of state of consciousness and it is not applicable to **TIVA**.

'MAC-BAR' (blocks adrenergic response) has also been studied; it refers to the minimum alveolar concentration of agent at which the increase in heart rate or BP (or both) provoked by skin incision is prevented in 50% of subjects.

The term 'MAC awake' has been used to describe the alveolar concentration of agent at which 50% of subjects no longer respond appropriately to command. The term has also been applied to the alveolar concentration at which 50% of subjects respond appropriately when recovering from anaesthesia, in the absence of other depressant drugs. It is often presented as the ratio of MAC awake/MAC; in general this ratio is in the order of 0.3–0.5 for the commonly used volatile agents. It has been suggested that MAC awake is the minimum alveolar concentration required to prevent **awareness** during anaesthesia, although this is disputed.

(For values of MAC, *see Table 27*; **Inhalational anaesthetic agents**).

James MFM, Hofmeyr R, Grocott MPW (2015). Br J Anaesth; 115: 824–6

Minimal blocking concentration (C_m). Lowest concentration of **local anaesthetic agent** that will block a nerve in vitro within (usually) 10 min. Temperature, pH and electrolyte composition are specified. Higher concentrations are required clinically, in order to achieve C_m at the axons. Dependent on the size of axon, not the site (although important clinically because of diffusion across membranes, drug absorption, etc.).

Minimal infusion rate (MIR). Application of the **MAC** concept to infusions of **iv anaesthetic agents**, e.g. in **TIVA**. Equals the minimal infusion rate of agent that prevents movement in response to skin incision in 50% of subjects studied. More complex than MAC of inhalational agents, because of the influence of pharmacokinetic factors associated with the use of iv infusions.

Minimal local anaesthetic concentration/dose/volume (MLAC/MLAD/MLAV). Measurement used to compare the effects of different **local anaesthetic** solutions and/or dosing regimens, typically for **epidural** or **spinal anaesthesia**. For example, for MLAD, it requires a series of patients to receive a standard concentration of local anaesthetic, the response of each patient according to a defined outcome (e.g. for labour analgesia, whether pain scores reach a 'target' reduction within a set time) affecting the dose that the subsequent patient receives (e.g. 'failed' analgesia results in the next patient receiving a 20% higher dose; 'successful' analgesia results in a 20% lower dose). Analysis of the fluctuating dosage requirements over a set number of patients allows calculation of the ED_{50} for that concentration and outcome. Thus akin to **MAC** for **inhalational anaesthetic agents**. Criticisms include the lack of usefulness of knowing the ED_{50} (ED_{90} or ED_{95} being more useful) and the arbitrariness of the defined outcomes. However, it has been useful for examining the effects of local anaesthetic dosage, concentration and volume independently, and of the addition of adjuncts, e.g. opioids.

Graf BM, Zausiq Y, Zink W (2005). Curr Opin Anesthesiol; 18: 241–5

Minimally invasive direct cardiac massage (MID-CM). Variant of open chest **cardiac massage** that does not require thoracotomy. Uses a hand-held device introduced via a small thoracostomy. The device consists of a 40 FG introducer and a flat umbrella-shaped 'plunger' that is collapsed and retracted during insertion. Once in the chest, the umbrella is opened, expanding to a diameter of 7.5 cm, and used to 'pump' the heart rhythmically from outside the pericardium.

Rozenberg A, Incagnoli P, Delpech P, et al (2001). Resuscitation; 50: 257–62

See also, Cardiac arrest; Cardiopulmonary resuscitation

Minitracheotomy. Commercially available device, enabling emergency **cricothyrotomy**. Also useful as a route for tracheobronchial suction when sputum retention is a problem, e.g. respiratory infection, impaired coughing or postoperatively. May thus avoid tracheal intubation or formal **tracheostomy**, e.g. in ICU.

The pack originally included a blade, 4-mm internal diameter tube and introducer, standard 15-mm connector, suction catheter and securing tapes. Because of difficulties inserting the device without a guide-wire, one was subsequently introduced into the pack along with a syringe, short 16 G needle and dilator. The needle and syringe are used to locate the trachea through a small vertical incision in the cricothyroid membrane and the guide-wire inserted into the trachea. The rest of the insertion proceeds using the **Seldinger technique**. Complications include haemorrhage, subcutaneous emphysema and misplacement.

Minoxidil. Antihypertensive drug causing peripheral vasodilatation. Reserved as third-line treatment after **diuretics** and **β-adrenergic receptor antagonists**, because of tachycardia and water and salt retention. Also causes increased hair growth. Taken orally, 2.5–25 mg od/bd.

Minute ventilation (Minute volume). Volume of air breathed per minute. Equals tidal volume × respiratory rate; i.e., includes **alveolar ventilation** and **dead space** ventilation. Normally 5–7 litres.

Minute volume dividers, *see Ventilators*

MIR, *see Minimal infusion rate*

Misoprostol. Analogue of naturally occurring **prostaglandin** E_1, licensed for gastric protection and healing of ulcers in patients taking **NSAIDs**. Has been used to increase uterine contractions (e.g. in therapeutic abortion) and to prevent and treat **postpartum haemorrhage**, for which doses of 200–800 µg have been given orally, vaginally and rectally. Serious side effects are rare, although shivering is common.

Misuse of Drugs Act 1971. Introduced in the UK as a replacement for the obsolete Dangerous Drugs Act. Defined three classes of drugs, according to the penalties for offences:

- Class A:
  - **opioid analgesic drugs**, e.g. **morphine, pethidine, fentanyl, alfentanil, diamorphine, methadone.**
  - **cocaine, methylenedioxymethamfetamine**, methylamfetamine, lysergide (LSD), phencyclidine.
  - parenteral forms of class B drugs.
- Class B:
  - opioids, e.g. **codeine, pentazocine.**
  - **amfetamines, barbiturates.**
  - **ketamine** (previously Class C) was upgraded to Class B in 2014.
  - **cannabis.**
  - others, e.g. glutethimide (sedative/hypnotic), phenmetrazine (appetite suppressant).
- Class C: includes **benzodiazepines**, anabolic steroids and certain amfetamine-related drugs.

The Misuse of Drugs Regulations 2001 (and subsequent amendments) specifies the requirements for handling, storage, record-keeping, etc.:

- Schedule 1: drugs not used therapeutically, e.g. lysergide.
- Schedule 2: opioids, including codeine, morphine, etc., ketamine, cocaine (**controlled drugs**). To be kept in locked cupboards (but not necessarily double-locked); details of patients are recorded in registers with practitioners' signatures and kept for 2 years.
- Schedule 3: barbiturates, **buprenorphine**, tramadol, pentazocine, **temazepam**. Registers and locked cupboards are not required (except for certain drugs including phenobarbital, midazolam, pentazocine, tramadol) but special prescription requirements are.
- Schedule 4: benzodiazepines other than temazepam and midazolam, zopiclone, anabolic steroids.
- Schedule 5: products containing low concentrations of substances otherwise in Schedule 2. Exempt from virtually all controlled drug requirements except for retention of invoices.

Misuse of Drugs Regulations, *see Misuse of Drugs Act 1971*

Mitral regurgitation. Most common valvular disease worldwide; usually due to degenerative disease associated with **mitral valve prolapse**; previously, most cases were due to **rheumatic fever**, when **mitral stenosis** usually coexisted. May also be due to papillary muscle dysfunction secondary to **MI** or degeneration; other causes include left ventricular dilatation in **cardiac failure, cardiomyopathy**, bacterial **endocarditis** and ruptured chordae tendinae. Results in an increased volume load to the left ventricle.

- Effects:
  - left atrial dilatation; **pulmonary oedema**, especially if acute. Regurgitant fraction increases if SVR rises.
  - left ventricular hypertrophy and increased stroke volume.
  - **AF** if severe. Ventricular filling is less reliant on atrial contraction than in mitral stenosis; thus cardiac output is usually maintained.
- Features:
  - left ventricular hypertrophy, with pansystolic murmur loudest at the apex on expiration and leaning forward, and radiating to the axilla. A thrill, third **heart sound** and diastolic flow murmur may be present. AF, left and later right ventricular failure may be present.
  - systemic embolism.
  - endocarditis.
  - **ECG** may reveal P mitrale, ventricular hypertrophy, and ventricular ectopics. **CXR** features may include cardiac enlargement, particularly of the left atrium, and pulmonary oedema. **Echocardiography** and **cardiac catheterisation** are useful.
- Anaesthetic management:
  - main principles are as for congenital and **ischaemic heart disease**. Drugs taken may include **diuretics, digoxin** and **anticoagulant drugs**. The following should be avoided: myocardial depression, **hypovolaemia**, bradycardia (which increases regurgitation; mild tachycardia is preferable), vasoconstriction, e.g. due

Table 32 American Heart Association/American College of Cardiology classification of mitral stenosis

	Mild	Moderate	Severe
Valve area (cm^2)	>1.5	1.0–1.5	<1.0
Mean gradient at heart rate 60–80 beats/min and sinus rhythm (mmHg)	<25	25–40	>40
Pulmonary arterial pressure (mmHg)	<30	30–50	>50

to sympathetic stimulation (pain, light anaesthesia), cold. If **pulmonary artery catheterisation** is done, large V waves are typically seen in the pulmonary **venous waveform.**

Badhwar V, Smith AJ, Cavalcante JL (2016). Trends Cardiovasc Med; 26: 126–34

See also, Heart murmurs; Valvular heart disease

Mitral stenosis. **Rheumatic fever** is by far the most common cause; others include congenital, infective and inflammatory causes. Has been classified according to valve area (Table 32). Symptoms are usually present if the valve area is reduced from the normal 4–5 cm^2 to <1.5 cm^2, although concurrent **anaemia**, **atrial fibrillation** or **pregnancy** may precipitate symptoms with less severe stenosis.

- Effects:
  - reduced left ventricular filling, with left atrial hypertrophy and dilatation.
  - increased pulmonary vascular pressures, with pulmonary congestion and reduced pulmonary compliance. Work of breathing is increased.
  - if prolonged, it may cause **pulmonary hypertension**, with right ventricular overload and/or tricuspid or pulmonary regurgitation. Progression may be rapid in 25%–30%; the reason is unknown.
  - **AF** occurs in up to 50%; ventricular filling is reliant on atrial contraction; thus AF may lead to **pulmonary oedema.**
- Features:
  - **cardiac failure** and dyspnoea. Haemoptysis may be caused by recurrent chest infection, pulmonary oedema or infarction, or blood vessel rupture.
  - AF and systemic embolism.
  - malar flush (mitral facies), parasternal heave and features of tricuspid valve regurgitation may be present.
  - 'tapping apex' (palpable first **heart sound**). The first sound is loud, with opening snap following the second sound. A low-pitched rumbling diastolic murmur follows, heard best at the apex on expiration with the stethoscope bell, leaning forward and to the left. Presystolic accentuation is heard before the first heart sound, due to atrial contraction; it disappears in AF. The opening snap may disappear if the valve is calcified. If pulmonary hypertension is present, the pulmonary component of the second heart sound (P2) may be loud.
  - **ECG** may reveal P mitrale (a widened, notched P wave), AF and right ventricular hypertrophy. **CXR** features may include cardiac enlargement, particularly of the left atrium, and pulmonary oedema. Mitral calcification and features of pulmonary hypertension may be present. **Echocardiography** and **cardiac catheterisation** are especially useful. In moderate and severe stenosis the area is reduced to <1.5 and <1 cm^2, respectively.
- Anaesthetic management:
  - main principles are as for congenital and **ischaemic heart disease.** Drugs taken may include **diuretics, digoxin, anticoagulant drugs.** The following should be avoided: myocardial depression; atrial fibrillation; tachycardia (reduces left ventricular filling time); **hypovolaemia** and vasodilatation (reduce atrial and thus ventricular filling); and increased **pulmonary vascular resistance**, e.g. due to **hypoxaemia.** In **pulmonary artery catheterisation, left ventricular end-diastolic pressure** estimation is inaccurate due to stenosis. Due to lower cost and morbidity, percutaneous catheter balloon valvuloplasty has become the treatment of choice in patients with suitable valve anatomy and/or high surgical risk.
  - postoperative IPPV may be required.

Nishimura RA, Vahanian A, Eleia MF, Mack MJ (2016). Lancet; 387: 1324–34

See also, Heart murmurs; Tricuspid valve lesions; Valvular heart disease

Mitral valve prolapse. Superior displacement of mitral valve leaflet tissue into the left atrium, above the mitral annular plane. Thought to occur in 2%–3% of the population, sometimes associated with autosomal dominant inheritance. Also associated with **Marfan's syndrome** and other collagen disorders (e.g. Ehlers–Danlos syndrome). Acquired causes are as for **mitral regurgitation.** Often asymptomatic, but may lead to mitral regurgitation, **cardiac failure**, bacterial **endocarditis**, systemic emboli and even sudden death.

- Signs:
  - mid-late systolic click, occurring at the onset of the carotid pulsation.
  - late systolic **heart murmur**, not always present.

Diagnosis is usually aided by **echocardiography** or angiography.

Perioperative complications are unlikely unless mitral regurgitation is severe or left ventricular dysfunction is present.

[Edvard Ehlers (1863–1927, Danish dermatologist; Henri-Alexandre Danlos (1844–1912), French physician]

Delling FN, Vasan RS (2014). Circulation; 129: 2158–70

See also, Heart sounds

Mivacurium chloride. Non-depolarising **neuromuscular blocking drug**, a benzylisoquinolinium ester (as is **atracurium**). Tracheal intubation is possible approximately 2 min after a dose of 0.07–0.25 mg/kg (doses above 0.15 mg/kg should be given over 30 s—more slowly in patients with asthma or CVS disease). Effects last 10–20 min. Supplementary dose: 0.1 mg/kg. May be given by iv infusion at 0.2–0.5 mg/kg/h. Causes little or no cardiovascular instability, although **histamine** release (with bronchospasm, urticaria and hypotension) may accompany high doses, especially if given rapidly. Metabolised by plasma **cholinesterase** (thus its action may be markedly prolonged in cholinesterase deficiency) to highly water-soluble metabolites, excreted rapidly via the urine; **half-life** is 2–5 min. Also undergoes some hepatic metabolism. More easily reversed than **atracurium** or **vecuronium.** Has been suggested as an alternative to **suxamethonium**, especially in children, in whom onset and recovery are faster than in adults.

Mixed venous blood. True mixed venous blood is obtained from the right ventricle or pulmonary artery, because superior and inferior vena caval blood is different in composition, and mixes during passage through the heart.

Mixed venous O_2 saturation ($S_{\bar{v}}O_2$) is related to arterial O_2 content, O_2 consumption and cardiac output; it may be monitored continuously via a fibreoptic bundle on a pulmonary artery catheter. ($S_{\bar{v}}O_2$) is used as an indicator of O_2 supply/demand in critically ill patients, and as an early indicator of imminent haemodynamic failure; tissue **O_2 delivery** is considered critical at ($S_{\bar{v}}O_2$) of under 50% (normally 75%). The measurement is non-specific, however, and is increased by peripheral shunting, e.g. in **septic shock**.

See also, Arteriovenous oxygen difference

MLAC/MLAD/MLAV, *see Minimal local anaesthetic concentration/dose/volume*

MMV, *see Mandatory minute ventilation*

MOC-etomidate, *see Etomidate*

Mode. Expression of the central tendency of a set of observations or measurements. Equals that observation, or group of observations, that occurs the most often. Equals the **mean** for a normal distribution.

See also, Median; Statistical frequency distributions; Statistics

Modified early warning score (MEWS). Scoring system used to aid identification of critically ill patients or those at risk of clinical deterioration. Uses six variables (systolic BP, heart rate, respiratory rate, temperature, neurological status and urine output) to score the degree of abnormality of a patient's physiology, with a possible composite score of 0 (normal) to 17. Used to 'trigger' calls for assistance from the patient's primary team, a **medical emergency team**, an **outreach team** or others. Thought to allow earlier detection of deterioration but a lack of uniformity of scoring and initiation of therapy makes this difficult to prove.

A similar concept (modified early obstetric warning score; MEOWS) has been applied to obstetric patients because analyses of maternal deaths and near-misses typically find that the severity of the mother's condition is not appreciated until late in the illness.

Alam N, Hobbelink EL, Tienhaven AJ, et al (2014). Resuscitation; 85: 587–94

See also, Acute life-threatening events—recognition and treatment; Early warning scores

MODS, *see Multiple organ dysfunction syndrome*

MOET, *see Managing Obstetric Emergencies and Trauma course*

Moffet's solution, *see Nose*

Molality. Number of **moles** of solute per kilogram of solvent. A molal solution contains 1 mole/kg.

Molarity. Number of **moles** of solute per litre of solution. A molar solution contains 1 mole/l.

Mole. SI **unit** of amount of substance. Defined as that quantity containing the same number of particles as there are atoms in 12 g of carbon-12. This number (**Avogadro's number**) equals 6.022×10^{23}.

Molecular adsorbents recirculation system, *see Liver dialysis*

Molecular weight (mw). Mass of a molecule, equal to the sum of atomic weights of its constituent atoms.

Molgramostim, *see Granulocyte colony-stimulating factor*

Monitoring. Adequate monitoring during anaesthesia and recovery is acknowledged to improve patient safety and reduce **anaesthetic morbidity and mortality**. Standards of minimal monitoring have been published in many countries, e.g. in the USA since 1986 and the UK since 1988. Failure to employ appropriate monitoring equipment is increasingly considered substandard. Devices should warn of adverse changes in the state of the patient, and of altered functioning of anaesthetic equipment.

- Most monitors involve electrical equipment. Technical considerations:
  - signal from patients may be:
    - primary electrical signals, e.g. **ECG**, **EEG**, power spectral analysis.
    - electrical signals derived from other energy forms, e.g. via pressure **transducers**.
    - evoked signals, e.g. **neuromuscular blockade monitoring**, **evoked potentials**.
  - skin electrodes are usually made of silver/silver chloride to reduce alterations in **impedance**, and to reduce the creation of interfering potentials within the electrode.
  - amplification/processing of the signal via intermediate components. Accuracy of reproduction is related to:
    - signal:noise ratio: improved by filtering, and averaging the signal so that background noise is cancelled out. Recording between two recording leads (differential input) also cancels out background noise, because the noise is in phase in both the leads.
    - baseline drift: may be random or due to the effect of temperature on semiconductors.
    - sensitivity of the **amplifier**: related to the voltage of the original signal (i.e., appropriate **gain**).
    - linearity of the response: distortion causes nonlinear response characteristics and **hysteresis**.
    - **damping**.
    - frequency range: related to the **harmonics** of the measured signal.
    - matched output/input voltage, current, etc., of components.
    - interference; may be caused by:
      - **capacitance** between the patient and electrical equipment.
      - **inductance** of current in the patient and monitor wires by electrical equipment.
      - other electrical equipment, e.g. **diathermy**, other monitors.
  - display of the signal, as, e.g. a waveform on **oscilloscopes**, numerical display, galvanometer and/or paper strip.
  - alarms are usually incorporated into monitors; limits are set to minimise inappropriate warnings without compromising sensitivity. Alarms of different devices are often of random pitch and frequency; standardisation of alarms has been suggested.

- risk of **electrocution and electrical burns** from electrical equipment.
- UK recommendations (**Association of Anaesthetists**):
  - presence of the anaesthetist is mandatory during the whole procedure, with adequate **record-keeping** and hand-over.
  - monitoring is instituted before induction and continued until **recovery**.
  - equipment monitoring: **O_2 failure warning device**, output and delivery O_2 analyser, and disconnection detection by expired tidal volume measurement, **capnography** and airway pressure measurement. Monitoring of volatile agent. All alarms set at appropriate values and enabled. Infusion devices checked and alarms set.
  - patient monitoring: clinical observation of colour, pupils, respiration, pulse and response to surgery, chest auscultation, **urine** output and **blood loss** when appropriate, plus:
    - for induction and maintenance: ECG, **arterial BP measurement**, pulse **oximetry**, capnography, oxygen and volatile agent analyser, a nerve stimulator whenever neuromuscular blocking drugs are used, and a means of **temperature measurement** available. Depth of anaesthesia monitoring (e.g. **bispectral index monitor**) should be used when using **TIVA**with neuromuscular blockade.
    - for recovery: oximetry and BP measurement (ECG, nerve stimulator, temperature measurement and capnography immediately available).
    - heart rate and BP recorded at regular intervals as appropriate. Waveforms are preferable to numeric displays. Trend displays/printouts recommended.
    - direct BP measurement, **CVP** measurement, pulmonary artery pressures, arterial **blood gas interpretation** and blood tests as appropriate.
    - for **sedation**, **regional anaesthesia**: at least ECG, oximetry and BP measurement, with capnography for those deeply sedated.
    - adequate monitoring (including easily accessible and visible displays) required for transfer of patients.

Checketts MR, Alladi R, Ferguson K, et al (2016). Anaesthesia; 71: 85–93

See also, Anaesthesia, depth of; Blood flow; Carbon dioxide measurement; Cardiac output measurement; Echocardiography; Gas analysis; Oxygen measurement; Pulmonary artery catheterisation; Pulmonary wedge pressure; Respirometer

Monoamine oxidase (MAO). **Enzyme** present in mitochondria of most tissues, especially liver, intestinal mucosa, lung, kidney and **catecholamine**-secreting nerve endings. Catalyses oxidative deamination of amines to aldehyde derivatives, e.g. $R–CH_2–NH_2 \rightarrow R–CHO$. Inactivates active amines, including catecholamines, whether circulating, absorbed from the gut, or at adrenergic/**5-HT** nerve endings. Many products are subsequently metabolised by **catechol-*O*-methyl transferase** (COMT), and many products of COMT metabolism are subsequently metabolised by MAO.

Two distinct types have been identified: type A, mainly inactivating **noradrenaline** and 5-HT, and type B, mainly inactivating tryptamine and phenylethylamine. **Dopamine** and tyramine are inactivated by both. Both are present in liver and brain; type B is thought to be predominant in certain CNS regions, e.g. basal ganglia.

Non-specific and type A-specific **MAO inhibitors** are used to treat depression; MAO type B inhibitors are used as **antiparkinsonian drugs**.

Monoamine oxidase inhibitors (MAOIs). The term usually refers to non-specific inhibitors of **monoamine oxidase**, used as **antidepressant drugs** and developed in the 1950s from anti-**TB** drugs. Examples include phenelzine, isocarboxazid, tranylcypromine and moclobemide. Recently increasing in use following a period of unpopularity. Inhibit **monoamine oxidase** irreversibly (except moclobemide), resynthesis of the enzyme taking at least 3 weeks.

- Anaesthetic relevance:
  - interaction with **pethidine**: may be:
    - excitatory: agitation, **hypertension**, tachycardia, hyperreflexia, hypertonus, pyrexia, **convulsions**, **coma**. Thought to be caused by excessive central **5-HT** activity, due to reduced 5-HT uptake. Treatment includes **α-adrenergic receptor antagonists**, **vasodilator drugs** and **chlorpromazine**. Steroids have been used.
    - depressive: may cause **hypoventilation**, **hypotension**, coma. Thought to be caused by impaired hepatic metabolism of opioid. **Naloxone** and directly acting vasopressors, e.g. **noradrenaline**, have been used for treatment.

    Morphine has been suggested as the opioid of choice, titrated to effect. Although **fentanyl** is related to pethidine, it has been safely used; however experience is limited. **Pentazocine** has also been used safely.
  - **sympathomimetic drugs** may produce exaggerated hypertensive responses, especially those acting indirectly via **catecholamine** release, e.g. **ephedrine**, **metaraminol**. Directly acting drugs (e.g. noradrenaline, **adrenaline** and **isoprenaline**) should be used in small amounts if required. Catecholamines and drugs increasing catecholamine levels should be avoided, e.g. **pancuronium**, **ketamine**, **cocaine** and adrenaline in local anaesthetic solutions (the last is controversial).
  - other iv and inhalational agents, **benzodiazepines** and non-depolarising neuromuscular blocking drugs are considered safe; **doxapram** is considered unsafe.
  - phenelzine may decrease plasma **cholinesterase** levels.

Crises may also follow oral ingestion of active amines or precursors (e.g. in tyramine-rich food such as cheese and red wine) because of inhibition of the enzyme in the gut wall.

Traditional advice, to stop taking MAOIs 2–3 weeks preoperatively, is rarely given now, because of risks of worsening depression, and possible inadequacy of this interval. Moclobemide is a reversible inhibitor of MAO type A (or RIMA), said to be less likely to interact with amines and drugs. No treatment-free period is required after stopping therapy. Selegiline is an MAO type B inhibitor used in **Parkinson's disease**; it increases central dopamine levels without exhibiting an exaggerated response to dietary amines.

Monro–Kellie doctrine. The cranial cavity is a rigid closed container; thus any change in intracranial blood volume is accompanied by the opposite change in **CSF** volume, if **ICP** remains constant.

[Alexander Monro (1733–1817) and George Kellie (1758–1829), Scottish anatomists]

Wilson MH (2016). J Cereb Blood Flow Metab; 36: 1338–50

Montelukast, *see Leukotriene receptor antagonists*

Morbidity and mortality, *see Anaesthetic morbidity and mortality; Mortality/survival prediction on intensive care unit*

Moricizine hydrochloride. Class I **antiarrhythmic drug**, structurally related to **phenothiazines**. Available on a named patient basis in the UK. Used to treat ventricular arrhythmias. **Half-life** is 3–6 h.

- Dosage: 200–300 mg orally tds or 400–500 mg followed by 200 mg tds for rapid control.
- Side effects: GIT disturbances, dizziness, arrhythmias, jaundice, thrombocytopenia.

Morphine hydrochloride/sulfate/tartrate. Opioid analgesic drug, in use for thousands of years as **opium** derived from poppy seeds. Isolated in 1803, and synthesised in 1952, although still obtained from poppies. The standard drug with which other opioids are compared.

Used for **premedication** and as an **analgesic drug**. Also useful in **pulmonary oedema**. Peak effect occurs 15–20 min after iv, and 60–90 min after im injection; action lasts 4–5 h. Undergoes significant **first-pass metabolism** when given orally. Undergoes hepatic dealkylation, oxidation and conjugation to morphine 3- and 6-glucuronide, excreted in urine. The latter is a highly active metabolite, and may be responsible for prolonged action, e.g. in renal impairment or chronic administration.

- Actions:
    - CNS:
        - depression of:
            - respiratory centre; rate is reduced more than tidal volume. **Neonates** and the **elderly** are particularly susceptible.
            - **cough** reflex.
            - **pain** sensation, especially dull, continuous pain. Most effective if given before the painful stimulus. Perception of painful stimuli is altered as well as pain sensation itself.
            - anxiety; morphine causes sedation and euphoria.
            - **ACTH** and prolactin secretion.
            - metabolic rate.
            - **vasomotor centre**; depression is now thought to be minimal, if it occurs at all.
        - stimulation of:
            - **chemoreceptor trigger zone**.
            - parasympathetic nucleus of the third **cranial nerve**, causing miosis.
            - **vasopressin** release.
            - vagus nerve, causing bradycardia.
            - higher centres causing euphoria or, less commonly, dysphoria.
        - muscle rigidity following high doses; may be caused by central interference with motor function, although the mechanism is unclear.
        - may cause addiction.
    - peripheral:
        - **histamine** release; may cause vasodilatation, bronchoconstriction, itching (typically of the nose), flushing. Hypotension may occur (partly a central effect).
        - **constipation**, delayed **gastric emptying** and reduced **lower oesophageal sphincter** tone. Increases the tone of biliary and genitourinary smooth muscle, including sphincters.
        - increases **catecholamine** release from the adrenal medulla.
- Dosage:
    - standard im, iv or sc dose: 0.1–0.15 mg/kg.
    - oral dose for: adults: 10–20 mg increased slowly up to 200 mg, 4-hourly; sustained-release preparation: from 10 mg bd.
    - has been given via buccal and rectal routes.

Doses and/or frequency of administration should be reduced at the extremes of age and in renal or hepatic failure.

[Morpheus, Greek god of dreams]

See also, Opioid receptors; Spinal opioids

Mortality and morbidity, *see Anaesthetic morbidity and mortality; Mortality/survival prediction on intensive care unit*

Mortality probability models (MPM). Scoring systems, similar to **APACHE** and **simplified acute physiology score**, for predicting outcome and length of stay of ICU patients. The latest version (MPM III) is based on multiple regression analysis applied to data from 125 000 patients at the time of admission to ICU and reflects changes in clinical management since the MPM II system was introduced. Scores are derived from weighting of variables related to physiology, acute and chronic disease, reason for admission, age and therapeutic interventions. A probability of hospital mortality can be calculated at 0, 24, 48 and 72 h after ICU admission. Individual versions of the MPM system are termed MPM_0 (calculation of risk of hospital death on entry to ICU), MPM_{24}, MPM_{48} and MPM_{72} (calculated after 24, 48 and 72 h of ICU care, respectively).

Salluh JI, Soares M (2014). Curr Opin Crit Care; 20: 557–65

See also Intensive care, outcome of; Mortality/survival prediction on intensive care unit

Mortality/survival prediction on intensive care unit. Many attempts have been made to develop methods of predicting outcomes in critically ill patients, to allow:

- estimation of prognoses for individual patients.
- comparison between different treatments, e.g. in clinical studies.
- comparison between different units (e.g. using the standardised mortality ratio: observed mortality divided by predicted mortality).
- allocation of resources.

Scoring systems may be based on a single set of data (static) or on repeated collections over time (dynamic). Many different systems exist, including:

- simple five-point scale according to clinical judgement, e.g. certain to die, likely to die, etc.
- **therapeutic intervention scoring system** (TISS): based primarily on treatment interventions.
- **acute physiology score** (APS), **simplified acute physiology score** (SAPS), **APACHE scoring systems, mortality probability models** (MPM), **logistic organ dysfunction system** (LODS): based mainly on the patient's physiological state ± therapeutic interventions.
- specific systems for certain conditions, e.g. **coma scales** such as the **Glasgow coma scale** (GCS), **trauma scales**, scoring systems for **sepsis**, **burns**, **subarachnoid haemorrhage, hepatic failure.**

None of the general systems has been shown to be superior to the others, although updated systems generally perform better than the original ones.

Salluh JI, Soares M (2014). Curr Opin Crit Care; 20: 557–65

See also, Intensive care, outcome of

Morton, William Thomas Green (1819–1868). US dentist, considered the founder of anaesthesia, despite being predated by **Clarke, Long** and **Wells.** Briefly practised with Wells in Boston in 1842–3, before entering Harvard Medical School in 1844, although he never completed his medical studies. Present at Wells' unsuccessful demonstration of N_2O at Harvard in 1844. Morton approached **Jackson** for advice on supplies of N_2O for further experiments. Jackson's suggestion of **diethyl ether** as a topical analgesic led to Morton's use of ether for inhalational anaesthesia for dental extraction on 30 September 1846. At the Massachusetts General Hospital on 16 October, he successfully anaesthetised Edward Gilbert Abbott, while **Warren** excised a mass from the latter's jaw. Became demoralised by subsequent battles against Jackson's claim to the discovery, and against widespread infringement of his patent (which he named **Letheon**). His contribution was recognised only posthumously.
[Edward Gilbert Abbott (1825–1855), US printer]
See also, Letheon

Motor neurone disease. Progressive degenerative disorder characterised by degeneration of **motor neurones** in the **brainstem** nuclei of the **cranial nerves** and anterior horn cells of the **spinal cord.** Prevalence is 5 per 100 000; mainly affects men aged 50–70. Death usually occurs within 3–5 years.

- Types:
  - amyotrophic lateral sclerosis: upper motor neurone lesions with spastic limb weakness.
  - progressive bulbar palsy: lower motor neurone lesions of the brainstem nuclei, causing dysarthria and dysphagia.
  - progressive muscular atrophy: lower motor neurone lesions of the anterior horn cells.
- Anaesthetic problems are related to:
  - possible laryngeal incompetence leading to **aspiration of gastric contents.**
  - respiratory muscle weakness, with greater sensitivity to respiratory depressant drugs.
  - increased sensitivity to **neuromuscular blocking drugs.** An exaggerated hyperkalaemic response to **suxamethonium** is theoretically possible but has not been reported.

ICU concerns include the above and also the ethical issues surrounding ventilatory support when **respiratory failure** occurs.

van Es MA, Michael A, Chio A, et al (2017). Lancet; 390: 2084–98

Motor neurone, lower. Term used to describe motor neurones that directly innervate **muscle,** i.e., without other neurones interposed. Lower motor neurone lesions therefore result in complete cessation of neural input to the muscle, resulting in characteristic clinical features:

- flaccid paralysis.
- visible **fasciculations,** thought to be caused by spontaneous firing of neighbouring **motor units** that have taken over the affected muscle.
- absent reflexes.
- muscular atrophy.
- **denervation hypersensitivity.** Thought to be the cause of invisible fibrillation of muscle fibres. An increased hyperkalaemic response to **suxamethonium** may occur from 4 days to 7 months after injury.

See also, Motor neurone, upper

Motor neurone, upper. Term used to describe neurones of the **motor pathways,** excluding lower motor neurones. Thus includes neurones of the motor cortex, cerebellar and extrapyramidal pathways, although the term commonly refers only to the former. Upper motor neurone lesions may thus occur at any level above the lower neurone cell bodies, producing characteristic features, after initial flaccid paralysis:

- increased tone and spastic paralysis. Typically, muscle exhibits 'clasp-knife' rigidity, possibly due to activity of **muscle spindles** without inhibitory higher input.
- increased reflexes and up-going plantar responses (Babinski reflex).
- no **fasciculation.**
- no atrophy.
- an increased hyperkalaemic response to **suxamethonium** may occur from 10 days to 7 months after injury, although the mechanism is unclear.

[Joseph Babinski (1857–1932), French neurologist]
See also, Motor neurone, lower

Motor pathways. Consist of the following systems:

- pyramidal pathways (Fig. 111): fibres arise from pyramidal cells of the motor cortex of the precentral gyrus and premotor area. Legs are represented uppermost, with the head at the lower part of the gyrus. Regions of densest innervation (e.g. face, hands) have a disproportionately greater representation. Fibres then pass via the internal capsule (legs represented behind, face anteriorly), and via the cerebral peduncle and pons to the medulla, forming the pyramids. Most of the fibres decussate in the lower medulla and pass within the lateral corticospinal tract of the **spinal cord.** Some pass within the anterior corticospinal tract without decussating; these cross within the spinal cord at their spinal levels. Some fibres pass to **cranial nerve** motor nuclei. Most of the fibres synapse with intermediate **neurones.**
- extrapyramidal pathways: less well defined than the above system. Fibres arise from the premotor area and corpus striatum, and pass via the basal ganglia, substantia nigra and nuclear masses of the midbrain and hindbrain. They descend within the rubroreticulospinal and vestibulospinal tracts. Other pathways pass from the tectum of the midbrain and olives of the medulla. Concerned with control of movement.
- cerebellar pathways: involve the thalamus, red nucleus, pons, medulla and cerebral cortex.
- pathways of the **autonomic nervous system.**

See also, Motor neurone, lower; Motor neurone, upper; Spinal cord lesions

Motor unit. One lower **motor neurone** and the **muscle** fibres it innervates. In muscles for fine movement (e.g. of the eye and hand) motor units are small, i.e., <10 fibres per neurone. Muscles involved in posture may have up to 1000 fibres per neurone. All fibres of a motor unit are of the same type, i.e., fast or slow; the type is thought to be determined by characteristics of the nerve itself.

Mountain sickness, *see Altitude, high*

Mouth, *see Larynx; Pharynx; Teeth; Tongue*

Mouth care. Important aspect of care of the unconscious patient. Involves regular inspection of the oral mucosa,

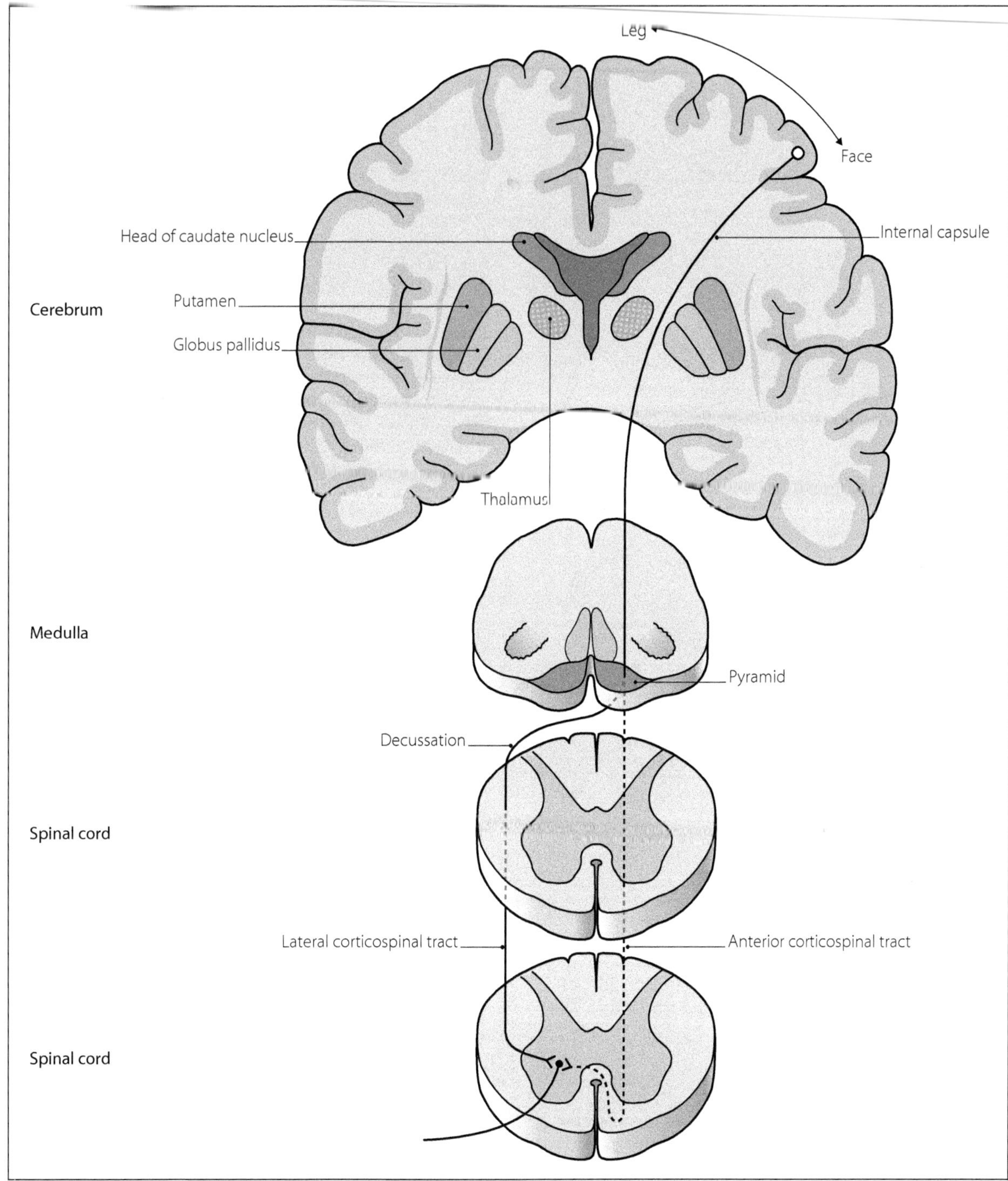

Fig. 111 Pyramidal (corticospinal) motor system

tongue, gums and teeth and their thorough cleansing. The teeth, tongue and palate are cleansed with toothpaste using a toothbrush or sponge-tipped swab. The mouth should be rinsed with water or a mouthwash solution. Meticulous mouth care reduces incidence of **ventilator-associated pneumonia**. Regular suction of the mouth is important to improve comfort and reduce the risk of aspiration. Immunocompromised patients or those receiving broad-spectrum antibiotics may develop oral candidiasis.

Tracheal or gastric tubes may exert pressure, leading to ulceration, unless they are adequately supported and moved to different parts of the mouth at regular intervals.

Mouth gags. Devices used to hold open the patient's mouth, e.g. during **dental surgery** (Fig. 112). The blade tips are usually covered with plastic or rubber to prevent dental damage, and are placed at the molars.
[Eugene L Doyen (1859–1916), French surgeon; Sir William Fergusson (1808–1877), Scottish-born London surgeon; Francis Mason (1837–1886), London surgeon]

Moxifloxacin hydrochloride. Broad-spectrum **4-quinolone** type **antibacterial drug**; acts by inhibiting bacterial DNA replication. More active against gram-positive organisms than **ciprofloxacin**, but is ineffective against **pseudomonas**

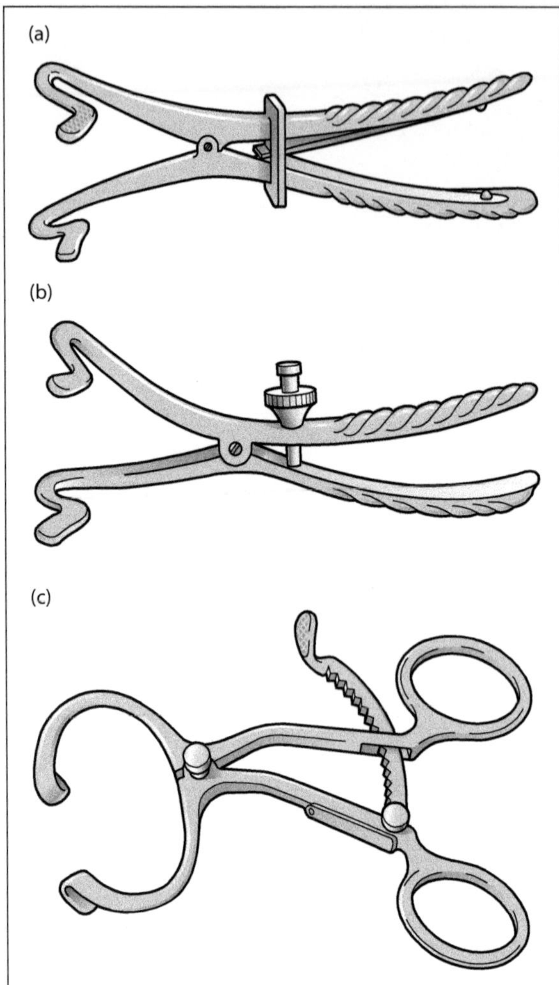

Fig. 112 Examples of mouth gags: (a) Fergusson; (b) Mason; (c) Doyen

infections. Due to potentially severe side effects, its use is restricted to specific infections (severe **chest infections**, complicated skin and soft tissue infections and pelvic inflammatory disease) that have failed to respond to other agents.

- Dosage: 400 mg orally or iv od.
- Side effects:
  - **prolonged Q–T syndromes** (contraindicated in patients with other risk factors for Q–T prolongation); fulminant **hepatitis; renal failure**; tendon inflammation/rupture; muscle weakness/**myoglobinuria**; uveitis; and convulsions.
  - may enhance the effects of **warfarin**.

Moxonidine. The first selective imidazoline receptor agonist, introduced as a centrally acting **antihypertensive drug**. Acts by stimulating imidazoline type 1 (I_1) receptors in the medulla, thereby reducing central and peripheral sympathetic activity. May also stimulate renal I_1 receptors, causing increased sodium and water excretion. Has minimal affinity for α_2-**adrenergic receptors** and thus causes fewer side effects than other centrally acting drugs. Peak plasma levels occur within 1 h of oral administration, with **half-life** of about 2 h. 90% is excreted unchanged in the urine.

- Dosage: 200 µg orally od, increased to 300 µg bd if required.
- Side effects: sedation, dry mouth, headache, dizziness, sleep disturbance.

MPM, *see Mortality probability models*

MRI, *see Magnetic resonance imaging*

MRSA, Meticillin-resistant *Staphylococcus aureus, see Infection control; Staphylococcal infections*

Mucolytic drugs. Used to reduce sputum viscosity (e.g. in **COPD, asthma**) via cleaving of disulfide bonds in mucus glycoprotein. Their use is controversial because no clear benefit has been shown when administered orally. Include carbocisteine, erdosteine and mecysteine. Inhaled dornase alfa, a genetically engineered DNA-ase (DNase), is indicated in **cystic fibrosis** but has been used in other lung conditions. ***N*-acetylcysteine** is used orally and by nebuliser in ICU, but the latter may cause severe bronchospasm. Other strategies to reduce sputum viscosity include instillation of saline and bicarbonate solutions.

MUGA, *see Multigated acquisition imaging*

Multigated acquisition imaging (MUGA imaging). Technique of **nuclear cardiology** in which information from each of many cardiac cycles is combined to assess regional ventricular wall function and left ventricular **ejection fraction** in **cardiac failure**. The subject's red blood cells are labelled with technetium-99m in vivo and time allowed for complete mixing of the marker throughout the circulating volume. Scanning then takes place over several cycles. Advantages over single-pass cardiographic techniques include less reliability on the injection technique (crucial in the single-pass method) and the ability to scan before and after exercise or drug administration. Disadvantages include the overlap of the heart chambers on the image and the inability to follow a tracer bolus through the chambers of the heart.

Mitra D, Bahu S (2012). World J Radiol; 4: 425–31

Multiple endocrine adenomatosis (MEA; Multiple endocrine neoplasia, MEN). Term encompassing three distinct syndromes of multiple endocrine tumours, all of which are inherited by autosomal dominant transmission:

- type I: parathyroid adenoma, pancreatic adenoma or carcinoma and anterior pituitary adenoma.
- type IIa: medullary thyroid carcinoma, **phaeochromocytoma** and parathyroid adenoma.
- type IIb: medullary thyroid carcinoma, phaeochromocytoma and mucosal neuromas.

Patients presenting for endocrine surgery may thus have other tumours and associated syndromes.

Marshm DJ, Gimm O (2011). Adv Otorhinolaryngol; 70: 84–90

See also, Apudomas; Hyperparathyroidism

Multiple organ dysfunction score. Scoring system for evaluating dysfunction of six organ systems: respiratory, renal, hepatic, cardiovascular, central nervous and haematological. Weighted scores (0–4 points) are given for increasing degrees of abnormality of six variables (arterial $P\text{O}_2$:$F_I\text{O}_2$ ratio, serum creatinine, serum bilirubin, platelet count, pressure-adjusted heart rate [heart rate × CVP:mean arterial BP ratio] and **Glasgow coma score**). Raw data are collected daily; the value recorded is a representative

value for the day (i.e., at a particular time and not necessarily the worst value).
Marshall JC, Cook DJ, Christou NV, et al (1995). Crit Care Med; 23: 1638–52

Multiple organ dysfunction syndrome (MODS). Syndrome of organ dysfunction affecting two or more organs, remote from the site of primary tissue injury or infection. Previously termed multiple organ failure. Thought to be caused by dysregulation of the innate inflammatory response, causing systemic inflammation, hypoperfusion and tissue injury. Mitochondrial dysfunction is also involved. Causes include: **sepsis**, **burns**, surgery and massive **blood transfusion**. Predominantly affects the respiratory, renal, hepatic, neurological, gastrointestinal, haematological and cardiovascular systems. A major cause of death in ICU; mortality increases as more organs are involved. The degree of organ dysfunction may be described by the **multiple organ dysfunction score** and the **sepsis-related organ failure assessment**.
Gustot T (2011). Curr Opin Crit Care; 17: 153–9

Multiple sclerosis, *see Demyelinating diseases*

Murphy eye, *see Tracheal tubes*

Muscarine. Alkaloid extracted from certain mushrooms; mimics some actions of **acetylcholine** (hence it is a **parasympathomimetic drug**) and was used to investigate the physiology of the **autonomic nervous system**. It stimulates postganglionic **acetylcholine receptors** (muscarinic receptors) at effector organs of the **parasympathetic nervous system**, and at sweat glands of the **sympathetic nervous system**. It also causes parkinsonian tremor, ataxia and rigidity; thus muscarinic receptors are thought to exist in the CNS. Other receptors may be involved in an inhibitory role at adrenergic nerve endings, e.g. in the heart and autonomic ganglia.

Muscle. Contractile tissue; may be:
- skeletal (striated; voluntary):
  - the most abundant form.
  - normally contracts only when stimulated.
  - no connections between individual fibres.
  - composed of elongated cylindrical fibres, each surrounded by its sarcolemma (muscle cell membrane). Each fibre contains myofibrils, containing **actin** and **myosin** filaments and surrounded by sarcoplasmic reticulum and mitochondria. The T-tubule system invaginates from the sarcolemma to connect all myofibrils with the extracellular space.
  - microscopically visible striations are due to myosin and actin arrangements, labelled for historical reasons (Fig. 113). The sarcomere (portion between adjacent Z lines) shortens during **muscle contraction**.
  - different types of fibre:
    - type I: red muscle; responds slowly with slow metabolism and high oxidative capacity (high **myoglobin**, mitochondria and capillary content). Suitable for prolonged contraction, e.g. postural muscles.
    - type IIB: white muscle, short contraction with low oxidative capacity. Suitable for rapid fine movements, e.g. eye and hand muscles.
    - type IIA: as for IIB but with high oxidative capacity, i.e., red. Uncommon in humans.

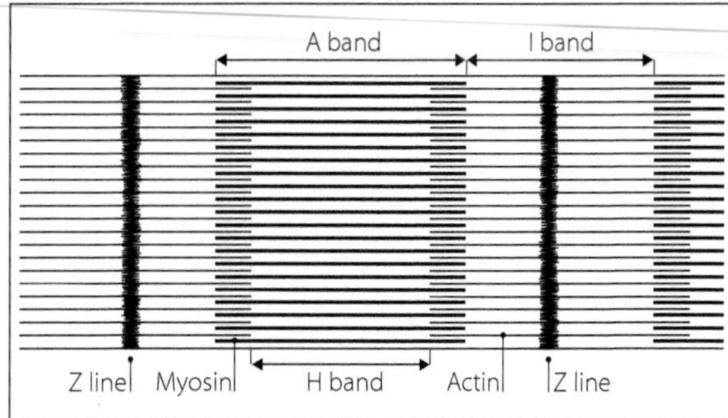

Fig. 113 Microscopic appearance of myofibril

- cardiac:
  - similar to slow striated muscle, but fibres are branched, and joined end to end by intercalated discs; also connected to adjacent fibres by gap junctions (i.e., forms a functional syncytium).
  - has spontaneous pacemaker activity, due to slow depolarisation between **action potentials**.
  - cannot exhibit **tetanic contraction**, due to a prolonged **refractory period**.
- smooth:
  - no striations; actin and myosin filaments arranged randomly.
  - occurs in sheets of interconnecting cells (e.g. visceral) or multiunits (e.g. iris).
  - exhibits slow spontaneous activity; also responsive to stimulation of the **autonomic nervous system**. Visceral muscle contracts if stretched.

See also, Motor unit; Muscle spindles; Neuromuscular junction

Muscle contraction. Involves the following steps:
- depolarisation of the postsynaptic **membrane** at the **neuromuscular junction**.
- area of depolarisation spreads across the **muscle** membrane and into the muscle bulk via the T-tubule system.
- depolarisation causes release and mobilisation of intracellular **calcium** ions from sarcoplasmic reticulum.
- calcium ions bind to the troponin component of the **actin** complex, causing displacement of the tropomyosin component from **myosin** binding sites.
- myosin can now bind to actin, with hydrolysis of **ATP**, structural alteration of myosin and shortening of muscle fibres. ATPase is present on myosin molecule heads. The process repeats with further muscle shortening. Histologically, contraction leads to shortening of the I band and H band (Fig. 113).
- further hydrolysis of ATP allows sequestration of calcium and muscle relaxation. ATP is derived from **glycolysis** and from dephosphorylation of phosphorylcreatine, stored during rest.

A single twitch caused by an **action potential** of 1 ms lasts up to 200 ms. Contraction may be isometric (force increases but muscle length remains constant) or isotonic (force is constant and muscle shortens). Repeated fast stimulation results in summation of contraction, because there is inadequate time for relaxation between stimuli. Above a certain frequency, **tetanic contraction** occurs.

Muscle relaxants, *see Neuromuscular blocking drugs*

Muscle spindles. Encapsulated structures present in and parallel to skeletal **muscle**. Contain up to 10 specialised muscle (intrafusal) fibres, attached to the ordinary muscle (extrafusal) fibres or to their tendons. **Muscle contraction** thus results in shortening of the spindles. Sensory **nerve** fibres from the spindles end on the motor **neurones** supplying the extrafusal muscle fibres of that muscle. They transmit impulses when stretched; thus passive muscle stretching causes reflex contraction, e.g. knee jerk **reflex arc**. Discharge in some afferent fibres is proportional to degree of stretch; discharge in others is also proportional to speed of stretch. Muscle contraction reduces tension within the spindle, reducing the afferent discharge. Activation of the reflex also inhibits contraction of opposing muscle groups (reciprocal innervation) via an inhibitory spinal interneurone.

Small γ-motor fibres innervate the ends of the intrafusal fibres, causing them to contract. This stretches the central portions, with reflex extrafusal fibre contraction as before, and increases the sensitivity of the spindles to passive stretching. γ-Motor activity is controlled by descending pathways in the spinal cord; thus muscle tone and posture are controlled at both spinal and supraspinal levels. Increased muscle tone and clonus seen in upper **motor neurone** lesions may result from overactive γ-activity due to interruption of inhibitory descending pathways. γ-Activity is also increased in anxiety, resulting in exaggerated tremor.

Increased passive stretching of a muscle eventually causes sudden relaxation, due to stimulation of Golgi tendon organs within the muscle tendons. This inverse stretch reflex is exaggerated in upper motor neurone lesions (clasp-knife effect).

[Camillo Golgi (1843–1926), Italian physician]

Muscular dystrophies. Hereditary disorders of **muscle**, involving progressive destruction of mainly skeletal, but also cardiac, muscle. Result from mutation of the gene for dystrophin, a cytoskeletal protein involved in the interaction between the sarcomeres and the extracellular matrix (via dystrophin-associated protein, DAP). Deficiency of dystrophin (and DAP) results in weakening of the muscle **membrane** with calcium influx and necrosis of muscle fibres; in Duchenne's dystrophy deficiency is severe whereas in Becker's a reduced amount of normal dystrophin still results in some activity. Plasma creatine kinase levels may be markedly increased. Classified according to inheritance: may be sex-linked (e.g. Duchenne's, Becker's), autosomal dominant (e.g. facioscapulohumeral, oculopharyngeal) or recessive (e.g. limb girdle):

- Duchenne's: most common (1 in 3500 live male births) and severe. Usually presents at 3–5 years of age; although death from respiratory failure previously occurred in late teens, life expectancy has improved with **non-invasive positive pressure ventilation** (NIV).
- Becker's, facioscapulohumeral, limb girdle: less severe, with later onset and death. Cardiac involvement is less common.

- Orthopaedic surgery is common for limb contractures, etc. Severe forms may present significant anaesthetic risk:
  - weak respiratory muscles and **kyphoscoliosis**: impaired ventilation and sputum clearance. Pre-existing and postoperative chest infection is more likely. Respiratory failure postoperatively is common and elective NIV is advocated.
  - rhabdomyolysis may follow **suxamethonium** or volatile anaesthetic agents, typically following prolonged exposure to the latter. Severe **hyperkalaemia** and **myoglobinuria** may result. An **MH**-like picture may develop as muscle metabolism increases (in the absence of true inherited MH). Total intravenous anaesthesia is the technique of choice.
  - cardiac involvement is common in Duchenne's; characteristically the **ECG** shows tachycardia, short P–R interval, deep Q waves laterally and tall R waves in V_1. **Cardiomyopathy, heart block** and **arrhythmias** (**VF** has occurred on induction of anaesthesia) may all be present. Bradycardia is common in facioscapulohumeral dystrophy.
  - delayed **gastric emptying** and impaired swallowing predispose to **aspiration of gastric contents**.

Plans for anaesthesia must take account of the above considerations. Regional techniques are popular when feasible. ICU concerns include the above and also the ethical issues surrounding respiratory support should **respiratory failure** occur.

[Guillaume Duchenne (1806–1875), French neurologist; Peter Becker (1908–2000), German geneticist]

Hayes J, Veyckemans F, Bissonnette B (2008). Paediatr Anaesth; 18: 100–6

MVV, Maximal voluntary ventilation, *see Lung function tests*

Myasthenia gravis. Autoimmune disease characterised by weakness and increased fatigability of skeletal **muscle**. Prevalence is 50–100 per million. More common in young women and older men. May also occur transiently in neonates born to affected mothers, and may be caused by drugs, e.g. **penicillamine**.

Caused by an immune response in which IgG autoantibodies are produced against the **acetylcholine receptors** of the **neuromuscular junction** postsynaptic membrane. The autoantibodies (detectable in 90% of patients) occupy receptors, leading to their destruction and reduction in receptor density. 50% of those without anti-acetylcholine receptor antibodies have antibodies directed at muscle-specific tyrosine kinase. The thymus gland is abnormal (either hyperplasia or thymoma) in 75% of cases and is thought to be the site of production of the autoantibodies. Often associated with other autoimmune conditions, e.g. thyroid disease.

- Characterised by muscle weakness (typically worse on exertion and improving with rest); may affect:
  - ocular muscles, causing ptosis and diplopia.
  - bulbar muscles, causing dysarthria and predisposing to **aspiration of gastric contents**.
  - respiratory muscles.
  - limb muscles (proximal > distal).

Myasthenic crises (suddenly worsening and spreading weakness requiring IPPV) may be provoked by drug omission, infection, stress, pregnancy or drugs (e.g. aminoglycosides).

- Classified according to severity:
  - grade I: confined to eye muscles (15% of cases).
  - grade IIa: generalised mild muscle weakness.
  - grade IIb: generalised moderate weakness and/or bulbar weakness.
  - grade III: acute fulminating: rapid and progressive and/or respiratory involvement.
  - grade IV: myasthenic crisis requiring IPPV.
- Diagnosis:
  - marked improvement following iv **edrophonium** 2 + 8 mg (Tensilon test).

- EMG shows reduced response to single twitch, fade on tetanic stimulation and **post-tetanic potentiation.**
- detection of anti-acetylcholine receptor antibodies.

- Treatment:
  - emergency intubation and IPPV for impending/actual respiratory failure or bulbar dysfunction. **Blood gas interpretation** is rarely useful in myasthenia for determining the need for IPPV; clinical indicators are best.
  - **acetylcholinesterase inhibitors**, e.g. **pyridostigmine** 30–90 mg 6-hourly, **neostigmine** 15–30 mg 4-hourly. Muscarinic side effects include miosis, colic, lacrimation, diarrhoea, salivation; **atropine** may be given to reduce these. May cause **cholinergic crisis** in overdosage; distinguished from myasthenic crises by injection of edrophonium 2 mg. Myasthenic crises may improve transiently, cholinergic crises do not.
  - immunosuppressive therapy includes **corticosteroids** (e.g. **prednisolone** 1 mg/kg on alternate days; usually started in hospital because of possible deterioration), **azathioprine**, **cyclophosphamide**, **ciclosporin**, **mycophenolate.**
  - treatment of any coexistent electrolyte abnormalities, especially **hypokalaemia**, **hypocalcaemia**, **hypermagnesaemia.**
  - **plasma exchange** and iv **immunoglobulin**, especially combined with immunosuppressive therapy, are used for short-term remission in severe cases.
  - thymectomy: benefits most myasthenic patients between 16 and 60 years old, producing either full remission or reduction in immunosuppressive therapy. Anaesthetic management:
    - preoperatively: assessment of respiratory function is important. Pyridostigmine is usually withheld on the morning of surgery. Preoperative plasma exchange or iv immunoglobulin has been used. Potassium abnormalities increase muscle weakness and should be corrected.
    - perioperatively: there is increased sensitivity to non-depolarising **neuromuscular blocking drugs** and relative resistance to **suxamethonium** with increased tendency to develop **dual block.** Tracheal intubation and IPPV are usually performed without neuromuscular blocking drugs, using e.g. **propofol** and/or a volatile agent. **Atracurium** in reduced doses (50%–60% of usual) has been suggested over other drugs. Surgery is performed via a suprasternal or trans-sternal route. Haemorrhage and pneumothorax may occur. The tracheal tube may be left in situ and ventilation monitored on ICU or HDU, although tracheal extubation is usually possible immediately postoperatively.
    - postoperatively: pyridostigmine may be restarted, usually in reduced dosage. Close respiratory monitoring and **physiotherapy** are required. Postoperative **atelectasis** and infection are common.

Anaesthetic management of patients with myasthenia gravis for other surgery should follow the above guidelines. Where feasible, regional techniques may be safer.

Gilhus NE (2016). N Engl J Med; 375: 2570–81

See also, Myasthenic syndrome

Myasthenic syndrome (Eaton–Lambert syndrome). Acquired disorder of the **neuromuscular junction** in which there is decreased quantal release of **acetylcholine** from the presynaptic nerve terminal. Caused by IgG autoantibodies interfering with voltage-gated calcium channels necessary for acetylcholine mobilisation and release. In 50% of cases it is associated with small cell bronchial carcinoma or **autoimmune disease** (e.g. **polyarteritis nodosa).**

- Distinguished from myasthenia gravis thus:
  - classically improves on exercise (**EMG** shows an increase in power on tetanic stimulation).
  - usually affects distal limb muscles.
  - autonomic nervous system involvement is common.
  - tendon reflexes are depressed or absent.
  - power is only slightly improved by **neostigmine**, despite possible improvement following **edrophonium.**

Treatment is of the underlying cause. Neuromuscular transmission may be improved by oral guanidine, 3,4-diaminopyridine or **pyridostigmine**; **corticosteroids**, iv **immunoglobulins** and **plasma exchange** have also been used.

General anaesthetic considerations are as for myasthenia gravis. There is increased sensitivity to non-depolarising and depolarising **neuromuscular blocking drugs. Atracurium** has been suggested as the drug of choice. Postoperative respiratory complications are more likely with severe weakness.

[LM Eaton (1905–1958), US neurologist; Edward H Lambert (1915–2003), US neurophysiologist]

Tarr TB, Wipf P, Meriney SD (2015). Mol Neurobiol; 52: 456–63

Mycophenolate mofetil. Cytotoxic **immunosuppressive drug** used in **organ transplantation**, especially in combination with **ciclosporin** and **corticosteroids.** Has also been used in **myasthenia gravis.** Metabolised to mycophenolic acid.

- Dosage: 1–5 mg/kg orally or iv od.
- Side effects: hypersensitivity reactions, myelosuppression, liver toxicity.

Mycoplasma infections. Caused by various species of mycoplasma, small bacteria that lack a cell wall (thus resistant to antibiotics that target cell wall synthesis). The most important infection is mycoplasma pneumonia (one type of 'atypical' pneumonia), caused by *Mycoplasma pneumoniae*:

- typically associated with initial headache, sore throat, fever, malaise and cough; the cough becomes productive and patchy chest signs may develop, although classic signs of consolidation are rare. Usually affects a single lower lobe only, although the clinical course is variable. **CXR** signs (patchy shadowing) often precede clinical features and persist after clinical recovery.
- extrapulmonary features include haemolytic **anaemia**, GIT upset, including hepatic and pancreatic involvement, rash, arthritis, CNS (**meningitis**, **encephalitis**, ascending paralysis, transverse myelitis, **cranial nerve** palsy) and cardiac (**myocarditis**, **pericarditis**) involvement.
- diagnosed by demonstration of a rising antibody titre, because culture of organisms is slow and difficult. Cold agglutinins may also be identified in blood.
- treatment with **clarithromycin**, **erythromycin** or **tetracycline.** Death is rare.

Other infections include GIT and genitourinary, such as non-specific urethritis, pelvic inflammatory disease, vaginitis and pyelonephritis. Most are caused by *Mycoplasma hominis* or *Ureaplasma urealyticum.*

Myelin. Lipoprotein derived from multiple layers of cell **membranes**, encasing the axons of myelinated **neurones**. Arises from Schwann cells in the peripheral nervous system (one cell to one axon portion), and from oligodendrocytes in the CNS (one cell to up to 40 axon portions). Deficient at 1-mm intervals (nodes of Ranvier). Unmyelinated peripheral nerves are merely encased in Schwann cell cytoplasm. Acts as an insulating sheath, increasing speed of **nerve conduction** in myelinated nerves by restricting membrane depolarisation to the nodes of Ranvier; depolarisation 'jumps' from node to node (saltatory conduction) instead of slower, smooth progression along unmyelinated nerves. Conditions affecting the myelin sheath include the **demyelinating diseases** and **Guillain–Barré syndrome**.
[Theodor Schwann (1810–1882), German physiologist; Louis Ranvier (1835–1922), French physician and pathologist]

Myocardial contractility. Ability of the myocardial muscle to contract at a particular length of fibre (i.e., independent of loading factors); thus a major determinant of **stroke volume**, **cardiac output** and myocardial O_2 demand.
- Increased by:
  - intrinsic mechanisms:
    - **Anrep effect.**
    - **Bowditch effect.**
  - extrinsic factors:
    - **sympathetic nervous system** activity.
    - **catecholamines** via β_1-**adrenergic receptors.**
    - **inotropic drugs.**
- Decreased by:
  - **parasympathetic nervous system** (slight effect).
  - **hypoxaemia** and **hypercapnia** (via direct effects; also cause increased sympathetic activity).
  - **acidosis** and **alkalosis.**
  - **sepsis**: release of **cytokines**, lysozymes and **endothelin**-1 has inhibitory actions on myocytes. Mitochondrial dysfunction also contributes.
  - cardiac disease, e.g. **ischaemic heart disease**, **cardiomyopathy**, **myocarditis.**
  - electrolyte disturbances, e.g. **hyperkalaemia**, **hypocalcaemia.**
  - drugs, e.g. most **iv** and **inhalational anaesthetic agents**, **antiarrhythmic drugs.**
- Assessment is difficult; indirect methods include measurement of:
  - stroke volume and **stroke work.**
  - speed of contraction.
  - cardiac output.
  - ratio of **left ventricular end-diastolic pressure** to **left ventricular end-diastolic volume.**
  - peak left ventricular pressure.
  - **ejection fraction.**

See also, Starling's law

Myocardial infarction (MI). Myocardial necrosis caused by unrelieved **myocardial ischaemia**, forming part of the spectrum of **acute coronary syndromes** (*see Acute coronary syndromes* for pathophysiology, classification, clinical features, investigations, differential diagnosis and management of MI). Usually starts at the endocardium, spreading outwards. Commonly affects the left ventricle, but may involve the right ventricle or atria. Classified according to **ECG** criteria into S–T segment elevation MI (STEMI) and non-S–T segment elevation MI (NSTEMI).

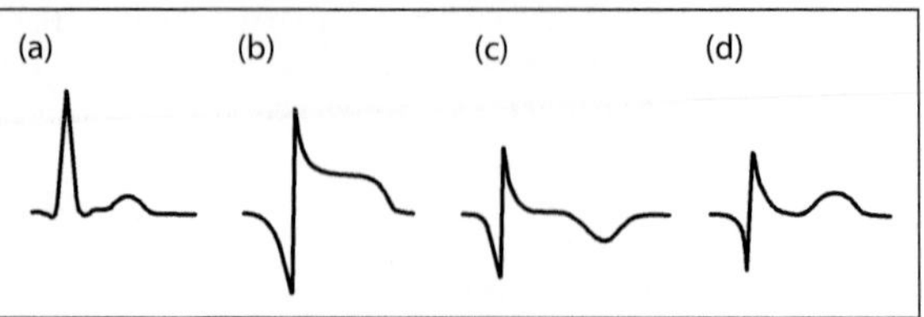

Fig. 114 Typical changes in ECG following MI: (a) normal; (b) immediate; (c) few weeks; (d) few months

- **ECG** changes in STEMI:
  - sequentially occurring **T wave** changes, **S–T segment** elevation and pathological **Q waves** in leads overlying the infarct are typical. Lead groupings and their corresponding cardiac territories:
    - II, III and aVF: inferior (diaphragmatic) surface.
    - V_{1-3}: interventricular septum.
    - V_{3-4}: anterior surface of the left ventricle.
    - V_{5-6}, I and aVL: lateral surface of the left ventricle.
    - V_{1-2}: posterior surface.
  - tall, widened ('hyperacute') T waves often precede S–T elevation. S–T elevation usually resolves in <2 weeks and T-wave inversion after several months, with Q waves often lasting for several years (Fig. 114).
  - persistent S–T elevation may indicate ventricular aneurysm or an area of dyskinetic myocardium. Q waves may be absent in subendocardial infarction.
  - other changes include abnormalities of the **P wave** and **P–R interval** in atrial infarction, conduction defects, e.g. **bundle branch block** and **heart block** and arrhythmias.
- Delayed complications include:
  - ventricular rupture, usually 5–8 days later.
  - ventricular aneurysm.
  - interventricular septum rupture, usually 4–6 days later.
  - papillary muscle damage and **mitral regurgitation.**
  - mural thrombus formation and systemic embolism.
  - **PE.**
  - Dressler's syndrome: **pericarditis**, pleurisy and pneumonitis, typically 4–6 weeks later.
- Perioperative MI has been investigated by several studies. Summary of findings:
  - postoperative MI is most common within the first 1–2 days, according to troponin levels.
  - with previous MI, overall reinfarction rate is 6%–7% (if no previous MI, infarction rate is 0.1%–0.2%).
  - quoted reinfarction rates are related to the time since the MI:
    - within 3 months of surgery: 20%–30%.
    - within 4–6 months: 10%–20%.
    - greater than 6 months: 4%–5%.
  - aggressive management (e.g. pulmonary artery catheterisation, use of inotropic and vasodilator drugs, admission to ICU) has been reported to lower the overall infarction rate to 2%, and the reinfarction rates as follows:
    - MI within 3 months: under 6%.
    - within 4–6 months: 2%–3%.
    - greater than 6 months: 1%–2%.

  However, the statistical analysis used has been criticised, and the value of routine intensive

monitoring and treatment remains controversial, especially when the increased cost is considered.
- perioperative reinfarction carries increased mortality (up to 70%).
- incidence of silent MI may be higher.
- risk factors include: unstable angina, perioperative hypotension, prolonged surgery and upper abdominal/thoracic or vascular surgery.
- risk is not increased by previous cardiac surgery.
- risk is not associated with the type of anaesthetic or drugs used.
- **cardiac risk index** has been developed for assessment of risk of death or severe perioperative cardiovascular complications. Presence of cardiac failure is the most important risk factor. Other factors are related to arrhythmias, age and general condition of the patient.
- reinfarction is often associated with perioperative myocardial ischaemia detected by S–T depression. It is not always associated with hypertension or hypotension.

- Risk of perioperative MI is thus reduced by:
  - postponement of elective surgery until >6 months after MI.
  - treatment of preoperative risk factors where possible.
  - avoidance of myocardial ischaemia as for **ischaemic heart disease**.

[William Dressler (1890–1969), US cardiologist]

Reed GW, Rossi JE, Cannon CP (2017). Lancet; 389: 3060–73

Myocardial ischaemia. Inadequate blood supply to the myocardium. Effects are related to myocardial O_2 supply/demand balance; largely dependent on:
- supply:
  - **coronary blood flow**:
    - aortic end diastolic pressure minus left ventricular end-diastolic pressure.
    - duration of diastole.
    - coronary vessels: calibre is usually maintained by **autoregulation**. Stenosis may be caused by atheroma, thrombosis and spasm. The subendocardial region is most at risk of ischaemia.
    - blood **viscosity**.
  - O_2 content.
- demand:
  - **stroke work** (determined by **preload**, **afterload** and **myocardial contractility**).
  - **heart rate**.

- Effects:
  - reversible increases in **hydrogen ion**, **potassium**, phosphate, **lactate** and **adenosine** concentrations. Unless ischaemia is corrected within about 30 min, **MI** ensues, with release of **cardiac enzymes** and **myoglobin**.
  - **ECG** changes: thought to be caused by ion leakage across the ischaemic myocardial membrane, altering membrane potentials and causing current flow between normal and ischaemic areas. **S–T segment** changes are most common; depression is due to subendocardial ischaemia, elevation due to transmural ischaemia. **Arrhythmias** may occur.
  - impaired myocardial contractility: first depressed, then absent, then myocardial lengthening with worsening ischaemia.
  - pain (angina): possibly due to increased potassium or **substance P**. Pain is typically constant, crushing and mid-sternal, radiating across the chest, to the neck or arms. Related to exertion, cold or emotion and relieved by rest, it may be absent (silent ischaemia). Dyspnoea and sweating may occur. Crescendo angina is characterised by increasing frequency of attacks with diminishing levels of exertion; unstable angina occurs at rest (diagnosed when MI has been excluded). Repeated small thromboses may be responsible; both types may herald imminent MI.

- Detection:
  - symptoms and signs as above.
  - detection of reduced supply/increased demand. Indices of supply include **diastolic pressure time index**. Indices of demand include **rate–pressure product** and **tension time index. Endocardial viability ratio** has been used to indicate the ratio between supply and demand.
  - ECG. Preoperative 'silent' ischaemia (i.e., without symptoms) has been found in up to 15% of patients over 40 years old; the significance of this in terms of outcome is unknown. The figure is higher for patients presenting for vascular surgery. Similar episodes of silent ischaemia have been found postoperatively, especially in those with risk factors. It has been suggested that patients who exhibit this are more likely to suffer postoperative MI.
  - **pulmonary capillary wedge pressure** monitoring.
  - **echocardiography**.
  - **nuclear cardiography**.
  - **coronary sinus catheterisation**.
- Management: as for **ischaemic heart disease**.

See also, Monitoring; Myocardial metabolism

Myocardial metabolism. Myocardial O_2 consumption is normally about 30 ml/min (10 ml/100 g/min). **Coronary blood flow** is directly proportional; the mechanism is unclear but may involve **adenosine**, CO_2, **potassium** ions, **prostaglandins**, **hydrogen ions** and **lactate**. O_2 extraction from blood is about 70%; thus increased demands are met mainly by increasing blood flow. The main energy substrate is free fatty acids; other substrates include glucose, pyruvate and lactate. Utilisation of the latter compounds increases in ischaemia.

O_2 requirements are reduced by volatile anaesthetic agents and other negative inotropes, e.g. **β-adrenergic receptor antagonists. Etomidate** and **propofol** may decrease demand; other iv agents may increase it if tachycardia occurs.

Myocardial preconditioning, *see Ischaemic preconditioning*

Myocarditis. Inflammation of the cardiac muscle; the definition is difficult because clinical diagnosis (acute **cardiac failure**, **arrhythmias** or **ECG** changes in a person with a previously normal heart) is often not supported by the results of biopsy or post-mortem histology (i.e., with lymphocytic infiltration).
- Caused by:
  - infective invasion of cardiac muscle, e.g. viruses (especially coxsackie B and echovirus), bacteria, rickettsia, fungi, trypanosomiasis. Myocarditis is thought to be a common feature of apparently mild viral upper respiratory tract infections. Features may be prompted by vigorous exercise or anaesthesia and especially if the diagnosis is unsuspected.

- post-infective inflammation: thought to represent a different mechanism to the above and includes post-viral, **HIV infection, rheumatic fever, diphtheria.** In the last case, bacterial toxins are thought to be responsible.
- primary autoimmune processes: rheumatic fever, **connective tissue diseases, sarcoidosis**, thyroid disorders, **diabetes mellitus** (microangiopathy may also be involved), amyloidosis.
- other allergic processes, e.g. drug-induced (e.g. penicillin, sulfonamides), rejection of cardiac transplants, serum sickness.
- direct drug toxicity, e.g. **lithium, cyclophosphamide, alcoholism.**
- physical trauma, e.g. radiation.
- other infiltration or inflammation, e.g. diabetic, myxoedema, haemochromatosis, connective tissue disease, drug-induced (e.g. cytotoxic drugs).

Treatment includes **corticosteroids, antiviral drugs** and supportive therapy.

Medical and anaesthetic management is as for cardiac disease in general; in acute disease surgery should be deferred if feasible, and as cardiostable an anaesthetic provided as possible. General treatment is supportive according to the presenting features.

Sagar S, Liu PP, Cooper LT (2012). Lancet; 379: 738–47

Myofascial pain syndromes. Dysfunction and usually **pain** in one or more muscles/muscle groups, associated with **trigger point** activity. May follow acute strain or repeated use. Typically associated with patterns of **referred pain**, e.g. trigger points in the neck with facial pain, trigger points in the shoulder with arm pain. Identified trigger points may be injected with local anaesthetic, treated with **acupuncture**, ultrasound and pressure, or the muscles passively stretched using a cold spray to allow adequate relaxation.

Myoglobin. Iron-containing molecule with mw 17000. Similar to **haemoglobin**, but binds only one molecule of O_2 per molecule. Its O_2 dissociation curve is to the left of that of haemoglobin, being a rectangular hyperbola with a steep rise to a plateau (Fig. 115). The **Bohr effect** does not occur. 95% saturated at Po_2 of 5.3 kPa (40 mmHg), falling below 65% saturation only at Po_2 below 1 kPa (7.5 mmHg). The P_{50} is 0.13 kPa (1 mmHg). Found in skeletal and heart **muscle**, where it binds O_2 from arterial haemoglobin, releasing it at O_2 tensions close to zero. Thus it acts as an O_2 transporter and reservoir for contracting muscle.

See also, Oxyhaemoglobin dissociation curve

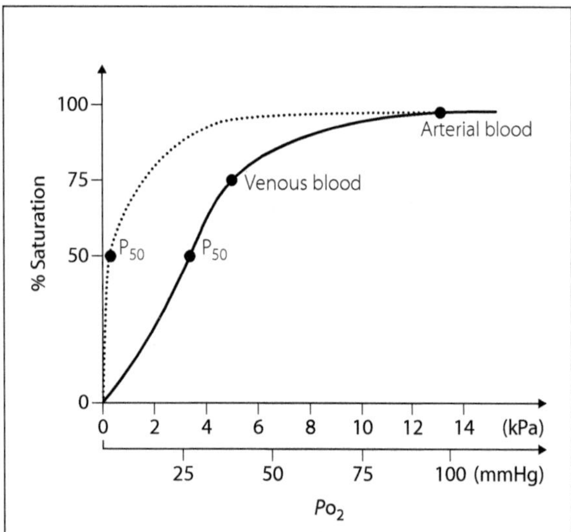

Fig. 115 Oxymyoglobin dissociation curve *(dotted line)* with oxyhaemoglobin dissociation curve *(solid line)* for comparison

Myoglobinuria. Presence of **myoglobin** in the urine, colouring it red. Results from skeletal muscle breakdown (rhabdomyolysis) due to:

- crush injury (**crush syndrome**).
- prolonged immobility/**hypothermia** from any cause, especially **poisoning and overdoses** (particularly **opioid, alcohol** and **cocaine** overdose).
- extreme exertion.
- polymyositis, myopathies, e.g. alcoholic, deficiency states, congenital conditions or associated with viral infections.
- toxins, e.g. of sea snakes, multiple wasp stings.
- **MH.**
- **neuroleptic malignant syndrome.**
- **carbon monoxide poisoning.**
- heatstroke.
- paroxysmal myoglobinuria: rare disorder of muscle pain, weakness, paralysis and myoglobinuria. Most common in young men/children. Affected muscles are classically painful and oedematous. Creatine kinase levels may be markedly raised.

Myoglobin is readily filtered by the kidneys because of its small size. May be associated with **renal failure**, thought to be caused by ferrihemate, a nephrotoxic breakdown product of myoglobin in acid conditions (myoglobin itself is not thought to be directly nephrotoxic). Tubular obstruction may also be involved. Maintenance of good hydration and urine output may prevent renal impairment. Administration of bicarbonate helps to increase urinary pH and reduce formation of ferrihemate.

David WS (2000). Neurol Clin; 18: 215–43

Myosin. Muscle protein (mw 520 kDa), consisting of two heavy and four light chains. Globular portions of the molecules contain ATPase and **actin** binding sites, and project sideways from myosin filaments.

See also, Muscle contraction

Myotomes. Inner parts of embryonic somites, differentiating into skeletal muscle and related to their corresponding **dermatomes.** Although the origins of certain skeletal muscle groups are controversial, they tend to retain their original somatic nerve supply; thus particular spinal nerves may be assessed clinically by testing specific muscles or groups (Table 33). Used to assess neurological lesions and the extent of spinal/epidural anaesthesia.

Myotonia congenita. Autosomal dominant or recessive disorder of skeletal muscle due to a chloride channelopathy. No systemic symptoms occur other than myotonia (involuntary sustained muscle contraction following stimulation), exacerbated by cold and rest, and relieved by exercise. A more common, milder form is inherited as autosomal recessive. Anaesthetic management is as for **dystrophia myotonica.** Hypothermia should be avoided. An association with **MH** has been suggested, although there are difficulties in interpreting the caffeine–halothane contracture test in myotonic patients.

Table 33 Segmental innervation of limb muscles

Movement	*Muscle(s)*	*Level*
Shoulder		
Abduction	Supraspinatus	C4–5
External rotation	Infraspinatus	C4–5
Adduction	Pectoralis	C6–8
Elbow		
Flexion/supination	Biceps	C5–6
Pronation	Pronators	C6–7
Extension	Triceps	C7–8
Wrist		
Extension/radial flexion		C6–7
Ulnar flexion		C7–8
Fingers		
Extension	Long extensors	C7
Flexion	Long flexors	C8
Spreading and closing	All short muscles of the hand	T1
Hip		
Flexion	Iliopsoas	L1–3
Extension	Gluteal	L5–S2
Knee		
Extension	Quadriceps	L3–4
Flexion	Hamstrings	L5–S2
Ankle		
Extension	Anterior tibial	L4–5
Flexion	Calf muscles	S1–2

Myotonic syndromes. Group of inherited muscle diseases including **dystrophia myotonica** and **myotonia congenita** characterised by an increase in muscle tone (myotonia) following muscular contraction. Myotonia may also be present in hyperkalaemic **periodic paralysis.** Anaesthetic considerations are related to systemic manifestations of the disease and the effects of certain anaesthetic drugs worsening myotonia, e.g. **suxamethonium.**

Myxoedema, *see Hypothyroidism*

N

Nabilone. Cannabinoid **antiemetic drug**, acting on CB_1 and CB_2 **cannabis** receptors, used in chemotherapy-induced nausea and vomiting. Has also been used in **palliative care**.
- Dosage: 1–2 mg orally bd/tds.
- Side effects: drowsiness, ataxia, visual disturbances, sleep disturbances, hypotension, tachycardia.

Nalbuphine hydrochloride. Opioid analgesic drug and **opioid receptor antagonist**, synthesised in 1968. Partial agonist at kappa and sigma **opioid receptors**, and partial antagonist at mu receptors. Active within 2–3 min of iv, or 15 min of im injection, with **half-life** about 5 h. Withdrawn from the UK market in 2003, but still available in the USA and other countries.
- Dosage: 0.1–0.3 mg/kg iv/im/sc. Up to 1.0 mg/kg iv has been used during anaesthesia.
- Sedation, increased sweating, nausea/vomiting, dizziness, dry mouth, headache.

Nalmefene hydrochloride. Opioid receptor antagonist, introduced in the USA in 1995 and approved within the European Union in 2013. Licensed in the UK for the reduction of **alcohol** consumption in patients with alcohol dependence who do not have physical withdrawal symptoms and who do not need to stop drinking immediately or achieve total abstinence. Longer **half-life** (10.8 h) than **naloxone**; thus less likely for opioid effects to recur following reversal.
- Dosage: 18 mg/day as required.
- Side effects: nausea, dizziness, insomnia, headache.

Nalorphine hydrochloride/hydrobromide. Opioid analgesic drug and **opioid receptor antagonist**, synthesised in 1941. Partial agonist at kappa and sigma **opioid receptors**, and antagonist at mu receptors. Psychomimetic effects are common at analgesic doses (5–10 mg). No longer available.

Naloxone hydrochloride. Opioid receptor antagonist, synthesised in 1961. *N*-Allyl derivative of **oxymorphone**. Although it has a high affinity for the mu receptor, it has no **intrinsic activity**. Used to reverse unwanted effects of **opioid analgesic drugs**, e.g. sedation, respiratory depression, biliary sphincter spasm, although it also reverses opioid-mediated analgesia. Has been used in **poisoning and overdoses** due to other depressant drugs, e.g. **alcohols**, **benzodiazepines**, **barbiturates**, although its efficacy is disputed. Has also been described as increasing BP and cardiac output in **septic shock**; the mechanism is unclear but increase of endogenous **catecholamine** release or antagonism of increased levels of **endorphins** has been suggested. Reverses the effects of **pentazocine** but not **buprenorphine**, and may reverse ventilatory depression and **pruritus** following **spinal opioids**, without reversing analgesia. Effective within 1–2 min of iv injection, with a **half-life** of 1–2 h; thus depressant effects of opioid analgesic drugs may recur after a few hours. Metabolised in the liver and excreted mainly renally.
- Dosage:
  - acute opioid overdose: 0.4–2.0 mg iv/im/sc; if no response, repeated every 2–3 min up to 10 mg. Administration by infusion (3–10 μg/kg/h) may be required.
  - opioid-induced respiratory depression/sedation in patients receiving palliative care/chronic opioid use: 0.1–0.2 mg (1.5–3 μg/kg); if inadequate response, 0.1 mg every 2 min with careful monitoring.
  - postoperatively: 1.5–3 μg/kg iv, followed by 1.5 μg/kg repeated every 2 min as required. Infusion or im injection may be used to prevent later resedation.
  - neonatal resuscitation: 10 μg/kg im, iv or sc repeated every 2–3 min or 60 μg/kg im as a single injection.
- Side effects: **hypertension**, **arrhythmias**, **pulmonary oedema** and **cardiac arrest** have followed rapid iv injection, possibly due to sudden catecholamine release secondary to reversal of sedation and analgesia.

Acute withdrawal may be precipitated in patients dependent on opioids.

NALS, Neonatal Advanced Life Support, *see Neonatal Resuscitation Program*

Naltrexone hydrochloride. Opioid receptor antagonist, synthesised in 1965. Derived from **naloxone**, with similar actions but longer duration (24 h after a single dose). Used as an adjunct to prevent relapse in formerly opioid- or alcohol-dependent patients.
- Dosage: 25–50 mg/day orally.
- Side effects: GIT upset, chest pain, anxiety, sleep disorders, headache, joint/muscle pain.

NAP, *see National Audit Projects*

Naproxen. NSAID derived from propionic acid. Longer acting than **ibuprofen**, with a slightly greater risk of peptic ulceration but the smallest cardiovascular risk among NSAIDs. Available over the counter for the treatment of primary dysmenorrhoea; otherwise, prescription-only in the UK.
- Dosage: 250–500 mg orally bd.
- Side effects: as for NSAIDs.

Narcotic drugs. Strictly, drugs that induce sleep, but the term usually refers to **morphine**-like drugs. Preferred terms include **opiates**, **opioids** and **opioid analgesic drugs**.

Nasal inhalers. Used instead of **facemasks** for **dental anaesthesia**. Designed to fit over the nose, leaving the mouth free. During **induction of anaesthesia**, the patient is instructed to breathe through the nose. During anaesthesia, a mouth pack prevents mouth breathing. Now rarely used.

- Different types:
  - Goldman's: black rubber, with an inflatable rim as for facemasks. Incorporates an **adjustable pressure-limiting valve**, and attaches to the breathing system over the patient's forehead. Held from behind the patient's head using both thumbs while the other fingers support the jaw. May also be held with a head harness using two studs incorporated into the sides.
  - **McKesson**'s: made of malleable black rubber; thus adjustable. Connected to the breathing system via two tubes that pass around the sides of the head to meet behind, helping to hold the inhaler in place. Incorporates an expiratory valve.
  - newer types are made of plastic, and may incorporate unidirectional gas flow, e.g. through inspiratory and expiratory tubes passing around the head. **Scavenging** of exhaled gases is thus aided.

[Victor Goldman (1903–1993), London anaesthetist]

Nasal positive pressure ventilation, *see Non-invasive positive pressure ventilation*

Nasogastric intubation. Performed for enteral **nutrition**, or gastric drainage. Fine-bore tubes are used for the former, usually inserted using a wire stylet that is removed after placement. Larger tubes (e.g. 10–16 Ch) are used for gastric drainage, e.g. following abdominal surgery or in intestinal obstruction. They may be placed in the awake patient (who aids placement by swallowing or sipping water) or the unconscious patient (e.g. after induction of anaesthesia, either before or after tracheal intubation). Placement can often be performed blindly, and may be aided by passage through a plain nasal tracheal tube placed into the pharynx. Placement may require direct vision using a laryngoscope and **forceps** (the oesophagus lies posterior to the **larynx** and to the left of the midline). Correct placement is confirmed by aspiration of gastric contents, which must be tested for acidity. If no fluid can be aspirated, correct placement must be confirmed with a chest x-ray showing the tube passing vertically in the midline or near midline to below the level of the carina, continuing to the level of the diaphragm with the tip of the tube visible on the left side of the abdomen ≥10 cm beyond the gastro-oesophageal junction. Auscultation over the left hypochondrium during injection of air is unreliable.

If already in place, withdrawal of the tube before induction of anaesthesia has been suggested, to avoid increasing gastro-oesophageal reflux or rendering **cricoid pressure** inefficient. However, its efficacy has been questioned and this is rarely done.

National Audit Projects (NAPs). Studies set up by the **Royal College of Anaesthetists**, now administered by the Health Services Research Centre on the College's behalf. The first two NAPs (2003–2004) were relatively limited and focused on consultant supervision and mortality/morbidity review meetings; subsequent NAPs were more extensive and resulted in important and influential reports:

- NAP3 (2006–2007): complications of central neuraxial block.
- NAP4 (2008–2009); with the Difficult Airway Society: complications of airway management.
- NAP5 (2012–2013); with the **Association of Anaesthetists of Great Britain and Ireland**: accidental **awareness** under general anaesthesia.
- NAP6 (2015–2016): **anaphylaxis**.

The NAP methodology suits uncommon outcomes for which large numbers of patients are required. Although there may be uncertainty over exact incidences (due to difficulty establishing accurate numerator/denominator data), the NAPs allow themes to be analysed and risk factors highlighted, such that recommendations for clinical practice and service provision can be made.

National Confidential Enquiry into Patient Outcome and Death (NCEPOD). Ongoing enquiry originally commissioned by the **Association of Anaesthetists of Great Britain and Ireland**, together with the Association of Surgeons of Great Britain and Ireland, and published in 1987 as the Confidential Enquiry into Perioperative Deaths (CEPOD). The first UK study to involve both anaesthetists and surgeons, it analysed all 4000 NHS deaths occurring within 30 days of surgery (excluding obstetric and cardiac surgery) in three regions during 1986. The first national Report (NCEPOD; 1989) focused on children under 10 years; subsequent Reports have focused on particular aspects, e.g. deaths following specific surgical or interventional procedures or in specific diseases or age groups, e.g. most recently, tracheostomy care, lower limb amputation (2014); GIT haemorrhage, sepsis (2015); acute pancreatitis (2016); non-invasive ventilation, mental health (2017); and cancer in young people, cerebral palsy, acute heart failure, perioperative diabetes (due 2018).

The scheme now includes independent hospitals and involves several Royal Colleges. The name changed in 2002 from 'Perioperative Death' to 'Patient Outcome and Death', reflecting extension of NCEPOD's remit to include physicians and primary care, and to review near misses as well as deaths. Although an independent body, NCEPOD is funded mainly by the UK Departments of Health.

- General findings and recommendations:
  - most deaths occur in elderly and/or the sickest patients.
  - overall care is good but there are identifiable deficiencies, involving:
    - staff: communication between and within specialties; training/supervision.
    - resources: availability of appropriate equipment and of emergency operating theatre, **ICU** and **HDU** facilities.
    - clinical care: **DVT** prophylaxis; use of protocols/guidelines; timely operating; preoperative resuscitation; transfer of critically ill patients.
  - the need for postmortem examination, **audit** and morbidity/mortality assessments has been repeatedly stressed.

National Halothane Study, *see Hepatitis*

National Institute of Academic Anaesthesia (NIAA). Established in 2008 by the **Royal College of Anaesthetists**, **Association of Anaesthetists of Great Britain and Ireland**, ***British Journal of Anaesthesia*** and ***Anaesthesia***, to further the academic profile of the specialty of anaesthesia and promote high-quality research. Co-ordinates the assessment and awarding by various funding bodies of anaesthetic research grants within the UK, and houses the Health Services Research Centre (HSRC), which co-ordinates national, outcome-based projects.

Mahajan RP, Reilly CS (2012). Br J Anaesth; 108: 1–3

National Institute for Health and Care Excellence (NICE). NHS Special Health Authority for England and Wales, established in 1999 (as the National Institute for Clinical Excellence) to provide authoritative, evidence-based and reliable guidance on current 'best practice'. Its guidance is derived from independent assessments of clinical evidence combined with cost-effectiveness analyses, and covers both individual health technologies (including medicines, medical devices, diagnostic techniques and procedures) and the clinical management of specific conditions. In 2005, NICE took on the functions of the Health Development Agency to become the National Institute for Health and Clinical Excellence and in 2013, became the National Institute for Health and Care Excellence (though still known as NICE), a non-departmental public body directly accountable to the Department of Health (of England). It is thus responsible for providing national guidance and quality standards for healthcare and social care.

National Patient Safety Agency (NPSA). NHS Special Health Authority, formed in 2001 to co-ordinate reports of adverse events or 'near misses' and their analysis. Operated three main services until its abolition in 2012:
- National Reporting and Learning Service (NRLS); collecting and analysing patient safety incidents in the NHS, now transferred to **NHS Improvement**.
- National Clinical Assessment Service (NCAS), providing advice and support to the NHS regarding concerns about the performance of individual doctors, dentists and pharmacists. This role transferred to **NICE** and in 2013, transferred to the NHS Litigation Authority.
- National Research Ethics Service (NRES), overseeing ethical review of research across the UK. This role transferred to the new Health Research Authority.

See also, Confidential Enquiry into Maternal Deaths; National Confidential Enquiry into Patient Outcome and Death

Natriuretic hormone, *see Atrial natriuretic peptide*

Nausea, *see Postoperative nausea and vomiting; Vomiting*

NCEPOD, *see National Confidential Enquiry into Patient Outcome and Death*

Near-drowning. Defined as initial survival following immersion in liquid, usually water; death at the time of immersion may be due to anoxia (drowning) or **cardiac arrest** caused by sudden extreme lowering of temperature (immersion syndrome). Secondary drowning refers to death following near-drowning after a period of relative well-being and is usually due to **ALI**.

Autopsy following drowning reveals little or no lung water in 15% of cases (dry drowning); **laryngospasm** following initial laryngeal contamination has been suggested. In 85% of cases, pulmonary aspiration of water occurs (wet drowning); this may involve:
- fresh water: systemic absorption may cause **haemolysis**, **haemodilution** and electrolyte disturbances.
- salt water: draws water into the lungs.

Both types cause **pulmonary oedema** and **hypoxaemia**. Haemodynamic changes due to fluid shifts are rare; thus in practice the type of water may have little clinical significance.

Other adverse factors include **hypothermia**, **aspiration of gastric contents** and predisposing conditions, e.g. **alcoholism** or drug abuse, **trauma**, **epilepsy**, **MI**, **stroke**.

Complications include **ALI**, **cerebral oedema**, **acute kidney injury**, pneumonia, **pancreatitis**, **acidosis** and **shock**. **Sepsis** is especially likely if the water is contaminated.
- Management:
  - **CPR**.
  - treatment of complications as appropriate.
  - rewarming.
  - antibiotics as appropriate. Use of **corticosteroids** is controversial and declining.
  - nasogastric aspiration to remove gastric water.

Recovery has been reported after up to 60 min immersion followed by prolonged CPR, especially in children and if hypothermic. **Cerebral hypoxic ischaemic injury** may occur.
Handley AJ (2016). BMJ; 348: bmj.g1734

Near infrared oximetry/spectroscopy (NIRS). Monitoring technique based on the principle that light in the near infrared spectrum (650–900 nm wavelength) transmits through biological tissues. Increasingly used to image biological events in the cerebral cortex. Photons produced by a **laser** photodiode are directed into the skull; while many are reflected and dispersed, a proportion is transmitted. Coloured compounds within the tissues (chromophores), especially oxyhaemoglobin, deoxyhaemoglobin and oxidised cytochrome oxidase, have characteristic absorption spectra. The emergent light intensity is detected and a computer converts the changes in light intensity into changes in chromophore concentration. Clinical applications include monitoring of cerebral oxygenation, metabolism and **cerebral blood flow** and volume, e.g. in **neurosurgery**, **cardiac surgery** and **head injury**, but its potential as a routine monitor has not yet been realised.
Ghosh A, Elwell C, Smith M (2012). Anesth Analg; 115: 1373–83
See also, Functional imaging

Nebulisers. Devices used to provide a suspension of droplets in a gas, for administration of inhaled drugs or **humidification**. Droplets of 5 µm are deposited in the trachea and bronchi; those of 1 µm pass to alveoli and may impair gas exchange, whereas those <0.5 µm may be exhaled before deposition. Thus the ideal droplet size is between 1 and 5 µm.
- Nebulisers may be:
  - gas-driven: water is entrained by the gas flow (**Venturi principle**) and broken into a spray; this may be directed against an anvil that breaks up the drops into smaller droplets. May be combined with a heater.
  - ultrasonic: droplets are formed from water lying on a vibrating plate, or from water dropped on to the plate. Water overload may occur, because the droplets are very small and the water content of the gas is high.
  - mechanical: water is dispersed into a mist by a spinning disc.

Gas-driven devices are used for drug delivery; all types may be used for humidification.

Neck, cross-sectional anatomy. At the level of C6, major anatomical structures within the layer of skin, fat and subcutaneous tissue may be described in terms of fascial layers (Fig. 116):
- superficial fascia: encloses platysma muscle and deep fascial layers.

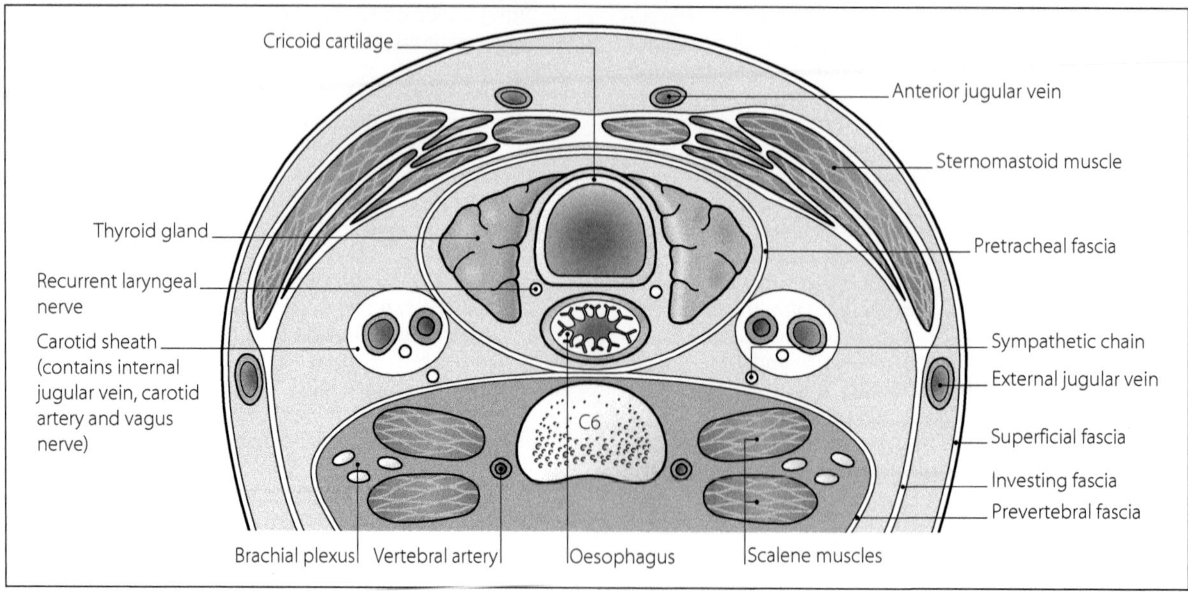

Fig. 116 Cross-section of neck at C6

- deep fascia: composed of three layers:
  - investing fascia: lies posterior to the anterior and external **jugular veins**. Splits to enclose sternohyoid, sternothyroid, omohyoid, sternomastoid and trapezius muscles.
  - prevertebral fascia: extends laterally on scalenus anterior and medius to form the floor of the posterior triangle of the neck, and passes downwards to form the axillary sheath. Separated from the oesophageal/pharyngeal junction in the midline by the retropharyngeal space.
  - pretracheal fascia: contains the trachea, oesophagus and **thyroid gland**.

See also, Carotid arteries; *Tracheobronchial tree*

Neck of femur, fractured, *see Fractured neck of femur*

Necrotising enterocolitis (NEC). Necrosis of GIT mucosa (especially terminal ileum, caecum and ascending colon) seen in **neonates**, usually within the first week of life. Prevalence is up to 8% in premature and low-birth-weight babies; predisposing factors include asphyxia, hypotension (or any cause of splanchnic hypoperfusion) and umbilical catheterisation. Mucosal damage follows hypoperfusion and ischaemia, leading to abdominal distension, vomiting, and faecal blood and mucus, although the onset may be insidious. Pallor, bradycardia, jaundice, intestinal perforation and **DIC** may occur. Plain abdominal x-ray shows dilated loops of bowel and intramural gas bubbles.

Management is largely supportive, with iv fluids, IPPV, correction of anaemia, **antibacterial drugs** (including anaerobic cover), probiotic agents and **TPN** (in place of enteral feeds). Surgery may be required if perforation occurs or there is no improvement despite medical therapy. Quoted mortality ranges from 10% to 50%. Survivors commonly exhibit neurological impairment with 20% having microcephaly.

Neu J, Walker WA (2011). N Engl J Med; 364: 255–64

Necrotising fasciitis. Uncommon deep-seated infection of subcutaneous tissue, resulting in destruction of fat and fascia. Predisposing factors include immunosuppression, alcoholism, diabetes, peripheral vascular disease, surgery, penetrating injuries (which may be minor) and varicella infection, although it may affect young, healthy individuals. Systemic upset is thought to result from bacterial toxins, endogenous **cytokines** and other inflammatory mediators. May be rapidly fatal unless aggressively treated. Classified as:

- type I: polymicrobial infection involving gram-negative bacilli, enterococci and mixed anaerobes. Infection involves fat and fascia, although the skin is usually spared. Includes Fournier's **gangrene** of the perineum.
- type II: caused by *Streptococcus pyogenes* or *Staphylococcus aureus*. Features include systemic toxicity, pain, necrosis of subcutaneous tissue and skin, gangrene, **shock** and **MODS**.

- Management:
  - prompt diagnosis; made on clinical grounds, although MRI and biopsy may help distinguish it from acute **cellulitis**.
  - early surgical debridement (the diagnosis is usually confirmed at surgery), with fasciotomy to prevent **compartment syndrome**.
  - **antibacterial drug** therapy and general supportive care; hyperbaric oxygen has been used.

[Jean A Fournier (1832–1914), Paris dermatologist]

Stevens DL, Bryant AE (2017). N Engl J Med; 377: 2253–65

Needles. Christopher Wren described injection via a quill and bladder in 1659. Metal tubes and stylets were subsequently used, but the hypodermic cannula and trocar were first described by Rynd in 1845. Different sizes and types are available for different uses, e.g. for iv/hypodermic use, **epidural** and **spinal anaesthesia**. Short-bevelled needles are traditionally preferred for **regional anaesthesia**. Hollow needles are not required for **acupuncture** or electrical stimulation/recording.

Needle size is described by a wire gauge classification (G; Stubs gauge; Birmingham gauge), which originally referred to the number of times the wire was drawn through

Table 34 Diameter of needles of different gauge number

Gauge number (G)	*Outside diameter (mm)*
36	0.10
30	0.30
29	0.33
28	0.36
27	0.41
26	0.46
25	0.51
24	0.56
23	0.64
22	0.71
21	0.81
20	0.90
19	1.08
18	1.27
17	1.50
16	1.65
15	1.83
14	2.11
13	2.41
12	2.77
11	3.05
10	3.40
9	3.76
8	4.19
7	4.57
6	5.16
1	7.62

the draw plate (Table 34). It differs slightly from the American and Standard wire gauges. Internal diameter varies according to different materials and needle strengths. The system is also used for iv cannulae. For hypodermic needles, colour-coding is mandatory in the UK for certain sizes: 26 G brown; 25 G orange; 23 G blue; 22 G black; 21 G green; 20 G yellow; 19 G cream.
[Sir Christopher Wren (1633–1723), English scientist and architect; Francis Rynd (1801–1861), Irish surgeon; Peter Stubs (1756–1806), English toolmaker and innkeeper]

Needlestick injury, *see Environmental safety of anaesthetists*

NEEP, *see Negative end-expiratory pressure*

Nefopam hydrochloride. Centrally acting **analgesic drug**, unrelated to **opioid analgesic drugs** and **NSAIDs**. Widely used in Europe. Inhibits reuptake of **5-HT**, **noradrenaline** and **dopamine** and blocks voltage-gated sodium channels. Has similar analgesic potency to NSAIDs. Peak action occurs 1–2 h after im injection. Drowsiness and respiratory depression may occur, but less than with opioids.

- Dosage: 30–90 mg orally tds.
- Side effects: nausea, headache, confusion, anticholinergic effects. Should be avoided in patients with epilepsy and those taking **monoamine oxidase inhibitors**.

Negative end-expiratory pressure (NEEP). Adjunct to **IPPV**, popular in the 1960s–1970s as a method of reducing the adverse cardiovascular effects of IPPV by maintaining a subatmospheric **airway pressure** at end-expiration. However, NEEP increases airway collapse, while reducing **FRC**. Thus no longer used.

Negligence. Civil charge in which the following must be established:

- duty of care owed to the patient by the practitioner or institution.
- failure in that duty.
- harm suffered as a result of that failure ('causation').

Although the first two may often be easy to demonstrate, establishing causation is usually more difficult. The 'burden of proof' for negligence and other civil claims is based on the 'balance of probabilities', as opposed to criminal charges, in which it is 'beyond reasonable doubt'.

A doctor's action (or lack thereof) is judged against that of a 'reasonable' body of medical opinion, even if that body is a minority (Bolam test); however, such an opinion must also be 'reasonable' and 'responsible' to be accepted by the courts (Bolitho test). In the UK, because negligence must be proved in order for compensation to be paid, there have been calls for no fault compensation schemes similar to those in other countries e.g. Sweden and other Scandinavian countries, and New Zealand, in which the fact that harm has occurred is enough to result in compensation without having to prove negligence.

Cases of negligence resulting in the death of a patient, in which the action or omission constitutes 'gross negligence', may lead to the criminal charge of **manslaughter**.
[John Hector Bolam, UK shipping assistant and psychiatric patient; suffered multiple fractures in 1954 during electroconvulsive therapy administered without paralysis or restraint. His claim of negligence was dismissed because withholding of anaesthesia was accepted medical practice at the time; Patrick Nigel Bolitho, died aged 2 years in 1984, following cardiac arrest after admission with croup.]

Neisserial infections. Mostly caused by two species of the gram-positive cocci genus:

- *Neisseria gonorrhoeae*: may cause acute **endocarditis**, urethritis, pelvic inflammatory disease and pelvic abscesses.
- *N. meningitidis* (meningococcus): causes **meningococcal disease**, including **meningitis**. The organism may be carried in the nasopharynx of about 5% of otherwise healthy subjects, increasing to about 30% during epidemics.

Neisserial infection is common in **complement** deficiency.
[Albert Neisser (1855–1916), German physician]

Neomycin sulfate. Aminoglycoside and **antibacterial** drug, used orally for **selective decontamination of the digestive tract**, specifically in **hepatic failure** and before bowel surgery. Also used topically for skin or mucous membrane infections.

- Dosage: 1 g orally, 4-hourly.
- Side effects: as for aminoglycosides. May be absorbed systemically in hepatic failure, resulting in toxicity.

Neonatal resuscitation, *see Cardiopulmonary resuscitation, neonatal*

Neonatal Resuscitation Program (NRP). Programme of training in neonatal **CPR**, established in 1988 in the USA and administered by the American Heart Association and American Academy of Pediatrics. Similar in concept to the **ATLS** and related courses. Unofficially referred to as 'NALS' (Neonatal Advanced Life Support).

Neonate. Child within 28 days of birth. Normally weighs 3–4 kg, with body surface area approximately 0.19 m^2.
- Major changes at birth include the following:
  - change from **fetal circulation** to adult circulation via transitional circulation. The fibrous left ventricle, which is of similar size to the right ventricle at birth, gradually increases in compliance and contractility.
  - expansion of fluid-filled alveoli; requires negative intrapleural pressures exceeding 70 cmH_2O. Increasing numbers of alveoli are expanded in successive breaths. Most fluid is rapidly expelled via the upper airway, with the remainder drained via capillary and lymphatic vessels over 1–3 days.

Anatomical and physiological features and principles of anaesthesia are as for **paediatric anaesthesia**. Perioperative risks are higher than for older children, especially in premature neonates; surgery is usually deferred if possible.
See also, Cardiopulmonary resuscitation, neonatal; Fetal haemoglobin; Fetal monitoring; Neurobehavioural testing of neonates; Obstetric analgesia and anaesthesia; Paediatric advanced life support; Paediatric intensive care; Surfactant

Neostigmine metilsulfate/bromide. **Acetylcholinesterase inhibitor**, first synthesised in 1931. Used to increase **acetylcholine** concentrations at the **neuromuscular junction**, e.g. reversal of **non-depolarising neuromuscular blockade** and **myasthenia gravis**. Also has a direct stimulatory effect on skeletal muscle **acetylcholine receptors**; in addition, it is thought to have significant presynaptic action, increasing the amount of acetylcholine released. May cause **depolarising neuromuscular blockade** in overdosage. Other effects are those of muscarinic stimulation, e.g. bradycardia, nausea/vomiting, increased GIT motility (resulting in diarrhoea) and bladder contractility (resulting in incontinence), sweating, salivation, miosis, bronchospasm. Has been used to treat urinary retention and ileus, e.g. postoperatively. Effects on autonomic ganglia are small, consisting of stimulation at low doses and depression at high doses. A quaternary ammonium compound, it crosses the **blood–brain barrier** poorly and has few CNS effects. Routinely given with **atropine** or **glycopyrronium** when administered iv to prevent muscarinic side effects. Active within 1 min of iv injection, with action lasting 20–30 min. Active for up to 4 h after oral administration. Excreted mainly renally, mostly unchanged. Elimination **half-life** is 50–90 min. May be administered parenterally (as metilsulfate [methylsulphate]) or orally (as bromide). Has also been given intrathecally; produces analgesia but with increased nausea and vomiting.
- Dosage:
  - reversal of non-depolarising blockade: 0.04–0.08 mg/kg iv with 0.02–0.04 mg/kg atropine or 10–20 μg/kg glycopyrronium.
  - myasthenia gravis: 15–30 mg orally or 1.0–2.5 mg sc/im, 2–4-hourly.
  - other uses: as for myasthenia gravis.
- Side effects: as above. **Cholinergic crisis** may occur in overdosage.

Neo-Synephrine, *see Phenylephrine*

Nephritic syndrome. Acute **glomerulonephritis** characterised by reduction of **glomerular filtration rate**, haematuria, proteinuria, salt and water retention, increased intravascular volume and **hypertension**. Most commonly a post-infectious condition, it is also seen in **SLE**. Usually mild; severe cases may result in **acute kidney injury**. Distinction between it and **nephrotic syndrome** has been overplayed in the past and both share common aetiologies.

Nephron. Basic renal unit; each **kidney** contains about 1.3 million.
- Structure (Fig. 117a):
  - glomerulus: formed by a 200-μm diameter invagination of capillaries into the blind end of the nephron (Bowman's capsule). Water is filtered from the blood across the glomerular membrane, together with substances under 4–8 nm in diameter. **GFR** equals about 120 ml/min (180 l/day).
  - tubule: 45–65 mm long. The site of reabsorption/secretion of substances from/into the filtrate, giving rise to the eventual composition of **urine**. Consists of:
    - proximal convoluted tubule: 15 mm long. Lies within the renal cortex. Lined by a brush border. Site of active reabsorption of **sodium** and **potassium** ions, **bicarbonate**, phosphate, **glucose**, uric acid and **amino acids**. Water moves passively from the tubule by osmosis. Up to 80% of filtered water and solutes is reabsorbed.
    - loop of Henle: about 15–25 cm long; length depends on whether the glomerulus lies within the outer or inner renal cortex (short in the former, long in the latter). A further 15% of filtered water is reabsorbed. 15% of loops extend into the medulla, where interstitial **osmolarity** is very high (up to 1200 mosmol/l). Water moves out of the descending limb, followed by sodium ions along a concentration gradient as the tubular fluid becomes more concentrated. In the ascending limb, which is impermeable to both water and sodium ions, sodium and chloride ions are actively co-transported from the tubule. The fluid thus becomes more dilute as it ascends. **Urea** is relatively free to pass across the tubular membranes. The solutes remain in the region of the medulla because of the countercurrent multiplier mechanism whereby the blood vessels supplying the loop pass close to those draining it. Solutes pass down concentration gradients from ascending vessels to descending vessels, and thus recirculate at the tip of the loop. Water passes from the descending vessels to the ascending vessels, and is thus removed from the area. This maintains the high osmolarity in the medullary region. The thick ascending segment forms part of the **juxtaglomerular apparatus** where it passes near the glomerulus.
    - distal convoluted tubule: 5 mm long. A further 5% of filtered water is reabsorbed. Sodium ions are reabsorbed in exchange for potassium or **hydrogen ions**, under the influence of **aldosterone**.
  - collecting ducts: 20 mm long. Each receives several tubules. Pass through the cortex and medulla, opening into the renal pelvis at the medullary pyramids. Some sodium/potassium/hydrogen ion exchange occurs at the cortical part. Water is reabsorbed depending on the amount of **vasopressin** present, which increases tubular permeability to water and thus increases urine concentration.
- Blood supply (Fig. 117b):
  - afferent and efferent arterioles supply and drain the capillaries to the glomerulus, respectively.

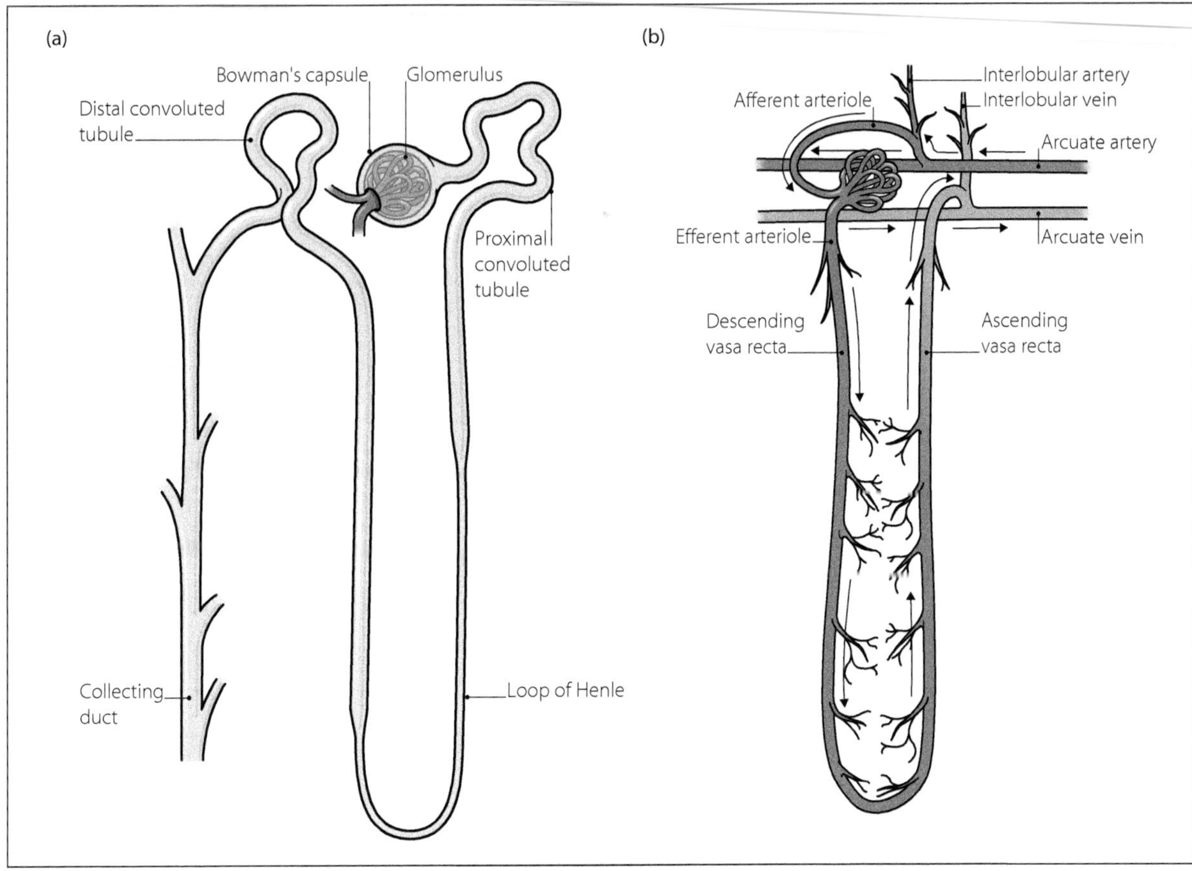

Fig. 117 Structure of nephron: (a) glomerulotubular system; (b) vascular system

- efferent arterioles subsequently divide to form peritubular capillaries or vasa recta (long loops that accompany the loop of Henle).
- peritubular capillaries and ascending vasa recta drain into interlobular veins.

[Sir William P Bowman (1816–1892), English surgeon; Friedrich GJ Henle (1809–1885), German anatomist]
See also, Acid–base balance; Clearance; Diuretics; Renin/angiotensin system

Nephrotic syndrome. Defined by daily urinary protein excretion >3.5 g/1.73 m^2 body surface area. May be primary due to glomerular disease (classified according to histology) or secondary (e.g. associated with **diabetes mellitus**, **pre-eclampsia**, **connective tissue disease**, post-viral **hepatitis** or **streptococcal infection**, drugs such as **NSAIDs** or **captopril**). Features include generalised **oedema**, susceptibility to infection and thromboembolism (especially renal vein thrombosis and **DVT**) and hyperlipidaemia. Hypoalbuminaemia may lead to altered drug binding.

Treatment includes a low-sodium diet and **diuretic** therapy to reduce oedema, and a low-protein diet and **angiotensin converting enzyme inhibitors** to reduce proteinuria. Other treatment is directed against the cause, e.g. **corticosteroids** in **glomerulonephritis**.
See also, Renal failure

Nernst equation. Equation for calculating the **membrane potential** at which an individual ion is at equilibrium across the **membrane** (assuming complete permeability to that ion). For ion X:

$$E = \frac{RT}{FZ} \ln \frac{[X]_o}{[X]_i}$$

where E = equilibrium potential
R = **universal gas constant**
T = absolute temperature
F = Faraday constant (coulombs per mole of charge)
Z = valence of the ion
$[X]_o$ = extracellular concentration of X
$[X]_i$ = intracellular concentration of X.

For chloride, potassium and sodium, E = –70 mV, –94 mV and +60 mV, respectively. Because the normal resting membrane potential is about –70 mV, other factors must affect potassium and especially sodium distribution (e.g. relative permeability and the **sodium/potassium pump**).
[Hermann W Nernst (1864–1941), German physicist; Michael Faraday (1791–1867), English scientist]
See also, Goldman constant-field equation

Nerve. Excitable tissue whose function is the transmission of nerve impulses. Typical peripheral nerves consist of several groups of fascicles. Each fascicle is surrounded by the perineurium and contains a group of **neurones**, the axons of which are encased in the endoneurium (Fig. 118).

Peripheral nerves originate in the **spinal cord**, and may be sensory, motor or mixed. Some also carry **autonomic nervous system** fibres.
See also, Motor pathways; Sensory pathways

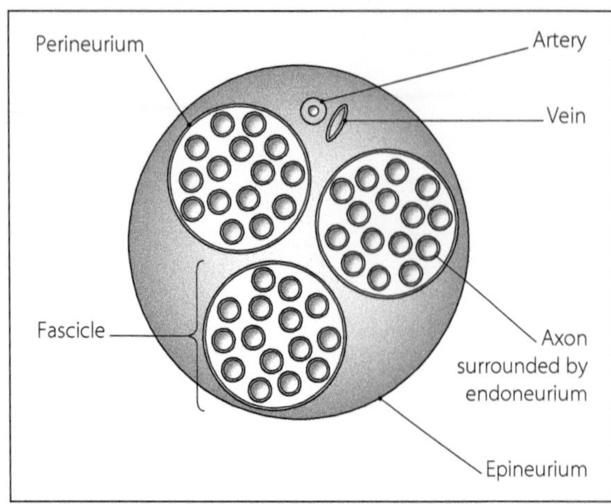

Fig. 118 Cross-section of a typical nerve

Nerve conduction. Passage of an **action potential** along **neurones**; involves waves of depolarisation and repolarisation that move longitudinally across the nerve **membrane**.

In unmyelinated **nerves**, impulses spread at up to 2 m/s. Positive charge flows into the depolarised area from the membrane just distally, altering the distal permeability to ions (especially sodium and potassium) as for action potential generation. When the threshold potential is reached, depolarisation occurs. Retrograde conduction is prevented by the **refractory period** of the membrane proximally.

The **myelin** sheath of myelinated nerves acts as an insulator that prevents the flow of ions across the nerve membrane. Breaks in the myelin (nodes of Ranvier), approximately 1 mm apart, allow ions to flow freely between the neurone and the ECF at these points. Depolarisation 'jumps' from node to node (saltatory conduction), a process that increases conduction velocity (up to 120 m/s) and conserves energy.

[Louis A Ranvier (1835–1922), French pathologist and physician]

Nerve growth factor (NGF). Protein produced by many cell types; taken up by small sensory and sympathetic nerve fibres via specific receptors and retrogradely transported to the cell body. Required for growth and survival of neurones in the fetus and neonate; released from connective tissue and inflammatory cells following tissue injury in response to cytokine stimulation. Causes **hyperalgesia** via both central and peripheral effects; thus thought to be important in acute and chronic pain states. Also involved in immune regulation and other non-neurological system function.

Nerve injury during anaesthesia. May occur during general, local or regional anaesthesia.

- Causes of neuronal injury include:
  - general anaesthesia:
    - poor **positioning of the patient**; thought to cause local nerve ischaemia.
    - ischaemia caused by **hypotension** or use of **tourniquets**.
    - **hypothermia**.
    - extravasation of drugs into perineural tissue.
    - toxicity of degradation products of anaesthetic agents, classically **trichloroethylene** with **soda lime**.
  - local/**regional anaesthesia**: positioning/ischaemia/hypothermia as discussed earlier plus:
    - direct trauma from a **needle** or catheter.
    - intraneural injection of **local anaesthetic agent**.
    - **cauda equina syndrome** following use of spinal catheters for continuous **spinal anaesthesia**.
    - infection.
    - haematoma formation.
    - chemical contamination of local anaesthetic, or injection of the wrong solution.
    - poor positioning of the anaesthetised limb with ischaemia as discussed earlier.
  - other:
    - **central venous cannulation**.
    - tracheal intubation.
- Classic division of nerve injuries:
  - neuropraxia: caused by compression. Typically incomplete, affecting motor more than sensory components (when present, touch and proprioception predominate). Usually recovers within 6 weeks. Damage during general anaesthesia is usually of this nature, and associated with positioning.
  - axonotmesis: axonal and **myelin** loss within the intact connective tissue sheath. Typically there is complete motor and sensory loss, with slow recovery due to nerve regeneration from proximal to distal nerve.
  - neurotmesis: partial or complete severance. Recovery is rare.

Electromyographic and nerve conduction studies may aid differentiation between types of injury, and are most useful 1–3 weeks after the event. 'Baseline' studies performed immediately after the injury are also useful to identify or exclude pre-existing deficit.

- Many specific neuropathies have been described, including lesions of the following:
  - **brachial plexus**: usually stretched, typically by shoulder abduction and extension, with supination. Stretch is exacerbated by bilateral abduction. Upper roots are usually affected; weakness lasts up to several months, although recovery usually occurs within 2–3 months. Lower roots may be damaged during sternal retraction in **cardiac surgery**. Compression may be caused by shoulder rests in the steep head-down position, resulting in temporary palsy.
  - **ulnar nerve**: may be compressed between the humeral epicondyle and the operating table or arm supports, or injured by stretcher poles if slid alongside the patient during transfer.
  - **radial nerve**: caused by the patient's arm hanging over the side of the operating table.
  - **median nerve**: may be damaged by direct needle trauma, or drug extravasation in the **antecubital fossa**.
  - facial nerve: compressed between the anaesthetist's fingers and the patient's mandible during mask anaesthesia.
  - abducens nerve: temporary lesions may follow **spinal** or **epidural anaesthesia**.
  - trigeminal nerve: typically damaged by the trichloroethylene/soda lime interaction.
  - supraorbital nerve: compressed by the tracheal tube connector, catheter mount, head **harness** or ventilator tubing.
  - common peroneal nerve: compressed between lithotomy pole and fibular head.
  - saphenous nerve: compressed between lithotomy pole and medial tibial condyle.

- sciatic nerve: damaged by im injections or compressed against the operating table in emaciated patients.
- pudendal nerve: compressed between a poorly padded perineal post and the ischial tuberosity.

Nerve injury may also be caused by surgical trauma/compression.

Similar concerns exist for patients undergoing prolonged treatment on ICU.

See also, Cranial nerves; Critical illness polyneuropathy; Eye care

Nerve stimulator, *see Neuromuscular blockade monitoring; Regional anaesthesia; Transcutaneous electrical nerve stimulation*

Netilmicin. **Aminoglycoside** and **antibacterial drug** with similar activity to **gentamicin** but less active against pseudomonas. Less ototoxic than gentamicin.

- Dosage: 4–6 mg/kg im/iv daily or up to 2.5 mg/kg im/iv bd/tds. Blood concentrations: 1 h post-dose <12 mg/l; predose <2 mg/l
- Side effects: as for aminoglycosides.

Neuralgia. **Pain** in the distribution of a defined nerve or group of nerves.

Neurally adjusted ventilatory assist (NAVA). Mode of partial ventilatory assist in which the **ventilator** delivers an inspiratory pressure using diaphragm electrical activity (EAdi) to control the timing and level of assist delivered. EAdi is measured using an oesophageal electrode placed at the level of the **diaphragm**. Said to improve patient-ventilator synchrony, especially at high levels of assist, and therefore useful for **weaning from ventilators**.

Navalesi P, Longhini F (2015). Curr Opin Crit Care; 21: 58–64

Neuritis. Inflammation of nerve(s).

Neurobehavioural testing of neonates. Investigation of the effects of **obstetric analgesia and anaesthesia** on the **neonate** is difficult because of many variables, e.g. obstetric details, fetal distress, method of delivery, type and route of drugs administered, methods of analysis of data. In many early studies, **aortocaval compression** was not avoided.

- Tests used:
    - neonatal behavioural assessment scale (NBAS): very detailed, taking up to 1 h to perform. More sensitive than the others.
    - early neonatal neurobehavioural scale (ENNS): directed more towards disorders of tone. Quicker and easier to perform.
    - neurological and adaptive capacity score (NACS): even more directed towards tone. Takes a few minutes to perform. The least sensitive test for subtle effects.
- Summary of results:
    - **pethidine**: reduces alertness and responsiveness before respiratory depression is evident. Greatest effect is at 2 days. Rapid placental transfer follows maternal iv injection.
    - anaesthetic agents: **thiopental** causes more neonatal depression than **ketamine** (but tone is increased by ketamine, giving higher scores). Low concentrations of volatile **inhalational anaesthetic agents** produce little, if any, effects. Regional techniques consistently produce higher scores.
    - **local anaesthetic agents**: concerns over hypotonia following **lidocaine** have now been refuted. All local anaesthetic drugs have similar effects, lowering scores only when very sensitive testing is employed. The significance of this is unknown.

Neurofibromatosis. Group of neurocutaneous diseases characterised by multiple tumours derived from the neurilemma sheath of cranial and peripheral **nerves**/nerve roots.

- Classified into:
    - neurofibromatosis 1 (NF-1; von Recklinghausen's disease). Autosomal dominant disease with gene locus at chromosome 17, with an incidence of 1:3000. Flat, brown 'café au lait' spots occur in all sufferers, six or more spots larger than 1.5 cm being diagnostic. Neurofibromata may be subcutaneous/cutaneous, or may occur in deeper peripheral nerves or autonomic nerves supplying viscera. They may also occur at the foramen magnum or within the theca, causing nerve root or **spinal cord** compression. **Pulmonary fibrosis** occurs in 20% of cases; hypertension is present in 6% of patients and may be associated with **phaeochromocytoma** (in 1%) or renal artery stenosis. Intracranial tumours occur in 5%–10% of cases, and skeletal abnormalities (including **kyphoscoliosis**) in 10%. Potential anaesthetic problems result from the distribution of neurofibromata and may include difficulty with tracheal intubation or regional blocks. Despite earlier reports, patients exhibit normal sensitivity to **neuromuscular blocking drugs**.
    - neurofibromatosis 2 (NF-2): very rare condition in which bilateral acoustic neuromas are present. Gene has been mapped to chromosome 22.

[Friedrich D von Recklinghausen (1833–1910), German pathologist]

Neurokinin-1 receptor antagonists. **Antiemetic drugs**, acting via inhibition at neurokinin-1 (NK1) receptors present in the GIT and CNS. **Aprepitant** is licensed for nausea and vomiting induced by cancer chemotherapy. Have also been studied in **PONV**.

See also, Tachykinins

Neurolepsis, *see Neuroleptanaesthesia and analgesia*

Neuroleptanaesthesia and analgesia. Use of very potent **opioid analgesic drugs** (e.g. **fentanyl** and **phenoperidine**) combined with **butyrophenones** (e.g. **droperidol** and **haloperidol**) to produce a state of reduced motor activity and passivity (neurolepsis). Introduced in 1959. The term neuroleptanaesthesia is usually restricted to the combination of opioid, butyrophenone and N_2O. Characterised by profound analgesia, **sedation** and antiemesis, with cardiovascular stability (although mild hypotension may occur). Has been used for **premedication**, sedation and as the sole anaesthetic technique for surgical procedures (now rarely employed for the latter because of prolonged recovery).

See also, Lytic cocktail

Neuroleptic malignant syndrome (NMS). Rare condition first described in 1960, characterised by altered consciousness, **hyperthermia**, autonomic dysfunction and muscle rigidity. Usually triggered by drugs (e.g. **butyrophenones**, **phenothiazines**, **metoclopramide**, **lithium**, **reserpine**), although it has been reported during withdrawal of L-dopa in patients with **Parkinson's disease**. The mechanism is thought to involve dopamine receptor blockade in the basal ganglia and **hypothalamus**. Occurs mostly in young males. Incidence is increased with dehydration, CNS disease and exhaustion.

- Features develop over 1–3 days:
  - hyperthermia and tachycardia (thought to be caused mostly by increased muscle metabolism, although a central component may be present).
  - extrapyramidal dysfunction: rigidity, dystonia, tremor.
  - autonomic dysfunction: labile BP, sweating, salivation, urinary incontinence.
  - increased creatine kinase (>1000 units/l) and white cell count.

Differential diagnosis is as for hyperthermia (in particular **MH**), Parkinson's disease, catatonia, **central anticholinergic syndrome**, **monoamine oxidase inhibitor** reaction, **serotonin syndrome** and infection, e.g. **tetanus**. Although similar to MH, NMS is generally considered an entirely separate entity.

- Management:
  - supportive: O_2, cooling, hydration, **DVT** prophylaxis.
  - increased central dopaminergic activity, e.g. with bromocriptine (dopamine agonist) 2.5–20 mg tds (orally only). **Amantadine** and L-dopa have also been used.
  - **dantrolene** and non-depolarising **neuromuscular blocking drugs** have been used to treat the peripheral muscle effects, reducing fever, rigidity and tachycardia. The latter drugs are effective in NMS, in contrast to MH.
  - **anticholinergic drugs** have also been used.

Mortality is 20%–30%, from **renal failure**, **arrhythmias**, **PE** or **aspiration pneumonitis**.

Tse L, Barr AM, Scarapichia V, Vila-Rodriguez F (2015). Curr Neuropharmacol; 13: 395–406

Neuromuscular blockade monitoring. Should be undertaken whenever non-depolarising **neuromuscular blocking drugs** are used, to reduce the risk of: (i) **awareness** e.g. if anaesthetic agents are discontinued at the end of a case without adequate reversal of neuromuscular blockade; and (ii) residual blockade/weakness in the recovery room (which may be common even after the use of intermediate-acting drugs such as **atracurium** and **vecuronium**). A nerve stimulator is used to stimulate a peripheral nerve via surface or needle electrodes; the muscle response is then assessed.

- Assessment may be:
  - qualitative i.e., visual/tactile: unreliable in practice because it is difficult to distinguish between degrees of neuromuscular blockade.
  - quantitative i.e., an actual figure (absolute, depending on the method of assessment, or expressed as a proportion of baseline): thought to be preferable in order to ensure detection of subtle degrees of blockade. May be:
    - mechanical: reflects both neuromuscular transmission and muscle contractility. May be assessed by:
      - measurement of tension developed in a muscle with a strain gauge or pressure **transducer**.
      - accelerometry: the transducer consists of a piezoelectric ceramic wafer with electrodes on both sides. Following changes in velocity, a voltage proportional to the acceleration is generated between the electrodes. Force = mass × acceleration; thus the muscle tension response may be evaluated.
    - electrical: registers the EMG response via two surface/needle electrodes. Only monitors transmission across the neuromuscular junction, and thus is more specific than mechanical assessment.
- Stimulation:
  - unipolar square waveform lasting 0.2–0.3 ms (ensures constant current during stimulation).
  - supramaximal stimulation is required to eliminate variation in muscle response caused by partial depolarisation of the nerve; this results in simultaneous depolarisation of all nerve fibres within the nerve. Required current may vary between 20 and 60 mA, and is minimised by placing the positive electrode proximally.
  - direct stimulation of the muscle should be avoided, because any response will be independent of neuromuscular blockade.
  - commonly used sites:
    - ulnar nerve: electrodes are placed along the ulnar border of the forearm, with assessment of thumb adduction. More sensitive than the diaphragm and vocal cords to neuromuscular blocking drugs.
    - facial nerve: electrodes are placed anterior to the tragus of the ear, with assessment of facial muscle contraction. Underestimation of the degree of blockade is common, because of direct muscle stimulation and relative insensitivity of the facial muscles to neuromuscular blocking drugs.
    - accessory nerve: one electrode is placed behind the mastoid process and the other at the posterior border of sternomastoid. Stimulation causes contraction of sternomastoid and trapezius muscles and is easier to see than following stimulation of the facial nerve. Asystole has followed tetanic stimulation when the upper electrode was placed anterior to the ear, attributed to stimulation of the vagus via the cranial root of the accessory nerve.
    - tibial nerve: electrodes are placed behind the medial malleolus, with assessment of big toe plantar flexion.
    - common peroneal nerve: electrodes are placed lateral to the neck of the fibula, with assessment of foot dorsiflexion.
  - patterns of stimulation:
    - single pulses (0.1–1.0 Hz).
    - tetanic stimulation (50–100 Hz) for 3–5 s. Painful in the awake patient. May be repeated every 5–10 min.
    - post-tetanic stimulation using single pulses.
    - train-of-four (TOF; four pulses at 2 Hz). TOF count is the number of palpable muscle twitches; TOF ratio is force of the fourth twitch divided by force of the first. May be repeated every 10–15 s.
    - post-tetanic count: used to assess intense blockade. Following 5 s tetanus at 50 Hz, the number of twitches produced by single pulses at 1 Hz is counted. Should not be performed more than once in 5 min.
    - double-burst stimulation: used to assess recovery from non-depolarising blockade. Two short tetanic stimulations (e.g. 50 Hz for 60 ms) are applied 750 ms apart. The second response is weaker than the first in non-depolarising blockade. More sensitive at detecting **fade** than TOF.

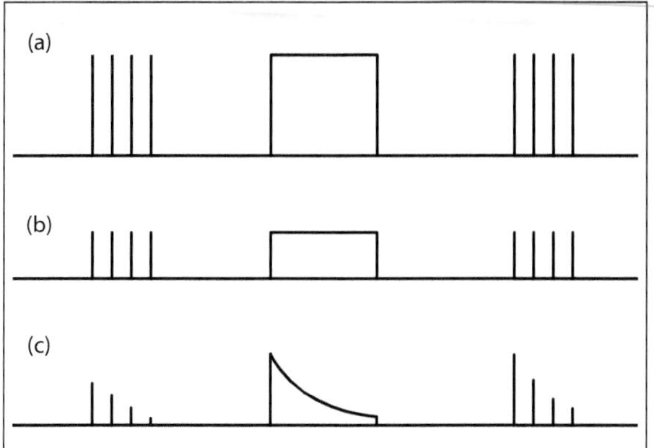

Fig. 119 EMG response to peripheral nerve stimulation in a train-of-four, tetanus, train-of-four pattern: (a) normal; (b) partial depolarising block; (c) partial non-depolarising block

- Observed responses:
  - normal neuromuscular function:
    - equal twitches in response to single pulses (Fig. 119a).
    - sustained **tetanic contraction**, with **post-tetanic potentiation** (PTP) revealed by mechanical assessment only.
  - **depolarising neuromuscular blockade**:
    - equal but reduced twitches in response to single pulses and TOF (Fig. 119b). TOF ratio thus equals 1.
    - sustained but reduced tetanic contraction, with neither fade nor PTP.
    - **dual block** may supervene if large amounts of **suxamethonium** are administered.
  - **non-depolarising neuromuscular blockade**:
    - progressively decreasing twitches in response to single pulses (Fig. 119c), with eventual disappearance.
    - tetanic contraction exhibits fade and PTP.
    - TOF: successive decrease in the four responses, with eventual disappearance of the fourth, third, second and first twitches at 75%, 80%, 90% and 100% blockade, respectively. During recovery, the twitches reappear in the reverse order. Suggested suitable values during anaesthesia:
      - TOF count of 1 for tracheal intubation.
      - TOF count of 1–2 for maintenance; deeper levels may be required for complete diaphragmatic paralysis.
      - TOF count of 3–4 before attempting reversal of blockade, especially with long-acting drugs.
      - TOF ratio (at the thumb) of 0.9 for adequate maintenance of spontaneous ventilation.
    - post-tetanic count and double-burst stimulation as above.
    - clinical assessments, e.g. the ability to sustain head lift >5 s, open the mouth, protrude the tongue, cough, maintain sustained hand grip, and achieve adequate tidal volume, vital capacity (15 ml/kg) and inspiratory pressure (–20 cm H_2O), have all been described. However, these are unreliable as they may all be possible at 50%–80% blockade (TOF ratio 0.5%–0.8%).

Naguib M, Brull SJ, Johnson KB (2017). Anaesthesia; 72(Suppl 1): 16–37

Neuromuscular blocking drugs. Drugs used to impair **neuromuscular transmission** and provide skeletal **muscle** relaxation during anaesthesia or critical care.

- May be one of two types:
  - non-depolarising: include **tubocurarine** (first used as **curare** in 1912), **gallamine** (1948), **dimethyl tubocurarine** (1948), **alcuronium** (1961), **pancuronium** (1967), **fazadinium** (1972), **atracurium** (1980), **vecuronium** (1983), **pipecuronium** (1990), **doxacurium** (1991), **mivacurium** (1993), **rocuronium** (1994), **cisatracurium** (1995) and **rapacuronium** (1999). Non-depolarising agents are competitive **antagonists** at postsynaptic **acetylcholine** (ACh) **receptors** of the **neuromuscular junction.** They are highly ionised at body pH, containing two quaternary ammonium groups (tubocurarine and vecuronium contain one each, but acquire a second following injection). Poorly lipid-soluble with variable protein binding. Following injection, the drugs are rapidly redistributed from blood to the **ECF** and other tissues, e.g. kidney, liver. The clinical effect depends on individual drug characteristics and drug concentration at the neuromuscular junction, which depends on the drug's pharmacokinetics.
  - depolarising: cause depolarisation by mimicking the action of ACh at ACh receptors, but without rapid hydrolysis by **acetylcholinesterase**. An area of depolarisation around the ACh receptor–drug complex results in local currents that open sodium channels before the continuing current flow inactivates them. Propagation of an **action potential** is prevented by the area of inexcitability that develops around the ACh receptors. Thus **fasciculations** occur before paralysis. Examples are **suxamethonium** (1951) and **decamethonium** (1948); only the former is available for clinical use in the UK.

Apart from the presence or absence of fasciculation, **non-depolarising** and **depolarising neuromuscular blockade** may be distinguished by **neuromuscular blockade monitoring**.

In general, suxamethonium is used for paralysis of rapid onset and short duration, e.g. to allow rapid tracheal intubation. The slower-acting non-depolarising drugs were traditionally used for prolonged paralysis when rapid intubation was not required, although atracurium and vecuronium, and especially rocuronium, have bridged the gap between these drugs and suxamethonium (Table 35).

See also, Interonium distance; Nicotine and nicotinic receptors

Neuromuscular junction. **Synapse** between the presynaptic motor **neurone** and the postsynaptic **muscle** membrane. On approaching the junction, the axon divides into terminal buttons that invaginate into the muscle fibre. The synaptic cleft is 50–70 nm wide and filled with ECF and a basement membrane containing high concentrations of **acetylcholinesterase.** The muscle **membrane** is folded into longitudinal gutters, whose ridges conceal orifices to secondary clefts. The orifices lie opposite the release points for **acetylcholine** (ACh) (Fig. 120).

- Three types of **acetylcholine receptor** have been identified at the neuromuscular junction:
  - postjunctional: involved in traditional **neuromuscular transmission.** Following activation of both α subunits, sodium and calcium move into the myocyte and potassium exits through specific ion channels (*see also Fig. 2b;* **Acetylcholine receptors**).
  - prejunctional: control an ion channel specific for sodium and respond to released ACh by mobilising

Table 35 Properties of neuromuscular blocking drugs

Drug	Onset time (min)	Half-life (min)	Vol. of distribution (l/kg)	Clearance (ml/kg/min)	Clinical duration of action (min)	Route of elimination	Histamine release	Autonomic effects
Alcuronium	3–5	180–200	0.1–0.3	1.5	20–40	Renal	±	–
Atracurium	1.5–2	20	0.16–0.18	5.5–6.0	20–30	Hofmann degradation + plasma hydrolysis	+	–
Cisatracurium	1–1.5	100	0.23	3.9	30–40	As for atracurium	–	–
Dimethyl tubocurarine (metocurine)	3–5	345	0.5	1.0	90–120	Renal	+	Weak ganglion blockade
Doxacurium	4–5	85–100	0.2	2.2–2.6	100–200	Renal + hepatic	–	–
Fazadinium	0.5–1.5	40–80	0.2	4.0	40–60	Renal	–	Muscarinic + ganglion blockade
Gallamine	1–2	160	0.25	1.2	20–30	Renal	–	Muscarinic blockade
Mivacurium	1.5–2	2–5	–	–	10–15	Plasma cholinesterase + hepatic	±	–
Pancuronium	2–3	120–140	0.25–0.3	1.8	40–60	Renal + hepatic	–	Weak muscarinic blockade + sympathomimetic action
Pipecuronium	2.5–3	140	0.3	2.5	90–120	Renal + hepatic	–	–
Rapacuronium	0.5–3.5	28	0.29	6–11	6–30	Renal + hepatic	++	–
Rocuronium	2	22–29	0.12–0.16	4.7–5.7	30	Hepatic	–	±
Tubocurarine	3–5	150–190	0.5–0.6	2–3	30–50	Renal + hepatic	++	Ganglion blockade
Vecuronium	1.5–2	55–70	0.27	5.2	20–30	Renal + hepatic	–	–
Suxamethonium	0.5–1.5	2.5	–	–	2–5	Plasma cholinesterase	+	Muscarinic + ganglionic stimulation

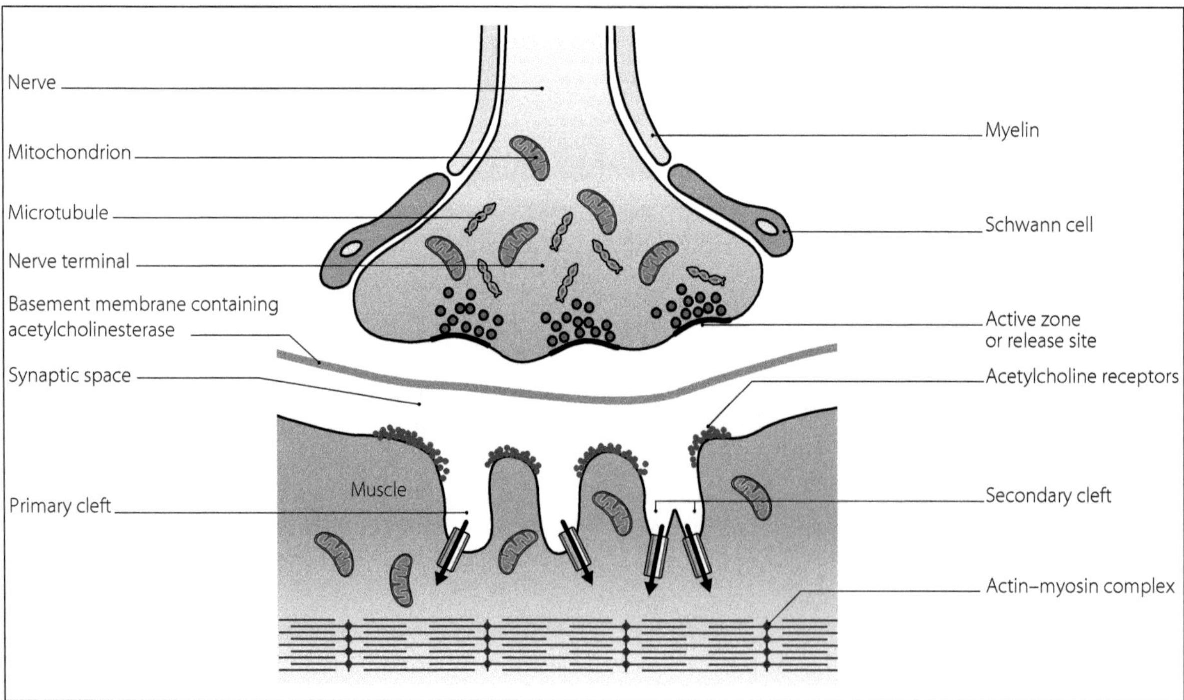

Fig. 120 Structure of neuromuscular junction

further ACh storage vesicles to the active zone of the junction, ready for release. Blockade of these receptors is thought to underlie the phenomenon of **fade** in **non-depolarising neuromuscular blockade**; activation during tetanic stimulation results in **post-tetanic potentiation**.

- extrajunctional: normally present in small numbers, but proliferate over the muscle membrane in **denervation hypersensitivity**, **burns** and certain muscle diseases.

See also, Neuromuscular blocking drugs

Neuromuscular transmission. Stages of transmission:

- depolarisation of the motor **nerve** leading to **action potential** propagation to the nerve endings at the **neuromuscular junction**.

- opening of presynaptic voltage-gated **calcium** channels. Resultant increase in intracellular calcium causes mobilisation of **acetylcholine** (ACh) vesicles to the active zone and subsequent release into the synapse.
- binding of ACh to postsynaptic nicotinic **ACh receptors**, allowing sodium and calcium ion influx and causing an **end-plate potential**. If the latter is large enough, depolarisation of the muscle membrane occurs.
- resultant action potential causing **muscle contraction**.
- hydrolysis of ACh by **acetylcholinesterase** within 1 ms.

- Transmission may be impaired by:
  - inhibition of ACh synthesis, storage or release, e.g. by **hemicholinium**, **β-bungarotoxin** and **botulinum toxins**, respectively. **Aminoglycosides** are also thought to impair ACh release, as does the **myasthenic syndrome**.
  - blockade of ACh receptors, e.g. by **neuromuscular blocking drugs**, α-bungarotoxin, receptor destruction in **myasthenia gravis**.
  - **acetylcholinesterase inhibitors**.

See also, Synapse

Neurone. Basic unit of the nervous system. Consists of:
- cell body: contains the nucleus and most of the cytoplasm. Usually at the dendritic end of the neurone. The dendritic zone is the site of integration of incoming impulses via dendrites, and of initiation of the **action potential**.
- axon: may exceed 1 metre in length. May be myelinated or unmyelinated (*see Myelin; Nerve conduction*). Anterograde and retrograde flow of organelles and proteins occurs along the axon.
- terminal buttons (**nerve** endings): situated near the cell body or dendrites of other neurones and contain **neurotransmitters**.

- Divided into classes in 1924 according to the compound action potential obtained when a mixed nerve is stimulated:
  - A: 1–20 μm diameter myelinated fibres. Subdivided into:
    - α: 70–120 m/s conduction; somatic motor and proprioception sensation.
    - β: 50–70 m/s; touch and pressure sensation.
    - γ: 30–50 m/s; motor fibres to **muscle spindles**.
    - δ: <30 m/s; **pain**, cold, touch sensation.
  - B: 1–3 μm diameter; <15 m/s conduction: myelinated preganglionic autonomic fibres.
  - C: <1 μm diameter; <2 m/s conduction: unmyelinated postganglionic autonomic fibres, and pain and temperature sensation.

Local anaesthetic agents block C fibres first, then B, then A fibres. Pressure blocks A, B and C fibres in order, and hypoxia B, A and C fibres.

- An alternative classification has been suggested:
  - I:
    - a: muscle spindles.
    - b: Golgi tendon organ.
  - II: muscle spindles, touch, pressure.
  - III: pain, cold, touch.
  - IV: pain, temperature, others.

[Camillo Golgi (1843–1926), Italian physician]

See also, Nociception

Neuropathic pain, *see Pain, neuropathic*

Neuropathy of critical illness, *see Critical illness polyneuropathy/myopathy*

Neuroradiology. Most neuroradiological procedures are painless and do not require anaesthetic intervention; sedation or anaesthesia may be required in children, unco-operative or neurologically impaired patients or for prolonged procedures. Principles are as for **radiology** and **neurosurgery**.
- Specific techniques:
  - **CT scanning.**
  - **MRI.**
  - **positron emission tomography.**
  - cerebral angiography: injection of **radiological contrast media** via femoral or carotid puncture. Hyperventilation improves the arteriogram quality by increasing cerebrovascular resistance. Complications include **stroke** (1% of patients), haemorrhage, haematoma, thrombosis, arterial spasm and bradycardia (especially during vertebral angiography).
  - myelography: injection of contrast into the thecal sac via lumbar puncture (occasionally via a cervical approach), to examine the spinal cord. Steep tilting is often required to aid spread of the contrast. Complications include headache, **convulsions** and **arachnoiditis**. Rarely performed nowadays with the widespread availability of the above imaging methods.
  - ventriculography and pneumoencephalography: injection of gas (usually air) into the ventricular system, with imaging in different positions. Bradycardia may occur. Rarely performed now.
  - therapeutic interventions:
    - embolisation: e.g. of cerebral and spinal arteriovenous malformations and cerebral aneurysms. Usually requires anticoagulation. Control of BP is essential to avoid rupture.
    - balloon angioplasty and stenting: e.g. of occlusive cerebral disease and vasospasm secondary to **subarachnoid haemorrhage**. Deliberate hypertension may be required to maintain **cerebral perfusion pressure** and avoid ischaemia.
    - carotid artery stenting for stenosis.
    - thrombolysis and thrombectomy of acute thromboembolic stroke. Cerebral haemorrhage may occur postoperatively.

Hayman MW, Paleologos MS, Kam PC (2013). Anaesth Intensive Care; 41: 184–201

Neurosurgery. Encompasses procedures involving the cranium, **brain**, **meninges**, **cranial nerves**, **spinal cord** and vertebral column, and those performed for **pain management**. Basic principles for intracranial surgery are related to maintenance of normal **cerebral perfusion pressure** and **cerebral blood flow**, with avoidance of **cerebral ischaemia**, **cerebral steal** and increased **ICP**. **Cerebral protection** techniques have been employed.
- Main considerations:
  - preoperatively:
    - **preoperative assessment** of neurological status, **hydrocephalus**, etc. Endocrine abnormalities may be present (e.g. **pituitary gland** surgery).
    - fluid and electrolyte imbalance may be present, especially if associated with reduced oral intake and **vomiting**.
    - **hypertension** may be present, especially in association with **subarachnoid haemorrhage**.

- drug therapy may include **anticonvulsant drugs** and **corticosteroids.**
- other injuries may accompany **head injury**.
- sedative **premedication** is usually avoided because of possible perioperative respiratory depression and decreased level of consciousness.

- perioperatively:
  - iv **induction of anaesthesia** is usual; most **iv anaesthetic agents** are suitable apart from **ketamine**. Smooth induction avoiding **hypoxaemia, hypercapnia**, hypertension and tachycardia is required. **Hyperkalaemia** has followed **suxamethonium** in certain upper and lower **motor neurone** lesions. **β-Adrenergic receptor antagonists** may be given to reduce the hypertensive response to laryngoscopy, whereas **lidocaine** 0.5–1.5 mg/kg may be given iv to reduce the increase in ICP. Adequate time should be allowed for full paralysis before tracheal intubation is attempted. Lidocaine spray may be employed during **laryngoscopy**. Use of a reinforced **tracheal tube** is usual, with thorough fixation. The eyes and face should be protected with padding.
  - a large-bore iv cannula is necessary, because blood loss may be considerable. **CVP** measurement may be required, especially if the patient is to be positioned sitting. **Arterial cannulation** is usual. End-tidal CO_2 measurement, pulse **oximetry, ECG** and **temperature measurement** are mandatory. **Neuromuscular blockade monitoring** is especially useful, because inadequate paralysis may have disastrous results. **ICP monitoring, evoked potentials** and **EEG** derivatives are sometimes employed.
  - permissive hypothermia (to 35°C) is increasingly popular in an attempt to reduce **cerebral metabolism.**
  - perioperative problems include:
    - those related to **positioning of the patient**. The supine position is common; others include:
      - lateral/prone: vena caval obstruction and damage to the face, eyes, etc., may occur.
      - sitting (for posterior fossa lesions): **gas embolism**, hypotension and obstruction of neck veins may occur. The first two may be reduced by the **antigravity suit, PEEP** and administration of iv fluids.
    - inaccessibility of the airway.
    - those of prolonged surgery, e.g. **heat loss**, fluid balance.
    - acute control of ICP.
    - **arrhythmias** and cardiovascular instability during manipulation of **brainstem** structures (posterior fossa lesions).
  - maintenance is usually with air/O_2 mixture with a volatile **inhalational anaesthetic agent** (e.g. **isoflurane** or **sevoflurane**) with or without a short-acting opioid, e.g. **fentanyl, remifentanil.** N_2O is usually avoided because it increases cerebral blood flow and ICP and because of the risk of expansion of a pneumoencephalocoele. **TIVA** is also used. An arterial $P\text{CO}_2$ of 4.5–5.0 (35–40 mmHg) is considered optimal.
  - **hypotensive anaesthesia** is sometimes employed, especially for vascular lesions.
  - bradycardia may follow application of suction to intracranial and extracranial drains.
  - some procedures involving **CT scanning** (e.g. stereotactic surgery) require moving the anaesthetised patient between operating and imaging rooms.
  - local anaesthetic techniques may also be used (e.g. for awake craniotomy). Once the skull and dura are opened, there is usually little discomfort and the patient's neurological state is easily monitored.
- postoperatively:
  - tracheal **extubation** is usually possible at the end of surgery and is performed under deep anaesthesia; coughing or straining should be avoided. Elective IPPV may be required, e.g. following prolonged operations and when ICP is critically raised. **Airway obstruction** caused by acute swelling of the tongue has been reported following posterior fossa surgery.
  - close observation is required, in case of bleeding, vasospasm, increased ICP, **convulsions**, hypotension or hypertension. The **Glasgow coma scale** is employed for monitoring progress. ICP monitoring may be used.
  - the patient should be kept normothermic to prevent postoperative **shivering.**
  - **morphine** is a suitable choice for postoperative analgesia.
  - **diabetes insipidus** or the **syndrome of inappropriate antidiuretic hormone secretion** may occur.
  - increased risk of **DVT** has been associated with neurosurgery. In the immediate postoperative period mechanical methods of prophylaxis are usually preferred to **heparin** due to the potentially catastrophic effects of postoperative bleeding.

See also, Spinal surgery

Neurotransmitters. Substances secreted from presynaptic nerve endings, which act at the postsynaptic **membrane** to cause excitatory or inhibitory effects. Act via specific receptors that elicit intracellular effects (e.g. by opening membrane ion channels, activating intracellular enzymes or altering DNA transcription). The same neurotransmitter may be excitatory at one **synapse**, and inhibitory at another.

- Examples:
  - amines, e.g. **noradrenaline, adrenaline, dopamine, 5-HT, histamine.**
  - **amino acids**, e.g. **glycine, glutamate, GABA**, aspartate.
  - polypeptides, e.g. **substance P, enkephalins.** Substances active as circulating hormones may also function as neurotransmitters, e.g. **vasopressin, oxytocin, vasoactive intestinal peptide, glucagon, somatostatin.**
  - others, e.g. **acetylcholine, nitric oxide.**

In general, acetylcholine and the amino acids are involved with fast point-to-point signalling whereas the polypeptides, amines and nitric oxide have a slower, more diffuse regulatory function. More than one neurotransmitter may be secreted by one neurone, e.g. vasoactive intestinal peptide is often secreted with acetylcholine, and is thought to potentiate the latter's actions. Amines are often secreted with peptide neurotransmitters.

See also, Neuromuscular junction; Receptor theory; Synaptic transmission

Neutral thermal range, *see Thermoneutral range*

Never Events. Defined as 'serious incidents that are wholly preventable as guidance or safety recommendations that provide strong systemic protective barriers are available at a national level and should have been implemented by all healthcare providers'. Although they may result in serious harm or death, these are not required for the incident to be categorised as a Never Event. Those with anaesthetic implications include:

- wrong-site surgery, regional anaesthetic block or line insertion.
- retained foreign object post-procedure, e.g. swabs, needles, guide-wires.
- accidental administration of strong **potassium**-containing solution.
- wrong-route administration of drug.
- overdose of **insulin** due to errors over units or incorrect syringe, etc.
- overdose of **midazolam** during sedation due to use of incorrect strength of solution.
- misplaced naso-/orogastric tubes (*see Nasogastric intubation*).

Never Events are reported and counted centrally, with possible financial and/or regulatory punishment of organisations responsible. The terminology and process have been criticised as Never Events may represent rare, random events, rather than an indicator of the quality of care.

Moppett IK, Moppett SH (2016). Anaesthesia; 71: 17–30

See also, Critical incidents

New injury severity score, *see Injury severity score*

New York Heart Association classification. Method of assessment of cardiac function, originally introduced in 1928 for classification of **cardiac failure** but now often used for functional classification of cardiac disease in general, e.g. in **preoperative assessment**:

- class I: no functional limitation.
- class II: slight functional limitation. Fatigue, palpitations, dyspnoea or angina on ordinary physical activity, but asymptomatic at rest.
- class III: marked functional limitation. Symptoms on less than ordinary activity, but asymptomatic at rest.
- class IV: inability to perform any physical activity, with or without symptoms at rest.

Newton. Unit of **force**. 1 N is the force required to accelerate a **mass** of 1 kg by 1 m/s^2.

[Sir Isaac Newton (1643–1727), English physicist]

Newtonian fluids, *see Fluids*

NGF, *see Nerve growth factor*

NIAA, *see National Institute of Academic Anaesthesia*

Nicardipine hydrochloride. Calcium channel blocking drug, used for treatment of hypertension (especially short-term) and ischaemic heart disease.

- Dosage:
  - angina: 20–30 mg orally tds (30–60 mg slow-release bd).
  - acute hypertensive crisis, e.g. postoperative: 3–5 mg/h for 15 min IV, increased by 0.5–1.0 mg/h every 15 min according to response up to 15 mg/h. Has been used in pregnancy: 1–5 mg/h adjusted by 0.5 mg/h after 30 min.
- Side effects: headache, vomiting, hypotension, tachycardia, oedema, GIT upset.

The iv preparation is incompatible with bicarbonate and Hartmann's solutions.

NICE, *see National Institute for Health and Care Excellence*

NiCO. Commercial non-invasive **cardiac output measurement** system that employs partial CO_2 rebreathing and the **Fick principle** to estimate cardiac output. A small rebreathing loop is inserted into the patient's breathing circuit and intermittently increases the volume of the circuit. Concentration and flow of CO_2 are measured by a sensor placed between the patient and the rebreathing loop. The change in cardiac output is proportional to the ratio of the change in CO_2 elimination and the resulting change in end-expiratory CO_2.

Nicorandil. Potassium channel activator with a nitrate component, used to prevent and treat angina. Causes arterial and venous vasodilatation. Peak plasma levels occur within 30–60 min of administration. Only slightly protein-bound.

- Dosage: 5–10 mg orally bd, increased up to 40 mg bd.
- Side effects: headache, vomiting, dizziness, hypotension.

Nicotine. Toxic alkaloid derived from tobacco; mimics certain actions of **acetylcholine**, and was used to investigate the physiology of the **autonomic nervous system**. At low doses, it stimulates postsynaptic nicotinic **acetylcholine receptors** of the **neuromuscular junction**, autonomic ganglia and adrenal medulla; at high doses, it blocks them. Also causes CNS stimulation, followed by depression.

See also, Smoking

Nifedipine. Dihydropyridine **calcium channel blocking drug**, affecting coronary and peripheral vascular smooth muscle more than myocardial muscle. Negative inotropic effect is usually insignificant because of **baroreceptor**-mediated tachycardia.

Has no antiarrhythmic action. Used in **hypertension**, **ischaemic heart disease** and Raynaud's phenomenon. Also used (unlicensed) as a tocolytic drug. Active within 20–30 min of oral administration, but a faster response follows sublingual retention of the capsule's contents (though not licensed for sublingual use). May thus be administered sublingually during anaesthesia. 95% protein-bound. **Half-life** is 3–5 h. Metabolised in the liver and excreted renally. A combined preparation with **atenolol** is also available.

- Dosage:
  - 5–20 mg orally bd/tds. Long-acting formulations are also available: 10–90 mg od.
  - 100–200 μg may be infused into the coronary arteries, e.g. for spasm during coronary angiography.
- Side effects: headache, flushing, dizziness, GIT disturbance, peripheral oedema.

[Maurice Raynaud (1834–1881), French physician]

Nimodipine. Dihydropyridine **calcium channel blocking drug**, preferentially affecting cerebral vascular smooth muscle. Increases **cerebral blood flow**, especially to poorly perfused areas, e.g. those affected by arterial spasm following **subarachnoid haemorrhage** (SAH). Prophylactic use following SAH decreases ischaemic neurological events

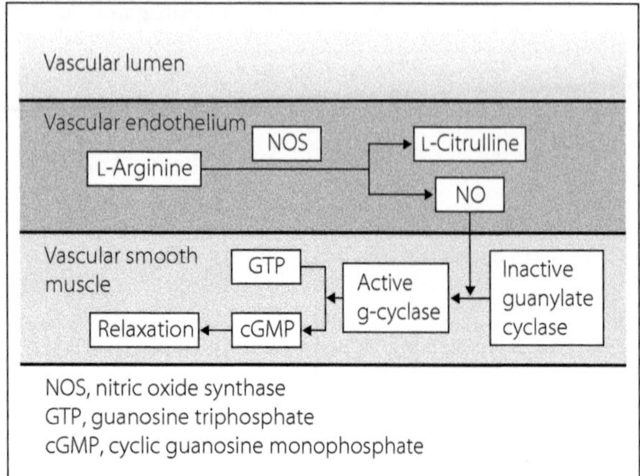

Fig. 121 Synthesis and action of nitric oxide (NO)

(probably by blocking calcium uptake into damaged neurones) and improves overall outcome.

- Dosage:
  - prophylactically following SAH: 60 mg orally 4-hourly for 21 days.
  - in established vasospasm: 0.5–1.0 mg/h iv, increased to 2 mg/h after 2 h if BP is stable. Continued for 5–14 days.
- Side effects: hypotension, flushing. Should be used with care in raised **ICP**.

Reacts with PVC infusion tubing; polypropylene and polyethylene are suitable. May be degraded by light.

NIPPV, *see Non-invasive positive pressure ventilation*

NIRS, *see Near infrared spectroscopy*

NISS, New injury severity score, *see Injury severity score*

Nitrazepam. **Benzodiazepine** widely used as a hypnotic drug. Has also been used as an anticonvulsant in childhood myoclonic **epilepsy**. Onset of sleep occurs within an hour; duration of action is 4–8 h. Extensively protein-bound; elimination **half-life** is up to 30 h, resulting in hangover effects during the day.

- Dosage: 5–10 mg orally at night.
- Side effects: disorientation, confusion, drowsiness. Dependence may occur.

Nitric oxide (NO). Oxide of **nitrogen**, active as a biological mediator throughout the body but especially in:

- vascular endothelium: responsible for vascular relaxation. Reduced production has been implicated in vasospasm associated with various disease states, e.g. **diabetes mellitus**, **hypertension** and following **subarachnoid haemorrhage**. NO is thought to be the effector molecule for all nitrate **vasodilator drugs**.
- brain tissue: acts as a **neurotransmitter**.
- macrophages: involved in the response to infection.
- **platelets**: involved in aggregation and adhesion.

Synthesised in endothelial cells during the oxidation of L-arginine to L-citrulline, the reaction being catalysed by NO synthase (NOS). The NO thus produced diffuses into vascular smooth muscle and converts inactive guanylate cyclase into the active form; the latter converts guanosine triphosphate into cyclic guanosine monophosphate, which causes vascular relaxation (Fig. 121). Two forms of NOS exist: the constitutive (endothelial) form, present in vascular and brain tissue, which produces small quantities of NO continuously (eNOS); and the inducible form, present in macrophages (iNOS).

NO has a biological **half-life** of <5 s, its action being terminated by combining with **haemoglobin** to form methaemoglobin.

In **sepsis**, activation of iNOS in various tissues results in overproduction of NO; although this increases bacterial destruction, it also leads to profound vasodilatation, activation of inflammatory cascades and decreased myocardial function. Although non-selective inhibitors of NOS increase mean arterial pressure, they tend to increase pulmonary artery pressure and reduce cardiac output; no overall survival benefits have been demonstrated.

Medical NO is produced by the reaction of nitric acid and sulfur dioxide ($2HNO_3 + 3SO_2 + 2H_2O \rightarrow 2NO + 3H_2SO_4$), followed by purification. It is supplied in aluminium cylinders containing 800 ppm. A colourless gas with a slight odour, ~2.5 times denser than air, NO is converted to the brown nitrogen dioxide (NO_2) on exposure to air; in water, it forms nitrous acid (HNO_3). It is administered clinically via specially designed gas delivery systems.

In neonatal, paediatric or adult **pulmonary hypertension**, inhaled NO (1–150 ppm) has been used to produce selective pulmonary vasodilatation without systemic effects. Rebound pulmonary hypertension may occur upon cessation (necessitating gradual weaning). A clear effect on outcome in **ALI** has not been conclusively demonstrated.

Measured in gaseous form using a chemiluminescence reaction (NO + ozone $\rightarrow O_2 + NO_2$ + light) or electroanalysis using a specific electrode. Levels in tissues are measured using electron paramagnetic resonance or fluorescence spectroscopy.

Occupational limits for exposure are limited to 25 ppm (30 mg/m^3) over 8 h.

See also, Nitrogen, higher oxides of

Nitrogen. Non-metallic element existing in the atmosphere as a colourless, odourless 'inert' gas (isolated in 1772). Forms 78.03% of atmospheric **air**. Atomic weight is 14; boiling point is –195°C. Obtained by fractional distillation of air. Reacts poorly with other substances. Blood/gas **solubility coefficient** is 0.014. Has anaesthetic properties at hyperbaric pressures (*see Inert gas narcosis*). Converted into organic compounds by nitrifying bacteria and plants, and present throughout the body in **amino acids** and **proteins**.

See also, Nitrogen balance; Nitrogen washout

Nitrogen balance. Difference between the amount of nitrogen ingested (as **amino acids** or **proteins**) and the amount of nitrogen excreted (mainly urinary). Usually measured within a 24-h period. Negative if losses exceed intake, e.g. **catabolism**, starvation; positive if intake exceeds losses, e.g. during recovery from severe illness.

- Estimated thus:
  - intake = the nitrogen content of all food/fluid intake.
  - output = the sum of nitrogen losses calculated from the following three components:
    - from urinary urea: nitrogen (g/24 h) = urea (mmol/24 h) × 6/5 because 1/6 is excreted as substances other than urea
      × 1/1000 to convert mmol to mol
      × 60 to convert mol urea to g
      × 28/60 to convert g urea to g nitrogen
      i.e., urea (mmol/24 h) × 0.0336.

- from blood urea: nitrogen (g/24 h) = change in urea (mmol/l/24 h) × 1/1000
  × 60
  × 28/60 as earlier
  × 60% × body weight (kg) because urea is distributed among total body water
  i.e., change in urea (mmol/l/24 h) × 0.0168 × body weight
- from other routes of loss, e.g. proteinuria: nitrogen loss (g/24 h) = protein loss (g/24 h)
  × 1/6.25 because 6.25 g protein contains 1 g nitrogen.

Other losses occur from sweat and faeces (e.g. 2–4 g/l GIT fistula fluid lost per 24 h).

Calculation is a useful guide to appropriate nutrition in critical illness. A normal adult requires about 0.15 g N/kg/day; this may double in severe sepsis.

See also, Energy balance

Nitrogen, higher oxides of. **Nitric oxide** (NO), nitrogen dioxide (NO_2) and nitrogen trioxide (N_2O_3); the latter decomposes to form NO and NO_2. NO reacts with O_2, forming NO_2, which dissolves in water to form nitrous and nitric acids. The gases are produced during some fires, during manufacture of **N_2O**, and in the metal industry. Irritant if inhaled, they cause mild upper airway symptoms initially but **pulmonary oedema** several hours after initial recovery. Severe pulmonary fibrotic destruction may follow 2–3 weeks later. Formation of nitrates in the body may result in vasodilatation and hypotension, and cause **methaemoglobinaemia.** Treatment is supportive. Contamination of some N_2O cylinders in 1967 in the UK led to their widespread recall. May be tested for using moistened starch iodide paper, which turns blue on exposure. NO is involved in intercellular signalling and control of vascular tone.

See also, Smoke inhalation

Nitrogen narcosis, *see Inert gas narcosis*

Nitrogen washout. Elimination of nitrogen from the lungs while breathing non-nitrogen containing gas. During successive breaths, the concentration of nitrogen exhaled falls as an **exponential process**, falling to about 2.5% after 7 min in normal patients. During anaesthesia using **circle systems**, 7–10 min high fresh gas flow is required to remove most body nitrogen. Elimination is prolonged if ventilation is distributed unevenly (*see later*).

- Tests employing nitrogen washout:
  - measure of **FRC**.
  - single-breath nitrogen washout (**Fowler's method**).
  - multiple-breath nitrogen washout: the patient breathes 100% O_2, with nitrogen measurement at the lips. Log nitrogen concentration is plotted against number of breaths. If lung ventilation is uniform, expired nitrogen concentration decreases by the same fraction with each breath, as demonstrated by a straight line on the graph. A curved line is obtained if ventilation is uneven, as nitrogen is quickly washed out from well-ventilated alveoli but only slowly from poorly ventilated ones (Fig. 122).

Nitroglycerin, *see Glyceryl trinitrate*

Nitroprusside, *see Sodium nitroprusside*

Nitrous oxide (N_2O). **Inhalational anaesthetic agent**, first isolated by **Priestley** in 1772. Suggested as being a

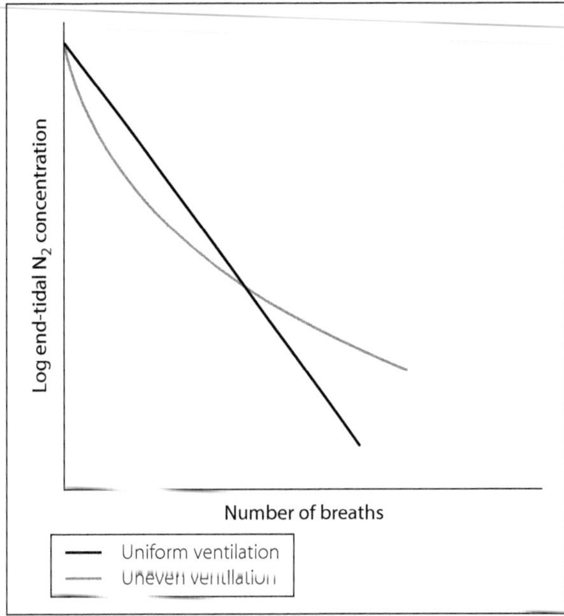

Fig. 122 Multiple-breath nitrogen washout

useful analgesic by **Davy** in 1799; first used for dental extraction by **Wells** in 1844 but superseded by **diethyl ether**. Reintroduced by **Colton** in 1863.

Manufactured by heating ammonium nitrate to 240°C and removing impurities (e.g. higher oxides of nitrogen, ammonia and nitric acid) by passage through scrubbers and washers. Water vapour is also removed.

- Properties:
  - colourless, slightly sweet-smelling gas, 1.53 times denser than air.
  - mw 44.
  - boiling point −88°C.
  - **critical temperature** 36.5°C.
  - **partition coefficients**:
    - blood/gas 0.47.
    - oil/gas 1.4.
  - **MAC** 105%.
  - non-flammable but supports combustion, breaking down to O_2 and nitrogen at high temperatures.
  - supplied as a liquid/gas in French blue **cylinders** with **pin index** positions 3 and 5: pressure is 40 bar at 15°C and 54 bar at room temperature. Ice often forms on the cylinder during use because of **latent heat** of vaporisation. Also supplied as gaseous **Entonox**.
- Effects:
  - CNS:
    - fast onset and recovery; strongly analgesic but weakly anaesthetic. Analgesic actions are through release of proenkephalin in the CNS.
    - increases **cerebral metabolism, cerebral blood flow** and **ICP** slightly.
    - has inhibitory effects at **NMDA receptors**; stimulatory at **opioid** and **adrenergic receptors**.
  - RS:
    - non-irritant. Depresses respiration slightly.
    - may cause diffusion hypoxia (**Fink effect**) at the end of surgery.
  - CVS: little effect on heart rate and BP usually, although it decreases myocardial contractility, especially when combined with volatile agents or opioids.

- GIT: the ENIGMA I trial showed N_2O causes significant **PONV**; possible causes include expansion of gas-containing bowel or inner ear cavities or a direct central effect (possibly via **opioid receptors**). It also showed an increased in risk in wound infection. The ENIGMA II trial showed that the increase in PONV can be largely negated by treatment with **antiemetic drugs**; it also contradicted the wound infection findings of the first trial.
- other:
  - does not affect hepatic or renal function, nor uterine or skeletal muscle tone.
  - interacts with **methionine** synthase by oxidising the cobalt ion in its cofactor vitamin B_{12}; prolonged use (12–24 h) may cause bone marrow depression, megaloblastic **anaemia** and **peripheral neuropathy**. Implicated in causing fetal abnormalities and spontaneous abortion, but no direct evidence exists. Generally considered as being safe during pregnancy.
  - expands air-filled cavities because it is over 40 times as soluble as nitrogen; thus passes from the blood into the cavity faster than the nitrogen can diffuse out. Can double the size of a **pneumothorax** in 10 min at 70%. Also expands **gas embolism** and may cause pneumoencephalocoele following **neurosurgery**.

Excreted unchanged from the lungs; a small amount diffuses through the skin.

Traditionally, commonly used for analgesia (above 20%) and as a carrier gas for other inhalational agents and O_2, usually in concentrations of 50%–66%. Although weakly anaesthetic and rarely adequate alone, it reduces the requirement for other agents. Its adverse effects and concern about its effects on the environment have led to a reduction in its use and replacement by air, although its recreational use is increasing.

Also used in the **cryoprobe**.

Brown SM, Sneyd JR (2016). BJA Educ; 16: 87–91

See also, Environmental safety of anaesthetists; Nitrogen, higher oxides of; Pollution; Relative analgesia

NIV, Non-invasive ventilation, *see Non-invasive positive pressure ventilation*

Nizatidine. **H_2 receptor antagonist** used in **peptic ulcer disease**; similar to **cimetidine** but does not cause **enzyme inhibition.** Well absorbed orally, it is 40% protein-bound, with 90% excreted by the kidneys.

- Dosage:
  - 150–300 mg orally od/bd.
  - 100 mg iv over 15 min tds, or 10 mg/h iv up to 480 mg/day.
- Side effects: as for **ranitidine**.

NMDA receptors, *see N-Methyl-D-aspartate receptors*

NMJ, *see Neuromuscular junction*

NMR, Nuclear magnetic resonance, *see Magnetic resonance imaging*

NO, *see Nitric oxide*

No reflow phenomenon. Reduction in organ blood flow following a period of ischaemia or infarction, without mechanical vessel obstruction. Has been observed affecting the heart and brain, e.g. after **MI/myocardial ischaemia** and **stroke/cerebral ischaemia**, respectively. The aetiology is unclear but small vessel vasospasm, endothelial oedema or extrinsic compression by tissue oedema, increased blood **viscosity**, **platelet** aggregation and venous congestion have all been suggested. Treatment has been aimed at all these factors, with varying degrees of success.

Durante A, Camici PG (2015). Int J Cardiol; 187: 273–80

Nociceptin, *see Orphanin FQ*

Nociception. The neural process of encoding noxious stimuli, i.e., associated with injury or threatened injury.

- Occurs via specialised **nerve** endings (nociceptors) of certain **neurones**:
  - C-fibres: respond to heat, mechanical and chemical stimuli, giving rise to **pain.** Action potentials generated by these stimuli are thought to be generated via the transient receptor potential vanilloid receptor-1 (TRPV1) receptor channels.

    They also respond to endogenous pain-producing substances, e.g. **bradykinin**, **histamine** and potassium ions. Because of their responsiveness to many stimuli, they are also known as 'polymodal nociceptors'.
  - Aδ-fibres:
    - type I: respond to heat and mechanical stimuli, with high threshold. Thought to give rise to pain from long-standing stimuli.
    - type II: respond to heat and mechanical stimuli, with fast response and low threshold. Thought to give rise to initial pain sensation.
    - receptors responding to cold and mechanical stimuli, thought to give rise to pain associated with cold.

Other types may also exist. Although initially described and most abundant in skin, they also exist in other tissues, e.g. muscle, joints, teeth. Injury increases their response and sensitivity.

Dubin AE, Patapoutian A (2010). J Clin Invest; 120: 3760–72

See also, Pain; Pain pathways

Nodal arrhythmias, *see Junctional arrhythmias*

Non-depolarising neuromuscular blockade. Caused by competitive antagonism of **acetylcholine** (ACh) by non-depolarising **neuromuscular blocking drugs** at the **ACh receptors** of the **neuromuscular junction.** The end-plate potential produced by ACh diminishes as receptor occupancy by the neuromuscular blocking drug increases; when it fails to reach the threshold for depolarisation, **neuromuscular transmission** fails. This only occurs when >80%–90% of ACh receptors are blocked, demonstrating the wide margin of safety of neuromuscular transmission.

- Features:
  - absence of **fasciculation** following administration of drug.
  - exhibits **fade** and **post-tetanic potentiation.**
  - antagonised by **acetylcholinesterase inhibitors.**
  - potentiated by **aminoglycosides**, volatile **inhalational anaesthetic agents**, **acidosis**, electrolyte disturbances (especially **hypokalaemia**, **hypermagnesaemia**, **hypocalcaemia**), **myasthenia gravis**, **myasthenic syndrome.**

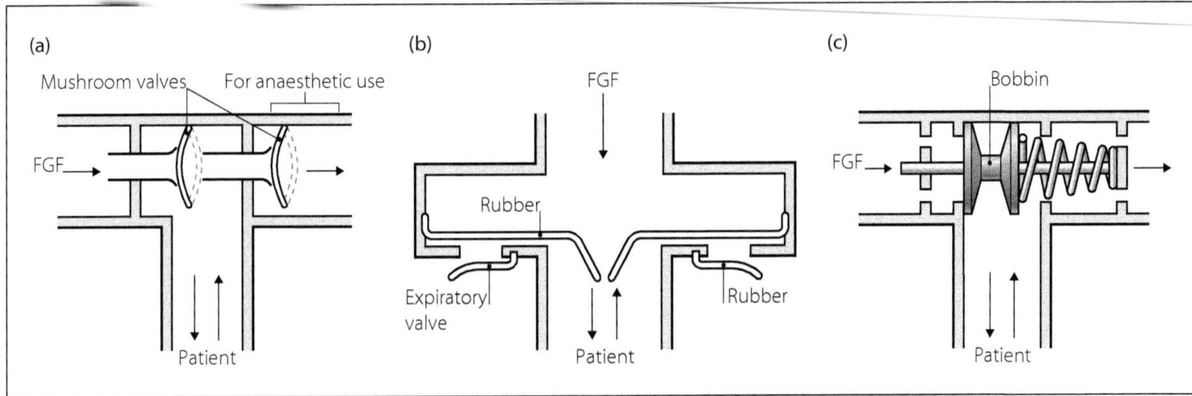

Fig. 123 Examples of non-rebreathing valves: (a) Ambu-E; (b) Laerdal; (c) Ruben. *FGF,* fresh gas flow

Blockade may also be potentiated by excess drug at the neuromuscular junction, e.g. caused by overdose, or reduced metabolism, excretion or muscle blood flow.
See also, Neuromuscular blockade monitoring; Priming principle

Non-invasive positive pressure ventilation. An alternative to **IPPV** via **tracheal tube**, positive pressure ventilation may be applied via a tightly fitting nasal mask, full facial mask, nasal 'pillows' that fit into the nostrils, or a 'helmet' that encloses the whole head. Ventilators may deliver a set volume or, more commonly, a set pressure. Uses include: ventilatory support in acute **respiratory failure** (especially exacerbations of **COPD** and cardiogenic **pulmonary oedema**); facilitation of extubation/**weaning from ventilators**; support for patients requiring nocturnal IPPV (e.g. central **sleep apnoea**, neuromuscular disorders); and palliation in end-stage respiratory disease.

- Indications for use in the acute setting:
  - increased dyspnoea, tachypnoea and **work of breathing**.
  - acute respiratory **acidosis**.
  - hypoxaemia despite conventional **oxygen therapy**.
- Contraindications:
  - inadequate mask fit, unco-operative patient.
  - haemodynamic instability, ongoing **myocardial ischaemia**.
  - inability to protect airway (e.g. reduced conscious level, bulbar failure).
  - recent upper GIT/respiratory tract surgery.

BIPAP (bi-level positive airway pressure) refers to a technique in which two levels of positive pressure are provided during inspiration and expiration. Airflow in the patient circuit is sensed by a **transducer** and augmented with a preset level of positive pressure. Cycling between inspiratory and expiratory modes may be triggered by the patient's spontaneous breaths or according to a preset rate (cycling either fully automatically or only if the patient fails to take a spontaneous breath within a certain time period). **CPAP** may also be delivered in either mode. BIPAP may also be administered via an oral mask.

Disadvantages and complications include discomfort, gastric distension, vomiting and **aspiration of gastric contents**, and pressure necrosis, e.g. to the bridge of the nose.

Non-parametric tests, *see Data; Statistical tests*

Non-rebreathing valves. Prevent exhaled gas from passing upstream from the patient in **anaesthetic breathing systems**, thus almost eliminating rebreathing (but reducing efficiency because **dead space** gas is wasted). Most commonly used in **draw-over techniques** and for **CPR** with **self-inflating bags**. Also used in **demand valves**. For use with a fixed fresh gas supply, a reservoir bag is required unless fresh gas flow rate exceeds peak inspiratory flow rate. Should be placed as near to the patient as possible, e.g. attached directly to the facemask/tracheal tube.

- Valves may be designed for either spontaneous ventilation or IPPV; commonly used ones may be used for both, and include:
  - Ambu-E valve (Fig. 123a): contains silicone rubber flaps (mushroom valves) within a clear plastic housing. Those designed for CPR contain one mushroom valve; those for anaesthetic use contain a second distal one to prevent in-drawing of room air.
  - Laerdal valve (Fig. 123b): contains a circular silicone rubber internal valve and a ring-shaped rubber expiratory valve.
  - Ruben valve (Fig. 123c): contains a bobbin that is held against the upstream port by a spring at rest and moved downstream by gas flow during inspiration.

Malfunction (e.g. due to condensation of water vapour) may cause sticking of the valve or rebreathing. **Barotrauma** may occur if high internal pressure holds the expiratory port closed, e.g. during apnoea with high fresh gas flow.
[Ambu: from ambulant, Danish for movable; Asmund S Laerdal (1913–1981), Norwegian businessman and manufacturer; Henning M Ruben (1914–2004), Danish anaesthetist]

Non-steroidal anti-inflammatory drugs (NSAIDs). Group of chemically dissimilar compounds with anti-inflammatory, antipyretic and analgesic actions. Widely used for mild pain (e.g. musculoskeletal disease, headache, dysmenorrhoea), inflammatory disorders and **postoperative analgesia** (reducing total opioid requirements). Individual responses to NSAIDs are variable.

- Classified into:
  - salicylic acids: e.g. **aspirin**, diflunisal.
  - propionic acids: e.g. **flurbiprofen, ibuprofen, ketoprofen, naproxen**, fenoprofen.
  - acetic acids: e.g. **diclofenac, indometacin**.
  - fenamates (anthranilic acid derivatives): mefenamic acid, tolfenamic acid.

 - oxicams (enolic acid derivatives): e.g. **piroxicam**, **tenoxicam**, meloxicam.
 - pyrroles: e.g. **ketorolac** (also included under acetic acids).

Effects are via inhibition of **cyclo-oxygenase**, resulting in reduced **prostaglandin**, **prostacyclin** and **thromboxane** production (*see Fig. 14;* **Arachidonic acid**). Inhibitors of cyclo-oxygenase-2 (COX-2) (e.g. **parecoxib**, celecoxib) have been produced for their relative lack of GIT side effects; several have since been withdrawn for their association with increased risk of MI in susceptible patients, thought to be due to unequal inhibition of prostacyclin and thromboxane synthesis (*see later*).

- Side effects:
  - GIT disturbance, e.g. nausea, discomfort, diarrhoea, bleeding and ulceration (for the non-selective NSAIDs, the risks are greatest with azapropazone (a pyrazolone, now obsolete) and least with ibuprofen; piroxicam, ketorolac, naproxen, indometacin and diclofenac are intermediate. The selective COX-2 inhibitors are associated with a lower risk than non-selective NSAIDs). If either type is to be used long term, NICE suggests concomitant use of **proton pump inhibitors**.
  - cardiovascular effects: both selective and non-selective agents are associated with an increased risk of myocardial infarction and coronary death. The risks appear highest for COX-2 inhibitors and diclofenac and increase with increasing dose. All NSAIDs cause a dose-dependent rise in blood pressure.
  - **stroke**: the most recent meta-analysis of randomised controlled trials shows no increased risk with either COX-2 or high-dose non-selective NSAIDs.
  - renal impairment (may occur with both selective and non-selective NSAIDs); may arise from:
    - renal hypoperfusion: especially common in patients with sodium depletion (e.g. those taking **diuretics**), **hypovolaemia** or pre-existing renal disease. Results from inhibition of protective prostaglandin-mediated renal vasodilatation; usually occurs soon after administration of the NSAID, in most cases with recovery following discontinuation. May progress to acute tubular necrosis.
    - acute interstitial nephritis: typically occurs after chronic administration, with slow recovery in most cases after discontinuation. Has also been reported after acute perioperative use. **Acute kidney injury** may result, usually associated with severe proteinuria. **Corticosteroids** have been suggested as being helpful.
    - systemic vasculitis (rare) leading to **glomerulonephritis** and papillary necrosis.
  - decreased **platelet** function and impaired **coagulation**. Although platelet dysfunction has been shown after perioperative use, bleeding problems are rare, although care is required if other drugs with anticoagulant actions are co-prescribed, e.g. prophylactic **heparin**. Selective COX-2 inhibitors may be associated with an increased incidence of cardiovascular side effects as above.
  - non-selective agents may exacerbate **asthma**.
  - **adverse drug reactions** are common (cross-sensitivity may occur between different drugs).
  - others, e.g. fluid retention, **hyperkalaemia** and metabolic **acidosis** (via inhibition of renin secretion with resultant hypoaldosteronism), rarely hepatotoxicity. NSAIDs have been implicated in reducing bone healing after fractures, leading some orthopaedic surgeons to suggest they should be avoided perioperatively, but the evidence is weak and they continue to be used widely.

Should be used cautiously if there is a risk of increased perioperative bleeding or renal impairment (the latter, for instance, in the elderly, diabetics, and after cardiac, hepatobiliary, renal or major vascular surgery) or sensitivity to aspirin.

Day RO, Graham GG (2013). Br Med J; 346: f3195

Noradrenaline (Norepinephrine). **Catecholamine**, the immediate precursor of **adrenaline** (differing by one methyl group on the terminal amine). A **neurotransmitter** in the **sympathetic nervous system**, **ascending reticular activating system** and **hypothalamus**. Also a hormone, forming about 20% of the catecholamines released from the adrenal medulla.

Predominantly stimulates **α-adrenergic receptors** (non-selectively), although with some β_1-receptor stimulation. After secretion, 80% is taken up by postganglionic sympathetic nerve endings for reuse (uptake$_1$); the remainder is metabolised by **catechol-*O*-methyltransferase** and **monoamine oxidase** or taken up by other cells, e.g. vascular smooth muscle (uptake$_2$).

Used as an **inotropic drug** when **SVR** is low, e.g. in **sepsis**. An extremely potent **vasopressor drug**, it increases both systolic and diastolic arterial BP via arterial and venous vasoconstriction. There may be compensatory bradycardia caused by **baroreceptor reflex** activation. Coronary perfusion is increased but with increased myocardial O_2 demand. **Cardiac output** may increase or decrease depending on clinical circumstances. **Cerebral blood flow** and O_2 demand may fall. Although hypotension may be corrected, renal and mesenteric vasoconstriction may reduce **renal blood flow**.

Supplied commercially as noradrenaline tartrate.

- Dosage: 0.03–0.2 μg/kg/min via a central vein, although higher doses may be needed in sepsis.

Tachyphylaxis may occur. Tissue necrosis may follow extravasation.

Norepinephrine, *see Noradrenaline*

Normal distribution, *see Statistical frequency distributions*

Normal solution. One containing 1 gram equivalent weight of substance per litre. So-called 'normal' **saline solution** (0.9%) is incorrectly described, being less than 1/6 normal.

See also, Equivalence

Noscapine, *see Papaveretum*

Nose. Entrance to the **pharynx** and thence **larynx** and **lungs**. Apart from its olfactory role, it filters, humidifies and warms inspired air with its extensive vascular surfaces (turbinates and septum). Filtering relies on the mucous lining, which traps particles larger than 4–6 μm, sweeping them back to the pharynx. Sneezing also rids the nose of irritants.

- Divided into:
  - external nose:
    - bones:
      - nasal part of frontal bones.
      - frontal process of maxillae.
      - nasal bones.

- cartilages (lower part and septum).
- fibrofatty tissue (ala).
- nasal cavity: subdivided by the septum into two separate compartments, opening anteriorly by the nares and posteriorly by the choanae. The small dilatation immediately within the nares (vestibule) is lined with stratified squamous epithelium bearing hairs and sebaceous and sweat glands. The remainder is lined with columnar ciliated cells and mucus-secreting goblet cells. Subdivided into:
  - roof: slopes upwards and backwards forming the bridge of the nose; it then has a horizontal part (cribriform plate of the ethmoid bone) and finally a downward sloping part (palatine bone).
  - floor: composed of the palatine process of the maxilla and horizontal plate of the palatine bone. A tissue flap (soft palate) extends into the nasopharynx, closing off the nasal passages during **swallowing**.
  - medial wall: nasal septum.
  - lateral wall: ethmoidal labyrinth, nasal surface of the maxilla and perpendicular plate of the palatine bone. The three scroll-like conchae hang down over the nasal meatus. The olfactory organ of the first **cranial nerve** lies above and beside the upper concha. The orifices of the maxillary, sphenoid, frontal and ethmoidal sinuses open on to the lateral nasal wall.

- Blood supply:
  - upper: anterior and posterior ethmoidal branches of the ophthalmic artery.
  - lower: sphenopalatine branch of the maxillary artery.
  - anteroinferior septum: septal branch of the superior labial branch of the facial artery.

Venous drainage is via a submucous plexus that drains into the sphenopalatine, facial and ophthalmic veins.

- Nerve supply is from branches of the ophthalmic (V_1) and maxillary (V_2) divisions of the trigeminal nerve:
  - skin:
    - supratrochlear branch of the frontal nerve (V_1).
    - anterior ethmoidal branch of the nasociliary nerve (V_1).
    - infraorbital branch of V_2.
  - maxillary antrum: V_2 via sphenopalatine ganglion.
  - frontal sinus: frontal nerve (V_1).
  - ethmoid region: anterior and posterior branches of the nasociliary nerve (V_1).
  - nasal cavities:
    - anterior: anterior ethmoidal branch of the nasociliary nerve (V_1).
    - posterior: short sphenopalatine and posterior nasal branches of V_2 (septum); long sphenopalatine branch (lateral wall).

Trauma to the nose may result from passage of a tracheal or nasogastric tube, or nasal airway. Resultant **epistaxis** may be severe, though may be reduced by prior administration of **cocaine** spray or paste, or other vasopressor solutions, e.g. **xylometazoline** 0.1%.

- For topical anaesthesia of the nose, many techniques have been described. Moffett's method is one of the best known:
  - solution consists of 2 ml 8% cocaine, 2 ml 1% sodium **bicarbonate** and 1 ml 1:1000 **adrenaline**.
  - one-sixth of the solution is instilled into each nostril and retained for 10 min in each of the following positions: right lateral head-down, face-down, and left lateral head-down.

Other techniques involve application of 8%–10% cocaine or other agent plus 1:200000 adrenaline swabs to the anterior septum and posterior nasal cavity.

Maxillary and **ophthalmic nerve blocks** may be used for operations on or around the nose.

[Arthur J Moffett (1904–1995), Birmingham otolaryngologist]

See also, Choanal atresia; Ear, nose and throat surgery

Nosocomial infection. **Infection** acquired as a result of a patient's admission to hospital. Occurs in up to 10% of patients, with mortality of up to 5%. More common in the acutely ill (e.g. on ICU).

- Aetiology may be related to:
  - hospital factors: widespread presence of pathogens, poor general hygiene and transfer between staff and patients.
  - patient factors: increasingly elderly population with reduced resistance, **immunodeficiency**, diabetes, smoking, **malnutrition**, **alcoholism**, **trauma** and drug therapy.
  - interventions: surgery, tracheal intubation, **catheter-related sepsis**, bladder catheterisation, use of broad-spectrum **antibacterial drugs** resulting in resistant organisms, **blood transfusion**, **TPN** or stress ulcer prophylaxis.

Sites of infection in order of decreasing frequency: **urinary tract infection**; surgical wound infection; **nosocomial pneumonia**; and **bacteraemia**. Organisms most commonly involved in order of decreasing frequency: *Staphylococcus aureus*; pseudomonas; coagulase-negative staphylococci; candida species; and *Escherichia coli*. **Fungal infection** is especially common in immunosuppressed patients.

- Management:
  - prevention:
    - effective **infection control**. Use of **care bundles**.
    - **selective decontamination of the digestive tract** may be appropriate in certain circumstances.
  - source control (e.g. debridement of infected wounds, removal of infected catheters).
  - treatment with appropriate anti-infective agents by the use of antimicrobial stewardship programmes.

See also, Ventilator-associated pneumonia

Nosocomial pneumonia. Hospital-acquired **chest infection** occurring >48 h after hospital admission; excludes infections incubating on admission. May occur in up to 25% of ICU patients and increases hospital mortality, length of stay and costs.

- Originates from:
  - microaspiration of oropharyngeal flora.
  - environment (air, water, food, etc.).
  - equipment (tracheal tubes, suction catheters, bronchoscopes, etc.).
  - other patients.
  - hospital staff (inadequate hygiene).
- Other contributing factors include:
  - patient's age and general condition.
  - drugs (e.g. **antacids**, **corticosteroids**, **H_2 receptor antagonists**, sedatives, broad-spectrum antibiotics).
  - supine position.
  - **aspiration of gastric contents**.
  - reintubation.
- Typical pathogens include:
  - *Streptococcus pneumoniae*.
  - *Haemophilus influenzae*.

- *Staphylococcus aureus.*
- gram-negative bacilli.

Often more than one organism is involved.

Approaches to clinical diagnosis vary but criteria include new, progressive or persistent CXR abnormalities, with evidence of infection (e.g. purulent sputum, hypo- or hyperthermia, and a low [<5000/mm^3] or raised [>10 000/mm^3] white cell count). Isolation of the responsible organism(s) is best undertaken using **bronchoalveolar lavage**, either blind or via fibreoptic bronchoscopy. Therapy should be organism-specific when possible, but broad-spectrum antibiotics are frequently necessary until the organism is identified.

- Prevention is assisted by:
    - vaccination, e.g. against *Haemophilus influenzae*, pneumococcus and influenza virus.
    - hygiene, e.g. hand-washing policies, removal of wristwatches, use of gloves.
    - avoidance of drug which increase gastric pH (e.g. H_2 receptor antagonists, **proton pump inhibitors**).
    - control of gastric volume and motility (distension risks reflux and aspiration).
    - **rotational therapy**.
    - good airway protocols, e.g. avoiding nasal intubation (risks **sinusitis**) and the supine position (patients should be nursed 30 degrees head-up), regular aspiration of subglottic secretions.
    - **selective decontamination of the digestive tract**, although this remains controversial except in trauma.

See also, Infection control; Nosocomial infection; Sepsis; Ventilator-associated pneumonia

Notifiable diseases. Diseases that are required by law to be notified to the government authorities, usually via communicable disease specialists or environmental/public health officers. Such a scheme allows epidemiological surveillance and early identification of potential epidemics. In the UK, the attending doctor is required to report the disease, and must not wait for laboratory confirmation of a suspected infection or contamination before notification. Similar schemes exist in several countries, with overlapping lists depending on historical and geographical factors (e.g. Table 36). In addition, diagnostic laboratories are required to notify the authorities if they confirm one of several notifiable organisms (60 in England and Wales, 71 in Scotland) that might pose a risk to public health. International agreements/regulations also exist for diseases that should be notified to the World Health Organization, particularly those that might threaten global public health via pandemics.

Similar lists exist for animal diseases, particularly livestock.

NovoSeven, *see Factor VIIa, recombinant*

NPSA, *see National Patient Safety Agency*

NRP, *see Neonatal Resuscitation Program*

NSAIDs, *see Non-steroidal anti-inflammatory drugs*

NSTEACS, non-S–T segment elevation acute coronary syndromes, *see Acute coronary syndromes*

NSTEMI. non-S–T segment elevation myocardial infarction, *see Acute coronary syndromes; Myocardial infarction*

Table 36 Notifiable diseases in (a) England and Wales and (b) Scotland

(a)	*(b)*
Acute encephalitis	Anthrax
Acute infective hepatitis	Botulism
Acute meningitis	Brucellosis
Acute poliomyelitis	Cholera
Anthrax	*E. coli* O157 infection
Botulism	Diphtheria
Brucellosis	Haemolytic–uraemic syndrome
Cholera	Haemophilus influenzae type b
Diphtheria	Measles
Enteric fever (paratyphoid or typhoid)	Meningococcal disease
Food poisoning	Mumps
Haemolytic–uraemic syndrome	Necrotising fasciitis
Infectious bloody diarrhoea	Paratyphoid fever
Invasive group A streptococcal disease Legionnaires' disease	Plague
Leprosy	Poliomyelitis
Malaria	Rabies
Measles	Rubella
Meningococcal septicaemia	Severe acute respiratory syndrome
Mumps	Smallpox
Plague	Tetanus
Rabies	TB
Rubella	Tularaemia
Severe acute respiratory syndrome	Typhoid fever
Scarlet fever	Viral haemorrhagic fever
Smallpox	West Nile fever
TB	Whooping cough
Tetanus	Yellow fever
Typhus	
Viral haemorrhagic fever	
Whooping cough	
Yellow fever	

Nuclear cardiology. Assessment of cardiac function using gamma cameras to trace **radioisotopes**. Technetium-99m-labelled blood may be followed through the heart during first pass of a bolus, or over many cardiac cycles linked to the ECG (**multigated acquisition imaging**; MUGA). Individual chamber movement and valve function may be observed, and **ejection fraction** calculated by recording the number of counts in systole and diastole. Alternatively, the uptake of thallium-201 by cardiac tissue may be observed (uptake by normal myocardium is proportional to blood flow). Thallium scanning may be enhanced by giving intravenous **dipyridamole** to precipitate ischaemia by causing **coronary steal**. Recently infarcted myocardium may be labelled with technetium-99m pyrophosphate. Other tracers used to identify areas of infarction, necrosis or inflammation include indium-111, gallium-67 citrate, and radiolabelled **myosin**-specific antibodies.

Nuclear magnetic resonance, *see Magnetic resonance imaging*

Null hypothesis. In **statistics**, the assumption that the observed frequency of an event equals the expected frequency. It may state that any observations are due to chance alone, or that the groups studied come from the same population; **statistical tests** aid the acceptance or rejection of this hypothesis (and whether an alternative

hypothesis, e.g. that observed differences are caused by a treatment under investigation, can be accepted). In traditional 'hypothesis testing', results are expressed in terms of the **probability** that the null hypothesis is true for the case concerned.
See also, Confidence intervals; Statistical significance

Number needed to treat (NNT). Indicator of treatment effect in **clinical trials**. The inverse of **absolute risk reduction**, it gives the number of patients that need to be given the treatment in question in order to prevent a specified undesirable outcome (e.g. PONV). For example, for an antiemetic with NNT for PONV of 5, one needs to treat five patients with the drug in order to prevent one patient suffering PONV. Combines both the efficacy of the drug and the incidence of the condition treated; for example, an antiemetic that is effective in 100% of patients will have NNT of 5 if the incidence of PONV is 1:5, but if it is only 50% effective (or the incidence of PONV falls to 1:10) the NNT will be 10. Number needed to harm (NNH) is a similar concept, indicating the number of patients needed to receive a drug before one suffers a complication.
See also, Meta-analysis; Odds ratio; Relative risk reduction

Nurse-controlled analgesia, *see Patient-controlled analgesia*

Nurses, prescription of drugs by. In the UK, specially trained nurses have been able to prescribe from a limited formulary since 1998; from 2006, regulations allowed nurse independent prescribers (and pharmacists) to prescribe any licensed drug (including opioids) so long as it is within their specific competence and local clinical governance frameworks. Other nurses and pharmacists are able to prescribe within specific management plans drawn up by a doctor for individual cases. Likely to have most relevance to acute and chronic pain management, premedication and intensive care.
See also, Midwives, prescription of drugs by

Nutrition. An adequately balanced daily supply of **carbohydrates, fats, proteins, vitamins**, electrolytes, trace elements and water is essential to maintain normal health.

- Average normal adult daily requirements:
  - water: 30–40 ml/kg.
  - nitrogen: 0.2 g/kg.
  - **energy**: 30–40 Cal/kg.
  - electrolytes:
    - **sodium**: 1 mmol/kg.
    - **potassium**: 1 mmol/kg.
    - chloride: 1.5 mmol/kg.
    - phosphate: 0.2–0.5 mmol/kg.
    - **calcium**: 0.1–0.2 mmol/kg.
    - **magnesium**: 0.1–0.2 mmol/kg.
  - trace elements:
    - iron: 0.2 mg/kg.
    - zinc: 0.2 mg/kg.
    - **selenium**: ~1 μg/kg.
  - vitamins: vary from under 0.1 g/kg to 1.0 mg/kg (*see Table 53*; **Vitamins**).

Energy requirements depend on the particular circumstances for each individual, e.g. they increase after **trauma** and **burns** (*see Catabolism*), and with pyrexia (by about 10% for every °C above normal). Patients should be fed via the oral route if possible, preferably with normal food.

The majority of patients in ICU are unable to eat for long periods and unchecked this leads to **malnutrition** with muscle wasting, susceptibility to infection, failure to wean from ventilation and overall, poorer outcomes. Early enteral feeding confers survival benefit but the energy requirement for critically ill patients remains controversial, with trials showing benefit from both restricted (trophic) and full energy feeding. It is not clear whether early parenteral feeding in those who cannot tolerate enteral feeding is beneficial. No evidence exists for supplementation of feeds with glutamine, arginine, n-6 fatty acids or micronutrients such as selenium, copper, manganese, zinc or iron.

Casaer MP, Van den Berghe G (2014). N Engl J Med; 370: 1227–36
See also, Metabolism; Nitrogen balance; Nutrition, enteral; Nutrition, total parenteral

Nutrition, enteral. Feeding via the GIT. Ideal route is by mouth using normal or liquidised food and calorific/protein supplements, if necessary. Commonly performed via fine-bore nasogastric tubes on ICU. Alternatives include a nasojejunal feeding tube (using a weighted tube or passed via endoscopy), **percutaneous endoscopic gastrostomy** or a jejunostomy tube placed at the time of surgery.

In patients with adequate GIT function, it is preferable to TPN as it is more physiological, provides protection against **stress ulcers**, maintains intestinal barrier integrity (thus reducing **bacterial translocation**) and promotes biliary flow, preventing the cholestasis commonly seen with TPN.

Principles are those of **nutrition** generally. **Carbohydrate** is the usual energy source in most enteral feeds, but high concentrations increase osmolality, causing diarrhoea. The **protein** source is usually whole protein, although preparations containing oligopeptides or **amino acids** are useful in pancreatic disease and malabsorption syndromes. Medium chain triglycerides are the usual source of **fat**. Most feeds also contain fibre.

- Complications:
  - mechanical, e.g. tube blockage, passage of the tube into the trachea, regurgitation.
  - nausea and vomiting: occur in 10% of cases; may require **antiemetic drugs** or **prokinetic drugs**.
  - diarrhoea: occurs in up to 60% of cases; may be caused by intolerance of high osmotic load, underlying bowel disorder, contaminated feed or concurrent **antibacterial drug** therapy. Administration of pre- and probiotic supplements may be beneficial.
  - **refeeding syndrome**.
  - electrolyte and liver function test abnormalities.

McClave SA, Taylor BE, Martindale REG, et al (2016). J Parenter Enteral Nutr; 40: 159–211
See also, Energy balance; Nutrition, total parenteral

Nutrition, total parenteral (TPN). Administration of total nutritional requirements by iv infusion; it may be required in patients who are hypercatabolic and/or have an abnormal GIT. Commonly required in critically ill patients on ICU with abdominal pathology or multiorgan failure. Only indicated if enteral **nutrition** fails to deliver requirements or is impossible to use. May also be used to support enteral nutrition.

Principles are those of nutrition generally, i.e., calculation of **nitrogen balance**, **energy** and fluid requirements. Nitrogen and the energy source should be given together, preferably continuously. 5–6 mmol potassium and 1–2 mmol magnesium are required per gram of nitrogen.

The nitrogen component is given as mixtures of essential and non-essential **amino acids** (the nitrogen content varies considerably between different solutions). Some amino acid solutions contain electrolytes and most are hypertonic. Some contain energy sources, e.g. **glucose** and fructose. **Carbohydrate** is usually given as glucose 10%–50%, and requires central venous infusion to avoid venous thrombosis. Other energy sources have also been used, e.g. sorbitol, xylitol and ethanol. **Insulin** is usually required to control **hyperglycaemia** associated with glucose-rich infusions. 'Tight' glycaemic control is no longer recommended as it is associated with greater morbidity secondary to hypoglycaemia. **Fat** is usually administered as 10% or 20% soya bean oil emulsions; allergic reactions may occur rarely with the 20% preparation. Trace elements and **vitamins** must be added.

Solutions are administered via a pump and a dedicated central venous cannula lumen, although a peripheral line is acceptable for temporary infusion of fat emulsion.

The patient should be encouraged to mobilise to prevent muscle breakdown.

- Complications:
  - those associated with **central venous cannulation**.
  - **sepsis**.
  - metabolic disorders:
    - hyperglycaemia.
    - **refeeding syndrome** with **hypophosphataemia**, **hypokalaemia** and **hypomagnesaemia**.
    - metabolic **acidosis**.
    - **hypernatraemia**.
    - lipaemia.
    - trace element or **vitamin deficiency**.
  - cholestasis resulting in acute **cholecystitis**.
- Routine monitoring should include:
  - clinical signs, weight and fluid balance daily. Skinfold thickness and arm circumference have been used.
  - plasma urea, creatinine, electrolytes and osmolarity daily. Glucose should be measured more frequently. Liver function and plasma calcium, phosphate and magnesium should be assessed at least twice a week.
  - urine urea and osmolarity daily.
  - full blood count every 1–3 days; prothrombin time once a week. Iron, folate and vitamin B_{12} should be measured at least weekly.

The benefits and adverse effects of parenteral nutrition are difficult to quantify as difficulties in assessing nutritional requirements often results in under- or overfeeding.

Berger MM, Pichard C (2014). Crit Care; 8: 478

See also, Energy balance; Nutrition, enteral

Nystatin. Polyene **antifungal drug**, principally used for treatment of *Candida albicans* infections of skin, mucous membranes and GIT. Not absorbed when administered by mouth and too toxic for parenteral use. Available as tablets, oral suspension, cream or pessaries.

- Dosage (adults and children): 400 000–600 000 units orally qds.
- Side effects: GIT upset, rash.

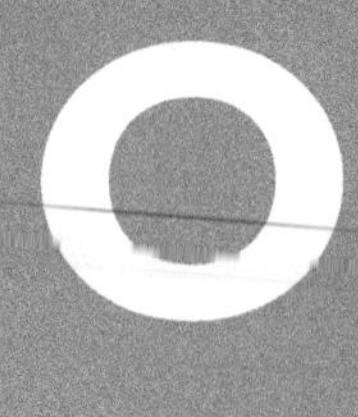

Obesity. Usually defined according to **body mass index** (*see Table 13; **Body mass index***). Approximately 40% of UK adults are obese and this number has doubled in the last 20 years, although the rate of increase has slowed over the last ~15 years. The prevalence of severe obesity ('morbid obesity'; **BMI** >40 kg/m^2) in the UK is 3%–4%. In the USA, the prevalence of obesity is ~40% and that of severe obesity is 5%–6%.

Obesity in children is classified according to growth reference charts; in the UK, ~12% of 2–10-year-olds and ~20% of 11–15-year-olds are obese.

An important cause of morbidity and mortality: a BMI of 30–35 kg/m^2 reduces an adult's life expectancy by ~3 years, whereas one of 40–50 kg/m^2 reduces it by 8–10 years, a similar reduction to that from lifelong smoking. Distribution of fat is thought to be more important than weight per se, with abdominal deposition particularly detrimental. Thus for a BMI ≥25 kg/m^2, a waist (just above the navel) circumference of ≥80 cm (women) and 94 cm (men) indicates increased risk; values ≥88 cm (women) and 102 cm (men) indicate substantially increased risk.

- Effects:
  - RS:
    - increased body O_2 demand and CO_2 production, because of increased tissue mass. Minute ventilation required to maintain normocapnia is thus increased, which further increases O_2 demand.
    - reduced **FRC** because of the weight of the chest wall. FRC is especially reduced in the supine position, due to the weight of the abdominal wall and contents. Thoracic **compliance** is thus reduced, increasing work of breathing and O_2 demand. ***$\dot{V}/\dot{Q}$* mismatch** results in **hypoxaemia**.
    - **hypoxic pulmonary vasoconstriction** increases work of the right ventricle and may lead to **pulmonary hypertension** and right-sided **cardiac failure**.
    - **obstructive sleep apnoea** and **obesity hypoventilation syndrome** may occur.
  - CVS:
    - cardiac output and blood volume increase, to increase **O_2 flux**.
    - **hypertension** occurs in 60%; thus left ventricular work is increased. Left ventricular hypertrophy and ischaemia may occur, with resultant left-sided cardiac failure. Arrhythmias are common.
    - **ischaemic heart disease** is common due to hypercholesterolaemia, hypertension, **diabetes mellitus** and physical inactivity.
  - other diseases are more likely, e.g. non–insulin-dependent diabetes mellitus (caused by insulin resistance and inadequate insulin production, the latter worsening with age), hypercholesterolaemia, gout and arthritis, gallbladder disease, hepatic impairment due to fatty liver and cirrhosis, **stroke**, and breast, endometrial, oesophageal, colorectal and prostate malignancies.

Patients may present for **bariatric surgery** or other procedures. The former is usually done laparoscopically and includes gastric banding, partial gastrectomy and gastric bypass, as single procedures or in combination.

- Anaesthetic considerations:
  - preoperatively:
    - **preoperative assessment** for the above complications and appropriate management. The **Obesity Surgery Mortality Risk Stratification score** has been used to identify patients at high risk of mortality after bariatric surgery. Patients may be taking **amfetamines** or other drugs for weight loss.
    - low-molecular-weight **heparin** prophylaxis is routine, because patients are less mobile and risk of **DVT** and **PE** is increased. The ideal prophylactic dose is not certain *(see later)* but the following have been suggested:
      - 100–150 kg: **enoxaparin** 40 mg bd; dalteparin 5000 units bd; tinzaparin 4500 units bd.
      - >150 kg: enoxaparin 60 mg bd; dalteparin 7500 units bd; tinzaparin 6750 units bd.

      Intermittent pneumatic calf compression should be used if possible.
    - im injection may be difficult because of subcutaneous fat, while anti-DVT stockings may not fit.
  - perioperatively:
    - venous cannulation may be difficult.
    - **hiatus hernia** is common, with risk of **aspiration of gastric contents**. Volume and acidity of gastric contents may be increased. In addition, tracheal intubation may be difficult: insertion of the laryngoscope blade into the mouth may be hindered, the neck may be short and movement reduced.
    - hypoxaemia may occur rapidly during **apnoea**, because FRC (hence O_2 reserve) is reduced, and O_2 consumption increased (the latter exacerbated by fasciculations caused by **suxamethonium**). FRC is improved if the patient is positioned head-up/ramped before induction of anaesthesia, with the tragus of the ear level with the sternum.
    - **airway** maintenance is often difficult, because of increased soft tissue mass in the upper airway. Spontaneous ventilation is often inadequate because of respiratory impairment, which worsens in the supine position (especially in the head-down position or with legs in the lithotomy position). Thus IPPV is usually employed; high inflation pressures may be required.
    - transferring and positioning the patient may be difficult. The typical maximum weight limit for manual operating tables is 135 kg, and for electrical operating tables is 250–300 kg. Two operating tables may be placed side by side if the patient is too wide for a single table. Air-hover mattresses assist transfer of the patient but care must be taken to control the patient's movement.

- **monitoring** may be difficult, e.g. BP cuff too small, small ECG complexes.
- surgery is more likely to be difficult and prolonged, with increased blood loss.
- drug use:
    - appropriate dosage may be difficult, because the proportion of body fat (with low blood flow i.e., 'vessel-poor') is increased. Thus **volume of distribution** and other pharmacokinetic indices may differ from those in non-obese patients. Most perioperative drugs (e.g. **propofol, thiopental, neuromuscular blocking drugs, morphine, paracetamol**) are given according to lean body weight, although for some (e.g. propofol by infusion, antibiotics, low-molecular-weight heparin, **alfentanil, neostigmine, sugammadex**), adjusted body weight is recommended (*see Table 14; **Body weight***).
    - increased metabolism of **inhalational anaesthetic agents** is thought to occur, e.g. increased **fluoride ion** concentrations after prolonged use of **enflurane**.
    - although regional techniques may have potential advantages over general anaesthesia, they are often technically difficult.

- postoperatively:
    - **atelectasis** and **hypoventilation** are common, with increased risk of infection, hypoxaemia and **respiratory failure**. Patients are often best nursed sitting. Elective **non-invasive positive pressure ventilation** may be beneficial. Difficulty mobilising may be a problem.
    - **postoperative analgesia, O_2 therapy** and **physiotherapy** are especially important. **CPAP** therapy for obstructive sleep apnoea should be restarted in the immediate postoperative period. **HDU** or **ICU** admission is often required.

Similar considerations apply to admission of obese patients to ICU for non-surgical reasons.

Nightingale CE, Margarson MP, Shearer E, et al (2015). Anaesthesia; 70: 859–76

Obesity hypoventilation syndrome (Pickwickian syndrome, after a character from Dickens' Pickwick Papers). **Obesity**, daytime hypersomnolence, **hypoxaemia** and **hypercapnia**, often in the presence of right ventricular failure. Causes are multifactorial:

- most patients have restrictive lung disease, resulting in poor **compliance**, increased work of breathing, alveolar hypoventilation and increased CO_2 production. **Pulmonary hypertension** is present in 60% of patients.
- patients often have coexisting **$\dot{V}/\dot{Q}$ mismatch**. Cyanosis and plethora are common, due to **polycythaemia** secondary to hypoxia.
- severe **obstructive sleep apnoea** is almost invariable. In addition there is a disordered central control of breathing, possibly due to leptin deficiency or resistance. Control is especially poor during sleep and sudden nocturnal death is common.

General and anaesthetic management is as for obesity and **cor pulmonale**. The F_IO_2 should be increased cautiously to avoid depression of the hypoxic ventilatory drive. CPAP may be useful to reduce hypercapnia and normalise O_2 saturations. Respiratory depressant drugs should also be used cautiously; postoperative respiratory failure may occur.

[Charles Dickens (1812–1870), English author]

Piper AJ, Grunstein RR (2011). Am J Respir Crit Care Med; 183: 282–8

Obesity Surgery Mortality Risk Stratification score. Scoring system for identifying patients undergoing **bariatric surgery** who are at high risk of perioperative mortality. One point is assigned for each of the following preoperative risk factors:

- age ≥45 years.
- male.
- **BMI** ≥50 kg/m^2.
- **hypertension.**
- risk factors for **PE** (previous PE/**DVT**, inferior vena cava filter, right heart failure or **pulmonary hypertension, obesity hypoventilation syndrome**).

Patients are categorised into class A (0–1 points; mortality risk ~0.3%), class B (2–3 points; mortality risk 1.0%–1.5%) and class C (4–5 points; mortality risk 2.5%–4.5%). Originally described in gastric bypass surgery, the scoring system has been applied to other bariatric operations and even as a general guide to non-bariatric surgery in patients with **obesity**.

Thomas H, Agrawal S (2012). Obes Surg; 22: 1135–40

Obstetric analgesia and anaesthesia. Pain during the first stage of labour is thought to be caused by cervical dilatation, and is usually felt in the T11–L1 **dermatomes**. Back and rectal pain may also occur. Pain often worsens at the end of the first stage. Pain during the second stage is caused by stretching of the birth canal and perineum.

Early attempts at pain relief included the use of abdominal pressure, **opium** and **alcohol. Simpson** administered the first obstetric anaesthetic in 1847, using **diethyl ether**. He used **chloroform** later that year, subsequently preferring it to ether. Moral and religious objections to anaesthesia in childbirth declined after **Snow**'s administration of chloroform to Queen **Victoria** in 1853. Regional techniques were introduced from the early 1900s, and have become increasingly popular since the 1960s.

Choice of technique is related to the physiological effects of **pregnancy** (especially risk of **aortocaval compression** and **aspiration pneumonitis**), and effects of drugs and complications on the fetus, **neonate** and course of labour. Anaesthesia has until the last 20–40 years been a major cause of maternal death in the UK, as revealed in the Reports on **Confidential Enquiries into Maternal Deaths.**

- Methods used:
    - non-drug methods, e.g. **TENS, acupuncture, hypnosis, psychoprophylaxis**, audioanaesthesia ('white noise'; high-frequency sound played through headphones), abdominal decompression (application of negative pressure to the abdomen): generally safe for mother and fetus, but of variable efficacy and thus rarely used, except for TENS and psychoprophylaxis.
    - systemic **opioid analgesic drugs**:
        - **morphine** was used with **hyoscine** to provide **twilight sleep** in the early 1900s. However, it readily crosses the **placenta** to cause neonatal respiratory depression. **Pethidine** was first used in 1940 and approved for use by UK midwives in 1950; it is the most commonly used opioid (e.g. 50–150 mg im up to two doses), but some units prefer **diamorphine**. 30%–75% of women gain no benefit from pethidine and there is little evidence that opioids actually reduce pain scores in labour. Nausea, vomiting, delayed **gastric emptying** and sedation

may occur, with neonatal respiratory depression especially likely 2–4 h after im injection. Neonatal respiratory depression is marked after iv injection. Subtle changes may be detected on **neurobehavioural testing of the neonate**.
  - other opioids have been used with similar effects. A lower incidence of neonatal depression has been claimed for partial agonists and agonist/antagonists (e.g. **nalbuphine**, **pentazocine**, **meptazinol**), but they are not commonly used.
  - **patient-controlled analgesia** has been used, e.g. pethidine 10–20 mg iv or nalbuphine 2–3 mg iv (10 min lockout), or **fentanyl** 10–25 μg following 25–75 μg loading dose (3–5 min lockout). More recently, **remifentanil** has been used (e.g. 30–40 μg bolus, 2–3 min lockout), though severe respiratory depression has been reported, requiring careful monitoring.
  - **opioid receptor antagonists**, e.g. **naloxone**, may be required if neonatal respiratory depression is marked.
- a variety of non-opioid sedative drugs were used in the past but these are now considered obsolete.
- **inhalational anaesthetic agents**:
  - ether and chloroform were first used in 1847. **Trichloroethylene** was used in the 1940s, and **methoxyflurane** in 1970; formerly approved for midwives' use with **draw-over techniques**, their use in the UK ceased in 1984.
  - **N_2O** was first used in 1880. **Intermittent-flow anaesthetic machines** were developed from the 1930s, using N_2O with air or O_2. **Entonox** was used in 1962 by Tunstall, and approved for use by midwives in 1965. It is usually self-administered using a facepiece or mouthpiece and **demand valve**. Slow, deep inhalation should start just before a contraction begins, in order to achieve adequate blood levels at peak pain. May cause nausea and dizziness; it is otherwise relatively safe with minimal side effects, although maternal arterial desaturation has been reported, especially in combination with pethidine. Useful in 50% of women but of no help in 30% and, like opioids, there is little evidence that it reduces pain scores. Addition of **isoflurane** has been studied (**Isoxane**) but this mixture is not commercially available.
  - **enflurane**, isoflurane, **desflurane** and **sevoflurane** have been used or studied with draw-over inhalation of air/oxygen, but none are widely used.
- general anaesthesia: no longer used for normal vaginal delivery. Problems are as for **caesarean section**.
- regional techniques: involve blockade of the nerve supply of:
  - **uterus**:
    - via sympathetic pathways in paracervical tissues and broad ligament to the **spinal cord** at T11–12, sometimes T10 and L1 also.
    - the cervix is possibly innervated via separate S2–4 pathways in addition.
  - birth canal and perineum: via pudendal nerves (S2–4), genitofemoral and ilioinguinal nerves and sacral nerves.

- Regional techniques used:
  - **epidural anaesthesia**/analgesia:
    - **caudal analgesia** was first used in obstetrics in 1909 by Stoeckel; a continuous technique was introduced in the USA in 1942.
    - continuous lumbar techniques were first used in 1946; they have become popular in the UK since the 1960s, with most units now providing a 24-h service. Uptake varies widely, with up to 70%–80% for primiparae in some centres. The overall epidural rate in the UK is around 20%–30%.
    - advantages:
      - reduces maternal exhaustion, **hyperventilation**, ketosis and plasma **catecholamine** levels.
      - avoids adverse effects of parenteral opioids.
      - reduces fetal **acidosis** and maintains or increases uteroplacental blood flow if hypotension is avoided.
      - may improve contractions in inco-ordinate uterine activity.
      - thought to reduce morbidity and mortality in breech delivery, multiple delivery, premature labour, **pre-eclampsia**, maternal cardiovascular or respiratory disease, **diabetes mellitus**, forceps delivery and caesarean section.
    - disadvantages:
      - risk of hypotension, extensive blockade, iv injection and other complications. **Post dural puncture headache** is more common in pregnant than in non-pregnant subjects following accidental **dural tap** (the maximum acceptable incidence of the latter has been set at about 1% in the UK). **Shivering** and urinary retention may occur.
      - motor block may be distressing, and if extensive may be associated with delayed descent of the fetal head.
      - requires iv cannulation (although routine administration of iv fluids may not be necessary if low-dose techniques are used and the mother is not dehydrated).
      - requires 24 h dedicated anaesthetic cover.
      - increased incidence of backache has been reported, but this has been shown to reflect selection of patients prone to backache (e.g. complicated labour, lower pain threshold), plus the tendency of patients to link back pain with any procedure performed on the back, rather than a result of regional analgesia or anaesthesia itself.
    - effect on labour:
      - temporary reduction in uterine activity has been reported following injection of solution, though this may be caused by the bolus of **crystalloid** traditionally given concurrently.
      - inco-ordinate uterine activity may improve.
      - no consistent effect on the first stage of labour has been found, but meta-analysis suggests prolongation of the second stage by an average of ~20 min, leading to an increased rate of ventouse delivery. The relative contributions of epidural analgesia per se (especially using modern low-dose techniques), and differences in obstetric management of mothers with epidurals, are uncertain.
    - technique:
      - standard techniques are used, but low doses of **local anaesthetic agent** are used to minimise motor block and risk of adverse effects. In general, smaller volumes are required than in non-pregnant women because venous engorgement reduces the volume of the **epidural space**.

Hypotension is common with higher doses of local anaesthetic, especially in the presence of **hypovolaemia**; it is reduced by preloading with iv fluid, usually crystalloid (e.g. 0.9% saline/Hartmann's solution, 500 ml). L2–3 or L3–4 interspaces are usually chosen, although, because identification of the lumber interspaces by palpation is not reliable (especially in pregnancy when the pelvis tilts), placement of the catheter at the lowest identifiable interspace is often advocated.

- **bupivacaine** is traditionally preferred, because fetal transfer is least. Others have been used, e.g. **lidocaine, chloroprocaine. Prilocaine** is rarely used because of the risk of **methaemoglobinaemia. Ropivacaine** is claimed to cause less motor block than bupivacaine when higher concentrations are used. Levobupivacaine has a better safety profile, but with low-dose regimens this difference becomes less relevant; it may be used as for bupivacaine, below.
- use of a **test dose** is controversial. With low-dose regimens, the first dose is also the test dose.
- suitable dose regimens:
  - bupivacaine 0.1% 10–15 ml with fentanyl 1–2 µg/ml as boluses. More concentrated solutions provide analgesia lasting slightly longer, but with more motor blockade. 0.75% solution is contraindicated in obstetrics. Manual top-up injections are usually given by midwives. Aspiration through the catheter should precede top-ups, which should be given in divided doses except for low-dose solutions. A maximum of 25 mg bupivacaine has been suggested for any single injection. Ropivacaine 0.2% is an alternative.
  - infusions: provide more consistent analgesia, with less motor block and hypotension than high-dose top-ups, and reduce the risk from accidental iv or subarachnoid injection. Bupivacaine 10–20 mg/h is usually employed, usually as a 0.1%–0.2% solution, and often combined with fentanyl 1–2 µg/ml. Large volumes of more dilute solutions have been used, supporting the concept of an 'extended sleeve' of anaesthetic solution over the appropriate segments. The height of the block must be regularly assessed, and the infusion adjusted accordingly.
  - patient-controlled epidural analgesia is also used, e.g. with 0.1%–0.125% bupivacaine with fentanyl 1–3 µg/ml, and boluses of 8–12 ml without a background infusion, or of 3–6 ml with a background infusion of 3–6 ml/min, and a lockout time of 10–20 min.
  - epidural opioids have been used alone, but rarely in the UK (*see Spinal opioids*). Fentanyl is usually added to weak solutions of bupivacaine as above. In the USA, **sufentanil** is often used. Epidural pethidine has also been used.
  - inadequate blockade includes: 'missed segment' (commonly in one groin; the cause is unclear); backache (especially with occipitoposterior presentation); rectal or perineal pain; and unilateral blocks. Remedial measures include further injection of solution, with the unblocked part dependent. Use of a stronger solution, a different local anaesthetic, or fentanyl 50–75 µg, may be helpful. The catheter should be withdrawn 1–2 cm if unilateral block occurs. Resiting of the catheter may be required. Suprapubic pain may result from a full bladder, and may be relieved by urinary catheterisation. Breakthrough pain in the presence of a uterine scar may indicate uterine rupture. Overall about 10% of epidurals require adjustment or extra doses.
- contraindications, complications and management are as for epidural analgesia/anaesthesia. Care should be taken in **antepartum haemorrhage** (*see later*). Extensive blockade and accidental iv injection of local anaesthetic are possible following catheter migration. All blocks should be regularly assessed and an anaesthetist should be readily available, with resuscitative drugs and equipment. Maximal doses of local anaesthetic agents should not be exceeded in a 4-h period.

  Backache and neurological damage may be caused by labour itself, although epidural analgesia is often blamed by the patient and non-anaesthetic staff.

- **spinal anaesthesia** was first used in 1900. Popular in the USA in the 1920s, it only increased in popularity in the UK towards the end of the 20th century. Technique and management are as standard, but with more rapid onset of hypotension and greater incidence of post-dural puncture headache and variable blocks (especially using plain bupivacaine) than in non-pregnant subjects. Dose requirements are reduced, possibly due to altered **CSF** dynamics, although changes in CSF pH, proteins and volume have been suggested. Effects are as for epidural anaesthesia. Mostly used for caesarean section, forceps and ventouse delivery and removal of retained placenta. Doses for vaginal procedures: 1.0–1.6 ml heavy bupivacaine 0.5%; lower doses with opioids have also been used.
- **CSE** has been advocated because of its rapid onset and intense quality of analgesia (from the spinal component, and possibly from increased efficacy of subsequent epidural doses via the dural hole). Its routine place in labour is controversial because of its increased cost, the increased risk of post-dural puncture headache, potential damage to the conus medullaris and (theoretical) concerns over increased risk of infection. In addition, the unreliability of identifying the lumbar interspaces by palpation may result in insertion of the needle at a higher vertebral level than intended. The lowest easily palpable interspace should therefore be chosen, and an epidural-only technique used above L3–4.

  A widely used starting intrathecal dose is 1 ml plain bupivacaine 0.25% mixed with fentanyl 25 µg, made up to 2 ml with saline. 3–5-ml boluses of the low-dose epidural mixture above are also used. Continuous spinal analgesia has been described, using the same low-dose solution.
- **paravertebral block**: bilateral blocks are required at either L2 (for sympathetic block) or T11–12 (somatic block).
- **paracervical block**: rarely performed because of fetal arrhythmias.

- **pudendal nerve block** and perineal infiltration/spraying with local anaesthetic: only of use for the second stage. Pudendal block (by the obstetrician) is used for forceps and ventouse delivery.
- local infiltration of the abdomen for caesarean section.

• Particular problems in obstetric anaesthetic practice:
  - obstetric conditions, e.g. pre-eclampsia, **placenta praevia, placental abruption, postpartum haemorrhage.** Haemorrhage may follow any delivery, and facilities for urgent transfusion should be available, including a cut-down set and O-negative uncrossmatched blood. **DIC** may also occur in septic abortion, intrauterine death, hydatidiform mole and severe **shock.**
  - maternal disease, e.g. cardiovascular, respiratory, diabetes. Epidural blockade is usually preferred.
  - fluid overload especially associated with **oxytocin** administration; **pulmonary oedema** associated with **tocolytic drugs**.
  - specific procedures/presentations:
    - premature labour: regional techniques are usually preferred, because they allow smooth, controlled delivery with or without forceps. The immature fetus may be especially susceptible to drug-induced depression. Tocolytic drugs may have been used.
    - twin delivery: epidural analgesia is usually employed for vaginal delivery. Caesarean section is required for delivery of the second twin in up to 10% of cases. Blood loss at delivery is greater than with a single fetus. The enlarged uterus is more likely to cause aortocaval compression.
    - breech presentation: most delivered by caesarean section nowadays because of evidence that neonatal outcome is better.
    - manual removal of placenta: spinal/epidural anaesthesia is usually considered preferable to general anaesthesia, because the latter risks aspiration of gastric contents, and inhalational agents cause uterine relaxation.
  - collapse on labour ward:
    - causes include: shock associated with abruption and DIC; postpartum haemorrhage; total spinal blockade; **sepsis**; overdosage or iv injection of local anaesthetic; **amniotic fluid embolism**; **PE**; eclampsia; inversion of the uterus; and pre-existing disease.
    - **CPR** is hindered by aortocaval compression, relieved by tilting the patient to one side or manually displacing the uterus laterally. Caesarean section should be undertaken within 5 min if there is no improvement in the mother's condition.

[Walter Stoeckel (1871–1961), German obstetrician; Michael E Tunstall (1928–2011), Aberdeen anaesthetist]

See also, Cardiopulmonary resuscitation, neonatal; Ergometrine; Fetal monitoring; Flying squad, obstetric; Labour, active management of; Midwives, prescription of drugs by; Obstetric intensive care

Obstetric intensive care. Required in 0.2–9 cases per 1000 deliveries, depending on the population served and the ICU admission criteria used. Most common reasons for admission are haemorrhage, **pre-eclampsia** and **HELLP syndrome**; a mortality of 3%–4% is reported in UK series but up to 20% has been reported elsewhere. Main problems are related to the risks to the fetus and the physiological changes of **pregnancy**: obstetric patients have increased oxygen demands and reduced respiratory reserves, and are more susceptible to **aspiration of gastric contents, aortocaval compression, ALI, DVT** and **DIC.**

General management is along standard lines, with attention to the above complications. Excessive fluid administration should be avoided, because ALI is a common feature of obstetric critical illness. **Fetal monitoring** should be ensured if antepartum, although the needs of the mother outweigh those of the fetus. Uteroplacental blood flow may be impaired by vasopressors and the mother may be too sick to receive **tocolytic drugs** should premature labour occur. Caesarean section may be required to improve the mother's condition. Breast milk may be unsuitable for use because of maternal drugs; if required, lactation can be suppressed with bromocriptine (although hypertension, **stroke** and MI have followed its use; hence it should be avoided in hypertensive disorders).

Guntupalli KK, Hall N, Karnad DR, et al (2015). Chest; 148: 1093–104 and 1333–45

See also, Placenta praevia; Placental abruption; Postpartum haemorrhage

Obstructive sleep apnoea (OSA). Most common form of **sleep-disordered breathing**, caused by decreased tone of the pharyngeal muscles during deep sleep, resulting in intermittent upper **airway obstruction**. Affects 5%–10% of the adult population.

• Risk factors:
  - male gender, **obesity**, age >50 years.
  - pharyngeal abnormalities (e.g. retrognathia, tonsillar hypertrophy, **acromegaly**) and other conditions (e.g. **hypothyroidism**, neuromuscular disorders).
  - sedative drugs (including alcohol) can precipitate or exacerbate the condition.

• Features:
  - loud snoring, associated with cycles of increasing partial airway obstruction (hypopnoea) leading to total obstruction (apnoea) followed by vigorous respiratory efforts and arousal to lighter planes of sleep and relief of obstruction. These cycles may occur up to 400 times/night. Associated with restlessness, morning headaches and daytime somnolence.
  - medical consequences of OSA include increased incidence of cognitive disorders, **hypertension, stroke, arrhythmias, MI** and **diabetes mellitus.**
  - severe OSA may result in **cor pulmonale** (**obesity hypoventilation syndrome**).

Screening questionnaires (e.g. **STOP-BANG score**) are used to identify those at high risk; formal diagnosis requires sleep studies, with polysomnography (monitoring of respiratory airflow, chest and abdominal movements, **EEG** and **oximetry**). OSA severity is classified according to the apnoea–hypopnoea index (number of apnoeas/hypopnoeas divided by the number of hours of sleep): 5–15 = mild; 15–30 = moderate; >30 = severe.

Treatment includes weight loss, nasal **CPAP** and removal of tonsils if enlarged. Uvulopharyngopalatoplasty (UVPP) is of dubious benefit. **Tracheostomy** may be indicated in severe cases.

• Anaesthetic implications:
  - of any predisposing cause.
  - patients may not satisfy criteria for **day-case surgery**.
  - sedative **premedication** may precipitate complete airway obstruction and should be avoided. If feasible, **regional anaesthesia** should be considered; if not, rapidly cleared anaesthetic agents should be used (e.g. **propofol, desflurane**).

- maintenance of the airway during **induction of anaesthesia** and tracheal intubation may be difficult. Tracheal extubation should only be when fully awake.
- patients are particularly sensitive to the depressant effects of sedatives and **opioid analgesic drugs**; airway obstruction, hypoventilation, **hypoxia** and **carbon dioxide narcosis** may readily occur postoperatively.
- patients are often nursed in ICU/HDU with nocturnal CPAP and maintenance of a 30-degree head-up tilt.

Chung F, Memtsoudis SG, Ramachandran SK, et al (2016). Anesth Analg; 123: 452–73

Obturator nerve block. Performed to accompany **sciatic nerve block** or **femoral nerve block**, or in the diagnosis and treatment of hip pain. The obturator nerve (L2–4), a branch of the **lumbar plexus**, passes down within the pelvis and through the obturator canal into the thigh, to supply the hip joint, anterior adductor muscles and skin of medial lower thigh/knee.

With the patient supine and the leg slightly abducted, an 8-cm needle is inserted 1–2 cm caudal and lateral to the pubic tubercle, and directed slightly medially to encounter the pubic ramus. It is then withdrawn and redirected laterally to enter the obturator canal, and advanced 2–3 cm. If a **nerve stimulator** is used, twitches in the adductor muscles are sought. Increasingly performed under **ultrasound** guidance. After careful aspiration to exclude intravascular placement, 10–15 ml **local anaesthetic agent** is injected.

In an alternative approach, the leg is externally rotated and abducted and an 8–10-cm needle inserted behind the adductor longus tendon near its pubic insertion, and directed posteriorly and slightly cranially and laterally. 5–10 ml solution is injected at a depth of 2–3 cm.

Occipital nerve blocks, *see Scalp, nerve blocks*

Octreotide. Long-acting **somatostatin** analogue, used in **carcinoid syndrome** and related GIT tumours and **acromegaly**. Also licensed for use in treating complications of pancreatic surgery. Has also been used in bleeding **oesophageal varices**, to reduce vomiting in palliative care, and in the management of chylothorax. Plasma levels peak within an hour of sc administration, and within a few minutes of iv injection. **Half-life** is 1–2 h. **Lanreotide** is a similar agent.

- Dosage:
  - 50 µg sc od/bd, increased to 200 µg tds if required (rarely up to 500 µg tds in carcinoid syndrome).
  - 50–100 µg iv in carcinoid crisis, diluted to 10%–50% in 0.9% saline.
  - 50 µg iv followed by 50 µg/h in bleeding varices.
- Side effects: GIT upset, glucose intolerance, hepatic impairment.

Oculocardiac reflex. Bradycardia following traction on the extraocular muscles, especially medial rectus. Afferent pathways are via the occipital branch of the trigeminal nerve; efferents are via the **vagus**. The reflex is particularly active in children. Bradycardia may be severe, and may lead to **asystole**. Other **arrhythmias** may occur, e.g. ventricular ectopics or junctional rhythm. Bradycardia may also follow pressure on or around the eye, fixation of facial fractures, etc. The reflex has been used to stop **SVT** with eyeball massage. Reduced by **anticholinergic drugs** administered as **premedication** or on induction of anaesthesia. If it occurs, surgery should stop, and **atropine** or **glycopyrronium** should be administered.

Retrobulbar block does not reliably prevent the reflex; **peribulbar block** may be more effective. Local infiltration of the muscles has also been used.

See also, Ophthalmic surgery

Oculogyric crises, *see Dystonic reactions*

Oculorespiratory reflex. **Hypoventilation** following traction on the external ocular muscles. Reduced respiratory rate, reduced tidal volume or irregular ventilation may occur. Thought to involve the same afferent pathways as the **oculocardiac reflex**, but with efferents via the respiratory centres. Heart rate may be unchanged, and the reflex is unaffected by **atropine**.

ODAs/ODPs, *see Operating department assistants/practitioners*

Odds ratio. Ratio of the odds of an event's occurrence in one group to its odds of occurring in another, used as an indicator of treatment effect in **clinical trials**. For example, in a trial of PONV with two antiemetic drugs:

	Drug A	Drug B
PONV	*a*	*b*
No PONV	*c*	*d*

The odds of PONV with Drug A are a/c, and the odds with Drug B are b/d

The odds ratio is therefore $a/c \div b/d = ad/bc$

Harder to understand (but more useful mathematically) than other indices of risk commonly used.

See also, Absolute risk reduction; Meta-analysis; Number needed to treat; Relative risk reduction

ODIN, Organ dysfunction and/or infection, *see Logistic organ dysfunction system*

O'Dwyer, Joseph (1841–1898). US physician; regarded as the introducer of the first practical intubation tube in 1885, although the technique had been described previously by others, e.g. **Kite**. His short metal tube, used as an alternative to **tracheostomy** in **diphtheria**, was inserted blindly into the **larynx** on an introducer; the flanged upper end rested on the vocal cords. He mounted his tube on a handle for use with Fell's resuscitation bellows in 1888; the Fell–O'Dwyer apparatus could be used for **CPR** or anaesthesia. Later modifications included addition of a **cuff**.

[George Fell (1850–1918), US ENT surgeon]

Baskett TF (2007). Resuscitation; 74: 211–14

Oedema. Generalised or localised excess **ECF**. Caused by:

- **hypoproteinaemia** and decreased plasma **oncotic pressure**.
- increased hydrostatic pressure, e.g. **cardiac failure**, venous or lymphatic obstruction; salt and water retention (e.g. renal impairment, drugs, e.g. **NSAIDs**, oestrogens, **corticosteroids**).
- leaky capillary endothelium, e.g. inflammation, allergic reactions, toxins.
- direct instillation, e.g. extravasated iv fluids, infiltration.

Several causes often coexist, e.g. hypoproteinaemia, portal hypertension and fluid retention in **hepatic failure**.

Characterised by pitting when prolonged digital pressure is applied, although fibrosis reduces this in chronic oedema. Generalised oedema occurs in dependent parts of the body, e.g. ankles if ambulant, sacrum if bed-bound. Treatment is directed at the cause. If localised, the affected part is raised above the heart.
See also, Cerebral oedema; Hereditary angio-oedema; Pulmonary oedema; Starling's forces

Oesophageal contractility. Used as an indicator of anaesthetic depth and **brainstem** integrity.
- Normal pattern of contractions:
  - primary: continuation of the **swallowing** process; propels the food bolus down the **oesophagus**.
  - secondary (provoked): caused by presence of food, etc., within the oesophageal lumen. Unrelated to swallowing.
  - tertiary (spontaneous): non-peristaltic; function is uncertain.

Measured by passing a double-ballooned probe into the lower oesophagus. The distal balloon is filled with water and connected to a pressure **transducer**; the other balloon (just proximal) may be inflated intermittently to study provoked contractions.
- Altered by:
  - anaesthesia: provoked contractions diminish in amplitude as depth increases, and spontaneous contractions become less frequent. Oesophageal contractility index ([70 × spontaneous rate] + provoked amplitude) is used as an overall measure of activity. Thought to be analogous to BP, heart rate, lacrimation and sweating during anaesthesia; i.e., suggestive of anaesthetic depth, but not reliable. Activity may be decreased by **atropine** and smooth muscle relaxants (e.g. **sodium nitroprusside**) and increased by **neostigmine**.
  - **brainstem death**: spontaneous contractions disappear, and provoked contractions show a low-amplitude pattern. Has been used to indicate the presence or absence of brainstem activity in ICU, but its role is controversial. Presently not included in UK brainstem death criteria.

See also, Anaesthesia, depth of

Oesophageal obturators and airways. Devices inserted blindly into the **oesophagus** of unconscious patients to secure the **airway** and allow **IPPV** when tracheal intubation is not possible, e.g. by untrained personnel. They have been used in failed intubation. Consist of a cuffed oesophageal tube, often attached to a **facemask** for sealing the mouth and nose and preventing air leaks. The cuff reduces gastric insufflation and regurgitation but may not prevent it.

The epiglottis is pushed anteriorly, creating an air passage for ventilation. An ordinary **tracheal tube** may be used to isolate the stomach and improve the airway in a similar way.
- Two main types are described:
  - blind-ended cuffed tube, perforated level with the hypopharynx for passage of air. Inflation is through the tube and via the perforations to the lungs.
  - open-ended tube, to allow gastric aspiration. Inflation is through a separate port of the facemask. If accidental tracheal placement occurs, IPPV may be performed through the tube.

The above features have been combined in a double-lumen device (Combitube), which may be placed in either the

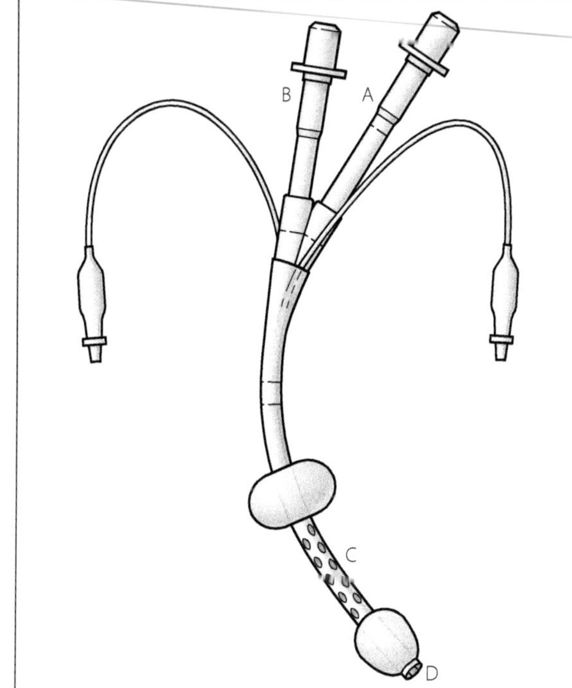

Fig. 124 The Combitube (*see text*)

oesophagus or trachea (Fig. 124). A distal cuff (15 ml) seals the oesophagus or trachea, whereas a proximal balloon (100 ml) seals the oral and nasal airways. IPPV may be performed through either tube depending on the device's position; it enters the oesophagus in over 95% of cases initially and ventilation via the longer proximal tube (A) will result in pulmonary ventilation via the proximal openings (C). The shorter distal tube (B) may then be used for gastric suction via the distal opening (D). If the device is tracheal, IPPV may be achieved via tube B and opening D. Has been suggested as a suitable device for non-medical personnel (e.g. for **CPR**), although trauma is more common than with available alternatives (e.g. **SADs**).

Oesophageal sphincter, *see Lower oesophageal sphincter*

Oesophageal stethoscope, *see Stethoscope*

Oesophageal varices. Dilated oesophagogastric veins occurring in portal hypertension, e.g. in hepatic cirrhosis; the veins represent one of the connections between the systemic and portal circulations. Account for up to a third of cases of massive upper **GIT haemorrhage**. Mortality is up to 30% if bleeding occurs, partly related to the underlying severity of liver disease.
- Management:
  - primary prophylaxis of variceal haemorrhage: treatment with non-selective **β-adrenergic receptor antagonists** e.g. **propranolol** or carvedilol is the management of choice. If β-blockade is contra-indicated, endoscopic variceal band ligation should be considered.
  - control of active variceal haemorrhage:
    - resuscitation and assessment (*see GIT haemorrhage*) as for acute **hypovolaemia**. Airway management is complicated by haematemesis and steps

to avoid aspiration of blood and gastric contents must be taken.
- prophylactic antibacterial drugs should be given.
- vasoconstrictor therapy should be started as soon as possible and continued until haemostasis is achieved:
  - **vasopressin** 20 U over 15 min iv or its analogue terlipressin 2 mg iv followed by 1–2 mg 4–6-hourly up to 72 h. Controls bleeding in 60%–70% of cases.
  - **somatostatin** 250 µg followed by 250 µg/h or its analogue **octreotide** 50 µg followed by 50 µg/h.
- following successful treatment of the acute bleeding, endoscopic variceal band ligation is the treatment of choice.
- if bleeding is uncontrollable, balloon tamponade using a **Sengstaken–Blakemore tube** should be attempted while awaiting transfer to a specialised centre, where early transjugular intrahepatic portosystemic shunting may be the most appropriate treatment.

Tripathi D, Stanley AJ, Hayes PC, et al (2015). Gut; 64: 1680–704

Oesophagus. Tubular organ connecting the **pharynx** and stomach. Consists of a mucosal lining, surrounded by connective tissue and internal circular and external longitudinal **muscle** layers (the latter consisting of smooth muscle in the lower third, skeletal muscle in the upper third, both types in the middle third). Approximately 25 cm long in adults, it extends from the level of C6 and descends at the back of the **mediastinum**, passing through the **diaphragm** with the vagus and gastric nerves and left gastric vessel branches at the level of T10. Thus lies behind the **trachea** in the **neck**, with the recurrent **laryngeal nerves** alongside, within the pretracheal fascia (*see Fig. 116*; **Neck, cross-sectional anatomy**), and behind the trachea and **heart** in the mediastinum, passing anterior to the thoracic aorta and posterior to the left main bronchus and right pulmonary artery. Has a muscular sphincter at the proximal (upper) end, mostly formed by the cricopharyngeus muscle, and the **lower oesophageal sphincter** at the distal end.

Afferent and efferent nerve supply is mainly vagal via oesophageal plexuses, but also via sympathetic nerves.

Blood supply is via the inferior thyroid artery (upper part), bronchial arteries (thoracic part) and left gastric/left inferior phrenic arteries (lower part including sphincter). Venous drainage is via azygos/hemiazygos veins (upper and lower parts) and left gastric vein (middle part).

Propels food from mouth to stomach by peristalsis (*see Oesophageal contractility*).

See also, Achalasia; Cricoid pressure; Gastro-oesophageal reflux; Oesophageal varices; Swallowing; Thoracic inlet; Vagus nerve

'Off-pump' coronary artery bypass graft, *see Coronary artery bypass graft*

Ofloxacin. **Antibacterial drug**, one of the **4-quinolones** related to **ciprofloxacin**. Used for respiratory and genitourinary tract infections.
- Dosage: 200–400 mg orally or iv (over 30–60 min) od/bd.
- Side effects: as for ciprofloxacin. Hypotension and thrombophlebitis may occur on iv administration.

Ohm's law. **Current** passing through a conductor is proportional to the potential difference across it, at constant temperature. Thus: voltage = current × **resistance** (i.e., V = IR). An analogous form exists for **flow** of a **fluid**: pressure = flow × resistance.
[Georg S Ohm (1787–1854), German physicist]

Old age, *see Elderly, anaesthesia for*

Oliguria. Reduced **urine** output; definition is controversial but usually described as under 0.5 ml/kg/h. Common after major surgery or in ICU.
- Caused by:
  - **urinary retention**, blocked catheter, etc.
  - poor renal perfusion, e.g. **hypotension**, **hypovolaemia**, low **cardiac output**. Urine formation usually requires MAP of 60–70 mmHg in normotensive subjects.
  - drugs, e.g. **morphine** causes **vasopressin** secretion.
  - increased intra-abdominal pressure (e.g. **abdominal compartment syndrome**): the mechanism is unknown but ureteric stents do not prevent it, suggesting mechanisms other than ureteric compression.
  - **renal failure**.
- Management:
  - exclusion of retention or blocked catheter.
  - urinary and plasma chemical analysis (e.g. sodium, **osmolality**) is useful in distinguishing renal from prerenal causes (*see Renal failure*). Management is according to the underlying cause.

Omeprazole. **Proton pump inhibitor** used to reduce gastric acidity. A prodrug converted to its active form by the acidic conditions of gastric parietal cell canaliculi.

Effects last for up to 24 h after single dosage.
- Dosage: 10–40 mg orally od. For reduction of risk from aspiration of gastric contents, 40 mg orally the night before, and 40 mg on the morning of surgery. May also be given iv: 40–80 mg over 40–60 min.
- Side effects: uncommon and usually mild: diarrhoea, rash, headache, rarely dizziness, hepatic enzyme and haematological changes.

Omphalocele, *see Gastroschisis and exomphalos*

Oncotic pressure (Colloid osmotic pressure). **Osmotic pressure** exerted by plasma proteins, usually about 3.3 kPa (25 mmHg). Important in the balance of **Starling forces**, and movement of water across capillary walls, e.g. in **oedema**. Although related to plasma protein concentration, the relationship is thought to be non-linear because of molecular interactions and effects of charge.
See also, Intravenous fluids

Ondansetron hydrochloride. **5-HT$_3$ receptor antagonist**, introduced in 1990 as an **antiemetic drug** following anaesthesia and chemotherapy. Does not affect **dopamine receptors** and unwanted central effects are rare, making it attractive compared with other antiemetics. Evidence suggests greater efficacy for treatment of **PONV** than for its prophylaxis. Has also been used to treat intractable **pruritus** following **spinal opioids**, and to prevent postoperative **shivering**, although evidence for its effectiveness in both of these is relatively weak. Only 70%–75% protein-bound. Undergoes hepatic metabolism and renal excretion. **Half-life** is 3 h.

- Dosage:
  - PONV:
    - prophylaxis: 4 mg slowly iv/im on induction, or 16 mg orally 1 h preoperatively. In children ≥1 month, 0.1 mg/kg slowly iv up to 4 mg.
    - treatment: 1–4 mg slowly iv/im (0.1 mg/kg up to 4 mg, in children).
  - nausea/vomiting due to radiotherapy or chemotherapy: doses of 8–24 mg (5 mg/m^2 in children, up to 8 mg) may be used, depending on the actual or anticipated severity of symptoms and the patient's age.

Because of the association with **prolonged Q–T syndrome**, a single iv dose should not exceed 16 mg (8 mg if >75 years) and should be infused over ≥15 min. Repeat doses should be ≥4 h apart.

An orodispersable film (4 mg) and a 'melt' preparation (4 and 8 mg) are also available; when placed on the tongue, they rapidly disintegrate into saliva, which can then be swallowed.

- Side effects: headache, constipation, flushing sensation, hiccups, occasionally hepatic impairment, visual disturbances, rarely convulsions. Prolongation of ECG intervals, including heart block, has been reported. May reduce the analgesic efficacy of **tramadol**.

Ondine's curse. **Hypoventilation** caused by reduced ventilatory drive, originally described following CNS surgery (classically to medulla/high cervical spine). Despite being awake, victims may breathe only on command, with apnoea when asleep. The term has also been applied to a congenital form of hypoventilation and to respiratory depression caused by **opioid analgesic drugs**.
[Ondine, German mythological sea nymph; the curse of having to remember when to breathe, and thus being unable to sleep for fear of dying, was inflicted on her unfaithful husband by her father, King of the Sea]
See also, Sleep-disordered breathing

One-lung anaesthesia. Deliberate perioperative collapse of one lung to allow or facilitate **thoracic surgery**, while maintaining ventilation and gas exchange on the other side. Requires the use of **endobronchial tubes** or blockers. Commonly performed for surgery to the lungs, oesophagus, aorta and mediastinum, but most operations are possible without it (sleeve resection of the bronchus being a notable exception). Its main problem is related to **hypoxaemia** caused by the **$\dot{V}/\dot{Q}$ mismatch** produced, exacerbated by the lateral position used for most thoracic surgery. Perioperative hypoxaemia increases postoperative risk of cognitive dysfunction, atrial fibrillation, renal failure and pulmonary hypertension.

- Effects of lateral positioning on gas exchange:
  - awake:
    - ventilation: **FRC** of the upper lung exceeds that of the lower lung, because of mediastinal movement to the dependent side, and pushing up of the lower hemidiaphragm by abdominal viscera. Thus the upper lung lies on a flatter part of the **compliance** curve (i.e., is less compliant) whereas the lower lung lies on the steep part of curve, i.e., is more compliant (Fig. 125a). In addition, the raised hemidiaphragm on the dependent side contracts more effectively. Thus most ventilation is of the lower lung.
    - perfusion: mainly of the lower lung because of gravity; i.e., is matched with ventilation.

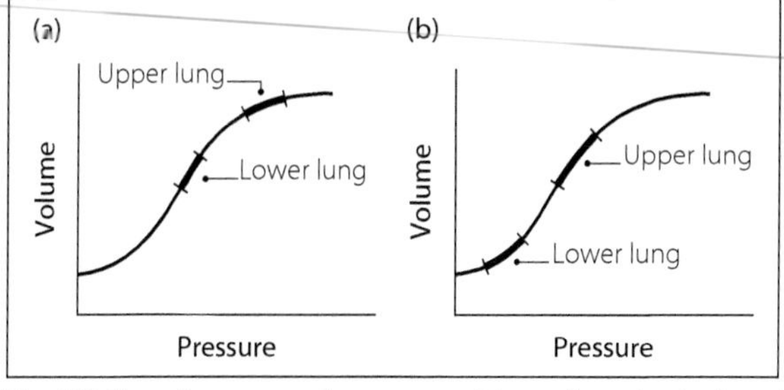

Fig. 125 Compliance curve for upper and lower lungs in the lateral position: (a) awake; (b) anaesthetised

  - anaesthetised:
    - FRC of both lungs is reduced; the upper lung now lies on the steep part of the curve and the lower lung on the flatter part (Fig. 125b). Thus the upper (more compliant) lung is ventilated in preference to the lower (less compliant) lung.
    - perfusion is still mainly of the lower lung, i.e., $\dot{V}/\dot{Q}$ mismatch occurs (usually of minor importance in normal patients, because both blood flow and ventilation usually differ by up to 10% between the two sides).
  - one-lung anaesthesia: all ventilation is of the lower lung, whereas considerable perfusion is still of the upper lung. Thus significant **shunt** occurs in the upper lung, with $\dot{V}/\dot{Q}$ mismatch usual in the lower lung.
    - CO_2 exchange increases via the lower lung; thus CO_2 elimination is thought to be maintained if minute ventilation is unchanged.
    - degree of hypoxaemia is affected by:
      - side of operation: as the right lung is larger than the left, oxygenation is often better during left thoracotomy.
      - pre-existing state of the lungs: decrease in oxygenation is greatest in normal lungs, e.g. during non-pulmonary surgery. Conversely, contribution to oxygenation by the diseased, operative lung is usually reduced; thus the drop in arterial P_{O_2} is smaller when it is collapsed.
      - F_IO_2: increases above 0.5 may not improve oxygenation, because pure shunt is not corrected by raising F_IO_2.
      - cardiac output: hypoxaemia worsens if cardiac output falls because of a decrease in the P_{O_2} of mixed venous blood passing through the shunt. The situation is complicated by altered distribution of pulmonary blood flow caused by changes in cardiac output.
      - **hypoxic pulmonary vasoconstriction**: whether it is attenuated by use of anaesthetic agents, or whether it contributes any protection against shunt, is unclear.
      - ventilation strategy: the optimum tidal volume and level of **PEEP** are controversial. To prevent atelectasis in the dependent lung, large tidal volumes (e.g. 12 ml/kg) have been used without PEEP (as PEEP may reduce cardiac output or increase shunt through the uppermost lung, exacerbating hypoxaemia). However, an alternative and increasingly common strategy is to use low tidal volumes (e.g. 6–7 ml/kg) with moderate PEEP to prevent atelectasis while reducing the risk of causing volutrauma and **ALI**.

- content of the collapsed lung: hypoxaemia worsens after about 10 min as contained O_2 is absorbed. Arterial PO_2 is increased by application of 5–7 cmH_2O CPAP using O_2, or by intermittent inflation, e.g. every 10–15 min.
- surgery: e.g. leaning on mediastinum, reduction of venous return. Tying the uppermost pulmonary artery stops shunt to the uppermost lung.

- Practical management:
  - **preoperative assessment** as for thoracic surgery; patients particularly at risk during one-lung anaesthesia may be identified.
  - close **monitoring** using **oximetry** and/or arterial **blood gas interpretation.**
  - F_IO_2 is usually set to 0.4–0.5.
  - surgical ligation of the pulmonary artery is performed early.
  - management of acute desaturation includes:
    - increasing F_IO_2 to 1.0.
    - use of fibreoptic **bronchoscopy** to check tube position and clear secretions.
    - administration of O_2 to the uppermost lung, e.g. with **CPAP** or intermittent inflation.
    - performing an **alveolar recruitment manoeuvre** on the dependent lung.
    - altering the ventilation strategy (i.e., changing tidal volume and/or PEEP).
  - suction is applied to the collapsed lung before reinflation, to remove accumulated secretions.
  - slow manual inflation is performed at the end of the procedure, to encourage expansion. The surgeon may request sustained pressures (e.g. 30–40 cmH_2O) to test the integrity of the bronchial suturing.

Lohser J, Slinger P, (2015). Anesth Analg; 121: 302–18

Open-drop techniques. Common and convenient techniques for administering **inhalational anaesthetic agents** in the 1800s/early 1900s. The volatile anaesthetic agent (e.g. **chloroform, diethyl ether, ethyl chloride**) was dripped on to a cloth (originally a folded handkerchief) on the patient's face from a dropper bottle. Concentration of agent depended on the rate of drop administration. Specially designed bottles and masks were later developed; the best-known mask is that of Schimmelbusch, although this was adapted from Skinner's earlier model. Some incorporated channels for O_2 insufflation, or gutters around the edge to catch liquid anaesthetic.

[Curt Schimmelbusch (1860–1895), German surgeon; Thomas Skinner (1825–1906), Liverpool obstetrician]

Operant conditioning. Type of learning in which voluntary behaviour is strengthened or weakened by rewards or punishments, respectively. May be involved in the development of certain behavioural aspects of pain syndromes. Has been used in chronic **pain management**, concentrating on behaviour secondary to pain instead of pain itself; now largely superseded by other behavioural therapies such as **cognitive behavioural therapy**.

Operating department assistants/practitioners (ODAs/ODPs). Non-medical anaesthetic support staff; the role arose from the requirements of military surgeons and anaesthetists for specialist non-nursing assistance during World War II, although 'box carriers' (so called because they carried the surgeon's instruments in a box) were in use in the UK in the early 1800s. Specific training in anaesthesia and surgery for ODAs without passage through the nursing training system was introduced in 1976, while the term 'ODP' was introduced in 1989, emphasising that adequately trained staff could equally come from nursing or traditional ODA backgrounds. Current training involves a 2-year diploma or 3-year degree course.

Compulsory registration of all ODPs was established in 2004. The professional body for ODPs is the College (formerly Association) of ODPs, an entity within the union UNISON; it has almost 5000 members and until 2015 published *The Journal of Operating Department Practice* (formerly *Technic*).

ODPs have an invaluable role in supporting most anaesthetic activity, e.g. preparing and ordering drugs and equipment, setting up the operating theatre for cases, helping to organise operating lists. They may also assist the surgical staff (including 'scrubbing') and the concept of 'multiskilling' supports their activity in various roles within the operating theatre suite and beyond, e.g. ICU, trauma teams. More extended practical roles are supported in some units (e.g. assisting at cardiac arrests, placing iv cannulae), although this is controversial.

Ophthalmic nerve blocks. Performed for procedures around the eye, **nose** and forehead, and certain intraoral procedures.

- Anatomy (*see Fig. 79*; **Gasserian ganglion block**):
  - ophthalmic division of the trigeminal nerve (V_1) is entirely sensory and passes from the Gasserian ganglion, where it divides into branches that pass through the superior orbital fissure:
    - lacrimal nerve: supplies the lateral upper eyelid and conjunctiva, lacrimal gland and skin of the lateral angle of the mouth.
    - frontal nerve: supplies the upper eyelid, frontal sinuses and anterior scalp via the supraorbital branch; upper eyelid and medial forehead via the supratrochlear branch.
    - nasociliary nerve: supplies the anterior dura, anterior ethmoidal air cells, upper anterior nasal cavity and skin of the external nose via the anterior ethmoidal branch; posterior ethmoidal and sphenoid sinuses via the posterior ethmoidal branch; medial upper eyelid, conjunctiva and adjacent nose via the infratrochlear branch; cornea, iris, ciliary body and dilator/sphincter pupillae via the long and short ciliary branches. Sympathetic fibres carried in short ciliary branches synapse in the ciliary ganglion
  - supraorbital foramen, pupil, infraorbital notch, infraorbital foramen, buccal surface of the second premolar and mental foramen all lie along a straight line.
- Blocks:
  - supraorbital nerve: 1–3 ml **local anaesthetic agent** is injected at the supraorbital notch.
  - supratrochlear nerve: 1–3 ml is injected at the superomedial part of the opening of the orbit.
  - both of these nerves may be blocked by subcutaneous infiltration above the eyebrow.
  - frontal nerve: 1 ml is injected at the central part of the roof of the orbit.
  - anterior ethmoidal nerve: 2 ml is injected at the superomedial side of the orbit, at a depth of 3–4 cm.

See also, Mandibular nerve blocks; Maxillary nerve blocks

Ophthalmic surgery. Historically, first performed without anaesthesia and then under topical anaesthesia (e.g. by **Koller**), because of the eye's accessibility and the disastrous effects of coughing during general anaesthesia. Subsequently, increasingly performed under general anaesthesia because of patients' expectations and the ability to control **intraocular pressure** (IOP), and then, with the development of effective and safe eye blocks, local anaesthesia has been favoured again, especially in the elderly. Children (for strabismus repair) and the elderly (for cataract extraction) form the largest groups of patients.

- Local anaesthesia:
  - cornea and conjunctiva: 4% **lidocaine** (with or without **adrenaline**) or 2%–4% **cocaine** is instilled into the conjunctival sac. Cocaine is not used in **glaucoma**, as it dilates the **pupil**.
  - **peribulbar block** or **sub-Tenon's block** (**retrobulbar block** less commonly performed now because of associated complications).
  - prevention of blepharospasm: infiltration between the muscles and bone parallel to the lower and lateral orbital margins from a point 1 cm behind the orbit's lower lateral corner; alternatively, local anaesthetic may be injected above the condyloid process of the mandible. These injections are rarely required with large-volume modern regional techniques.
  - **sedation** may be used. Close **monitoring** is required as the patient's head is covered by drapes. Supplementary O_2 should be delivered.
- General anaesthesia:
  - preoperatively:
    - **preoperative assessment** of children with strabismus for muscle disorders and **MH** susceptibility. Cataracts may occur in **dystrophia myotonica**, **inborn errors of metabolism**, chromosomal abnormalities, **diabetes mellitus**, **corticosteroids** therapy or following trauma. Lens subluxation may occur in **Marfan's syndrome** and inborn errors, e.g. homocystinuria. The elderly should be assessed for other diseases, e.g. diabetes, **hypertension** (*see Elderly, anaesthesia for*).
    - drugs used in eye drops may be absorbed and active systemically, e.g. **ecothiopate**, timolol.
    - opioid **premedication** is usually avoided because of its emetic properties. **Benzodiazepines** are popular.
  - perioperatively:
    - procedures include the above operations, repair of retinal detachment, vitrectomy, repair of eye injuries (*see Eye, penetrating injury*) and operations on the lacrimal system.
    - the **airway** is usually not easily accessible to the anaesthetist.
    - for children, considerations include those for **paediatric anaesthesia**, the very active **oculocardiac** and **oculorespiratory reflexes**, and the increased incidence of **PONV** after strabismus repair (thought also to be associated with traction on extraocular muscles). **Atropine** or **glycopyrronium** should be available; some advocate routine administration to all patients preoperatively or on induction of anaesthesia. Standard techniques are employed, with tracheal intubation or **SAD** and spontaneous or controlled ventilation.
    - for adults, standard agents and techniques are used. Control of IOP is usually achieved by iv induction, IPPV and **hyperventilation**, and use of a volatile **inhalational anaesthetic agent** (*for effects of specific drugs, use of sulfur hexafluoride, etc., see Intraocular pressure*). Administration of iv **acetazolamide** may be required. Spontaneous ventilation may be suitable for extraocular procedures. A SAD is often used, because coughing and straining are less pronounced than with tracheal intubation. The oculocardiac reflex may still occur in adults.
    - systemic absorption of topical solutions, e.g. adrenaline, cocaine, may occur.
    - coughing, straining and vomiting may increase IOP; especially undesirable if the globe is open.
  - postoperatively: avoidance of straining and vomiting is desirable. Postoperative pain tends to be mild.

Opiates. Strictly, substances derived from **opium**. Formerly used to describe agonist drugs at **opioid receptors**; the terms **opioids** and **opioid analgesic drugs** are now preferred.

Opioid analgesic drugs. **Opium** and **morphine** have been used for thousands of years; morphine was isolated in 1803 and **codeine** in 1832. **Diamorphine** was introduced in 1898, **papaveretum** in 1909. Other commonly used drugs include: **pethidine** (1939); methadone (1947); phenoperidine (1957); **fentanyl** (1960); **alfentanil** (1976); **tramadol** (1977); **sufentanil** (1984) and **remifentanil** (1997). Drugs with **opioid receptor antagonist** properties include **pentazocine** (1962), **nalbuphine** (1968), **meptazinol** (1971) and **buprenorphine** (1968).

May be divided into naturally occurring alkaloids (e.g. morphine, codeine), semisynthetic drugs (slightly modified natural molecules, e.g. diamorphine, **dihydrocodeine**) and synthetic opioids (e.g. pethidine, fentanyl, alfentanil, remifentanil). May also be classified according to their **opioid receptor** specificity and actions, or according to their onset and duration of action.

Each drug has slightly different effects on the body's systems, but their general effects are those of morphine. The 'purer' drugs, e.g. fentanyl, alfentanil, sufentanil, do not cause **histamine** release, and may be used in very high doses with relative cardiostability, e.g. for **cardiac surgery**. In lower doses, they are used to provide intra- and **postoperative analgesia**, and to prevent the haemodynamic consequences of tracheal intubation and surgical stimulation. Also used as general **analgesic drugs** and for **premedication**, anxiolysis, cough suppression and treatment of chronic diarrhoea.

See also, Opioid...; Spinal opioids

Opioid detoxification, *see Rapid opioid detoxification*

Opioid-induced hyperalgesia. Enhanced pain sensitisation in patients receiving therapy with **opioid analgesic drugs**. Has been observed in patients on chronic opioid therapy, in postoperative patients and in experimental models of pain. Some clinical studies have reported an increase in postoperative analgesic requirements and pain scores in patients given high-dose opioids at induction of anaesthesia, and small studies of healthy volunteers have implicated **remifentanil** infusion in the development of mechanical hyperalgesia. The mechanism is unclear but may involve central, descending and peripheral **pain pathways**, although those involving **NMDA receptors** in particular have been implicated. Weaning from opioids altogether, and rotation to different drug classes, have been suggested as management options.

Fletcher D, Martinez V (2016). Br J Anaesth; 116: 447–9

Opioid poisoning. Presents with nausea and **vomiting**, respiratory depression, **hypotension**, pinpoint **pupils** and **coma**. Depressant effects are exacerbated by **alcohol** ingestion. **Hypothermia**, **hypoglycaemia** and, rarely, **pulmonary oedema** and rhabdomyolysis may occur. **Convulsions** may occur with **pethidine**, **codeine** and **dextropropoxyphene**. Drug combinations containing opioids include **atropine**–diphenoxylate for diarrhoea and **paracetamol**–dextropropoxyphene/codeine/**dihydrocodeine** for pain. The former combination may cause convulsions, tachycardia and restlessness (hence it has been withdrawn from US and UK markets); the latter may cause delayed **hepatic failure**.

- Management:
  - supportive: includes **gastric lavage**, **iv fluids**, O_2 **therapy** and **IPPV**. Activated **charcoal** may be helpful if oral opioids have been recently ingested.
  - **naloxone** 0.4–2.0 mg iv repeated after 2–3 min as required to a total of 10 mg; infusion may be necessary as its duration of action is short. Respiratory depression due to **buprenorphine** may not be responsive.

Boyer EW (2012). N Engl J Med; 367: 146–55

Opioid receptor antagonists. Different types:

- pure antagonists, e.g. **naloxone**, **naltrexone**: antagonists at all **opioid receptor** subtypes. **Methylnaltrexone** is a peripherally acting mu antagonist, used as a treatment for opioid-induced constipation.
- agonist–antagonists: agonists at some receptors but antagonists at others, e.g.:
  - **pentazocine**: agonist at kappa and sigma, antagonist at mu receptors.
  - **nalorphine**: partial agonist at kappa and sigma, antagonist at mu receptors.
  - **nalbuphine**: as for nalorphine, but a less potent sigma agonist.
- partial agonists, e.g. **buprenorphine**, **meptazinol** (mu receptors); may antagonise mu effects of other opioids (e.g. morphine).

Their main clinical use is to reverse effects of **opioid analgesic drugs**, e.g. in **opioid poisoning**. Those with agonist properties are also used as **analgesic drugs**; some have been used to reverse unwanted effects of other opioids (e.g. respiratory depression) while still maintaining analgesia. In practice, this is very difficult to achieve. Also used in diagnosis and treatment of opioid addiction. Receptor-specific compounds have been developed for research and identification of receptor subtypes.

Many result from modification or substitution of the side chain on the nitrogen atom of parent analgesic drugs, e.g. *N*-allyl group substitution for the *N*-methyl group (hence the name, nal…).

Opioid receptors. Naturally occurring receptors to **morphine** and related drugs, isolated in the 1970s. Each is the product of a single gene. All are **G protein-coupled receptors** and activation results in opening of potassium channels and closure of voltage-gated calcium channels; this leads to membrane hyperpolarisation, reduced neuronal excitability and thus reduced nociceptive transmission. This effect is enhanced by reduction of **cAMP** by inhibition of **adenylate cyclase**. Found mainly in the CNS but also GIT; thought to be involved in central mechanisms involving **pain** and emotion. Three primary subgroups are now recognised (each subdivided into two or more putative subtypes), although others have been suggested in the past. More recently, data from transgenic mice lacking a single opioid receptor (e.g. MOP) have called into question the validity of further subtype classification.

- Subgroups:
  - mu (MOP):
    - activation causes analgesia, respiratory depression, euphoria, hypothermia, pruritus, reduced GIT motility, miosis, bradycardia, physical dependence; i.e., the classic effects of morphine.
    - responsible for 'supraspinal analgesia'; i.e., drugs act at brain level.
    - the mu_1 receptor subtype is thought to be responsible for supraspinal analgesia; the mu_2 for most of the other effects; and mu_3 receptors have been identified on immune cells.
    - endogenous ligands: **β-endorphins**.
    - agonists: all **opioid analgesic drugs**.
    - partial agonists: **buprenorphine**, **meptazinol** (thought to be specific at mu_1 receptors).
    - antagonists: **nalorphine**, **nalbuphine**, **pentazocine**.
  - delta (DOP):
    - distributed throughout the CNS. Located presynaptically, they inhibit the release of neurotransmitters.
    - activation has been experimentally shown to produce analgesia and cardioprotection.
    - endogenous ligands: **enkephalins**.
  - kappa (KOP):
    - activation causes analgesia, miosis, sedation, different sort of dependence.
    - responsible for 'spinal analgesia'; i.e., drugs thought to act at spinal level.
    - endogenous ligand: **dynorphin** A.
    - agonists: experimental agents spiradoline and enadoline cause analgesia but adverse effects, including diuresis, sedation and dysphoria, preclude clinical use.

Sigma receptors, previously considered opioid receptors, are not considered so now because the effects of their stimulation are not reversed by naloxone. They bind to phencyclidine and its derivatives, e.g. **ketamine**. All subtypes are antagonised by naloxone and naltrexone (mu and kappa more than delta).

The nociceptin/orphanin FQ peptide (NOP) receptor (previously termed the 'orphan' receptor) is related to the above receptors but its lack of sensitivity to naloxone makes it difficult to classify in the original opioid taxonomy. It is found throughout the brain and spinal cord, binds endogenous orphanin FQ, and produces antanalgesia supraspinally and analgesia at spinal level.

McDonald J, Lambert DG (2015). BJA Educ; 15: 219–24

Opioids. Substances that bind to **opioid receptors**; include naturally occurring and synthetic drugs, and endogenous compounds.

Opium. Dried juice from the unripe seed capsules of the opium poppy *Papaver somniferum*. Contains many different alkaloids, including **morphine** (9%–20%), **codeine** (up to 4%) and **papaverine**. Used for thousands of years as a recreational drug and for analgesia, especially in the Far East. Use as a therapeutic drug is rare now, purer drugs and extracts being preferred.

Oral rehydration therapy. Method of treating **dehydration** when mild or where facilities for **iv fluid administration** are lacking, e.g. in the community or developing countries. Particularly useful in gastroenteritis and in children; it has also been used in less serious

burns. Various commercial mixtures exist; all contain **glucose**, the presence of which in the intestinal lumen facilitates the reabsorption of sodium ions and thus water. A simple version can be made by adding 20 g glucose (or 40 g sucrose because only half becomes available as glucose after ingestion), 3.5 g sodium chloride, 2.5 g sodium bicarbonate and 1.5 g potassium chloride per litre of water. Suitable solutions have been made by taking three 300-ml soft drink bottles of water and adding a level bottle capful of salt and eight capfuls of sugar, or 6 level teaspoons of sugar and ½ level teaspoon of salt dissolved in a litre of clean water.

Orbeli effect. Increase in strength of contraction of fatigued **muscle** following sympathetic nerve stimulation. [Leon A Orbeli (1882–1958), Russian physiologist]

Orbital cavity. Cavity containing the eye and extraorbital structures. Roughly pyramidal with the apex posteriorly, its roof is formed by the orbital plate of the frontal bone (and lesser wing of the sphenoid posteriorly); its floor by the maxilla and zygoma; its medial wall by the frontal process of the maxilla and lacrimal bone anteriorly and orbital plate of the ethmoid and body of the sphenoid posteriorly; and its lateral wall by the zygoma and greater wing of the sphenoid (Fig. 126). Has three openings posteriorly:

- superior orbital fissure: transmits the third, fourth and fifth (the three branches of the ophthalmic division) **cranial nerves**. Also transmits branches of the middle meningeal and lacrimal arteries, ophthalmic veins and sympathetic fibres.
- inferior orbital fissure: transmits the maxillary nerve.
- optic canal: transmits the optic nerve and ophthalmic artery. The extraocular muscles are supplied by the third, fourth and sixth cranial nerves and have the following actions on the pupil:
  - superior rectus: elevates.
  - inferior rectus: lowers.
  - medial and lateral rectus: moves medially and laterally, respectively.
  - superior oblique: moves downwards and laterally.
  - inferior oblique: moves upwards and laterally.

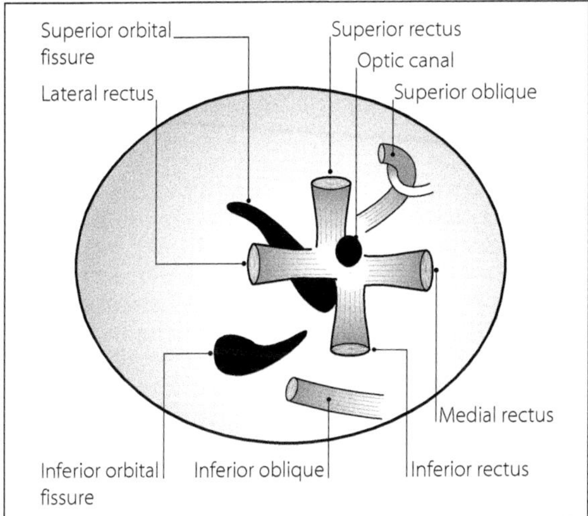

Fig. 126 Frontal view of right orbital cavity

The rectus muscles attach posteriorly to a common tendinous ring surrounding the optic canal and part of the superior orbital fissure; they attach anteriorly to the sclera of the eyeball in front of the equator. The superior oblique muscle attaches posteriorly above the tendinous ring, hooking round the pulley-like trochlea before attaching posterolaterally to the eyeball, behind the equator. The inferior oblique attaches posteriorly to the floor of the orbit and attaches to the posterolateral surface of the eyeball, behind the equator.

See also, Peribulbar block; Retrobulbar block; Skull; Sub-Tenon's block

Oré, Pierre-Cyprien (1828–1889). French physician; Professor of Physiology at Bordeaux. Investigated **blood transfusion** and the effects of iv injection of drugs. Produced general anaesthesia with iv **chloral hydrate** in 1872, thus becoming the first to employ **TIVA**. Also treated **tetanus** with the drug.

Orexins (Hypocretins). Excitatory neuropeptides derived from an amino acid precursor, prepro-orexin, secreted from the lateral and posterior hypothalamus. Involved in arousal, maintenance of the waking state, neural control of food intake and neuroendocrine function, including energy metabolism and reproduction. Deficiency results in a form of narcolepsy.

Organ donation. Demand for organs outstrips supply; in the UK, >7000 people are on the national transplant waiting list, with >3000 transplants per year. In many countries, e.g. the USA, Germany and most of the UK, members of the public identify themselves as potential donors by joining a national registry (an 'opt-in' system). In some countries (e.g. Spain, Austria, Belgium), an 'opt-out' system operates in which permission is assumed unless specified otherwise; such a scheme results in the availability of more organs for transplantation, and this was introduced in Wales in 2015.

- Organ donation may be:
  - living, e.g. liver, kidney, bone marrow: the main issue concerns the undertaking of anaesthesia and surgery (with their attendant risks) by a healthy patient for altruistic reasons.
  - dead, e.g. kidney, heart, lung, liver, small bowel, pancreas, skin and cornea: the main issue is around assent and the diagnosis of **death**:
    - donation after **brainstem death**.
    - donation after circulatory death (DCD): donors are classified according to the Maastricht system of 1995 into patients who:
      - arrive in hospital dead (I).
      - suffer a witnessed cardiac arrest outside hospital and in whom CPR is instituted within 10 min but is unsuccessful (II).
      - are awaiting cardiac arrest after withdrawal of treatment (III).
      - suffer cardiac arrest after brainstem death (IV).
      - suffer cardiac arrest as a hospital inpatient (V; added 2000).

In the UK, about 40% of all donors are from DCD, mostly in group III. Treatment is withdrawn once the surgical team is ready; death is pronounced 2 min after asystole, and surgery to retrieve organs begins 5–10 min after asystole.

Maintenance of tissue oxygenation, organ function and metabolic and cardiovascular stability should be pursued as for critically ill patients, until and during organ removal. Endocrine therapy with methylprednisolone, triiodothyronine and control of blood sugar with insulin may improve donor organ function.

Citero G, Cypel M, Dobb GJ, et al (2016). Int Care Med; 42: 305–15

Organe, Geoffrey Stephen William (1908–1989). English anaesthetist, born in India. A major influence on the development of anaesthesia in the UK and abroad, and involved in much research, particularly into the newly introduced **neuromuscular blocking drugs**. Professor of Anaesthesia at Westminster Hospital, London, and knighted in 1968.

Organophosphorus poisoning. An important worldwide cause of death due to acute poisoning, organophosphorus compounds are **acetylcholinesterase inhibitors**, commonly used as insecticides but also manufactured as **chemical weapons**. One, **ecothiopate**, is used in glaucoma. Those used in insecticides are usually ester, amide or thiol derivatives of phosphoric or phosphonic acids, or their mixtures. They may be absorbed via the GIT, lungs or skin, and are rapidly distributed to all tissues, especially liver and kidney. **Half-lives** vary from minutes to hours, with metabolism by oxidation, ester hydrolysis and combination with glutathione, and excretion in faeces or urine.

- Toxic effects:
  - peripheral **enzyme** inhibition:
    - phosphorylation of **acetylcholinesterase**: may be irreversible depending on the compound involved. Features are those of **cholinergic crisis** and include muscarinic effects (bronchospasm, sweating, increased secretions, abdominal cramps, bradycardia, miosis) and nicotinic effects (muscle twitching, weakness, hypertension and tachycardia). Enzyme 'reactivation' may be induced by **pralidoxime** if administered within 24–36 h.
    - phosphorylation of other enzymes, e.g. lipases, GIT enzymes.
  - myopathic effects: weakness may occur within 24 h of poisoning, with recovery taking up to 3 weeks. Muscle paralysis in humans may occur after recovery from the initial cholinergic crisis, 24–96 h after poisoning. Mainly affecting proximal muscles, it is thought to involve postsynaptic dysfunction at the **neuromuscular junction**.
  - delayed polyneuropathy: usually follows poisoning with non-insecticide compounds. Develops 2–4 weeks after the cholinergic crisis, with weakness and paraesthesiae. Pyramidal signs may be present. Recovery is variable.
  - CNS effects: anxiety, tremor, confusion, **coma** and **convulsions** may occur, with EEG abnormalities.

Respiratory failure may result from peripheral weakness, central depression and increased tracheobronchial secretions.

Diagnosis is based on history, tolerance to **atropine** therapy, **acetylcholine** assay and measurement of blood and urine organophosphorus and metabolite levels.

- Treatment:
  - supportive measures as for **poisoning and overdoses** in general. Care should be taken to avoid self-contamination.
  - drug therapy:
    - atropine 2 mg (20 µg/ml in children) iv each 5–10 min until dry flushed skin, dilated pupils and tachycardia.
    - pralidoxime 30 mg/kg diluted in 10–15 ml water, iv over 5–10 min. May be repeated up to twice if no improvement is seen within 30 min, up to a usual maximum of 12 g/24 h. Rarely, iv infusion of up to 500 mg/h may be required.

Orphanin FQ (OFQ; nociceptin), *See Opioid receptors*

Orthopaedic surgery. Anaesthetic considerations may be related to:

- indication for surgery:
  - **trauma**: presence of other injuries, risks of **emergency surgery** (e.g. **aspiration of gastric contents**). Adequate resuscitation is important preoperatively, especially in the **elderly**, e.g. following **fractured neck of femur** (NOF). Cases with risk of infection, ischaemia or nerve damage are particularly urgent.
  - hip/knee joint degeneration requiring replacement: problems are mainly related to co-morbidity associated with age or **obesity**, or both.
  - systemic musculoskeletal disease, e.g. **rheumatoid arthritis**, **connective tissue diseases**, muscular abnormalities. There may be a higher than normal incidence of **MH** susceptibility in young patients with musculoskeletal abnormalities.
  - congenital malformations: may be accompanied by other system involvement, e.g. cardiac lesions.
  - risk of massive **hyperkalaemia** following **suxamethonium** if neurological or muscle lesions are present.
- surgical procedure:
  - may involve repeated anaesthesia.
  - use of **tourniquets**.
  - use of methyl methacrylate cement (*see Bone cement implantation syndrome*).
  - problems of specific procedures, e.g. **kyphoscoliosis**.
  - increased risk of **DVT** and **PE**, especially after hip surgery; prophylactic measures should be taken. **Fat embolism** may occur after long bone fractures.

Oscilloscope. Device for displaying recorded signals, particularly those of high frequency and when analysis of their shape is required, e.g. **ECG** or **arterial waveform**. May also be used without the time-base to plot two signals with respect to each other, e.g. **flow–volume loops**.

The earliest oscilloscopes utilised a cathode ray tube to generate, accelerate and focus an electron beam on to a fluorescent screen, the beam visible as a bright dot. The signal potential was applied vertically across the beam, causing vertical deflection; a spatial reconstruction of the signal against time was then seen on the screen. The pattern could be made to persist by altering the characteristics of the fluorescent material, or by using a second cathode system. These are now termed analogue oscilloscopes, to distinguish them from the modern digital devices that have replaced them in medical practice. These utilise an analogue-to-digital converter to translate measured voltages (sampled at close, regular time intervals) into digital information that is then displayed on liquid crystal or light-emitting diode panels. Digital devices benefit from greater portability and the option to apply processing algorithms to recorded signals (e.g. for **S–T segment** analysis and detection of **arrhythmias**).

Oscillotonometer. Obsolete device for indirect **arterial BP measurement**, using one (upper) cuff for occluding the brachial artery and a second (lower) cuff for detecting pulsations, often incorporated into a double cuff. Both cuffs are inflated by hand to above systolic BP and then allowed to deflate slowly, using a lever to switch the dial to a sensitive 'indicator' mode by which increased and then decreased oscillations of the dial needle indicate systolic and then diastolic pressures, respectively. At each of these points, the lever is used to return the indicator dial to a 'recording' mode to allow actual cuff pressure to be displayed. Has been replaced by automated devices, which employ similar principles but are more accurate, more reliable and easier to use.

Osmolality and osmolarity. Expressions of concentration of osmotically active particles in solution:

- osmolality = the number of osmoles per kilogram solvent.
- osmolarity = the number of osmoles per litre solution.
- osmoles = the mw of a substance divided by the number of freely moving particles liberated in solution.

Thus 1 mmol of a salt that dissociates completely into two ions provides 2 mosmol. In the body, the solvent is water, with density 1 kg/l; thus osmolality and osmolarity are often used interchangeably, although proteins and fats in plasma give rise to a small difference.

Osmolality of plasma is maintained at 280–305 mosmol/kg. Regulatory mechanisms include stimulation of thirst by **osmoreceptors, baroreceptors** and the **renin/angiotensin system.** Osmoreceptors also stimulate **vasopressin** release. Most contribution to plasma osmolality arises from **sodium** and its anions, **glucose** and **urea**; thus plasma osmolality may be estimated thus:

$$\text{mosmol/kg} = [\text{glucose}] + [\text{urea}] + (2 \times [\text{Na}^+])\ (\text{all in mmol/l}).$$

Alcohols, **proteins**, triglycerides and **mannitol** are not accounted for. Proteins usually contribute little because, despite their high concentration, few particles are liberated in solution because of their high mw.

Osmolality/osmolarity is determined by measuring ionic concentration with a flame photometer, measuring **osmotic pressure** or by employing the **colligative properties of solutions** (e.g. depression of freezing point, lowering of vapour pressure).

Urinary and plasma osmolality measurement is useful in investigating **oliguria** and **renal failure**.

See also, Fluid balance; Hyperosmolality; Hypo-osmolality; Osmolar gap; Tonicity

Osmolar gap (Osmolality gap). Difference between calculated and measured plasma **osmolality**. Normally 10–15 mosmol/kg; increased in the presence of low-molecular-weight substances not included in the formula for calculating plasma osmolality, e.g. **alcohols, mannitol, glycine** (in the **TURP syndrome**). May also be applied to **urine** osmolality, e.g. to indicate the presence of osmotically active substances such as ammonium ions.

Osmoreceptors. Cells in the anterior **hypothalamus**, outside the **blood–brain barrier**; respond to changes in plasma **osmolality**. Control thirst and secretion of **vasopressin**, possibly via separate groups of osmoreceptors.

Osmosis. Movement of solvent molecules across a semipermeable **membrane** from a dilute solution to a concentrated one, tending to equalise the concentrations on both sides. Thus water moves across cell membranes from the **ECF** following **dextrose** infusion, once the dextrose has been metabolised. Similarly, water in very hypotonic **iv fluids** may move into red blood cells after infusion, causing **haemolysis**.

Osmotic clearance, *see Clearance, osmotic*

Osmotic diuretics, *see Diuretics*

Osmotic pressure. **Pressure** required to prevent movement of solvent molecules by **osmosis** across a semipermeable **membrane**.

$$\text{equals } \frac{nRT}{V} \text{ as for the ideal gas law,}$$

where n = number of particles
R = **universal gas constant**
T = absolute temperature
V = volume.

Thus proportional to the number of osmotically active particles per unit volume, not mw. Ideal ionic solutions dissociate completely in solution, whereas in the body incomplete dissociation and interactions between ions result in lower osmotic pressure than predicted. Plasma osmotic pressure is approximately 7.3 atmospheres.

See also, Oncotic pressure; Osmolality and osmolarity; Tonicity

Ouabain. Plant-derived **cardiac glycoside**, traditionally used as an arrow poison in East Africa. Poorly absorbed from the GIT and administered iv. Faster acting than **digoxin**; thus was used when rapid action is required. No longer commercially available in the UK.

Outreach team. Similar in role to the **medical emergency team**: improving the identification and care of acutely ill patients throughout hospitals but especially on general wards. Usually nurse-led, but may also contain experienced medical and physiotherapy staff, often from ICUs, who may provide the following services: rapid response to acutely ill patients in general ward areas; critical care education for ward clinicians; facilitation of early admission to ICU/HDU; early recognition of patients for whom CPR and/or ICU admission is inappropriate; and early post-ICU follow-up. Referral criteria include specific clinical scenarios or the results of **early warning scores**. Although popular and widely adopted, there is little robust evidence that such teams improve hospital mortality.

Goldhill DR (2005). Br J Anaesth; 95: 88–94

See also, Acute life-threatening events—recognition and treatment

Ovarian hyperstimulation syndrome. Condition caused by pharmacological stimulation of the ovaries with human chorionic gonadotropin (hCG) in assisted conception programmes. Characterised by ovarian enlargement,

pleural effusion, raised haematocrit and white blood cell count, oliguria, **acute kidney injury**, hepatic impairment and **ascites**; the last in particular may be massive and unrelenting. Clinical features range from abdominal discomfort/swelling and nausea/diarrhoea to hypovolaemic **shock**, renal failure and **ALI**. **DVT** may also occur. Mild symptoms occur in up to a quarter of cases of induced ovulation, whereas the severe form occurs in 1%–2%. Prevented by use of gonadotropin-releasing hormone agonists instead of hCG.

Treatment is mainly supportive, with correction of **hypovolaemia**, careful attention to fluid balance and correction of metabolic disturbances. DVT prophylaxis is recommended. Abdominal **paracentesis** and pleural drainage are usually performed in severe cases; ultrafiltration and re-infusion of the ascitic fluid iv have been used to replace the protein-rich fluid otherwise lost.

Overdoses, *see Poisoning and overdoses*

Oximetry. Determination of arterial **O_2 saturation** of **haemoglobin** (S_aO_2) by measuring absorbance of light by blood. Described in 1934 using open blood vessels, and in 1940 using ear/hand probes, but the technique was cumbersome and difficult to perform. Modern **pulse oximeters** became widespread from the 1980s following advances in microchip technology, allowing manipulation of the recorded signal. Included in the UK/Ireland minimal monitoring standard for anaesthesia since 1987.

Relies on the principle that absorbance of light energy by haemoglobin varies with its level of oxygenation. Oxygenated and deoxygenated haemoglobin (HbO and Hb, respectively) have different absorbance spectra (Fig. 127). **Isosbestic points** occur where the lines cross. Thus comparison of absorbance at different wavelengths allows estimation of the relative concentrations of HbO and Hb (i.e., S_aO_2). Earlier machines used two wavelengths, including one isosbestic point as a reference; modern pulse oximeters may use two or more wavelengths, not necessarily including an isosbestic point.

Blood gas machines estimate S_aO_2 from arterial samples, whereas pulse oximeters read from ear or finger probes measuring light passing through tissue. Analysis of reflected light has also been used to determine S_aO_2; surface probes have been developed that may be stuck on to skin at any site, e.g. the head of a fetus. Other applications/derivations include retinal oximetry, in which a digital camera image of the retina is split according to wavelength and analysed for HbO/Hb components, and **near infrared spectroscopy**.

Oximeters are calibrated using data measured from human volunteers; saturations <80% are therefore estimated from extrapolated data, and may be inaccurate.
See also, Beer–Lambert law

Oxpentifylline, *see Pentoxifylline*

Oxycodone hydrochloride. **Opioid analgesic drug**, described in 1916. Oral preparations are twice as potent as oral **morphine** due to higher oral **bioavailability**. Intravenous oxycodone is roughly equivalent to iv morphine.

- Dosage: initially 5 mg orally 4–6-hourly, or 10 mg slow-release 12-hourly, increased to a maximum of 400 mg/day. May also be given sc/slowly iv: 1–10 mg 4-hourly.

Also available as suppositories (as the pectinate) by special order.

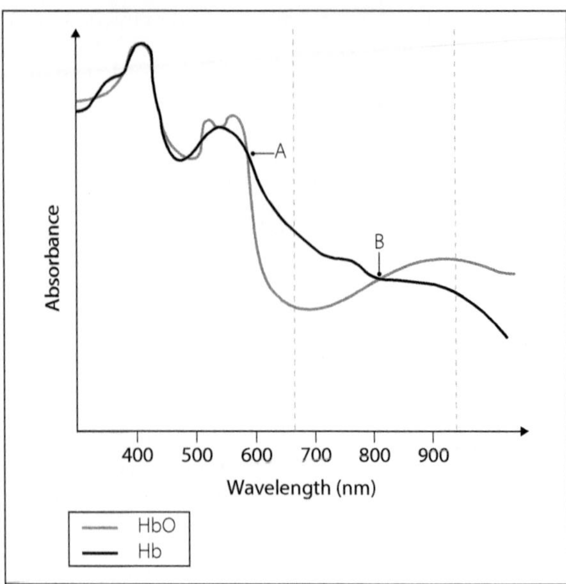

Fig. 127 Absorbance of light by oxygenated (HbO) and deoxygenated (Hb) haemoglobin: *A* and *B* are isosbestic points. The vertical dashed lines indicate the wavelengths (660 nm and 940 nm) most often used by modern pulse oximeters

Oxygen. Non-metallic element existing as a colourless, odourless diatomic gas (O_2) in the lower atmosphere, and as triatomic oxygen (O_3, ozone) and monatomic oxygen (O) in the upper atmosphere. The most plentiful element in the Earth's crust (as opposed to nitrogen, the most plentiful in the atmosphere), it makes up 21% of **air** by volume. Discovered independently in 1771 by Scheele and **Priestley**, the latter calling it 'dephlogisticated air'. Recognised as a gas by **Lavoisier**, who named it and explained the process of combustion. Combines with many other elements and molecules, and most abundant as water.

Essential for cellular respiration in animals and lower plants; higher plants take in CO_2 and release O_2 during photosynthesis. Boiling point is −183°C; melting point is −218°C; **critical temperature** is −118°C. Atomic weight is 16; **specific gravity** is 1.1 for liquid O_2 and 1.4 for gaseous O_2.

Commercial O_2 is supplied in liquid form, manufactured by the fractional distillation of air. Available in hospitals by **piped gas supply**, **O_2 concentrators** or in **cylinders** at 137 bar.
[Carl W Scheele (1742–1786), Swedish chemist]
See also, Oxygen...; Phlogiston; Vacuum insulated evaporator

Oxygen cascade. Series of 'steps' of PO_2 from atmospheric **air** to mitochondria in cells:

- dry atmospheric gas: 21 kPa (160 mmHg): influenced by barometric pressure and inspired O_2 concentration.
- humidified tracheal gas: 19.8 kPa (150 mmHg).
- alveolar gas: 14 kPa (106 mmHg): influenced by alveolar ventilation and O_2 consumption.
- arterial blood: 13.3 kPa (100 mmHg): influenced by **$\dot{V}/\dot{Q}$ mismatch**.
- capillary blood: 6–7 kPa (45–55 mmHg): influenced by blood flow and haemoglobin concentration.
- mitochondria: 1–5 kPa (7.5–40 mmHg).

Reduction in PO_2 at any stage, e.g. due to **hypoventilation**, lung disease, causes reduction in subsequent steps, risking

inadequate mitochondrial Po_2 for aerobic metabolism (below the **Pasteur point**).
See also, Hypoxia; Oxygen, tissue tension; Oxygen transport

Oxygen concentrator. Device for extracting **O_2** from atmospheric **air**. Air is passed under pressure through a column of **zeolite**, which acts as a molecular sieve, trapping nitrogen and water vapour while leaving O_2 and trace gases. Nitrogen is removed by depressurising the column. Two columns are used, each alternatively adsorbing or expelling nitrogen. Produces a continuous supply of over 90% O_2, suitable for most medical uses. Range in size from small units for home use to large ones supplying whole hospitals.

Oxygen delivery ($\dot{D}o_2$). Calculated **O_2 flux**. Used with O_2 consumption ($\dot{V}o_2$) to optimise treatment in critical illness.

$$\dot{D}o_2 = \textbf{cardiac output}\ (CO) \times \text{arterial } O_2 \text{ content}$$
$$= 850\text{–}1200\ \text{ml/min}\ (500\text{–}700\ \text{ml/min/m}^2)$$
$$\dot{V}o_2 = CO \times (\text{arterial } O_2 \text{ content} - \text{mixed venous } O_2 \text{ content})$$
$$= 240\text{–}270\ \text{ml/min}\ (120\text{–}160\ \text{ml/min/m}^2)$$

May be used to supplement other measured cardiovascular variables, e.g. BP, CVP, CO. As $\dot{D}o_2$ falls, a critical point is reached, after which $\dot{V}o_2$ also falls, representing tissue anaerobic respiration. Maintenance of $\dot{D}o_2$ above 600 ml/min/m^2, and $\dot{V}o_2$ above 170 ml/min/m^2, was previously suggested to increase survival in critical illness, but this is no longer considered to be the case.

O_2 extraction ratio has also been used (normally 22%–30%):

$$\frac{\text{arterial} - \text{mixed venous } O_2 \text{ contents}}{\text{arterial } O_2 \text{ content}}$$

See also, Oxygen extraction ratio; Oxygen, tissue tension; Regional tissue oxygenation; Shock

Oxygen extraction ratio. Ratio of oxygen uptake ($\dot{V}o_2$) to **oxygen delivery** ($\dot{D}o_2$), expressed as a percentage. Normally 22–30%, it increases during periods of increased tissue demand, e.g. exercise. Also varies according to the tissue involved; thus myocardial extraction ratio is about 70%.

Oxygen failure warning device. Device attached to (or incorporated into) the **anaesthetic machine**; designed to alert anaesthetists to failure of the O_2 supply. Earlier models were often unreliable, e.g. Bosun device (required batteries to power a warning light, which could be switched off, and only operated when the N_2O supply was connected).

- Ideal features of mechanical devices:
  - audible warning activated when O_2 pressure falls below a certain value; powered by O_2 itself.
  - warning continues when O_2 is exhausted; powered by N_2O.
  - delivery of N_2O turned off.
  - breathing system opened to atmosphere, allowing inhalation of air.
  - cannot be switched off.

Most consist of a spindle, kept at one end of its casing by the normal working O_2 pressure; a spring moves the spindle towards the other end as O_2 pressure falls, allowing O_2 to pass to a whistle via a port previously blocked by the spindle. Further movement as O_2 pressure continues to fall allows N_2O to flow to a whistle, stops N_2O delivery to the patient and opens the system to air. Many have a visual indicator too, e.g. producing a colour change.

Modern devices are electronic rather than gas-powered.

Oxygen flux. Amount of O_2 delivered to the tissues per unit time.

Equals:

$$CO \times \text{arterial } \mathbf{O_2} \text{ content}$$
$$= (CO \times O_2 \text{ bound to } \textbf{haemoglobin} + O_2 \text{ dissolved in plasma})$$
$$= CO \times [(Hb \times S_aO_2 \times 1.34) + (10 \times P_aO_2 \times 0.0225)]$$

where CO = **cardiac output** in l/min
Hb = haemoglobin concentration in g/l
S_aO_2 = arterial **O_2 saturation** of haemoglobin
1.34 = **Hüfner constant**
P_aO_2 = arterial Po_2 in kPa
0.0225 = ml of O_2 dissolved per 100 ml plasma per kPa (0.003 ml per mmHg)

Normally 850–1200 ml/min, or 500–700 ml/min/m^2 if **cardiac index** is used.

The tissues cannot utilise all of the transported O_2: the last 20%–25% remains bound to haemoglobin. Tissue O_2 supply can increase during times of extra demand via increases in cardiac output, e.g. during exercise. If the O_2 carrying capacity of blood is reduced (e.g. in **anaemia**) cardiac output must increase at rest in order to maintain O_2 flux, and reserves are less. Myocardial depression during anaesthesia in this situation is thus particularly hazardous.
See also, Oxygen delivery; Oxygen extraction ratio; Oxygen, tissue tension; Oxygen transport

Oxygen, hyperbaric. O_2 therapy at greater than atmospheric pressure, usually 2–3 atmospheres. Increases the amount of dissolved O_2 in blood, according to **Henry's law**. In 100 ml blood, 0.3 ml O_2 dissolves at Po_2 of 13.3 kPa (100 mmHg). Thus for 100% O_2 at 3 atmospheres, dissolved O_2 = 5.7 ml. Because **haemoglobin** is always saturated, even in venous blood, its binding capacity for CO_2 and buffering capacity are reduced, and pH falls. The resultant **hyperventilation** may result in **hypocapnia**.

Used in the treatment of **carbon monoxide poisoning**, **gas embolism**, **gas gangrene**, **decompression sickness** and chronic wounds, and has been investigated as an adjunct to **radiotherapy** and in multiple sclerosis. Single-patient chambers filled with 100% O_2 may be used, or large, pressurised chambers containing patient and attendants, with a tightly fitting mask applied to the patient.
See also, Oxygen transport

Oxygen measurement. Methods include:

- **gas analysis**:
  - chemical, e.g. conversion to non-gaseous compounds, with reduction in overall volume of gas mixture (**Haldane apparatus**).
  - physical:
    - O_2 electrode (Clark electrode; polarographic cell): silver/silver chloride anode and platinum cathode in potassium chloride solution inside a cylinder, with a gas-permeable plastic membrane covering its end. 0.6 V potential

is applied across the electrodes. O_2 diffuses to the cathode, reacting with electrons and water to form hydroxide ions and causing current flow proportional to the O_2 concentration. Thus:

$$O_2 + 2H_2O + 4e^- \rightarrow 4OH^-$$

The following reactions occur at the anode:

$$4\,Ag \rightarrow 4\,Ag^+ + 4e^-$$

$$4\,Ag^+ + 4\,Cl^- \rightarrow 4\,AgCl$$

May be used with gas or liquid samples. Maintained at 37°C. Falsely high readings caused by **halothane** are prevented by using a membrane impermeable to halothane.

- fuel cell: similar to the O_2 electrode but produces its own potential. Consists of lead anode and gold mesh cathode within potassium hydroxide solution. Hydroxide ions are produced at the cathode as above; they combine with lead at the anode to form lead oxide and give up electrons. Thus current flows, proportional to the number of O_2 molecules diffusing through the plastic membrane. No external power source is required, but lifespan is limited. May be affected by **N_2O** unless special cells are used.
- paramagnetic cell: most gases are diamagnetic, i.e., repelled by magnetic fields. O_2 and nitric oxide are paramagnetic, i.e., attracted. The cell contains two nitrogen-filled glass spheres joined by a bar that is suspended on a vertical wire within a magnetic field. O_2 introduced into the cell is attracted into the magnetic field, displacing the spheres and rotating the bar against the torque of the wire. Degree of rotation is proportional to the number of O_2 molecules. It may be measured by observing the deflection of a beam of light reflected by a mirror mounted on the wire, or by measuring the current required to prevent rotation when passing through a coil mounted on the bar. A rapid response paramagnetic device employs an alternating magnetic field applied to two streams of gas, one sample and the other reference; the O_2 concentration in the sample gas is represented by a difference in pressure between the two streams. Alternatively, an alternating magnetic field is applied to the gas, producing a sound wave; its amplitude is proportional to the concentration of O_2 (magnetoacoustic technique). Accuracy of these techniques is high.
- non-specific methods, e.g. **mass spectrometer**, ultraviolet light absorption.

- measurement of arterial $P\text{O}_2$:
  - O_2 electrode as above. Tiny intravascular probes have been developed for continuous arterial measurement.
  - transcutaneous electrode: similar to the O_2 electrode, but with a heating coil to cause vasodilatation, increase rate of O_2 diffusion, and reduce the difference between arterial and skin $P\text{O}_2$. Inaccurate, especially in adults, and with slow response time; they may also cause burns.
  - fibreoptic sensor placed intravascularly; measures intensity or wavelength of reflected light.
- measurement of arterial O_2 content: e.g. liberation of gas from blood with chemical analysis (**van Slyke apparatus**) or use of an O_2 electrode.
- measurement of **oxygen saturation** of haemoglobin.

[Leland C Clark (1918–2005), US biochemist]

Oxygen radicals, *see Free radicals*

Oxygen saturation. Refers to percentage saturation of **haemoglobin** with O_2; equals

$$\frac{O_2 \text{ content of haemoglobin}}{O_2 \text{ capacity of haemoglobin}}$$

May be calculated for whole blood, and the dissolved O_2 component subtracted, or measured using **oximetry**. Normal range in arterial blood at 37°C, pH 7.40 and normal barometric pressure is 97%–100%. Reduced in cardiac or respiratory disease.

Oxygen therapy. Used to:

- correct **hypoxaemia** due to **$\dot{V}/\dot{Q}$ mismatch**, **hypoventilation** or impaired alveolar gas **diffusion**. Only partially corrects hypoxaemia due to **shunt**.
- increase pulmonary O_2 reserves, e.g. in case of **apnoea**, **hypoventilation**, **preoxygenation**.
- increase the amount of dissolved oxygen, e.g. in **anaemia**, **cyanide poisoning** and **carbon monoxide poisoning** (also increases rate of carboxyhaemoglobin dissociation).
- other uses include reduction of **pulmonary hypertension**, reduction of air-filled cavities (e.g. subcutaneous emphysema, **pneumothorax**, **gas embolism**, intestinal distension), and special uses of hyperbaric O_2 (*see Oxygen, hyperbaric*).

The effects of breathing 100% O_2 compared with air are shown in Table 37.

- Methods of administration:
  - fixed performance devices; i.e., $F_{I}O_2$ is constant, despite changes in inspiratory flow rate:
    - O_2 tent.
    - **anaesthetic breathing system**.
    - **Venturi** devices or high air flow O_2 enrichers (HAFOE): the facemask feed connector incorporates holes designed to allow entrainment of atmospheric air into the O_2 stream by **jet mixing**.

      Specific connectors produce set $F_{I}O_2$ values at certain O_2 flow rates, assuming the patient's peak inspiratory flow rate does not exceed the total gas flow rate (if this occurs, air will be entrained via the side-holes in the facemask, and the $F_{I}O_2$ will fall). Devices that deliver lower $F_{I}O_2$ entrain more air and deliver higher total gas flow, and so deliver the stated $F_{I}O_2$ more reliably; e.g. the 0.28 $F_{I}O_2$ device delivers a total flow of 45 l/min to the patient, while the 0.6 $F_{I}O_2$ delivers 30 l/min total flow.
  - variable performance devices; i.e., $F_{I}O_2$ depends on inspiratory flow rates:
    - nasal cannulae. A nasal catheter, with a foam cuff to aid placement in the nostril, is also available.
    - plastic masks, e.g.:
      - moulded hard plastic.
      - Edinburgh: soft plastic.
      - MC: soft plastic with foam-padded edges.

      All perform similarly, delivering approximately 25%–30% O_2 at 2 l/min O_2 flow, and 30%–40% at 4 l/min flow.

Table 37 Effects of breathing air or 100% O_2

	Air	100% O_2
Alveolar PO_2 (kPa [mmHg])	14 [106]	88 [667]
Arterial blood		
PO_2 (kPa [mmHg])	13.3 [100]	84 [638]
O_2 saturation	99%	100%
O_2 content (ml/100 ml blood):		
bound to haemoglobin	19.7	20.1
dissolved	0.3	1.9
Venous blood		
PO_2 (kPa [mmHg])	5.3 [40]	7 [53.2]
O_2 saturation	75%	85%
O_2 content (ml/100 ml blood):		
bound to haemoglobin	14.9	17.2
dissolved	0.1	0.2

 - other means of administration include **IPPV** and its variations, **CPAP**, **apnoeic oxygenation** (including **THRIVE**) and hyperbaric therapy. Transtracheal administration has also been used in chronic lung disease requiring continuous O_2 therapy, via a narrow-bore catheter inserted above the sternal notch.
- Problems of O_2 therapy:
  - reduction of hypoxic ventilatory drive in a small group of patients who have chronic CO_2 retention, e.g. **COPD**. Apnoea may result if chronic hypoxaemia is reversed, thus necessitating controlled O_2 therapy. 24% O_2 is administered initially; if arterial PCO_2 has not risen by more than 1–1.5 kPa (7.5–10 mmHg), and PO_2 has not improved adequately, 28% O_2 is administered, then 30%, etc., until satisfactory PO_2 and PCO_2 have been achieved. It has recently been suggested that this phenomenon is related to an acute decrease in pulmonary vascular resistance following O_2 administration, rather than a reduction in hypoxic ventilatory drive itself.
  - it is recognised that patients in ICU have in the past received high levels of oxygen supplementation resulting in hyperoxaemia. This can result in cerebral vasoconstriction, neuronal cell damage, seizures, decreased cardiac output and vasoconstriction,. Pulmonary **O_2 toxicity** may also occur. F_IO_2 is now titrated to produce normal P_aO_2 levels.
  - absorption **atelectasis**.
  - increased risk of **explosions and fires**.
  - **retinopathy of prematurity**.

[MC: Mary Catterall (1939–2009), London physician]

Oxygen, tissue tension (P_TO_2). Partial pressure of O_2 in tissues; represents the balance between local supply and consumption of O_2. Most often measured in subcutaneous tissue because of its ease of measurement and relative stability (normally 1 ml/kg/min). Measured using an O_2 electrode mounted on a microcatheter or a fibreoptic probe placed under the skin. Has been used to indicate tissue perfusion; thought to be important in wound healing and susceptibility to infection.

De Santis V, Singer M (2015). Br J Anaesth; 115: 357–65

Oxygen toxicity. May be:
 - respiratory: pulmonary toxicity is related to actual PO_2, not concentration. Tracheobronchial irritation and substernal discomfort are noticed by healthy volunteers after 12–24 h breathing 100% O_2. Reduced **vital capacity, compliance** and **diffusing capacity**, and increased arteriovenous **shunt** and **dead space**, may occur after 24–36 h. Changes include endothelial damage, reduced mucus clearance and infiltration by inflammatory cells. **Surfactant** levels may decrease and capillary permeability increase. Eventually fibrosis may occur, although maximal safe concentrations and duration of **O_2 therapy** are unclear. Up to 48 h breathing 100% O_2 is thought not to be associated with permanent damage; up to 50% is considered safe for any period. Certain **cytotoxic drugs** increase the incidence and severity of fibrosis, e.g. **bleomycin. Free radical** formation is the most likely mechanism. Free radical scavengers, surfactant and **leukotriene** blocking drugs have been investigated as protective or therapeutic agents, but prevention is considered more effective. The lowest F_IO_2 that produces an acceptable arterial PO_2 should be used whenever O_2 is administered.
 - neurological: visual disturbances, tinnitus, nausea, twitching, irritability/anxiety/confusion, dizziness. At above 2–3 atmospheres, **convulsions** may occur (**Bert effect**).
 - ocular: exposure to high arterial PO_2 for long periods may lead to **retinopathy of prematurity**.

Oxygen transport. In a normal person with a haemoglobin concentration of 150 g/l breathing air, arterial blood carries approximately 20 ml O_2 per 100 ml:
 - 19.7 ml combined with **haemoglobin**.
 - 0.3 ml dissolved in plasma.

In venous blood, 15 ml is carried per 100 ml blood:
 - 14.9 ml combined with haemoglobin.
 - 0.1 ml dissolved.

Normally, the amount carried by haemoglobin is only slightly increased with **O_2 therapy**, because haemoglobin is already over 97% saturated; the dissolved O_2 is increased in proportion to the arterial PO_2: 0.0226 ml per kPa per 100 ml blood (0.3 ml per 100 mmHg).

See also, Oxygen flux

Oxygenation index. Indicator of the degree of impairment of oxygenation, often used in studies of neonatal respiratory support as a means of assessing severity of respiratory failure when comparing different respiratory therapies:

$$\text{equals} \frac{F_IO_2\ (\%) \times \text{mean airway pressure } (\text{cmH}_2\text{O})}{P_aO_2\ (\text{mmHg})}$$

Values above 40 are associated with about 80% mortality with conventional treatment.

Oxygenators, *see Cardiopulmonary bypass*

Oxyhaemoglobin dissociation curve. Plot of **oxygen saturation** of **haemoglobin** against PO_2, for normal haemoglobin and PCO_2 at 37°C (Fig. 128a). The curve is sigmoid-shaped because of the increasing affinity of haemoglobin for successive O_2 molecules after the first.
- Important points on the curve:
  - P_{50}: PO_2 at which saturation is 50%; normally about 3.5 kPa (27 mmHg).

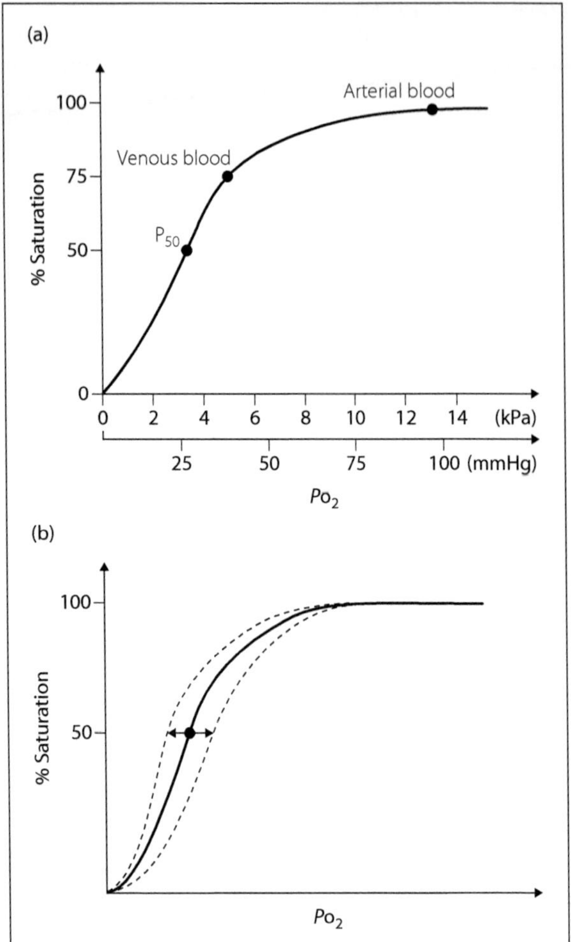

Fig. 128 Oxyhaemoglobin dissociation curve: (a) normal; (b) shift to right or left

- venous blood: normally corresponds to 75% saturation and Po_2 of 5.3 kPa (40 mmHg).
- arterial blood: normally corresponds to 97% saturation and Po_2 of 13.3 kPa (100 mmHg).

Thus a small drop in Po_2 from normal levels causes only slight reduction in arterial saturation, because the curve is flat at this point. If Po_2 is already reduced, e.g. in lung disease, the same small drop may cause significant desaturation, corresponding to the steep part of the curve.

The curve is shifted to the right (i.e., P_{50} >3.5 kPa) by **acidosis**, **hyperthermia**, **hypercapnia (Bohr effect)** and increased **2,3-DPG** levels (Fig. 128b). Saturation becomes lower for any given Po_2; i.e., O_2 is bound less avidly. Thus O_2 unloading to the tissues is favoured.

The curve is shifted to the left (i.e., P_{50} <3.5 kPa) in the opposite situations, and in **fetal haemoglobin**, **methaemoglobinaemia** and **carbon monoxide poisoning**. Saturation becomes greater for any given Po_2; i.e., O_2 is bound more avidly. Thus fetal haemoglobin can bind O_2 from maternal haemoglobin.

See also, Myoglobin

Oxymorphone hydrochloride. **Opioid analgesic drug**, derived from **morphine** and 6–8 times as potent. Developed in 1955. Available in the USA for parenteral and rectal use. Action lasts 4–5 h.

Oxytocin. Hormone secreted by the posterior **pituitary gland**, causing smooth muscle contraction in the **uterus** and milk ducts. Used to stimulate uterine contraction, e.g. during labour, postpartum or post-abortion. Less effective in early pregnancy. Acts within 2–3 min of iv injection. Synthetic preparation (Syntocinon) is free of **vasopressin**, and thus preferable to pituitary extract.

Causes less nausea/vomiting than **ergometrine** and does not cause hypertension (*but see later*). Available as 5 U and 10 U, and as 5 U in combination with ergometrine 500 µg.

- Dosage:
  - to stimulate labour: 1–4 mU/min iv, increased in at least 30-min steps up to 20 mU/min.
  - at **caesarean section** or after vaginal delivery: 2.5–5 U slowly iv (may also be given im, although not licensed by this route). Often given as an infusion after caesarean section (typically 40 U/500 ml, given over 4 h).
  - to treat **postpartum haemorrhage**: 5–10 U slowly iv followed by 5–40 U/500 ml crystalloid, infused as required.
- Side effects:
  - uterine hyperstimulation and fetal distress.
  - reduction in SVR and BP and increased cardiac output results from vasodilatation (thought to be due at least partly to the preservative/vehicle rather than to the drug itself), together with autotransfusion from the uterus to the systemic circulation. Tachycardia may also occur. These changes may be severe, especially when a single bolus of oxytocin is given rapidly, in doses >5 U and following **ephedrine** administration. Severe hypotension may occur when oxytocin is given to patients with cardiac disease.
  - severe **hyponatraemia** has followed prolonged infusion if diluted in dextrose solutions, exacerbated by a direct antidiuretic effect of the hormone itself.
  - rashes, nausea, allergic reactions.

P_{50}, *see Oxyhaemoglobin dissociation curve*

P value, *see Probability*

P wave. Component of the **ECG** representing atrial depolarisation. Normally positive (i.e., upwards) in lead I, and best seen in leads II and V_1 (*see Fig. 60b;* **Electrocardiography**). Maximal amplitude is normally 2.5 mm in lead II, and its duration 0.12 s (three small squares). In right atrial enlargement, the P wave is tall and peaked (P pulmonale); in left atrial enlargement, it is wide and notched (P mitrale).
See also, P–R interval

PA(A)s, *see Physicians' assistants (anaesthesia)*

Pacemaker cells. Cardiac muscle cells that undergo slow spontaneous depolarisation to initiate **action potentials**. Their activity results from a slow decrease in **membrane** potassium ion permeability, resulting in a gradual increase in intracellular calcium (via T-type calcium channels). Rate of discharge depends on the slope of phase 4 depolarisation, resting **membrane potential** and threshold potential. Pacemaker cells exist in the sinoatrial (SA) node, atrioventricular (AV) node, bundle of His and ventricular cells. Spontaneous rates of discharge for the different sites: SA node 70–80/min, AV node 60/min, His bundles 50/min and ventricular cells 40/min. Impulses from the faster SA node usually reach and excite the slower pacemaker cells before the latter can discharge spontaneously.
See also, Heart, conducting system

Pacemakers. Devices implanted subcutaneously, usually outside the thorax, that provide permanent **cardiac pacing** (to distinguish them from temporary pacing devices).

Modern devices consist of a titanium casing, containing the pulse generator and lithium iodide battery (the latter lasting >10 years). Electrodes are usually unipolar; i.e., one intracardiac electrode, with current returning to the pacemaker via the body. The heart electrode is usually endocardial, passed via a central vein; epicardial electrodes have been used. Leads may be steroid-eluting to reduce inflammation at the site of contact. Modern pacemakers are checked and adjusted via radiofrequency programming without requiring removal, and recorded data downloaded for analysis of cardiac function.

Indicated if an **arrhythmia** is associated with syncope, dizziness and **cardiac failure**, e.g. in **sick sinus syndrome**, **heart block** or post-**MI**. Prophylactic use is controversial.

A generic pacemaker code identifies function (Table 38), the first three positions indicating basic pacing function. Thus VVI denotes ventricular pacing and sensing, with inhibition of pacing if any spontaneous ventricular complex occurs (e.g. as would apply in temporary transvenous pacing). DDD denotes pacing and sensing of both chambers, with inhibition or triggering to maintain sequential atrial and ventricular contraction, allowing spontaneous activity if it occurs. Rate modulation implies the ability to alter the heart rate in response to the patient's level of activity; rate-adaptive devices respond to physiological parameters normally associated with changes in heart rate (e.g. body movement, **Q–T interval**, respiration, temperature, pH, myocardial contractility, haemoglobin saturation) by increasing the pacing rate. The fifth position is allocated to multisite pacing, which refers to stimulation of different sites either within one chamber (e.g. right ventricle) or within two chambers of the same type (e.g. both ventricles). With the development of implantable cardioverter defibrillators, much of the latter functions are covered within the defibrillator codes (*see Defibrillators, implantable cardioverter*).

- Anaesthesia for patients with pacemakers:
  - preoperatively:
    - **preoperative assessment** is particularly directed towards coexisting **cardiovascular disease**.
    - pacemaker type and indication are ascertained. Ideally patients should carry a European Pacemaker Patient identification card which provides all necessary details. Pacemakers are usually checked regularly (e.g. every 3 months).
    - if pacing spikes occur on the ECG before all or most beats, heart rate is pacemaker-dependent.
    - although traditional advice was to convert older demand pacemakers to fixed rate by placing a magnet over the pulse generator, this is no longer recommended outside specialist cardiac pacing units because the effect on the device's programming is unpredictable.
    - CXR: pulse generator and lead position may be identified.
  - perioperatively:
    - potential electrical interference or pacemaker damage by **diathermy** is more likely if the latter

Table 38 North American Society of Pacing and Electrophysiology/British Pacing and Electrophysiology Group generic pacemaker code

Position 1: chamber paced	*Position 2: chamber sensed*	*Position 3: response*	*Position 4: rate modulation*	*Position 5: multisite pacing*
0 = None	0 = None	0 = None	0 = None	0 = None
A = Atrium	A = Atrium	T = Triggered	R = Rate modulation	A = Atrium
V = Dual	V = Ventricle	I = Inhibited		V = Ventricle
D = Dual	D = Dual	D = Dual		D = Dual

is applied near the device. Sensing may be triggered, with resultant chamber inhibition, or arrhythmias induced. Diathermy may also reprogramme the pacemaker to a different mode.
    - if diathermy must be used, risks are reduced by using bipolar diathermy, or placing the plate distant from the pacemaker if unipolar diathermy is used. Current should not be applied across the chest, and its strength and duration of use should be minimal.
    - care should be taken with CVP/pulmonary artery catheters because they may dislodge the electrodes.
    - temporary pacing facilities (or non-invasive transthoracic pacing) and an external defibrillator should be available.
    - **isoprenaline** may be required if pacemaker failure occurs.
    - **MRI** may be hazardous because the pacemaker may be switched to asynchronous mode, may fail altogether or may move within the chest.
  - postoperative pacemaker checking may be required.

Healey JS, Merchant R, Simpson C, et al (2012). Can J Anaesth; 59: 394–407

Packed cell volume, *see Haematocrit*

PADP, Pulmonary artery diastolic pressure, *see Pulmonary artery pressure*

Paediatric Advanced Life Support (PALS). Course set up in the USA by the American Heart Association and the American Academy of Pediatrics. Intended for healthcare professionals caring for acutely ill children (e.g. those working in paediatric, anaesthetic, intensive care and emergency departments). Course objectives include:
  - recognition of the infant or child at risk of cardiopulmonary arrest and the application of strategies for its prevention.
  - identification of the cognitive and psychomotor skills necessary for resuscitating and stabilising the neonate, infant or child in respiratory failure, shock or cardiopulmonary arrest (e.g. drug dosages, airway and ventilation techniques, identification of normal and abnormal cardiac rhythms, defibrillation, vascular access).

The course is predominantly practical with an emphasis on 'hands-on' training. Technical skills and cognitive processes are first taught separately in small group sessions. Practical application of these skills and knowledge in critical situations is then emphasised by using case presentations.
See also, Advanced Paediatric Life Support

Paediatric anaesthesia. Main considerations are related to the anatomical and physiological differences between adults and children, especially **neonates** (defined as <1 month old; infants are <1 year old).
- Thus in children compared with adults:
  - RS:
    - the **tongue** is large and the **larynx** situated more anteriorly and cephalad (C3–4). The epiglottis is large and U-shaped. A straight **laryngoscope blade** may thus be preferred for intubating small babies, and the head should be in the neutral position (as opposed to the 'sniffing position' in adults).
    - the cricoid cartilage is the narrowest part of the upper airway up to 8–10 years of age (cf. glottis in adults). A small decrease in diameter (e.g. caused by oedema or stricture formation following prolonged tracheal intubation) may lead to **airway obstruction**.
    - the left and right main bronchi arise at equal angles from the trachea. At birth, the **tracheobronchial tree** is developed as far as the terminal bronchioles. Alveoli number 20 million, increasing to 300 million by 6–8 years.
    - respiration is predominantly diaphragmatic, and sinusoidal and continuous instead of periodic. Neonates are obligatory nose breathers. Respiratory rate is higher. **Tidal volume** is about 7 ml/kg as in adults. The infant lung is more susceptible to **atelectasis** because the chest wall is more compliant and therefore pulled inwards by the lungs, decreasing **FRC**. **Closing capacity** may exceed FRC during normal respiration in neonates and infants. **Surfactant** may be deficient in premature babies.
    - response to CO_2 is reduced at birth, and irregular breathing may also occur. Premature babies may suffer from apnoeic episodes; they are at risk of postoperative apnoea up to about 60 weeks postconceptual age. **Gasp** and **Hering–Breuer reflexes** are active.
    - **basal metabolic rate** and O_2 consumption are high (the latter is 5–6 ml/kg/min, compared with about 3–4 ml/kg/min in adults). **Hypoxaemia** thus occurs more rapidly than in adults.
    - the **oxyhaemoglobin dissociation** curve of **fetal haemoglobin** is shifted to the left (P_{50} of 2.4 kPa [18 mmHg]). **Haemoglobin** concentration falls from 180 g/l (1–2 weeks of age) to 110 g/l (6 months–6 years).
  - CVS:
    - in order to meet metabolic oxygen demand, **cardiac output** is relatively higher than in adults, achieved largely by increased **heart rate**. **Arterial BP** is lower (Table 39).
    - the immature heart is less compliant; **stroke volume** is relatively fixed and cardiac output highly rate dependent and particularly sensitive to increases in **afterload**.
    - **blood volume** at birth is up to 90 ml/kg (or 50 + **haematocrit**). It falls to 80 ml/kg for children and 70 ml/kg by 14 years.
    - veins may be more difficult to cannulate.
  - CNS:
    - the **spinal cord** ends at L3 at birth, receding to L1–2 by adolescence.
    - the immature **blood–brain barrier** results in increased sensitivity to centrally depressant drugs, particularly **opioid analgesic drugs**.
    - vagal reflexes are particularly active in children. Bradycardia readily occurs in hypoxaemia.
    - subependymal vessels are fragile in premature neonates, with risk of rupture if BP and **ICP** increase.

Table 39 Normal heart rate and BP at different ages

Age	Heart rate (beats/min)	BP (mmHg)
0–6 months	120–180	80/45
3 years	95–120	95/65
5 years	90–110	100/65
10 years	80–100	110/70

The potential neurotoxicity of anaesthetic drugs in the developing brain is an active area of research, with a number of in vitro and animal studies demonstrating neuronal loss with long-term neurocognitive deficits. Human studies (mostly retrospective observational studies) have yielded conflicting results; several prospective, randomised trials are in progress, with initial data suggesting that a single general anaesthetic in infancy has no impact on early development or cognition.

- **temperature regulation** is impaired. Ratio of body **surface area** to body weight is greater than in adults and there is less body fat. Thus heat loss is rapid, compounded by impaired shivering and increased metabolic rate. **Brown fat** is metabolised to maintain body temperature. **Insensible water loss** is increased in premature babies.
- prolonged fasting may cause **hypoglycaemia** in small children. Recommended fasting times: solid food and formula milk, 6 h, breast milk, 4 h. Although clear fluids have traditionally been withheld for 2 h preoperatively, they are increasingly being allowed up to 1 h before induction.
- **fluid balance** is delicate, because a greater proportion of body water is exchanged each day. Total body water is normally increased, with a higher ratio of **ECF** to **intracellular fluid** (ECF exceeds intracellular fluid in premature babies). The kidneys are less able to handle a water or solute load, or to conserve water or solutes. Thus **dehydration** may readily occur. Approximate maintenance fluid requirements (using glucose/saline) may be calculated thus:
  - 4 ml/kg/h for each of the first 10 kg, plus
  - 2 ml/kg/h for each of the next 10 kg, plus
  - 1 ml/kg/h for each kg thereafter.

  More recently, because of the risk of perioperative **hyponatraemia** (children being at particular risk from resultant encephalopathy), and because perioperative hypoglycaemia is less of a problem than traditionally thought, there has been a move away from hypotonic solutions such as glucose/saline, with maintenance fluids given as 0.45%–0.9% saline or Hartmann's solution, and isotonic fluids avoided if plasma sodium concentration is under 140 mmol/l. In acute **hypovolaemia**, 10 ml/kg **colloid** is a suitable initial bolus dose.

  Red cell transfusion should be given to maintain adequate **oxygen delivery**, taking into account underlying physiology (e.g. cyanotic heart disease) and potential for ongoing bleeding. 4 ml/kg of packed red cells increases **haemoglobin** concentration by approximately 10 g/l.
- actions of drugs may be affected by the above factors, or by lower plasma **albumin** levels (up to 1 year of age), resulting in greater amounts of free drug. Renal and hepatic immaturity may contribute to reduced **clearance**. The **MAC** of **inhalational anaesthetic agents** is increased in neonates, but may be reduced in premature babies. Neonates and infants are more sensitive to non-depolarising **neuromuscular blocking drugs**, probably due to altered pharmacokinetics. They require higher doses of **suxamethonium** (up to twice the adult dose) due to the larger **volume of distribution**.

- Practical conduct of anaesthesia:
  - children are placed first on the operating list, to minimise fasting time.
  - most standard drugs are used, administered according to weight. If the exact weight is unavailable, it may be estimated thus:
    - <1 year old, (age in months)/2 + 4;
    - 1–6 years old, 2 × (age in years) + 8;
    - >6 years old, 3 × (age in years) + 7.
  - sedative **premedication** may be given by the buccal/oral route (e.g. **midazolam**) or intranasally (e.g. **dexmedetomidine**). Intramuscular **atropine** may be given to reduce excessive secretions and vagal reflexes.
  - **induction of anaesthesia**:
    - a calm induction is the aim, with various techniques used to reduce anxiety, e.g. distraction, involving parents in their child's care, the use of toys and cartoons, etc.
    - **sevoflurane** (± **nitrous oxide**) is considered the agent of choice, as it leads to rapid induction with little airway irritation. Inhalational induction is rapid because of increased alveolar ventilation, a low **FRC** and a high **cerebral blood flow**.
    - standard **iv anaesthetic agents** are suitable. Administration im (e.g. **ketamine**) is also used. **EMLA** or topical **tetracaine** (amethocaine) is routinely used before iv induction.
  - appropriately sized **laryngoscope** handles and blades are employed. Uncuffed **tracheal tubes** are commonly used (usually until ~10 years), with a small air leak at 15–25 cmH_2O airway pressure, to avoid subglottic stenosis. Cuffed tubes are increasingly being used in younger children, on the basis that a smaller tube with a low-pressure, high-volume cuff is better able to provide an adequate conduit for ventilation while minimising pressure on the cricoid cartilage (from the tube itself) and the trachea (from the cuff). Several formulae have been suggested for estimating appropriate tube diameter and length (see Table 40). All formulae are merely guides, and appropriate sizing/length should be confirmed clinically and by observing the length of the tube at the glottis.
  - **dead space** and resistance should be minimal in **anaesthetic breathing systems**; adult forms are suitable if the child weighs over 20–25 kg but the Bain system is often avoided because of increased resistance to expiration. Ayre's T-piece is suitable up to 25 kg. Spontaneous ventilation via a **facemask** or **SAD** is usually suitable for short procedures in

Table 40 Paediatric tracheal tube sizes: (a) uncuffed and (b) cuffed

(a)				(b)	
Age	*Internal diameter (mm)*	*Length oral (cm)*	*Length nasal (cm)*	*Age*	*Internal diameter (mm)*
Neonate (>2 kg)	3.0–3.5	Weight in kg + 6	(Weight in kg + 6) × 1.2	Neonate (>2 kg)	2.5–3.0
6 months to 1 year	4.0–4.5	(Weight in kg ÷ 2) + 8	(Weight in kg ÷ 2) + 9	6 months to 1 year	3.0–4.0
>1 year	(Age in years ÷ 4) + 4.5	(Age in years ÷ 2) + 12	(Age in years ÷ 2) + 15	>1 year	(Age in years ÷ 4) + 3.5

children older than 3 months. Below this, tracheal intubation and IPPV are traditionally performed, although SADs are preferred by some.
    - for IPPV using a T-piece, the following fresh gas flows have been suggested, producing slight hypocapnia:
        - 10–30 kg: 1000 ml + 100 ml/kg per min.
        - >30 kg: 2000 ml + 50 ml/kg per min.

      Set minute volume should equal twice fresh gas flow.
    - routine **monitoring**, including **temperature measurement**.
    - anaesthetic rooms and operating theatres should be warmed. Warming blankets and reflective coverings should also be used, with **humidification** of inspired gases.
    - tracheal **extubation** may be performed with the child awake or anaesthetised, depending on the clinical context.
    - **emergence phenomena** such as **laryngospasm** and agitation/delirium may occur; the latter is particularly common after sevoflurane anaesthesia and in pre-school age children.
    - a multimodal approach to **postoperative analgesia** is used, where possible combining regional techniques (e.g. **caudal analgesia**), **paracetamol**, **NSAIDs** and **opioid analgesic drugs** (e.g. **morphine** or **fentanyl**). Intravenous opioids may be administered via nurse-controlled analgesia. **Ketamine** is often useful in severe postoperative pain, and may be added to morphine infusions. **Codeine** was previously widely used in children, but this has been restricted since 2013 because of the risk of excessive sedation/respiratory depression; it is now contraindicated in children <12 years and all children undergoing adenoidectomy or tonsillectomy for **obstructive sleep apnoea**.
    - **PONV** is common, particularly in children >3 years; prophylactic **antiemetic drugs** (e.g. **ondansetron**, **dexamethasone**) are routinely given.
- Other specific problems are related to the procedure performed, e.g.:
    - repair of congenital defects, e.g. **tracheo-oesophageal fistula, pyloric stenosis, gastroschisis, diaphragmatic hernia, congenital heart disease**.
    - related to **trauma**.
    - **ENT, dental** and **ophthalmic surgery**.

Paediatric intensive care. Classified into levels 1, 2 and 3, primarily on the basis of interventions undertaken. Level 1 is high dependency care; level 3 is almost always provided in tertiary paediatric centres. In general, differs from adult intensive care by virtue of anatomical and physiological differences between adults and children (*see Paediatric anaesthesia*) and the range of conditions seen.
- Main clinical problems encountered include:
    - acute respiratory failure:
        - upper **airway obstruction**:
            - neonates: **choanal atresia**, congenital **facial deformities**, laryngeal/tracheal abnormalities.
            - infants/children: inhaled **foreign body**, tonsillar/adenoidal hypertrophy, **croup**, **epiglottitis** and **angio-oedema**.
        - lung disorders:
            - neonates: meconium aspiration, **respiratory distress syndrome**, **diaphragmatic hernia**, **pneumothorax**, **chest infection**.
            - infants/children: pneumonia, **asthma**, **bronchiolitis**, **cystic fibrosis**, **congenital heart disease**, **trauma**, **near-drowning**, **burns**.
            - in neonates, respiratory impairment may result in the development of a persistent **fetal circulation**.
    - neurological disease:
        - neonates: birth asphyxia, central apnoea, **convulsions**.
        - infants/children: **meningitis**, **encephalitis**, **status epilepticus**, **Guillain–Barré syndrome**.
    - trauma: the leading cause of death in children under a year old and the third leading cause in older children (after sudden infant death syndrome and congenital abnormalities). Non-accidental injury must always be considered.
        - **TBI** occurs in 50% of cases of blunt trauma. A modified **Glasgow coma scale** is used for assessment; otherwise, management is along similar lines to that of adults.
        - **spinal cord injury** and thoracic/abdominal trauma is usually caused by road traffic accidents.
    - **poisoning and overdoses**.
- Specific attention must be paid to:
    - smaller equipment, drug doses and fluid volumes; specialised equipment.
    - **nutrition** and electrolyte/**fluid balance**.
    - **temperature regulation**.
    - **sedation** and analgesia.
    - educational and psychological needs.
    - the risk of **retinopathy of prematurity** in neonates.

In 1997, the Department of Health recommended that level 3 paediatric intensive care should be primarily delivered in lead centres supported by district general hospitals (capable of initiating intensive care), major acute general hospitals (large adult ICUs already managing critically ill children at level 2 or 3) and specialist hospitals (e.g. those caring for children with burns or requiring cardiac or neurosurgery). Each centre must comply with specific standards relating to training, equipment, the experience of medical and nursing staff, access to specialist services and advice, treatment protocols, facilities for families and audit. Regional paediatric retrieval teams have also been established.

Overall mortality ranges from 5% to 10% depending on admission criteria. Scoring systems such as the **paediatric trauma score**, **injury severity score** and **paediatric risk of mortality score** attempt to predict outcome and allow **audit** of care within and between units.

See also, Brainstem death; Cardiopulmonary resuscitation, neonatal; Cardiopulmonary resuscitation, paediatric; Necrotising enterocolitis

Paediatric logistic organ dysfunction score (PELOD). Scoring system for the severity of multiple organ dysfunction in **paediatric intensive care**. Based on 12 variables relating to six organ systems (neurological, cardiovascular, renal, respiratory, haematological and hepatic). Has been used as daily indicator of organ dysfunction. The modified PELOD-2 score takes account of mean arterial pressure and lactaemia while dispensing with hepatic dysfunction.

Leteurtre S, Duhamel A, Salleron J, et al (2013). Crit Care Med; 41: 1761–73

Paediatric risk of mortality score (PRISM). Scoring system used in **paediatric intensive care** to help predict mortality. Originally used weighted scores for 14 variables related to acute physiological status; the latest version (PRISM III) has 17 and includes additional risk factors,

including acute and chronic diagnosis. Has been validated for most categories of paediatric ICU.
Pollack MM, Holbkov R, Funai T, et al (2016). Pediatr Crit Care Med; 17: 2–9

Paediatric trauma score. **Trauma scale** designed to allow **triage** of paediatric patients. Six variables (weight, patency of airway, systolic BP, level of consciousness, presence of skeletal injury and skin injuries) attract scores of 2 (normal), 1 or –1 (severely compromised); scores under 8 indicate increased morbidity and mortality and require referral to a paediatric trauma centre.

PAF, *see Platelet-activating factor*

Pain. Classically defined as an unpleasant sensory and emotional experience resulting from a stimulus causing, or likely to cause, tissue damage, or expressed in terms of that damage. Pain is a subjective experience that can be influenced by various emotional factors, making **pain evaluation** difficult. Chronic pain is often referred to as pain lasting >3 months (*see Pain, chronic*).
See also, Allodynia; Dysaesthesia; Hyperaesthesia; Hyperalgesia; Hyperpathia; Hypoalgesia; Myofascial pain syndromes; Nociception; Pain, neuropathic; Pain clinic; Pain management; Postoperative analgesia

Pain, central. Neuropathic pain resulting from damage to the central nervous system. May be spontaneous (either continuous or paroxysmal) or evoked by nociceptive stimuli. Usually burning in nature. Most commonly follows a **stroke** anywhere in the spinothalamic pathway but especially involving the thalamus (hence formerly called thalamic syndrome). Tends to occur within 6 months of the stroke. Proven treatments include **amitriptyline**, **selective serotonin reuptake inhibitors** and **lamotrigine**. Intravenous **lidocaine** can produce temporary analgesia. **Opioid analgesic drugs** are largely ineffective. Deep brain stimulation may be effective in drug-resistant patients.
Klit H, Finnerup NB, Jensen TS (2009). Lancet Neurol; 8: 857–68
See also, Pain, neuropathic

Pain, chronic. Persistent or recurring **pain** lasting longer than 3 months. Diagnoses can be classified as chronic:
- cancer pain.
- postsurgical or post-traumatic pain.
- neuropathic pain.
- headache or orofacial pain.
- visceral pain.
- musculoskeletal pain.
- primary pain (not fitting into the other categories, e.g. chronic widespread pain).

Treede RD, Rief W, Barke A, et al (2015). Pain; 156: 1003–7
See also, Analgesic drugs; Pain evaluation; Pain management; Pain, neuropathic; Pain pathways; Postoperative pain

Pain clinic. Outpatient clinic run by consultants (often anaesthetists) with a special interest in the management of chronic **pain**. Its role includes diagnosis of the underlying condition and management directed at reducing subjective pain experiences, reducing drug consumption, increasing levels of normal activity and improving quality of life. Requires appropriate facilities for consultation and interventions, which may include drugs, nerve blocks, surgical procedures, physiotherapy and psychological programmes. Ideally, services are multidisciplinary and include anaesthetists, physicians, psychologists, specialist nurses, occupational therapists, pharmacists and physiotherapists. Primary referrals to the clinic are usually from general practitioners or hospital consultants.
See also, Pain, chronic; Pain management

Pain evaluation. The gold standard of **pain** assessment is patient self-reporting because pain is a subjective experience. Should include exploration of the pain's characteristics, duration, location, intensity, time relations, any modifying factors (e.g. food, exercise) and associated symptoms.
- Methods used:
  - acute pain, e.g. postoperative:
    - self-reported assessment of pain, e.g. **linear analogue scale**, discrete rating scales (numerical or verbal rating scale) indicating the degree/severity of pain. Specific image-based scales have been used in children (e.g. Wong-Baker faces scale, consisting of happy/unhappy cartoon faces).
    - behavioural assessment, used in patients unable to self-report, e.g. behavioural pain scale in sedated critically unwell patients, FLACC (face, legs, activity, cry, consolability scale) in paediatrics, Abbey Pain Scale in patients with dementia and unable to verbalise.
  - chronic pain:
    - characterisation of pain plus examination/investigation as appropriate.
    - linear analogue/rating scales as above.
    - more complicated questionnaires that may include evaluation of disability, affect and the pain experience are often used (e.g. Brief Pain Inventory, McGill questionnaire).

Functional MRI allows imaging of pain pathways and the processes involved in pain perception.
[Donna Lee Wong (1948–2008), US paediatric nurse; Connie Baker, US child life specialist; Jennifer Abbey, Australian nurse]

Pain management. Acute **pain**, e.g. postoperative, is usually treated with systemic analgesics and regional techniques (*see Postoperative analgesia*).
- **Chronic pain** management may involve the following, after **pain evaluation**:
  - simple measures, e.g. exercise, heat and cold treatment, vibration.
  - systemic drug therapy:
    - **analgesic drugs**: different drugs, dosage regimens and routes of administration may be chosen, depending on the severity and temporal pattern of the pain, and efficacy and side effects of the drugs. Drugs used range from **paracetamol** and mild **NSAIDs** to **opioid analgesic drugs**. The latter are usually reserved for severe pain of short duration, or pain associated with malignancy. Implantable devices may be used for intermittent iv, epidural or subarachnoid injection or continuous infusion of opioids.
    - other drugs used include:
      - psychoactive drugs, e.g. **antidepressant drugs**, **anticonvulsant drugs** (e.g. **pregabalin**, **gabapentin**, **carbamazepine**). Of these, **amitriptyline**, pregabalin and **duloxetine** are suitable first-line agents for chronic/neuropathic pain.

- **corticosteroids**, either by local injection or oral therapy. Often injected with **local anaesthetic agents**, e.g. epidurally for back pain.
- muscle relaxants, e.g. **baclofen, dantrolene**; may be useful if muscle spasm is problematic.
- others, e.g. **antimitotic drugs**, calcitonin in bony pain, **β-adrenergic receptor antagonists, clonidine.**

▸ local anaesthetic nerve blocks: may be diagnostic, prognostic (to allow assessment before destructive lesions) or therapeutic. Include:
- injection of **trigger points** in **myofascial pain syndromes.**
- **facet joint injection.**
- **caudal analgesia, epidural anaesthesia, spinal anaesthesia.**
- **paravertebral nerve blocks.**
- **sympathetic nerve blocks**, e.g. **stellate ganglion, coeliac plexus** and **lumbar sympathetic blocks**, iv **guanethidine** block.

▸ neurolytic procedures: usually reserved for severe pain associated with malignancy, because relief may not be permanent and severe side effects may occur, e.g. **anaesthesia dolorosa.** X-ray guidance is usually employed to aid percutaneous neurolysis. Methods include:
- regional techniques as above, using phenol or absolute alcohol.
- extremes of temperature, e.g. **cryoprobe**, radio-frequency probe. The latter delivers a high-frequency alternating current, producing up to 80°C heat. It is used at peripheral nerves, facet joints, dorsal root ganglia and trigeminal ganglion, and for percutaneous **cordotomy.**
- surgery: includes peripheral neurectomy, dorsal rhizotomy or lesions in the dorsal root entry zones (DREZ), commissurotomy (sagittal division of the **spinal cord**), mesencephalotomy and thalamotomy.

▸ electrical stimulation:
- **TENS** and electroacupuncture.
- **spinal cord stimulation.**
- stimulation of deep brain structures has also been used, e.g. via electrodes implanted in the periventricular grey matter or thalamus.

▸ **acupuncture.**

▸ psychological techniques, e.g. psychotherapy, **cognitive behavioural therapy, operant conditioning, hypnosis, biofeedback**, relaxation techniques.

▸ physiotherapy and graded exercise programmes.

▸ multidisciplinary pain management programmes.

The World Health Organization has suggested a 'pain ladder' for cancer pain, which is often used as a guide for managing non-cancer pain: mild pain is treated by a non-opioid ± adjuvant; moderate pain by a mild opioid ± non-opioid ± adjuvant; and severe pain with a strong opioid ± non-opoid ± adjuvant.

Pain, neuropathic. Chronic pain arising from a lesion or disease of the somatosensory system. Affects ~8% of the UK population and is more common in women. May be:

▸ peripheral:
- diabetic neuralgia.
- **trigeminal neuralgia.**
- **complex regional pain syndrome.**
- immune-mediated neuralgia e.g. due to **Guillain–Barré syndrome**, chronic inflammatory demyelinating neuropathy.
- infection-related eg. **postherpetic neuralgia**, HIV-associated sensory neuropathy
- chemotherapy-induced neuropathy.

▸ central:
- post-stroke pain (*See also, Pain, central*).
- **multiple sclerosis.**
- post-**spinal cord injury.**

Signs and symptoms are diverse but often include reduced thermal or mechanical sensation in the area supplied by the affected nerve, or **hyperalgesia** and dynamic **allodynia.**

Although notoriously difficult to treat, management usually consists of first-line agents such as **anticonvulsant drugs** (e.g. **gabapentin, carbamazepine**) and **antidepressant drugs** (e.g. **amitriptyline, duloxetine**). Early referral to specialist multidisciplinary teams should be a priority, for consideration of further assessment and other treatment options, e.g. topical agents (**capsaicin** or **lidocaine** patches) or interventional techniques (e.g. **spinal cord stimulation**). Opioids are usually only a third-line treatment option in neuropathic pain.

Finnerup NB, Attal N, Haroutounian S, et al (2015). Lancet Neurology; 14: 162–73

See also, Pain evaluation; Pain management; Pain pathways

Pain, paradoxical. Term describing **pain** that does not respond to **opioid analgesic drugs** in the usual way. Typically described in patients with cancer pain on large doses of analgesics, especially **opioid analgesic drugs.** Now thought to represent **opioid-induced hyperalgesia** rather than a distinct entity itself.

Pain pathways. Most **pain** arises from stimulation of specialised receptors (mechanoreceptors for touch, thermoreceptors for temperature and chemoreceptors for chemical stimulation) on specific primary sensory neurons (nociceptors) that are widely distributed in the skin and musculoskeletal system. Myelinated Aδ fibres convey sharp pain sensation from thermo- or mechanoreceptor stimulation and are responsible for rapid pain transmission and reflex withdrawal. Receptors responding to pressure, heat, chemical substances (e.g. **histamine, prostaglandins, acetylcholine**) and tissue damage (polymodal receptors) are associated with unmyelinated C-fibre endings, and are responsible for dull pain sensation and immobilisation of the affected part.

- Afferent impulses pass centrally thus:
  ▸ first-order neurones have cell bodies within the dorsal root ganglia of the **spinal cord.** Aδ fibres synapse with cells in laminae I and V of the cord, while C fibres synapse with cells in laminae II and III (substantia gelatinosa).
  ▸ most second-order neurones synapse with Aδ fibres in the posterior horn, crossing to the opposite side immediately or within a few segments. They ascend within the anterolateral columns (spinothalamic tract) to the ventroposterior nucleus of the thalamus and periaqueductal grey matter.

  The substantia gelatinosa does not project directly to higher levels, but contains many interneurones involved in pain modulation (e.g. described by the **gate control theory of pain**). Some fibres project to deeper layers of the spinal grey matter, giving rise to the spinoreticular tract, which projects to the ascending reticular activating system (ARAS). Fibres are then relayed to the thalamus and **hypothalamus**

(some fibres reach the thalamus without passing to the ARAS, via the palaeospinothalamic tract).
- third-order neurones transmit from the thalamus to the somatosensory cortex.

Pain sensation may thus be modified by ascending or descending pathways at many levels.
See also, Nerves; Nociception; Sensory pathways

Pain, postoperative, *see Postoperative analgesia*

Palliative care. General approach to care of patients with advanced, progressive illness (often **malignancy** but also neurological, inflammatory, etc.), aimed at achieving the best quality of life within the time remaining to the patient rather than just prolonging life per se. Recognised as a separate specialty in the UK since 1987. Includes not only symptom control but also psychological, spiritual and social support of the patient and his/her family. Requires a multidisciplinary approach, including the expertise of general physicians, oncologists, surgeons, nursing staff, physiotherapists and religious advisers. Anaesthetists are often involved as they have expertise in controlling symptoms such as pain, anxiety, nausea and vomiting; they also care for patients with terminal disease in the ICU.
See also, Ethics; Euthanasia; Withdrawal of treatment in ICU

Palonosetron. **5-HT$_3$ receptor antagonist** licensed as an **antiemetic drug** in chemotherapy-induced nausea and vomiting.
- Dosage: single dose of 250 µg iv 30 min before, or 500 µg orally 1 h before, chemotherapy treatment.
- Side effects include GIT upset, arrhythmias, angina and peripheral neuropathy.

PALS, *see Paediatric advanced life support*

Pancreatitis. Acute pancreatitis is an autodigestive process caused by unregulated activation of trypsin in pancreatic acinar cells; this in turn leads to release of other enzymes and activation of complement and kinin pathways. Inflammatory processes also occur with the release of other harmful enzymes. Ischaemic changes, together with generation of **free radicals**, cause ischaemia and haemorrhagic necrosis of the pancreatic parenchyma. Although the condition is mild in 80% of patients, mortality is high in the remainder because of resulting **sepsis**, **respiratory failure**, **shock** and **acute kidney injury**.

Associated with biliary tract disease or **alcoholism** in about 80% of cases. May occasionally follow upper abdominal surgery, pancreatic ductal obstruction (e.g. by carcinoma), **trauma**, mumps, **hepatitis**, **cystic fibrosis**, **hypothermia**, **hypercalcaemia**, hyperlipidaemia, **diuretics** or **corticosteroids**. More common in smokers and those with type 2 **diabetes mellitus**.
- Features:
  - severe epigastric pain (typically radiating through to the back), nausea and vomiting, fever, occasionally mild jaundice.
  - epigastric tenderness, progressing to features of peritonitis.
  - discoloration in flanks caused by tracking of blood from the retroperitoneal space (Grey Turner's sign) or via the falciform ligament to the umbilicus (Cullen's sign).
  - **hypotension**, **oliguria**, respiratory failure.

Investigations reveal raised serum and urinary **amylase** (secondary to leakage from the pancreas), leucocytosis, **hyperglycaemia**, **hypocalcaemia** (secondary to calcium sequestration in areas of fat necrosis), **hypoproteinaemia** and hyperlipidaemia. Because many other disorders also result in increased amylase levels, measurement of the more specific marker serum lipase is increasingly used for diagnosis. Abdominal x-ray may reveal a 'sentinel loop' of small bowel overlying the pancreas. **CXR** may show a raised hemidiaphragm, **pleural effusion**, **atelectasis** or **ALI**. CT scanning may be helpful in confirming the diagnosis and assessing the severity of pancreatic damage.

Poor prognosis may be indicated by: age >55 years; systolic BP <90 mmHg; white cell count >15 × 10^9/l; temperature >39°C; blood glucose >10 mmol/l; arterial $P\text{O}_2$ <8 kPa (60 mmHg); plasma urea >15 mmol/l; serum calcium <2 mmol/l; haematocrit reduced by over 10%; abnormal **liver function tests**.
- Management:
  - supportive, e.g. **O_2 therapy**, **iv fluid administration**, electrolyte replacement (especially calcium and magnesium), insulin therapy and **nutrition** (via nasogastric or nasojejunal routes). **MODS** is treated along conventional lines. Early fluid resuscitation with appropriate volumes of Ringer's lactate solution is associated with reduced organ failure. Similarly, early enteral nutrition (within 48 h) improves outcome.
  - effective pain relief is essential.
  - **aprotinin**, **peritoneal lavage**, **glucagon**, **calcitonin** and **somatostatin** have been used, but with little evidence of efficacy.
  - prophylactic antibacterial agents to prevent infection of the necrotic pancreas are no longer advocated.
  - evidence of necrosis on CT imaging may merit fine-needle aspiration to diagnose localised infection and guide antibiotic therapy.
  - early endoscopic retrograde cholangiopancreatography (ERCP) with sphincterotomy is recommended in patients with biliary obstruction/sepsis.
  - surgery may be required for drainage of an abscess or pseudocyst or for relief of biliary obstruction. Resection of necrotic pancreas has been performed but mortality from surgery in early disease is high.

Chronic pancreatitis usually occurs in alcoholics, and is characterised by pancreatic calcification and impaired enzyme secretion with malabsorption, and repeated episodes of pain. Surgery may be required; anaesthetic considerations are related to alcohol abuse, and the consequences of malabsorption and **malnutrition**.
[George Grey Turner (1877–1951), English surgeon; Thomas S Cullen (1868–1953), Canadian-born US gynaecologist]
Lankisch PJ, Apte M, Banks PA (2015). Lancet; 386: 85–96

Pancuronium bromide. Synthetic non-depolarising **neuromuscular blocking drug**, first used in 1967. Bisquaternary amino-steroid, but with no steroid activity. Initial dose is 0.05–0.1 mg/kg, with tracheal intubation possible after 2–3 min. Effects last 40–60 min. Supplementary dose: 0.01–0.02 mg/kg. **Histamine** release is extremely rare. May cause increases in heart rate, BP and cardiac output, caused by vagolytic and sympathomimetic actions. The latter may be due to release of **noradrenaline** from sympathetic nerve endings or blockade of its uptake. Pancuronium is strongly bound to plasma gammaglobulin after iv injection, and metabolised mainly by the kidney but also by the liver. Elimination is delayed in renal and hepatic impairment.

Pandemic. Outbreak of an infectious disease affecting human populations across a wide region (e.g. multiple continents or worldwide).
See also, Influenza

Pantoprazole sodium. **Proton pump inhibitor**; actions and effects are similar to those of **omeprazole.**
- Dosage: 40–80 mg orally or iv od.
- Side effects: as for omeprazole.

Papaveretum. **Opioid analgesic drug**, first prepared in 1909 and consisting of **opium** alkaloids: **morphine** 47.5–52.5%, **codeine** 2.5%–5.0%, noscapine (narcotine) 16%–22%, **papaverine** 2.5%–7.0% and others, e.g. thebaine <1.5%. Widely popular for many years, especially as **premedication.** In response to a warning issued by the **Committee on Safety of Medicines** that noscapine may be genotoxic, a new formulation was made available in 1993, consisting of morphine, papaverine and codeine alone. Confusion over dosage regimens has led to many anaesthetists abandoning papaveretum in favour of morphine.
- Dosage: 7.7–15.4 mg sc, im or iv 4-hourly as required. Also available in combination with **hyoscine.**

Papaverine. Benzylisoquinoline **opium** alkaloid, without CNS activity. Used for its relaxant effect on smooth muscle, e.g. GIT and vascular. Has been used to treat cerebral and coronary vasospasm. May be injected iv or applied directly during surgery. Its use has been advocated following intra-arterial injection of **thiopental.**
- Dosage: up to 30 mg slowly iv (may cause **histamine** release). Also used in combination oral preparations to relieve GIT spasm.

Paracelsus (1493–1541). Swiss philosopher and physician; his real name was Theophrastus Bambastus von Hohenheim. Lectured at the University of Basle. Revolutionised the theory of medicine, encouraging the science of research and experimentation. Described the effects of **diethyl ether** on chickens in 1540 and advocated its use in epilepsy. He is also credited with introducing the use of bellows for ventilating the lungs.
Davis A (1993). J R Soc Med; 86: 653–6

Paracentesis. Puncture of any hollow organ or cavity for removal or instillation of material; however, the term usually refers to drainage of **ascites** from the peritoneum, e.g. in **hepatic failure.** Removal of large volumes improves cardiac output and respiratory function, decreasing portal venous pressure. It also reduces weight, improving comfort and mobility. However, rapid aspiration may be followed by cardiovascular collapse and oliguria, possibly due to sudden release of the splinting effect of the intra-abdominal fluid.

With the patient supine and with the bladder emptied, a needle is inserted through the abdominal wall, usually in the left and right upper and lower quadrants, after infiltration with local anaesthetic. The avascular linea alba below the umbilicus is also commonly used. Insertion of the needle along a Z-shaped path through the layers has been suggested, to reduce subsequent persistent leakage.
See also, Peritoneal lavage

Paracervical block. Used to provide analgesia during the first stage of labour, or for gynaecological procedures, e.g. dilatation and curettage. First performed in 1926.

With the patient's legs apart, a special sheathed needle (with tip protected) is directed into the lateral vaginal fornix by the operator's fingers. The needle tip is advanced 0.5–1 cm to point cranially, laterally and dorsally, and 5–10 ml **local anaesthetic agent** injected into the parametrial tissue on either side, blocking the uterine nerves that form a plexus at the base of the broad ligament. Vaginal, vulval and perineal sensation is unaffected.

Seldom used in modern obstetrics, because of the high incidence of fetal arrhythmias (especially bradycardia), thought to be caused by alterations in uteroplacental blood flow or absorption of local anaesthetic.
See also, Obstetric analgesia and anaesthesia

Paracetamol (Acetaminophen). **Analgesic drug**, derived from *para*-aminophenol; introduced in 1956. Inhibits central **prostaglandin** synthesis and has a central antipyretic action. Purported to have minimal peripheral anti-inflammatory effects, although this has been disputed. Also inhibits **cyclo-oxygenase** pathways in the brain, but less so peripherally. Does not cause gastric irritation or affect **platelet** adhesion. Used in isolation to treat minor pain, and as part of a multimodal strategy for **postoperative analgesia.**

Rapidly absorbed after oral administration, with peak plasma levels within 60 min. Minimally protein-bound in plasma. Conjugated with glucuronide and sulfate in the liver; <10% is oxidised by the hepatic P_{450} system to form *N*-acetyl-*p*-benzoquinone imine, a potential cellular toxin. Normally, this is safely conjugated with glutathione, but it may cause hepatic necrosis in **paracetamol poisoning,** when the glucuronide and sulfate pathways are saturated and glutathione stores are depleted. **Half-life** is about 2 h, but its effects last longer.
- Dosage:
  - 0.5–1.0 g orally/rectally 4-hourly, up to 4 g maximum daily.
  - in children, traditionally recommended dosage of 10–15 mg/kg 4-hourly × 4/day has been challenged based on pharmacokinetic data; an initial loading dose of 20 (oral) or 40 (rectal) mg/kg may be followed by doses of 10–15 mg/kg 4–6-hourly up to 40 (premature), 60 (<3 months old) or 90 (>3 months) mg/kg/day for up to 48 h (72 h if >3 months).
  - an iv preparation was introduced in the UK in 2004:
    - adult/child >50 kg: 1 g 4–6-hourly up to 4 g daily.
    - adult/child 10–50 kg: 15 mg/kg 4–6-hourly up to 60 mg/kg daily.
    - adult/child <10 kg: 7.5 mg/kg 4–6-hourly up to 30 mg/kg daily.
- Side effects: nausea, vomiting, rashes. Transient rises in alanine transaminase are unlikely to reflect significant liver damage.

Available in combination with other analgesics, e.g. **codeine.** Over-the-counter sale of 500-mg tablets/capsules in the UK is limited to packs of 32 (packs of 100 tablets/capsules may be purchased from pharmacists in special circumstances).

Paracetamol poisoning. The commonest cause of acute **hepatic failure** in the UK and USA. Hepatocellular necrosis may occur if >75 mg/kg is taken, due to saturation of the normal metabolic pathways for **paracetamol** and exhaustion of hepatic glutathione stores. Lower doses may also be toxic, especially in the presence of pre-existing hepatic **enzyme induction** (e.g. in patients on **phenytoin, barbiturates, carbamazepine** or **rifampicin** therapy), or in malnourished, alcoholic or **HIV**-positive patients.

Patients may be asymptomatic for 24 h after ingestion. Early features include nausea and vomiting, anorexia and right upper quadrant pain. Early impaired consciousness suggests concurrent depressive drug ingestion, e.g. **alcohol, opioid analgesic drugs. Liver function tests** become abnormal after about 18 h, with prolonged prothrombin time and raised bilirubin at 36–48 h. Hepatotoxicity peaks at about 3–4 days, with hepatic failure if severe. **Lactic acidosis, hypoglycaemia** and **acute kidney injury** may also occur. Prognostic factors include the presence of acidaemia (mortality ~95% if pH <7.3), renal impairment, severe hepatic encephalopathy and a factor V level <10% (~90% mortality).

- Treatment:
  - as for **poisoning and overdoses. Activated charcoal** is given if >75 mg/kg has been ingested and if the patient presents within 2 h of the overdose. Gastric lavage and **ipecacuanha** are no longer recommended. Ingestion of opioid/paracetamol combinations (e.g. containing **codeine, dextropropoxyphene**) should be considered if level of consciousness is depressed on presentation, and **naloxone** given.
  - replenishment of hepatic glutathione stores with glutathione precursors:
    - ***N*-acetylcysteine**: first-line antidote, previously thought to be effective only within 16 h of poisoning, but evidence now also supports later administration. 150 mg/kg is given in 200 ml 5% dextrose iv over 1 h, followed by 50 mg/kg in 500 ml dextrose over 4 h, then 100 mg/kg in 1 l dextrose over 16 h (maximum of 110 kg body weight used for obese patients).
    - methionine: animal studies suggest lower efficacy than *N*-acetylcysteine. Can be given within 10–12 h of poisoning if the patient is not vomiting. 2.5 g is given orally, followed by 2.5 g 4-hourly for 12 h. Nausea and vomiting are common side effects.
  - **liver transplantation** may be required (*see Hepatic failure*).

A single measurement of plasma paracetamol concentration taken more than 4 h after ingestion (earlier measurements are unreliable) identifies patients at risk of hepatic damage and thus requiring treatment. Previously, treatment was initiated at different blood levels according to risk factors (Fig. 129); in 2012 the Commission on Human Medicines advised that treatment should be given regardless of risk factors (and if there was doubt over the timing of ingestion).

Buckley NA, Dawson AH, Isbister GK (2016). Br Med J; 353: i2579

Paradoxical pain, *see Pain, paradoxical*

Paraesthesia. Abnormal sensation similar to 'pins and needles', occurring when neural tissue is irritated (e.g. peripheral nerve, **spinal cord**, sensory cerebral cortex). May be produced accidentally or intentionally during **regional anaesthesia** (a technique now largely replaced by **ultrasound** guidance or use of a nerve stimulator). Elicitation of paraesthesia may increase the chances of successful nerve block but also of neurological damage.

Paraldehyde. Obsolete hypnotic and **anticonvulsant drug**, introduced in 1882. Has an offensive smell, and is irritant and flammable. Decomposes with heat and light to acetic acid, and dissolves plastic. Has been used in the treatment of psychiatric disturbance, **status epilepticus** and for **premedication**.

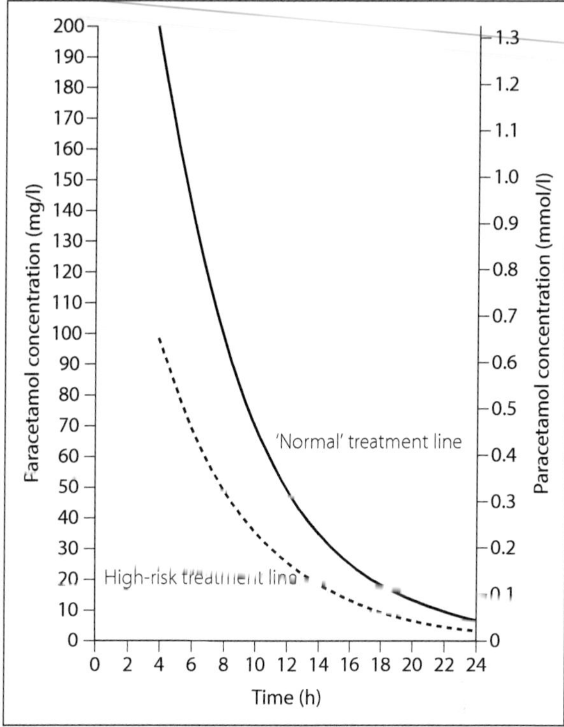

Fig. 129 Treatment lines for 'normal' and high-risk patients after paracetamol poisoning; 2012 guidance dispensed with this distinction and advises treatment with acetylcysteine for blood levels above a line joining 100 mg/l at 4 hours and 15 mg/l at 15 hours (approximating to the dotted line)

Paralysis, acute. May result in paraplegia (diplegia) with paralysis of the legs and lower part of the trunk or quadriplegia (tetraplegia) with paralysis of all four limbs and trunk. The suffix 'plegia' denotes complete paralysis; 'paresis' denotes partial paralysis. 'Hemiplegia' refers to unilateral paralysis, e.g. associated with **stroke** and other neurovascular conditions including **migraine**.

- May be caused by lesions affecting the:
  - cerebrum/**brainstem**:
    - neoplastic, e.g. frontal lobe or brainstem tumours.
    - vascular, e.g. bilateral carotid or basilar artery thrombosis.
    - **demyelinating disease**, e.g. multiple sclerosis, **central pontine myelinolysis**.
    - **hydrocephalus**, cerebral palsy.
  - **spinal cord**:
    - **spinal cord injury**.
    - neoplastic (primary or metastatic).
    - vascular, e.g. arteriovenous malformations, anterior spinal artery thrombosis, epidural haematoma.
    - inflammatory, e.g. transverse myelitis, multiple sclerosis.
    - infectious, e.g. viral myelitis (e.g. herpes, **poliomyelitis, HIV infection**), epidural abscess, **syphilis, TB**.
    - degenerative, e.g. **motor neurone disease**, bone disease affecting the spinal column.

- nutritional, e.g. **vitamin B_{12}** and E deficiency.
- hereditary, e.g. **Friedreich's ataxia.**

- peripheral nerve:
  - inflammatory, e.g. **Guillain–Barré syndrome, diphtheria.**
  - metabolic, e.g. acute intermittent **porphyria.**
  - poisoning, e.g. **heavy metal poisoning.**
- **neuromuscular junction:**
  - poisoning, e.g. **botulism, organophosphorus poisoning,** aquatic toxins (e.g. **tetrodotoxin**).
  - **bites and stings,** e.g. snakes.
  - immunological, e.g. **myasthenia gravis, myasthenic syndrome.**
- **muscle:**
  - inflammatory, e.g. **polymyositis.**
  - congenital, e.g. **periodic paralysis.**
  - electrolyte imbalance, e.g. **hypo-/hyperkalaemia, hypercalcaemia, hypermagnesaemia, hypophosphataemia.**

Diagnosis is based largely on history, examination and investigations (e.g. MRI, CSF examination, nerve conduction studies). The commonest cause of acute paralysis is Guillain–Barré syndrome followed by spinal cord injury caused by fracture dislocation of the **cervical spine.** Thoracic and lumbar spine damage is less common but may also cause paraplegia. In the absence of trauma, vascular insult to the spinal cord may produce paralysis that may be sudden or evolve over several hours. This usually follows thrombosis of a spinal segmental artery and results in the **anterior spinal artery syndrome.** Spinal subarachnoid haemorrhage similarly causes rapid paralysis, as does basilar artery thrombosis causing pontine infarction (often resulting in the **locked-in syndrome**). Peripheral causes usually produce subacute paralysis, with the exception of periodic paralysis (may occur over minutes).

- Anaesthetic/ICU implications:
  - **respiratory failure** requiring ventilatory support, e.g. **IPPV**; this may be exacerbated by **aspiration of gastric contents** if the pharyngeal and laryngeal muscles are affected. Prolonged support is likely to be required because most conditions resolve slowly.
  - control of the airway: **suxamethonium** may cause severe hyperkalaemia depending on the age of the lesion or whether the process is ongoing. Alternative methods include use of rapidly acting non-depolarising drugs, e.g. **rocuronium,** awake intubation, **tracheostomy.** The latter is often used in the long term.
  - there may also be autonomic disturbance depending on the cause.
  - other features of the primary disease.
  - long-term supportive care includes **nutrition** and **fluid balance,** regular turning and prevention of **decubitus ulcers,** prophylaxis against **DVT** and **nosocomial infection,** prompt treatment of infection and psychological support.

See also, Intubation, awake

Paramagnetic oxygen analysis, *see Oxygen measurement*

Paramedic. Person trained to assist a doctor or provide healthcare (usually emergency first aid) in the absence of a doctor. Most paramedics in the NHS work for ambulance services (other ambulance personnel include 'emergency care assistants'), but paramedics may also work in other areas within hospitals and primary care. Extended skills training for ambulance personnel in the UK was introduced in certain areas in the early 1970s, with a national training programme adopted in 1984. Currently, the only route to becoming registered as a paramedic is either via a student paramedic position with an ambulance service trust, or passing an approved university course in paramedic science. Trainee paramedics attend local hospitals and are required to perform tracheal intubations and iv cannulations under supervision, often involving anaesthetists.

Parametric tests, *see Data; Statistical tests*

Paraplegia, *see Paralysis, acute*

Paraquat poisoning. A widely used herbicide (though restricted or banned in many countries including within Europe), paraquat is rapidly absorbed when ingested orally, peak plasma levels occurring in 1–2 h. Can also be absorbed through the skin. Industrial preparations contain 10%–20% paraquat; those for home use contain 2.5%. Lethal dose is 3–5 g; mortality is up to 75%.

- Features:
  - corrosive burns to mouth, pharynx and oesophagus.
  - dyspnoea, **pulmonary oedema, ALI,** rapidly progressive **pulmonary fibrosis.** Lung damage is exacerbated by high inspired O_2 concentrations.
  - cardiac, hepatic and renal impairment.
- Management:
  - general support as for **poisoning and overdoses.**
  - oral administration or gastric instillation of an adsorbent such as activated **charcoal** 100 g followed by 50 g 4-hourly, or **fuller's earth** 1000 ml 15% aqueous suspension (or 500 ml 30%) 2-hourly, together with 200 ml 20% **mannitol** or magnesium sulfate as a laxative; administration is repeated until the charcoal or fuller's earth is seen in the stool. **Gastric lavage** is not recommended.
  - **haemoperfusion** has been advocated but paraquat's large **volume of distribution** limits its usefulness.

Paraquat concentrations can be measured in the serum or (more easily) in the urine.

Garawammana IB, Buckley NA (2011). Br J Clin Pharmacol; 72: 745–57

Parasympathetic nervous system. Part of the **autonomic nervous system.** Myelinated preganglionic efferent fibres emerge with **cranial nerves** III, VII, IX and X, and **spinal nerves** S2–4. They pass to their target organs, where they synapse with short non-myelinated postganglionic fibres (cf. **sympathetic nervous system**). The **vagus nerves** carry about 75% of all parasympathetic fibres and innervate the **heart, lungs, oesophagus,** stomach, other viscera and GIT as far as the splenic flexure. The sacral nerves run as the pelvic splanchnic nerves to the pelvic viscera (*see Fig. 20;* **Autonomic nervous system**). Afferent fibres travel in cranial nerves IX and X and in the sacral nerves.

- Effects of parasympathetic stimulation:
  - pupillary and ciliary muscle contraction, increased lacrimal secretion.
  - bradycardia, reduced velocity of cardiac conduction. Vasodilatation occurs in skeletal muscle, abdominal viscera, and coronary, pulmonary and renal circulations.
  - bronchoconstriction and increased secretions.
  - increased GIT motility, relaxation of sphincters and increased secretions (profuse watery secretion from salivary glands). Increased **insulin** and **glucagon** secretion.
  - bladder contraction and relaxation of sphincter.

- variable effect on the **uterus**.
- penile erection.

Acetylcholine is the **neurotransmitter** at all synapses. Its actions are divided into nicotinic (at ganglia) and muscarinic (at postganglionic synapses).
See also, Acetylcholine receptors; Muscarine; Nicotine

Parasympathomimetic drugs. Drugs producing the effects of stimulation of the **parasympathetic nervous system**. Include:
- drugs that stimulate **acetylcholine receptors**:
  - **acetylcholine**: has widespread actions, therefore not used therapeutically.
  - synthetic choline esters, e.g. carbachol, methacholine: the former has nicotinic and muscarinic actions, the latter mainly muscarinic. Both are resistant to hydrolysis by cholinesterases. Carbachol is used in **glaucoma** and urinary retention. Bethanechol is a similar drug, and used in urinary retention and as a laxative.
  - cholinomimetic alkaloids, e.g. pilocarpine: used in glaucoma.
- **acetylcholinesterase inhibitors**.

Paravertebral block. Blocks nerves as they pass through the intervertebral foramina into the paravertebral space; may be performed in the thoracic or lumbar region, e.g. for breast or abdominal surgery, respectively. Solution may track medially through the foramina into the **epidural space**, or laterally into the **intercostal space**.

With the patient sitting or in the lateral position, a skin wheal is raised 3–5 cm lateral to the most cephalad aspect of the appropriate spinous processes. An 8-cm needle is inserted approximately 3–4 cm perpendicular to the skin until the transverse process is encountered, then walked off the cephalad border and advanced a further 1–2 cm. 5 ml **local anaesthetic agent** is then injected. May be performed bilaterally.

A loss-of-resistance technique may be used to confirm correct needle placement, as for **epidural anaesthesia**. **Ultrasound** may also be used. A catheter may be passed into the paravertebral space for prolonged analgesia. Complications include epidural, subarachnoid and iv injection.

Parecoxib. **NSAID** acting preferentially on **cyclo-oxygenase**-2, licensed for short-term (<2 days) treatment of postoperative pain. Onset of action is 7–13 min, with effects lasting up to 12 h. A **prodrug** of valdecoxib, to which it is rapidly converted (**half-life** 22 min); valdecoxib itself has a half-life of 8 h.
- Dosage: 40 mg iv/deep im injection followed by 20–40 mg bd/qds up to 80 mg/day.
- Side effects: as for NSAIDs. Hyper- or hypotension and peripheral oedema may also occur. Has been associated with severe hypersensitivity reactions, especially in patients allergic to sulfonamides.

Parenteral nutrition, *see Nutrition, total parenteral*

Parkinsonism, *see Parkinson's disease*

Parkinson's disease. Idiopathic degenerative disorder of the CNS involving the basal ganglia and extrapyramidal motor system, with loss of **dopamine** leading to an imbalance between acetylcholine and dopamine in the substantia nigra. Secondary causes include **carbon monoxide poisoning**, **encephalitis**, **stroke**, **heavy metal poisoning**, or drugs that antagonise **dopamine receptors** (e.g. **phenothiazines**); secondary disease is termed 'parkinsonism'. Affects 3% of the population >65 years old; the aetiology is in most cases unknown but may include genetic, toxic and environmental factors.
- Features:
  - bradykinesia, rigidity ('lead-pipe' or 'cogwheel'), rest tremor (4–6 Hz). Initiation, speed, strength and precision of movement are impaired. The face is typically expressionless and the gait shuffling.
  - upper airway and vocal cord dysfunction can result in laryngospasm.
  - in so-called 'parkinson plus' syndromes, features of parkinsonism are accompanied by those of other multisystem degeneration, e.g. certain forms of dementia and autonomic failure.
  - a restrictive ventilatory defect may occur.
- Treatment is aimed at restoring the dopaminergic/cholinergic balance, and includes:
  - increasing brain levels of dopamine by administering its precursor levodopa (dopamine does not cross the **blood–brain barrier**). Conversion of levodopa to dopamine outside the CNS with resultant side effects is prevented by concurrent administration of carbidopa or benserazide. These inhibit dopa decarboxylase peripherally, as they do not cross into the brain. Bradykinesia and rigidity are improved more than tremor. Side effects include involuntary movements, nausea, vomiting, and psychiatric disturbances. Improvement may be intermittent (on–off effect).
  - **anticholinergic drugs: benzatropine**, trihexyphenidyl (benzhexol), orphenadrine: improve tremor and rigidity more than bradykinesia.
  - other drugs: bromocriptine, **apomorphine** and lisuride (dopamine agonists), selegiline (type B **monoamine oxidase inhibitor**), **amantadine**, pergolide.
  - stereotactic surgery (especially stimulation of the globus pallidus and subthalamic nucleus) may be successful. Fetal tissue implantation has been performed experimentally.
- Anaesthetic considerations:
  - pre-existing restrictive lung disorders and postural hypotension. Excessive salivation and dysphagia may result in aspiration of secretions.
  - levodopa is continued up to surgery, because its **half-life** is short. It has been given iv.
  - symptoms may be exacerbated by dopamine antagonists, e.g. phenothiazines and **butyrophenones** (including **antiemetic drugs**).
  - the risk of **hyperkalaemia** following **suxamethonium** is controversial.
  - postoperative **sleep apnoea** has been reported, especially in the postencephalitic disease.

[James Parkinson (1755–1824), London physician]

Paroxysmal nocturnal haemoglobinuria. Rare acquired chronic haemolytic **anaemia**, resulting from blood cell **membrane** abnormality and increased sensitivity to lysis by **complement**. Haemoglobinuria is classically noticed on waking.

Haemolysis may be precipitated by infection, **hypoxaemia**, **hypercapnia**, **acidosis** and hypoperfusion, all of which should be avoided during anaesthesia. Steroids may help reduce haemolysis. **Platelet** destruction may lead to bleeding, or abnormal function may lead to venous thrombosis. Renal impairment is common. Drugs causing complement activation should be avoided, and red blood cells washed before **blood transfusion**.

PART team, Patient-at-risk team, *see Outreach team*

Partial liquid ventilation, *see Liquid ventilation*

Partial pressure. Pressure exerted by each component of a **gas** mixture. For a gas dissolved in a liquid (e.g. blood) the term '**tension**' is used, although denoted by the same symbol (P).
See also, Dalton's law; Respiratory symbols

Partial thromboplastin time, *see Coagulation studies*

Partition coefficient. Ratio of the amount of substance in one phase to the amount in another phase at stated temperature, with the two phases being of equal volume and in equilibrium with each other. Depends on the relative **solubility** of the substance in the two phases. May refer to solids, liquids or gases; when the phases are liquid and gas it equals the Ostwald **solubility coefficient**. Blood/gas and oil/gas partition coefficients of **inhalational anaesthetic agents** are related to speed of uptake and potency, respectively.

Pascal. SI **unit** of **pressure**. 1 pascal (Pa) = 1 N/m^2.
[Blaise Pascal (1623–1662), French physicist]

Pasteur point. Critical mitochondrial Po_2 below which aerobic **metabolism** cannot occur. Thought to be 0.15–0.3 kPa (1.4–2.3 mmHg).
[Louis Pasteur (1822–1895), French scientist and microbiologist]
See also, Oxygen cascade

Patent ductus arteriosus, *see Ductus arteriosus, patent*

Patient-at-risk team, *see Outreach team*

Patient-controlled analgesia (PCA). Technique whereby intermittent boluses of analgesic drugs (e.g. **opioid analgesic drugs**) are self-administered by patients according to their own requirements, used widely for **postoperative analgesia**. Usually iv but other routes include epidural, sc and intranasal. Systems usually consist of infusion devices that deliver on-demand bolus injections, with or without a continuous background infusion. Bolus volume and rate and the minimum time between boluses (lockout interval) may be altered. These controls must be inaccessible to the patient (or relatives), and the infusion connected downstream from a non-return valve if attached to another iv infusion (to prevent retrograde flow into the second infusion set with subsequent overdosage when the latter is flushed).

Has been shown to provide more consistent plasma drug levels when compared with standard im techniques. The usefulness of background infusions is controversial, the risk of overdosage balanced by possibly improved analgesia. Preoperative explanation of the technique is desirable.

Drugs with relatively short half-lives are usually employed. Widely varying dosage regimens have been described; individual adjustment may be required (Table 41). Complications are related to incorrect programming and setting-up, patients' misunderstanding of the technique, equipment malfunction and administration of additional conventional 'on demand' opioid analgesia leading to overdose. Patients require adequate **monitoring**, because respiratory depression may still occur. Nausea and **vomiting** may be a problem if regular antiemetics are not prescribed, firstly because drug levels remain constant, and secondly because the 'as required' antiemetics that would be routinely given along with im opioids tend not to be given if 'as required' opioids themselves are no longer being given. PCA is also used (epidural and iv) for analgesia in labour (*see Obstetric analgesia and anaesthesia*).

Nurse-controlled analgesia (NCA) is used in paediatric patients unable to use PCA appropriately due to young age or developmental delay; similar equipment and drugs are used, usually with a longer lockout interval (e.g. 20 minutes), with or without a background infusion. Administration of bolus doses is guided by regular **pain evaluation**.

Table 41 Dosage regimens for different opioids for iv patient-controlled analgesia

Drug	Bolus dose (mg)	Lock-out interval (min)
Diamorphine	0.5–1.5	3–5
Fentanyl	0.02–0.05	3–10
Morphine	0.5–2.0	5–15
Nalbuphine	1–5	5–15
Oxycodone	0.5–2.0	5–10
Pethidine	5–20	5–15

PAV, *see Proportional assist ventilation*

PCA, *see Patient-controlled analgesia*

PCV, Packed cell volume, *see Haematocrit*

PCWP, *see Pulmonary capillary wedge pressure*

PDA, Patent ductus arteriosus, *see Ductus arteriosus, patent*

PDPH, *see Post-dural puncture headache*

PE, *see Pulmonary embolism*

PEA, *see Pulseless electrical activity*

Peak expiratory flow rate (PEFR). Maximal rate of air flow during a sudden **forced expiration**. Most conveniently measured with a **peak flowmeter**; may also be measured from a **flow–volume loop**, or with a **pneumotachograph**. Highly dependent on patient effort. Reduced by obstructive airways disease, e.g. **asthma**, **COPD**. Normal values: 450–700 l/min (males), 250–500 l/min (females).

Peak flowmeters. Simple and inexpensive hand-held **flowmeters** for measuring **peak expiratory flow rate** (PEFR). The Wright peak flowmeter is a constant pressure, variable orifice device, able to measure peak flow rates of up to 1000 l/min. It has a flat circular body, with a handle and mouthpiece. Exhaled air is directed by a fixed baffle within the body on to a movable vane that is free to rotate around a central axle against the force of a small spring. There is a circular slot in the base of the chamber, through which expired air escapes. As the vane moves, the slot is uncovered, thus increasing the effective orifice size. The vane reaches its furthest excursion according to PEFR, and is held there by a ratchet. PEFR is read from a dial on the face of the meter, according to a pointer attached to the vane. It slightly underreads in comparison with a **pneumotachograph**.

A simpler, cheaper version consists of a cylindrical tube, employing a piston that is blown along its length. As it does so, it uncovers a linear slot along the tube. A ratchet mechanism operates as before. PEFR is read from a scale at the top of the cylinder.

[B Martin Wright (1912–2001), London engineer]

Pecs block. Regional anaesthetic technique used for breast surgery. Involves placement of **local anaesthetic agent** into the interfascial plane between pectoralis major and minor muscles, under **ultrasound** guidance, blocking the medial and lateral pectoral nerves (pecs I). Additional local anaesthetic may be placed under pectoralis minor to provide more extensive analgesia (pecs II). May partly overlap with **serratus anterior plane block**.

PEEP, *see Positive end-expiratory pressure*

PEFR, *see Peak expiratory flow rate*

PEG, *see Percutaneous endoscopic gastrostomy*

Pelvic trauma. Usually caused by blunt **trauma** (e.g. road accidents or falls) and often associated with **abdominal trauma**, **chest trauma** and **head injury**.

- Damage may involve:
  - pelvic ring: disruption causes pain on movement. Diagnosis is confirmed with x-ray or CT scanning.
  - bladder: rupture occurs in 10%–15% of pelvic trauma cases. Suggested by lower abdominal peritonism and inability to pass urine. IV urography (or cystography if a urinary catheter is in place) shows extravasation of contrast from the torn bladder wall.
  - urethra: damage is suggested by disruption of the pubis symphysis on x-ray, perineal bruising, blood at the meatus, inability to pass urine and a high-riding prostate on pr examination in males. IV urography should be performed to exclude total disruption.
  - vaginal and bowel perforation from bony fragments.
  - pelvic blood vessels: arteriography may be necessary for diagnosis.
  - pelvic nerves.
- Management:
  - resuscitation as for trauma generally.
  - simple pelvic fractures require bed rest only, whereas complicated fractures require early operative fixation. External fixation is now common.
  - intraperitoneal bladder rupture requires laparotomy and drainage of the bladder with both suprapubic and urethral catheters. Extraperitoneal rupture requires drainage via a urethral catheter with subsequent confirmation of healing using cystography. Broad-spectrum **antibacterial drugs** should be given.
  - urethral injuries generally should be treated by suprapubic catheterisation and drainage; however, if pelvic x-ray shows no disruption of the symphysis and there is no blood at the meatus, a urethral catheter may be passed cautiously.
  - pelvic vessels may require embolisation if haemorrhage is severe.

Arvieux C, Thony F, Broux C, et al (2012). J Visc Surg; 149: e227–38

Pendelluft. Phenomenon originally believed to cause the **hypoxaemia** occurring in **flail chest**. The theory suggested that air is drawn from the affected side into the unaffected lung during inspiration, due to disrupted chest wall integrity on the damaged side. During expiration, air passes from the normal lung back into the affected lung; thus air moves to and fro between the two sides, instead of in and out of the chest via the trachea. **Hypoventilation** and **$\dot{V}/\dot{Q}$ mismatch** due to pain, lung contusion and sputum retention are now thought to be more important.

[German: 'oscillating breath']

Penicillamine. Degradation product of **penicillin** used as a **chelating agent**, especially in copper, lead, gold, mercury and zinc poisoning. Also used in the treatment of **rheumatoid arthritis** and chronic active **hepatitis**.

- Dosage: from 125 to 250 mg/day orally for chronic inflammatory conditions to 1–2 g/day in divided doses for chronic copper overload or lead poisoning.
- Side effects: blood dyscrasias, convulsions, neuropathy, nausea and vomiting, colitis, renal and hepatic impairment, bronchospasm, **myasthenia gravis**, systemic lupus erythematosus-like syndrome, rashes. Blood counts and urine testing for proteinuria should be performed regularly.

Penicillins. Group of natural and synthetic bactericidal **antibacterial drugs** with a **β-lactam** structure. Act by interfering with formation of peptidoglycan cross-links within the bacterial cell wall, resulting in osmotic damage. Penetrate body tissue and fluids well except for the CNS (unless the meninges are inflamed). Excreted renally by active tubular secretion. **Bacterial resistance** is caused by production of β-lactamases that hydrolyse the β-lactam ring.

- May be classified into:
  - **benzylpenicillin** and **phenoxymethylpenicillin**.
  - penicillinase-resistant penicillins: **flucloxacillin**, temocillin.
  - broad-spectrum penicillins: **ampicillin**, **amoxicillin**, **co-amoxiclav**, **co-fluampicil**.
  - antipseudomonal penicillins: **piperacillin**, **ticarcillin**.

Problems include hypersensitivity (related to the basic penicillin structure—thus all penicillins may cross-react; only 7%–23% of 'allergic' patients are truly allergic), cerebral irritation (causing encephalopathy), especially in high dosage or renal failure, and excessive administration of sodium or potassium in parenteral preparations.

Penile block. Used to provide peri- and **postoperative analgesia** for circumcision and other procedures on the penis, especially in children.

The dorsal nerves of the penis (terminal branches of the pudendal nerves, S2–4) travel medial to the ischiopubic rami into the deep perineal pouch, and pierce the perineal membrane to pass to the penis. They may be blocked within a triangular space bounded by the symphysis pubis above, corpora cavernosa below and superficial fascia anteriorly. The penile vessels lie in the midline. Some innervation of the skin at the base of the penis arises from the genital branch of the genitofemoral nerve.

A needle is introduced at right angles through a skin wheal in front of the symphysis, and passed below its caudal edge. It is inserted up to 3–5 mm deeper than the symphysis (a click may be felt). After negative aspiration for blood, 1–2 ml **local anaesthetic agent** is injected for children up to 3 years old, 3–5 ml for older children and 5–10 ml for

adults. **Adrenaline** may cause ischaemia and necrosis and must not be used. Solution diffuses to block both sides following midline injection, but risk of haematoma is greater; therefore two injections may be performed, one either side of the midline. 1–5 ml solution is also injected around the base of the penis.
See also, Lumbar plexus; Sacral plexus

Pentamidine isetionate. Antiprotozoal agent used in the treatment and prophylaxis of **pneumocystis pneumonia**. Because of its side effects, used as a second-line drug if infection is resistant to **co-trimoxazole**. Has also been used to treat leishmaniasis and trypanosomiasis.
- Dosage:
  - pneumocystis treatment: 4 mg/kg/day slowly iv for at least 14 days or 300 mg by inhalation of nebulised solution, every 4 weeks (or 150 mg every 2 weeks).
  - pneumocystis prophylaxis: 300 mg every 4 weeks (or 150 mg every 2 weeks) by nebulised solution.
  - other infections: 3–4 mg/kg iv/im every 1–7 days.
- Side effects: severe, sometimes fatal hypotension, hypoglycaemia and ventricular arrhythmias, pancreatitis, renal failure, blood dyscrasias, bronchospasm, nausea, vomiting.

Pentastarch, *see Hydroxyethyl starch*

Pentazocine hydrochloride/lactate. Agonist–antagonist **opioid analgesic drug** described in 1962. Benzomorphan derivative, with agonist activity at kappa and sigma **opioid receptors**, and antagonist activity at mu receptors. Used for moderate to severe pain; has been used to reverse the respiratory depression caused by **morphine** or **fentanyl** while maintaining analgesia.

Undergoes extensive **first-pass metabolism**; conjugated with glucuronides and excreted renally. **Half-life** is about 2–3 h.
- Dosage: 0.5–1.0 mg/kg, iv/im/sc. 50–100 mg orally, 3–4-hourly.
- Side effects:
  - sedation, dizziness.
  - hallucinations and dysphoria, especially in the elderly.
  - sweating, hypertension, tachycardia.
  - precipitation of withdrawal reactions in opioid addicts.

Its side effects have limited its popularity.
See also, Opioid receptor antagonists

Pentolinium tartrate. Obsolete long-acting **ganglion blocking drug** used to treat hypertension and in **hypotensive anaesthesia**.

Pentoxifylline (Oxpentifylline). **Xanthine** used in peripheral vascular disease and vascular dementia. Reduces blood **viscosity**. Also inhibits tumour necrosis factor production by macrophages; has thus been studied as a potential therapeutic agent in **sepsis**.
- Dosage: peripheral vascular disease: 400 mg orally bd/tds.
- Side effects: nausea, headache, GIT disturbances, thrombocytopenia.

See also, Cytokines

PEP, Pre-ejection period, *see Systolic time intervals*

Peptic ulcer disease. Ulceration due to an imbalance between the action of gastric acid and the normal protective mechanisms of the upper GIT mucosa. May occur at any site exposed to gastric acid, e.g. oesophagus, stomach, duodenum. Abnormal **gastric emptying**, **gastro-oesophageal reflux**, drugs (e.g. **NSAIDs**, **corticosteroids**), alcohol, psychological and epidemiological factors are thought to contribute. Infection with *Helicobacter pylori* has a fundamental role in the development of chronic gastritis and peptic ulcer disease; the persistence of serum antibodies against the organism reflects the chronicity of the infection. About 70% of patients with non-NSAIDs-induced gastric ulcers have evidence of *H. pylori* infection that can be detected with the ^{13}C-urea breath test. Infected patients have an increased rate of GIT bleeding in the ICU.
- Treatment:
  - neutralisation of existing acid with **antacids**.
  - increased surface protection:
    - **sucralfate**.
    - bismuth compounds.
    - carbenoxolone.
  - reduction of acid production:
    - **H_2 receptor antagonists**.
    - **proton pump inhibitors**.
    - **anticholinergic drugs**, e.g. pirenzepine.
    - eradication of *H. pylori* infection. Recommended therapy includes PAC regimen (double dose **proton pump inhibitor**, **amoxicillin**, **clarithromycin**) or PCM regimen (amoxicillin is replaced by **metronidazole**) for 1 week. Effective in <90%.
  - surgery: indications include failed medical treatment, malignant change, or complications as above. Surgery may involve highly selective vagotomy or vagotomy and drainage procedure (duodenal ulcer), or partial gastrectomy (gastric ulcer). Anaesthesia in chronic disease requires no special precautions unless gastro-oesophageal reflux or **anaemia** is present. Acute haemorrhage or perforation may present with vomiting, **shock** and **hypovolaemia**.

Lanas A, Chan FKL (2017). Lancet; 390: 613–24

Percentile. Value that indicates the percentage of a distribution equal to or below it; e.g. 97% of measurements are equal to or less than the 97th percentile. Often used in charts, e.g. of children's height against age. The 3rd, 50th and 97th percentiles plotted on the chart indicate the heights that include 3%, 50% and 97% of the population, respectively, at each age. May thus be used to follow a child's growth, because height would be expected to remain within the same percentile during normal development. The 3rd and 97th percentiles approximate to ±2 **standard deviations** from the **mean**, for normally distributed data.

The 25th and 75th percentiles are often used to indicate variability (scatter) around the **median** for ordinal **data**; the measurements between the two values (the interquartile range, IQR) include the middle 50% of all the data points.

Percutaneous coronary intervention (PCI). Group of percutaneous endovascular techniques for treating **ischaemic heart disease**. Considerably cheaper than surgical **coronary artery bypass graft** (CABG), with a similar risk of death and **MI** in selected patients; CABG is more effective at relieving angina and less likely to require repeat intervention, but carries higher procedural risk of **stroke**.

Techniques include:
- balloon dilatation of stenosed coronary arteries (coronary angioplasty).
- rotational excision atherectomy.
- laser ablation atherectomy.
- insertion of endoluminal stents.

Due to a high restenosis rate (30%–50% within 6 months), balloon angioplasty has been replaced as the standard of care by insertion of self-expanding mesh stents, the latter either bare metal or drug-eluting. Bare metal stents (BMS) still carry a 20%–25% risk of restenosis due to neointimal hyperplasia; drug-eluting stents (DES) release an anti-proliferative agent (e.g. sirolimus [rapamycin], everolimus) that inhibits stent endothelialisation and reduces 1-year restenosis rate to 5%. However, drug-eluting stents carry a higher risk of potentially catastrophic late stent thrombosis (*see later*).

- Indications:
  - elective revascularisation for patients with stable angina.
  - urgent treatment for those with non S–T elevation **acute coronary syndromes.**
  - emergency treatment for S–T elevation **MI** if readily available.

Patients are pretreated with **antiplatelet drugs** to prevent in-stent thrombosis, and may also receive **calcium channel blocking drugs** to reduce coronary vasospasm. Those with BMS require ongoing dual antiplatelet therapy (e.g. **clopidogrel** and **aspirin**) for 6 weeks; those with DES require two agents for 1 year (as the poorly endothelialised stent surface is highly thrombogenic). All PCI patients should receive aspirin therapy for life.

- Anaesthetic considerations (for non-cardiac surgery):
  - as for ischaemic heart disease generally.
  - timing of surgery: risk of stent thrombosis is highest within 30 days of PCI. Elective surgery should be postponed for >6 weeks or >12 months in those with BMS or DES, respectively.
  - if surgery cannot be postponed, premature cessation of clopidogrel markedly increases risk of adverse cardiovascular events, particularly in those with DES. Some therefore recommend that in most cases these patients continue dual therapy perioperatively. For procedures where risks of bleeding are very high (e.g. intracranial surgery), dual therapy may be temporarily stopped and a rapidly reversible 'bridging therapy' (e.g. **tirofiban** or **heparin**) should be considered. These decisions should be made in conjunction with a cardiologist.

Percutaneous endoscopic gastrostomy (PEG). Technique for establishing enteral **nutrition** that avoids the discomfort and complications of long-term **nasogastric intubation.** Useful for patients with neurological dysphagia. After passing a gastroscope into the stomach, the stomach is inflated so that its anterior wall makes contact with the anterior abdominal wall. Using the light from the gastroscope, an appropriate site (usually 2 cm below the left costal margin and 2 cm from the midline) is marked on the skin. Under local anaesthesia, a trocar is introduced into the stomach and a thread fed through it into the stomach. This is grasped by the endoscope and pulled out through the mouth; the PEG tube is attached to the thread and pulled through the mouth into the stomach. The PEG is secured to the anterior abdominal wall with a clip. In patients unable to lie flat due to diaphragmatic failure, a radiologically inserted gastrostomy (RIG), in which the gastrostomy is inserted following a barium meal, may be safer.

Percutaneous endoscopic jejunostomy (PEJ). Technique for enteral nutrition, similar to **percutaneous endoscopic gastrostomy.** Used to administer **nutrition** and drugs directly to the small bowel (e.g. in cases where the stomach has been removed).

Percutaneous tracheostomy, *see Tracheostomy, percutaneous*

Percutaneous transluminal coronary angioplasty (PTCA), *see Percutaneous coronary intervention*

Perfluorocarbons (PFCs). Chemically inert organic compounds in which all the hydrogen atoms have been replaced by fluorine. Clear liquids, they dissolve O_2 and CO_2 to an extent directly proportional to the gas concentration to which they are exposed (i.e., according to **Henry's law**), and have therefore been investigated as artificial blood substitutes. Insoluble in water, they require emulsification (e.g. with egg phospholipids) for use in the circulation. PFCs can dissolve about 20 times as much O_2, and four times as much CO_2 as plasma. Their use in humans has been limited by side effects, e.g. **stroke, thrombocytopenia**, flu-like illness.

They have also been investigated as a suitable medium for **liquid ventilation**, because their high density means they displace exudate from the airways and alveoli while their low surface tension is thought to increase lung **compliance.** Also used in eye surgery as a temporary replacement for vitreous humour.

See also, Blood, artificial

Perfusion pressure. Represents the pressure head for **blood flow** to an organ or tissues. Equals **MAP** minus mean venous pressure; e.g. **cerebral perfusion pressure** equals MAP minus **ICP.**

Peribulbar block. Used in **ophthalmic surgery** as an alternative to **retrobulbar block**, because the risk of complications (e.g. retrobulbar haemorrhage) is lower. **Facial nerve block** is not required. Involves injection of **local anaesthetic agent** outside the muscle cone.

Several techniques have been described. In one, a needle is inserted through the lid margin between the superior orbital notch and the medial canthus, and directed upwards between the globe and orbital roof. 3–4 ml solution is injected at a depth of 2.0–2.5 cm. The needle is then inserted through the lid margin at the junction of the outer one-third and inner two-thirds of the lower orbital rim, and directed downwards between the globe and orbital floor. 4–5 ml solution is injected at a depth of 2.0–2.5 cm. Gentle pressure is applied to the eye for 10 min. Alternatives include a more superficial injection (anterior peribulbar block) and the use of a single injection through either the upper or the lower lid. A mixture of **lidocaine** 2% and **bupivacaine** 0.5%–0.75% in equal proportions with or without **adrenaline** 1:400 000 is suitable; alternatives include **prilocaine** 3% or **ropivacaine. Hyaluronidase** 5 units/ml promotes spread of solution.

See also, Orbital cavity

Pericardiocentesis Removal of fluid from within the pericardium. Usually performed to relieve acute **cardiac tamponade**, although may also be used for diagnostic purposes. If ultrasonography is available, needle aspiration may be performed from any reasonable area on the chest wall. For blind pericardiocentesis, the subxiphoid approach is most commonly used:

- a long 18–22 G needle attached to a syringe is introduced between the xiphisternum and the left

costal margin, and directed towards the left shoulder at 35–40 degrees to the skin. Aspiration is performed as the right ventricle is approached, until pericardial fluid is obtained. A three-way tap is used. Pericardial sanguinous effusions do not clot, whereas intracardiac blood does.
  - an **ECG** chest lead may be attached to the needle; S–T elevation and ventricular ectopics may indicate contact with the ventricle.
  - trauma to myocardium and coronary vessels is reduced by inserting a plastic iv cannula over the needle into the pericardial space.
- Alternative approaches:
  - in the fifth intercostal space just lateral to the left sternal edge (approaches the left ventricle).
  - one intercostal space lower, and 1–2 cm lateral to the apex beat, directed towards the right shoulder (approaches the apex).

Pericarditis. Inflammation of the **pericardium**. May be:
  - acute:
    - caused by infections, **connective tissue diseases**, **renal failure**, **hypothyroidism**, **MI**, **trauma**, drugs, radiation and tumours. Post-viral pericarditis (often with coxsackie B virus) is the most common form.
    - features include sudden central chest pain, worse lying down or on moving, often with fever and tachycardia. Auscultation may reveal a pericardial friction rub. **ECG** may reveal **S–T segment** elevation, possibly with **T wave** inversion later.
    - **NSAIDs** are the first-line treatment; adjunctive colchicine therapy reduces recurrence rates by 50%. **Corticosteroids** may be useful in pericarditis secondary to autoimmune disease.
    - pericardial fluid may accumulate, with disappearance of the rub. Slow accumulation may cause little cardiovascular disturbance, whereas rapid accumulation may cause **cardiac tamponade**.
  - chronic constrictive:
    - the pericardium becomes fibrous or calcified, and thus rigid.
    - usually follows radiation, chronic renal failure, **rheumatoid arthritis** or **TB**, or is idiopathic.
    - resembles cardiac tamponade, with restriction of diastolic cardiac filling. A sharp drop in right atrial pressure ('y' descent) occurs just before right ventricular filling, due to rapid blood flow across the tricuspid valve (cf. tamponade, where atrial pressures remain high throughout diastole). The **heart sounds** may be quiet, and ECG complexes small. Pericardial calcification may be present on the **CXR**.
    - management: as for cardiac tamponade. Surgery may be required.

Imazio M, Gaita F, LeWinter M (2015). JAMA; 314: 1498–506

Pericardium. Sac enclosing the **heart** and roots of the great vessels. The outer fibrous pericardium fuses below with the central tendon of the **diaphragm**, and above and superiorly with the adventitia of the great vessels. The inner serous pericardium has visceral and parietal layers, enclosing the pericardial cavity. The visceral layer covers the heart and is termed the epicardium.

See also, Mediastinum; Pericardiocentesis; Pericarditis

Peridural, *see Epidural*

Periodic paralysis. Group of diseases, usually inherited in an autosomal dominant pattern, characterised by episodic skeletal muscle weakness.
- Classified into different types:
  - hypokalaemic: caused by point mutations in skeletal muscle calcium channels. Weakness may be generalised and severe and is usually precipitated by strenuous exercise or a carbohydrate load. May result in respiratory failure. Treatment of acute attacks is with iv or oral potassium; prophylaxis is with **acetazolamide.**
  - hyperkalaemic/normokalaemic: caused by point mutations in muscle sodium channels. Occurs in first decade of life and results in episodic mild weakness to total paralysis. May be precipitated by exercise, cold or potassium ingestion. Treatment is with acetazolamide or **thiazide diuretics**. Anaesthesia may result in prolonged paralysis, especially if **suxamethonium** is used.

Bandschapp O, Iaizzo PA (2013). Paediatr Anaesth; 23: 824–33

Perioperative medicine. Term used to describe the care of patients undergoing surgery, and increasingly used to emphasise the anaesthetist's role in the whole process (which, strictly, extends from discussion of surgery as a treatment option to full postoperative recovery), rather than just the intraoperative part; thus there have been calls for anaesthetists to be called 'perioperative physicians' instead of 'anaesthetists' and to lead this process, although this is controversial. The perioperative 'journey' includes:
  - preoperative counselling (including discussion of risks/benefits), optimisation (e.g. **prehabilitation**, cessation of **smoking**) and investigation.
  - short-term preoperative management, e.g. **premedication**, management of concurrent morbidity and drug therapy (e.g. **insulin**, **warfarin**).
  - intraoperative anaesthesia.
  - immediate/early postoperative care, including **recovery** from anaesthesia, acute **pain management**, etc.
  - long-term recovery, including follow-up, chronic/long-term medication, etc.

At each point in the process, the importance of multidisciplinary consultation, input and co-operation is emphasised.

Cannesson M, Ani F, Mythen MM, Kain Z (2015). Br J Anaesth; 114: 8–9

See also, Recovery, enhanced

Peripheral neuropathy. Term encompassing any disorder affecting the peripheral nerves (motor and/or sensory).
- Divided into:
  - polyneuropathy: generalised process characterised by widespread and symmetrical degeneration of the:
    - axon, e.g. drugs, metabolic disorders.
    - **myelin** sheath, e.g. **diphtheria**, **Guillain–Barré syndrome**.
    - **neurone** cell body, e.g. **motor neurone disease**.
  - focal and multifocal neuropathies: asymmetrical involvement of one or more peripheral nerves, e.g. by ischaemia, trauma (including **nerve injury during anaesthesia**), vasculitis, infiltration (e.g. by tumour).

Diabetes mellitus is the most common cause of chronic peripheral neuropathy (causing both polyneuropathy and focal neuropathy), followed by carcinoma, vitamin B_1 and B_{12} deficiency (e.g. in **alcoholism**) and drug therapy (e.g. **isoniazid**, **amiodarone**, **cimetidine**). Other causes include

renal failure, **hypothyroidism**, **connective tissue diseases**, **HIV**, leprosy, amyloidosis, **porphyria** and **heavy metal poisoning**.

Clinical features include weakness and sensory disturbance, usually initially distal in polyneuropathies. **Autonomic neuropathy** may occur.

- Anaesthetic and ICU considerations:
  - underlying disease.
  - bulbar involvement.
  - autonomic involvement.
  - risk of severe **hyperkalaemia** following administration of **suxamethonium** in motor neuropathy.
  - difficulty **weaning from ventilators**.

See also, Critical illness polyneuropathy/myopathy

Peripheral vascular resistance, *see Systemic vascular resistance*

Peritoneal dialysis (PD). **Dialysis** technique used primarily in chronic **renal failure** and less commonly in **poisoning and overdose**. Following insertion of an intraperitoneal PD catheter through the lower anterior abdominal wall (surgically or percutaneously), prewarmed dialysate fluid is introduced into the peritoneal cavity. The peritoneum acts as a semipermeable membrane between blood and dialysate; the latter is allowed to remain within the cavity for a period ('dwell time') to allow equilibration between the two compartments. The speed and degree of equilibration depend on the frequency and volume of exchanges and dwell time (2 l dialysate is usually exchanged over 1 h), the permeability and blood supply of the peritoneum and the tonicity of the dialysate (contains sodium, chloride, calcium, magnesium, lactate and a variable amount of glucose and potassium; osmolality is 346–485 mosmol/kg depending on the glucose content, which varies from 1.3% to 4.5%; potassium free solutions are also available).

Advantages of PD are its simplicity, lack of requirement for vascular access and anticoagulation, and haemodynamic stability; disadvantages include its inefficiency and slowness. Complications include pain, bleeding, visceral perforation, **peritonitis**, **hyperglycaemia**, hypoproteinaemia and respiratory embarrassment if large volumes of dialysate are used. As with **haemodialysis**, drugs are removed from the plasma during PD and alterations in dosage may be required. Contraindications include previous abdominal surgery, drains, ileus and adhesions. PD may be performed continuously (e.g. in ICU) to improve its efficacy and reduce respiratory embarrassment.

Peritoneal lavage. Technique for diagnosis of intra-abdominal bleeding following blunt **abdominal trauma**. Following bladder drainage and decompression of the stomach using a nasogastric tube, a peritoneal lavage catheter is introduced under local anaesthesia into the abdominal cavity, 1–2 cm below the umbilicus in the midline. A **Seldinger** or cut-down technique may be used. If no fluid is aspirated, 10 ml/kg (up to 1000 ml) of warm saline is introduced into the cavity and then drained by gravity. The resultant aspirate is sent for analysis; the presence of significant numbers of white (>500/ml) or red cells (>100 000/ml), or bacteria, indicates the need for diagnostic laparoscopy or laparotomy. Introduction of blood during the procedure itself may lead to a false-positive result. Abdominal ultrasound is used as a less invasive diagnostic method.

Continuous peritoneal lavage has been used in acute **pancreatitis**, **peritonitis** and postoperatively in **intra-abdominal sepsis** in an attempt to wash away bacteria and toxins.

See also, Paracentesis

Peritonitis. Inflammation or infection of the peritoneum. Infection is usually with bacteria, most commonly involving mixed anaerobic and aerobic organisms, although 'spontaneous' (primary) peritonitis is caused by a single species (usually streptococci, pneumococci or haemophilus).

- Caused by:
  - perforation of part of the GIT.
  - penetrating **trauma** (including postoperative infection from drains).
  - direct spread from an infected organ, e.g. appendicitis, **cholecystitis**.
  - haematogenous spread in **bacteraemia**.

Clinical features include fever (or hypothermia in severe **sepsis**), tachycardia, pain (worse on movement and breathing), guarding and rigidity. Bowel sounds may be sparse or absent, with abdominal distension. Untreated, **shock** may occur. Diagnosis may be aided by **paracentesis**; imaging may reveal an underlying cause. If the diagnosis remains in doubt, exploratory laparotomy may be indicated as for **intra-abdominal sepsis**.

- Treatment:
  - general resuscitative measures: iv fluids, inotropes, respiratory support.
  - nasogastric tube.
  - broad-spectrum **antibacterial drug** therapy, e.g. a **cephalosporin**, **metronidazole** and **aminoglycoside**.
  - surgical correction of the underlying cause.
  - **peritoneal lavage** with or without antibiotics has been used, especially postoperatively.

Complications include **MODS**, GIT obstruction caused by adhesions and persistent **ileus**. **TPN** may be required. Overall mortality is approximately 10%, although rates of 50%–70% may occur in faecal peritonitis in high-risk patients (e.g. elderly).

Permissive hypercapnia. Acceptance of **hypercapnia** in patients undergoing **IPPV**, e.g. for **respiratory failure** especially **asthma** and **ALI**. Used as part of a **lung protective strategy**, when ventilation to a normal P_{CO_2} may result in excessive **airway pressure**, **barotrauma** and volutrauma.

Permissive hypotension, *see Damage control resuscitation*

Peroneal nerve block, *see Ankle, nerve blocks; Knee, nerve blocks*

Persistent vegetative state, *see Vegetative state*

PET, Pre-eclamptic toxaemia, *see Pre-eclampsia*

PET scanning, *see Positron emission tomography*

Pethick's test, *see Checking of anaesthetic equipment*

Pethidine hydrochloride. Synthetic **opioid analgesic drug**, developed in Germany in 1939. One-tenth as potent as **morphine**, with duration of action of 2–4 h and **half-life** of about 3–4 h. Approximately 60% protein-bound in plasma. 5%–10% is excreted unchanged in urine, more if the urine is acidic. 90% undergoes hepatic metabolism to norpethidine, an active substance (half-life 20–40 h) that may cause hallucinations and **convulsions**.

Table 42 Corresponding values for pH and hydrogen ion concentration

pH units	*[H⁺] (nmol/l)*
6.8	158
6.9	126
7.0	100
7.1	79
7.2	63
7.3	50
7.4	40
7.5	32
7.6	25
7.7	20
7.8	16
7.9	13
8.0	10

Has similar effects to morphine, but also has local anaesthetic and anticholinergic actions. May cause bronchodilatation, but may also cause **histamine** release. May relax contracted GIT and urinary smooth muscle. High doses may cause convulsions and myocardial depression.

Indications for use are as for morphine.

- Dosage: 50–150 mg orally or 25–50 mg iv 4-hourly. Also used in **obstetric analgesia and anaesthesia** (50–150 mg im, max 400 mg/day), and has been given by subarachnoid injection (50–100 mg).

Has been used as a component of the **lytic cocktail.**

Should be avoided in patients taking **monoamine oxidase inhibitors.**

PFA-100, *see Coagulation studies*

pH. Negative logarithm to base 10 of **hydrogen ion** concentration (lower case 'p' being the symbol for $-\log_{10}$); i.e., pH = $-\log [H^+]$. Used as an indication of acidity; the more acid a solution, the lower the pH (Table 42). pH of normal arterial blood is 7.34–7.46, corresponding to $[H^+]$ of 34–46 nmol/l.

See also, Acid–base balance

pH measurement. Relies on the principle that, when two electrolyte solutions are separated by a semipermeable membrane, an electrical potential difference is generated across the membrane that is proportional to the **hydrogen ion** concentration gradient across it.

The **pH** electrode uses H^+-sensitive glass as the membrane; this separates the sample solution (e.g. blood), from the silver/silver chloride measuring electrode immersed in an internal buffer solution of constant pH. Thus, the potential difference across the glass is dependent on the $[H^+]$ of the sample. A mercury/mercurous chloride/potassium chloride electrode system also makes contact with the blood (via a membrane to prevent contamination), acting as a reference electrode. The potential difference between the reference and measuring electrodes is amplified and displayed.

The system is maintained at 37°C; potential output is linear at approximately 60 mV per pH unit.

See also, Blood gas interpretation

Phaeochromocytoma. Rare tumour secreting **catecholamines**, originating from chromaffin tissue. 90% occur in the **adrenal gland**, 10% at other sites within the **sympathetic nervous system.** 10% are bilateral and 10% malignant. May occur as part of **multiple endocrine adenomatosis** 2A or 2B or in association with **neurofibromatosis.**

Usually presents with headache, psychosis, palpitations, sweating and **hypertension** (episodic or sustained). Tumours secreting mainly **adrenaline** cause tachyarrhythmias; those secreting **noradrenaline** cause vasoconstriction, ischaemia and hypertension. Some tumours secrete both these **catecholamines** and also **dopamine. Glucose** intolerance and **cardiomyopathy** may occur.

- Diagnosis is confirmed by:
  - measuring plasma catecholamines or urinary catecholamine metabolites (e.g. metanephrine, normetanephrine, hydroxymethylmandelic acid; HMMA).
  - suppression tests (e.g. using **clonidine**) with measurement of plasma catecholamines.
  - provocation tests (e.g. using **histamine**, tyramine or **glucagon**). Rarely used now, because dangerous hypertension may occur.

Tumours may be located using selective venous catheterisation and catecholamine assays, arteriography (may provoke hypertensive crises), CT scanning, **MRI** and radioactive *meta*-iodobenzyl guanidine (MIBG) scintigraphy. **Positron emission tomography** has also been used.

Definitive treatment is with surgical excision, traditionally by open laparotomy but increasingly by **laparoscopy.** Anaesthetic considerations:

- preoperatively:
  - chronic hypertension may lead to hypertrophic or dilated **cardiomyopathy**, the latter associated with **cardiac failure.** Preparation includes several weeks' oral therapy with **α-adrenergic receptor antagonists** (e.g. traditionally **phentolamine** or **phenoxybenzamine** but more recently with α_1-selective antagonists, e.g. **prazosin** or doxazosin). With the older non-selective α-receptor antagonists, **β-adrenergic receptor antagonists** are administered when α-receptor blockade is complete, but doxazosin may be used without β-receptor antagonists because it does not block presynaptic α_2-receptors and thus is not associated with increased cardiac sympathetic activity (unless tumours are predominantly adrenaline-secreting). Initiation of β-receptor blockade before α-receptor blockade is contraindicated as it may exacerbate hypertension because of antagonism of β_2-mediated vasodilatation in muscle. Labetalol and atenolol are often used. **α-Methyl-*p*-tyrosine** and **calcium channel blocking drugs** have also been used.
  - fluid therapy may be required; this may be aided by **central venous cannulation.**
- perioperatively:
  - drugs causing minimal cardiovascular disturbance are used for anaesthesia.
  - direct **arterial BP measurement** and CVP with or without **pulmonary capillary wedge pressure** monitoring are required.
  - catecholamines may be released in response to surgical stress, anaesthetic drugs and handling of the tumour. **Sodium nitroprusside**, phentolamine, **GTN**, prazosin, calcium channel blocking drugs and **magnesium sulfate** have been used to control perioperative hypertension. β-Receptor antagonists or other **antiarrhythmic drugs** may be used to control tachycardia.

- following the tumour's removal, **iv fluids** and occasionally **phenylephrine** or dopamine may be required to maintain BP.
- postoperatively:
  - ICU care is required.
  - **hypoglycaemia**, cardiovascular instability and fluid imbalance may occur.
  - bilateral adrenalectomy will require replacement of **corticosteroids**.

Rarely, phaeochromocytoma may present for the first time during incidental surgery, pregnancy or labour; morbidity and mortality are higher in this context.

Connor D, Boumphrey S (2016). BJA Educ; 16: 153–8

Phantom limb. Sensation of the continued presence of an amputated limb, occurring in around 65% of amputees after six months and commonly described as throbbing, aching or burning. The 'limb' may also be felt to be in an abnormal position. Risk factors include upper limb amputation, pain before amputation and female gender. Putative mechanisms include the peripheral afferent theory (ectopic firing and lowered stimulation thresholds in the neuroma or damaged afferent) and the central nervous theory (neuroplastic changes in the dorsal horn as a result of prolonged stimulation, causing decreased sensitivity to descending inhibitory pathways and reorganisation of the somatosensory cortex). Treatment includes **anticonvulsant drugs**, **ketamine**, **opioid analgesic drugs**, local somatic and **sympathetic nerve blocks**, **spinal cord stimulation**, mirror therapy (in which the remaining limb is placed into a mirror box that gives the illusion that two limbs are present) and biofeedback therapy.

Epidural anaesthesia has been claimed to prevent the development of phantom limb pain when instituted before surgical amputation, but the evidence for this is weak.

Pharmacodynamics. Describes the effects of drugs on the body. Drugs may act by physical interactions (e.g. **antacids**, general anaesthetics), or by interacting with receptors (**receptor theory**) or **enzymes**.

See also, Dose–response curves; Gender differences and anaesthesia; Pharmacogenetics; Pharmacokinetics

Pharmacogenetics (Pharmacogenomics). Describes variations in the **pharmacodynamics** and/or **pharmacokinetics** of a drug that are attributable to the genetic make-up of the individual. Examples include a prolonged action of **suxamethonium** due to variations of plasma **cholinesterase**, and variation in metabolism of opioid drugs, benzodiazepines, paracetamol and other NSAIDs due to genetic variation in the **cytochrome** P_{450} enzyme system. Easiest to characterise if single nucleotide polymorphism (SNP) is involved, in which variation in a single nucleotide of the genome leads to different responses; a number of SNPs may be relevant to differences in response to a particular drug or drug group. Potential applications include the 'tailoring' of drug therapy to individual patients based on their genotype, which could be analysed from a single blood sample. Current obstacles include the incomplete understanding of many drugs' mechanism of action, the involvement of multiple genes in a given response to a drug, and the difficulty in predicting actual patients' responses from genotype alone.

Landau R, Bollag LA, Kraft JC (2012). Anaesthesia; 67: 165–79

See also, Gender differences and anaesthesia

Pharmacokinetics. Describes the absorption, distribution, metabolism and elimination of drugs, i.e., effects of the body on drugs. These factors determine how the effector site concentration of a drug varies over time. Population differences in pharmacokinetic characteristics may arise from general individual variations and genetic factors (*see Pharmacogenetics*).

- Absorption:
  - may be via oral, sublingual, buccal, inhalational, iv, im, sc, rectal or topical routes.
  - rate of absorption affects the maximum concentration and duration of drug action. Most drugs are absorbed by simple **diffusion**; i.e., rate depends on drug **solubility**, tissue permeability, surface area and vascularity of the absorption site. Lipid solubility depends on the degree of **ionisation** of the drug, which depends on the **p*K*** of the drug in solution and body **pH**. Some drugs are absorbed by **active transport**, e.g. L dopa, **α-methyldopa**.
  - absorption from the GIT also depends on drug characteristics, gut motility, vomiting, destruction of drug by digestive enzymes, interaction with food or other drugs, GIT disease and intestinal microflora. **First-pass metabolism** reduces the **bioavailability** of many orally administered drugs, e.g. **opioid analgesic drugs**. Other routes of administration avoid this.
  - absorption occurs via the lungs for **inhalational anaesthetic agents**.
- Distribution:
  - related to lipid solubility, p*K*, body fluid pH, **protein-binding**, regional blood flow, and specific properties of the drug (e.g. iodine taken up by thyroid tissue).
  - protein-binding limits both the amount of free drug and redistribution of drugs from the blood. **Volume of distribution** and **clearance** of a drug are inversely proportional to its protein-binding.
  - initial redistribution may reduce blood levels of a drug with recovery from its effects, although the total amount in the body has hardly changed, e.g. **thiopental** and other **iv anaesthetic agents**.
  - compartment models have been described to explain the distribution of drugs in the body:
    - one-compartment model: plasma concentration declines as a simple negative **exponential process** after a bolus injection (first-order kinetics; Fig. 130a), i.e.:

$$C_t = C_0 e^{-kt}$$

where C_t = concentration at time t
C_0 = concentration at time zero
k = rate constant
$e \approx 2.718$

A straight line is obtained when it is plotted using a semi-logarithmic scale (Fig. 130b).

$$\text{The slope of the line} = \frac{k}{2.303}, \text{ and } \textbf{half-life} = \frac{0.693}{k}$$

$$\text{Clearance} = k \times \text{volume of distribution} = \frac{D}{\text{AUC}}$$

where AUC = area under the plasma concentration/time curve
D = dose of drug at time zero

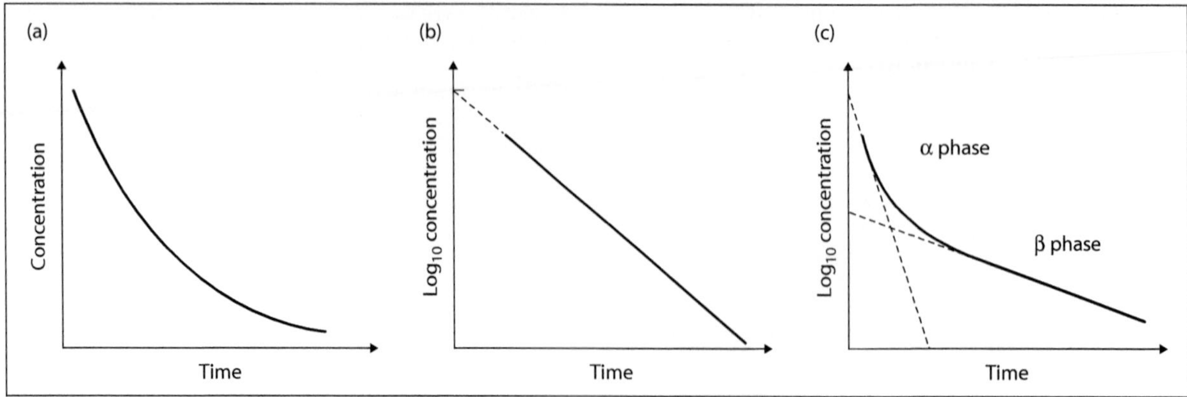

Fig. 130 Drug concentration against time: (a) and (b) one-compartment model; (c) two-compartment model

- two-compartment model: bi-exponential decline in plasma level; an initial rapid α distribution phase is followed by a slower β elimination phase (Fig. 130c). Each component of the curve may be analysed separately.

  Drug is distributed from a central compartment (i.e., blood, brain, lungs) to a peripheral one (e.g. **ECF**, tissues). The central compartment does not necessarily correspond to an anatomical volume, but is defined in terms of its apparent volume. Elimination occurs from the central compartment.
- three-compartment distribution: one central and two peripheral compartments are assumed.

- Metabolism:
  - drug activity may be enhanced (e.g. **morphine** metabolised to morphine-6-glucuronide), decreased (most drugs) or unaltered (e.g. certain **benzodiazepines**).
  - usually occurs in two phases in the **liver**. Phase I involves oxidation, reduction or hydrolysis, often involving the cytochrome P_{450} enzyme system. Phase II reactions involve conjugation with glucuronic acid, glycine, glutamine and sulfate, increasing water solubility. Rate of metabolism may be altered by **enzyme induction/inhibition**.
  - other sites may be involved, e.g. plasma cholinesterase (**suxamethonium**), kidney (e.g. **dopamine**).
- Elimination:
  - may occur via lungs, bile, urine, GIT, saliva or breast milk. Renal excretion depends on **GFR**, water solubility and extent of active tubular secretion and reabsorption.
  - most drugs are eliminated by first-order kinetics, whereby rate of elimination is proportional to the amount of drug in the body (i.e., simple exponential decay).
  - in zero-order kinetics, a constant amount of drug is eliminated per unit time (e.g. alcohol, **phenytoin**). Zero-order kinetics may replace first-order kinetics when elimination pathways are saturated, i.e., at high drug concentrations.

These analyses allow prediction of drug kinetics for calculation of appropriate dosage regimens or incorporation into the software of computer-controlled infusion pumps. For a continuous drug infusion, 50% of steady-state levels are reached after one half-life, 75% after two half-lives, 87.5% after three, 93.75% after four, 96.875% after five, etc. A loading dose achieves steady-state levels more quickly, but is limited by adverse effects if a large dose is given, depending on the drug's **therapeutic ratio/index**. At steady state, the infusion rate equals the rate of elimination of drug for a one-compartment model, or the rate of transfer to a peripheral compartment for a multi-compartment model.

Rigby-Jones AE, Sneyd JR (2012). Anaesthesia; 67: 5–11

See also, Drug interactions; Gender differences and anaesthesia; Pharmacogenetics; Michaelis–Menten kinetics; Target-controlled infusions

Pharynx. Common upper end of the respiratory and alimentary tracts, extending from the base of the **skull** to the level of C6.

- Divided into:
  - nasopharynx: lies behind the nasal cavities, above the soft palate. Contains the adenoids, and a Eustachian tube orifice on each lateral wall.
  - oropharynx: lies behind the mouth and **tongue**, below the soft palate. Bounded anteriorly by the anterior pillars of the fauces (with buccal cavity anteriorly), superiorly by the palate and inferiorly by the tip of the epiglottis. Contains the tonsils, lying between the anterior and posterior pillars (containing palatoglossus and palatopharyngeus muscles, respectively).
  - laryngopharynx: lies behind and around the **larynx**, extending from the level of the epiglottic tip to the C6 level. The larynx projects into the laryngopharynx, leaving a deep recess (piriform fossa) on each side.

Composed of mucosa (ciliated columnar type in the nasopharynx; stratified or squamous elsewhere), submucosa, muscle layer and loose areolar sheath. The muscles (superior, middle and inferior constrictors) are arranged so that the upper parts of each overlap the lower fibres of the muscle above. They arise thus:
  - superior: from the pterygomandibular raphe, and bony points at either end.
  - middle: from the hyoid bone and stylohyoid ligament.
  - inferior: from the thyroid and cricoid cartilages.

Their anterior borders are open to form the nasal, buccal and laryngeal cavities. Their posterior borders insert into a median raphe along the length of the pharynx.

- Blood supply:
  - arterial: via superior thyroid and ascending pharyngeal branches of the external **carotid artery**.
  - venous: via pharyngeal plexus to the internal **jugular vein**.

• Nerve supply: ninth and 10th **cranial nerves**, with additional nasal innervation via the fifth nerve.

[Bartolomeo Eustachio (1513–1574), Italian physician]

See also, Nose

Phase II block, *see Dual block*

Phase shift. Delay between the arrival of a signal at a **monitoring** device (e.g. **transducer**) and the latter's output. Distortion of the signal is minimised by applying the same delay to all components of the **waveform**, thus maintaining the phase relationship between **harmonics**. This is achieved by adjusting the **damping** of the system to about two-thirds critical damping, at which there is a linear relationship between phase lag and the frequency of the wave.

Phenobarbital/Phenobarbital sodium (Phenobarbitone). Long-acting **barbiturate** and **anticonvulsant drug**, introduced in 1912. Used as a secondary agent in all types of **epilepsy** except absence attacks. Also used in the treatment of **status epilepticus**. Although absorbed slowly after oral administration, it has an oral **bioavailability** of 90% with duration of action up to 16 h. Elimination **half-life** is about 90 h. 20%–45% protein-bound, and 75% metabolised by hepatic microsomal enzymes; 25% is normally excreted unchanged in urine.

- Dosage:
  - 60–180 mg orally od (5–8 mg/kg/day in children).
  - for status epilepticus: 15–18 mg/kg.
- Side effects include sedation and ataxia. Paradoxical excitation may occur in children.

Hepatic **enzyme induction** may reduce the effectiveness of other drugs, e.g. **warfarin**, oral contraceptives, **corticosteroids**.

Phenol (Carbolic acid). Organic compound with the chemical formula C_6H_5OH. Widely used in manufacturing, including drug production. Medically, used as a neurolytic agent in chronic **pain management**. Thought to spare large myelinated fibres while damaging unmyelinated C pain fibres by protein denaturation. Hyperbaric 5% solution in glycerine is used for subarachnoid neurolysis of posterior nerve roots; 0.5–2.0 ml has an effect lasting up to 14 weeks. 6%–7% solution in water is used for **sympathetic nerve blocks**.

Also used for sclerotherapy of haemorrhoids, and as a throat gargle. 1%–5% solution (carbolic acid) is also used for disinfection of equipment. Irritant to the skin. Used for surgical antisepsis by Lister in Glasgow in 1865.

[Joseph Lister (1827–1912), English surgeon]

Phenoperidine hydrochloride. Obsolete synthetic **opioid analgesic drug** related to **pethidine**; discontinued in the UK in 1997.

Phenothiazines. Group of sedative and **antipsychotic drugs**. Also have antimuscarinic, antiemetic, antihistamine, antidopaminergic and **α-adrenergic receptor antagonist** properties. Some may potentiate the effects of **opioid analgesic drugs**. Different drugs have varying degrees of these properties, depending on the side chains of the molecule. Act mainly on the **ascending reticular activating system**, **limbic system**, basal ganglia, **hypothalamus** and **chemoreceptor trigger zone**. Cause sedation, with reduced muscular, GIT and cardiovascular activity. Effect on respiration is variable. Central temperature regulatory mechanisms, shivering, and peripheral vasoconstriction are impaired, but metabolic rate is unaffected. Highly lipid-soluble and extensively protein-bound. Metabolised in the liver to mostly inactive metabolites.

- Side effects:
  - extrapyramidal symptoms, e.g. tardive dyskinesia, dystonia, tremor, facial grimacing.
  - drowsiness, insomnia, depression, hypothermia, prevention of shivering.
  - anticholinergic effects, e.g. tachycardia, **arrhythmias**, dry mouth, urinary retention, blurring of vision.
  - galactorrhoea, menstrual irregularity, gynaecomastia, weight gain.
  - blood dyscrasias, **haemolysis**.
  - photosensitivity, contact dermatitis, rash.
  - obstructive **jaundice**.
  - hypotension.
  - **neuroleptic malignant syndrome**.
  - potentiation of other depressant drugs.

Chlorpromazine is the standard phenothiazine; others include **alimemazine** (trimeprazine), **promethazine**, perphenazine, promazine, thioridazine, fluphenazine and trifluoperazine.

Phenoxybenzamine hydrochloride. Irreversible non-selective **α-adrenergic receptor antagonist**, chemically related to the nitrogen mustards; forms covalent bonds with **α-adrenergic receptors**. Used mainly to control **hypertension** caused by **phaeochromocytoma**. Has also been used in **complex regional pain syndrome** type 1. More active at α_1-receptors than at α_2-receptors. Onset of action may be up to 1 h after iv injection, due to conversion to an active form. Effects last for several days, although its elimination **half-life** is about 24 h.

- Dosage:
  - 10 mg orally od, increased by 10 mg/day as required.
  - 1 mg/kg in 200 ml saline over 2 h od (profound hypotension may occur).
- Side effects: postural hypotension, tachycardia, inhibition of ejaculation, nasal congestion, miosis, rarely GIT disturbances.

See also, Vasodilator drugs

Phenoxymethylpenicillin (Penicillin V). Natural **penicillin** used especially in **streptococcal infections** and in **rheumatic fever** prophylaxis. Also used for pneumococcal prophylaxis after splenectomy or in **sickle cell anaemia**. Similar to **benzylpenicillin** but less active and more acid-stable; thus suitable for oral administration, following which peak serum levels occur in about 60 min (although somewhat variably, hence the recommendation that it not be used for severe infections). 80% of the drug is protein-bound. Excreted in urine (the dose should be reduced in renal impairment) and faeces. Elimination **half-life** is 40 min.

- Dosage:
  - 500–1000 mg orally bd/qds.
  - for prophylaxis, 250 mg (rheumatic fever) or 500 mg (splenectomy, sickle cell) bd.
- Side effects: as for benzylpenicillin.

Phentolamine mesylate. Non-selective **α-adrenergic receptor antagonist**, with an additional direct relaxant action on vascular smooth muscle. Used in **hypotensive anaesthesia** and to control **hypertensive crisis**, e.g. caused by **phaeochromocytoma**, **monoamine oxidase inhibitor** interactions and **clonidine** withdrawal. An oral preparation is used for the treatment of erectile dysfunction. Previously used for diagnosing phaeochromocytoma and in the assessment of **complex regional pain syndromes**. Acts within 2 min of iv injection, with duration of action 10–15 min.

- Dosage: 2–5 mg iv repeated as required; 0.1–2.0 mg/min by infusion.
- Side effects: postural hypotension, tachycardia, abdominal pain, diarrhoea, nasal congestion.

See also, Vasodilator drugs

Phenylephrine hydrochloride. Synthetic selective α_1-adrenergic receptor agonist, used as a **vasopressor drug**, e.g. in spinal anaesthesia. Causes intense vasoconstriction and compensatory bradycardia. Popular in obstetric regional anaesthesia, because it appears more effective than **ephedrine**, and fetal acid–base profile is better than if large doses of ephedrine are used. Has been administered topically to the nasal mucosa and eye to cause vasoconstriction and mydriasis, respectively, and as a vasoconstrictor agent for local anaesthesia. Has also been used to treat **SVT**. Of similar structure to **adrenaline**, lacking only the 4-hydroxyl group.

- Dosage:
  - 2–5 mg im or sc.
  - 100–500 µg iv (5–10 µg/kg in children); 30–180 µg/min by infusion. Boluses of 25–100 µg (or increasingly, 25–50 µg/min infusion) are used to treat hypotension in obstetric regional anaesthesia.
  - 2.5–5 mg added to 100 ml local anaesthetic solution.
- Side effects: hypertension, bradycardia, vomiting.

Phenytoin/phenytoin sodium. Hydantoin **anticonvulsant drug**, introduced in the late 1930s. Used to treat all types of **epilepsy** except petit mal, in chronic **pain management**, and previously as a class Ib **antiarrhythmic drug** (especially for **digoxin**-induced **arrhythmias**). Has membrane-stabilising effects on all neuronal cells, including peripheral nerves and cardiac muscle; acts by blocking voltage-gated sodium channels.

A poorly water-soluble weak acid, with **pK_a** ~ 8.3. Variably absorbed from the GIT, it may cause gastric irritation. Erratically absorbed after im injection, probably due to local precipitation. About 90% protein-bound, and metabolised in the liver to inactive metabolites that are excreted renally. Elimination follows first-order kinetics at plasma levels below 10 mg/l; zero-order kinetics occur above 10 mg/l, due to saturation of enzyme systems (*see Pharmacokinetics*). Elimination **half-life** is about 24 h but varies. Susceptible to hepatic **enzyme induction**, and is itself an enzyme inducer.

- Dosage:
  - 3–4 mg/kg daily as one or two oral doses, increased up to 600 mg/day.
  - for **status epilepticus**: 20 mg/kg (up to 2 g) iv slowly, with ECG monitoring, followed by 100 mg tds/qds.
  - to prevent/treat seizures after **neurosurgery** or **head injury**: 2.5 mg/kg orally bd up to 4–8 mg/kg/day.

Plasma levels should be monitored; therapeutic range is 10–20 mg/l (40–80 µmol/l). IV administration should be via a large vein at no more than 1 mg/kg/min (up to 50 mg/min). Flushing with saline should follow as the solution is strongly alkaline and irritant. Arrhythmias and hypotension may occur.

- Side effects:
  - headache, vomiting, confusion, tremor. Ataxia, nystagmus and blurred vision may indicate overdosage.
  - skin eruptions, lymphadenopathy, hirsutism, fever, hepatitis, gingival hyperplasia. The purple glove syndrome (blue/purple discoloration followed by oedema and necrosis) may occur around the site of iv administration.
  - osteomalacia.
  - rarely, megaloblastic anaemia (due to impaired folate absorption and storage), other blood dyscrasias.
  - fetal neural tube defects and neonatal bleeding may follow its use in pregnancy.

Chronic usage may cause resistance to non-depolarising **neuromuscular blocking drugs**.

Available as a **prodrug, fosphenytoin.**

PHI, *see Prehospital index*

Phlogiston. Imaginary substance proposed in the 1720s, thought to separate from combustible material during burning. Following experiments in the 1770s, **Priestley** concluded that 'dephlogisticated air' (O_2) and 'dephlogisticated nitrous air' (N_2O) were deficient in phlogiston and could thus support combustion, whereas 'nitrous air' (NO_2) was saturated with it and was unable to do so. The phlogiston theory was subsequently disproved by **Lavoisier**.

Phonocardiography. Technique employing contact microphones placed on the chest, for amplification and recording of **heart sounds**. Used to obtain an objective record of heart sounds and **heart murmurs**. May be performed simultaneously with **ECG** and **arterial waveform** recording, allowing calculation of **systolic time intervals**. A similar technique is employed in **fetal monitoring**.
See also, Cardiac cycle

Phosphate. Total body content is about 25 000 mmol, most of which is intracellular. 80% is in bone, 15% is in soft tissues and only 0.1% is in **ECF**. Most intracellular phosphate is in the organic form. Normal plasma inorganic phosphate levels: 0.8–1.45 mmol/l. Dietary phosphate is absorbed mainly in the duodenum and jejunum via active and passive transport mechanisms.

Involved in cell **membranes** (phospholipids), **enzyme** regulation, energy storage (**ATP**), **O_2 transport (2,3-DPG)** and acid–base buffering.

Levels are controlled by renal excretion; most of the filtered phosphate is reabsorbed in the proximal tubule of the **nephron**. Excretion is increased by parathyroid hormone, **calcitonin, adrenaline** and increased phosphate intake. Decreased excretion occurs when intake is low or in response to thyroxine or **growth hormone. Hyperphosphataemia** causes no specific clinical sequelae but may disturb **calcium** metabolism. **Hypophosphataemia** is common in ICU patients, especially associated with **TPN** and **ketoacidosis.**

Phosphodiesterase inhibitors. Substances that prevent conversion of **3′,5′-adenosine monophosphate** (cAMP) to 5′-adenosine monophosphate, or 3′,5′-guanosine monophosphate (cGMP) to 5′-guanosine monophosphate by the enzyme phosphodiesterase (PDE; *see Fig. 5;* **Adenosine monophosphate, *cyclic***). Both cAMP and cGMP are important intracellular messengers. Many isoenzymes of PDE exist; PDE3 inhibitors include **amrinone, milrinone, enoximone**, piroximone and pimobendan; PDE4 inhibitors include ibudilast (asthma), apremilast (psoriasis) and roflumilast (COPD); and PDE5 inhibitors include **sildenafil** and **dipyridamole.**

Aminophylline, papaverine and **caffeine** are non-selective PDE inhibitors.

Phrenic nerve pacing. Intermittent electrical stimulation of the **phrenic nerves** (usually bilaterally), to pace the **diaphragm** in chronic **hypoventilation** due to brainstem, medulla or upper cervical cord lesions. Has also been used in **COPD**. Described in the 1960s, it requires intact phrenic nerves and diaphragm function, thus excluding its use in lower **motor neurone** lesions and myopathies.

Platinum electrodes are implanted around the nerves in the neck or thorax and connected to a subcutaneous radio receiver, which is triggered by an external power source. Respiratory rate, inspiratory time and sighs may be adjusted. Neck electrodes risk inadvertent stimulation of the brachial plexus. Nerve trauma at surgery, infection and poor contacts may cause failure. Diaphragmatic fatigue may also occur. Obstructive apnoea may be precipitated in some cases of central alveolar hypoventilation.

Implantation of electrodes directly into the diaphragm has also been used, thus not requiring intact phrenic nerves.

Pimpec-Barthes F, Legras A, Arame A, et al (2016). J Thorac Dis; 8 (suppl 4): S376–86

Phrenic nerves. Originate from the ventral rami of C3–5 on each side, supplying the motor innervation of the **diaphragm.** Also convey sensory fibres from the diaphragm; hence the shoulder-tip **referred pain** caused by diaphragmatic irritation. Sensory fibres from the mediastinal **pleura**, fibrous **pericardium** and parietal serous pericardium are also conveyed.

Descend vertically on the scalenus anterior muscles, which they cross from lateral to medial sides. Each nerve passes to the root of the neck beneath the sternomastoid muscle, inferior belly of omohyoid, internal **jugular vein** and (on the left) the thoracic duct. The right phrenic nerve enters the thorax behind the subclavian/internal jugular venous junction, descending subpleurally next to the right brachiocephalic vein, superior and inferior venae cavae and pericardium. Some of its branches pass through the caval foramen of the diaphragm, spreading over its peritoneal surface. The remainder pierce the diaphragm just lateral to the caval orifice. The left nerve enters the thorax between the subclavian artery and vein. It passes superficially to the aortic arch, to pierce the diaphragm anteriorly and to the left of the caval opening. Some of the divisions of each nerve cross to the other side.

Local anaesthetic block has been advocated as a treatment for chronic **hiccups.** 10 ml **local anaesthetic agent** is injected 1–2 cm deep at a point 2 cm above the sternoclavicular joint and for 5 cm laterally.

Phrenic paralysis may complicate **brachial plexus block**, trauma, tumour, neurological disease and cardiac surgery. Clinically, paradoxical inward abdominal movement is seen on inspiration, with a raised hemidiaphragm on **CXR**.

See also, Phrenic nerve pacing

Physicians' assistants (anaesthesia). Non-medically qualified personnel able to deliver anaesthesia under supervision by a qualified anaesthetist. In the UK, the term is specific to graduates of 2-year programmes (plus 3 months' supervised practice) approved by the Royal College of Anaesthetists, set up as pilots initially in 2003, in response to predicted shortfalls in manpower. The scheme mirrors those introducing other support roles within the NHS, taking on some of the activities and duties traditionally exclusive to qualified doctors. The original term 'Anaesthesia Practitioners' was replaced by the new title in 2008 to bring it into line with Physicians' Assistants (now 'Physician Associates') in other areas/specialties within the NHS, and to aid understanding of the role.

Physiological and operative severity score for the enumeration of mortality and morbidity (POSSUM). Scoring system described in 1991 as a method of predicting outcome (morbidity and mortality) for surgical patients. Patients are scored before operation (using measures of physiological derangement) and at operation (using an operative severity score) to give predictions of morbidity and hospital mortality. The original POSSUM model has been modified for specific subspecialties to provide greater accuracy (e.g. P-POSSUM for general surgery, CR-POSSUM for colorectal cancer surgery, V-POSSUM for vascular surgery).

Moonesinghe SR, Mythen MG, Das P, et al (2013). Anesthesiology; 119: 959–81

Physiotherapy. Treatment and prevention of disease using passive and active movement, vibration, massage and application of heat. Used for neurological, musculoskeletal and respiratory disorders. Has an important role in the ICU in preventing stiffness of limbs and joints during prolonged immobility, and in helping the patient mobilise during recovery.

Chest physiotherapy aims to maintain clear airways, increase lung expansion and thus reduce **atelectasis** and sputum retention. Often beneficial pre- and postoperatively in patients with respiratory disease, helping to optimise respiratory function. It is also valuable in the ICU management of patients with **respiratory failure**, before, during and after **IPPV**. It is thought to be most useful when excessive sputum is present; its place in uncomplicated **COPD**, **chest infection** without sputum production, and routine postoperative management is unclear. Thought to be of little benefit if disease is mainly peripheral; thus it is most effective if secretions are within the bronchi.

- Techniques include:
  - postural drainage: positioning according to the anatomy of the **tracheobronchial tree**, with or without breathing exercises.
  - breathing exercises, e.g. **incentive spirometry**, coughing. **Forced expirations** may be more effective than cough alone, especially if combined with postural drainage.
  - intermittent lung inflations using **ventilators**, to increase lung expansion.
  - chest wall percussion and vibration: their efficacy has also been questioned.
  - upper airway suction: usually combined with the above.

Administration of nebulised **bronchodilator drugs** before physiotherapy may produce a better sputum yield. Nebulised saline, humidified O_2 and mucolytics are also commonly used.

May be painful, especially postoperatively, and adequate analgesia is essential.

Physostigmine salicylate/sulfate. Acetylcholinesterase inhibitor, derived from the West African Calabar bean. Causes reversible inhibition of **acetylcholinesterase** by binding to its esteratic site, lasting 1–2 h. Readily crosses the **blood–brain barrier** because of its tertiary amine structure. Used to treat the **central anticholinergic syndrome**, and topically in **glaucoma**. Has also been used in **γ-hydroxybutyric acid** poisoning. Formerly used as a general CNS stimulant, e.g. in **tricyclic antidepressant drug**

poisoning and to reverse opioid-induced respiratory depression. No longer available in the UK.

- Dosage: 0.04 mg/kg slowly iv.
- Side effects: nausea, hypertension, tachycardia. Large doses may result in **cholinergic crisis**.

PiCCO. Commercial non-invasive **cardiac output measurement** system made available in 1997, combining the principles of transpulmonary thermodilution, in which the 'cold' transverses the lungs after injection, and arterial pulse contour analysis. Requires injection of a single bolus injection of cold saline through a central venous catheter and its detection by a specially modified cannula placed in a large artery (e.g. femoral/brachial). Permits continuous estimation of **cardiac output**, intrathoracic blood volume, left ventricular **afterload**, **extravascular lung water** and **stroke volume** variation. Provides cardiac output measurements with similar accuracy to that obtained from **pulmonary artery catheterisation**, although frequent calibration may be required in unstable patients (e.g. in **sepsis** or **haemorrhage**).

PiCCO 2 uses a more refined algorithm and was released in 2008.

Litton E, Morgan M (2012). Anaesth Intensive Care; 40: 393–409

Pickwickian syndrome, *see Obesity hypoventilation syndrome*

Pierre Robin syndrome, *see Facial deformities, congenital*

Pin index system. International system introduced in 1952, preventing accidental connection of a gas **cylinder** to the wrong **anaesthetic machine** yoke. The cylinder valve block bears holes into which fit pins protruding from the yoke. A flush connection is only achieved if the holes and pins align correctly. The positions of the holes on the valve block (and corresponding pins on the yoke) are specified by an international standard (Fig. 131):

- O_2: positions 2 and 5.
- N_2O: positions 3 and 5.
- **air**: positions 1 and 5.
- CO_2: positions 1 and 6.
- **Entonox**: position 7.

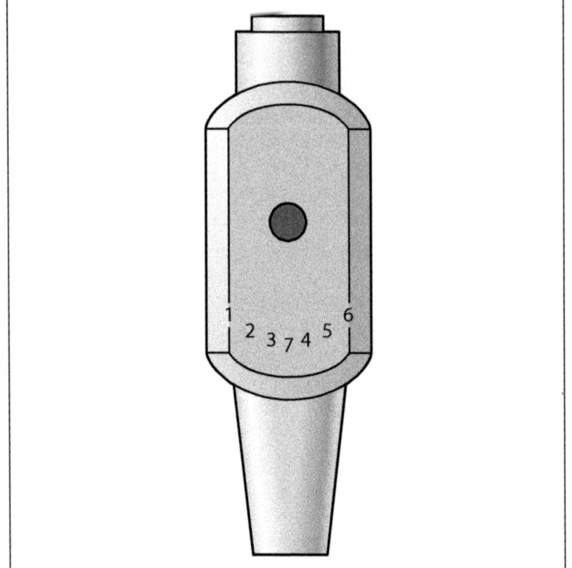

Fig. 131 Position of holes (1–7) in pin index system

The system may be circumvented, e.g. by removing pins or using several **Bodok seals**. When piped gas supplies were first introduced, pin-indexed fittings were attached to the pipelines; these could be inserted upside-down into the cylinder yokes, allowing incorrect gas connection. The positions for **cyclopropane** were 3 and 6.

Pipecuronium bromide. Non-depolarising **neuromuscular blocking drug**, related to **pancuronium**, synthesised in Hungary in the late 1970s and made available in the USA in 1990 (and withdrawn in 1999).

Piped gas supply. Networks of pipes and socket outlets that distribute medical gases from a central source to points of use. In the UK, only O_2, N_2O, **Entonox**, CO_2 (rarely) and compressed air may be distributed by such systems. All are supplied at 4 bar except air, which may be required at 7 bar for surgical instruments. Medical vacuum is also supplied by a pipeline system.

- Essential features include:
  - indexing system to prevent cross-connection.
  - prevention of contamination of gases.
  - automatic function, especially when switching over supplies.
  - anti-combustion and anti-explosion controls.
- Systems consist of:
  - central gas source: either a large primary source and small reserve supply, or large primary and secondary sources used alternately with a small reserve supply. The primary source may be a manifold of **cylinders**, **vacuum insulated evaporator**, air compressor or O_2 **concentrator**.
  - pipeline distribution network: made of phosphorus deoxidised non-arsenical copper, greased and specially cleaned with steam, shot and medical air. Joints are usually made with a silver alloy, although some are threaded. They should be colour-coded and marked with the name of the gas contained. Isolation valves should be supplied.
  - terminal distribution system: includes self-closing sockets, probes, **flowmeters**, and hoses and their connections with **anaesthetic machines**. The probes and sockets should be specific for the service supplied, the probe of one gas fitting only the socket for the same gas.

    Some probes (e.g. for ward use) may incorporate flowmeters. Connecting hoses to probes should only be possible if specialised equipment is used, reducing the risk of misconnection. Hose connections to anaesthetic machines are made specific for each service by non-interchangeable screw-thread connectors. UK colour coding of hoses:
    - N_2O: French blue.
    - O_2: white.
    - air: black/white.
    - Entonox: French blue/white.
    - vacuum: yellow.
  - system failure alarms: predominantly low-pressure alarms, they sound when secondary and reserve systems are in use. Usually situated at hospital telephone switchboards.

Howell RS (1980). Anaesthesia; 35: 676–98

See also, Suction equipment

Piperacillin. Semisynthetic **penicillin** derivative with broad-spectrum antibacterial activity; has greater activity against gram-negative organisms than narrow-spectrum penicillins, with slightly reduced effectiveness against certain gram-positive organisms (e.g. *Streptococcus pneumoniae*). Especially effective against pseudomonas infections, although **bacterial resistance** is a growing problem. Often given with an **aminoglycoside** in severe pseudomonas infections because the combination is synergistic (but the two drugs should not be mixed in the same syringe). Only available combined with the β-lactamase inhibitor tazobactam. Piperacillin is 20% protein-bound with **volume of distribution** 15–20 l. Excreted via urine and faeces. Elimination **half-life** is approximately 1 h.

- Dosage: 4.5 g iv tds (qds in neutropenic patients).
- Side effects: as for **benzylpenicillin**. The high sodium content of the preparation may result in **hypernatraemia**.

Pirbuterol. **β-Adrenergic receptor agonist**, developed for the treatment of **asthma** but has been investigated as an orally active **inotropic drug**. Active at **β_1-adrenergic receptors**, with some activity at β_2-receptors. Thus increases **cardiac output** and causes vasodilatation; BP may fall. Tachycardia is uncommon.

Piritramide. **Opioid analgesic drug**, developed in 1960. Of faster onset than **morphine**, with similar duration of action and ~75% as potent. Not available in the UK.

Pirogoff, Nicholai Ivanovich (1810–1881). Russian surgeon at St Petersburg, a pioneer of battlefield trauma surgery, also known for introducing rectal **diethyl ether** for surgery in 1847. Also studied the effects of ether, designed apparatus for its rectal and inhalational administration, and published the first book on the subject in 1847.

Secher O (1986). Anaesthesia; 41: 829–37

Piroxicam. Oxicam **NSAID**. Rapidly absorbed after oral administration, it is 99% protein-bound and has a long (50 h) **half-life**; thus can be given once daily. Due to a high incidence of cutaneous and GIT adverse reactions, its use is now restricted to analgesia in chronic inflammatory or rheumatoid conditions.

- Dosage: 10–20 mg orally, od/bd.
- Side effects: as for NSAIDs (though see above).

Pituitary gland. Lies in the pituitary fossa of the sphenoid bone, above the sphenoid air sinuses and below the optic chiasm. Composed of anterior and posterior lobes, connected to the **hypothalamus** by the infundibular stalk, which contains nerve fibres and the hypophyseal portal blood system. The infundibulum pierces the diaphragma sellae, a dural sheet that covers the gland.

- Function:
  - anterior lobe:
    - contains cells formerly classified by their staining properties (chromophobe, eosinophil and acidophil cells); now identified on an immunocytochemical basis into five cell types:
    - somatotrophs: secrete **growth hormone**.
    - lactotrophs: secrete prolactin.
    - corticotrophs: secrete **ACTH**.
    - thyrotrophs: secrete thyrotropin.
    - gonadotrophs: secrete luteinising and follicle-stimulating hormones.
    - secretion is controlled by hypothalamic inhibitory or releasing factors, carried to the anterior pituitary by the portal blood system and by negative feedback control by circulating end-organ hormones.
  - posterior lobe: secretes **vasopressin** and **oxytocin**.

Pituitary gland disease may be associated with over- or under-secretion of hormones (usually the latter). Enlargement may cause visual field defects, optic atrophy and raised **ICP**.

See also, Acromegaly; Cushing's disease; Diabetes insipidus; Hypopituitarism

pK. Negative logarithm (to base 10) of the dissociation constant for a weak acid or base in aqueous solution. The law of mass action states that for a weak acid (HA) dissociating in solution, HA ⇌ $H^+ + A^-$:

$$\text{dissociation constant } K_a = \frac{[H^+][A^-]}{[HA]}$$

$$\text{Thus} -\log[H^+] = -\log K_a + \log\frac{[A^-]}{[HA]}$$

Substituting **pH** for $-\log [H^+]$, and pK_a for $-\log K_a$:

$$pH = pK_a + \log\frac{[A^-]}{[HA]}$$

For a weak base (B):

$$pH = pK_b + \log\frac{[B]}{[BH^+]}$$

The pK represents the pH value at which the solute is 50% dissociated; i.e., $[A^-] = [HA]$ or $[B] = [BH^+]$.

While pK_a strictly refers to an acidic substance and pK_b to a basic one, by convention pK_a is used to refer to both acids and bases.

The stronger an acid, the lower its pK_a, and the stronger a base, the higher its pK_a. Thus important when considering **ionisation of drugs** and passage of drugs or other substances across **membranes**.

Placenta. Structure dividing the fetal and maternal circulations. Approximately 5–6 days after conception the fertilised egg (now a mass of uniform cells) attaches to the endometrium. The endometrium is invaded by the outer layer of the trophoblast of the egg, the syncytiotrophoblast. Further proliferation of the trophoblast forms finger-shaped masses of tissue, the chorionic villi, between which spaces (lacunae) appear. The tips of the villi erode the walls of the endometrial spiral arteries so that the lacunae expand to form large spaces filled with maternal blood within which float the villi. Primitive blood vessels appear in the villi from about 18 days after fertilisation, eventually joining the fetal umbilical vessels. Densely packed masses of fetal villi (fetal cotyledons) are supplied by branches of the umbilical arteries, distributed radially as end-arteries. Several cotyledons form a single placental lobe. Thus the barrier between fetal and maternal circulations is two cells thick, consisting of the fetal capillary endothelium and its covering of syncytial trophoblast.

- Blood supply:
  - fetal: blood arrives via two umbilical arteries and leaves by a single umbilical vein. Umbilical blood flow is up to 100 ml/min at 22 weeks and 300 ml/min

at term, of which about 20% does not participate in exchange with maternal blood.
- maternal: delivered via the uterine arteries. Uterine blood flow (UBF) at term is 500–700 ml/min, 80% of which passes to the placenta. There is no autoregulation in the placental circulation and therefore flow is directly related to mean uterine perfusion pressure and inversely related to uterine vascular resistance. UBF may be reduced by maternal hypotension, hyperventilation and stress, and by **vasopressor drugs**.

Placental function is related to its total surface area (~15 m^2) and UBF. Impaired function causes fetal **hypoxaemia** and **acidosis** if acute, and may lead to delayed fetal growth if chronic.

- Functions:
  - gas exchange: O_2 and CO_2 exchange is favoured by **fetal haemoglobin** and the double **Bohr effect**, respectively.
  - nutrient exchange: all energy substrates, water, minerals and electrolytes enter the fetus via the placenta by facilitated or **active transport**.
  - hormone synthesis and release: hormones include chorionic gonadotrophin, human placental lactogen, oestrogens, progesterone, prolactin, somatomammotrophin and renin. Several corticosteroid hormones are synthesised by the fetoplacental unit, e.g. placental pregnenolone is metabolised by the fetus before further placental metabolism to form oestrogens.
  - drug transfer across the placenta depends on placental surface area, metabolism, UBF and the pH of maternal and fetal blood; drug characteristics influencing transfer include molecular weight (drugs <500 Da readily diffuse), lipid solubility, pK_a, protein binding and concentration gradient across the placenta. Type 1 drugs (e.g. thiopental) completely transfer; type 2 drugs (e.g. ketamine) cross the placenta to reach greater concentrations in the fetus compared with the mother; type 3 drugs (e.g. suxamethonium) are incompletely transferred to the fetus.

See also, Fetus, effect of anaesthetic agents on; Obstetric analgesia and anaesthesia; Placenta praevia; Placental abruption

Placenta praevia. Encroachment of the **placenta** upon the cervical os. Overall risk is about 0.25%, increased if there has been previous **caesarean section** (CS), e.g. up to 10% after four previous CS. May coexist with **placental abruption** in 10% of cases.

- Classified into:
  - grade 1: the placenta is low-lying, i.e., within the lower uterine segment; the placenta does not reach the internal os.
  - grade 2: the placenta reaches the os.
  - grade 3: the placenta covers the whole of the os but most of the placenta is positioned to one side.
  - grade 4: the placenta is placed squarely over the os.

Grades 1 and 2 are sometimes called ‘minor’, and grades 3 and 4 ‘major’.

- Problems:
  - may cause **antepartum haemorrhage** with cardiovascular collapse and fetal distress.
  - requires CS, especially in the higher grades, because the presenting part will compress the placenta and obstruct blood flow during labour and vaginal delivery. Malpresentation is more common.
  - associated with **postpartum haemorrhage** because the lower uterine segment is unable to contract as effectively as the upper segment, being less muscular.
  - may be associated with placental invasion (placenta accreta) or even penetration of the uterine wall (placenta percreta); delivery of the placenta may be accompanied by torrential haemorrhage that may require hysterectomy, uterine artery embolisation or iliac artery ligation. Placenta accreta occurs in about 0.04% of all pregnancies, increased to 5%–10% in mothers with placenta praevia and up to 40%–50% if there have been 2–3 previous CS.
- Anaesthetic management:
  - standard techniques, as for **obstetric analgesia and anaesthesia.**
  - choice of anaesthetic according to standard criteria; in emergency CS general anaesthesia is usually preferred unless the amount of bleeding is small and there is no cardiovascular instability. Traditionally, general anaesthesia has been preferred for elective CS because of the impaired compensatory CVS reflexes during extensive regional block and the difficulty managing an awake patient should severe haemorrhage occur. More recently, opinion has shifted to accept regional anaesthesia even in grades 3/4 placenta praevia, although many obstetric anaesthetists would prefer general anaesthesia if there has been previous CS and/or suspicion of placenta accreta.
  - for grades 3 and 4, at least two large-bore iv cannulae (plus blood warmer), immediately available cross-matched blood and appropriate senior staff should be ensured. Coagulopathy is uncommon unless massive transfusion is required; thus CS can usually wait until these facilities and back-up are present.

See also, Placental abruption

Placental abruption. Complete or partial separation of the **placenta** before delivery, causing retroplacental haemorrhage; thought to occur to some degree in up to 4%–5% of all pregnancies, although only 10%–50% of these present clinically. More common in smokers, **pre-eclampsia**, multiparity, abdominal **trauma**, and those with a previous history of placental abruption. May coexist with **placenta praevia** in 10% of cases. Has been classified into asymptomatic (grade 0), vaginal bleeding without maternal or fetal distress (grade 1), fetal distress present (grade 2), and fetal and maternal distress (grade 3), although this classification is not used as commonly as that for placenta praevia.

- Problems:
  - a cause of **antepartum haemorrhage**; presents with abdominal pain and, usually, fetal distress. The amount of vaginal bleeding (if present) may underestimate the extent of haemorrhage, which may be visible on ultrasound as retroplacental clot.
  - associated with **DIC** (in up to 10%) and renal cortical necrosis (although renal impairment more often results from acute tubular necrosis caused by hypovolaemia). The extent of DIC may be out of proportion to the amount of bleeding; it may worsen (or develop if not already present) if caesarean section (CS) is delayed. Thus, urgent CS is required in significant abruption, although mild cases may be managed expectantly.
- Anaesthetic management:
  - standard techniques as for **obstetric analgesia and anaesthesia.**

- general anaesthesia is usually preferred for CS because of the risk of **hypovolaemia** and DIC. **Coagulation studies** are mandatory before regional anaesthesia is performed, if chosen.
- at least two large-bore iv cannulae (plus blood warmer), cross-matched blood and appropriate senior staff should be arranged. Because coagulopathy may worsen unless delivery is achieved, CS should not be delayed.

Plasma. Non-cellular portion of **blood**; represents the **ECF** component within the vascular space. A clear, yellowish fluid.

- Normal composition:
  - water.
  - **proteins**:
    - **albumin** (35–50 g/l).
    - globulins, including **immunoglobulins** (25–35 g/l).
  - electrolytes:
    - main cations:
      - **sodium** (135–145 mmol/l).
      - **potassium** (3.5–5.5 mmol/l).
      - **calcium** (2.12–2.65 mmol/l).
      - **magnesium** (0.75–1.05 mmol/l).
    - main anions:
      - chloride (95–105 mmol/l).
      - **bicarbonate** (24–33 mmol/l).
      - **phosphate** (0.8–1.45 mmol/l).
      - **lactate** (0.6–1.8 mmol/l).
  - others, e.g. **urea** (2.5–7.0 mmol/l), **creatinine** (60–130 μmol/l), **fats**, **carbohydrates**, e.g. **glucose** (4.0–6.0 mmol/l), **amino acids**, **enzymes**, **vitamins**, hormones, bilirubin.

Osmolality is 280–305 mosmol/kg.

Plasma clots on standing; the supernatant solution is termed serum. Plasma volume is about 3.5 l in adults (5% of body weight), and measured by **dye dilution techniques**, using dyes or radioactive markers.

Available for transfusion as fresh frozen plasma.

See also, Blood products; Coagulation

Plasma exchange. The removal of a patient's **plasma** in order to remove high molecular weight substances (e.g. autoantibodies, antigens, immune complexes, drugs). Typically 30–40 ml/kg (1–1.5 plasma volumes) is removed at each procedure and replaced with human **albumin** solution to prevent a fall in plasma **oncotic pressure**. Partial substitution with **colloids** or **crystalloids** is often used.

One volume plasma exchange removes ~66% of a plasma constituent and two exchanges ~85%. Five exchanges in total are usually performed, either daily or alternate days. Selective removal of small volumes (up to 600 ml) of plasma from the body is termed plasmapheresis; replacement with **iv fluids** is not required. Exchange requires intermittent extracorporeal centrifugation or continuous filtration. Practical considerations and complications are as for **extracorporeal circulation** and **iv fluid administration**.

Evidence-based uses:

- neurological diseases: **myasthenia gravis**, **myasthenic syndrome**, **Guillain–Barré syndrome**, acute exacerbations of multiple sclerosis, autoimmune **encephalitis**, cerebral **SLE**, neuropathy associated with hyperparaproteinaemia.
- haematological diseases: **thrombotic thrombocytopenic purpura**, pure red cell aplasia.
- renal diseases: **Goodpasture's syndrome**, rapidly progressive **glomerulonephritis**, antibody-mediated renal transplant rejection.
- poisoning with mushrooms and **digoxin**.

Nguyen TC, Kiss JE, Goldman JR, Carcillo JA (2012). Crit Care Clin; 28: 453–68

Plasma expanders. **Intravenous fluids** that increase plasma volume by an amount greater than that infused, because of indrawing of water from the extracellular and intracellular spaces by **osmosis**. The term is usually reserved for **colloids**, although **hypertonic iv solutions** act as short-term plasma expanders.

Plasma, fresh frozen, *see Blood products*

Plasma substitutes, *see Colloids*

Plasmapheresis, *see Plasma exchange*

Plasmin and plasminogen, *see Fibrinolysis*

Plastic surgery. Anaesthetic considerations:

- related to the reason for surgery, e.g. **burns**, **trauma**, **facial deformities** (*see Ear, nose and throat surgery*).
- possible requirement for **hypotensive anaesthesia**.
- problems of prolonged surgery, e.g. **heat loss**, **blood loss**, **positioning of the patient**.
- skin grafts may be taken from trunk or limbs, reducing sites of access to the patient.
- regional techniques may be useful for graft donor sites, e.g. **femoral nerve block**, **lateral cutaneous nerve of the thigh block**.
- a low **haematocrit** is thought to improve perfusion and healing of grafts. **Dextran** solutions may be used to improve perfusion of grafted areas.
- **tourniquets** may be required.

Platelet-activating factor (PAF). Phospholipid autacoid produced by **platelets**, polymorphonuclear leucocytes and other blood cells. Thought to be a major mediator (along with **cytokines**) in **sepsis**. Natural and synthetic PAF antagonists have been investigated as possible treatment for sepsis, with mixed results. PAF has also been shown to modulate CNS activity (e.g. neuronal differentiation) and increased levels are associated with neuronal injury.

Platelet function analysers, *see Coagulation studies*

Platelets. Non-nucleated, smooth, disc-shaped **blood** cells derived from cytoplasmic fragments of megakaryocytes (bone marrow stem cells). Maturation of megakaryocytes, and thus platelet production, is controlled by a feedback mechanism involving the humoral agent thrombopoietin. The latter is produced by the liver and kidneys at a constant rate; an inducible form of thrombopoietin is produced by the spleen and bone marrow in response to a low platelet count. Measure 2–4 μm in diameter and 5–8 fL in volume, with a circulatory life span of 8–14 days. Normal adult count is 150–400 × 10^9/l blood; 10%–20% of the total platelet population lies within the spleen. Platelet deficiency and excess are termed **thrombocytopenia** and thrombocytosis, respectively.

Essential for normal **coagulation**, spontaneous haemorrhage occurring at counts below 20–30 × 10^9/l. Cytoplasmic granules within platelets contain many substances, including **ATP**, ADP, **5-HT**, **adrenaline**, **calcium**, fibronectin, fibrinogen, β-thromboglobulin and thrombospondin, which contribute to platelet aggregation, blood coagulation, local vasoconstriction, chemotaxis and vessel repair.

Thromboxane synthase is also present, and is activated when platelets contact damaged vascular endothelium. Release of thromboxane A_2 stimulates platelet aggregation via increased ADP levels, the ADP binding to specific receptors and activating the glycoprotein IIb/IIIa complex (at which fibrinogen, **von Willebrand** factor and adhesive proteins bind). Aggregation leads to further ADP release and release of the other substances, eventually resulting in formation of a plug. During this process, the platelets become more spherical and extend pseudopodia. Conversely, **prostacyclin**, present in the vascular endothelium, stimulates production of platelet cAMP and reduces release of ADP, inhibiting aggregation. Thus a fine balance exists between the two processes.

Apart from **coagulation disorders** arising from abnormal platelet numbers, prolonged bleeding may arise from abnormal function despite normal counts, e.g. **renal failure**, **hepatic failure**, **pre-eclampsia** and use of **antiplatelet drugs**. Platelet function may be assessed using the bleeding time and **thromboelastography**.
See also, Coagulation studies; Platelet-activating factor

Plethysmography. Recording of volume changes of an organ, part of the body or the whole body.

- Clinical applications:
  - **body plethysmograph.**
  - non-invasive **arterial BP measurement.**
  - **impedance plethysmography.**
  - measuring limb blood flow:
    - recording pressure changes in a circumferential cuff or strain gauges.
    - inflating a proximal cuff to between venous and arterial pressures, and recording volume changes by immersing the limb in water.

Pleura. Double-layered sac enclosing the **lungs**. The outer parietal layer attaches to the **diaphragm**, **mediastinum** and chest wall. The inner visceral layer is closely applied to the lung surface and enters its fissures. The layers meet at the lung hila. They are held together by the negative **intrapleural pressure** within the pleural cavity, which normally contains a small amount of serous fluid.

- Surface markings:
  - apex: 3.5 cm above the clavicular midpoint.
  - medial border: passes behind the sternoclavicular joint, meeting the opposite pleura level with the second costal cartilage. Descends to the costoxiphoid angle on the right; deflects laterally to the lateral sternal edge on the left.
  - inferior border: lies level with the eighth rib in the midclavicular line, 10th rib in the midaxillary line, and passes up to the spine of T12 posteriorly.

Pleural effusion. Serous fluid between the parietal and visceral layers of **pleura** (interpleural pus and blood are called empyema and haemothorax, respectively). May be unilateral or bilateral. Divided according to the protein content into:

- transudates (<30 g/l), e.g. **cardiac failure**, **hypoproteinaemia.**
- exudates (>30 g/l), e.g. tumours, inflammatory disease (e.g. **connective tissue diseases**), infection (e.g. **TB**), **PE**, abdominal disease (e.g. subphrenic abscess, **pancreatitis**, ovarian carcinoma).

Features include dyspnoea, usually related to the size of the effusion. Chest wall movement and breath sounds are reduced over the effusion, with percussion typically 'stony dull'. Large unilateral effusions may displace the mediastinum (and thus the trachea) towards the opposite side. Confirmed by **CXR**, **ultrasound** or **CT scanning**; examination of the fluid aids the underlying cause.

Treatment includes **chest drainage** and is otherwise directed towards the cause.

Large pleural effusions may hinder lung expansion and should be drained preoperatively. Other anaesthetic considerations are related to the underlying cause.
Bhatnagar R, Maskell N (2015). Br Med J; 351: h4520

Pneumatics, *see Fluidics*

Pneumocystis pneumonia (PCP). **Chest infection** caused by the fungus *Pneumocystis jirovecii* (formerly *P. carinii*), particularly common in patients with **immunodeficiency** associated with **HIV infection**, chemotherapy or organ **transplantation**. The organism produces an acute interstitial **pneumonitis** that is rapidly followed by **pulmonary fibrosis** and impaired pulmonary diffusion and decreased lung **compliance**. Features include **hypoxaemia**, dyspnoea and dry cough. Often, patients have an associated picture of systemic **sepsis**. The **CXR** typically shows subtle diffuse interstitial shadowing, but may be normal or occasionally grossly abnormal. The diagnosis is confirmed by obtaining specimens, in most cases by using **bronchopulmonary lavage**. The incidence has decreased recently with more effective prophylaxis and treatment with **co-trimoxazole** and **pentamidine**. **Corticosteroids** are recommended in moderate-to-severe disease, initiated at the same time as antimicrobial therapy. Mortality is 20%–50%.
Siegel M, Masur H, Kovacs J (2016). Semin Respir Crit Care Med; 37: 243–56

Pneumonia, *see Chest infection*

Pneumonitis. Inflammation of the lung caused by physical or chemical agents, e.g. inhalation of toxic or irritant substances and fumes, **radiation**. Clinical features vary from mild **dyspnoea** to those of severe **ALI**. Inflammation caused by infection is termed pneumonia; that caused by an allergic reaction is termed alveolitis.
See also, Aspiration pneumonitis

Pneumotachograph. Constant orifice, variable pressure **flowmeter**, used widely in anaesthetic and respiratory research. Measures the pressure gradient across a fixed resistance using pressure **transducers**; using the **Hagen–Poiseuille equation**, if **flow** is laminar, the pressure difference is proportional to flow. In the Fleisch pneumotachograph, the resistance is produced by an array of tubes 1–2 mm in diameter, the number of tubes being matched for the desired flow range. The resistor is enclosed within an electrical coil to prevent condensation. In other devices, the resistance consists of a layer of metal or plastic gauze, the latter less likely to cause condensation.

The instrument head should be appropriately sized to avoid turbulence, and the gas flow spread evenly over the resistance unit. The pressure gradient depends not only on the gas flow but also on its composition, viscosity and temperature; thus difficulties may arise if gas composition varies between breaths.
[Alfred Fleisch (1892–1973), Swiss physiologist]

Pneumothorax. Free gas, usually air, within the pleural cavity.

- Has been classified as:
  - simple: the gas is not under tension. May be:
    - open: continuing communication between the source of the gas and the pleural cavity. Intrapleural and atmospheric pressures are equal and lung expansion is poor, causing marked **hypoxaemia. Pendelluft** may occur. Mediastinal shift may occur in phase with respiration, causing cardiovascular collapse. Gas exchange may improve with **IPPV**, which increases expansion of the collapsed lung (but tension pneumothorax may develop if gas is forced into the pleural cavity and is unable to escape).
    - closed: no continuing communication with the gas source; lung collapse is proportional to the volume of gas introduced into the pleural cavity. Gas exchange is unaltered by IPPV, if there is no risk of further gas leakage.
  - tension: gas flow into the pleural cavity is unidirectional and a 'valve' mechanism prevents its escape. The pressure within the pleural cavity increases, with worsening pulmonary collapse, hypoxaemia, **hypercapnia**, mediastinal shift and obstruction to venous return. Tension is increased by IPPV.
- May occur by three mechanisms:
  - intrapulmonary rupture: retrograde perivascular dissection of gas towards the lung hilum, which may result in mediastinal emphysema. May follow use of high inflation pressures during IPPV, or severe cough or Valsalva manoeuvre. May also occur spontaneously if the alveolar septum is weakened by infection or chronic lung disease.
  - injury to the visceral **pleura**: air escapes through the hole into the pleural cavity; the lung collapses and the hole may seal or act as a valve. Causes include spontaneous rupture of an emphysematous bulla, fractured **ribs**, regional anaesthetic techniques or **central venous cannulation, tracheostomy** and lung biopsy.
  - injury to the parietal pleura: gas enters from the atmosphere (e.g. open chest wound, during central venous cannulation) or from adjoining structures:
    - peritoneal cavity: gas passes upwards through the retroperitoneal tissue and ruptures through the mediastinal parietal pleura, or passes through defects in the **diaphragm**.
    - mediastinum: gas ruptures through the pleura as above; it may arise following oesophageal perforation and procedures such as tracheostomy and thyroidectomy.
- Features:
  - range from mild dyspnoea and pleuritic chest pain to respiratory distress. If the pneumothorax is very large or under tension, severe hypoxaemia and cardiovascular collapse may occur.
  - clinical signs may be absent in small pneumothoraces (<15% of the hemithorax), but there may be: subcutaneous emphysema; ispilateral reduction of chest wall movement and breath sounds; and increased resonance to percussion. There may be audible wheezing, or a 'crunch' caused by air in the mediastinum (Hamman's sign). Inflation pressures may rise during anaesthesia with IPPV.
  - erect **CXR** in expiration may reveal absent lung markings beyond the edge of the collapsed lung, with the characteristic lung edge usually visible. Diagnosis may be difficult from a supine film. Pleural gas under tension causes marked lung collapse, hyperexpansion of the ipsilateral lung and mediastinal shift.

Treatment depends on the size of the pneumothorax; small ones often resolve spontaneously. If symptomatic, or if IPPV is planned, **chest drainage** should be performed. A tension pneumothorax may be life-threatening and requires urgent relief, e.g. with a needle or iv cannula. **N_2O**, being more soluble than atmospheric nitrogen, may rapidly expand a pneumothorax (by 100% in 10 min at an inspired concentration of 70%); it should therefore not be used unless a chest drain has been placed.

[Louis Hamman (1877–1946), US physician]

See also, Chest trauma; Flail chest

POCD, *see Postoperative cognitive dysfunction*

Poise. Unit of **viscosity** in the **cgs system of units.** 1 P = 1 dyne s/cm^2

[Jean Poiseuille (1797–1869), French physiologist]

Poiseuille's equation, *see Hagen–Poiseuille equation*

Poisoning and overdoses. May be deliberate, or may follow accidental exposure or ingestion. Substances responsible include those found in the home, industrial or agricultural chemicals, plant or animal toxins, and therapeutic drugs.

- Principles of management:
  - removal of the patient from the source of the toxic substance, e.g. from scene of a fire, chemical spillage. Medical staff should be adequately protected, because absorption through skin and lungs may occur.
  - **CPR** and standard management of the unconscious patient, including **monitoring**.
  - blood and urine analysis for drug, glucose and electrolyte levels, specific organ function tests, etc.
  - prevention of further absorption of ingested substances, e.g. using activated **charcoal** (**gastric lavage** and **emetic drugs** are no longer routinely recommended). **Whole bowel irrigation** may be useful after poisoning with extended-release drug preparations.
  - specific antidotes and treatments, e.g. **naloxone, flumazenil, chelating agents, digoxin** antibody fragments, thiosulfate in **cyanide poisoning**.
  - **lipid emulsion** has been used to treat overdose with a variety of lipid-soluble drugs.
  - increasing elimination of ingested substances, e.g. **forced diuresis, haemoperfusion, dialysis**, activated charcoal.

Common problems include respiratory depression, **hypotension, arrhythmias, coma, convulsions** and disturbances of **temperature regulation. Pulmonary oedema, ALI, hepatic failure** and **renal failure** may also occur.

Regional or national poisons units provide information and advice.

See also, Alcohol poisoning; Barbiturate poisoning; Carbon monoxide poisoning; Chemical weapons; Opioid poisoning; Organophosphorus poisoning; Paracetamol poisoning; Salicylate poisoning; Smoke inhalation; Tricyclic antidepressant drug poisoning

Polarographic oxygen analysis, *see Oxygen measurement*

Poliomyelitis. Disease caused by one of three small RNA enteroviruses transmitted by the respiratory or faeco-oral routes. Now rare in developed countries following successful immunisation programmes. Following 7–14 days' incubation period, an acute febrile illness occurs, with upper respiratory or GIT symptoms lasting a few days. Over 90% of cases of infection are subclinical. Pyrexia may recur with features of acute viral **meningitis.** Asymmetrical lower **motor neurone** weakness develops in 1% of cases of infection, caused by destruction of the anterior horn cells of the **spinal cord** and **cranial nerve** nuclei. Ventilatory support is required during the acute illness in approximately 30% of cases, because of intercostal or diaphragmatic involvement. Bulbar involvement may impair swallowing, cough reflexes and vocal cord function. Rarely, medullary involvement may cause cardiovascular instability or **sleep apnoea.**

Most patients have residual disability, but improvement may continue for up to 2 years after the acute episode. Progressive weakness may occur 20–30 years later (post-polio syndrome). 10%–30% of those requiring ventilatory support acutely require long-term support.

Pollution. Traditionally, most attention has been paid to the effects of **inhalational anaesthetic agents** on the well-being of nearby staff, e.g. in the operating theatre. More recently the contribution of anaesthetic agents to atmospheric ozone depletion and global warming has been a concern. Both **N_2O** and volatile agents are degraded in the atmosphere by ultraviolet light to form radicals and halogen atoms, respectively; these damage the ozone layer. Both N_2O and volatile agents also contribute to the greenhouse effect. Anaesthetic use has been estimated to contribute ~1% of atmospheric N_2O. Recent international agreements on reduction of atmospheric pollutants have included agents such as these, leading to renewed interest in alternative anaesthetic agents such as **xenon.**

Other concerns include the effect of plasticisers (e.g. phthalates) in polyvinyl chloride (PVC) tubing and other equipment; they have been implicated in causing multiple health issues, particularly involving the endocrine system.
See also, COSHH regulations; Environmental safety of anaesthetists; Scavenging

Polyarteritis nodosa. Connective tissue disease characterised by a necrotising arteritis affecting small and medium-sized arteries causing aneurysm formation, haemorrhage and infarction in major organs. Incidence peaks at 40–50 years, with men affected twice as commonly as women.
- Features:
  - malaise, fever, weight loss, myalgia.
  - arthralgia, rash, **peripheral neuropathy. Myasthenic syndrome** may occur rarely.
  - GIT involvement including haemorrhage, **pancreatitis,** intestinal and gallbladder infarction.
  - renal impairment (may be part of a triad of haematuria, haemoptysis and asthma); includes **nephritic syndrome** or **nephrotic syndrome.**
  - CVS involvement: **hypertension, ischaemic heart disease, cardiac failure, pericarditis.**
  - CNS involvement: cerebral ischaemia, blindness, **subarachnoid haemorrhage,** encephalopathy, seizures.
- Anaesthetic considerations include any pre-existing organ damage as described above, plus possible drug therapy that may include **corticosteroids** and **immunosuppressive drugs.**

See also, Vasculitides

Polycythaemia. General term for a **haemoglobin** concentration above 160–170 g/l, red cell count above 5.6–6.4 × 10^{12}/l, or **haematocrit** above 0.47–0.54 (all values female–male, respectively).
- May be:
  - relative (reduced plasma volume, e.g. **burns, dehydration**).
  - absolute (increased red cell volume):
    - primary (polycythaemia rubra vera, PRV): myeloproliferative disorder, occurring mainly in men over 50 years. Features are caused mainly by hypervolaemia and hyperviscosity (headaches, plethora, pruritus, dyspnoea, visual disturbances, reduced cardiac output, thrombotic and haemorrhagic episodes) and a high metabolic rate (night sweats, weight loss). Hepatosplenomegaly may occur. White cell and **platelet** counts may also be increased; platelet function may be abnormal.

      The main perioperative risks are haemorrhage (caused by abnormal platelets) and thrombosis. Elective surgery should be delayed to allow treatment; **emergency surgery** should proceed only after venesection and volume replacement. Treatment is directed at keeping the haematocrit below 0.5, usually with repeated venesection, radioactive phosphorus or myelosuppressive drugs (busulfan). PRV progresses to myelosclerosis in 20%–30% of cases.
    - secondary to raised **erythropoietin** levels, e.g. in response to chronic **hypoxaemia** (e.g. pulmonary disease, cyanotic **congenital heart disease,** high **altitude**) or inappropriate secretion (e.g. renal carcinoma, hepatocellular carcinoma, haemangioblastoma). Risks are related to increased blood viscosity and thrombosis as above.

Polymyositis. Group of idiopathic autoimmune inflammatory diseases, including dermatomyositis, affecting muscle and skin. May involve multiple systems. Usually presents with myalgia, muscle tenderness and weakness (mainly proximal). Bulbar weakness may lead to dysphagia, dysphonia and regurgitation. Intercostal and diaphragmatic weakness may result in **respiratory failure,** exacerbated by interstitial pneumonitis that is also a feature of the disease. Cardiac manifestations include **arrhythmias,** conduction defects, **myocarditis** and **cardiomyopathy.** In dermatomyositis, there is a characteristic erythematous rash of the face and neck. **Malignancy** is common, especially in older men.

Creatine kinase is raised; muscle biopsy is confirmatory. Treatment includes **corticosteroids** and other **immunosuppressive drugs.**

An abnormal sensitivity to **neuromuscular blocking drugs** has been suggested but is unproven.

Findlay AR, Goyal NA, Mozaffar T (2015). Muscle Nerve; 51: 638–56

Polymyxins. Group of **antibacterial drugs** active against gram-negative organisms, including pseudomonas. Include polymyxin E (**colistin**) and polymyxin B, which is used in otitis externa. May enhance the action of non-depolarising **neuromuscular blocking drugs** via their postsynaptic blocking action at the **neuromuscular junction.**

Polyneuropathy, acute post-infective, *see Guillain–Barré syndrome*

Polyneuropathy of critical illness, *see Critical illness polyneuropathy/myopathy*

Polystyrene sulfonate resins. Ion exchange resins used to treat mild or moderate **hyperkalaemia**. Available as calcium (calcium resonium) or sodium (resonium A) preparations. Given orally, they remain in the GIT without renal or hepatic excretion. Decrease in plasma potassium occurs 2–24 h after administration. Electrolytes must be monitored closely during therapy. Contraindicated in **hyperparathyroidism**, multiple myeloma, sarcoidosis, metastatic bone disease (calcium resins) and cardiac failure (sodium resins).

- Dosage: 15 g orally tds/qds; 30 g rectally retained for 9 h.
- Side effects: cardiac failure, headaches, encephalopathy, metabolic alkalosis, fluid retention, nausea, vomiting, constipation, colonic necrosis, GIT obstruction.

PONV, *see Postoperative nausea and vomiting*

Popliteal fossa. Diamond-shaped space behind the knee joint, bounded inferiorly by the two heads of gastrocnemius muscle and superiorly by biceps femoris (laterally) and semimembranosus/semitendinosus muscles (medially).

- Contents (medially to laterally):
  - popliteal artery: continues from the **femoral artery**, and divides into anterior and **posterior tibial arteries** at or below the lower part of the fossa. The popliteal vein lies superficially.
  - tibial nerve: arises from the sciatic nerve, usually at the upper pole of the fossa. Lies superficial to the popliteal vessels. The common peroneal nerve passes laterally around the fibular head, lateral to the fossa.
  - fat pad.

See also, Knee, nerve blocks

Pop-off valve, *see Adjustable pressure-limiting valve*

Populations. In **statistics**, any group of similar objects, events or observations. Usually contains too many individuals to be studied as a whole; thus **samples** are studied and any conclusions drawn are applied to the whole population. A population may be described by its:

- shape, i.e., **statistical distribution curve**, e.g. normal, binomial.
- central tendency, e.g. **mean**, **median**, **mode**.
- scatter, e.g. **standard deviation**, **percentiles**.

Porphyria. Group of diseases characterised by overproduction and excretion of porphyrins (intermediate compounds produced during haemoprotein synthesis) and their precursors. Caused by specific **enzyme** defects within the haem metabolic pathway. Several forms exist, divided into hepatic and erythropoietic varieties. Only three forms affect the conduct of anaesthesia, all of them hepatic varieties transmitted by autosomal dominant inheritance with incomplete penetrance:

- acute intermittent porphyria (AIP): results in increased amounts of urinary porphobilinogen and δ-aminolaevulinic acid (D-ALA) during attacks. May present with acute abdominal pain, vomiting, acid–base disturbances, motor and sensory **peripheral neuropathy**, autonomic dysfunction, **cranial nerve** palsies, mental disturbances, **convulsions** and **coma**. Diagnosed by urinalysis.
- variegate porphyria: may present with similar features to AIP. Photosensitivity is common. Diagnosed by stool examination for copro- and protoporphyrin.
- hereditary coproporphyria: photosensitivity may occur.

Acute attacks may be precipitated by drugs, stress, infection, **alcohol** ingestion, menstruation, **pregnancy** and starvation, although not at every exposure. Information about drugs is obtained from case reports, animal studies and analysis of drug effects on cell cultures.

- Effects of drugs:
  - definite precipitants: include **barbiturates**, **phenytoin** and **sulfonamides**.
  - implicated in laboratory or animal studies but not in humans: **etomidate**, **lidocaine**, chlordiazepoxide.
  - considered safe to use: **opioid analgesic drugs**, **N_2O**, **diazepam**, **suxamethonium**, **tubocurarine**, **gallamine**, **atropine**, **neostigmine**, **bupivacaine**, **prilocaine**, **procaine**, **propranolol**, **chlorphenamine**, **droperidol**, **chlorpromazine**, **chloral hydrate**, **aspirin**, **paracetamol**, **insulin**.
  - controversial: **halothane**, **corticosteroids**, **ketamine**, **propofol**. All have been used safely despite conflicting evidence.

See also, Inborn errors of metabolism

Poseiro effect. Decrease in arterial BP during uterine contraction; thought to be caused by exacerbations of **aortocaval compression**.

[JJ Poseiro (described 1967), Uruguayan obstetrician]

See also, Obstetric analgesia and anaesthesia

Positioning of the patient. Undertaken to:

- facilitate surgery, imaging, etc.
- encourage venous drainage (for surgery) or distension (for **central venous cannulation**).
- allow the performance of and control the extent of **regional anaesthesia**.
- protect the **airway** (e.g. **recovery position**).
- improve oxygenation (**prone ventilation**).
- reduce **ICP**.
- encourage drainage of sputum, e.g. postural drainage.
- relieve **aortocaval compression**.

Often performed when the patient is anaesthetised; damage to limbs, joints, pressure areas and nerves may occur unless care is taken. Tracheal tube, iv lines, etc., may be displaced during movement.

- Specific problems associated with certain positions:
  - supine: **$\dot{V}/\dot{Q}$ mismatch** may occur, especially if **closing capacity** exceeds **FRC**. **Regurgitation** of **gastric contents** may occur. The calves should be raised off the bed to reduce risk of **DVT**. In **pregnancy**, aortocaval compression may occur.
  - prone: similar considerations to the supine position apply. Chest wall and abdominal movement during respiration may be hindered. Supports should be positioned under the iliac crests and shoulders, leaving the abdomen free. **Venous return** may be impeded if the abdomen is compressed. Acute **hepatic failure** has been reported in a small number of patients following prolonged surgery in the prone position; intraoperative hepatic ischaemia related to positioning has been implicated, though not proven; nevertheless, monitoring of acid–base status and plasma **lactate** concentration has been advised. The face and eyes should be carefully padded (*see Eye*

care). Particular care is required to prevent undue extension or rotation of the neck; the fully neutral position has been suggested, because neurological lesions have been reported, especially after long procedures.
- lateral: $\dot{V}/\dot{Q}$ mismatch occurs (*see One-lung anaesthesia*). The lower arm may be compressed and its venous drainage impaired.
- Trendelenburg: originally described as supine with steep head-down tilt, with the knees flexed over the 'broken' end of the table. Diaphragmatic movement is limited by the weight of the abdominal viscera, reducing FRC and increasing **atelectasis**. Risk of regurgitation is increased. Venous engorgement of the head and neck may be accompanied by raised **ICP** and **intraocular pressure. Brachial plexus** injury may occur if shoulder supports are used.
- reversed Trendelenburg: hypotension may occur if the head-up tilt is achieved rapidly.
- lithotomy position: similar considerations to the Trendelenburg position. Injury to the lower back, hips and knees may occur. Common peroneal or saphenous nerves may be compressed against the lithotomy poles. Sciatic nerve injury has been reported after prolonged procedures. DVT may follow calf compression against the poles.
- sitting: difficult to position the unconscious patient. Hypotension and **air embolus** may occur (*see Dental surgery; Neurosurgery*).

Neurological lesions or those relating to tissue ischaemia (e.g. bald areas on the scalp, **compartment syndrome**) are thought to be more likely if there is prolonged hypotension associated with long procedures.
[Friedrich Trendelenburg (1844–1924), German surgeon]
See also, Nerve injury during anaesthesia

Positive end-expiratory pressure (PEEP). Adjunct to **IPPV**, introduced in 1967. Produced by maintaining a positive airway pressure during expiration: usually 5–20 cmH_2O, although higher levels have been used ('super-PEEP'). Minimises airway and alveolar collapse and increases **compliance**, by increasing **FRC**. Thus improves oxygenation and reduces pulmonary **shunt**. High levels may increase **dead space** and exacerbate the adverse effects of IPPV related to intrathoracic pressure; **barotrauma** and reduced cardiac output are more likely. Urine output is reduced, and **vasopressin** secretion and **ICP** increased.

Used to reduce O_2 requirement and improve oxygenation in **respiratory failure**, except where its adverse effects are especially dangerous, e.g. **asthma**. The following terms have been used to describe the adjustment of PEEP:
- best PEEP: produces the least shunting without significant reduction of cardiac output.
- optimum PEEP: produces maximal **O_2 delivery** with the lowest dead space/tidal volume ratio.
- appropriate PEEP: that with the least dead space.

Auto-PEEP (intrinsic PEEP) is the difference between alveolar pressure and airway pressure at end-expiration, and exists when expiration continues right up to inspiration (i.e., no expiratory pause). It may occur in **airway obstruction**, asthma, **COPD**, **ALI**, and in forced expiration.

Positron emission tomography (PET). Technique for imaging the distribution of inhaled or injected positron-emitting **radioisotopes**, e.g. ^{15}O, ^{13}N, ^{11}C and ^{18}F. Tomographic techniques similar to those used for **CT scanning** are used. Provides information about regional blood flow, O_2 and glucose metabolism; thus particularly useful for detecting malignancy.

POSSUM, *see Physiological and operative severity score for the enumeration of mortality and morbidity*

Post-dural puncture headache (PDPH). Headache occurring after dural puncture, e.g. **spinal anaesthesia** or diagnostic **lumbar puncture**. First described by **Bier** in 1899. May rarely develop after **epidural anaesthesia** without an obvious dural tap. More common in obstetrics and in young patients. Reported incidence varies but is <1% with pencil-point 25–29 G needles in non-pregnant patients, and up to 75% with 16 G epidural needles in **obstetric analgesia and anaesthesia**.

Thought to be due to **CSF** leaking through the dural hole, with caudal shift of the **brain** and stretching of intracranial nerves, dura and blood vessels in the upright position. The most likely cause is thought to be cerebral venous dilation. The incidence is increased by using large-gauge needles, especially if the longitudinal dural fibres are cut transversely by the needle bevel instead of being split longitudinally, e.g. by non-cutting pencil-point spinal needles.

Headaches usually occur within 1–3 days of dural puncture, normally lasting for 1–2 weeks but occasionally for months. They are classically severe, frontal or occipital, and exacerbated by sudden movement, getting up from the supine position, and coughing and straining. Neck stiffness, visual disturbance and altered hearing may occur. Diagnosis is from the history and on clinical grounds. Typically, manual pressure over the right hypogastrium causes lessening of the headache, possibly via epidural venous congestion secondary to hepatic compression. MRI and CT scanning have been used to demonstrate CSF leaks. Rarely, **cranial nerve** palsies, convulsions and subdural or intracranial haemorrhage have been reported.
- Treatment:
  - avoidance of dehydration.
  - simple analgesics, e.g. **paracetamol**, **NSAIDs**.
  - specific therapy: **caffeine** 150–200 mg orally tds/qds has been shown to reduce the severity of headache. Sumatriptan 6 mg sc od (*see Triptans*); caffeine/ergotamine mixture 100 mg/1 mg; **ACTH** 1.5 μU/kg iv in 1–2 l saline over 1 h or its synthetic analogue Synacthen 1 mg im have also been used, although the evidence is relatively weak and the putative mechanism of action unclear.
  - epidural administration of fluids, e.g. saline, **dextran**, blood: thought to displace CSF cranially and possibly reduce further leakage across the dura. Epidural **blood patch** is effective, but is generally reserved for when headache is persistent.

Prophylactic bed rest after dural puncture is no longer considered helpful.

Posterior tibial artery. Arises (with the anterior artery) from the popliteal artery at the lower border of the **popliteal fossa**. Runs distally on the surface of the posterior tibial muscle deep to soleus; lower down it becomes superficial and lies medial to tendo calcaneus. Divides into lateral and medial plantar arteries. The artery can be palpated between the medial malleolus and the prominence of the heel and may be used for **arterial cannulation**.

Postherpetic neuralgia. Persistent **pain** in the distribution of one or more peripheral nerves following shingles (reactivation of dormant varicella-zoster virus seeded during an earlier episode of primary chickenpox. The virus lies dormant in the dorsal root ganglia but may multiply and invade the corresponding sensory nerves). Usually defined as pain lasting for >3 months. Occurs in up to ~20% of cases of shingles, with ~2% of patients having persistent pain 5 years after acute infection. It usually affects adults and occurs spontaneously, although predisposing factors include age >55 years and **immunodeficiency** (especially associated with **HIV infection** and leukaemia).

Most commonly affects the T5 and T6 **dermatomes.** Pain usually precedes the appearance of cutaneous vesicles, although no rash may appear (zoster sine herpete). In 10% of cases, scarring and pain persist; the latter may be severe and intractable, triggered by contact, draughts and stress.

Treatment may be disappointing, but includes **tricyclic antidepressant drugs, anticonvulsant drugs** and topical **lidocaine** and **capsaicin.** Use of **aciclovir** during acute infection may reduce pain duration. Less evidence exists for the use of **TENS**, **acupuncture**, repeated **epidural anaesthesia** and peripheral or **sympathetic nerve block.**

Johnson RW, Rice ASC (2014). N Engl J Med; 371: 1526–33

Post-intensive care syndrome (PICS). New or worsened impairments in physical, cognitive and mental wellbeing of the ICU survivor. Include:

- pulmonary complications e.g. decreases in lung volumes and diffusing capacity: related to the duration of IPPV and tend to improve in the first year following discharge from ICU.
- neuromuscular weakness following **critical illness neuromyopathy/myopathy** and general atrophy: results in poor physical function that may persist for >5 years. Known risk factors include **sepsis**, **MODS**, immobility, use of **corticosteroids**, poor glycaemic control, increased age and poor pre-existing physical function.
- cognitive dysfunction: occurs in 30%–80% of patients and includes problems with memory and executive functions (e.g. planning, processing, visual-spatial awareness). Risk factors include those associated with **confusion in the intensive care unit**.
- psychological problems including depression, anxiety, **post-traumatic stress disorder** (in 10%–50%): may persist for many years. Psychological sequelae are also common in families of patients nursed in ICU and are termed post-intensive care syndrome in families (PICS-F). Depression is seen in 10%–35% and post-traumatic stress disorder in 8%–40% (50% if the patient dies).

Methods to reduce the prevalence of PICS include those aimed at reducing length of ICU stay and duration of IPPV, early treatment of sepsis, etc., while promoting early mobilisation and optimising environmental conditions within ICU. Meticulous **intensive care follow-up** and early psychological support (e.g. with **cognitive behavioural therapy**) are vital. PICS-F can be reduced by frequent and realistic communication regarding the patient's condition, shared decision-making, family-centred care programmes and psychological support.

Harvey MA, Davidson JE (2016). Crit Care Med; 44: 381–5

Postoperative analgesia. Increasingly managed by acute pain teams; duties include education of medical and nursing staff, **audit**, research, and visiting postoperative patients specifically to monitor and adjust analgesia regimens.

Analgesic requirements vary according to the type of surgery, fitness of the patient, psychological factors and interindividual differences.

- Techniques available:
  - **opioid analgesic drugs**:
    - im: painful to administer, and result in variable plasma drug levels. The time from the patient's expressing pain to the drug's administration depends on the patient's persistence, the level of nursing staffing and the procedures for obtaining and checking controlled drugs. Commonly used, however, because of its convenience and low cost.
    - iv: more reliable; methods include:
      - incremental small boluses titrated against effect; reduces accidental overdosage but still may allow periods of inadequate analgesia.
      - continuous infusion: may be adjusted to the minimal effective rate with minimal side effects. Steady-state plasma levels may be slow to achieve, and overdosage may still occur.
      - **patient-controlled analgesia**: less demanding on the nursing staff, and the patient's sense of being in control may be beneficial.
    - **spinal opioids**: although analgesia is usually extremely good, large interpatient variability exists. Side effects include urinary retention, nausea, **pruritus** and respiratory depression; careful monitoring is required to detect the latter.
    - sc: useful if iv access is limited but confers no advantage over iv administration.
    - oral: use may be restricted by inability to drink, nausea and **vomiting**, delayed **gastric emptying** and **first-pass metabolism.**
    - transdermal: slow-release patches are stuck to the skin; does not require cannulae or catheters, but adjustment of the release rate is impossible. **Fentanyl** and **buprenorphine** are available in transdermal preparations.
    - sublingual/buccal: avoids injection but suffers the disadvantages of intermittent administration. Fentanyl and buprenorphine are available in buccal formulations.
    - rectal: drug absorption may be variable; the technique is less common in the UK.
  - **NSAIDs**: popular as a method of reducing opioid requirements, particularly after **day-case surgery**, **dental surgery** and **orthopaedic surgery.** May be given parenterally, orally or rectally. They may cause GIT upset and impair renal and **platelet** function. Increased perioperative bleeding has been reported, but this is rarely clinically significant.
  - other drugs: **ketamine** reduces opioid requirements and may be particularly useful in postoperative neuropathic pain (e.g. after limb amputation). **Clonidine** and **gabapentin** may also be useful adjuncts, the former particularly if hypertension is a problem.
  - **local anaesthetic agents:** provide excellent analgesia but with the risk of motor blockade and toxicity of local anaesthetics, and variable duration of action (depending on the technique and drug chosen). Duration may be prolonged by the use of repeated injections or infusions via catheters. Methods:
    - infiltration or nerve block: performed before or after surgery.
    - **caudal analgesia**, **epidural anaesthesia** or **spinal anaesthesia**: limited by hypotension and motor paralysis. May be combined with opioids.

IV infusions of lidocaine (1–3 mg/kg/h) have been shown to reduce pain/opioid requirements after major surgery; however, this is not widely used because of the low **therapeutic ratio** of lidocaine and the risk of toxicity.
- **inhalational anaesthetic agents**: some postoperative benefit is derived from the agents used perioperatively. **Entonox** is the only agent used postoperatively, e.g. for **physiotherapy** or changes of dressings, and is limited by its adverse effects on the haematological system.
- nerve destruction (e.g. **cryoanalgesia**) has been used in thoracic surgery, but has limited application elsewhere.
- other methods less widely used include **TENS**, **acupuncture** and **hypnosis**.

See also, Analgesic drugs; Pain; Pain evaluation; Pain management

Postoperative care team. Proposed system of comprehensive postoperative care that includes regular rounds and a team of specialist 'postoperative care' nurses to support ward nursing and medical staff by providing additional expertise and equipment. An extension of the role of acute pain teams and incorporated into the concept of **perioperative medicine**. Aims include better maintenance of vital organ function, decreased postoperative complications, reduced postoperative mortality, greater comfort and satisfaction and a shorter hospital stay.

Goldhill DR (1997). Br Med J; 314: 389

See also, Care of the critically ill surgical patient; Medical emergency team; Outreach team; Safe transport and retrieval team

Postoperative cognitive dysfunction (POCD). Reduced cognitive function following anaesthesia and surgery, without altered level of consciousness, as distinct from florid postoperative delirium/**confusion**. Requires neurocognitive testing for diagnosis. Occurs in up to 25% of elderly patients in the first week after non-cardiac surgery, and in 10%–15% at 3 months. Patients with pre-existing cognitive problems and those undergoing cardiac surgery are especially at risk. The contribution of perioperative factors such as sedative drugs, intraoperative hypotension/hypoxaemia/hypocapnia and sleep disturbance is unclear, although all have been implicated. Possible pathophysiological factors include:
- poor control of postoperative delirium.
- neuronal and synaptic loss due to sedative/anaesthetic agents or hypoxic/ischaemic injury.
- cytokine release triggered by tumour necrosis factor alpha.
- deposition of neurotoxic proteins (similar to those found in Alzheimer's disease) in brain cells following anaesthesia.
- neuroinflammatory changes due to surgical trauma.

It has been suggested that preoperative cognitive function testing may identify those patients at risk.

[Alois Alzheimer (1864–1915), German neurologist and pathologist]

Steinmetz J, Rasmussen LS (2016), Anaesthesia; 71: 58–63

Postoperative nausea and vomiting (PONV). Consistently rated by patients as one of the most feared/unpleasant aspects of undergoing surgery. Apart from its unpleasantness, it may also increase pain, disturb dressings/surgical repairs, increase bleeding and increase the risk of **aspiration of gastric contents**. May lead to electrolyte imbalance and **dehydration** if prolonged.
- In the absence of prophylaxis, PONV occurs after up to 90% of surgical procedures, the following increasing the risk:
  - patient factors:
    - young age.
    - female gender. Incidence increases during menstruation and decreases after the menopause, i.e., is presumably hormonally mediated.
    - anxiety, especially in patients who 'always vomit'. Increases in circulating **catecholamine** levels may be important.
    - previous history of PONV or motion sickness.
    - non-smoking.
    - early postoperative mobilisation, eating and drinking.
  - surgical factors:
    - gynaecological/abdominal/ENT/squint surgery.
    - laparoscopic procedures.
    - severe pain.
  - anaesthetic factors:
    - use of **opioid analgesic drugs**, including **premedication**.
    - use of certain anaesthetic drugs, e.g. **diethyl ether**, **trichloroethylene**, **cyclopropane**, **etomidate**, **N_2O** (the last via a direct central effect, GIT distension and/or expansion of middle ear cavities).
    - possibly prolonged anaesthesia and the use of **neostigmine** (though these are disputed).
    - physical factors, e.g. gastric insufflation, pharyngeal stimulation.
  - other factors:
    - **hypoxaemia/hypotension**.
    - dehydration.

Various scores have been devised for predicting the likelihood of PONV in a particular case, based on the presence or absence of the following factors: female gender; history of PONV/travel sickness; non-smoker; postoperative opioids; ± prolonged procedure.
- Reduced by:
  - avoidance of triggers where possible, e.g. anxiety, opioids, N_2O, vigorous pharyngeal suction, and possibly general anaesthesia altogether.
  - use of specific **antiemetic drugs** and procedures (e.g. **acupuncture** at the wrist), especially in combination.
  - use of drugs, techniques and procedures associated with low incidence of nausea and vomiting, e.g. **propofol**.
  - administration of iv fluids.

With prophylaxis the incidence is usually under 30% in high-risk cases. The most effective approach for preventing PONV is thought to be the use of multiple strategies and different drugs.

See also, Vomiting

Postpartum haemorrhage (PPH). Divided by the Royal College of Obstetricians and Gynaecologists into minor (blood loss <500 ml that has settled) and major (blood loss 500–1000 ml + ongoing bleeding or clinical shock, often divided into moderate (<2000 ml) and severe (>2000 ml). N.B smaller volumes may be clinically significant in women of smaller size). A common cause of maternal morbidity and mortality, it is associated with a number of predisposing factors, including multiple pregnancy, multiparity, **pre-eclampsia**, **placenta praevia** and prolonged augmented labour. The only intervention shown to be effective in reducing PPH is the administration of **oxytocic drugs** following delivery. Problems include not identifying women at risk (even though risk factors are well known), not recognising significant **hypovolaemia** when it occurs and a lack of timely resuscitation. The problems of **DIC** and dilutional coagulopathy may rapidly be superimposed upon the underlying condition.

- Caused by:
  - obstetric factors, e.g. uterine atony, retained placenta, uterine/vaginal tears, uterine inversion, instrumentation or intrauterine manipulation.
  - non-obstetric factors, e.g. **coagulation disorders**.

Typically, PPH presents with tachycardia and other features of **haemorrhage**, although because most cases are fit young women, cardiovascular compensation is usually very effective until severe hypovolaemia occurs, when sudden collapse may ensue. Uterine inversion may be associated with profound hypotension and bradycardia.

Initial management consists of basic fluid resuscitation. Specific treatment is aimed at the underlying cause, e.g. **oxytocin** and **carboprost** for uterine atony, evacuation of the uterus for retained products, surgical repair of tears, reduction of uterine inversion. Anaesthetic management for obstetric intervention depends on the state of the circulation, whether there is an epidural catheter already in situ and the possibility of coagulopathy. The risks of regional anaesthesia must be weighed against the risks of general anaesthesia in each case.

See also, Caesarean section; Obstetric analgesia and anaesthesia

Post-resuscitation care. Following successful resuscitation with return of spontaneous circulation (ROSC), most patients will show signs of the post-**cardiac arrest** syndrome consisting of:

- **cerebral hypoxic ischaemic injury**: includes **coma**, **seizures**, myoclonus, cognitive dysfunction and **brain death**. Brain injury accounts for 60% of out-of-hospital and 25% of in-hospital deaths following cardiac arrest with ROSC. Death often follows **withdrawal of treatment in ICU** following prediction of poor outcome.
- myocardial dysfunction accounts for the majority of deaths occurring within the first three days following cardiac arrest and ROSC, often reflecting the underlying cause of the cardiac arrest.
- systemic ischaemia/reperfusion response producing immune and **coagulation disorders** and resulting in **MODS** and an increased risk of **sepsis**.

The severity of the syndrome depends on the duration of circulatory arrest but is worsened by **hypotension**, **hypoxaemia**, **hypercarbia**, loss of organ **autoregulation**, poor glycaemic control, **pyrexia** and seizures.

- Management:
  - ventilation and oxygenation: all patients, except those with immediate ROSC, require tracheal intubation and IPPV. Oxygen should be titrated to achieve an arterial saturation of 94%–98%. Hypoxaemia and hypercapnia increase the risk of further cardiac arrest and secondary brain injury. The latter is worsened by hyperoxaemia due to the release of **free radicals**.
  - circulation:
    - early **percutaneous coronary intervention** following ROSC may improve survival and neurological outcome, especially if ST elevation is present on the ECG.
    - hypotension and low cardiac output are common and result from systemic vasodilatation; treatment is with iv fluids and inotropes (usually **noradrenaline** ± **dobutamine**).
    - arrhythmias are often due to **hypokalaemia** and potassium levels should be kept at 4–4.5 mmol/l. Implantable cardioverter defibrillators may be useful for those with severely impaired left ventricular function (*see Defibrillators, implantable cardioverter*).
  - glucose levels should be maintained at ≤10 mmol/l and hypoglycaemia avoided.
  - neurological support:
    - following ROSC, cerebral autoregulation is impaired in 40% of patients but **cerebral oedema** and raised **ICP** are usually not prominent; therefore, mean arterial pressure should be maintained at the patient's normal level.
    - seizures and **status epilepticus** should be treated aggressively. Myoclonic seizures may require treatment with **propofol** to prevent ventilator asynchrony.
    - **targeted temperature management**.

    prognostication allows a realistic measure of outcome that will help dictate the probability of a successful outcome i.e., in terms of quality of life, dependency, etc. (*see Cerebral hypoxic ischaemic injury*).

There is some evidence that regional centres specialising in post-cardiac arrest care may improve outcome.

Nolan JP, Soar J, Cariou A, et al (2015). Resuscitation; 95: 201–21

See also, Advanced life support, adult; Cardiopulmonary resuscitation

Post-tetanic count, *see Neuromuscular blockade monitoring*

Post-tetanic potentiation (PTP; post-tetanic facilitation). Increased response to a single pulse stimulus following **tetanic contraction**. Seen during **non-depolarising neuromuscular blockade** and in **myasthenia gravis**; thought to be caused by increased presynaptic mobilisation and release of **acetylcholine** in response to increased frequency of **action potentials**. Absent in **depolarising neuromuscular blockade**. Mechanical PTP occurring in normal subjects without neuromuscular blockade is thought to be caused by **calcium** ion accumulation resulting in increased **muscle** strength. **EMG** recording does not exhibit PTP in unblocked muscle.

See also, Neuromuscular blockade monitoring

Post-traumatic stress disorder. Psychological disorder following a severe physical or mental trauma, e.g. accident or natural disaster; has also been reported after **awareness** during anaesthesia and as a component of the **post-intensive care syndrome**. In order to make the diagnosis the following must exist:

- the stressor is considered exceptional, e.g. severe trauma or accident.
- onset within 6 months of the event.
- prominent memories: often distressing, intrusive, recurrent and causing the sufferer to relive the experience.
- avoidance behaviour, e.g. refusing to undergo anaesthesia.
- hyperarousal, e.g. irritability or anxiety.

Management includes psychological support and counselling, with specific psychological treatment according to the individual requirements. Drug therapy may also be required. The advice of a psychologist or psychiatrist with a specific interest is recommended.

Has also been recognised in staff, e.g. after a clinical catastrophe such as a patient's unexpected death (hence the concept of the 'second victim'), a major external incident (e.g. dealing with multiple severe trauma cases after an accident), or an internal incident (e.g. a hospital fire).

Shalev A, Liberzon I, Marmar C (2017). New Engl J Med; 376: 2459–69

Potassium. Principal intracellular cation, present at 135–150 mmol/l. Present in the **plasma** at 3.5–5.0 mmol/l. Total body content is about 3200 mmol, of which 90% is intracellular, 7.5% within bone and dense connective tissue and 2.5% in **interstitial fluid**, transcellular fluid and plasma. About 90% is exchangeable. Essential for maintenance of the cell **membrane potential** and generation of **action potentials**.

Filtered potassium is reabsorbed mainly at the proximal convoluted tubule of the **nephron**. It is secreted at the distal tubule, in effect in exchange for **sodium** and **hydrogen ions** under the influence of **aldosterone**.

- Daily requirement: about 1 mmol/kg/day.

Gumz ML, Rabinowitz L, Wingo CS (2015). N Engl J Med; 373: 60–72

Potassium channel activators. Class of antianginal drugs that act by opening potassium channels primarily in smooth muscle but also in other excitable tissues, causing arterial and venous dilatation. Result in improved blood flow to post-stenotic areas of myocardium. **Nicorandil** was the first to be developed.

Potency. Ability of a drug to produce a certain effect at a given dose; thus potent drugs are effective in small doses. Influenced by the drug's absorption, distribution, metabolism, excretion and **affinity** for its receptor.

See also, Dose–response curves

Potentiation, post-tetanic, *see Post-tetanic potentiation*

Power (in Physics). Rate of performing **work**. SI **unit** is the **watt**: 1 W = 1 J/s.

Power (in Statistics). The ability of **statistical tests** to reveal a difference of a certain magnitude. Power analysis is performed before a **clinical trial** to determine the sample size required to show a certain difference, or retrospectively when analysing a statistically insignificant result. Increased if groups are equally sized and large, and if the difference between them is large. Power equals $1 - \beta$, where β = type II **error**; power of 80%–90% (β = 0.1–0.2) is usually considered acceptable.

Choi SW, Tran DHD (2016). Anaesthesia; 71: 462–4

Power spectral analysis. **Fourier analysis** of 2–16 second sections (epochs) of the **EEG**, with graphical representation of the distribution of frequencies within each epoch. The frequency distribution of successive epochs may be plotted consecutively on continuous paper as a series of peaks and troughs (compressed spectral array) representing frequencies of high and low activity, respectively. Has been used to monitor depth of anaesthesia. The technique has also been applied to beat-to-beat variability of heart rate and BP to determine the relative influence of sympathetic and parasympathetic activity, e.g. perioperatively.

More recently, the technique has been combined with analysis of the relationship between different frequency components and the degree of burst suppression to give the **bispectral index**.

See also, Anaesthesia, depth of

Poynting effect. Dissolution of gaseous O_2 when bubbled through liquid N_2O, with vaporisation of the liquid to form a gaseous O_2/N_2O mixture.

[John H Poynting (1852–1914), English physicist]

See also, Entonox

PPF, Plasma protein fraction, *see Blood products*

PPH, *see Postpartum haemorrhage*

P–R interval. Represents atrial depolarisation. Measured from the beginning of the **P wave** to the beginning of the **QRS complex** of the **ECG**, irrespective of whether the QRS complex starts with a **Q wave** or an **R wave** (*see Fig. 60b;* **Electrocardiography**). Normally 1.2–2.0 ms. Shortened in **junctional arrhythmias**, **Wolff–Parkinson–White syndrome** and **Lown–Ganong–Levine syndrome**. Prolonged in **heart block** and **hypothermia**.

Pralidoxime mesylate/chloride. **Acetylcholinesterase** reactivator, used with **atropine** to treat **organophosphorus poisoning**. Has three main actions:

- converts the **acetylcholinesterase inhibitor** to a harmless compound.
- protects acetylcholinesterase transiently against further inhibition.
- reactivates the inhibited acetylcholinesterase.

Does not reverse the muscarinic effects of organophosphorus compounds, but highly active at nicotinic sites. Must be given within 24–36 h of poisoning to be effective. Its effects usually occur within 10–40 min of administration.

- Dosage: 30 mg/kg iv over 20 min, followed by iv infusion of 8 mg/kg/h, up to a maximum of 12 g/24 h.
- Side effects: drowsiness, visual disturbances, nausea, tachycardia, muscle weakness.

Prasugrel hydrochloride. Thienopyridine **antiplatelet drug**, used in combination with **aspirin** in patients with **acute coronary syndromes** undergoing **percutaneous coronary intervention**. More effective than **clopidogrel** at reducing the risk of ischaemic events, coronary stent thrombosis and all-cause mortality, but is associated with a higher incidence of fatal haemorrhage. Like clopidogrel, it is an inactive prodrug, rapidly converted to an active metabolite by the CYP3A4 subtype of the cytochrome P_{450} enzyme system; however, unlike clopidogrel, there is no clinically relevant effect of **pharmacogenetic** variations in enzyme expression. Cessation 7 days before elective surgery is recommended.

- Dosage: 60 mg orally initially followed by 10 mg od (5 mg od if body weight <60 kg or age >75 years).
- Side effects: bleeding, rash, rarely **thrombotic thrombocytopenic purpura**.

Prazosin hydrochloride. **α-Adrenergic receptor antagonist**, highly selective for **α_1-adrenergic receptors**. Used as a **vasodilator drug** (e.g. in **hypertension** and **cardiac failure**) and as a bladder smooth muscle relaxant in outflow obstruction. Rarely causes compensatory tachycardia. 97% protein-bound, with a **half-life** of 2–3 h. Excreted mainly via bile and faeces. Doxazosin and terazosin are related drugs.

- Dosage: 0.5 g orally bd–qds, increasing to 3–4 (rarely up to 20) mg/day in divided doses.
- Side effects: postural hypotension (especially after the first dose), nausea, drowsiness, headache.

Predictive value. In **statistics**, a test to predict or exclude a condition. May be:

- positive: proportion of patients with positive test results who have the condition.
- negative: proportion of patients with negative test results who do not have the condition.

Incorporates the **sensitivity** and **specificity** of a test as well as how common the condition is; for example, a test for predicting failed intubation may have a reasonably high sensitivity and specificity, but because the condition (failed intubation) is rare, the positive predictive value will always tend to be low.

Altman DG, Bland JM (1994). Br Med J; 309: 102

See also, Errors; Sensitivity, Specificity

Prednisolone. **Corticosteroid** with predominantly **glucocorticoid** activity, used in the long-term suppression of allergic, autoimmune and inflammatory disease. Four times as potent as **hydrocortisone**.

- Dosage: initially 10–60 mg orally od, usually reduced after a few days but occasionally longer. Maintenance dose: 2.5–15 mg daily. The acetate preparation may be given im (25–100 mg once or twice weekly) or into inflamed joints (5–25 mg).
- Side effects: as for corticosteroids.

Pre-eclampsia (Pre-eclamptic toxaemia, PET). Defined by **NICE** as the following occurring after the 20th week of **pregnancy**:

- **hypertension**: divided into mild (diastolic BP 90–99 mmHg/systolic BP 140–149 mmHg), moderate (diastolic BP 100–109 mmHg/systolic BP 150–159 mmHg) and severe (diastolic BP ≥110 mmHg/systolic BP ≥160 mmHg).
- proteinuria (defined as **urinary protein:creatinine ratio** >30 mg/mmol or 24-hour urine >300 mg protein.

Represents a multisystem disease with many other manifestations; hence the move in definition away from the classic 'triad of PET' (hypertension, **oedema** and proteinuria), towards the definition of gestational hypertension as above, with or without other features. Gestational hypertension occurs in 10%–12% of pregnancies whereas PET itself has an incidence of 2%–3%. Commoner in: first pregnancies with a particular partner (typically the features are less severe or present later in subsequent pregnancies); older age; family or previous history; pre-existing hypertension, kidney disease or **diabetes mellitus**; polyhydramnios; **obesity**; black race; and multiple pregnancy. Perinatal mortality is increased. Usually improves rapidly following delivery of the fetus, although the clinical picture may first worsen before recovery.

Pathogenesis is unclear but is thought to involve impaired trophoblastic invasion of myometrial arteries, with reduced placental perfusion and increased placental oxidative stress. This leads to release of inflammatory mediators from the placenta, resulting in a generalised inflammatory response with systemic endothelial dysfunction.

- Maternal features:
    - cardiovascular: thought to involve increased sensitivity to angiotensin II (sensitivity is normally decreased in pregnancy) and **catecholamines**, with vasoconstriction, reduced plasma volume, oedema and increased arterial BP. Ventricular function may be impaired.
    - renal: **renal blood flow**, **GFR** and **urine** output are decreased, with proteinuria.
    - haematological: fibrinogen, fibrin and platelet turnover is increased. **HELLP syndrome** (haemolysis, elevated liver enzymes, low platelets) may occur. Platelet function may be impaired.
    - neurological: hyperexcitability and hyperreflexia; visual symptoms and headache may forewarn of impending **convulsions (eclampsia)**.

Severe PET is defined as PET with severe hypertension and/or symptoms, biochemical and/or haematological impairment. It may progress to **oliguria**, **DIC**, **pulmonary oedema**, neurological symptoms and epigastric pain (thought to be due to stretching of the hepatic capsule).

Consistently one of the commonest causes of maternal mortality, especially in the developing world; death may result from **aspiration of gastric contents**, **stroke**, hepatorenal failure or **cardiac failure**. In the UK, most deaths are now caused by stroke (previously by **ALI**).

- Treatment includes bed rest, control of hypertension, prevention of convulsions and delivery of the fetus if possible:
    - **antihypertensive drugs** used include **α-methyldopa**, **labetalol**, **hydralazine** and **calcium channel blocking drugs** orally. Severe hypertension may require iv treatment with:
        - labetalol 5–10 mg increments, or 10–200 mg/h infusion.
        - hydralazine 5–10 mg increments, or 5–50 mg/h infusion.
        - **sodium nitroprusside** or **GTN** 0.1–5.0 µg/kg/min.

      Concurrent administration with **iv fluids** is important because the intravascular compartment is generally depleted; **central venous cannulation** may be required (**pulmonary artery catheterisation** is now rarely performed as evidence of its benefit is lacking). Administration of fluids (by consensus, preferably colloids) should begin before iv vasodilators to avoid precipitous falls in BP and/or placental perfusion. Oliguria is common, and it is relatively easy for inexperienced staff to overload the circulation in an attempt to improve urine output. As oliguria usually resolves spontaneously 1–2 days after delivery, it is generally accepted that tolerating a degree of transient renal impairment is preferable to causing pulmonary oedema. If the latter does occur, **furosemide** iv and **CPAP** may avoid the need for intubation and **IPPV**.
    - **anticonvulsant drugs**: **magnesium sulfate** reduces the incidence of eclampsia by almost 60%, although the **number needed to treat** is large (60–90; even higher in developed countries where the disease tends to be less aggressive) and side effects are relatively common, albeit mild. Magnesium has also been shown to be superior to **diazepam** and **phenytoin** at preventing recurrent convulsions after eclampsia.

Anaesthetic involvement may be required for analgesia during labour, **caesarean section** or assistance with management of fluids and BP.

- Anaesthetic techniques:
    - **epidural anaesthesia**:
        - prevents the increases in catecholamines associated with pain, thus increasing placental blood flow.
        - avoids the risks of general anaesthesia.

- contraindicated if there is a coagulopathy or low platelet count (<50 × 10^9/l is an absolute contraindication; 50–80 × 10^9/l has been suggested as acceptable if laboratory **coagulation studies** are normal, depending on clinical circumstances).
- careful fluid management and local anaesthetic administration are required to avoid cardiovascular instability following blockade. Sensitivity to **sympathomimetic drugs** is increased.
- avoidance of **adrenaline** in local anaesthetic solutions has been suggested but this is controversial.

▸ **spinal anaesthesia** has previously been avoided because of the fear of sudden severe hypotension, but this can be prevented if there is adequate volume expansion and BP control.

▸ general anaesthesia:
- risks include difficult intubation (because of airway oedema), the hypertensive response to intubation and cardiovascular instability. Administration of antihypertensive drugs or **opioid analgesic drugs** (e.g. **alfentanil** 7–10 μg/kg or **fentanyl** 1–4 μg/kg, especially in combination with magnesium) before intubation has been used.
- the anticonvulsant effect of **thiopental** may be beneficial.
- magnesium sulfate may result in increased sensitivity to **neuromuscular blocking drugs**.

Monitoring, BP control and eclampsia prophylaxis (if appropriate) should continue after delivery.

Mol BWJ, Roberts CT, Thangaratinam S, et al (2016). Lancet; 387: 999–1011

See also, Obstetric analgesia and anaesthesia

Pre-ejection period, *see Systolic time intervals*

Pre-emptive analgesia, *see Preventive analgesia*

Pregabalin. **Anticonvulsant drug**, related to **gabapentin**. Licensed for adjunctive therapy of partial seizures and also treatment of neuropathic **pain**.

- Dosage:
  - ▸ pain: 150 mg orally/day in 2–3 doses, increased after 1–2 weeks to 300–600 mg/day.
  - ▸ **epilepsy**: 25 mg orally bd, increased by 50 mg/week up to 600 mg/day.
- Side effects: dry mouth, GIT upset, CNS impairment, weight gain; rarely neutropenia, heart block, pancreatitis.

Pregnancy. Usually lasts 40 weeks. Most physiological changes occur in response to the increased metabolic demands of the **uterus**, **placenta** and fetus, and include alterations in the following systems:

▸ cardiovascular:
- increased intravascular volume from the first trimester, returning to normal within 2 weeks of delivery. Plasma expansion (50%) exceeds red cell expansion (20%), resulting in the 'physiological **anaemia**' of pregnancy. **Haemoglobin** concentration is usually about 120 g/l at term. White cell count increases throughout and peaks after delivery.
- increased **heart rate**, peaking at 28–36 weeks, when it may exceed normal rate by 10–15 beats/min.
- increased **cardiac output** from 10 weeks, reaching 140% of normal at term with further increases during labour. **Stroke volume** increases by 30%. Ejection systolic **heart murmurs** are common, and third or fourth **heart sounds** may occur.
- decreased **SVR** as a result of the smooth muscle relaxation caused by progesterone. Engorgement of cutaneous and epidural veins, the latter presumed to affect height of block in **epidural anaesthesia**.
- reduced **MAP**, being lowest at the time of maximal cardiac output.
- **aortocaval compression** in the supine position.
- **ECG** changes caused by cephalad displacement of the **diaphragm** by the uterus include left axis deviation and inverted **T waves** in leads V_2 and V_3.

▸ respiratory:
- increased minute ventilation (by 50% in the first trimester), mainly caused by increased **tidal volume** (thought to be a central effect of progesterone).
- reduced arterial $P\text{CO}_2$ to about 4 kPa (30 mmHg) with resulting respiratory alkalosis by the 12th week of pregnancy; arterial $P\text{O}_2$ increases by about 1.3 kPa (10 mmHg). Arterial pH remains normal due to renal excretion of **bicarbonate**.
- reduced **FRC** (both **expiratory reserve volume** and **residual volume** decrease) from the 20th week onwards, caused by the upward displacement of the diaphragm by the uterus.
- increased O_2 consumption throughout pregnancy, but especially in the third trimester (up to 20%).
- increased risk of **hypoxaemia** during anaesthesia results from reduced FRC and increased O_2 demand.
- venous engorgement of the upper **airway**, predisposing to spontaneous epistaxis or haemorrhage on instrumentation.

▸ gastrointestinal: **gastric emptying** is probably normal apart from during labour, when it may be reduced (markedly if opioids are given). Gastric acidity is probably normal. **Gastro-oesophageal reflux** occurs in at least 80% of women, caused by the effects of progesterone on the **lower oesophageal sphincter**, and the uterus pushing the stomach into a horizontal position. The time after conception at which the GIT effects occur, and the time after delivery at which they revert to normal, are unknown. 16–20 weeks has been suggested as the time of onset; progesterone levels fall to non-pregnant levels by 24 h of delivery, and reflux usually resolves by 36 h.

▸ **coagulation**: increased levels of fibrinogen and all clotting factors except XI and XIII, predisposing towards thromboembolism. Platelet count falls slightly. Systemic fibrinolytic activity is depressed, but localised activity (i.e., ability to lyse clots from within) is maintained. Thus the level of **fibrin degradation products** increases as pregnancy progresses. However, in normal pregnancy neither bleeding nor clotting times are increased.

▸ renal: dilatation of the renal pelvises and ureters from the end of the first trimester. **Renal blood flow** and **GFR** increase by 40%. Increased **renin/angiotensin system** activity increases sodium and water retention, with falls in serum creatinine and urea; glycosuria may occur.

▸ endocrine: peripheral insulin resistance due to antagonism by hormones (e.g. human placental lactogen) may aggravate or precipitate gestational diabetes.

- hepatic: blood flow is unaltered. Serum **albumin** and **cholinesterase** levels fall, while hepatic enzyme levels may increase.

Non-urgent surgery is usually delayed until the second trimester, because of the possible risk (although never proven) of teratogenic effects on the fetus. Conditions requiring abdominal surgery are associated with increased risk of miscarriage or premature labour.
See also, Fetus, effect of anaesthetic agents on; Obstetric analgesia and anaesthesia

Prehabilitation. Component of enhanced recovery programmes in which preoperative **exercise testing** and encouragement of physical exercise and other methods of increasing physical fitness are used to improve perioperative outcomes, based on the observation that less fit patients tend to have higher incidences of postoperative morbidity and mortality after major surgery. The evidence from randomised trials that prehabilitation programmes may counter this trend is supportive but relatively weak, possibly due to the small number of trials, the need to individualise prehabilitation, and the limited time available before surgery ± adverse effect of adjunct treatments, e.g. in cancer surgery.
Levett DZ, Grocott MP (2015). Can J Anesth; 62: 131–42
See also, Perioperative medicine; Recovery, enhanced

Prehospital index (PHI). Scoring system used to assess **trauma** according to BP, pulse rate, respiratory status, level of consciousness and mechanism of injury. Now rarely used.

Preload. End-diastolic ventricular wall tension. May be inferred from ventricular end-diastolic pressure, itself approximating to **pulmonary capillary wedge pressure** (left) or **CVP** (right). Related to **myocardial contractility** and **cardiac output** by **Starling's law. Fluid responsiveness** is a measure of a patient's response to an increase in preload.

Also refers to prophylactic administration of **iv fluids** to reduce hypotension, e.g. before **spinal** or **epidural anaesthesia**; administration of fluid as the block develops is sometimes referred to as 'co-load'.

Premedication. Administration of medication before anaesthesia.

- Aims:
  - anxiolysis.
  - analgesia.
  - smooth **induction of anaesthesia** and reduction of anaesthetic agent requirements.
  - reduced upper airway and salivary secretions.
  - reduced risk of **awareness**.
  - reduced **PONV**.
  - reduced risks of specific complications associated with anaesthesia/surgery or the patient's pre-existing condition, e.g.:
    - bradycardia, e.g. in **ophthalmic surgery**.
    - hypertensive response to **tracheal intubation**.
    - **aspiration pneumonitis**.
    - **adverse drug reactions**.
    - **bronchospasm**.
    - **DVT**.
- Drugs that have been used for premedication include:
  - **opioid analgesic drugs**, e.g. **morphine**.
  - **benzodiazepines** (e.g. **midazolam, temazepam**) and other sedatives, e.g. **dexmedetomidine**.
  - **barbiturates**, e.g. pentobarbital.
  - **butyrophenones**, e.g. **droperidol**.
  - **phenothiazines**, e.g. **alimemazine** (trimeprazine), **promethazine**.
  - **anticholinergic drugs**, e.g. **atropine**, **hyoscine**, **glycopyrronium**.
  - other **antiemetic** or **prokinetic drugs**, e.g. **metoclopramide**.
  - **H_2 receptor antagonists**, e.g. **ranitidine**, cimetidine.
  - **antacids**, e.g. sodium citrate.

In addition, certain drugs already taken regularly by the patient are usually continued up to and including the day of surgery, e.g. **antiarrhythmic drugs, antihypertensive drugs**, drugs used in **ischaemic heart disease** and **asthma, anticonvulsant drugs**.

In modern practice, premedication with oral benzodiazepines (most commonly) or im opioids is most often used for sedation, although many anaesthetists do not routinely prescribe sedative premedication at all because of disadvantages such as:
  - excessive sedation.
  - difficulty with timing of drug administration.
  - pain from im injections.
  - nausea and vomiting (with opioids).
  - dry mouth with anticholinergic drugs.
  - unnecessary drug administration.
  - **antanalgesia** and restlessness.
  - delayed **recovery**.

Preoperative assessment. Main objectives include assessment of:
  - the risk of perioperative morbidity or death.
  - whether the patient's condition may be improved before surgery, e.g. by changing medication, treating pre-existing disease, administering fluids.
  - how otherwise to minimise the perioperative risk, e.g. by enlisting more experienced help, rescheduling the time of surgery, using special anaesthetic or analgesic techniques, booking a bed on ICU or HDU.

Preadmission clinics (involving assessment by an anaesthetist, surgeon or nurse) attempt to reduce the rate of delay and cancellation of surgical procedures caused by inadequate preparation of patients. Protocols may support non-anaesthetic staff in assessing patients.

- Assessment is directed towards the individual patient's circumstances but in general is divided into:
  - history:
    - medical and surgical history, including the nature of the proposed surgery.
    - previous anaesthetic history, including adverse reactions, **PONV** and other problems.
    - family history of medical or anaesthetic problems.
    - drug history (past and present).
    - **smoking** and **alcohol** intake.
    - known allergies and **atopy**.
    - weight of the patient (especially children).
    - presence of capped, crowned, chipped or loose **teeth**.
    - anxiety.
    - time of last oral intake.
    - systems review, in particular:
      - CVS: hypertension, features of ischaemic heart disease, cardiac failure, arrhythmias.
      - RS: recent **chest infection**, features of **COPD** or **asthma**.

- GIT: hiatus hernia or other risk factors for **aspiration of gastric contents**.
- CNS: **epilepsy**, pre-existing neurological lesions.

- examination:
  - **airway**, teeth, **cervical spine** (including assessment for possible difficult tracheal intubation or mask ventilation).
  - CVS: for **hypovolaemia**, **dehydration**, **cyanosis** and **anaemia**; **pulse**, BP, **JVP**, cardiac impulse, **heart sounds**, lung bases, periphery (for **oedema**).
  - RS: for clubbing and cyanosis, position of the trachea, chest expansion, air entry, **respiratory sounds**.
  - CNS: **cranial nerves**, **spinal cord** and peripheral nerves, including **dermatomes** and **myotomes**.
  - suitable veins for cannulation.
  - suitability for regional techniques where intended.
- preoperative **investigations**.

Scoring systems may be used to classify patients according to preoperative status, e.g. **ASA physical status**, **cardiac risk index**, **New York Heart Association classification**, **Glasgow coma scale**, **subarachnoid haemorrhage** and **hepatic failure** scoring systems.

Cardiopulmonary exercise testing is increasingly used to predict outcome in high-risk surgical cases. The need for **blood compatibility testing** and **premedication** is also assessed.

The assessment period is also an opportunity to explain the forthcoming anaesthesia and confirm the patient's **consent**.

See also, individual diseases and drugs; Emergency surgery

Preoperative fasting, *see Gastric emptying*

Preoperative optimisation. Term referring to the technique of short-term preoperative improvement of physiological variables with iv fluids, **inotropic** and **vasodilator drugs** to produce supranormal levels of **oxygen delivery** ('goal-directed therapy') in patients undergoing major surgery. Has been claimed to reduce morbidity and mortality in certain groups of patients, e.g. those undergoing major vascular surgery. Because it requires preoperative admission to the ICU and invasive monitoring, the process has implications in terms of costs and utilisation of ICU beds. Now considered part of the spectrum of possible treatment options within **perioperative medicine**.

Preoxygenation. Administration of 100% O_2 before **induction of anaesthesia**. Increases the O_2 reserve in the lungs (by replacing N_2 in the **FRC**) and thus the time to **hypoxaemia** during subsequent **apnoea**, e.g. during tracheal intubation. The size of the FRC (and therefore the oxygen store) is increased if patients are positioned head-up, particularly if the patient is obese.

Particularly useful when airway difficulties are anticipated, or in patients at risk from **aspiration of gastric contents**. Thus a vital part of 'rapid sequence induction'.

A tightly fitting **facemask** (to prevent entrainment of room air) and adequate flow of O_2 are essential. Monitoring of end-expiratory O_2 concentration may be a useful guide during preoxygenation; **washout** of nitrogen from the lungs is indicated by an increase in expired O_2 concentration towards steady state (near 100% in ideal conditions with no gas leaks or mixing). The time required to achieve >95% nitrogen washout is determined by the alveolar minute ventilation and size of the FRC (*see Exponential process*); in an adult undertaking normal tidal breathing, 3–5 min is usually sufficient, and can be shortened by asking the patient to take **vital capacity** breaths.

Nimmagadda U, Salem MR, Crystal GJ (2017). Anesth Analg; 124: 507–17

See also, Induction, rapid sequence

Pressure. **Force** per unit area. SI **unit** is the **pascal**: 1 Pa = 1 N/m^2.

Pressure generators, *see Ventilators*

Pressure measurement. May be:

- direct:
  - liquid manometers that measure:
    - absolute pressure, e.g. mercury barometer.
    - pressure relative to atmospheric pressure (gauge pressure), e.g. U tube. The sensitivity may be increased by using liquid of low density, inclining the manometer tube or using a different non-miscible liquid in each of the limbs of the U tube (differential liquid manometer).
  - aneroid gauge (one in which there is no liquid). In one form, a sealed metal bellows changes size with changes in external or applied pressure, moving a pointer on a scale (e.g. aneroid barometer). In the Bourdon gauge used in anaesthesia, a coiled tube of oval cross-section uncoils as it becomes circular on cross-section, due to the high pressure of the gas inside it, and this moves the pointer.
  - pressure **transducers**.
- indirect, e.g. in **arterial BP measurement**.

[Eugene Bourdon (1808–1884), French engineer]

Pressure-regulated volume control ventilation. Ventilatory mode combining the benefits of pressure-controlled **IPPV** with a decelerating inspiratory flow pattern and a guaranteed tidal volume. The ventilator automatically monitors the lung's properties and modifies the inspiratory pressure level to deliver a predetermined volume. Maximum inspiratory pressure permitted is just below the preset upper pressure limit and, if the tidal volume cannot be delivered with this pressure, the ventilator alarms, indicating that the breath has been pressure-limited. Useful mode where lung/chest **compliance** alters during inspiration, e.g. **atelectasis**, **bronchospasm**. Achieves a set tidal/minute volume with the lowest possible inspiratory pressure. The maximum pressure change between two breaths is preset by the ventilator (approximately 3 cmH$_2$O).

Pressure regulators. Formerly called reducing valves, devices for reducing the high pressures delivered by **cylinders** to **anaesthetic machines**, and maintaining the reduced pressure at a constant level that is easier to use. Also reduce the requirement for high-pressure tubing.

- May be:
  - direct (Fig. 132a): cylinder pressure P tends to open the valve.
  - indirect (Fig. 132b): cylinder pressure P tends to close the valve.

The diaphragm moves according to p and the tension in the springs. As p falls, the diaphragm bulges into the regulator, allowing more gas flow into the upper half and thus maintaining p. If p increases, the diaphragm is pushed upwards, decreasing gas flow and again maintaining p. Thus pressure is maintained despite changes in demand. If cylinder pressure P falls, p is likewise maintained.

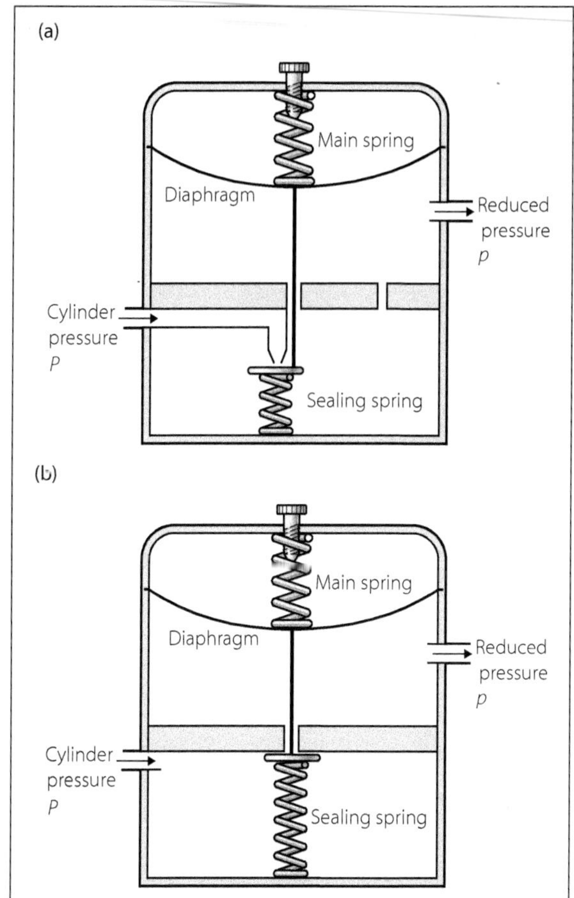

Fig. 132 Diagram of pressure regulators: (a) direct; (b) indirect. See text

The regulators are specific to each gas, and should be labelled accordingly. Pressure relief valves are incorporated in case of excessive pressures. Pressure gauges may also be incorporated.

Two-stage regulators are often used, to reduce wear and tear on the diaphragm and reduce pressure fluctuations, especially if high gas flows are required. The output of one stage is the input of the second. **Demand valves** may be based on this principle.

Slave regulators are those whose output depends on the output of another regulator. For example, the output of an O_2 regulator may be applied above the diaphragm of an N_2O regulator, keeping the latter's valve open. If the O_2 pressure fails, the N_2O valve closes.

Pressure sores, *see Decubitus ulcers*

Pressure support, *see Inspiratory pressure support*

Preventive analgesia. Intervention during the perioperative period with the aim of reducing postoperative pain and/or analgesic consumption. Distinct from the concept of 'pre-emptive analgesia', which refers solely to an intervention given before surgical incision with the intention to provide greater analgesia than if it were given post-incision. 'Preventive analgesia' incorporates all perioperative methods used to reduce postoperative pain and arose as a result of an appreciation that several mechanisms (such as premorbid psychological factors, perioperative immobilisation and postoperative inflammation) can contribute to central sensitisation and long-term postoperative pain, rather than just surgical incision, and that the nature and duration of therapy are more important than the timing per se.

Clarke H, Poon M, Weinrib A, et al (2015). Drugs; 75: 339–51

Priestley, Joseph (1733–1804). English scientist and theologian, best known for his work on various gases. A major proponent of the **phlogiston** theory, he isolated ammonia (as 'alkaline air'), sulfur dioxide ('vitriolic acid air'), O_2 ('dephlogisticated air'), N_2O ('dephlogisticated nitrous air'), nitrogen dioxide ('nitrous acid air') and methane. Also investigated electrical conduction. Emigrated to the USA in 1794.

Prilocaine hydrochloride. Amide **local anaesthetic agent**, introduced in 1959. Slower in onset than **lidocaine**, but lasts about 1.5 times as long and less toxic. pK_a is 7.9. 55% protein-bound. Undergoes hepatic and renal metabolism. Maximal safe dose: 5 mg/kg alone, 8 mg/kg with **adrenaline**. Used as 0.5%–1.0% solutions for infiltration, 1%–2% for nerve blocks and 0.5% for **IVRA**. Also available as a 4% plain or 3% solution with **felypressin** for dental infiltration, and in **EMLA** cream. May cause **methaemoglobinaemia** in doses above about 600 mg in adults, due to its metabolite *ortho*-toluidine.

A preservative-free hyperbaric 2% solution (with 6% glucose) for **spinal anaesthesia** was introduced in the UK in 2011.

Priming principle. Shortening of the time of onset of **non-depolarising neuromuscular blockade** by administration of a non-depolarising **neuromuscular blocking drug** in divided aliquots. The priming dose (15%–20% of the usual intubating dose) is followed by the remainder of the intubating dose 4–8 min later, depending on the drug used.

- Suggested explanatory theories:
  - the priming dose occupies a proportion of postsynaptic receptors at the **neuromuscular junction**; the main dose can thus occupy more rapidly the critical mass of receptors for neuromuscular blockade.
  - the priming dose occupies presynaptic receptors, reducing mobilisation and release of acetylcholine; the main dose thus acts faster.

Initially thought to answer the need for rapid tracheal intubation without using **suxamethonium**. However, the priming dose itself may cause unpleasant symptoms (e.g. diplopia and weakness) and serious complications, e.g. **hypoventilation** and **aspiration of gastric contents**.

Jones RM (1989). Br J Anaesth; 63: 1–3

PRISM, *see Paediatric risk of mortality score*

Proarrhythmias. Arrhythmias caused or exacerbated by **antiarrhythmic drugs**. May occur even with standard dosage and normally therapeutic plasma drug levels. Common examples include **VT** and **torsade de pointes**.

Probability (*P*). In **statistics**, the likelihood that the observed result is a chance occurrence. Analogous to, but distinct from, the chance of a type I **error**. **Statistical significance** is usually denoted by a *P* value <0.05, indicating that the observed result might be expected to occur by chance alone, ≤5 times in 100 occasions.

Probability limits, *see Confidence intervals*

Procainamide hydrochloride. Class Ia **antiarrhythmic drug**, chemically related to **procaine**. Effective against ventricular and supraventricular arrhythmias. Has 85% oral **bioavailability** and 15% protein-bound. Undergoes hepatic metabolism (largely via acetylation to *N*-acetylprocainamide) and renal excretion, although 40%–50% is excreted unchanged. Rarely used in the UK and available only via 'special order'.

- Dosage:
  - up to 50 mg/kg/day orally in 4–8 doses.
  - 20 mg/min slowly iv up to 17 mg/kg, with ECG monitoring for widened **QRS complex** or **P-R interval** prolongation. 2–6 mg/min may follow.
- Side effects: hypotension with iv usage, GIT upset, rash, agranulocytosis, SLE-like syndrome (especially in slow acetylators).

Procaine hydrochloride. Ester **local anaesthetic agent**, introduced in 1904, now seldom used. The first synthetic local anaesthetic. Less lipid-soluble than **lidocaine**, with slower onset of less intense anaesthesia, and shorter duration of action. pK_a is 8.9; 6% protein-bound. Poorly absorbed from mucous membranes; thus not useful as a topical anaesthetic. Used in 0.25%–1.0% solutions for infiltration anaesthesia, and 1%–2% for nerve blocks, usually with **adrenaline** 1:200 000. Maximal safe dose: 12 mg/kg. Also used in **cardioplegia** solutions.

Procalcitonin. Propeptide of **calcitonin**, produced by the C cells of the **thyroid gland** but not normally released into the circulation (except in low concentrations) in health. Systemic procalcitonin levels rise significantly during severe infection (especially bacterial); hence interest in its use as a marker of infection and antibiotic treatment, most studies using cut-off levels of 1.0–2.0 μg/l for initiation of, and 0.1–0.5 μg/l for stopping, antibiotic therapy. **Half-life** is 25–30 h.

Liu D, Su L, Han G, et al (2015). PLoS One; 10: e0129450

Prochlorperazine maleate/mesylate. Piperazine **phenothiazine** with antiemetic, α-adrenergic agonist and weak sedative properties. Used mainly as an **antipsychotic drug** and perioperatively, as an **antiemetic drug**. Active within 10–20 min of im administration and 30–40 min of oral administration. Action lasts 3–4 h.

- Dosage:
  - 12.5 mg orally bd increased to up 100 mg daily if required, or 12.5–25 mg im bd/tds. Not licensed for iv use in the UK, although it has been safely given by that route.
- Side effects: as for phenothiazines. Extrapyramidal reactions are more likely than following **chlorpromazine**, especially in children.

Procyclidine hydrochloride. Anticholinergic drug, used in the treatment of **Parkinson's disease** and drug-induced extrapyramidal symptoms, e.g. acute **dystonic reaction**. Acts by reducing the effect of acetylcholine in the basal ganglia.

- Dosage:
  - 2.5–10 mg orally tds.
  - 5–10 mg im, repeated after 20 min up to 20 mg/day.
  - 5 mg iv repeated as necessary; relief is usual after a single dose and within 5 min but may take 30 min.
- Side effects: dry mouth, GIT disturbance, urinary retention, dizziness, blurred vision.

Prodrug. Inactive substance metabolised to active drug within the body, e.g. **clopidogrel, diamorphine**.

Prokinetic drugs. Group of drugs that increase GIT activity. Include **metoclopramide** and **domperidone**, their prokinetic actions mediated via enhancement of GIT cholinergic activity (although **dopamine** antagonism may contribute). Used in oesophageal reflux, gastric stasis and non-ulcer dyspepsia. **Erythromycin** has a powerful prokinetic effect via GIT motilin receptors and has been used in **ileus**. General **parasympathomimetic drugs** also increase GIT motility but are rarely used for this purpose.

Prolonged Q–T syndromes. Conditions in which the **Q–T interval** of the ECG exceeds 0.44 s.

- May be:
  - congenital: due to mutation of genes coding for cardiac sodium or potassium ion channels. At least 15 specific gene loci have been identified. Most forms are autosomal dominant; the autosomal recessive form is often associated with sensorineural deafness. Syncope may be provoked by physical exercise and stress.
  - acquired:
    - myocardial disease, e.g. **MI, rheumatic fever**, third-degree **heart block, cardiomyopathy**.
    - electrolyte disturbance, e.g. **hypocalcaemia, hypokalaemia, hypomagnesaemia.**
    - drugs, e.g. class Ia, Ic and III **antiarrhythmic drugs, phenothiazines, tricyclic antidepressant drugs, selective serotonin reuptake inhibitors, ondansetron** and related drugs (at high doses), and some antibacterial agents, e.g. **erythromycin, ciprofloxacin.**
    - severe **TBI.**

Both forms are associated with the development of ventricular arrhythmias, including **torsade de pointes** and **VT**, causing recurrent syncope or sudden death. This has been associated with anaesthesia. The risk may be greater if there is also increased **Q–Tc dispersion**. Avoidance of the above drugs and those that increase sympathetic tone, and use of **β-adrenergic receptor antagonists**, are generally recommended; **phenytoin** and **verapamil** have been used to treat acute arrhythmias. Long-term treatment is with β-blockers or an implantable cardioverter defibrillator.

Staikou C, Chondrogiannis K, Mani A (2012). Br J Anaesth; 108: 730–44

Promethazine hydrochloride/teoclate. Phenothiazine and **antihistamine drug**, with sedative, anticholinergic and antiemetic properties. Used for antiemesis, allergic reactions, sedation and **premedication**, especially in children. Also used topically to relieve pruritus. One component of the **lytic cocktail**. Well absorbed orally but undergoes extensive **first-pass metabolism**. Excreted renally following hepatic metabolism.

- Dosage:
  - 10–20 mg orally bd/tds; 0.5–1.0 mg/kg for paediatric premedication.
  - 25–50 mg im or by slow iv injection.
- Side effects are those of phenothiazines and **anticholinergic drugs**.

Prone ventilation. Technique in which patients are turned prone while receiving **IPPV**; used in **ALI**. Improves oxygenation in up to 80% of patients; although initial studies failed to show survival benefits, recent **meta-analysis**

suggests improved survival in those with severe **hypoxaemia**.

Proposed mechanisms for improved oxygenation include increased **FRC** (via redistribution of secretions, interstitial oedema and **atelectasis** away from the posterior areas), changes in regional diaphragmatic excursion and redistribution of perfusion away from more oedematous lung regions. Patients may be turned regularly, e.g. for up to 8 h every 24 h. Disadvantages during turning include accidental displacement of tubes and catheters/cannulae, injury to eyes/face/limbs, stimulation of coughing and cardiovascular instability; once turned, the main problems are inaccessibility and care of pressure areas. These problems may be reduced by using **rotational therapy** instead.

Scholten EL, Beeitler JR, Prisk GK, Malhotra A (2017). Chest; 151: 215–24

Propafenone hydrochloride. Class Ic **antiarrhythmic drug**, affecting atria, conducting system and ventricles. Has slight β-adrenergic antagonist properties. Used for preventing and treating SVT and VT. Undergoes hepatic metabolism and renal excretion. Should not be given to patients with known ischaemic or structural heart disease.

- Dosage: 150–300 mg orally tds.
- Side effects; arrhythmia, hypotension, dizziness, GIT disturbances, blurred vision, blood dyscrasias, hepatic impairment.

Propanidid. **Intravenous anaesthetic agent**, first used in 1956 and withdrawn in 1984. Eugenol (oil of cloves) derivative, prepared in **Cremophor EL** or polyoxyethylated castor oil. Hydrolysed by plasma and liver esterases. Rapidly acting, with rapid recovery. Hypotension, apnoea following initial hyperventilation, venous thrombosis and **adverse drug reactions** were common.

Propofol. 2,6-Diisopropylphenol (Fig. 133). **Intravenous anaesthetic agent**, first used in 1977 and introduced into clinical practice in 1986. Exact mechanism of action is unknown, but may involve binding to **GABA$_A$ receptors**, potentiating the action of endogenous **GABA**.

Originally formulated in **Cremophor EL**, but reformulated before commercial release because of allergic reactions. Now presented as an oil–water emulsion: 1% (presented in 20-ml ampoules, 50/100-ml vials and 50-ml prefilled syringes) or 2% (for infusion only and presented in 50-ml vials and 50-ml prefilled syringes), containing 10% soya bean oil, 1.2% egg phosphatide and 2.25% glycerol. A new formulation containing medium-chain triglycerides causes less pain on injection; in addition some formulations contain either 0.005% EDTA or sulfite as a preservative. Fospropofol is the phosphate **prodrug** of **propofol** and as such has a slower onset of action; it is licensed in the USA for 'light sedation'. Aquafol is a newly developed emulsification of propofol in water, which has similar properties to the parent agent but causes more pain on injection.

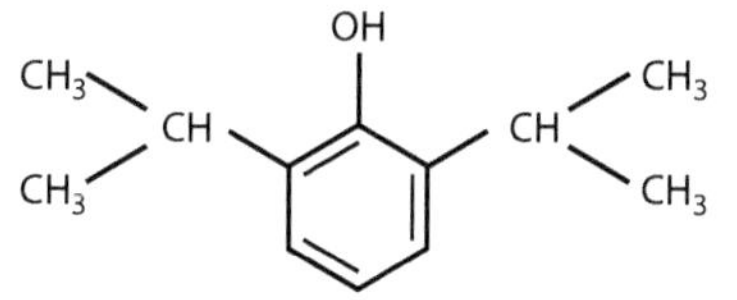

Fig. 133 Structure of propofol

pK_a is 11. Distribution and elimination half-lives are 1–2 min and 1–5 h, respectively; context-sensitive **half-life** is approximately 20 min after 2 h infusion, 30 min after 6 h infusion and 50 min after 9 h infusion. 98% protein-bound after iv injection. Metabolised in the liver and excreted renally. Extrahepatic metabolism is suggested by a plasma **clearance** (25–30 ml/kg/min) that exceeds hepatic blood flow. There are no active metabolites. Thus recovery is rapid with minimal residual effects, making it particularly suited to short cases, e.g. in **day-case surgery**. These properties also make it suitable for **TIVA** and iv **sedation**.

- Effects:
  - induction:
    - smooth and rapid, with only occasional movements. Loss of response to verbal command may be a better indication of adequate dosage than loss of eyelash reflex.
    - pain on injection is common; it may be reduced by prior injection of, or mixing with, **lidocaine**, administration of **opioid analgesic drugs**, or injecting into a large vein.
  - CVS/RS:
    - hypotension is common, although whether caused by direct myocardial depression, reduced SVR, or both is controversial. Normo- or bradycardia is common; resetting of the **baroreceptor reflex** has been suggested. Reduces the hypertensive response to tracheal intubation.
    - respiratory depression is marked.
    - tends to obtund upper airway reflexes, thus allowing manipulation/instrumentation more readily than **thiopental**. Thus particularly useful when placing **SADs**. Tracheal intubation may be possible after propofol induction without neuromuscular blocking drugs, especially if opioids are also given.
  - CNS:
    - **antanalgesia** has not been reported.
    - has an antiemetic effect. Increased appetite has been suggested but may reflect the excellent quality of recovery rather than a direct effect.
    - involuntary movements have been reported following propofol, but these are not thought to be epileptiform convulsions. Has been used successfully in intractable **epilepsy**.
    - reduces **cerebral blood flow**, **ICP** and **intraocular pressure**.
    - dreams may occur. Claims by patients of sexual assault while anaesthetised have been made.
  - other: allergic phenomena have been reported although suggested cross-reactivity with allergy to peanuts, soy or eggs has been disproved.
- Dosage:
  - 1.5–2.5 mg/kg for induction (increased to 2.5–5 mg/kg in children).
  - for maintenance, several regimens have been suggested, based on pharmacokinetic studies, including the Bristol regimen (applies to concurrent use of 66% **N_2O**, or infusion of **alfentanil** 30–50 µg/kg/h):
    - 10 mg/kg/h for 10 min.
    - 8 mg/kg/h for 10 min.
    - 6 mg/kg/h thereafter, adjusted if required according to clinical response.

  In modern practice, more precise anaesthesia is achieved by using **target-controlled infusion** (TCI) pumps that automatically adjust infusion rates according to the patient's age, weight, volume infused

and target plasma propofol concentration (in healthy patients, 4–8 µg/ml for induction of anaesthesia and 3–6 µg/ml for maintenance).
- 1.0–4.0 mg/kg/h for sedation.

Contamination during preparation for infusion has led to iatrogenic bacteraemia; hence the development of the EDTA preparation.

Contains the same energy content as 10% fat emulsion (900 Cal/l). Plasma lipid levels should be monitored in all patients receiving propofol infusions for longer than 3 days.

The 1% solution is licensed for induction/maintenance of anaesthesia and sedation for short procedures in children over 1 month (the 2% solution should not be used in children <3 years). Not approved for sedation of children <16 years in ICU (neurological, cardiac, renal and hepatic impairment have been reported after its use in this setting). Myocardial failure and acidosis have been reported after prolonged infusion of high doses in adults, leading to the description of a distinct metabolic syndrome, the **propofol infusion syndrome**.

Propofol infusion syndrome. Progressive myocardial failure (often with refractory bradycardia), metabolic **acidosis**, **hyperkalaemia** and evidence of muscle damage in the absence of other causes, in patients receiving infusions of **propofol**. Originally described associated with hyperlipaemia and high infusion rates of propofol (>4 mg/kg/h) for prolonged periods (>2 days), but it has also been reported after lower infusion rates and total doses. Thought to be related to exacerbation of poor tissue oxygenation and impaired cellular utilisation of **glucose**, due to impairment of mitochondrial oxidative phosphorylation. Inhibition of fatty acid oxidation may also be involved. Treatment is supportive and includes withdrawal of propofol; **haemodialysis** has been used successfully. Mortality is around 50% overall.

Krajčová A, Waldauf P, Anděl M, Duška F (2015). Crit Care; 19: 398

Proportional assist ventilation (PAV). Mode of partial ventilatory support in which the **ventilator** generates an instantaneous inspiratory pressure in proportion to the instantaneous effort of the patient (i.e. does not use preset pressure or volume targets). Intended to facilitate normal neuroventilatory coupling by allowing the patient to control all aspects of breathing (i.e. **tidal volume**, inspiratory and expiratory durations, and flow patterns), while the ventilator functions as an extension of the patient's respiratory muscles. Changes in lung and chest wall **impedance** may prevent PAV from being fully effective. Has several potential benefits:
- greater patient comfort and lower sedation requirements.
- reduced ventilator asynchrony and improved sleep quality.
- reduction of peak airway pressures.
- preservation and enhancement of the patient's own homeostatic control mechanisms.
- may have a non-invasive role in **COPD**.

Moerer O (2012). Curr Opin Crit Care; 18: 61–9

Propranolol. **β-Adrenergic receptor antagonist** (the first to be introduced, in 1964). Non-selective, and without **intrinsic sympathomimetic activity**. 90%–95% protein-bound. Its primary metabolite, 4-hydroxypropanolol, has β-blocking activity. Uses and side effects are as for β-adrenergic receptor antagonists in general.
- Dosage:
  - hypertension, portal hypertension, angina, migraine, phaeochromocytoma: 30–80 mg orally bd, increased up to 120–320 mg/day.
  - arrhythmias, hypertrophic obstructive cardiomyopathy, anxiety, thyrotoxicosis: 10–40 mg orally bd/tds.
  - **acute coronary syndromes**: 40 mg orally qds for 2–3 days, then 80–160 mg/day.
  - acute iv administration: 1 mg over 1 min, repeated as required up to 5–10 mg.

Propylene glycol. Diol **alcohol** ($CH_3.CHOH.CH_2OH$), used as a solvent in drugs, e.g. **etomidate, GTN, lorazepam**. Has been associated with hypotension, **lactic acidosis**, **pulmonary hypertension** and **haemolysis**; these effects are independent of the drug infused.

Prostacyclin. **Prostaglandin** PGI_2 produced by the intima of blood vessels via the **cyclo-oxygenase** limb of the **arachidonic acid** metabolism pathway. The most potent inhibitor of **platelet** aggregation, acting via an increase in **cAMP** levels. At high doses, may disperse circulating platelet aggregates. Thought to have vital importance in preventing **coagulation** within normal blood vessels. Also a potent **vasodilator drug**. Increases renin production and blood glucose levels.

Provided commercially as synthetic epoprostenol sodium, which is reconstituted in saline and glycerine to produce a clear, colourless solution of pH 10.5. Used to prevent platelet aggregation during renal **dialysis** or other forms of **extracorporeal circulation**; has also been used in **pre-eclampsia**, **pulmonary hypertension**, **haemolytic–uraemic syndrome** and **septic shock**. **Half-life** is 2–3 min, with cessation of platelet effects within 30 min of stopping an infusion. Its main metabolite is 6-keto-prostaglandin $F_{1\alpha}$.
- Dosage: 2–35 ng/kg/min iv.
- Side effects: flushing, headache, hypotension.

Prostaglandins (PGs). Unsaturated fatty acids containing 20 carbon atoms and a five-membered carbon ring (cyclopentane ring) at one end. Derived from **arachidonic acid**, and thought to be synthesised in most tissues, although originally isolated from seminal fluid in the 1930s. Named according to the configuration of the cyclopentane ring (e.g. PGA, B, C, etc. to PGI [**prostacyclin**]), with subscript numbers denoting the number of side-chain double bonds.
- Functions include:
  - immune and inflammatory responses.
  - **platelet** aggregation.
  - temperature regulation by action on the **hypothalamus**.
  - exocrine/endocrine and reproductive function.
  - **renal blood flow** and renin production.
  - CNS neurotransmission.
  - pain perception and local sensitisation of tissues to inflammatory mediators.

Have varying effects on smooth muscle: PGE_2, PGI_2 and PGA_2 cause arteriolar dilatation, whereas $PGF_{2\alpha}$ causes vasodilatation in some vascular beds and vasoconstriction in others. $PGF_{2\alpha}$ and PGD_2 cause bronchoconstriction, whereas PGE_2 causes bronchodilatation. PGE_2 and $PGF_{2\alpha}$ cause uterine contraction and are used (as dinoprostone and **carboprost**, respectively) in obstetrics.

PGE_1 (as **alprostadil**) is used iv to maintain patency of the **ductus arteriosus** in **congenital heart disease** before corrective surgery. Tachy- or bradycardia, hypotension, pyrexia, DIC and convulsions may occur. It has been studied in the treatment of **ALI**. The analogues gemeprost and misoprostol are used in obstetrics (misoprostol is also used to prevent gastric ulcers associated with **NSAIDs**).

Half-life is a few minutes, with local metabolism of circulating PGs via the pulmonary, hepatic and renal circulations.

Many of the effects of NSAIDs involve inhibition of PG synthesis.

Protamine sulfate. Mixture of low-molecular-weight, cationic, basic proteins originally prepared from the sperm of salmon and other fish but now produced using recombinant technology. Used as a **heparin** antagonist (both unfractionated and low-molecular-weight heparin), and in the preparation of protamine zinc **insulin**. Has an anticoagulant effect when given alone in high doses, via inhibition of formation and action of thromboplastin. Binds and inactivates anionic, acidic heparin, forming a stable salt.

- Dosage: 1 mg iv neutralises 80–100 U heparin if given within 15 min of the latter's administration; less is required after longer intervals. Dosage is usually adjusted according to the patient's coagulation status. Should be given slowly (i.e., over 5 min); rapid administration may cause severe hypotension.
- Side effects: myocardial depression, bradycardia, pulmonary hypertension, **histamine** release, **complement** activation, **anaphylaxis**. These effects are more likely following rapid administration. Chronic exposure in diabetics, previous vasectomy or allergy to fish may predispose to allergic reactions.

Protein-binding. Occurs for many blood-borne substances, e.g. bilirubin, mineral ions, hormones, and many drugs. Important in drug **pharmacokinetics** because only the free unbound fraction is available to cross membranes, produce its effects, or be metabolised or excreted. Free fraction of drug is affected by plasma protein levels, drug concentration, pH and presence of other substances or drugs that compete for the same binding sites. The drug–protein complex may act as an **antigen** in **adverse drug reactions**.

- The main proteins involved are:
  - **albumin**: binds certain ions (e.g. **calcium**) and acidic drugs, e.g. **thiopental**, **phenytoin**, **warfarin**, **salicylates**.
  - α_1-acid glycoprotein: binds basic drugs, e.g. **local anaesthetic agents**, **propranolol**, **quinidine**.
  - globulins: bind e.g. **tubocurarine**.

See also, Anaesthesia, mechanism of; Drug interactions; Hypoproteinaemia

Protein C. Plasma protein that promotes **fibrinolysis** and inhibits thrombosis and inflammation. The circulating inactive form is activated by the enzyme complex of thrombin coupled with thrombomodulin (an endothelial surface membrane protein). Activated protein C blocks the activated forms of **coagulation** factors V and VIII, thereby inhibiting prothrombinase and factor Xase complexes. Activation of protein C may be impaired during **sepsis** and protein C may also be consumed. Reduced levels of protein C are associated with increased mortality. Inherited protein C abnormalities include protein C deficiency and activated protein C resistance (most commonly factor V Leiden), both of which predispose to venous thrombosis.

A recombinant form of activated protein C, drotrecogin alfa, was previously recommended by **NICE** in the treatment of severe **sepsis**; it was withdrawn from use worldwide in 2011 following a number of trials showing no benefit compared with placebo.

[Leiden; city in Netherlands where the factor was first identified in 1993]

Protein:creatinine ratio (PCR). Ratio of protein to creatinine in a random urine sample, used as a more accurate quantitative indicator of proteinuria than simple stick testing while not requiring a 24-h urine collection. A value >30 mg/mmol is usually taken to indicate significant proteinuria. Albumin:creatinine ratio has also been used.

Proteins. Polypeptide chains of **amino acids** (usually defined as over 50–500). May incorporate **carbohydrates** or **fats**. Present in all cell protoplasm and required for growth and healing. Involved in:

- cellular structure, e.g. collagen, **myosin**, **actin**, **membranes**
- **enzymes**.
- hormones and precursors.
- blood components, e.g. **immunoglobulins**, **haemoglobin**, **albumin**.

See also, Nitrogen balance; Nutrition

Prothrombin complex concentrate. Preparation derived from human plasma, containing a combination of **coagulation** factors II, VII, IX and X plus **protein C** and S. Used in major bleeding or before emergency surgery to reverse anticoagulation caused by **warfarin** and related drugs or in patients with congenital coagulation factor deficiency. Thrombotic events and **DIC** have been reported. Available as a dried powder requiring reconstitution; an adult dose costs £500–600. Dosage is estimated according to the pre-existing international normalised ratio (INR):

- 25 U/kg for INR 2 to <4, up to 2500 U
- 35 U/kg for INR 4–6, up to 3500 U
- 50 U/kg for INR >6, up to 5000 U

('U' referring to units of factor IX activity, which varies between vials).

Should be given at 0.12–8.4 ml/kg/min (~3–210 units/min). Blood should not be aspirated into the syringe in case of fibrin clot formation. Coagulation usually corrects within ~30 min and may remain so for up to 12–24 h.

Prothrombin time, *see Coagulation studies*

Proton pump inhibitors. Group of drugs that selectively inhibit the H^+/K^+-ATPase enzyme located on the luminal surface of the gastric parietal cells, thus virtually abolishing gastric acid production. Used to treat **peptic ulcer disease** and severe **gastro-oesophageal reflux** and to decrease the risk from **aspiration of gastric contents** in high-risk patients. Should be used with caution in liver disease. Include **omeprazole**, **lansoprazole**, **pantoprazole** and **rabeprazole**.

Pruritus. Itch-like sensation in the absence of a normal stimulus; can arise from cutaneous, neurological or psychological triggers. Afferent pathways involve a number of inflammatory mediators, e.g. **histamine** peripherally and **5-HT** centrally.

- Causes may be:
  - cutaneous:
    - release of histamine, e.g. due to drugs (**morphine**, **cyclizine**, antibiotics, **anaphylaxis**) or other cutaneous stimuli, including trauma, infections/infestations, systemic inflammatory conditions.

  - deposition of other irritant substances, e.g. bile salts, calcium.
  - other skin diseases.
- neurological:
  - interaction with central **neurotransmitters** (e.g. epidural/**spinal opioids**).
  - cerebral lesions.
  - **peripheral neuropathy**.
- psychological.

Often seen after administration of anaesthetic or related drugs. Although many drugs (e.g. **propofol, ondansetron**) have been studied as possible prophylactic or therapeutic agents, supporting evidence for most is weak. For systemic opioid-induced pruritus, **antihistamine drugs** may be used, while **opioid receptor antagonists** are effective following epidural/spinal opioids.

Pseudocholinesterase, *see Cholinesterase, plasma*

Pseudocritical temperature. Temperature at which gas mixtures separate into their component parts. Varies with pressure: for **Entonox**, highest (–5.5°C) at 117 bar, and decreases above and below this pressure. Thus equals –7°C for Entonox cylinders (135 bar) and –30°C for pipelines (4 bar).

Pseudomembranous colitis, *see Clostridial infections*

Pseudomonas infections. Commonly seen in hospitals, systemic effects occur via release of **endo-** and **exotoxins**. Manifestations include **catheter-related sepsis**, severe **chest infection** (especially in those receiving IPPV), **meningitis** and general features of **sepsis**. Infection typically results in a characteristic odour. Treatment following culture and sensitivity testing consists of an antipseudomonas **penicillin** (or third-generation **cephalosporin**) combined with an **aminoglycoside**.
See also, Nosocomial infection

Psoas compartment block. Regional anaesthesia technique used to block components of the **lumbar plexus** (specifically, femoral, obturator and lateral femoral cutaneous nerves) and part of the **sacral plexus**, which lie between psoas major anteriorly and quadratus lumborum posteriorly, e.g. for hip and femoral shaft surgery.

With the patient in the lateral position with the operative side uppermost and hips partly flexed, a skin wheal is raised 3–5 cm lateral to the lower border of the spinous process of L4. A 10–15-cm needle is inserted perpendicular to the skin until it contacts the transverse process, then withdrawn and redirected slightly caudad to pass the process. A nerve stimulator may be used to identify the optimal injection point (eliciting quadriceps twitch with a threshold of 0.3–0.5 mA). Alternatively, a loss-of-resistance technique may be used to identify the psoas compartment (usually at 10–12 cm) as for **epidural anaesthesia. Ultrasound** has also been used. 30–40 ml **local anaesthetic agent** is injected.

Complications include subarachnoid, epidural and intravascular injection.

Psychological aspects of intensive care, *see Confusion in the intensive care unit; Intensive care follow-up; Post-intensive care syndrome; Post-traumatic stress disorder*

Psychoprophylaxis. Technique used in **obstetric analgesia and anaesthesia** to increase comfort and relaxation during labour. Requires antenatal education about pregnancy and labour, and training in relaxation and breathing techniques.

PT, Prothrombin time, *see Coagulation studies*

PTS, *see Paediatric trauma score*

PTT, Partial thromboplastin time, *see Coagulation studies*

Pudendal nerve block. Used bilaterally to provide analgesia during/after gynaecological surgery and in **obstetric analgesia and anaesthesia**, especially for forceps and ventouse delivery. In obstetrics, requires adequate time between performance of the block and attempted delivery to be useful.

The pudendal nerve (S2–4) arises from the **sacral plexus** and leaves the pelvis through the greater sciatic foramen, passing behind the ischial spine and sacrospinal ligament to re-enter the pelvis through the lesser sciatic foramen. It supplies the perineum, vulva and lower vagina.

- Techniques:
  - transvaginal approach: with the patient in the lithotomy position, two fingers palpate the ischial spine from within the vagina. A 12.5-cm guarded needle is introduced 1.2 cm beyond the spine, into the sacrospinal ligament, and the needle point extended. After negative aspiration for blood, 10 ml **local anaesthetic agent** is injected.
  - transperineal approach: a needle is introduced through a point midway between the anus and ischial tuberosity, and directed as above by a finger in the vagina.

Ultrasound has also been used. Local infiltration of the labia is required to block cutaneous branches of the genitofemoral and ilioinguinal nerves.

Pugh, Benjamin (1715–1798). Shropshire-born surgeon and apothecary; practised in Essex. Early advocate of vaccination against smallpox and author of *A Treatise of Midwifery* in 1754. Advocated the use of an air pipe, inserted into the larynx, to maintain the airway of neonates during delayed breech extraction.
See also, Cardiopulmonary resuscitation, neonatal

Pulmonary artery catheterisation. Performed using flow-directed balloon-tipped pulmonary artery catheters, introduced into clinical practice in the early 1970s by Swan and Ganz (after whom one commercial device is named), among much controversy.

- Catheters may have some of the following features:
  - 70 cm long, marked every 10 cm.
  - channels/lumina:
    - distal (opens at the tip).
    - proximal (opens 30 cm from the tip).
    - for inflating the balloon (1–1.5 ml air used).
    - connections to a thermistor, a few cm from the tip.
    - fibreoptic bundles for continuous **oximetry**.
    - others include those for cardiac pacing and Doppler imaging.
- Insertion:
  - as for **central venous cannulation**, usually employing the **Seldinger technique**. The right internal jugular vein is most commonly used. The catheter is threaded down an 8 G introducer sheath, with continuous visible pressure monitoring from the distal lumen.

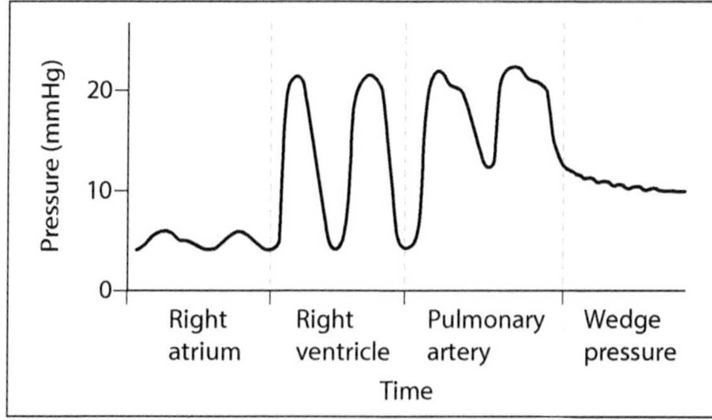

Fig. 134 Pressure trace obtained during placement of a pulmonary artery catheter

The balloon is inflated in the right atrium and directed by the flow of blood into the pulmonary artery via the right ventricle. **Pulmonary capillary wedge pressure** is displayed when the balloon occludes a pulmonary vessel; the catheter tip is now separated from the left atrium by a continuous column of blood. Placement is confirmed by the changes in the pressure trace obtained (Fig. 134).
   - once inserted, the balloon is left deflated until wedge pressure measurement is required, to reduce risk of pulmonary artery damage and infarction. The distal lumen pressure should always be displayed, to alert to accidental wedging.
- Information gained:
   - mixed venous, right atrial and ventricular gas tensions and O_2 saturations; e.g. for estimation of cardiac **shunt**. Continuous monitoring of mixed venous O_2 saturation is possible via fibreoptic bundles.
   - measurement of right atrial and ventricular pressures, **pulmonary artery pressure** and pulmonary capillary wedge pressure. By convention, measured at end-systole and end-expiration.
   - measurement of right ventricular **ejection fraction**.
   - **cardiac output measurement**.
   - derived data:
      - **systemic** and **pulmonary vascular resistance**.
      - **cardiac index**, **stroke volume**/index.
- Uses:
   - investigating cardiac shunts.
   - monitoring the above pressures and optimising fluid therapy; particularly useful when right atrial pressures do not reflect left heart function; e.g. left ventricular failure or infarction, severe **bundle branch block**, **pulmonary hypertension**, **cardiac tamponade** and constrictive **pericarditis**, valvular heart disease (*for interpretation, etc., see Pulmonary capillary wedge pressure*).
   - measuring cardiac output and derived data.
   - monitoring mixed venous O_2 saturation as a continuous indicator of cardiac output and tissue perfusion, e.g. in ICU.
   - as a route for **cardiac pacing**.
   - infusion of drugs into the pulmonary circulation, e.g. **prostacyclin** in pulmonary hypertension.
- Complications:
   - as for central venous cannulation.
   - catheter knotting or coiling.
   - damage to valves, myocardium, etc.
   - pulmonary artery damage or rupture.
   - pulmonary infarction.
   - incorrect positioning, measurement and interpretation.

Although previously widely used in critically ill patients, its use has been associated with increased mortality, and has declined since the widespread introduction of alternative methods of cardiac output monitoring.

[Harold JC Swan (1922–2005), Irish-born US cardiologist; William Ganz (1919–2009), Los Angeles cardiologist]

Gidwani UK, Goel S (2016). Cardiol Rev; 24: 1–13

Pulmonary artery pressure (PAP). Typically one-fifth of systemic circulatory pressure; normal ranges are 15–30 mmHg systolic, 0–8 mmHg diastolic and 10–15 mmHg mean. Usually measured by right-sided cardiac catheterisation. Changes may indicate changes in **pulmonary capillary wedge pressure** and **pulmonary vascular resistance**.

Pulmonary capillary wedge pressure (PCWP; Pulmonary wedge pressure, PWP; Pulmonary artery occlusion pressure, PAOP). Pressure measured within the pulmonary arterial system during **pulmonary artery catheterisation**, with the tip of the catheter 'wedged' in a tapering branch of one of the pulmonary arteries. In most patients, represents left atrial filling pressure and thus left **ventricular end-diastolic pressure** (LVEDP). Thus an indirect indicator of left ventricular end-diastolic volume and myocardial fibre length (*see Starling's law*). Also indicates the likelihood (with measurement of plasma colloid **osmotic pressure**) of **pulmonary oedema** formation, assuming normal pulmonary capillary permeability.
- Normal range: 6–12 mmHg; usually 1–4 mmHg less than pulmonary artery diastolic pressure (PADP). Traditionally measured at end-expiration.
- Values should be interpreted with caution in:
   - left ventricular failure: LVEDP may exceed PCWP.
   - mitral valve disease: in stenosis PCWP may exceed LVEDP; in regurgitation large 'v' waves interfere with the PCWP waveform.
   - raised intrathoracic pressure, e.g. **PEEP**: LVEDP may exceed PCWP.
   - non-compliant left ventricle: LVEDP may exceed PCWP.
   - aortic regurgitation: LVEDP may greatly exceed PCWP.

Gradients between PADP, PCWP and LVEDP may be increased in tachycardia and increased **pulmonary vascular resistance**. The position of the catheter tip is also important; a continuous column of blood between the catheter and the left ventricle only occurs if the tip lies in zone 3 of the lung (*see Pulmonary circulation*). Although the catheter usually flows to zone 3, especially in the supine position, repositioning of the patient may alter the zonal distribution.

The waveform resembles the **venous waveform**, with 'a', 'c' and 'v' waves, and swings with respiration. PCWP should not exceed PADP.

As with **CVP** interpretation, trends are more useful than single values. Response of PCWP to drug or iv fluid administration may be used to indicate intravascular volume status and cardiac function, and guide therapy. Pulmonary oedema is likely at PCWP above 18–20 mmHg, with normal colloid osmotic pressure.

Pulmonary circulation. Low-pressure/low-resistance system in series with the systemic circulation, receiving the whole cardiac output. The pulmonary artery divides into right and left main pulmonary arteries. Pulmonary arteries are thin-walled and easily distensible, lying close to the corresponding airways in connective tissue sheaths, eventually dividing to form capillaries with a total gas exchange interface of about 70 m^2. Venules run close to the septa that separate the **lung** segments and drain into four main pulmonary veins, which deliver oxygenated blood to the left atrium.

The separate bronchial circulation supplies the lower airways down to the respiratory bronchioles, local connective tissue and the visceral pleura; it arises from the aorta and eventually drains via the azygos system into the pulmonary veins, i.e., representing an anatomical **shunt**.

The diameter of 'extra-alveolar' vessels (those running through lung parenchyma) is affected by lung volume, via the pull of lung parenchyma on their walls. That of 'alveolar' pulmonary vessels (predominantly capillaries) depends on the difference between arterial (P_a), venous (P_v) and alveolar (P_A) pressures, and thus on gravity. Four zones have been described by West, from above downwards:
- zone 1: lung apex; P_A exceeds both P_a and P_v; thus no flow occurs. Does not occur at normal BP in normal lungs.
- zone 2: $P_a > P_A > P_v$; thus flow depends on the difference between P_a and P_A, and not on P_v.
- zone 3: $P_a > P_v > P_A$; i.e., flow depends on the difference between P_a and P_v, as usually occurs in other tissues.
- zone 4: suggested as existing at lung bases; pulmonary interstitial pressure exceeds P_a, thus impairing blood flow.

The vessels are supplied by sympathetic vasoconstrictor (α-receptors) and vasodilator (β_2-receptors) fibres, and by parasympathetic vasodilator fibres. However, resting vascular tone is minimal, with vessels almost maximally dilated in the resting state. Other factors affecting vessel calibre include vascular responses to local changes, e.g. **hypoxic pulmonary vasoconstriction** and other factors affecting **pulmonary vascular resistance**.

The pulmonary circulation contains about 10%–20% of the total blood volume (i.e., 0.5–1.0 l). It changes during respiration (especially **IPPV**) and may increase by 25%–40% in moving from the erect to the supine position.

[John B West, Australian-born Californian physiologist]

See also, Starling resistor; Ventilation/perfusion mismatch

Pulmonary embolism (PE). Mechanical obstruction of a pulmonary artery/arteriole; usually refers to blood-borne thrombus. The most common cause of death within the first 10 postoperative days. Thrombus usually arises from a **DVT** in the legs/pelvis, although the venae cavae and right side of the heart are sometimes sources. The effects depend on the size and distribution of the PE; release of vasoactive mediators (e.g. **prostaglandins**) may contribute to resultant vasospasm. Massive PEs cause rapid respiratory and cardiovascular collapse, and death. Smaller PEs may cause few haemodynamic effects, but may result in infarction of a section of lung tissue if collateral blood flow is inadequate. Multiple PEs may cause widespread pulmonary vascular obstruction and lead to **pulmonary hypertension**.

Risk factors are as for DVT.
- Features:
    - pleuritic chest pain, haemoptysis, dyspnoea and mild pyrexia in small PEs.
    - cyanosis, tachypnoea, hypotension, tachycardia, raised JVP and bronchospasm. Third and fourth **heart sounds** may be present. A pleural rub may develop.
    - arterial **blood gas interpretation** reveals **hypoxaemia** and hypocapnia, with subsequent metabolic acidosis in severe PE. During anaesthesia, end-tidal CO_2 concentration may fall dramatically because of increased **dead space** and reduced cardiac output.
    - right axis deviation, right **bundle branch block** and T inversion in leads V_{1-4} may occur in the **ECG**; both a normal ECG and the 'classic' $S_1Q_3T_3$ pattern are rarely seen.
    - **CXR** may show enlarged proximal pulmonary arteries with peripheral oligaemia, but is usually non-specific. Wedge-shaped infarcts (Hampton's hump), elevation of the ipsilateral diaphragm and **pleural effusion** may subsequently develop.

Definitive diagnosis is usually made by CT angiography or ventilation–perfusion scan (if the former is unavailable). MRI and echocardiography imaging techniques are also used.

Features of DVT may be present. A normal D-dimer concentration reliably excludes PE.
- Management:
    - immediate **CPR** if required. A precordial thump may break up a large PE and improve circulation.
    - O_2 therapy, **iv fluids**, **inotropic drugs**, analgesia.
    - anticoagulation: **fondaparinux**, **rivaroxaban**, **dabigatran** or **heparin** (low mw is recommended except in severe renal impairment and/or if the ability to reverse it readily is required) in the acute phase; maintenance can be provided with **warfarin** or one of the direct oral anticoagulant drugs as for DVT. **Fibrinolytic drugs** are indicated in the presence of **shock** or sustained hypotension.
    - surgical or catheter embolectomy may be required for large PEs. Ligation of the inferior vena caval/superficial femoral vein, or insertion of a vena caval filter, may be required for recurrent PEs.

[Aubrey Otis Hampton (1900–1955), US radiologist]

Di Nisio M, van Es N, Büller HR (2017). Lancet; 388: 3060–73

See also, Gas embolism; Amniotic fluid embolism; Fat embolism

Pulmonary fibrosis. Thickening and infiltration of alveolar walls and perialveolar tissue.
- May result from:
    - localised loss of lung parenchyma, e.g. following infection, infarction or aspiration of irritant substances (e.g. **aspiration of gastric contents**). May also follow treatment with **cytotoxic drugs**, e.g. **bleomycin**. Causes decreased movement and breath sounds, dullness to percussion and increased vocal resonance. Neighbouring structures (e.g. trachea) may be pulled towards the affected portion.
    - generalised **alveolitis**: a degree of fibrosis may remain following **ALI**.
    - idiopathic interstitial pneumonitis: progressive, irreversible and usually lethal.

Loss of the pulmonary vascular bed may lead to **pulmonary hypertension** and **cor pulmonale**. Typically, there is hypoxaemia with hypocapnia due to hyperventilation. **$\dot{V}/\dot{Q}$ mismatch** is now thought to be responsible for the hypoxaemia, rather than alveolar membrane thickening, as previously suspected. **Diffusing capacity**, **compliance** and lung volumes are reduced, with normal **FEV_1/FVC** ratio.

Work of breathing is increased; rapid, shallow breathing is common. **CXR** may reveal diffuse nodular/reticular shadowing, with local contraction in focal disease.

Treatment is of the underlying cause; **corticosteroids** are often used.

- Anaesthesia: although the pulmonary defect is restrictive instead of obstructive, principles are as for **COPD**.

Pulmonary function tests, *see Lung function tests*

Pulmonary hypertension (PH). Defined as mean **pulmonary artery pressure** (PAP) >25 mmHg at rest, measured by **cardiac catheterisation**. Prevalence is ~100 per million in the UK. Prognosis varies widely according to clinical subtype, patient characteristics and response to treatment. Absolute PAP values are not usually of prognostic value; clinical features are more useful for assessing severity. High-risk features (implying a 1-year mortality of >10%) include rapid progression of symptoms, signs of right ventricular (RV) failure and repeated syncope.

Anaesthesia presents significant risk to patients with PH, who should ideally be managed in specialist centres. Patients with PH requiring intensive care support have a mortality of ~40%. PH also carries a very high maternal mortality (~40%–50%) and pregnancy is actively discouraged.

- Previously described as either 'primary' or 'secondary', now classified by the World Health Organization into 5 groups according to pathology, clinical features and treatment strategies (although individual patients may overlap multiple groups):
    - group 1: pulmonary arterial hypertension (PAH). Characterised by PH with **pulmonary capillary wedge pressure** (PCWP) <15 mmHg and **pulmonary vascular resistance** (PVR) of >3 **Wood units**. Causes include: idiopathic (previously termed 'primary'); heritable; drug-induced (e.g. by **amfetamines**); connective tissue diseases (e.g. **systemic sclerosis**); portal hypertension; schistosomiasis; and **congenital heart disease** (commonly left-to-right shunt lesions, e.g. **ASD**, **VSD**, patent **ductus arteriosus**). Also includes pulmonary veno-occlusive disease and persistent pulmonary hypertension of the newborn (PPHN).
    - group 2: PH due to left heart disease resulting in pulmonary venous/capillary hypertension, e.g. in left ventricular failure, left heart inflow/outflow tract obstruction (e.g. **mitral stenosis**).
    - group 3: PH due to lung diseases that result in chronic **hypoxaemia**, e.g. **COPD**, **pulmonary fibrosis**, **sleep-disordered breathing**.
    - group 4: PH due to chronic **PE** or other pulmonary artery obstruction.
    - group 5: PH with unclear/multifactorial mechanisms.

Pathological mechanisms are complex and variable, but include: vascular remodelling of the pulmonary arteries with medial hypertrophy and intimal thickening; impaired production of **nitric oxide** and **prostacyclin**; localised inflammation and fibrosis; and **hypoxic pulmonary vasoconstriction**. The increased RV **afterload** causes progressive hypertrophy and dilatation as ventricular failure supervenes; biventricular failure may then ensue, owing to ventricular interdependence.

- Features:
    - fatigue, dyspnoea, angina, syncope, haemoptysis.
    - low cardiac output, cyanosis, features of right ventricular enlargement/failure, e.g. sternal heave, peripheral oedema.
    - **ECG** findings: right axis deviation, right bundle branch block, **prolonged Q–T syndromes**, right atrial and ventricular hypertrophy.
    - **CXR**: right atrial and ventricular enlargement, large pulmonary arteries with peripheral pruning.
- Diagnosis and assessment:
    - **echocardiography** is used initially to assess the probability of PH; suggestive features include peak tricuspid regurgitation velocity of >3.4 m/s, RV/RA enlargement and significant diastolic pulmonary valve regurgitation. If PH is suspected, high resolution chest **CT**, **lung function tests** ± $\dot{V}/\dot{Q}$ scans are then performed, and cardiac catheterisation considered.
    - definitive diagnosis requires right heart catheterisation, which is always performed before commencing specific treatment for PH.
- Treatment:
    - supportive treatment includes oral **anticoagulant drugs**, **diuretics**, and **oxygen therapy**.
    - specific drug therapy includes **calcium channel blocking drugs**, prostacyclin analogues, **endothelin receptor antagonists** and type 5 **phosphodiesterase inhibitors**, alone or in combination.
    - treatment of the underlying cause where possible.
    - **lung-transplantation** (or rarely, **heart-lung transplantation**).
- Anaesthetic management:
    - centres around supporting right ventricular output by optimising **preload** and **contractility** and avoiding factors that increase PVR (e.g. hypoxia, acidosis).
    - **SVR** should be proactively maintained and tachycardia avoided to protect **coronary blood flow** to the right heart.
    - combinations of **midazolam**, **fentanyl**, and **etomidate** may be used for induction. A balanced technique with volatile agent and opioids may be used for maintenance. N_2O is often avoided as it may increase PVR.
    - direct **arterial blood pressure measurement** is usual.
    - **transoesophageal echocardiography** may be used to direct intraoperative management.
    - an acute rise in PVR ('PVR crisis') is managed with 100% oxygen, adequate anaesthesia/neuromuscular blockade, hyperventilation (to achieve respiratory alkalosis) and pulmonary vasodilators (e.g. inhaled nitric oxide).

Galie N, Humbert M, Vachiery JL, et al (2016). Eur Heart J; 37: 67–119

See also, Cor pulmonale

Pulmonary irritant receptors. Receptors situated between airway epithelial cells, responsible for initiating bronchospasm and hyperpnoea in response to inhaled noxious gases, smoke, dust and cold air. Afferent impulses pass via the vagi to the medulla. May be involved in initiating **asthma** attacks.

Pulmonary oedema. Increased pulmonary **ECF** (normally minimal). Small amounts of fluid normally pass through the capillary wall into the interstitial space of the lung. The junctions between alveolar epithelial cells are relatively resistant to fluid, which is removed by the lymphatic system at about 10 ml/h. Lymphatic removal may increase dramatically if transudation into the interstitial space increases. Net flux into the interstitial space is governed by **Starling forces**.

- Mechanisms of formation of pulmonary oedema:
  - alteration of Starling forces:
    - increased hydrostatic pressure, e.g. hypervolaemia, left ventricular failure, **mitral stenosis**.
    - decreased plasma **oncotic pressure**, e.g. **hypoproteinaemia**.
    - acute severe subatmospheric airway pressure, e.g. upper **airway obstruction**.
  - damage to the alveolar–capillary membrane, e.g. **ALI**.
  - impairment of lymphatic drainage, e.g. lymphangitis carcinomatosis, silicosis.
  - causes of uncertain aetiology:
    - neurogenic: thought to involve sudden **catecholamine** release following **TBI**, with vasoconstriction increasing lung capillary pressures and capillary permeability.
    - following **naloxone** administration: also thought to involve catecholamine release.
    - in **opioid poisoning**, possibly related to decreased vascular permeability.
    - following pulmonary surgery or re-expansion of a **pneumothorax**: probably involves local changes in capillary pressures and permeability.
    - after exposure to high altitude, possibly via pulmonary vasoconstriction.

As fluid clearance mechanisms are overwhelmed, interstitial oedema increases, until alveolar oedema occurs. Eventually, frothy oedema fluid fills the airways, impairing gas exchange. Airways and pulmonary vessels become narrowed by interstitial oedema, and **FRC** and **compliance** decrease.

- Features:
  - dyspnoea, tachypnoea, cough with pink frothy sputum, and tachycardia. Respiratory distress is worse lying flat (orthopnoea).
  - wheeze and basal crepitations on auscultation.
  - features of **respiratory failure**.
  - arterial **blood gas interpretation** usually reveals **hypoxaemia**, with hypocapnia secondary to hyperventilation. Metabolic acidosis may be present in severe cases.
  - **CXR** features include those of the underlying condition. Lung oedema itself appears as fluffy shadowing, typically perihilar ('bat's wing') in left ventricular failure and patchy ('cotton-wool') and peripheral in ALI. Bronchial and vascular markings may appear thickened due to interstitial oedema. **Kerley's** (B) **lines** and fluid in the transverse fissure may be present.

Differentiation between hydrostatic and other causes may be aided by measurement of **pulmonary capillary wedge pressure**. Alveolar fluid protein content may also be measured. Total lung water content has been measured using radioactive or dye dilution techniques.

- Treatment of severe acute pulmonary oedema:
  - of the underlying condition.
  - O_2 therapy. **CPAP** may be useful.
  - sitting the patient, with the legs over the edge of the bed.
  - **diuretics**, e.g. **furosemide** 20–120 mg iv (causes vasodilatation and diuresis).
  - opioids, e.g. **morphine**, **diamorphine** 1–5 mg iv (for anxiolysis and vasodilatation).
  - **inotropic** and **vasodilator drugs**.
  - **IPPV** may be required. Gas exchange is usually improved by **PEEP**.
  - venesection may be performed for pulmonary oedema due to volume overload, with removal of 200–500 ml blood.

Pulmonary stretch receptors. Mechanoreceptors within the smooth muscle of the lower airways; transmit impulses via the vagi to the dorsal medulla. Excitation limits inspiration during pulmonary overinflation (**Hering–Breuer reflex**). Sensitivity is increased by decreased arterial $P\text{CO}_2$ and increased pulmonary venous pressure. May also be involved in other pulmonary reflexes, e.g. **gasp** and **deflation reflexes**.

Pulmonary valve lesions. Include:

- pulmonary stenosis (PS): may occur at the valve (90%), infundibulum or within the artery. Almost always congenital, accounting for 5%–10% of **congenital heart disease**. Other causes include **rheumatic fever** and **carcinoid syndrome**. Usually asymptomatic; if severe, PS may cause fatigue, dyspnoea and angina secondary to decreased cardiac output. Right ventricular (and later atrial) hypertrophy may occur, with associated diastolic dysfunction. May be associated with right-to-left **shunt** and cyanosis, e.g. **Fallot's tetralogy**.

  Features: ejection systolic murmur at the upper left sternal edge, heard best during inspiration. Splitting of the second **heart sound** is increased, with a quiet pulmonary component in severe PS. Right ventricular and atrial enlargement may be suggested by the **ECG** and **CXR**; a prominent pulmonary artery and pulmonary oligaemia may appear on the latter.

  During anaesthesia, increased right ventricular O_2 consumption (e.g. caused by tachycardia and increased contractility) should be avoided.
- pulmonary regurgitation (PR): usually a feature of **pulmonary hypertension**, and results from dilatation of the valve ring. Other causes include congenital absence of the valve, **endocarditis** (usually in iv drug abusers) and surgical valvotomy. Causes right ventricular hypertrophy with subsequent dilatation if persistent and severe.

  Features: high-pitched blowing diastolic murmur at the upper left sternal edge.

Pulmonary vascular resistance (PVR). **Resistance** in the **pulmonary circulation**, analogous to **SVR**. May be calculated using the principle of Ohm's law:

$$\underset{(\textbf{dyne}\ \text{s/cm}^5)}{\text{PVR}} = \frac{\text{mean pulmonary artery pressure} - \text{left atrial pressure (mmHg)} \times 80}{\textbf{cardiac output}\ \text{(l/min)}}$$

where 80 is a correction factor.

Normally 20–120 dyne s/cm^5 (N.B. 1 dyne s/cm^5 = 100 N s/m^5). May also be expressed as **Wood units**.

Resistance is distributed more evenly than in the systemic circulation, with approximately 50% residing in the arteries and arterioles, 30% in the capillaries and 20% in the veins. The pulmonary arteries are thin-walled, large in diameter and easily distensible. The pulmonary circulation is therefore more dependent on gravity, posture and the relationship between alveolar and intravascular pressures than on vascular muscular tone.

- PVR is affected by:
  - passive factors:
    - lung expansion: at lung volumes below **FRC**, the radial forces holding the extra-alveolar vessels

open are reduced, thus increasing PVR. However, at high lung volumes, the increased airway pressures associated with hyperexpansion may compress the vessels, also increasing PVR. PVR is thus lowest at lung volumes around FRC.
- intravascular pressures: PVR falls when either pulmonary artery pressure or pulmonary venous pressure increases, because of recruitment of previously closed vessels or distension of individual capillary segments.
- cardiac output: as pulmonary blood flow increases, vessel diameter increases, thus reducing PVR.
- **haematocrit** and blood **viscosity**.

- active factors via changes in vascular tone:
  - **hypoxia** (*see Hypoxic pulmonary vasoconstriction*), **hypercapnia** and **acidosis** increase PVR, especially in combination, whereas their opposites decrease PVR.
  - drugs and biological mediators, e.g. **vasoconstrictor drugs, 5-HT** and **histamine** increase PVR whereas **vasodilator drugs**, **nitric oxide**, **prostacyclin** and **acetylcholine** decrease it. Drugs may also affect PVR via changes in cardiac output and lung volumes.
  - neural control: **sympathetic nervous system** supplies vasoconstrictor (**α-adrenergic receptor**) and vasodilator (β-adrenergic receptor) fibres to the pulmonary vessels, while the **parasympathetic nervous system** supplies cholinergic vasodilator fibres.

In addition, local vascular resistance may be increased by **PE**, **atelectasis**, **pleural effusions** and surgery.

PVR may be corrected for differences in body size by multiplying by body **surface area** (PVR index).

See also, Lung; Pulmonary artery catheterisation; Pulmonary hypertension

Pulse. Traditionally palpated at the wrist, but commonly palpated at the head and neck during anaesthesia (*see Carotid arteries*).

- May be assessed for:
  - **heart rate**: speed, rhythm, regularity.
  - volume and character, i.e., reflecting **pulse pressure** and **arterial waveform**. **Pulsus alternans** and **pulsus paradoxus** are two specific abnormalities.
  - simultaneous pulsation at upper and lower limb arteries; femoral delay occurs in **coarctation of the aorta**.

Pulse deficit. Difference between the auscultated heart rate and palpated pulse rate. Occurs when one heart beat follows another so quickly that ventricular filling is insufficient for a palpable pulsation, e.g. in **ventricular ectopic beats** and **AF**.

Pulse detector. Several devices have been used to detect the **pulse**, e.g. to monitor heart rate or to aid in **arterial BP measurement**. Each utilises a small **transducer** positioned over a peripheral artery or attached to a digit:

- microphone or **Doppler** probe.
- finger probe containing a light source and photocell that detects changes in reflected or transmitted light due to arterial pulsation.

Simple devices emit a noise or flashing light in time with the pulse, or register the pulse rate on a meter. These have been largely replaced by more sophisticated devices displaying a waveform, e.g. **pulse oximeter**.

Pulse oximeter. Device used to determine arterial O_2 **saturation** using **oximetry**. Consists of the following components:

- two light-emitting diodes (LEDs) within the probe emit monochromatic light at red (660 nm) and infrared (940 nm) wavelengths.
- a photodiode on the opposite side of the probe detects the transmitted light; because it is unable to differentiate between the wavelengths, each LED is alternately switched on and off, the timing of which allows identification of red and infrared pulses. The periods when both LEDs are off allow compensation for ambient light conditions.
- the signal is converted to a DC component representing tissue background, venous blood and the constant part of arterial blood flow, and an AC component representing pulsatile arterial blood flow. The former is discarded, the latter amplified and averaged over a few seconds.
- the ratio of pulsatile transmitted red to infrared light is calculated and compared with stored calibration curves (derived from healthy human volunteers) to give an estimated S_pO_2 (suggested as appropriate notation of S_aO_2 measured by a pulse oximeter).
- the signal is displayed ideally as a continuous trace, showing quality of signal and a numerical value of S_pO_2. Most modern machines automatically adjust gain to maintain a constant size of trace.

An important part of routine **monitoring** during anaesthesia/sedation and on intensive care. Oximetry is also used to monitor **sleep apnoea** during sleep studies, in cardiac and respiratory function testing, **CPR** and assessment of peripheral circulation. It has been shown to detect desaturation in patients when clinical assessment reveals no abnormality, e.g. during anaesthesia, **recovery** and transport of patients.

- Inaccuracy may result from excessive ambient light, movement artefact, poor peripheral perfusion, electrical interference, venous congestion, and when S_aO_2 is less than 80% (as calibration data below this level are extrapolated). Response time to detecting desaturation varies with probe location (e.g. up to 30–60 s with a finger probe). Coloured nail polish may produce inaccuracies (tends to increase readings). Effects of other pigments:
  - carboxyhaemoglobin: most is counted as HbO; thus S_pO_2 is falsely high.
  - methaemoglobin and bilirubin: counted as Hb; thus S_pO_2 is falsely low (but may be falsely high if true saturation is very low, i.e., <70%).
  - methylthioninium chloride (methylene blue), indocyanine green, etc.: may temporarily decrease S_pO_2 for a few minutes after iv injection.
  - **fetal haemoglobin, polycythaemia**: no effect.

Machines are calibrated during manufacture. Some are preset for low values of carboxyhaemoglobin and methaemoglobin. More recent designs use multiple wavelengths of light to allow estimation of carboxy- and methaemoglobin levels, as well as Hb concentration.

Burns and pressure sores have been reported following prolonged use, especially with finger probes on children.

Pulse pressure. Difference between systolic and diastolic blood pressures, normally about 35–45 mmHg.

A narrow pulse pressure is usually caused by reduced stroke volume, e.g. due to **cardiac failure** or **aortic stenosis**.

Pulse pressure may be widened by: increased cardiac output (e.g. **exercise, pregnancy, anaemia**); reduced arterial compliance (e.g. **atherosclerosis**); **aortic regurgitation.** It also widens as the **arterial waveform** moves peripherally.
See also, Pulse

Pulseless electrical activity (PEA). Cardiac state in which there is electrical activity adequate to produce myocardial contraction but contractions either do not occur or they do not produce a detectable cardiac output. Distinguished from **electromechanical dissociation** (EMD), in which there are no contractions despite apparently adequate electrical activity. The term pseudo-EMD has been proposed for PEA in which flow is so low it cannot be detected by non-invasive means.
See also, Cardiac arrest

Pulsus alternans. Alternating weak and strong **pulses** reflecting similar alterations in left ventricular filling and output. Common in left ventricular failure.
See also, Arterial waveform

Pulsus paradoxus. Defined as an abnormally large inspiratory decrease in **arterial BP** (e.g. greater than 10 mmHg). The 'paradox' lies in the observation that the radial pulse may disappear during inspiration despite the continued presence of the cardiac impulse at the precordium. **Cardiac output** and BP fall due to reduced left ventricular filling. Proposed mechanisms for this include: pooling of blood in the **pulmonary circulation** due to increased negative intrathoracic pressure (e.g. in **COPD** or **upper airway obstruction**); and impaired LV filling due to inspiratory RV filling within a restricted pericardium (e.g. **cardiac tamponade**, constrictive **pericarditis**).
See also, Pulse

Pumping effect. Increased **vaporiser** output when pressure within the breathing system/back bar increases intermittently, e.g. during IPPV or use of the O_2 flush. During the pressure increase, gas within the back bar (i.e., containing the set concentration of volatile agent) is compressed back into the vaporiser chamber, where it becomes saturated with the volatile agent. When the downstream pressure falls, this gas re-expands into the back bar, thus increasing the concentration of volatile agent within the back bar. In addition, saturated vapour in the vaporiser chamber may be forced retrogradely into the vaporiser bypass, increasing the delivered concentration of volatile agent further.

The effect is greatest at low vaporiser settings and low gas flows, and may be minimised by:
- increasing resistance to flow through the vaporiser and bypass.
- lengthening the path through which the retrograde flow must pass before reaching the bypass.
- minimising the volume of the vaporiser chamber.
- placing a non-return valve downstream of the vaporiser.

Pupil. Central orifice of the iris; normally 1–8 mm in size. Contraction (miosis) is caused by parasympathetic stimulation, drugs including **opioid analgesic drugs** and anaesthetic agents, and pontine lesions. Dilatation (mydriasis) is caused by sympathetic stimulation and **anticholinergic drugs.** Dilated pupils may occur during **awareness** or **hypercapnia** during anaesthesia.

- Abnormal pupils and **pupillary reflex** may occur in particular lesions, e.g.:
  - ipsilateral fixed dilatation in **head injury**, followed by bilateral dilatation due to herniation of the brain through the tentorium, causing compression of the third **cranial nerve.**
  - **Horner's syndrome.**
  - Argyll Robertson pupil: small and irregular, fixed to light but responsive to accommodation. Classically occurs in tertiary **syphilis** but may occur in **diabetes mellitus** and brainstem **encephalitis.**
  - Holmes–Adie pupil: large and regular, with sluggish light reflex. Often associated with loss of knee reflexes but no other pathology.

[Douglas Argyll Robertson (1837–1909), Scottish surgeon; Gordon M Holmes (1876–1965), Irish-born English neurologist; William J Adie (1886–1935), Australian-born English neurologist]

Pupillary reflex. Easily tested reflex arcs involving the pupils:
- light reflex (Fig. 135): pupillary constriction normally follows direct or contralateral (consensual) illumination. Occasionally, phasic contraction and dilatation occur (hippus). Pathway: from retina via optic nerve to the optic chiasma, thence to both lateral geniculate bodies via the optic tracts. Fibres then pass to the Edinger–Westphal nuclei of the third **cranial nerve.** Efferent parasympathetic fibres pass to the ciliary ganglia, then via oculomotor and short ciliary nerves to the iris sphincter muscles of both sides. The cerebral cortex is not involved in the reflex.
- accommodation reflex: constriction normally occurs when the eyes converge. Fibres from the lateral geniculate bodies pass to the visual areas of the cerebral cortex; impulses then pass via superior

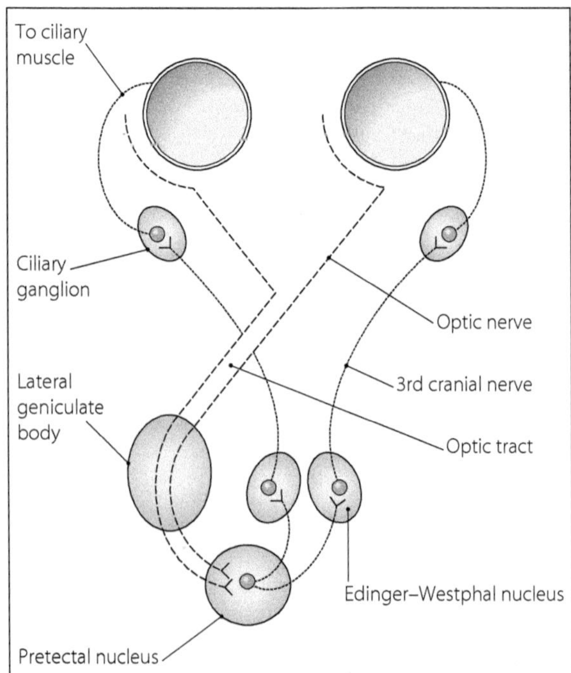

Fig. 135 Pupillary light reflex, showing pathways from one side of the visual field. The right lateral geniculate body and pretectal nucleus have been omitted

longitudinal fasciculus and internal capsule to the oculomotor nuclear mass next to the Edinger–Westphal nucleus. When both medial recti are adducted, the pupils constrict.

Impaired reflexes are caused by lesions anywhere along their paths.

[Ludwig Edinger (1855–1918) and Karl FO Westphal (1833–1890), German neurologists]

PVS, Persistent vegetative state, *see Vegetative state*

Pyloric stenosis. Stenosis of the gastric outflow. May be:

- congenital:
  - hypertrophy of the circular pyloric muscle; cause is unknown. Occurs in 1:500 births, 80% in males (usually first-born).
  - usually presents within 3–12 weeks of age, with persistent projectile vomiting, failure to gain weight and hunger. A mass may be palpable in the right hypochondrium. The diagnosis is confirmed by **ultrasonography**.
  - marked **dehydration** and metabolic **alkalosis** may be present. Resultant **aldosterone** secretion causes exchange of potassium and hydrogen ions for sodium in the urine, resulting in **hypokalaemia** and hypochloraemia with paradoxical acid urine.
  - treated initially by nasogastric drainage and restoration of electrolyte/fluid balance.
  - corrective surgery (pyloromyotomy; Ramstedt's procedure) should only be performed following adequate resuscitation, as indicated by clinical examination, good urine output, and normal acid–base and electrolyte (especially chloride) status. Anaesthetic management is as for **paediatric anaesthesia**, taking measures to avoid **aspiration of gastric contents**.
- acquired: usually results from gastric carcinoma or ulcer. Metabolic features are similar to those above. Residual gastric contents may be voluminous.

[Wilhelm C Ramstedt (1867–1963), German surgeon]

Pyrazinamide. Bactericidal **antituberculous drug** used in combination with other drugs. Effectiveness lasts 2–3 months. Useful in tuberculous meningitis because of good penetration into CSF.

- Dosage: 1.5–2.0 g daily for 2 months.
- Side effects: hepatotoxicity, anaemia, vomiting.

Pyrexia (Fever). Increased core body temperature, usually taken as ≥38°C (100.4°F), although definitions vary. The term implies intact homeostatic mechanisms, whereas **hyperthermia** refers to thermoregulatory failure. Common in ICU patients, it is a feature of the general inflammatory response and brought about by **cytokines** (especially interleukin-6) and other mediators.

- Caused by:
  - infection, including **chest infection, urinary tract infection, catheter-related sepsis** and **sinusitis.**
  - others: primary inflammatory diseases (e.g. **connective tissue disease**), drugs (e.g. **antibacterial drugs**), **MI**, **PE**, endocrine disorders (e.g. **hyperthyroidism**), acute **adrenocortical insufficiency**, **MH** and many others. May occur postoperatively, especially in children (in whom it has been reported in up to 40% of cases).

Management includes careful examination and investigation (including blood culture and culture of sputum, urine, wound; x-rays, etc.), removal/replacement of catheters, and review of drug therapy. Symptomatic treatment includes surface or core cooling and simple antipyretics. However, some suggest that antipyretics should not be administered, as they may have deleterious effects (they deny the patient an important host defence mechanism and eliminate an important diagnostic aid). Empirical use of antibiotics to treat isolated pyrexia is rarely advocated.

Pyridostigmine bromide. Acetylcholinesterase inhibitor. Pyridine analogue of **neostigmine**, with slower onset and longer duration of action. Also has weaker nicotinic action on voluntary muscle and less muscarinic action on viscera. Used in **myasthenia gravis** but less useful than neostigmine for reversing **non-depolarising neuromuscular blockade. Half-life** is 3–4 h.

- Dosage: 30–120 mg orally 4–12-hourly, up to 1.2 g/day.
- Side effects: as for neostigmine.

Q

Q wave. Initial downward deflection of the **QRS complex** of the **ECG** (*see Fig. 60b;* **Electrocardiography**). Small (q) waves are normal in leads aVL and I when left axis deviation is present, and in leads II, III and aVF with right axis deviation. They may be large in aVR. Pathological (Q) waves are wide (e.g. >30–40 ms) and deep (e.g. >2–4 mm, or more than a quarter of the height of the R wave in the same lead). In the absence of left **bundle branch block** they suggest **MI**, which may be old or of new onset; in acute S–T elevation MI, Q waves are associated with poorer outcomes.

QRS complex. Represents ventricular depolarisation; normally follows the **P wave** of the **ECG** (*see Fig. 60b;* **Electrocardiography**). Upper-case letters are used if a particular wave is considered large, lower-case if small. The initial deflection is termed the **q (Q) wave** if downward, and **R wave** if upward. The downward **S wave** follows an R wave. The QRS complex may be used to calculate the electrical axis. Normally has rS pattern in V_1, qR pattern in V_6. The initial small deflection represents left-to-right septal depolarisation; the larger subsequent deflection represents (mainly left) ventricular depolarisation. Normal duration: <0.12 s. Abnormalities may represent **arrhythmias, heart block, bundle branch block** or **MI**.

qSOFA, *see Sepsis-related organ failure assessment*

Q–T interval. Represents the duration of ventricular systole; varies with age, sex and heart rate. Measured from the beginning of the **QRS complex** to the end of the **T wave** of the **ECG** (*see Fig. 60b;* **Electrocardiography**). Corrected for heart rate by dividing by the square root of the preceding R–R interval in seconds (Bazett's formula). Normal range is 0.35–0.43.

Shortened in **hypercalcaemia, hyperkalaemia** and **digoxin** therapy. **Prolonged Q–T syndromes** may be caused by **hypocalcaemia, hypothyroidism** and **hypothermia**, and are associated with recurrent syncope or sudden death due to ventricular arrhythmias, including **VT** and **torsade de pointes**.
[H Cuthbert Bazett (1885–1950), English-born US physiologist]

Q–Tc dispersion. Difference between the longest and shortest measurable corrected **Q–T interval** on the 12-lead **ECG**. Originally described using manual calculation, although automatic measuring methods have been described. Has been shown to be a powerful predictor of **arrhythmias** and sudden cardiac death in several cardiac conditions.

Suggested explanations for Q–Tc dispersion include patchy myocardial fibrosis and left ventricular dilatation, although the exact mechanism is unclear.
Sahu P, Lim PO, Rana BS, Struthers AD (2000). Q J Med; 93: 425–31

Quadratus lumborum block, *see Transversus abdominis plane block*

Quality assurance/improvement (QA/QI). Systematic processes by which the quality of a 'product' (in this case, healthcare) is examined and deficiencies analysed, using methods often translated from industry or commercial business. Quality *assurance* is the older term and is based on meeting a defined threshold (e.g. compared with benchmarks derived from pooled data or an accepted standard of care), typically involving retrospective analysis (e.g. **audit**) in three areas:

- structure, i.e., the system in place, e.g. assessment of staffing levels, equipment, type of patients.
- process, i.e., how the care is delivered, e.g. anaesthetic techniques, monitoring.
- outcome, i.e., use of quality indicators, e.g. death rates, pain scores, patient satisfaction.

Quality *improvement* may involve similar methodology but may be retrospective or prospective and has a focus on continuous improvement of quality i.e., with no upper boundary. May be seen as an extension of traditional quality assurance in that an organisation (or individual) meeting the required QA standard is still obliged to strive to improve. Continuous QI may involve a number of established tools, e.g.:

- PDSA: plan (plan a change in the system); do (carry out the plan and collect data); study (analyse before/after data); act (formulate action plan to improve outcomes, including repeating the cycle).
- statistical process control: use of statistical methods of monitoring and control, the latter often by the use of control charts that plot outcomes, with or without 'action thresholds'. The CUSUM (cumulative sum) chart is one form that focuses on detecting changes, based on sequential analysis of outcome; they have been used to indicate when e.g. trainees are likely to have achieved competence in specific procedures or require remedial action.
- six sigma (Motorola): the term refers to a manufacturing standard relating to standard deviation (σ) such that a 'six sigma' process is equivalent to 3.4 defects or errors per million. Includes DMAIC (define, measure, analyse, improve, control) for existing processes and DMADV (define, measure, analyse, design, verify) for new processes. Often combined with the 'Lean' approach (Toyota), that focuses on the flow of systems and elimination of waste.
- FADE: focus (define the process to be improved); analyse (collect and analyse data to establish baselines and identify root causes/possible solutions); develop (develop action plans for implementation, communication, measuring/monitoring, etc.); execute (implement action plans); evaluate (establish ongoing measuring/monitoring system).

The drive for QA/QI programmes has come from clinical, administrative and political quarters.
See also, Clinical governance; National Institute for Health and Care Excellence; Risk management

Quantal theory. Widely accepted theory proposed in the 1950s to explain miniature **end-plate potentials** recorded from the **neuromuscular junction** postsynaptic membrane, at approximately 2 Hz. Postulates that small 'quanta' (packets) of **acetylcholine** are released randomly from the nerve cell membrane, even in the absence of motor nerve activity. Each quantum is thought to be one vesicle's content, about 10000 acetylcholine molecules. During single motor nerve activation about 200 quanta are released into the synaptic cleft.

Quantiflex apparatus. Continuous-flow **anaesthetic machines** that can deliver preset mixtures of O_2 and N_2O, adjusted by a percentage control (minimum of 30% O_2). A single dial adjusts total gas flow delivered. Individual **flowmeters** indicate flow of O_2 and N_2O; the O_2 flowmeter is usually on the right, and N_2O flowmeter on the left. They are sometimes used in **dental surgery**.

Quincke, Heinrich Irenaeus (1842–1922). German physician; described and standardised **lumbar puncture** in 1891, originally as a treatment for **hydrocephalus**. Used the paramedian approach and suggested 24 hours' bed rest afterwards. His bevelled needle design is still used for lumbar puncture and **spinal anaesthesia**. Quincke's sign is pulsation in the nail capillary bed and is seen in aortic regurgitation. Also first to describe **angio-oedema**.
Minagar A, Lowis GW (2001). J Med Biogr; 9: 12–15

Quinidine. Class Ia **antiarrhythmic drug**. An isomer of **quinine**. Used to treat **SVT** and **VT**, but rarely used now because of side effects including include ventricular arrhythmias (e.g. **torsade de pointes**), anticholinergic effects; CNS effects (cinchonism) including tinnitus and visual changes, and hypersensitivity reactions. Unavailable in the UK although still licensed in a number of other countries. May possibly have a role in reducing the frequency and severity of arrhythmias in Brugada syndrome, as a far cheaper alternative to implantable cardioverter-defibrillators, especially in resource-poor countries.
[Pedro and Josep Brugada, Spanish-born cardiologists]

Quinine sulfate/dihydrochloride. Antimalarial drug, reserved for treatment (but not prophylaxis) of falciparum **malaria**. Also used to treat nocturnal leg cramps.

- Dosage
  - malaria:
    - 600 mg orally tds for 5–7 days.
    - 20 mg/kg over 4 h iv as initial dose (unless a related drug has been given within 24 h), then 10 mg/kg over 4 h tds until able to complete the 7-day course with oral therapy.
  - leg cramps: 200–300 mg orally at night.
- Side effects: tinnitus, headache, visual disturbances (cinchonism), GIT disturbances, hypersensitivity (including thrombocytopenia and DIC), arrhythmias, renal failure, hypoglycaemia, convulsions.

4-Quinolones. Class of broad-spectrum **antibacterial drugs**, which include **ciprofloxacin, levofloxacin, moxifloxacin, ofloxacin** and norfloxacin. More effective against gram-negative than gram-positive bacteria, they have limited activity against anaerobes. Side effects include **prolonged Q–T syndromes**, spontaneous tendon rupture and muscle weakness. May also induce convulsions in susceptible individuals, especially if **NSAIDs** are taken concurrently. They should be used with caution in hepatic or renal impairment.

Quinupristin/dalfopristin. Synergistic combination of **antibacterial drugs** that inhibits the 50S bacterial ribosomal unit. Used for serious skin infections (e.g. severe **cellulitis**) caused by *Staphylococcus aureus* or *Streptococcus pyogenes*. Has short **half-life** (0.8 h) and excreted mainly through faeces.

- Dosage: 7.5 mg/kg iv by infusion over 1 h, 12-hourly.
- Side effects: pain and inflammation over infusion site, hyperbilirubinaemia, GIT upset, rash.

R on T phenomenon. Arises when the **R wave** of a **ventricular ectopic beat** falls on the **T wave** of the preceding beat. At the middle of the T wave, the myocardium is partly depolarised and partly repolarised, and thus vulnerable to establishment of re-entrant and circulatory conduction, leading to **VF** or **VT**.

R wave. First upward deflection of the **QRS complex** of the **ECG** (*see Fig. 60b;* **Electrocardiography**). Tends to increase in size from V_1 to V_6, with an accompanying reduction in size of **S wave** across these leads. Loss of this 'R wave progression', with a sudden increase in R wave size in V_5 or V_6, may indicate old anterior **MI**. In V_{1-6}, at least one normally exceeds 8 mm, but none exceeds 27 mm.

Rabeprazole sodium. Proton pump inhibitor; actions and effects are similar to those of **omeprazole**.
- Dosage: 20 mg orally od.
- Side effects: as for omeprazole.

Rabies. Infection caused by a lyssavirus of the rhabdovirus family, eradicated from Britain in 1902; however, occasional cases thought to have originated outside the UK have occurred in animals, e.g. dogs and bats. Fewer than five cases occur annually in Europe and the USA. Dogs are the source of infection in 99% of cases but bats and other wildlife are occasionally responsible. Transmitted via infected saliva penetrating broken skin or intact mucosa; it has also been reported following organ transplantation from a person who has died of the disease. The virus replicates in local muscle then migrates proximally along peripheral nerves to dorsal root ganglia and the CNS, eventually causing lethal **encephalitis**. Incubation period is usually 20–90 days in humans, but may be 4 days to several years.

Malaise, fever, depression and psychosis may be followed by laryngeal spasm, and extreme anxiety on drinking fluids. Respiratory and autonomic failure occurs early and cardiac involvement, including myocarditis, is common.

Treatment of established rabies includes injection of human antirabies immunoglobulin, early IPPV, sedation and paralysis, with careful maintenance of acid–base and fluid balance. Almost inevitably fatal once established (death typically occurs 7–10 days after symptoms appear), it may be prevented by wound cleaning and active and passive immunisation.

Crowcroft NS, Thampi N (2015). Br Med J; 350: g7827

Radford nomogram. Diagram showing the relationship between **tidal volume**, patient's weight and respiratory frequency. Used to aid appropriate selection of ventilator settings for children and adults. Now rarely used.

[Edward P Radford (1922–2001), US physiologist]

Radial artery. Terminal branch of the **brachial artery**. Arises in the **antecubital fossa**, level with the radial neck, and runs distally on the tendons and muscles attached to the radius (biceps tendon, supinator, pronator teres, flexor digitorum superficialis, flexor pollicis longus, pronator quadratus). Lies deep to brachioradialis muscle in the upper forearm, but subcutaneous in the lower forearm and easily palpable, especially over the distal quarter of the radius. Runs deep to abductor pollicis longus and extensor pollicis brevis tendons at the radial styloid, entering the anatomical snuffbox. Then enters the palm between the first and second metacarpals, forming the deep palmar arch. Branches include a superficial palmar branch (enters the palm superficial to the flexor retinaculum), which supplies the muscles of the thenar eminence before anastomosing with the superficial palmar arch. At the wrist, it is a common site for palpation of the **pulse** and for **arterial cannulation**.

See also, Ulnar artery

Radial nerve (C5–T1). Terminal branch of the posterior cord of the **brachial plexus**. Descends in the posterior upper arm, passing laterally behind the middle of the humerus in the radial groove. Crosses the **antecubital fossa** anterior to the elbow joint, between brachialis and brachioradialis. Descends under brachioradialis lateral to the **radial artery** in the forearm, passing posteriorly proximal to the wrist to end on the dorsum of the hand as digital branches.
- Branches:
  - axillary: to deltoid, teres minor and skin of the posteromedial upper arm.
  - upper arm:
    - to triceps, brachioradialis and extensor carpi radialis longus.
    - skin of the lower posterolateral arm.
  - forearm:
    - to the elbow joint.
    - posterior interosseous nerve arising at the elbow joint: passes posteriorly round the radial neck to supply the elbow, wrist and intercarpal joints, and all extensor muscles of the forearm apart from extensor carpi radialis longus.
    - via digital branches to the lateral side of the dorsum of the hand and posterior aspects of the lateral 2.5 digits up to the distal phalanx.

May be blocked at the elbow, wrist, and at mid-humerus with the elbow flexed (the nerve is palpable in the radial groove).

See also, Brachial plexus block; Elbow, nerve blocks; Wrist, nerve blocks

Radiation. Emission of **energy** in the form of waves or particles. Includes emission of electromagnetic waves (e.g. light), most of which is non-ionising (does not have sufficient energy to overcome electron binding energy). Ionising radiation may result in displacement of electrons in organic material with the potential for tissue damage, and includes:

- α particles: helium nuclei consisting of two protons and two neutrons. Have high energy but penetrate matter poorly.
- β particles: electrons or positrons with variable energy and velocity. Those with high energies are more penetrating than α particles but much less than γ-rays and x-rays.
- γ-rays and x-rays: electromagnetic waves emitted from (γ-rays) or outside (x-rays) the nuclei of excited atoms. Have extremely high penetration of matter and thus pose a health hazard requiring radiation safety precautions. γ-Rays are used in **radiotherapy** and imaging, and x-rays in imaging.

Exposure to ionising radiation is kept to a minimum with appropriate storage and handling of **radioisotopes**, minimal use of x-rays and appropriate use of shielding. Formal training is required for those performing or directing radiology procedures.
See also, Environmental safety of anaesthetists

Radiography in intensive care. Increasingly used as the range and quality of techniques and equipment available increase. Consultation with radiologists aids the proper selection and interpretation of many imaging techniques. In most cases, the use of mobile equipment results in less than optimal results but may be acceptable given the difficulty of transporting critically ill patients from the ICU; subtle changes between sequential films may be misleading if this is not taken into account. Investigations include **CXR**, **ultrasound** (including **echocardiography**) and **CT** and **MRI** scanning; bedside CT scanners are now available but not widespread; therefore CT and MRI require transport to the imaging department. MRI scanning times are often long and therefore CT imaging is favoured in critically ill patients. **Radioisotope scanning** requires transfer from the ICU, often to a specialist centre.

Practical considerations include the requirement for **sedation** and adequate **monitoring** during transport or the procedure itself, the interference of the procedure with background therapy including the requirement for moving the patient (e.g. to place films underneath), and the potentially adverse effects of **radiological contrast media**.
See also, Imaging in intensive care

Radioisotope scanning. Use of **radioisotopes** to label certain parts of the body in order to investigate organ function, either directly or attached to circulating cells. Includes the following:

- assessment of blood flow: **cerebral blood flow**, **renal blood flow**, lung perfusion scans (e.g. combined with ventilation scans in suspected **PE**).
- **nuclear cardiology**.
- localisation of lesions: PE, bone metastases/infection/ fracture, **intra-abdominal sepsis**.

The **radiation** contained within the body after scanning is negligible, posing no risk to staff.

Radioisotopes. Isotopes of elements that undergo disintegration; i.e., the nucleus emits α, β or γ **radiation** either spontaneously or following a collision. Used clinically as labels to determine fluid compartments, blood flow, pulmonary $\dot{V}/\dot{Q}$ distribution and sites of infection. Technetium-99m and xenon-133 are often suitable because they are easy to use and their **half-lives** are short. Also used to label metabolically active substances that are taken up by certain tissues, allowing imaging of the tissue concerned, e.g. fibrinogen labelled with iodine-123 accumulates in a clot and may be used to detect **DVT**. Therapeutic use includes **radiotherapy**.
See also, Radioisotope scanning

Radiological contrast media. Contain large molecules that absorb x-rays (e.g. barium [enteral] or iodine [enteral or iv]) or have paramagnetic properties (e.g. gadolinium) for MRI scanning. Adverse reactions may follow iv injection:

- related to high **osmolality** (up to 7× that of plasma):
  - initial hypervolaemia followed by osmotic diuresis and hypovolaemia.
  - damage to red blood cells and vascular endothelium.
- immunological:
  - reactions range from mild symptoms to cardiovascular collapse and death.
  - adverse reactions are most likely to be due to direct **histamine** release or **complement** activation. 'True' **anaphylaxis** (involving previous exposure to the antigen) is not thought to occur.
- direct toxicity: myocardial depression and systemic vasodilatation.

Thus initial hypertension may be followed by prolonged hypotension. **Renal failure** may result from cardiovascular changes plus direct toxicity.

Incidence of reactions and renal failure is decreased by using low osmolar, non-ionic media. Other measures to prevent renal injury include adequate hydration and administration of ***N*-acetylcysteine**. Resuscitation equipment and drugs must always be available.
Pasternak JJ, Williamson EE (2012). Mayo Clin Proc; 87: 390–402
See also, Adverse drug reactions

Radiology, anaesthesia for. Most radiological procedures require neither general anaesthesia nor **sedation**. Anaesthesia may be required for the very young, confused or agitated patients and those with movement disorders. Procedures include **CT scanning**, **MRI**, angiography and invasive procedures, e.g. embolisation of vascular lesions in **neuroradiology**.

- Main anaesthetic considerations:
  - underlying disease process.
  - remote location, often cramped conditions, with poor lighting.
  - old or incomplete anaesthetic/**monitoring** equipment.
  - poor access to the patient.
  - adverse effects of **radiological contrast media**.
  - specific problems of MRI.

Preoperative assessment and preparation should be as for any anaesthetic procedure.

Radiotherapy. Use of ionising **radiation** to treat neoplasms. May involve:

- external radiation.
- implantation of internal sources (brachytherapy), e.g. in gynaecological or CNS tumours.
- administration of radioactive **radioisotopes**, e.g. iodine-131 in hyperthyroidism, phosphorus-32 in polycythaemia.

- General anaesthesia is rarely required, except when patients are unco-operative, i.e., mainly children and patients with movement disorders. Anaesthetic considerations:

- general condition of the patient: features of **malignancy**, site and nature of the neoplasm and drug therapy. Haematological abnormalities are common.
- repeated anaesthetics: multiple treatments are required, e.g. daily for several weeks. Considerations include fear of injections and repeated periods of starvation (especially important in children). IV cannulation may be difficult, although long-term catheters are often sited.
- immobilisation of the head may be required, e.g. for CNS tumours; clear plastic casts that cover the whole face are often used, with risks of airway obstruction. Head-down positioning may be required.
- treatments usually consist of short periods of radiation (e.g. a few minutes), during which the anaesthetist cannot be present. Monitoring is usually visible via remote-control cameras, but may be restricted.

Techniques used include **sedation** or general anaesthesia using **TIVA** with **propofol**, or intermittent boluses of **ketamine** (especially in children).

Patients formerly treated by radiotherapy may have inflammatory or fibrotic changes in the irradiated area. Pulmonary, cardiac, neuroendocrine, renal and hepatic involvement may be present. Tissue fibrosis around the airway may make tracheal intubation difficult.

Kolker A, Mascarenhas J (2015). Curr Opin Anaesthesiol; 28: 464–8

Randomisation. Technique for allocating subjects (e.g. patients to treatment groups in **clinical trials**) that reduces allocation bias when **samples** are compared. Ensures that both known and unknown factors affecting the outcome (e.g. baseline characteristics, environmental exposure) are randomly distributed among the groups; i.e., any difference in these factors is due to chance alone.

- Randomisation may be:
  - simple: no restriction on allocation. Groups may be unequally sized.
  - block: allocation is performed in blocks, so that groups are equally sized within each block.
  - stratified: factors such as age and sex are randomised separately, so that they are equally distributed among the groups. A more sophisticated method, minimisation, involves the distribution of successive subjects to the groups by taking into account the number of subjects already allocated who have these various factors, using a scoring system. For example, if age, weight and female sex are felt to be important prognostic factors in a particular study, an obese subject may still be allocated to a group that already has several obese subjects in it, if there are fewer older subjects and females than in the other groups.

Computer-generated random numbers are usually employed. Use of coins or dice is tedious and presents the temptation to repeat an allocation if the result is not liked. Other methods have also been used, e.g. allocation of alternate patients, or according to patients' birthdays or record numbers. However, these methods cannot always be guaranteed free of hidden bias.

Ranitidine hydrochloride. **H_2 receptor antagonist**; better absorbed and more potent than **cimetidine**, with fewer side effects. Does not inhibit hepatic enzymes or interfere with metabolism of other drugs. Oral **bioavailability** is about 50%. Plasma levels peak within 15 min of im injection and 2–3 h after oral administration; effect lasts about 8 h. **Half-life** is about 2 h. Undergoes hepatic metabolism and is excreted via urine; hence the dose is reduced in **renal failure**.

- Dosage:
  - 50 mg iv/im tds. Effective if given 45–60 min preoperatively. If administered iv, 50 mg should be diluted into 20 ml and injected over at least 2 min, because severe bradycardia may occur. May also be given by continuous infusion: 125–250 μg/kg/h.
  - 150–300 mg orally bd. For prophylaxis against **aspiration pneumonitis**, 150 mg orally qds (e.g. in labour), or 2 h preoperatively (preferably preceded by 150 mg the night before).
- Side effects: blood dyscrasias, impaired liver function and confusion; all are rare.

Ranking, *see Statistical tests*

Ranolazine. Antianginal drug, licensed as adjunctive therapy. Inhibits the late inward sodium current in cardiac muscle, reducing intracellular **calcium** concentration and thus wall tension and oxygen demand.

- Dosage: 375–750 mg orally bd.
- Side effects: GIT upset, headache, dizziness, hypotension, prolonged Q–T interval, oedema, confusion.

Raoult's law. The addition of a solute to an ideal solution reduces the vapour pressure of the solvent in proportion to the molar concentration of the solute.

[François M Raoult (1830–1901), French scientist]

See also, Colligative properties of solutions

RAP, Right atrial pressure, *see Cardiac catheterisation; Central venous pressure*

Rapacuronium bromide. Non-depolarising **neuromuscular blocking drug**, introduced in the USA in 1999 and withdrawn in 2001 just before its introduction in the UK, because of reports of fatal bronchospasm. Chemically related to **vecuronium**, it causes rapid onset of neuromuscular blockade (tracheal intubation possible within 60 s) with fast recovery (6–30 min depending on dosage) and was thus suggested as an alternative to **suxamethonium**.

Rapid opioid detoxification. Technique for treating opioid addiction by precipitating withdrawal using **opioid receptor antagonists**, e.g. **naloxone** or **naltrexone**, supposedly reducing relapse rates compared with conventional management. Ultrarapid opioid detoxification refers to administration of general anaesthesia or heavy sedation for prolonged periods to reduce awareness or recall of unpleasant withdrawal symptoms while the opioid antagonists are given. The technique is controversial (especially the ultrarapid form) because deaths have occurred and supportive evidence for its efficacy is poor, leading many authorities to abandon its use.

Rapid sequence induction, *see Induction, rapid sequence*

Rate–pressure product (RPP). Product of heart rate and systolic BP, used as a rough indicator of myocardial workload and O_2 consumption. It has been suggested that RPP should be maintained below 15 000 in patients with **ischaemic heart disease** during anaesthesia. Its usefulness has been questioned, because a proportional increase in rate may increase myocardial O_2 demand more than the same increase in BP. A pressure–rate quotient (MAP/rate) of <1 has been suggested as being a better predictor of **myocardial ischaemia**.

RBBB, Right bundle branch block, *see Bundle branch block*

RDS, *see Respiratory distress syndrome*

Reactance. Portion of **impedance** to flow of an alternating current not due to **resistance**; e.g. due to **capacitance** or inductance. Given the symbol X, and measured in ohms. [Georg S Ohm (1787–1854), German physicist]

Rebreathing techniques, *see Carbon dioxide measurement*

Receiver operating characteristic (ROC) curves. Curves drawn to indicate the usefulness of a predictive test, originally derived from analysis of radar signals between the World Wars (i.e., did a deflection represent a real signal or just random noise; and if the former, with what degree of certainty?). For the test to be analysed (e.g. the usefulness of **ASA physical status** to predict mortality after anaesthesia), each cut-off level is examined in turn, and **sensitivity** and **specificity** calculated for it. Thus, for example, an ASA grade of 1 has high sensitivity (all deaths have an ASA grade of 1 or above) but low specificity (most patients with a grade of 1 or above do not die). For an ASA grade of 2, sensitivity is a little lower (some patients who die have a grade of 1, and will not be predicted by a grade of 2) while specificity is higher, although still poor (a grade of 2 is better at predicting death than a grade of 1, although most patients achieving 2 or above still do not die). The process continues until grade 5, which has low sensitivity (few of the deaths have a grade of 5) but high specificity (most patients who are graded 5 do, by definition, die). Sensitivity is plotted against (1 – specificity) and a curve obtained (Fig. 136); the area under the curve (AUC) represents the usefulness of the test: a perfect test includes 100% of the available area and one where prediction is no better than chance, 50%.

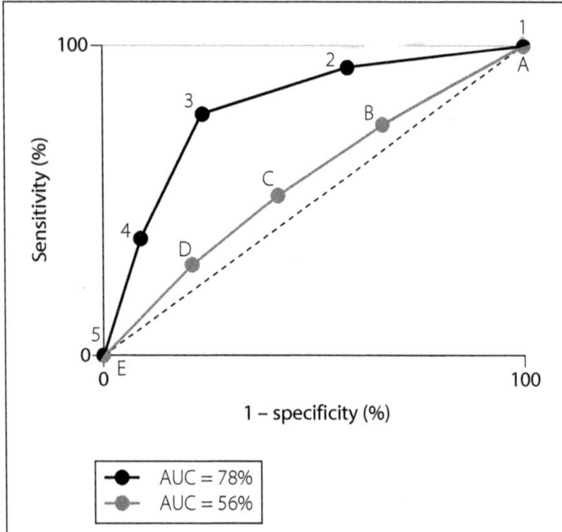

Fig. 136 Examples of two receiver operating characteristic curves for the usefulness of two different five-point scales (1–5 and A–E) for predicting an outcome. The 1–5 scale performs better than the A–E scale. The dotted line denotes the curve for a test where prediction is no better than chance

ROC curves may be drawn using continuous (e.g. **C-reactive protein** to predict infection), ordinal (e.g. ASA system) or nominal (e.g. presence of different features on the **ECG** to diagnose **MI**) scales. They may also be drawn for different tests in the same plot, allowing comparison between the tests. They also allow selection of the best cut-off to use clinically, usually the uppermost and most left-hand part of the curve, being the best compromise between sensitivity and specificity. Commonly used to analyse the usefulness of tests or scoring systems in anaesthesia and intensive care, including difficult tracheal intubation and other outcomes.

Receptor theory. States that receptors are specific proteins or lipoproteins located on cell **membranes** or within cells that interact selectively with extracellular compounds (**agonists**) to initiate biochemical events within cells. The structures of the agonist and receptor determine the selectivity and quantitative response. Drugs that interact with the receptor and inhibit the effect of an agonist are antagonists. Degree of binding to receptors is **affinity**; ability to produce a response is **intrinsic activity**.

Initial assumptions that the degree of response is proportional to the number of receptors occupied are not universally accepted. Other suggestions include:

- reduced occupancy is required for a potent agonist compared with a less potent agonist, to produce the same response.
- degree of response is proportional to the rate of receptor–agonist interaction and dissociation.

Interaction of drug and receptor may resemble **Michaelis–Menten kinetics**. Covalent, ionic and hydrogen bonding, and **van der Waals forces** may be involved.

- Different types of receptor:
  - ligand-gated ion channels: direct opening of membrane pores allowing passage of ions (e.g. Na^+, K^+, Ca^{2+}, Cl^-) across the membrane, e.g. nicotinic **acetylcholine receptor**. Typically fast responses (<1 ms).
  - **G protein-coupled receptors**: binding to the receptor causes a change in the guanine binding properties of the neighbouring G protein, which then leads to the intracellular response, e.g. **adrenergic receptors**. Typically of the order of many milliseconds to seconds.
  - ligand-activated tyrosine kinases: binding at the cell surface causes activation of tyrosine kinase at the inner surface of the cell, which catalyses phosphorylation of target proteins via **ATP**, e.g. **insulin** receptors. Typically minutes to hours.
  - nuclear receptors: the lipid-soluble agonist passes through the cell membrane to interact with the receptor, leading to alteration of DNA transcription, e.g. **corticosteroid** and thyroid hormones. Typically up to several hours.

Expression of receptors varies. Chronic stimulation (e.g. asthmatics taking β_2-adrenergic receptor agonists) results in a decreased number of receptors (downregulation) whereas understimulation (e.g. following spinal cord injury) leads to an increased number of receptors (upregulation).

See also, Dose–response curves; Pharmacodynamics

Recommended International Non-proprietary Names (rINNs), *see Explanatory Notes at the beginning of this book*

Record-keeping. The first anaesthetic chart was devised by Codman and **Cushing** in 1894 at the Massachusetts

General Hospital, for recording of respiration and pulse rate. BP charting was included in 1901 at Cushing's insistence. F_IO_2 was included by **McKesson** in 1911.

Careful record-keeping is now recognised as essential to chart preoperative risk factors, the perioperative course of anaesthesia and postoperative events/instructions. It is particularly useful when taking over another anaesthetist's anaesthetic, and for providing information to those administering anaesthesia subsequently. Similarly, ICU records should chart physiological data, therapy and instructions relating to the stay of any patient in an ICU. Record-keeping is also important for teaching, research and **audit**, and is extremely important in **medicolegal aspects of anaesthesia**. Although tending to include similar information, anaesthetic and intensive care charts are not standardised nationally, although this has been suggested.

Automated anaesthetic record systems are increasingly used, sometimes incorporated into anaesthetic machines or ICU **monitoring** systems. They provide accurate, legible and complete documents for data acquisition and subsequent scrutiny. Data from monitoring devices are incorporated with information provided by the anaesthetist/intensive care staff (e.g. drug or other interventions).

Postoperative **recovery** and progress may be recorded on separate charts, or on the anaesthetic chart.

[Ernest A Codman (1869–1940), US surgeon]

Recovery, enhanced (Fast-track/multimodal/rapid/accelerated recovery). Approach to **recovery from anaesthesia** and surgery based on evidence-based, multimodal perioperative care, particularly for patients undergoing major surgery. Aims to improve surgical outcomes and speed of recovery by increasing patients' preoperative fitness for surgery where possible (**prehabilitation**), delivering optimal intraoperative care, and providing postoperative support/rehabilitation beyond just early **postoperative analgesia** and treatment of **PONV** and other short-term problems.

Includes preoperative optimisation of **nutrition** and cessation of **smoking**, minimisation of surgical stress by use of minimal access (e.g. laparoscopic, endovascular) techniques where possible, avoidance of excessive fluid administration and nasogastric tubes/urinary catheters, multimodal prevention and management of postoperative pain, and early postoperative mobilisation, **physiotherapy** and self-care.

Special issue (2015). Can J Anesth; 62: 99–235

Recovery from anaesthesia. Period from the end of surgery to when the patient is alert and physiologically stable. Definition is difficult because some drowsiness may persist for many hours. **Recovery testing** is used for more precise investigation. Time to recovery depends on the patient's condition, drugs given, their doses, and the patient's ability to eliminate them. For **inhalational anaesthetic agents**, similar considerations as for uptake are involved, plus length of operation and degree of redistribution to fat. Thus blood gas **solubility** is the most important factor initially, but more potent agents (e.g. **isoflurane**) are more extensively bound to fat after prolonged anaesthesia than less potent ones, e.g. **desflurane**. For **iv anaesthetic agents**, initial recovery is due to drug redistribution from vessel-rich to vessel-intermediate tissues; subsequent course is related to the rate of clearance from the body. Thus **propofol** characteristically results in rapid clear-headed emergence, whereas **thiopental** is more likely to produce drowsiness lasting several hours, especially after repeated dosage. Recommendations for provision of recovery care (**Association of Anaesthetists**):

- designated **recovery rooms** or areas should be used.
- during transfer to the recovery area O_2 should be administered, and appropriate **monitoring** performed.
- the anaesthetist should formally hand over the patient's care to properly trained staff, giving details of the operation, anaesthetic technique, preoperative morbidity, perioperative problems, including blood loss, and drugs given.
- all patients should be observed by at least one member of staff until there is a clear airway and cardiovascular stability, and the patient is able to communicate (at least two members of staff should be present when there is a patient in the recovery room who does not meet the discharge criteria). The anaesthetist is responsible for removal of tracheal tubes, the presence of which requires continuous **capnography**.
- O_2 should be administered at least until awake.
- level of consciousness, arterial O_2 saturation, BP, heart rate, respiratory rate, pain intensity, iv infusions and drugs administered (including O_2) should be recorded, along with other variables as appropriate (e.g. temperature, urine output).
- there should be written criteria for discharge, including full consciousness, clear airway, respiratory and cardiovascular stability, adequate **postoperative analgesia** and control of **PONV**, stable temperature and prescription of postoperative drugs, including O_2 and iv fluids as appropriate. There should be adequate handover during discharge from the recovery area.
- children should be recovered in a designated area.

Patients are often placed on their side, e.g. the **recovery position**. In the 'tonsillar position', the pillow is placed under the loin and the trolley tipped head-down.

- Problems during recovery:
  - respiratory, e.g. **hypoventilation**, **hypercapnia**, **hypoxaemia**, **airway obstruction**, **bronchospasm**, **aspiration of gastric contents**.
  - cardiovascular, e.g. **hypotension**, **hypertension**, **arrhythmias**, **myocardial ischaemia**.
  - confusion and agitation. Pain and bladder distension are common causes of restlessness and hypertension postoperatively. The above causes must also be excluded.
  - related to anaesthetic drugs, e.g. inadequate reversal of **non-depolarising neuromuscular blockade**, **adverse drugs reactions**, **MH**, **dystonic reactions**, **emergence phenomena**, **central anticholinergic syndrome**.
  - **hypothermia**, PONV, **shivering**.
  - related to surgery, e.g. pain, bleeding.

The speed and quality of recovery from anaesthesia have been proposed as a possible measure of quality of anaesthesia.

See also, Anaesthetic morbidity and mortality; Recovery, enhanced

Recovery position. Position recommended for unconscious but spontaneously breathing subjects, assuming no contraindication, e.g. **cervical spine** injury. Encourages a clear airway and drainage of vomit, secretions and blood away from the airway. Often used during **recovery from anaesthesia**.

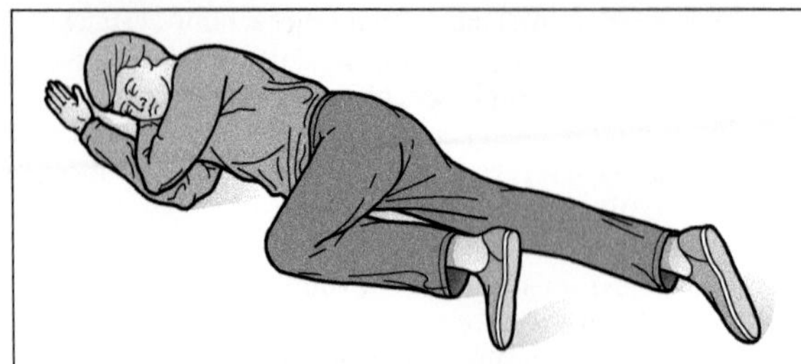

Fig. 137 Recovery position

Any recovery position is a compromise between the full prone position (better airway and drainage but more diaphragmatic splinting) and the full lateral position (less diaphragmatic splinting but less effective for the airway and less stable; also may be harmful in neck injury). Classically includes flexion of both arms with the upper hand placed under the jaw to support the airway (Fig. 137). The actual position adopted should reflect the particular circumstances of the case and the need to protect the airway, stabilise the neck and allow unhindered ventilation. It should be possible to observe the patient at all times and to turn him/her supine easily when required.

Recovery room (Post-anaesthesia care unit; PACU). An area reserved for postoperative care was described by Florence Nightingale in 1863, but the first dedicated recovery room was opened in the USA in 1923. Many more were introduced there after experiences in World War II and the Korean War. First introduced in the UK in 1955.

- Features:
  - staffed by fully trained personnel.
  - placed near the operating suite, if possible near ICU.
  - open ward, allowing good patient observation.
  - at least two bays per operating theatre are recommended.
  - each bay is equipped for monitoring (ECG, BP, O_2 saturation) and patient care (suction, O_2).
  - a supply of iv equipment and fluids, blankets and airways should be available.
  - resuscitation equipment, ventilator and drugs should be readily available, with an emergency call system.
  - adequate ventilation is required to remove exhaled anaesthetic gases.
- Drugs available should include:
  - analgesics, antiemetics, sedatives, anticonvulsants, naloxone, flumazenil.
  - doxapram, bronchodilators, corticosteroids, antihistamines.
  - anticholinergics, antiarrhythmics, antihypertensives, diuretics, heparin.
  - antibiotics, anticholinesterases, neuromuscular blocking drugs, insulin, dextrose, dantrolene.
  - local anaesthetics, lipid emulsion.

Recovery units should have an effective and regularly tested emergency call system. If used for temporary care of critically ill patients, guidelines stress that the primary responsibility for the patient lies with the hospital's critical care team.

[Florence Nightingale (1820–1910), English nurse]

See also, Recovery from anaesthesia

Recovery testing. Ranges from simple clinical assessment to more sophisticated methods, e.g. used for experimental comparison between anaesthetic techniques and drugs. Routine testing is usually limited to assessment of general alertness and orientation, and ability to respond, drink, dress and walk where appropriate.

- Sophisticated techniques used include tests of:
  - psychomotor function:
    - assessing speed and number of errors made while performing set tasks:
      - moving pegs from one set of holes in a board to another set.
      - deleting every letter 'p' from a page of text.
      - connecting dots on a page.
    - reaction testing:
      - being faced with four light sources, and pressing the correct switch (out of four choices) when one of them flashes.
      - tracking moving targets with a pen or light.
  - perception:
    - noting the frequency at which a flashing light appears to be continuous (critical flicker–fusion threshold).
    - perception of auditory stimuli in a similar fashion, including discrimination between left and right ears.
  - memory:
    - recall or recognition of objects, pictures, words or word associations shown a short time before.
    - orientation in time and space.
  - cognitive function, e.g. adding/subtracting numbers, or adding values of different coins.
  - physiological function, e.g. divergence of eyes caused by reductions in extraocular muscle tone.

Problems of detailed recovery testing are related to the time taken, cumbersome equipment required, fatigue, boredom and learning if tests are repeated. Critical flicker–fusion, reaction testing, letter deletion and memory tests are most widely used and thought to be reasonably efficient, the first two especially so. General advice to patients is usually to avoid potentially dangerous activities (e.g. driving, cooking, using machinery) for 24 h following day-case anaesthesia, although subtle changes may persist beyond this period; 48 h has been suggested.

Bowyer A, Jakobsson J, Ljungqvist O, Royse C (2014). Anaesthesia; 69: 1266–78

Rectal administration of anaesthetic agents. Results in effective absorption of drugs because of a rich blood supply provided by communicating plexuses formed by the superior, middle and inferior rectal arteries and veins. Drugs undergo minimal **first-pass metabolism**, because the plexuses are anastomoses between portal and systemic circulations. The technique is usually restricted to children. Traditionally used more in continental Europe, e.g. France. Drugs used have included **diazepam** 0.4–0.5 mg/kg (widely used for treatment of convulsions in children), **methohexital** 15–25 mg/kg and **thiopental** 40–50 mg/kg as 5%–10% solutions. Opioids and **ketamine** have also been given in this way. **Diethyl ether** was administered rectally by **Pirogoff. Bromethol** and **paraldehyde** were used in the 1920s to produce unconsciousness (basal narcosis).

Rectus sheath block. Performed as part of **abdominal field block** or alone to reduce pain from abdominal incisions. Abdominal contents are not anaesthetised.

With the patient supine, a blunted needle is introduced 3–6 cm above and lateral to the umbilicus. A gentle 'scratching' motion may aid identification of the tough anterior layer of the sheath, puncture of which is accompanied by a click. The needle is advanced up to the resistance offered by the posterior layer of the sheath, and 15–20 ml **local anaesthetic agent** injected after negative aspiration. Deposition of solution between rectus muscle and posterior layer allows spread up and down, blocking the lower 5–6 intercostal nerves within the sheath. Spread between the muscle and anterior layer is limited by the tendinous intersections along its length. Multiple injections have been suggested between intersections, to improve spread, but the posterior layer is deficient below a point halfway between the umbilicus and pubis, and peritoneal puncture is more likely below this level. Has also been done using ultrasound guidance although the additional benefit is uncertain.

Recurarisation. Recurrence of **non-depolarising neuromuscular blockade** after apparent reversal with **acetylcholinesterase inhibitors**. Originally described with **tubocurarine** in patients with impaired renal function, where the duration of action of the neuromuscular blocking drug exceeds that of the acetylcholinesterase inhibitor. Has been described with other **neuromuscular blocking drugs**.

Red cell concentrates, *see Blood products*

Reducing valve, *see Pressure regulators*

Refeeding syndrome. Clinical syndrome seen after reintroduction of **nutrition** to previously starved patients, often seen on ICU. First noted after World War II, when malnourished prisoners of war inexplicably died of **cardiac failure** after receiving a normal diet. Associated with any condition leading to malnutrition (e.g. **anorexia nervosa**, **alcoholism**, **intra-abdominal sepsis**).

- Pathophysiology:
  - restoration of **carbohydrates** as a dietary substrate leads to increased **insulin** secretion and activation of anabolic pathways. **Hypophosphataemia**, **hypomagnesaemia**, **hypokalaemia** and **vitamin deficiency** (particularly thiamine) may follow due to increased intracellular uptake on a background of whole body depletion.
  - depletion of **ATP** and **2,3-DPG** leads to tissue hypoxia and mitochondrial dysfunction.
- Clinical features:
  - **hyperglycaemia** and electrolyte disturbances as above.
  - sodium and fluid retention.
  - cardiac failure, **arrhythmias**.
  - muscle weakness, contributing to respiratory failure and difficulty weaning from ventilators.
  - Wernicke's encephalopathy due to thiamine deficiency.
- Prevention and treatment:
  - correction of electrolyte deficiencies before reintroducing feeding.
  - gradual introduction and escalation of caloric intake, with close monitoring of electrolytes and replacement as required. Vitamin supplementation.
  - close attention to fluid balance to prevent fluid overload.

Karl Wernicke (1848–1904), German neurologist

Referred pain. **Pain** felt in a site remote from the source of pain. The pain is often of visceral origin with the referred pain felt in a somatic site, e.g. diaphragmatic pain is felt in the shoulder tip. The aetiology is obscure, but is thought to be related to the embryological segment from which the organ arose, e.g. diaphragm from the neck region, and heart from the same region as the arm.

- Theories include:
  - convergence: afferent fibres from different tissues converge on to common spinal neurones. The spinal cord then misinterprets the signal as originating from another structure to the actual source.
  - facilitation: input from visceral afferents increases sensitivity of neurones receiving somatic afferents, thus promoting somatic sensation.

Effects of local anaesthetic injected at referred areas are inconsistent, supporting both theories (should ease the pain if facilitation is responsible, but not if convergence is responsible).

Reflex arc. Involves predictable, repetitive stereotypic responses to a particular sensory stimulus. Consists of sense organ, afferent **neurone**, one or more **synapses**, efferent neurone and effector. The afferent neurones enter the **spinal cord** via dorsal roots or **brain** via **cranial nerves**; the efferent neurones leave via ventral nerve roots or corresponding motor cranial nerves. Also involved in autonomic functions. The simplest reflex arc is monosynaptic, e.g. knee jerk and other stretch reflexes involving **muscle spindles**. Polysynaptic reflex arcs (two or more synapses) include the withdrawal reflex. Widespread effects may result from activation of a single reflex arc because of ascending, descending, excitatory and inhibitory interneurones.

Reflex sympathetic dystrophy, *see Complex regional pain syndrome*

Reflux, *see Gastro-oesophageal reflux*

Refractometer, *see Interferometer*

Refractory period. Period during and following the **action potential** during which the neurone is insensitive to further stimulation. Subdivided thus:

- absolute: excited by no stimulus, however strong.
- relative: excitation may follow stronger stimuli than normal.

Refrigeration anaesthesia. Use of cold to reduce pain sensation. Used by **Larrey** in 1807, although the effect of cold on pain has been recognised for centuries. Up to 3 h packing in ice was recommended for operations through the thigh. The principle is still used today, e.g. **ethyl chloride** spray to enable minor procedures.

Regional anaesthesia. Term originally coined by **Cushing** to describe techniques of abolishing pain using **local anaesthetic agents** as opposed to general anaesthesia. Pioneers included **Halsted**, **Corning** and **Labat** in the USA, **Bier**, **Braun** and **Lawen** in Europe and **Anrep** in Russia.

- Techniques include:
  - **topical anaesthesia**.
  - **infiltration anaesthesia**, **Vishnevisky technique** and **tumescent anaesthesia**.
  - peripheral nerve blocks: plexus and single nerve blocks.
  - central neuraxial blockade: **epidural** and **spinal anaesthesia**.

  - **IVRA** and **intra-arterial regional anaesthesia.**
  - **sympathetic nerve blocks.**
  - others, e.g. **interpleural analgesia.**
- Advantages of regional anaesthesia:
  - conscious patient, able to assist in positioning, and warn of adverse effects (e.g. in **carotid endarterectomy** and **TURP**). There is less interruption of oral intake, especially beneficial in **diabetes mellitus.**
  - good **postoperative analgesia.**
  - reduction of certain postoperative complications, e.g. **atelectasis** and **DVT**, possibly myocardial ischaemia.
- Contraindications:
  - absolute: patient refusal and localised infection.
  - relative: abnormal anatomy or deformity, **coagulation disorders**, previous failure of the technique, and neurological disease or other medicolegal considerations.

  Specific contraindications may exist for specific techniques.
- Management:
  - preoperatively:
    - **preoperative assessment** and preparation as for general anaesthesia.
    - full explanation of the procedure, and **consent.**
    - preparation of drugs and equipment for general anaesthesia and resuscitation, in addition to those required for the regional technique chosen.
  - perioperatively:
    - **monitoring** applied as for general anaesthesia, i.e., before and during the procedure.
    - aseptic technique should be observed.
    - for nerve or plexus blocks, short-bevelled **needles** are traditionally used to minimise nerve contact, although nerve damage may be greater should the nerve be impaled. Nerve stimulators (using 0.3–1.0 mA current lasting 1–2 ms and delivered at 1–3 Hz) increase the success of many blocks and may reduce damage further. A distant ground electrode is required. The needle (preferably sheathed) is placed near the target nerve and stimulated until twitches are elicited; the output is reduced, the needle repositioned and the process repeated. Optimal positioning is suggested by a twitch threshold of ~0.3 mA.

      Ultrasound imaging is now widely used to guide needle placement. Addition of colour Doppler imaging identifies blood vessels. Advantages include: more accurate placement of the needle, especially if anatomy is abnormal; reduced volume of injectate required; greater success rate; and reduced complication rate.
    - a single injection of local anaesthetic, repeated boluses (using repeated injections or a catheter) or continuous infusions may be used.
    - the extent of the block should be assessed (e.g. by response to pinprick or cold) before allowing surgery to start.
    - if **sedation** is used, care should be taken to ensure that respiratory and cardiovascular depression does not occur. Analgesic drugs (e.g. N_2O or **opioid analgesic drugs**) may be used to supplement incomplete blockade. General anaesthesia may be used as a planned part of the technique, or if the technique is unsuccessful.
  - postoperatively:
    - monitoring and supervision should continue as for general anaesthesia.
      - patients should be advised to protect insensate limbs e.g. using a sling for upper limb blocks.
      - patients should be warned of potentially unpleasant paraesthesia as the block recedes.
    - neurological complications may only become apparent once the block has worn off.
- Complications:
  - technical: direct trauma to nerves, blood vessels and pleura; breakage of needles or catheters.
  - associated with **positioning of the patient**, e.g. compression of an anaesthetised limb.
  - local anaesthetic toxicity: intravascular injection or systemic absorption.
  - excessive spread, e.g. total spinal block during epidural anaesthesia, or phrenic nerve block during **brachial plexus block.**
  - failure of the technique.
  - those of specific techniques, e.g. hypotension following spinal anaesthesia.
  - others, e.g. injection of the wrong solution through catheters.

See also, specific blocks; Nerve injury during anaesthesia

Regional tissue oxygenation. Important because **shock** and **hypoxaemia** cause redistribution of blood flow and alter the metabolic properties of cells; global measurements thus fail to detect areas of local ischaemia. Measurement of regional tissue oxygenation may be useful in critically ill patients because deficiencies may be involved in the development and continuation of **MODS.** Lack of evidence of benefit and technical difficulties have hindered the more intricate techniques from becoming routine practice. Methods of assessment include:
  - blood **lactate** levels (>2 mmol/l suggests insufficient oxygen delivery): a late marker.
  - mixed venous O_2 saturation ($S_{\bar{v}}O_2$), measured using repeated blood sampling or continuous **oximetry** via a pulmonary artery catheter. Regional $S_{\bar{v}}O_2$ (e.g. hepatic = $S_{h\bar{v}}O_2$; jugular = $S_{j\bar{v}}O_2$) can be determined using indwelling catheters.
  - intestinal regional capnography (i.e., **gastric tonometry**). Measures PCO$_2$ in an air- or saline-filled tonometric balloon, placed in the GIT.
  - surface or tissue O_2 electrodes: based upon the Clark electrode (*see Oxygen measurement*), they are formed of a noble metal (e.g. gold, silver, platinum). Change in voltage between the anode and cathode is proportional to the amount of O_2 reduced at the cathode.
  - optode sensors: use the change in the optical properties (e.g. absorbance or fluorescence) of indicator substances generated by photochemical reactions to measure the concentration of a substance (e.g. O_2) in tissues. Can be mounted in intravascular catheters (e.g. Paratrend monitor).
  - **near infrared spectroscopy.**
  - reflectance spectrophotometry. Measures the absorption of reflected visible light on a tissue surface, e.g. gut wall, fetal scalp.
  - nicotinamide adenine dinucleotide (NADH) fluorescence: during tissue hypoxia, NADH accumulates in tissues. The absorption properties of NADH, and its reduced state, NAD$^+$, are different. Tissue catheters have been used in both animal and human models.
  - imaging using online microscopic observation of the microcirculation.

Regression, *see Statistical tests*

Regurgitation. Term usually describing passive passage of **gastric contents** into the pharynx. May be silent; thus **aspiration of gastric contents** may occur unnoticed. Normally prevented by the **lower oesophageal sphincter**; however, swallowed dyes have been found to stain areas of the pharynx and larynx during/after anaesthesia in normal patients.

Relative analgesia. Technique used in **dental surgery** involving nasal administration of subanaesthetic concentrations of $\mathbf{N_2O}$, e.g. 10% in O_2, slowly increased to 30%–50%. Verbal contact is maintained at all times, and the concentration of N_2O reduced if excessive drowsiness occurs. Performed by the dentist, it depends partly on suggestion.

Relative risk reduction. Indicator of treatment effect in **clinical trials**. For a reduction in incidence of events from a% to b%, it equals $([a - b] \div a)$%. Gives an overestimated impression of treatment effect if events are rare, and an underestimate if events are common.
See also, Absolute risk reduction; Meta-analysis; Number needed to treat; Odds ratio

Relatives of critically ill patients. Present particular challenges to ICU staff because of the serious nature of the patient's condition, unfamiliarity with the ICU environment and the natural behavioural responses to extreme stress, including fear, anger and guilt. The suddenness of many severe conditions may exacerbate relatives' distress. Up to 70% of relatives develop psychological problems including anxiety, sleep disruption and **post-traumatic stress disorder**. Risk factors include pre-existing psychiatric illness, female sex, the underlying diagnosis (e.g. **trauma**) and death of the patient. Worries about adequacy of ICU care and poor communication compound the problem. When sustained, psychological difficulties may form the family component of the **post-intensive care syndrome**.

Relatives must be kept regularly informed about the patient's progress, preferably by a consistent single senior doctor accompanied by a member of the nursing staff; they should also feel included in discussions about treatment (including its withdrawal).

Honest and clear explanations, avoiding technical language, may need repeating several times and the potential frustration felt by the medical team must not be transmitted to the relatives; enough time, free of interruptions, must be allocated. Most ICUs have a separate room for interviews with patients' families and friends, which is preferable to the open ward or corridor. It is vital to acknowledge relatives' concerns and address them with clarity. A detailed plan of what the ICU team is trying to achieve should be provided.

In general, few restrictions are placed on visiting times, and most relatives appreciate and respect the need for staff to perform basic care and procedures during which they may be asked to leave the unit. However, some may choose to stay and participate in some aspects of their relative's care, e.g. washing or shaving. Counselling and religious support may be required and is often best arranged via the ICU staff.

Whether relatives should witness attempts at resuscitation (e.g. in casualty departments) has attracted debate, with some welcoming the opportunity for relatives to see that appropriate attempts to save the patient are being made, while others argue that their presence may be stressful for medical and nursing staff.

Warrillow S, Farley KJ, Jones D (2015). Int Care; 41: 2173–76

Remifentanil. Ultra-short-acting synthetic **opioid analgesic drug**, 2000 times more potent than **morphine**, introduced in the UK in 1997. Available as a white powder for reconstitution to a 0.1% solution that is stable for 24 h at room temperature. Further diluted for administration; in adults a 50-µg/ml solution is recommended by the manufacturer. Approximately 70% protein-bound. Rapidly metabolised by non-specific plasma and tissue esterases to remifentanil acid (very low potency) and excreted renally. Its context-sensitive **half-life** is about 3 min regardless of the duration of infusion; thus provides a rapid recovery when stopped.

Because it is cleared so rapidly and completely, patients very soon experience pain postoperatively unless longer-acting analgesics are given. In addition, **opioid-induced hyperalgesia** may occur following remifentanil infusion. Has been used via **patient-controlled analgesia** during labour (*see Obstetric analgesia and anaesthesia*). Not recommended for epidural or spinal use because the formulation contains glycine. Postoperative respiratory depression may occur if any drug is left in the dead space of iv lines and subsequently flushed with other drugs or fluids.

- Dosage:
  - to supplement induction of anaesthesia: 30–60 µg/kg/h, ± initial bolus of 0.25–1.0 µg/kg over at least 30 s.
  - during anaesthesia: 3–120 µg/kg/h during IPPV; 2.4 initially then 1.5–6 µg/kg/h during spontaneous ventilation. For target-controlled infusions, a plasma concentration of 3–8 ng/ml will generally achieve adequate intraoperative analgesia (very stimulating procedures may require up to 15 ng/ml).
  - sedation on ICU: 6–9 µg/kg/h initially then 0.36–44.4 µg/kg/h (recommended for ≤3 days).

Remote ischaemic preconditioning, *see Ischaemic preconditioning*

Renal blood flow (RBF). Normally 1200 ml/min (400 ml/100 g/min); i.e., 22% of **cardiac output**.

- Measurement:
  - direct: circumferential **electromagnetic flow measurement**, **Doppler** or thermodilution techniques.
  - indirect:
    - **clearance** methods: a substance neither metabolised nor taken up by the kidney, and completely cleared, is required, e.g. *para*-amino hippuric acid (PAH). Clearance then equals renal plasma flow. RBF = plasma flow divided by (1 – haematocrit). Continuous iv infusion of PAH is required; inaccuracies may occur because clearance of PAH is only 90% in humans. Radioactive markers have been used; almost 100% cleared, they require only a single injection.
    - digital subtraction angiography and radioactive inert gas washout techniques have also been used, the latter indicating regional blood flow.
- Affected by:
  - arterial BP: maintained by **autoregulation** at MAP between 70 and 170 mmHg in normal subjects.
  - **sympathetic nervous system**: stimulation causes vasoconstriction and reduction of RBF, and also increases release of renin and **prostaglandins**. **Dopamine** may increase RBF by vasodilatation via **dopamine receptors**.
  - **renin/angiotensin system**: angiotensin II decreases RBF via vasoconstriction, and increases **aldosterone**

secretion. The latter increases fluid retention, which inhibits further renin release.
- **vasopressin**: causes renal vasoconstriction, especially cortical.
- intravascular volume: in **haemorrhage**, autoregulation is overridden, with vasoconstriction and intrarenal redistribution of blood away from the cortex.
- prostaglandins: increase cortical blood flow, and reduce medullary blood flow.
- **atrial natriuretic peptide**: causes vasodilatation, although effects on RBF are unclear. May alter blood flow distribution.

RBF and **GFR** are reduced by most anaesthetic agents, mainly via reduced cardiac output and BP. Volatile agents are also thought to interfere with autoregulation, although some benefit may arise from the vasodilatation they cause, maintaining blood flow. **Urine** output therefore often falls perioperatively.

Other factors include pre-existing renal disease or conditions predisposing to **renal failure** or impairment, e.g. vascular surgery, toxic drugs, **trauma**, **jaundice**, **hypovolaemia**.

Renal failure. Loss of renal function causing abnormalities in electrolyte, fluid and **acid–base balance** with increases in plasma **urea** and **creatinine**. Divided into acute and chronic renal failure.

- Acute renal failure (*see Acute kidney injury for definitions, diagnosis and management*).
- Chronic renal failure (CRF):
  - irreversible, and often follows **acute kidney injury**.
  - glomerulonephritis is the most common cause, with others, including pyelonephritis, diabetes, polycystic disease, vascular disease and hypertension, drugs and familial causes.
  - classified according to GFR into different stages:
    - normal: healthy with GFR ≥90 ml/min.
    - stage 1: damage with GFR ≥90 ml/min.
    - stage 2 (mild): GFR 60–89 ml/min.
    - stage 3 (moderate): GFR 30–59 ml/min.
    - stage 4 (severe): GFR 15–29 ml/min.
    - stage 5 (established failure): GFR <15 ml/min or on dialysis.
  - features (may not be present until in established failure):
    - malaise, anorexia, confusion leading to convulsions and coma. Peripheral and **autonomic neuropathy** may occur.
    - oedema, **pericarditis**, hypertension (in 80%; thought to result from increased **renin/angiotensin system** activity, sodium and water retention and secondary **hyperaldosteronism**), peripheral vascular disease, **cardiac failure. Ischaemic heart disease** is 20 times more common in CRF patients.
    - nausea, vomiting, diarrhoea.
    - osteomalacia, muscle weakness, bone pain, **hyperparathyroidism, hyperphosphataemia**.
    - amenorrhoea, impotence.
    - pruritus, skin pigmentation, poor healing, increased susceptibility to infection.
    - normocytic normochromic **anaemia**: caused by reduced **erythropoietin** production, shortened red cell survival and bone marrow depression. Impaired **platelet** function may cause bruising and bleeding.
    - **hypernatraemia** or **hyponatraemia** may occur. Hyperkalaemia is usual, but **hypokalaemia** may follow diuretic therapy. Acidosis is common.
  - management:
    - reduction of dietary protein.
    - control of hypertension and cardiac failure.
    - erythropoietin is increasingly used for anaemia.
    - **dialysis**.
    - **renal transplantation**.
- Anaesthesia in renal failure:
  - preoperatively:
    - features of the underlying disease must be assessed, e.g. diabetes, hypertension.
    - assessment for the above features of renal failure, in particular cardiovascular complications, fluid and electrolyte and acid–base derangements. Dialysis may be required; if it has been recently performed, patients are often hypovolaemic, and therefore vulnerable to perioperative hypotension. Anaemia rarely requires transfusion because of its chronicity with compensatory mechanisms. Patients may be at risk from **aspiration of gastric contents** if autonomic neuropathy is present.
    - drugs taken commonly include antianginal and **antihypertensive drugs, insulin** and **corticosteroids**.
    - pre-existing arteriovenous fistulae or **shunts** should be noted.
    - **premedication** as required.
  - perioperatively:
    - iv cannulae should not be sited near arteriovenous fistulae, which should be loosely padded for protection.
    - potassium-containing iv fluids should be avoided.
    - drugs whose actions are not terminated by renal excretion are preferred. Thus a common technique consists of **propofol** followed by **atracurium** and **isoflurane, sevoflurane** or **desflurane**.
    - drugs that accumulate in renal failure (e.g. **morphine**) should be used with caution. Patients are more sensitive to many iv agents, including opioids, because of smaller volumes of distribution and reduced plasma protein levels.
    - **suxamethonium** is not contraindicated unless there is pre-existing peripheral neuropathy or hyperkalaemia.
    - nephrotoxic drugs (e.g. NSAIDs) should be avoided. **Enflurane** has been avoided because of **fluoride ion** formation, although the need for this is controversial. Previous concerns regarding **sevoflurane** and compound A formation are not considered relevant in humans.
    - regional techniques are often suitable, e.g. **brachial plexus block** for fistula formation.
  - postoperatively: close attention to fluid balance is required.

Webster AC, Nagler EV, Morton RL, Masson P (2017). Lancet; 389: 1238–52

Renal failure index, *see Renal failure*

Renal replacement therapy, *see Dialysis*

Renal transplantation. First performed in 1950, and now widespread but limited mainly by the supply of kidneys, which may be from either cadaveric or live donors. Graft survival at 2 years is >80% for cadaveric donors and >90%

for live donors. Indicated for patients with stage 4 or 5 **renal failure**. Previously considered an emergency and performed on unprepared patients, but the importance of proper **preoperative assessment** and preparation is now generally accepted. Major contraindications include active malignancy and infection. Most patients are already on **dialysis** although transplantation may be done before this is needed (pre-emptive transplant). If on dialysis, this is usually performed within 24 h of surgery.

- Anaesthetic problems and techniques are as for chronic renal failure and **transplantation**. Additional points:
  - general anaesthesia is preferred, although **epidural** and **spinal anaesthesia** have been successfully used.
  - direct **arterial blood pressure measurement** is not necessarily required (although **ischaemic heart disease** and **cardiac failure** are common in these patients); **CVP** monitoring is routinely used to guide perioperative fluid therapy.
  - adequate perioperative hydration is vital to optimise intravascular volume and BP in order to avoid acute tubular necrosis in the transplanted kidney.
  - the patient should be kept normothermic.
  - **mannitol**, **furosemide** and **dopamine** are sometimes given before the vessels to the new kidney are unclamped, in order to increase BP, stimulate urine production and improve graft function.
  - transient hypertension may follow unclamping of the renal vessels.
  - postoperatively, **PCA** may be used with care. **NSAIDs** are avoided.
  - there is an increased incidence of kidney rejection in patients who have received blood transfusion during transplantation; preoperative correction of anaemia with **erythropoietin** should be considered.
  - donors should be well hydrated to optimise perfusion of the kidney before harvesting.

Ricaurte L, Vargas J, Lozano E, Díaz L (2013). Transplant Proc; 45: 1386–91

See also, Organ donation

Renal tubular acidosis. Group of conditions characterised by decreased ability of each **nephron** to excrete **hydrogen ions** (cf. **renal failure**, where the overall number of functioning nephrons is reduced, but those that remain excrete more hydrogen ions than normal). Characterised by normal GFR, metabolic acidosis, hyperchloraemia and a normal **anion** gap. May be associated with distal tubule dysfunction (type 1), proximal tubule dysfunction (type 2; usually associated with other abnormalities of proximal tubule function, e.g. Fanconi's syndrome), or **aldosterone** deficiency or resistance (type 4). Type 3 is now considered a combination of types 1 and 2 and not a separate entity. **Acidosis** may be severe, and accompanied by marked **hypokalaemia** (**hyperkalaemia** in type 4). Treatment includes alkali (e.g. oral sodium bicarbonate) in types 1 and 2, thiazides in type 2 and mineralocorticoid therapy in type 4.

[Guido Fanconi (1892–1979), Swiss paediatrician]

Renin/angiotensin system. Renin, a proteolytic enzyme (mw 37 kDa), is synthesised and secreted by the **juxtacapillary apparatus** of the renal tubule. Formed from two precursors, prorenin and preprorenin, its **half-life** is about 80 min. Secretion is increased in **hypovolaemia**, **cardiac failure**, cirrhosis and renal artery stenosis. Secretion is decreased by angiotensin II and **vasopressin**. Renin cleaves the circulating glycoprotein angiotensinogen with subsequent production of the peptides angiotensin I, II and III, involved in **arterial BP** control and **fluid balance** (Table 43). Angiotensin I is a precursor for angiotensin II, a powerful vasoconstrictor with a half-life of a few minutes. It causes **aldosterone** release from the adrenal cortex, and **noradrenaline** release from sympathetic nerve endings. It also stimulates thirst and release of vasopressin, and acts directly on renal tubules, resulting in sodium and water retention. Some may also be produced in the tissues. Angiotensin III also causes aldosterone release and some vasoconstriction.

Table 43 Peptides of the renin/angiotensin system

Substance	*Converted to*	*By the action of*	*Site*
Angiotensinogen	Angiotensin I	Renin	Plasma
Angiotensin I	Angiotensin II	Angiotensin converting enzyme	Mainly in lungs
Angiotensin II	Angiotensin III	Aminopeptidase	Many tissues

Angiotensin converting enzyme inhibitors and **angiotensin II receptor antagonists** are used to treat hypertension. Aliskiren, a direct renin inhibitor, has recently been introduced for the treatment of essential hypertension; it has been associated with renal impairment, stroke, hypotension and **hyperkalaemia**, and avoidance of its combination with the above inhibitors/antagonists has been recommended.

Angiotensin II or its analogues have been used as **vasopressor drugs** when α-agonists are unable to correct severe hypotension, e.g. during surgery for hepatic tumours secreting vasodilator substances.

Reperfusion injury. Tissue injury resulting from restoration of blood flow after a period of ischaemia. Mechanisms include intracellular **calcium** excess, cellular oedema and **free radicals**. Although any tissue may be affected, most work has focused on cardiac function following hypoxic insult or hypoperfusion. Arrhythmias and myocardial stunning (reversible impairment of cardiac function) may also follow reperfusion.

See also, Isoprostanes, No reflow phenomenon

Reptilase time, *see Coagulation studies*

Reserpine. **Antihypertensive drug**, no longer available in the UK. Depletes central and peripheral post-ganglionic adrenergic neurones of **noradrenaline** by irreversibly preventing its reuptake from axoplasm into storage vesicles. Side effects include bradycardia and postural hypotension, depression, sedation and extrapyramidal signs.

Reservoir bag. Usually 2 l capacity in most adult **anaesthetic breathing systems** and 0.5–1.0 l for paediatric use; its volume must exceed tidal volume. Movement indicates ventilation, but estimation of tidal volume from the degree of movement is inaccurate. Made of rubber (usually latex-free), distending when under pressure; maximal pressure is thus prevented from rising above about 60 cmH_2O (**Laplace's law**).

Residual volume (RV). Volume of gas remaining in the lungs after maximal expiration. About 1.5 l in the average

70-kg male; measured as for **FRC**. Increased RV accounts for most cases of increased FRC.
See also, Lung volumes

Resistance. In electrical terms, the ratio of the potential difference across a conductor to the current flowing through it (**Ohm's law**). Measured in ohms (Ω). Resistance to **flow** of a fluid through a circular tube is analogous to this; it equals the ratio of the pressure gradient along the tube to the flow through it.

Resistance vessels. Term given to those blood vessels involved in regulation of **SVR**. 50% of resistance to blood flow occurs in the arterioles, which are thus the main regulators of SVR and therefore distribution of cardiac output.

Resonance. Situation in which an oscillating system responds with maximal amplitude to an alternating external driving force. Occurs when the driving force frequency coincides with the natural oscillatory frequency (resonant frequency) of the system. May occur in pressure transducer systems if long, compliant tubing is used. May give rise to artefacts in the **arterial waveform** during direct **arterial BP measurement**.
See also, Damping

Resonium, *see Polystyrene sulfonate resins*

Respiration, *see Breathing...; Lung...; Metabolism*

Respirators, *see Ventilators*

Respiratory centres, *see Breathing, control of*

Respiratory depression, *see Hypoventilation*

Respiratory distress syndrome (RDS; Hyaline membrane disease). Occurs in approximately 1% of all live births, almost exclusively in premature babies. Caused by deficiency of **surfactant**, normally detectable in the fetal lung at 24 weeks' gestation, although reversal of amniotic fluid lecithin/sphingomyelin ratio (related to fetal lung maturity) only occurs at 30 weeks. Decreased lung **compliance**, increased work of breathing and alveolar collapse may lead to **respiratory failure**, with characteristic granular appearance of the CXR.

Treatment is directed towards preventing **hypoxaemia** with **CPAP** initially, although IPPV is usually necessary, while trying to avoid **O_2 toxicity**, **barotrauma** and **retinopathy of prematurity**. Exogenous surfactant given immediately after birth decreases mortality. **Extracorporeal membrane oxygenation** has been used.

Respiratory exchange ratio. Estimation of **respiratory quotient** derived from expired CO_2/inspired O_2 measurements; thus dependent on ventilation.

Respiratory failure. Defined as an arterial $P\text{O}_2$ <8 kPa (60 mmHg) breathing air at sea level, and at rest, without intracardiac shunting.

- Divided into:
  - type I failure: **hypoxaemia** with normal or low arterial $P\text{CO}_2$. Usually due to **$\dot{V}/\dot{Q}$ mismatch**, with intrapulmonary right-to-left shunt if severe. Causes include **chest infection, asthma, pulmonary embolus**, pulmonary **oedema, PE, ALI, aspiration pneumonitis. O_2 therapy** improves hypoxaemia due to $\dot{V}/\dot{Q}$ mismatch but not shunt; the response to breathing 100% O_2 may indicate the degree of shunt. $P\text{CO}_2$ is often low because of hyperventilation in response to hypoxaemia.
  - type II failure (ventilatory failure): hypoxaemia accompanied by arterial $P\text{CO}_2$ >6.5 kPa (49 mmHg). Causes are as for **hypoventilation**. Acute exacerbation of **COPD** is a common cause.

Diagnosis is made by arterial **blood gas interpretation**, but may be suspected clinically by signs of hypoxaemia and **hypercapnia**, with tachypnoea and use of accessory **respiratory muscles**.

- Treatment:
  - of underlying cause.
  - sitting the patient up increases **FRC** and often improves oxygenation.
  - **oxygen therapy**: should be titrated cautiously in type II failure if chronic hypercapnia is suspected.
  - respiratory stimulant drugs (e.g. **doxapram**) have been used to avoid **IPPV**, e.g. in COPD, but are rarely used now.
  - **CPAP** or **non-invasive positive pressure ventilation** may improve oxygenation and ventilation, avoiding the need for tracheal intubation.
  - IPPV may be required if $P\text{CO}_2$ is rising or the patient is exhausted. Criteria similar to those used in **weaning from ventilators** have been suggested for institution of IPPV. **Tracheostomy** may be necessary to aid weaning from mechanical ventilation.
  - **intravenous oxygenator, extracorporeal oxygenation** and **extracorporeal CO_2 removal** have been used.

Respiratory function tests, *see Lung function tests*

Respiratory muscle fatigue. Inability of the respiratory muscles to sustain tension with repeated activity. May be caused by:

- decreased central drive, e.g. caused by CNS depressant drugs (e.g. **opioid analgesic drugs**).
- increased ventilatory load caused by increased **airway resistance** and reduced **compliance** (e.g. **asthma**, **COPD**) or increased demand (e.g. **exercise**, fever, hypoxaemia).
- respiratory muscle weakness (e.g. following prolonged IPPV, malnutrition, electrolyte imbalance, thyroid disorders, neuromuscular disease, hypoxaemia, sepsis).

Causes hypercapnic **respiratory failure** and difficulty in **weaning from ventilators**. Treatment is directed at the underlying cause.

Respiratory muscles. Muscle actions during:

- quiet inspiration:
  - **diaphragm** (the most important muscle of respiration) flattens and moves 1–2 cm caudally.
  - external intercostal muscles (fibres pass downwards and forwards) lift the upper ribs and sternum up and forwards, and the lower **ribs** mainly up and outwards. The first rib remains fixed.
- forced inspiration: as above, with the diaphragm descending up to 10 cm, plus accessory muscles:
  - scalene muscles.
  - sternomastoid.
  - serratus anterior.
  - pectoralis major.
  - ala nasi.

- quiet expiration: passive recoil of chest and abdomen.
- forced expiration:
  - mainly abdominal muscles (internal and external oblique, rectus abdominis).
  - internal intercostal muscles (pass downwards and backwards); opposite action to the external intercostals, and prevent intercostal bulging.

Respiratory quotient (RQ). Ratio of the volume of CO_2 produced by tissues to the volume of O_2 consumed per unit time. At rest, it depends on the type of substrate being utilised: RQ of carbohydrate is 1, RQ of fat 0.7 and that of protein about 0.82. Also depends on the ratio of aerobic to anaerobic respiration that is occurring; after strenuous **exercise** RQ may rise transiently to up to 2 (due to excess lactic acid reacting with available **bicarbonate**).

Whole body RQ calculated by measurement of expired CO_2 and inspired O_2 only approximates to true RQ, because these volumes are affected by respiration. The term **respiratory exchange ratio** (R) is therefore becoming more commonly used for this measurement.

Respiratory sounds. Traditionally assessed with a **stethoscope**, more recently analysed by digital processing using microphones or accelerometers placed on the chest wall. Sounds arise from vibration of airways and movement of fluid films within them. The nature of the sounds depends on the tissue through which they pass, e.g. quiet or absent in **pleural effusion** and **pneumothorax**, increased transmission in consolidation. The pitch is related to the size of the airway involved and the density of the gas.

- Classification:
  - basic sounds: arise from:
    - central airways of the lung. Normally audible throughout inspiration and the beginning of expiration, with a gap between the two.
    - large airways and trachea. Typically audible throughout both inspiratory and expiratory phases, with no gap. Usually audible only over the trachea, this 'bronchial breathing' sound may be heard over the chest if transmitted to the stethoscope via abnormally solid tissue (e.g. consolidated lung).

    Range from under 100 Hz to over 1000–3000 Hz.
  - adventitious sounds:
    - **wheezing**: arises from the central/lower airways with a sinusoidal frequency (polyphonic), ranging from 100 Hz to over 1000 Hz.
    - rhonchi: snore-like, arise from the larger airways. Typically under 300 Hz and rapidly damped, but lasting over 100 ms. Occur in small airway collapse and secretions.
    - crackles: fine; arise from the lower airways. Rapidly damped, typically lasting under 20 ms. Occur in secretions, oedema and fibrosis.

Other sounds may occur (e.g. **stridor**), although not from the lung itself.

Respiratory stimulant drugs, *see Analeptic drugs; Opioid receptor antagonists*

Respiratory symbols. By convention, standardised as in Table 44. Thus, e.g. F_IO_2 = inspired fractional concentration of O_2; P_aO_2 = arterial O_2 tension.

S_pO_2 has been suggested as representing haemoglobin saturation as measured by pulse **oximetry**.

Table 44 Notation of respiratory symbols

General variables (N.B. a dash above a symbol indicates mean value)

V = gas volume, Q = volume of blood } with a dot above = volume per unit time
P = pressure or tension
F = fractional concentration in dry gas mixture
f = respiratory frequency
C = content of a gas in blood
D = diffusing capacity
R = respiratory exchange ratio
S = saturation of haemoglobin with O_2 or CO_2

Localisation (in subscript):

I = inspired gas
E = expired gas
A = alveolar gas
T = tidal gas
D = dead space gas
B = barometric
a = arterial blood
c = pulmonary capillary blood
v = venous blood

Respirometer. Device for measuring expiratory gas volumes. Examples:

- Wright's anemometer (axial turbine flowmeter): a design commonly integrated into **ventilators**. Expired gas is passed into its chamber through oblique slits, creating circular gas flow that causes rotation of a double-vaned turbine within the chamber. Rotation is measured and displayed as the volume of gas passing through the device, using an indicator needle attached to the vane, and a dial. Electrical versions are also available; rotations of a disc attached to the vane interrupt passage of light between an emitter and photosensitive cell mounted astride the disc. Less prone to inertia inaccuracies than the Wright's respirometer.
- Wright's respirometer: measures gas volume passing in one direction only; thus it may be placed in the two-way portion of a breathing system. It tends to underestimate at low volumes and overestimate at high volumes, due to inertia/momentum of the vane.
- others: include **flowmeters**, whose signals may be integrated to indicate volume.

[B Martin Wright (1912–2001), London engineer]
See also, Spirometer

Resuscitation, *see Cardiopulmonary resuscitation*

Resuscitation Council (UK). Multiprofessional group formed in 1981 to facilitate education of lay and professional members of the population in the most effective methods of resuscitation. Aims of the Council include: encouraging research and study of resuscitation techniques; the promotion of training and education in resuscitation; and the establishment and maintenance of standards. The Council has published guidelines for **CPR** and has set up a series of advanced courses in adult and paediatric resuscitation (i.e., **ALS**, **ILS**).
See also, European Resuscitation Council

Resuscitators, *see Self-inflating bags*

Reteplase. Recombinant plasminogen activator, used as a **fibrinolytic drug** in management of **acute coronary syndromes.** Has a longer **half-life** (13–16 min) than **alteplase.**

- Dosage: 10 U iv in under 2 min, repeated after 30 min.
- Side effects: as for fibrinolytic drugs. May precipitate with heparin solutions.

Reticular formation/activating system, *see Ascending reticular activating system*

Retinopathy of prematurity (Retrolental fibroplasia). Abnormal proliferation of retinal vessels in response to high arterial PO_2 for long periods. Very premature infants of low birth weight are the most susceptible, remaining so until 44 weeks' post-conceptual age. O_2 therapy should therefore be monitored closely (e.g. when treating **respiratory distress syndrome**). Precise mechanisms are unclear, as it may occur in infants who have not received additional O_2. Genetic factors appear to be important. The role of O_2 administered during neonatal anaesthesia is controversial, but F_IO_2 is generally thought to be best restricted to 0.3 unless higher concentrations are required to maintain arterial PO_2 of 8.5–11 kPa (60–80 mmHg).

Retrobulbar block. Obsolete technique, performed to allow surgery to the globe of the eye, e.g. cataract extraction. **Cranial nerves** III and VI, and long and short ciliary nerves (branches of V_1) are blocked within the cone formed by the extraocular muscles. Now rarely used due to its relatively high frequency of complications, including retrobulbar haemorrhage, intravascular and subarachnoid injection and globe perforation. **Peribulbar block** and **sub-Tenon's block** are safer and equally effective alternatives.

With the patient supine and looking straight ahead, a 3.0-cm needle is inserted through the conjunctiva at the lower lateral orbital rim. It is passed backward and 10 degrees upward until its tip has passed the mid-globe, then angled medially and upward to reach a point behind the globe at the level of the iris. After aspiration, 2–4 ml **lidocaine** with **hyaluronidase** 5 U/ml is injected.

See also, Orbital cavity

Retrolental fibroplasia, *see Retinopathy of prematurity*

Retzius cave block. Used to supplement anaesthesia for prostatectomy and bladder surgery. The cave of Retzius is the space between the bladder and pubic symphysis, containing nerves of the **sacral plexus** and a venous plexus. After subcutaneous infiltration 2–3 cm above the pubis, an 8-cm needle is directed to the back of the symphysis. After negative aspiration for blood, 10 ml **local anaesthetic agent** with adrenaline is injected in the midline, with a further injection on each side.

[Anders Retzius (1796–1860), Swedish anatomist]

Reuben valve, *see Non-rebreathing valves*

Revised trauma score (RTS). **Trauma scale** derived from the **trauma score** but simplified and with greater emphasis on the presence of **head injury**. Uses the **Glasgow Coma Scale**, systolic BP and respiratory rate, each assigned a value of 0–4, with 0 representing the most severe. The values are added to give a total RTS, with a normal of 12. Superior to the trauma score at predicting outcome; an RTS of <4 suggests the need for transfer to a specialist trauma unit.

Gilpin DA, Nelson PG (1991). Injury; 22: 35–7

Reye's syndrome. Rare condition of unknown aetiology, characterised by vomiting, depression of consciousness and **hepatic failure. Jaundice** is typically absent or minimal. Usually occurs in children, typically following a viral illness; **aspirin** has been implicated in epidemiological studies and is thus contraindicated as an **analgesic drug** in those under 16 years of age (it may be used in children for other specific indications, e.g. as an **antiplatelet drug** after cardiac surgery). Thought to be due to an acquired mitochondrial abnormality. Treatment is mainly supportive, with correction of metabolic disturbances, **cerebral oedema** and raised **ICP**. Thought to be improved by administering up to a third of the fluid intake as 10% dextrose.

[R Douglas Reye (1912–1977), Australian pathologist]

Reynolds' number (*Re*). Dimensionless number predicting when **flow** of a **fluid** becomes turbulent:

$$Re = \frac{\text{density} \times \text{velocity} \times \text{diameter of tube}}{\textbf{viscosity}}$$

Turbulent flow occurs at *Re* >2000, laminar flow at <2000.

[Osborne Reynolds (1842–1912), Irish-born English engineer]

Rhabdomyolysis, *see Myoglobinuria*

Rhesus blood groups. System of **blood group** antigens first described in 1939 following work on rhesus monkeys. Includes many antigens but the terms Rhesus (Rh)-positive and -negative usually refer to the D antigen, as it is the most immunogenic. Rh-negative individuals have no D antigen, and form anti-D antibodies when injected with Rh-positive blood. 85% of Caucasians are Rh-positive, as are 99% of Orientals.

- Clinical importance:
  - **blood transfusion** reactions: administration of Rh-positive blood to Rh-negative individuals who have anti-D antibodies following previous exposure to Rh-positive blood.
  - haemolytic disease of the newborn: occurs in Rh-positive fetuses of Rh-negative mothers. Passage of fetal blood cells into the maternal circulation during pregnancy or labour causes formation of maternal anti-D antibodies. These may pass into subsequent Rh-positive fetuses, causing haemolysis, which may be fatal. Incidence of primary immunisation in primigravidae is about 15%. Uncommon now with widespread availability of anti-Rh immunoglobulin, which is administered to Rh-negative mothers at delivery, and after abortion or amniocentesis. Routine administration of anti-Rh to all Rh-negative pregnant women has been suggested as a way of reducing the problem further.

Rheumatic fever. Acute systemic autoimmune disease occurring after infection by certain serotypes of group A streptococci. Most common between 5 and 15 years of age; now rare in the West but still common in developing countries and in indigenous populations of Australia and New Zealand. Typically occurring 2–6 weeks after a sore throat, features include fever, flitting asymmetrical arthritis, carditis, chorea and erythema marginatum (erythema spreading out from a central macule while the centre returns to normal). Subcutaneous nodules (Aschoff bodies) may occur over the extensor surfaces of the wrists, elbows and knees. Epistaxis and abdominal pain are common.

Diagnosed clinically and by evidence of recent **streptococcal infection**. Traditionally treated with rest, **penicillin, aspirin** and **corticosteroids**; the effect of drugs on valve disease has been controversial although prolonged (>5–10 years) monthly injections of long-acting penicillin are now thought to prevent recurrence and progressive heart disease. 50% of patients with carditis progress to valvular heart disease, which may not present until later in life. Mitral and aortic valves are most commonly affected.

Anaesthetic management of patients previously affected is directed towards any existing valve disease and associated complications (e.g. **cardiac failure, pulmonary hypertension**).

[Karl Albert Ludwig Aschoff (1866–1942), German pathologist]

Webb RH, Grant C, Harnden A (2015). BMJ, 351: h3443

See also, individual valve lesions

Rheumatoid arthritis (Rheumatoid disease). Systemic inflammatory disease with many features of **connective tissue diseases**. Characterised by symmetrical polyarthropathy, but affects other organs too. Three times more common in females; peak incidence is at ages 30–50 years. Up to 5% of females over 60 years are affected in the UK. Aetiology is unclear but may involve an immunological process triggered by infectious agents coupled with a genetic predisposition. Recent advances in treatment, including early therapy with disease-modifying antirheumatic drugs (DMARDS), including biological agents that block tumour necrosis factor, appear to improve the course and severity of the condition.

- Anaesthetic considerations:
    - systemic effects:
        - skeletal: **temporomandibular joint** involvement, atlantoaxial subluxation, reduced mobility of the lumbar/**cervical spine**.
        - neuromuscular: nerve entrapment, sensory/motor neuropathy, myopathy.
        - respiratory: restrictive defect due to **pulmonary fibrosis** and costochondral disease, pulmonary nodules, **pleural effusions**, cricoarytenoid arthritis.
        - cardiovascular: **ischaemic heart disease** (often with 'silent' **MI**), **pericarditis, heart block**, coronary arteritis, peripheral vasculitis.
        - haematological: **anaemia** (usually normochromic normocytic), leucopenia. Felty's syndrome consists of rheumatoid arthritis, splenomegaly and leucopenia; **thrombocytopenia**, malaise and fever may occur.
        - renal: amyloidosis, pyelonephritis, drug-related impairment.
        - others: ophthalmic complications, including Sjögren's syndrome, and atrophic skin and subcutaneous tissues.
    - drug therapy: may include **NSAIDs, corticosteroids** and **immunosuppressive drugs**. Gold may cause blood dyscrasias, peripheral neuritis, pulmonary fibrosis, hepatic and renal impairment. **Penicillamine** may cause blood dyscrasias, renal impairment, neuropathy and a **myasthenia gravis**-like syndrome.
    - practical considerations:
        - airway maintenance difficulties: caused by involvement of the temporomandibular joint, cervical spine and larynx. Clinical evidence of laryngeal involvement should prompt a preoperative nasendoscopy to assess degree of laryngeal stenosis. The value of preoperative cervical spine x-rays is uncertain; flexion/extension radiographs may worsen atlantoaxial subluxation, are often diagnostically inadequate, and may not alter anaesthetic technique (although proven cervical instability mandates minimal neck manipulation).
        - venous cannulation may be difficult; skin and veins are fragile, and joints may have reduced mobility.
        - discomfort lying flat; skeletal involvement may make regional techniques unsuitable. Careful positioning and padding are required. Skin is easily damaged.
        - wrist and hand arthritis may preclude the use of **patient-controlled analgesia**.

[Augustus R Felty (1895–1963), US physician; Henrik SC Sjögren (1899–1986), Swedish ophthalmologist]

Smolen JS, Aletaha D, McInnes IB (2016). Lancet; 388: 2023–38

See also, Intubation, difficult

Ribavirin (Tribavirin). **Antiviral drug**; a nucleoside, it inhibits DNA synthesis and is active against many RNA and DNA viruses, although usually reserved for treatment of respiratory syncytial viral infection and Lassa fever. Also used in combination with interferon alfa for the treatment of chronic hepatitis C.

- Dosage: nebulisation or aerosol inhalation of 20 mg/ml solution for 12–18 h for 3–7 days. For hepatitis C, 400–600 mg orally bd.
- Side effects are rare but include anaemia and worsening respiratory function.

Rib fractures. Middle **ribs** are most commonly affected. Fracture usually occurs at the posterior axillary line, the point of maximal stress. If the first three ribs are affected, injury to the aorta and tracheobronchial tree should be considered. If the lower ribs are involved, damage to liver, spleen and kidneys may occur. **Pneumothorax** and haemothorax may be present. Morbidity and mortality are related to the number of ribs involved; fractures of seven or more ribs have a mortality of ~ 30%.

Rib fractures cause pain on breathing, with splinting of the chest wall, inability to cough and atelectasis. Multiple fractures may cause flail chest. The mainstay of treatment is good analgesia; this may involve systemic analgesics, epidural anaesthesia or regional blocks, e.g. **intercostal nerve block, serratus anterior plane block.** If pain persists, surgical rib fixation may be necessary.

General management is as for **chest trauma** and **abdominal trauma.**

May L, Hillermann C, Patil S (2016). BJA Educ; 16: 26–32

Ribs. Exist in 12 (thoracic) pairs, with occasional additional cervical or lumbar ribs. Attached to thoracic vertebrae posteriorly and costal cartilage anteriorly. Ribs 2–8 are typical (Fig. 138a), consisting of:

- head: bears two facets for articulation with adjacent vertebrae.

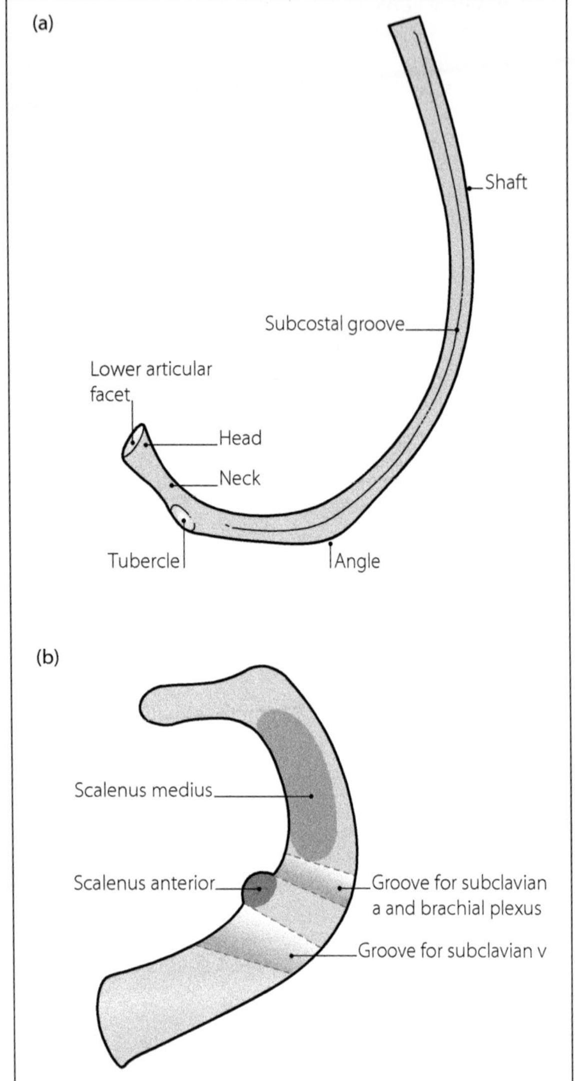

Fig. 138 Anatomy of (a) a typical rib, seen from undersurface; (b) the first rib, seen from above

- neck.
- tubercle: articulates posteriorly with the transverse process of the corresponding vertebra.
- shaft: flattened in the vertical plane. Curves forwards and inwards from the angle, lying lateral to the tubercle. The intercostal neurovascular bundle runs in the subcostal groove at the inferior border.

- The first rib is of particular anaesthetic importance because of its relationship to the **brachial plexus** and other structures (Fig. 138b). Features:
  - short, wide and flattened in the horizontal plane.
  - lower surface is smooth and lies on pleura.
  - upper surface is grooved for the subclavian vessels and brachial plexus.
  - sympathetic chain, superior intercostal artery and upper branch of the first intercostal nerve lie anterior to its neck, between it and the pleura.
  - scalenus anterior and medius attach to the scalene tubercle and body of the rib, respectively.

See also, Intercostal nerve block; Intercostal space

Table 45 RIFLE criteria for renal failure

Stage	*GFR*	*Urine output*
Risk	Creatinine >1.5 × baseline or GFR >25% decrease	<0.5 ml/kg/h for 6 h
Injury	Creatinine >2 × baseline or GFR >50% decrease	<0.5 ml/kg/h for 12 h
Failure	Creatinine >3 × baseline or >355 µmol/l (with a rise of >44) or GFR >75% decrease	<0.3 ml/kg/h for 24 h or anuria for 12 h
Loss	Complete loss of renal function for >4 weeks	
End-stage renal disease	Complete loss of function for >3 months	

Rifabutin. **Antituberculous drug** used for prophylaxis against *Mycobacterium avium* in immunocompromised patients.

- Dosage: prophylaxis: 300 mg orally od; treatment: 150–450 mg od.
- Side effects: blood dyscrasias, nausea, vomiting, hepatic impairment, orange discoloration of body secretions.

Rifampicin. **Antibacterial drug**, used primarily as an **antituberculous drug** but also in brucellosis, **Legionnaires' disease**, severe **staphylococcal infection**, leprosy and as prophylaxis against **meningococcal disease** (thus may be given to ICU staff after caring for an infected patient or to household contacts). Causes hepatic **enzyme induction** and thus decreases the efficacy of oral contraceptives, anticoagulants and phenytoin.

- Dosage: 300 mg orally (iv in severe infections) bd–qds.
- Side effects: GIT upset, haemolytic anaemia, dyspnoea, renal and hepatic impairment, rashes, myopathy. Colours body secretions orange.

RIFLE criteria. Consensus staging classification of **acute kidney injury** described in 2004, consisting of five stages of increasingly severe impairment graded according to plasma **creatinine** level, **GFR** and/or **urine** output (Table 45):

Limitations of the classification include: frequent disparity between creatinine and urine output criteria; requirement for knowledge of baseline creatinine/GFR; poor sensitivity of the 'Risk' criteria, i.e., less severe renal impairment is also associated with worse outcome.

A modified version, the AKIN (Acute Kidney Injury Network) classification, includes the following changes:

- stages 1–3 corresponding to RIF categories; removal of 'Loss' and 'End-stage' categories.
- addition of an absolute increase in creatinine of 26.5 µmol/l to stage 1.
- 48-h timeframe specified for period of deterioration.
- patients receiving renal replacement therapy automatically classed as stage 3.
- diagnostic criteria to be applied only after fluid optimisation.

Lopes JA, Jorge S (2012). Clin Kidney J; 6: 8–14

Right atrial pressure, *see Cardiac catheterisation; Central venous pressure*

Right ventricular function. The right ventricle (RV) receives blood from systemic and coronary veins, and pumps it into the left ventricle (LV) across the pulmonary vascular bed. The pulmonary bed is of low resistance, therefore RV pressures (15–25/8–12 mmHg) are lower than systemic. The low intraventricular pressure permits right **coronary blood flow** to be continuous throughout the **cardiac cycle**. The output of the right heart is influenced by its **preload**, contractility and **afterload**.

The RV is very compliant and, when afterload increases (e.g. because of **pulmonary vascular resistance** secondary to lung injury), the RV dilates. The end-diastolic volume may increase to a greater extent than the preload; consequently, the RV **ejection fraction** will decrease markedly with increasing afterload. Changes in the geometry of the RV affect the function of the LV, and vice versa (ventricular interdependence), e.g. impaired RV function (whether acute or chronic) may hinder LV function via RV distension and deviation of the interventricular septum.

Although the RV is analogous to the LV in terms of control mechanisms, it is more difficult to assess; e.g. the relationship between RV preload, RV volume and RV filling pressures is not always constant. In addition, attempts to study RV function are hindered by the greater effect of respiratory excursions on the RV because the pressures involved are less than those on the left side of the heart.

RV function may be altered in acute **respiratory failure**, **sepsis**, **chest trauma**, **ischaemic heart disease**, and after **cardiac surgery**. The possibility of RV ischaemia or infarction in critically ill patients as a cause of RV dysfunction is increasingly recognised. During **IPPV**, decreased **venous return** due to the increased intrathoracic pressure results in decreased RV end-diastolic volume and thus **cardiac output**. RV impairment may result in the classic features of right-sided **cardiac failure**, but may present as a general poor perfusion state.

Vandenheuval MA, Bouchez S, Wouters PF, DeHert SG (2013). Eur J Anaesthesiol; 30: 386–94

Ringer's solution. Developed as an in vitro medium for tissues and organisms, emphasising the importance of inorganic ions in maintaining cellular integrity. Exact constitution varies between laboratories, but approximates to sodium 137 mmol/l, potassium 4 mmol/l, calcium 3 mmol/l and chloride 142 mmol/l. Modifications include Ringer's lactate (**Hartmann's solution**) and Ringer's acetate (similar to Hartmann's solution but with acetate instead of lactate).

[Sydney Ringer (1834–1910), English physician]

Lee JA (1981). Anaesthesia; 36: 1115–21

rINNs, Recommended International Non-proprietary Names, *see Explanatory notes*

Risk management. Process for reducing the frequency and overall cost of adverse events, e.g. complications of anaesthesia. Consists of:

- analysis of risks (e.g. morbidity/mortality meetings, **critical incident** reporting schemes). Risks are often categorised into:
  - individual-based (e.g. arising from human error), e.g. wrong drug given.
  - environment-based (e.g. arising from the interaction between anaesthetists and the operating theatre), e.g. disconnection of breathing system.
  - system-based (human actions superimposed on inherent flaws in a system or process), e.g. because of alterations to the operating list caused by cancellations due to lack of beds, a patient arrives in the anaesthetic room without the diseased limb marked and has the wrong leg amputated.
- prevention of risks associated with routine activities (e.g. proper training and supervision, provision of trained anaesthetic assistants, implementing the **World Health Organization Surgical Safety Checklist**).
- avoidance of particularly high-risk activities (e.g. wider use of regional anaesthesia for caesarean section).
- minimising the severity of adverse events should they occur (e.g. training in defibrillation, maintenance of emergency drugs and equipment).
- risk financing (e.g. indemnity).
- having a system for dealing with disasters and complaints, to reduce both psychological and legal sequelae.

Audit is an integral part of a risk management programme, the costs of which may be considerable, although the avoidance of litigation is a strong incentive. Protocols may contribute to risk management by standardising care.

See also, Clinical governance; Quality assurance/improvement

Ritodrine hydrochloride. **β-Adrenergic receptor agonist**, used as a tocolytic drug in premature labour but discontinued because of its side effect profile including arrhythmias, pulmonary oedema, and blood dyscrasias after prolonged use.

Rivaroxaban. Orally active direct **factor Xa inhibitor**, licensed in adults for **DVT** prophylaxis after elective hip or knee replacement surgery, **stroke** prophylaxis in non-valvular **AF**, and prevention of thrombotic events after acute coronary syndromes. More effective than **enoxaparin** at preventing **DVT** and **PE**, with comparable risks of haemorrhagic side effects. Also used off-license for treatment of DVT/PE and **acute coronary syndromes**.

Rapidly absorbed via the oral route (peak plasma concentration within 2–4 h) with 80%–100% oral **bioavailability**. 70% undergoes hepatic metabolism (by the cytochrome P_{450} system) to inactive products; 30% is excreted unchanged in urine. Thus, caution is required in patients with **renal failure**, and those taking drugs that cause hepatic **enzyme induction/inhibition**.

- Dosage:
  - prevention of DVT after knee or hip replacement surgery: 10 mg orally od, starting 6–10 h after surgery and continued for 2 or 5 weeks, respectively.
  - treatment of DVT/PE: 15 mg orally bd for 21 days, then 20 mg od.
  - prevention of stroke: 20 mg orally od.
  - following acute coronary syndromes: 2.5 mg orally bd, with aspirin ± clopidogrel.
- Side effects: nausea, haemorrhage.

Rivastigmine, *see Acetylcholinesterase inhibitors*

ROC curves, *see Receiver operating characteristic curves*

Rocuronium bromide. Non-depolarising **neuromuscular blocking drug**, introduced in 1994. Chemically related to vecuronium, with similar lack of cardiovascular effects, although tachycardia may accompany very large doses. Has been suggested as an alternative to **suxamethonium** in rapid sequence induction. Good intubating conditions occur 60 s after an initial dose of 0.6 mg/kg; relaxation lasts for about 30–40 min (about 20 min after 0.45 mg/kg). During a **rapid sequence induction**, an intubating dose of 1–1.2 mg/kg is advocated by some; it produces better intubating conditions in a shorter time. Supplementary dose: 0.15 mg/kg; effects last for about 15 min. May be infused iv at 0.3–0.6 mg/kg/h after a loading dose. Primarily excreted by the liver. Cumulation is unlikely at recommended doses. Reversed by **sugammadex**.

Ropivacaine hydrochloride. Amide **local anaesthetic agent**, introduced in 1997. Chemically related to **bupivacaine** (a propyl group replacing a butyl group) but less lipid-soluble and less toxic, being associated with less severe CNS and CVS adverse effects. pK_a is 8.1. Presented as the (S)-enantiomer (*see Isomerism*). Used in 0.2%–1.0% concentrations; initially reported to be approximately equipotent to bupivacaine in terms of analgesia while producing less motor block, e.g. for **epidural anaesthesia**. However, this is disputed, the reduced motor block seen with ropivacaine being related to its lower potency and thus selection of non-comparable solutions in comparative studies. In addition, comparable concentrations contain slightly less ropivacaine than bupivacaine.

Has vasoconstrictor properties; thus relatively unaffected by addition of **vasoconstrictor drugs**. About 94% protein-bound; undergoes hepatic metabolism with 1% excreted unchanged in the urine. Has about 40% greater **clearance** than bupivacaine. Maximal safe dose is estimated at 3.5 mg/kg.

Rotameter. The trade name of a type of **flowmeter** commonly used on **anaesthetic machines**; first used in the 1930s and still in common use.

- Features include:
    - constant pressure, variable orifice.
    - consists of a needle valve, below a bobbin within a tapered tube. Gas flow rates are marked along the tube's length. Readings are taken from the top of the bobbin. Tubes are arranged in banks at the back of the anaesthetic machine, traditionally for O_2, CO_2 and cyclopropane (the last two on older machines only), N_2O, and air, from left to right in the UK (*see later*).
    - accurate to within 2%.
    - bobbins are made of light metal alloy; each is individually matched to its particular tube, and is specific for a certain gas.
    - the tube's taper is narrower at the bottom to allow accurate measurement of low flow rates, and wider above to measure higher flows.
    - the space between the bobbin and walls of the tube is narrow at the bottom of the tube; gas **flow** behaves as through a tube, i.e., is largely laminar. Thus gas **viscosity** is important at low flow rates. Higher up the tube, the space between the bobbin and tube is wide compared with the length of the bobbin, because of the tube's taper. Gas flow behaves as through an orifice, i.e., is turbulent. Thus gas density is important at high flow rates.
    - inaccuracies may result from sticking of the bobbin against the sides of the tube. This is reduced by:
        - keeping the tube vertical to reduce friction between bobbin and tube.
        - angular notches in the bobbin, causing it to rotate when gas flows.
        - regular cleaning to prevent dirt accumulating within the tube.
        - reduction of static charge building up within the tube. Many are internally coated with a thin layer of gold. Alternatively, regular spraying with antistatic solution may be performed.
    - the O_2 control knob is larger than the others and differently shaped to aid recognition. All are colour-coded as for **cylinders**.
    - on some older machines, the CO_2 bobbin could be hidden at the top of the tube if the CO_2 valve was accidentally left fully open.
    - with the traditional arrangement of rotameters, i.e., O_2 upstream, O_2 may be lost if there is a leak from a tube downstream. This may be prevented by placing the O_2 inlet downstream from the others, e.g. by fitting a baffle across the top of the rotameter tubes so that N_2O enters first, and O_2 last.
    - in modern machines, N_2O and O_2 rotameters are mechanically linked such that less than 25% O_2 cannot be delivered.

Rotational therapy (Kinetic therapy). Technique in which critically ill patients are turned laterally from the horizontal to an angle of about 40 degrees, often several times per hour on a programmable bed. Shown to reduce the incidence of **nosocomial pneumonia** and possibly **decubitus ulcers**, **DVT** and **PE**. Also reported to shorten duration of both IPPV and ICU stay. May share mechanisms of action with **prone ventilation** techniques. Compared with the prone position, it has less chance of accidental displacement of tubes and catheters/cannulae, damage to eyes/face/limbs, stimulation of coughing and cardiovascular instability. Accessibility to the patient remains good.

Staudinger T, Bojic A, Holzinger U, et al (2010). Crit Care Med; 38: 486–90

Rowbotham, Edgar Stanley (1890–1979). English pioneer of anaesthesia. With **Magill**, developed tracheal intubation, including blind nasal intubation, and endotracheal anaesthesia. Also pioneered **basal narcosis** with rectal **paraldehyde**, and local and intravenous techniques. The first anaesthetist in the UK to use **cyclopropane**. Designed several pieces of apparatus, including a **vaporiser**, airway, local anaesthetic needles and other equipment.

Condon HA, Gilchrist E (1986). Anaesthesia; 41: 46–52

Royal College of Anaesthetists. Arose from the granting of a Charter to the **College of Anaesthetists** by Queen Elizabeth II in March 1992. Regulates and promotes research, training, education and maintenance of standards in anaesthesia. Administers the **FRCA examination.** Has around 17 000 members in various categories, of whom ~14 000 are UK-based (~5000 of whom are trainees without the Final FRCA). Created the **Faculty of Pain Medicine** in 2007 and the **Faculty of Intensive Care Medicine** in 2010. The ***British Journal of Anaesthesia*** has been its official journal since 1990.

Spence AA (1992). Br J Anaesth; 68: 457–8

R–R interval. Time between successive **R waves** on the **ECG**. Thus heart rate =

$$\frac{60}{\text{R–R interval(s)}}$$

Normally varies by less than 0.16 s at rest (**sinus arrhythmia**). Useful in the diagnosis of **autonomic neuropathy**.

RT, Reptilase time, *see Coagulation studies*

RTS, *see Revised trauma score*

Rule of nines. Guide to the percentage of body **surface area** represented by various parts of the body; used in assessment and treatment of **burns**:

- head: 9%.
- arms: 9% each.
- trunk: 18% front; 18% back.
- legs: 18% each.
- perineum: 1%.

For small areas, the patient's palmar surface of the hand and fingers represents about 1% of surface area. For children, proportions of body parts vary with age, with the head comprising up to 18% in infants (and the lower limbs contributing proportionally less); for accurate assessment specialised charts should be used.

S-100β protein. **Calcium**-binding protein present in glial cells, studied as an early marker of damage to the **blood–brain barrier**, e.g. after **stroke**, **TBI**, **cardiac surgery** and **neurosurgery**. A normal level reliably excludes significant CNS injury. After moderate or severe TBI, raised levels reliably predict poor short- and long-term prognosis. Metabolised in the kidney with a **half-life** of ~25 min, the serum concentration is usually negligible but increases after brain injury, although it is thought that S-100β may also be produced from other tissues and its relationship with functional impairment is uncertain.
Cata JP, Abdelmalak B, Farag E (2011). Br J Anaesth; 107: 844–58

S wave. Downward deflection following the **R wave** of the **ECG** (*see Fig. 60b;* **Electrocardiography**). Its size usually decreases from V_2 to V_6; the deepest wave is normally less than 30 mm. Prominence in standard leads I, II and III ($S_1S_2S_3$ pattern) may be normal in young people but may be associated with right ventricular hypertrophy. May also be seen in **MI** along with other changes.
See also, QRS complex

SA node, Sinoatrial node, *see Heart, conducting system*

Sacral canal. Cavity, 10–15 cm long and triangular in section, running the length of the sacrum, itself formed from five fused sacral **vertebrae** (Fig. 139). Continuous cranially with the lumbar **vertebral canal**. The anterior wall is formed by the fused bodies of the sacral vertebrae, and the posterior walls by the fused sacral laminae. Due to failure of fusion of the fifth laminar arch, the posterior wall is deficient between the cornua, forming the sacral hiatus, which is covered by the sacrococcygeal membrane (punctured during **caudal analgesia**). Congenital variants of fusion are common, e.g. deficient fusion of several laminae; this is thought to be a contributing cause of unreliability of caudal analgesia. The canal contains the termination of the dural sac at S2, the sacral nerves and coccygeal nerve, the internal vertebral venous plexus and fat. Its average volume in adults is 32 ml in females and 34 ml in males.
Crighton IM, Barry BP, Hobbs GJ (1997). Br J Anaesth; 78: 391–5

Sacral nerve block, *see Caudal analgesia*

Sacral plexus. Supplies the pelvic and hip muscles, and the skin of the buttock and posterior thigh. Lies on piriformis muscle on the posterior wall of the pelvis, deep to the pelvic fascia, and is formed from the anterior primary rami of L4–S4 (Fig. 140). Its major branches are the sciatic, pudendal and gluteal nerves.
See also, Sciatic nerve block

SAD, *see Supraglottic airway device*

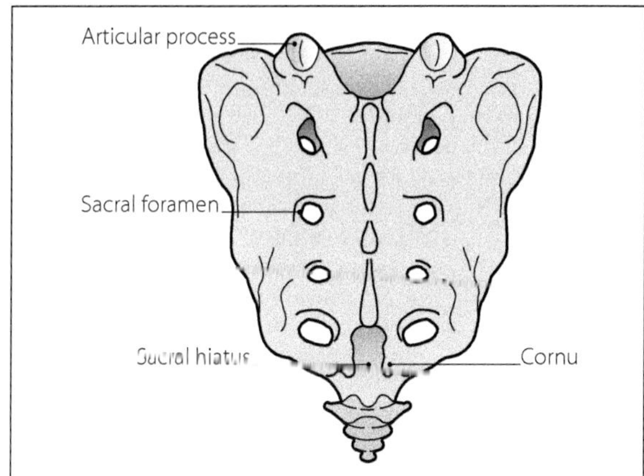

Fig. 139 Anatomy of the sacrum (posterior view)

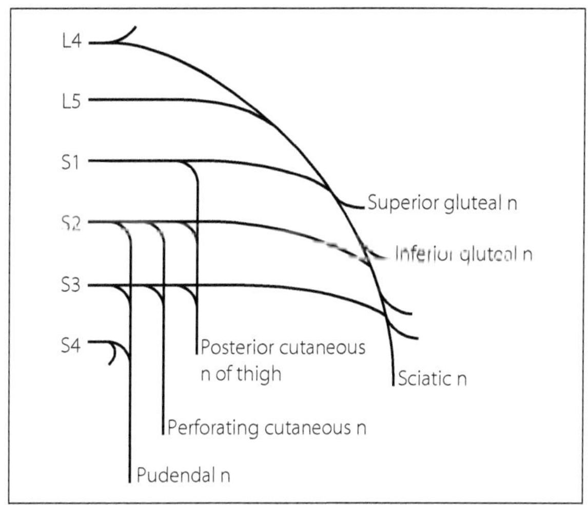

Fig. 140 Plan of the sacral plexus

Saddle block, *see Spinal anaesthesia*

Safe transport and retrieval (STaR). Course conceived by the Advanced Life Support Group and first run in 1998. Teaches a systematic approach to the safe transfer and retrieval of critically ill and injured patients. Aimed at doctors, nurses and paramedics.
See also, Transportation of critically ill patients

Salbutamol. **β-Adrenergic receptor agonist**, used mainly as a **bronchodilator drug**. Relatively selective for β_2-receptors, although it does cause β_1-receptor stimulation. Undergoes extensive **first-pass metabolism** if given orally; thus usually administered by inhalation or iv. Produces bronchodilatation within 15 min; effects last 3–4 h. May also reduce the release of **histamine** and inflammatory mediators from **mast cells** sensitised with IgE; hence its particular use in **asthma**.

Also used as a **tocolytic drug** in premature labour and to improve cardiac output in low perfusion states, via β_2-receptor-mediated smooth muscle relaxation in the **uterus** and blood vessels, respectively.

- Dosage:
  - 2–4 mg orally tds/qds.
  - 500 µg im/sc, 4-hourly as required.
  - 250 µg iv slowly, repeated as required. 3–20 µg/min infusion may be used. IV injection may be more effective than inhalation in severe asthma, but this is controversial. Up to 45 µg/min may be required in premature labour.
  - 1–2 puffs by aerosol (100–200 µg) tds/qds. 200–400 µg is recommended for dry powder inhalation, because **bioavailability** for the latter is lower.
  - 2.5–5 mg by nebulised solution, 4–6-hourly.
- Side effects: tachycardia, tremor, headache. **Hypokalaemia** may occur with prolonged use. **Pulmonary oedema** and **MI** may occur after use for tocolysis; iv infusion should therefore not be used >48 h, and oral administration not used at all as the evidence for benefit is small.

Salicylate poisoning. Usually acute but may be chronic, especially in children.

- Features:
  - nausea, vomiting, haematemesis, sweating, tinnitus, deafness, confusion, hallucinations. Loss of consciousness is uncommon unless poisoning is severe.
  - **hyperventilation** results from direct respiratory centre stimulation, possibly via central uncoupling of oxidative phosphorylation. Respiratory **alkalosis** results. Compensatory renal excretion of **bicarbonate** results in urinary water and potassium loss with **dehydration** and **hypokalaemia**.
  - metabolic **acidosis** is caused by the salicylic acid, and its metabolic effects (increased production of **ketone bodies**, **lactic acid** and pyruvic acid, **hyperglycaemia** or **hypoglycaemia**). Thus the urine, initially alkaline, becomes acid.
  - **arrhythmias**, hypotension.
  - **convulsions**, **pulmonary oedema**, **hyperthermia** and **acute kidney injury** may occur.
  - impaired **coagulation** is rarely significant.
- Treatment:
  - general measures as for **poisoning and overdose**, e.g. O_2 **therapy**, **iv fluid administration.** Activated **charcoal** (1 mg/kg up to 50 mg) should be given within an hour of ingesting >125 mg/kg.
  - increased elimination may be indicated if plasma levels exceed 500 mg/l (3.6 mmol/l) in adults or 300 g/l (2.2 mmol/l) in children. Techniques include **dialysis** (preferred if plasma levels exceed 700 mg/l [5.1 mmol/l]), **haemoperfusion** and forced alkaline diuresis (monitoring potassium levels closely to avoid hypokalaemia).

Mortality of acute overdose is approximately 2%; mortality of chronic overdose about 25%.

Pearlman BL, Gambhir R (2009). Postgrad Med; 121: 162–8

See also, Forced diuresis

Salicylates. Group of **NSAIDs** derived from salicylic acid. **Aspirin** (acetylsalicylic acid) is the most commonly used; others are available but are less potent, e.g. sodium salicylate. Have anti-inflammatory and antipyretic effects; they inhibit both central and peripheral synthesis of **prostaglandins**. Inhibit **platelet** and vascular endothelial **cyclo-oxygenase**; at low dosage, they selectively inhibit platelet cyclo-oxygenase. They are thus used as **antiplatelet drugs**. Effects on platelets are irreversible, lasting until new platelets are synthesised (7–10 days).

Used for mild-to-moderate **pain**, **pyrexia**, **rheumatic fever**, **rheumatoid arthritis**, and peripheral and coronary artery disease. Contraindicated in gout as they may impair excretion of uric acid.

Absorbed rapidly from the upper GIT after therapeutic dosage, with peak plasma levels within 2 h of ingestion. Absorption is determined by the composition of tablets, intestinal pH and **gastric emptying**. About 90% protein-bound, they compete with other substances for protein binding sites, e.g. thyroxine, penicillin, phenytoin. Metabolised in the liver and excreted mainly in the urine, especially if the latter is alkaline. **Half-life** is about 15 min, but is very dependent on the dose taken.

- Side effects: as for NSAIDs and **salicylate poisoning**. Implicated in causing **Reye's syndrome** in children. Contraindicated in children <16 years and patients with **peptic ulcer disease**; used with caution in those with **coagulation disorders** or taking **anticoagulant drugs**.

Saline solutions. **Intravenous fluids** containing sodium chloride, used extensively to replace **sodium** and **ECF** losses, e.g. in **dehydration**, and perioperatively. A 0.9% solution is most commonly used ('physiological saline'; often erroneously called 'normal saline'); other saline-containing solutions include **Hartmann's solution, Ringer's solution** and dextrose/saline mixtures. Hypertonic saline (e.g. 3%) is used in the treatment of symptomatic **hyponatraemia** and raised **intracranial pressure**.

Administration of large volumes of saline may result in hyperchloraemic acidosis, the clinical significance of which is unclear.

See also, Hypertonic intravenous solutions; Normal solution

Samples, statistical. Parts of **populations**, selected for **statistical tests** or analysis. In order to represent the true population, samples should be as large as possible to ensure appropriate **power**, and free of bias; i.e., should be random. Matched samples refer to groups matched for possible confounding variables, allowing better comparison of the desired measurements. Optimum matching occurs when subjects act as their own controls (i.e., measurements are paired).

See also, Clinical trials; Randomisation; Statistics

Sanders oxygen injector, *see Injector techniques*

Saphenous nerve block, *see Ankle, nerve blocks; Knee, nerve blocks*

SAPS, *see Simplified acute physiology score*

Sarcoidosis. Systemic disease, possibly caused by immunological derangement secondary to an infective agent, characterised by non-necrotising granuloma formation. The lungs or hilar lymph nodes are affected in 90%–95% of patients, but the disease may involve the eyes, skin, musculoskeletal system, abdominal organs, heart or nervous system. Often acute in onset and self-limiting, with ~85% undergoing spontaneous remission within 2 years. Most common in women, with peak incidence at 20–30 years.

Diagnosed on clinical grounds, supported by tissue biopsy, CXR, **hypercalcaemia** (due to derangement of vitamin D metabolism), raised angiotensin converting enzyme levels; the Kveim test (granuloma formation following intradermal injection of sarcoid tissue suspension) is no longer used in the UK.

Anaesthetic and ICU considerations include the possibility of **pulmonary fibrosis**, **cardiac failure**, **heart block**, laryngeal fibrosis, **renal failure** and **hypercalcaemia**. **Corticosteroids** are often prescribed.

[Morten A Kveim (1892–1967), Norwegian pathologist]

Valeyre D, Prasse A, Nunes H, et al (2014). Lancet; 383: 1155–67

SARS, *see Severe acute respiratory syndrome*

Saturated vapour pressure (SVP). Pressure exerted by the vapour phase of a substance, when in equilibrium with the liquid phase. Indicates the degree of volatility; e.g. for **inhalational anaesthetic agents**, **diethyl ether** (SVP 59 kPa [425 mmHg]) is more volatile and easier to vaporise than **halothane** (SVP 32 kPa [243 mmHg]). SVP increases with temperature, therefore SVPs of volatile agents are quoted at a specified temperature (usually 20°C). At **boiling point**, SVP equals atmospheric pressure.
See also, Vapour pressure

Scalp, nerve blocks. Local anaesthetic infiltration is usually performed with added **adrenaline**, because of the rich vascular supply of the scalp. Injection is performed first in the subcutaneous tissue above the aponeurosis (where nerves and vessels lie), then below. Infiltration in a band around the head, above the ears and eyebrows, provides anaesthesia of the scalp. Individual branches of the **maxillary nerve** may also be blocked. The occipital nerves supplying the posterior scalp may be blocked by infiltrating between the mastoid process and occipital protuberance on each side.

Scavenging. Removal of waste gases from the expiratory port of **anaesthetic breathing systems**; desirable because of the possible adverse effects of exposure to **inhalational anaesthetic agents**. Adsorption of volatile agents using activated **charcoal** (Aldasorber device) has been used but does not remove $\mathbf{N_2O}$.

- Scavenging systems consist of:
  - collecting system: usually a shroud enclosing the **adjustable pressure limiting valve**. For paediatric breathing systems, several attachments have been described, including various connectors and funnels.
  - tubing: standard plastic tubing is usual; all connections should be 30 mm to avoid improper connection to the breathing system.
  - receiving system: incorporates a reservoir to enable adequate removal of gases, even if the volume cleared per minute is less than peak expiratory flow rate. May use rubber bags or rigid bottles. If the system is closed, a **dumping valve** and pressure-relief valve are required to prevent excess negative or positive pressure, respectively, being applied to the patient's airway. Vents are often present in rigid reservoirs. Requirements:
    - negative pressure: maximum 0.5 cmH_2O at 30 l/min gas flow.
    - positive pressure: maximum 5 cmH_2O at 30 l/min gas flow, and 10 cmH_2O at 90 l/min. Ideally, the relief valve should be as near to the expiratory valve as possible.
  - disposal system: may be:
    - passive: no external energy supply; the gases pass through wide-bore tubing to the roof of the building, terminating in a ventile. Maximal resistance should be 0.5 cmH_2O at 30 l/min. The least efficient system, because it depends on wind direction. Requires a water trap to remove condensed water vapour.
    - assisted passive: employs the air-conditioning system's extractor ducts.
    - active: uses a dedicated fan system or **ejector flowmeter**. Requires a low-pressure, high-volume system (able to remove 75 l/min with a peak flow of 130 l/min); thus, hospital suction equipment is unsuitable.

Workplace exposure limits set out in **COSHH regulations** for Great Britain and Northern Ireland are 100 ppm N_2O, 50 ppm enflurane/isoflurane and 10 ppm halothane (each over an 8-h period). Maximum permitted levels vary between countries; e.g. in the USA, the National Institute for Occupational Safety and Health has recommended an 8-h time-weighted average limit of 2 ppm for halogenated anaesthetic agents in general (0.5 ppm together with exposure to N_2O).
See also, Environmental safety of anaesthetists; Pollution

SCCM, *see Society of Critical Care Medicine*

Schimmelbusch mask, *see Open-drop techniques*

Sciatic nerve block. Used for surgery to the lower leg, often combined with **femoral nerve block**, **obturator nerve block** and **lateral cutaneous nerve of the thigh block** (*see Fig. 69;* **Femoral nerve block**). May also be performed to provide analgesia after fractures, or **sympathetic nerve block** of the foot.

The sciatic nerve (L4–S3) arises from the **sacral plexus**, leaving the pelvis through the greater sciatic foramen beneath the piriformis muscle, and between the ischial tuberosity and the greater trochanter of the femur. It becomes superficial at the lower border of gluteus maximus, and runs down the posterior aspect of the thigh to the **popliteal fossa**, where it divides into tibial and common peroneal nerves. It supplies the hip and knee joints, posterior muscles of the leg and skin of the leg and foot below the knee, except for the medial calf. The posterior cutaneous nerve of the thigh runs close to it and is usually blocked by it.

- Four different approaches are commonly used:
  - posterior: with the patient lying with the side to be blocked uppermost, and the uppermost hip and knee flexed, a line is drawn between the greater trochanter and posterior superior iliac spine. At the line's midpoint, a perpendicular is dropped 3 cm, and a 12-cm needle introduced at this point, at right angles to the skin. The nerve lies on the ischial spine and is identified using a **nerve stimulator** (seeking contraction of the hamstrings and muscles of the back of the lower leg and foot). 15–30 ml **local anaesthetic agent** is injected. Onset of blockade may take 30 min.
  - anterior: with the patient lying supine, a line is drawn between the pubic tubercle and anterior superior iliac spine, and divided into thirds. A perpendicular line is dropped from the junction of the medial and middle thirds. Another line, parallel with the original line, is drawn from the greater trochanter; its intersection with the perpendicular marks the site of needle

insertion. A 12-cm needle is directed slightly laterally to encounter the femur, then withdrawn and directed medial to the femur to a depth of 5 cm from the femur's anterior edge. 15–30 ml solution is injected. This approach is particularly useful if movement is painful, e.g. fractured femur.
- lithotomy: with the hip and knee on the side to be blocked flexed to 90 degrees, a needle is inserted perpendicular to the skin at the midpoint of a line between the greater trochanter and the ischial tuberosity. 15–20 ml solution is injected at a depth of 4–8 cm. The posterior cutaneous branch (supplying the posterior thigh) may be missed.
- lateral: with the patient lying supine, a needle is inserted horizontally at a point 2–3 cm below and 4–5 cm distal to the greater trochanter. When the femur is encountered the needle is withdrawn and redirected posteriorly ~30 degrees and cranially ~30–45 degrees to reach the nerve at 8–10 cm. 20–30 ml solution is injected.

See also, Regional anaesthesia

Scleroderma, *see Systemic sclerosis*

Scoliosis, *see Kyphoscoliosis*

Scopolamine, *see Hyoscine*

Scribner shunt, *see Shunt procedures*

SCUF, Slow continuous ultrafiltration, *see Ultrafiltration*

SDD, *see Selective decontamination of the digestive tract*

Second. SI **unit** of time; defined according to the frequency of radiation emitted by caesium-133 in its lowest energy (ground) state.

Second gas effect. Increased alveolar concentration of one **inhalational anaesthetic agent** caused by uptake of a second inhalational agent. Most marked when the second gas occupies a large volume, e.g. N_2O. Analogous but opposite to the **Fink effect** at the end of anaesthesia.

Second messenger. Intracellular substance (e.g. **cAMP**, **calcium** ions) linking extracellular chemical messengers (first messengers) with the physiological response. **G protein-coupled receptors** are often involved in second messenger systems.

Sedation. State of reduced consciousness in which verbal contact with the patient may be maintained. Used to reduce discomfort during unpleasant procedures, e.g. **regional anaesthesia**, **dental surgery**, endoscopy, **cardiac catheterisation**, and on **ICU**. For short procedures, drugs of short duration of action causing minimal cardiorespiratory depression are preferable. Best control is usually achieved with iv administration, although other routes may be used, e.g. oral **premedication**. Routine **monitoring** should be employed during procedures as for general anaesthesia. Drugs may be given by intermittent bolus, or by continuous infusion; the latter is easier to titrate. The level of sedation required depends on the individual patient and the procedure performed. Patient-controlled sedation has been used during procedures performed under local or regional anaesthesia; the patient uses a **PCA** device containing, e.g. **propofol** as required.

On ICU, there has been a shift towards light sedation following the recognition that early deep sedation is consistently associated with increased morbidity and mortality, prolonged hospital and ICU stay, haemodynamic instability, long-term cognitive decline and psychological problems including **confusion in the intensive care unit**. Although deep sedation is necessary for some patients (e.g. those with severe **ALI**, **TBI**, **status epilepticus**), most can be managed with low levels, especially as new ventilatory modes can reduce patient-ventilator asynchrony. Most modern minimal sedation guidelines aim to allow patients to be comfortable, calm and able to co-operate with staff and interact with family.

- Achieving adequate comfort involves consideration of the following:
  - pre-existing conditions, e.g. continuing treatment of chronic neuropathic pain with **gabapentin**.
  - acute pain, e.g. opioid analgesic drugs for trauma/surgery.
  - ICU intervention-related discomfort, e.g. tracheal intubation/IPPV, physiotherapy, chest drains.
- Drugs used include:
  - morphine 2.5–5-mg boluses (20–60 µg/kg/h infusion). Accumulation of metabolites may occur after prolonged infusion, especially in renal failure. Increased susceptibility to infection has been shown in experimental animals receiving very large doses.
  - fentanyl 1–5 µg/kg/h; accumulation readily occurs after prolonged infusion, because its short duration of action initially is due to redistribution, and clearance is slower than that of morphine.
  - alfentanil 30–60 µg/kg/h; accumulation is less likely than with fentanyl.
  - remifentanil 0.025–0.1 mg/kg/min.
  - NSAIDs and regional techniques may also be used.

Light sedation equates to a Richmond Agitation Sedation Scale of -1/0 (*see Sedation scoring systems*). There is a move away from **benzodiazepines**, which are associated with increased duration of IPPV and length of ICU stay. Propofol, **clonidine** or **dexmedetomidine** are considered the drugs of choice in adults. A continuous low-level infusion of sedation appears to be as effective as intermittent daily sedation interruptions. Daily sedation checks should be carried out to ensure the minimal sedation necessary is employed.

Reade MC, Finfer S (2014). N Engl J Med; 370: 444–54

Sedation scoring systems. Used in intensive care to assess the level of **sedation** of patients in order to balance its beneficial (reduced stress, cardiovascular stability, ventilator synchrony) and adverse effects (increased risk of **ventilator-associated pneumonia**, **deep vein thrombosis**). Facilitates titration of sedation against predefined endpoints (e.g. assessments of consciousness, agitation and/or ventilator synchrony). Other parameters assessed include pain, anxiety, muscle tone and response to tracheal suction. Most systems use single numerical scores:
- Ramsay scale: described in 1974. Has three levels of 'awake' states (1–3) and three of 'asleep' states (4–6). Although widely used in the UK, it lacks discrimination between sedation levels. A score of 2 represents an ideal sedation level.
- Sedation–Agitation Scale (SAS): described in 1999. Ranges from +3 (agitated) to −3 (unrousable) with an optimal score of 0. Has good reliability and is well validated against other systems.

- Motor Activity Assessment Scale (MAAS): system based on observed levels of motor activity developed in surgical patients in 1999. Ranges from 0 (unresponsive) to 6 (dangerously agitated and unco-operative). Optimum sedation level is 3. Not widely used.
- Richmond Agitation Sedation Score (RASS): reliable and well validated system increasing in popularity. A 10-point scoring system ranging from +4 (agitated and combative) to -5 (unrousable). Optimum level is 0.
- Adaptation to the Intensive Care Environment (ATICE): more complex system that scores level of consciousness, comprehension and tolerance (assessing calmness, ventilator synchrony and facial relaxation).

[Michael AE Ramsay, US anaesthetist; Richmond, Virginia, city where the scale was developed]

Seebeck effect, *see Temperature measurement*

Seldinger technique. Method for percutaneous cannulation of a blood vessel (e.g. **central venous cannulation**), described in 1953. A needle is inserted into the vessel, and a guide-wire passed through it. After removal of the needle, the cannula is introduced into the vessel over the wire, which is then removed. Refinements include the use of a dilator passed over the wire to enlarge the hole made by the needle, before the cannula is inserted.

Also used to cannulate other body cavities, e.g. the trachea in percutaneous **tracheostomy** formation, the chest for insertion of a **chest drain** or the abdominal cavity in **paracentesis**.

[Sven-Ivar Seldinger (1921–1998), Swedish radiologist]

Selective decontamination of the digestive tract (SDD; Selective parenteral and enteral antisepsis regimen, SPEAR). Selective oropharyngeal decontamination (SOD) and SDD are prophylactic antibiotic regimens aimed at preventing **nosocomial infection** in ICU patients. During SOD, antibiotics are exclusively applied to the oropharynx throughout the ICU stay. In SDD, antibiotics are not only applied to the oropharynx but also to the GIT throughout the stay, in combination with iv **cefotaxime** for the first 4 days. Non-absorbable **antibacterial drugs** (e.g. **tobramycin, colistin, amphotericin, neomycin**) are administered to the pharynx/mouth/upper GIT. Although studies show SDD and SOD reduce rates of **ventilator-associated pneumonia,** mortality and ICU length of stay appear to be unaffected. The technique has not been widely adopted due to concerns about **bacterial resistance.**

Plantinga NL, Bonten MJ (2015). Crit Care; 19: 259

Selective serotonin reuptake inhibitors (SSRIs). **Antidepressant drugs** introduced in 1987 and largely replacing **tricyclic antidepressant drugs**. Inhibit the presynaptic reuptake of **5-HT** in the CNS, leading to an increase in 5-HT activity. Include citalopram, escitalopram, fluoxetine, fluvoxamine, paroxetine and sertraline; they have similar actions and are metabolised in the liver with **half-lives** of about a day (4–6 days for fluoxetine).

Have fewer side effects than tricyclic antidepressants because muscarinic, dopamine, histamine and noradrenergic receptors are unaffected. However, GIT upset, insomnia and agitation may occur; the **syndrome of inappropriate antidiuretic hormone secretion** and impaired **platelet** function have been reported. In overdose, severe adverse effects are uncommon, although the **serotonin syndrome** may occur if tricyclics or **monoamine oxidase inhibitors** are also taken.

May cause hepatic **enzyme inhibition** (by competing with other drugs for the same metabolic pathways), thus increasing the action of certain tricyclics, type Ic **antiarrhythmic drugs** (especially lipid-soluble **β-adrenergic receptor antagonists**), **phenytoin** and **benzodiazepines**. Increased bleeding may occur in **warfarin** therapy. Concurrent administration of drugs that have 5-HT reuptake blocking effects (e.g. **pethidine**) may provoke the serotonin syndrome.

Selenium. Trace element found in meat, chicken and fish; normal intake ~60–75 μg/day. Selenoproteins are antioxidants and are involved in certain biological reactions, e.g. conversion of thyroxine to triiodothyronine. Low blood selenium levels have been recorded in ICU patients, especially those with septic shock, and are associated with a high ICU mortality; however, the evidence that supplementation with selenium decreases nosocomial infection and mortality is disputed.

Self-inflating bags. Rubber or silicone bags used for IPPV that reinflate when released after compression. Thus may be used for IPPV without requiring an external gas supply, e.g. during **draw-over anaesthesia**, transfer of ventilated patients or **CPR**. May be thick-walled or lined with foam rubber. Usually assembled with a **non-rebreathing valve** at the outlet and a one-way valve at the inlet; thus fresh air is drawn in during refilling. O_2 may be added through a port at the inlet; a reservoir bag may also be added to the inlet to increase F_IO_2. Available in adult and paediatric sizes. **Bellows** may be used in a similar way, but are less convenient to use.

Sellick's manoeuvre, *see Cricoid pressure*

Semon's law, *see Laryngeal nerves*

Sengstaken–Blakemore tube. Double-cuffed gastric tube designed to compress **gastro-oesophageal varices**, thereby controlling bleeding. Passed via the mouth into the stomach; the distal balloon is then inflated with 150–250 ml air, preventing accidental removal. The proximal balloon is then inflated to 30–40 mmHg (4–5 kPa), compressing the varices. Traction has been advocated but is rarely used. Newer versions include channels for aspiration of gastric and oesophageal contents (Fig. 141); the latter may be

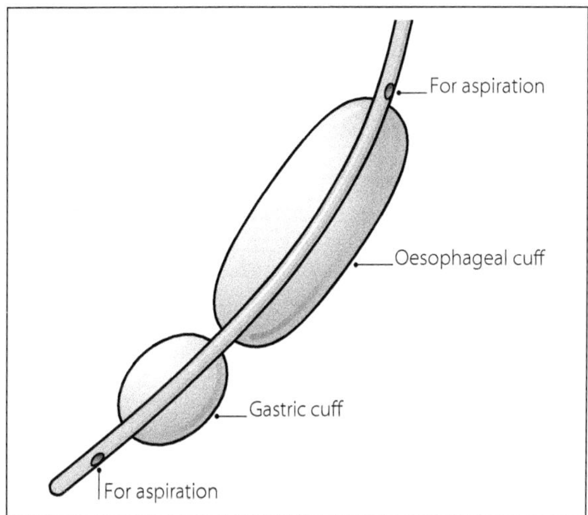

Fig. 141 Distal end of Sengstaken–Blakemore tube

aspirated continuously to reduce pulmonary soiling. Thus four lumens may be present:
- for aspiration above the oesophageal balloon.
- for aspiration from the stomach.
- for inflation of each balloon.

Usually kept inflated for 12–24 h; the oesophageal balloon is deflated first. Careful placement is essential to avoid airway obstruction, pulmonary aspiration, ischaemic necrosis of gastric mucosa or oesophageal rupture. The tubes are very uncomfortable.

[Robert W Sengstaken (1923–1978) and Arthur H Blakemore (1879–1970), US surgeons]

Sensitivity. In **statistics**, the ability of a test to exclude false negatives. Equals:

$$\frac{\text{the number correctly identified as positive}}{\text{total with the condition}}$$

See also, Errors; Predictive value; Specificity

Sensory evoked potentials, *see Evoked potentials*

Sensory pathways. The sensory system includes the special senses, visceral sensation and general somatic sensation. The latter is divided into:
- exteroreceptive sensation: provides information about the external environment and includes modalities such as touch, pressure, temperature and **pain**.
- proprioceptive sensation: provides information about body position and movement.

Free nerve endings may be associated with **nociception**. Some nerve endings are 'specialised', e.g. Meissner's corpuscles (touch), Pacinian corpuscles (vibration and joint position) and Ruffini corpuscles (joint position). The last two may be involved with **muscle spindles**.

The sensory fibres enter the **spinal cord** through the dorsal root, their cell bodies lying in the dorsal root ganglia. Subsequent pathways (Fig. 142):
- dorsal columns: carry impulses concerned with proprioception (movement and joint position sense), vibration and discriminative touch:
  - first-order **neurones** turn medially and ascend in the ipsilateral posterior columns (the fasciculus gracilis and cuneatus) to the lower medulla, where they synapse with cells in the cuneate or gracile nuclei.
  - second-order neurones cross (decussate) to the contralateral side of the medulla and ascend in the medial lemniscus to the ventral posterior nucleus of the thalamus.
  - third-order neurones project to the somatosensory cortex.
- spinothalamic tract: carries impulses concerned with pain, temperature, non-discriminative touch and pressure:
  - first-order neurones synapse in the dorsal horn of the spinal cord (most nociceptive Aδ- and C-fibres terminate in laminae I–II whereas Aβ fibres terminate in laminae III–IV).
  - second-order neurones carrying pain and temperature cross within one segment of their origin, whereas those carrying touch and pressure may ascend for several segments before crossing. They ascend in the spinothalamic tract; in the medulla, this forms the spinal lemniscus, which ascends to the ventral posterior nucleus of the thalamus.
  - third-order neurones project to the somatosensory cortex.

The primary somatosensory area of the cerebral cortex is in the postcentral gyrus, although there is a large distribution of sensory fibres in other areas. Regions of greatest importance (e.g. face, mouth, hands) have a disproportionately greater representation than other areas.
- Signs of sensory pathway loss:
  - peripheral nerve lesion: complete loss of sensation in the nerve's distribution (although the zone of loss may be limited because of overlap between nerves).
  - posterior root lesion: pain and paraesthesia are experienced in the dermatomal distribution. If the root involves a **reflex arc**, the reflex will be diminished or lost.
  - posterior column lesion: ipsilateral loss of position and vibration sense with preservation of pain, touch and temperature sensation.
  - spinothalamic tract lesion: contralateral loss of pain and temperature sensation.
  - **brainstem** and thalamus lesions: upper brainstem or thalamic lesions may cause complete hemisensory disturbance with loss of postural sense, light touch and pain sensation. 'Pure' thalamic lesions may result in **central pain**.
  - sensory cortex lesions: paraesthesia may be felt, with or without impaired sensation, e.g. inability to distinguish between heat and pain, or inability to identify objects by touch.

[Georg Meissner (1829–1905), German anatomist; Filippo Pacini (1812–1883), Italian anatomist; Angelo Ruffini (1864–1929), Italian histologist]

See also, Dermatomes; Spinal cord injury

Sepsis. Life-threatening organ dysfunction caused by a dysregulated host response to infection (Sepsis-3 2016 definition); characterised by an acute increase in the **sepsis-related organ failure assessment** (SOFA) score of 2 or more. The latest definition eliminates the term **systemic inflammatory response syndrome**, the features of which are inadequate and non-specific for the accurate diagnosis of sepsis. Similarly, the terms 'severe sepsis' and **septicaemia** are now considered redundant, the former being replaced by the term **septic shock**. Although the definitions are supported by evidence from large databases, these data apply to adults in high-income countries and may be less able to predict morbidity and mortality in other populations. In addition, data used to provide the definitions are derived from groups of patients with highly heterogeneous conditions and therefore may be limited when applied to individual patients.

Sepsis is a major cause of organ failure in **ICU**, being directly or indirectly responsible for 75% of all ICU deaths.

Most ICU infections are endogenous, caused by colonisation of the patient's GIT by pathogenic organisms that gain access to the systemic circulation through **bacterial translocation**. Gram-negative bacteria (e.g. *Escherichia coli*, klebsiella, pseudomonas, acinetobacter and proteus species) have traditionally been most commonly responsible, because of their widespread presence, their tendency to acquire resistance to **antibacterial drugs** and their resistance to drying and disinfecting agents. Gram-positive bacteria (e.g. streptococci, staphylococci) are increasingly common, especially associated with invasive cannulation;

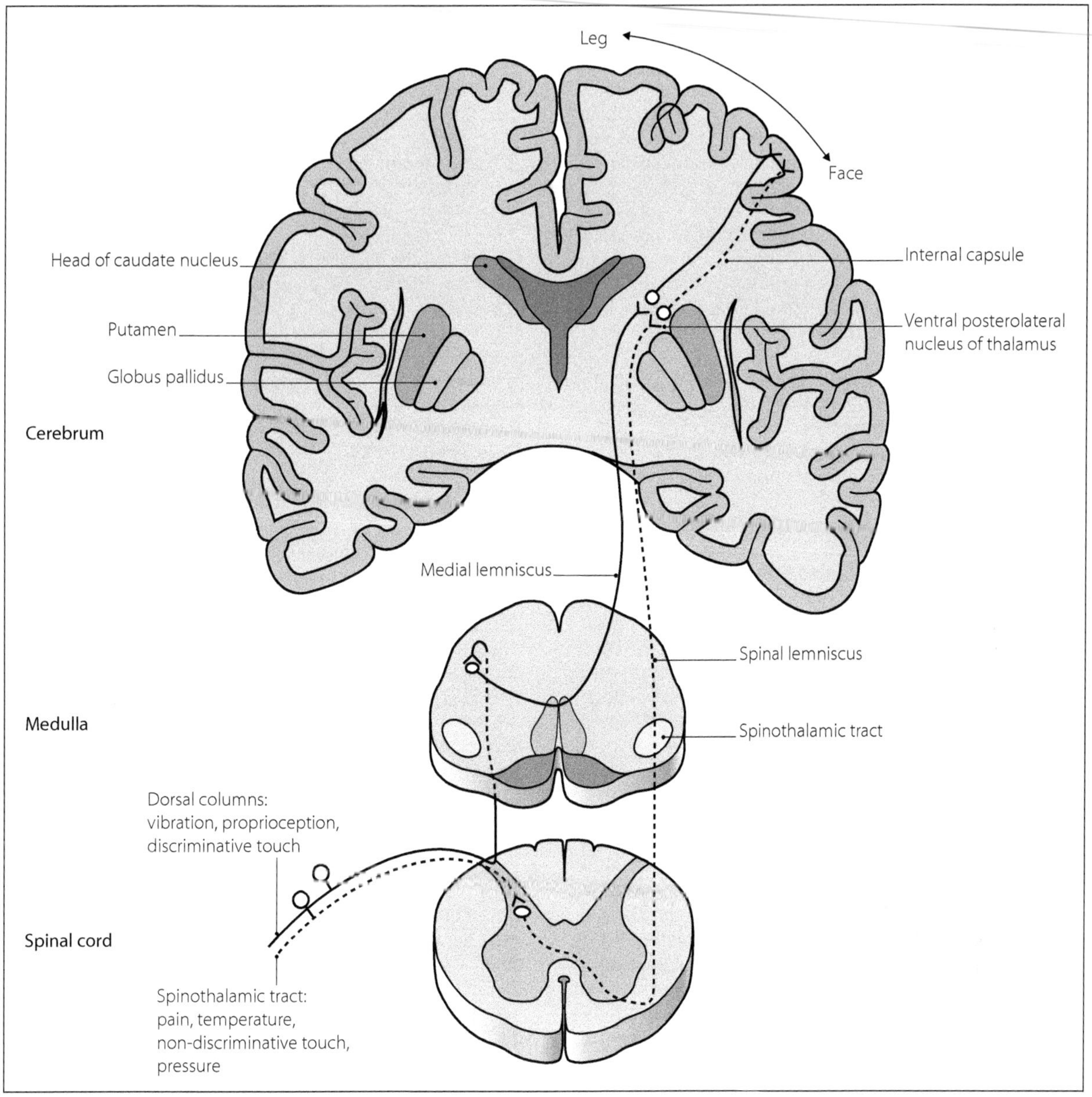

Leg
Face
Head of caudate nucleus
Internal capsule
Putamen
Ventral posterolateral nucleus of thalamus
Globus pallidus
Cerebrum
Medial lemniscus
Spinal lemniscus
Medulla
Spinothalamic tract
Dorsal columns: vibration, proprioception, discriminative touch
Spinal cord
Spinothalamic tract: pain, temperature, non-discriminative touch, pressure

Fig. 142 Anatomy of sensory pathways

other organisms (e.g. fungi) may also be responsible. The inflammatory response involves **cytokines**, **nitric oxide**, **thromboxanes**, **leukotrienes**, **platelet activating factor**, **prostaglandins** and **complement**. Endothelial and neutrophil **adhesion molecule** expression increases, resulting in cellular infiltration into the tissues.

- Critically ill patients are susceptible to sepsis because of:
    - impaired local defences, e.g. anatomical barriers, **ciliary activity**, coughing, gastric pH. Tracheal tubes, indwelling catheters and cannulae provide routes for infection.
    - impaired immunity. Contributory factors include drugs, **malnutrition**, **diabetes mellitus**, old age, **malignancy**, organ failure and infection itself. Patients receiving systemic cancer treatment or immunological therapy are susceptible to neutropenic sepsis (i.e., sepsis in the presence of a white cell count <0.5 × 10^9/l).
- Prevention:
    - **infection control** programmes.
    - antibacterial drug prophylaxis (e.g. with **ciprofloxacin** for patients at risk of neutropenic sepsis).
- Management:
    - early recognition and low threshold for suspecting sepsis in patients presenting with infection or organ dysfunction even in the absence of a systemic host response. The q(quick)SOFA score has been used as a simple and useful system, particularly for ward-based patients (*see Sepsis-related organ failure assessment*).
    - **O_2 therapy**, monitoring, iv access, urinary catheterisation.
    - the **Surviving Sepsis Campaign** emphasises the importance of the first 6 h of resuscitation as being critical to the outcome:
        - management in the first hour:
            - to counteract sepsis-induced organ hypoperfusion, give at least 30 ml/kg of iv crystalloid,

with further fluid resuscitation dictated by assessment of haemodynamic status, preferably using dynamic assessment of **fluid responsiveness**. A balanced salt solution (e.g. **Hartmann's solution**) is preferable to 0.9% saline, which may produce hyperchloraemic **metabolic acidosis**. **Albumin** solutions should be considered if large volumes of crystalloid are ineffective. **Hydroxyethyl starch** should not be used as it is associated with increased mortality and need for renal replacement therapy. Effectiveness of resuscitation should be guided by **lactate** levels; although lactate-directed therapy does not influence outcome, levels are indicative of the severity of sepsis.
- obtain **blood cultures** and samples of urine, sputum and CSF as indicated, before starting antimicrobial therapy.
- administer appropriate doses of iv broad-spectrum antibacterial drugs within 1 hour of recognition of sepsis or septic shock. Delay is associated with increased mortality and organ dysfunction. Antifungal and antiviral cover may also be indicated. A combination of two classes of antibacterial agents is indicated for septic shock but not for 'uncomplicated' or neutropenic sepsis. Once bacterial sensitivities have been obtained, the antibacterial drug spectrum may be narrowed. Therapy for 7–10 days is recommended for most infections, but **procalcitonin** levels may be used to guide duration.
- management to be completed within 6 h: if MAP <70 mmHg (<80 mmHg if the patient has pre-existing hypertension) following resuscitation, **inotropic drugs** should be given. **Noradrenaline** is the drug of choice; **vasopressin** or **adrenaline** may be added if necessary to reduce the dose of noradrenaline. **Dobutamine** may have a role if there is persistent hypoperfusion despite the use of vasopressor agents. 'Renal' doses of **dopamine** are no longer recommended.

- haemoglobin levels >70 g/l are acceptable in the absence of myocardial ischaemia, severe hypoxaemia or active bleeding. **Coagulation disorders** should only be corrected if active bleeding occurs or invasive procedures are planned. **Platelet** transfusion is indicated when counts are $<10 \times 10^9$/l; higher counts ($>50 \times 10^9$/l) are needed for bleeding, planned surgery or invasive procedures.
- source control: e.g. surgical drainage, debridement, removal of infected lines and catheters.
- **corticosteroids** (i.e., iv hydrocortisone 200 mg/day) are only indicated if the BP does not respond to fluid resuscitation and vasopressor drugs (*see Septic shock*).
- newer immunomodulatory treatments (e.g. **anti-endotoxin antibodies**, activated **protein C**, anti-cytokine products) have been investigated, with disappointing clinical results. This may represent the heterogeneous patient population and/or the complex pathophysiology of sepsis.
- iv **immunoglobulin** and blood purification (e.g. with haemofiltration, haemoperfusion or haemoadsorption) are not currently recommended.
- early enteral **nutrition** is important, as hypercatabolism is inevitable. **Prokinetic drugs** may be necessary, as may jejunal feeding. Supplements such as selenium, omega-3 fatty acids, arginine and glutamine are not currently recommended. Early parenteral nutrition (i.e., in the first 7 days) for those who cannot tolerate enteral feeding is not recommended, as it does not improve mortality and increases risk of infection.
- intensive **glycaemic control** is not recommended because of the risks of hypoglycaemia. Blood glucose levels of 8–12 mmol/l are suitable.
- **DVT** prophylaxis should be given unless contraindicated.

Complications include septic shock and multiple organ failure, including **ALI**, **acute kidney injury**, **hepatic failure**, **pancreatitis** and diabetes mellitus, **DIC**, **cardiac failure** and **coma**. GIT haemorrhage is common, especially in patients with **peptic ulcer disease**; this group requires prophylaxis with **proton pump inhibitors** or **H_2 receptor antagonists**.

Rhodes A, Evans LE, Alhazzani W, et al (2017). Intensive Care Med; 43: 304–77

Sepsis-related organ failure assessment (SOFA). Scoring system devised in 1994 to describe quantitatively and objectively the degree of organ dysfunction in **sepsis** over time. Intended to improve the understanding of organ dysfunction/failure and to assess the effect of particular therapies on its progression. The function of six different organ systems (respiratory, cardiovascular, central nervous, coagulation, hepatic and renal systems) is weighted (each scored 1–4) according to the degree of derangement observed clinically or measured in the laboratory. Minimum SOFA score is 6; maximum 24 (Table 46). SOFA has a superior predictive validity for in-hospital mortality compared with the **systemic inflammatory response syndrome** criteria; it has a similar validity to **LODS** but is less complex to use.

A related system, the quickSOFA (qSOFA: one point assigned for systolic BP ≤100 mmHg, one for respiratory rate ≥22 breaths/min, and one for **Glasgow coma scale** <15), has been validated as a convenient bedside assessment tool, a score ≥2 identifying patients at greater risk of prolonged ICU stay or in-hospital death. However, its general applicability is disputed.

Singer M, Deutschman CS, Seymour CW, et al (2016). JAMA; 315: 801–10

Sepsis score. Index of severity of **sepsis**, devised in 1983; assigns scores according to local infection, pyrexia, systemic response and laboratory results. Now rarely used.

Elebute EA, Stoner HB (1983). Br J Surg; 70: 29–31

Sepsis severity score. Index of severity of **sepsis**, devised in 1983 by assigning scores of 1–5 according to the degree of impairment of each of the following organ systems: lung, kidney, coagulation, CVS, liver, GIT and neurological. The three highest (worst) scores are then squared to produce the final score.

Stevens LE (1983). Arch Surg; 118: 1190–2

Sepsis syndrome. Obsolete term for the systemic response to infection.

See also, Sepsis; Septic shock; Septicaemia; Systemic inflammatory response syndrome

Septic shock. A subset of **sepsis** in which particularly profound circulatory, cellular, and metabolic abnormalities are associated with a greater risk of mortality than with sepsis alone (Sepsis-3 definition 2016). Clinically, identified

Table 46 Sepsis-related organ failure assessment

System		Score				
		0	1	2	3	4
Respiratory	P_aO_2/F_iO_2 (kPa [mmHg])	≥53.3 [400]	<53.3 [400]	<40 [300]	<26.7 [200] with respiratory support	<13.3 [100] with respiratory support
Coagulation	Platelets (×10⁹/l)	≥150	<150	<100	<50	<20
Liver	Bilirubin (μmol/l [mg/dl])	<20 (1.2)	20–32 (1.2–1.9)	33–101 (2.0–5.9)	102–204 (6.0–11.9)	>204 (12.0)
CVS	MAP (mmHg)	≥70	<70	Dopamine <5 μg/kg/min or any dose of dobutamine for ≥1 h	Dopamine 5.1–15 μg/kg/min, or adrenaline/noradrenaline ≤0.1 μg/kg/min, for ≥1 h	Dopamine >15 μg/kg/min, or adrenaline/noradrenaline >0.1 μg/kg/min, for ≥1 h
CNS	Glasgow coma scale	15	13–14	13–12	6–9	<6
Renal	Creatinine (μmol/l [mg/dl])	<110 (1.2)	110–170 (1.2–1.9)	171–299 (2.0–3.4)	300–440 (3.5–4.9)	>440 (5.0)
	Urine output (ml/day)				<500	<200

by the requirement for **vasopressor drugs** to maintain MAP ≥65 mmHg and plasma **lactate** level >2 mmol/l (>18 mg/dl) in the absence of **hypovolaemia**. Initial features include hyperthermia, tachycardia, tachypnoea, hypotension and vasodilatation with a hyperdynamic circulation and increased cardiac output. In later stages, or if hypovolaemia or poor myocardial function is present, hypotension with vasoconstriction supervenes. Mortality is 40%–50%, although it varies with patients' characteristics and the nature of the sepsis. Most cases are caused by **bacteria** (approximately equally split between gram-positive and gram-negative, although traditionally associated with gram-negative organisms); other organisms may also be responsible.

Risk factors include: age (<10 years and >70 years); **diabetes mellitus**; alcoholic liver disease; **ischaemic heart disease**; **malignancy**; immunosuppression; prolonged hospital stay; invasive monitoring; tracheal intubation; and prior use of antibacterial agents. The underlying pathophysiology is as for sepsis; microvascular abnormalities supervene, including impaired **autoregulation**, altered blood cell morphology, increased endothelial permeability and opening of arteriovenous shunts.

- Cardiovascular features include:
  - reduced **SVR** with relative hypovolaemia.
  - increased **pulmonary vascular resistance**.
  - increased capillary permeability.
  - reduced **myocardial contractility** caused by circulating depressant factors, **acidaemia** and **hypoxaemia**.
  - O_2 consumption may be normal but O_2 extraction and utilisation are reduced.
- Management:
  - as for sepsis.
  - high-dose **corticosteroids** are associated with increased mortality; however, recent evidence suggests that at lower doses (e.g. **hydrocortisone** 50 mg iv qds) they may reduce vasopressor requirements and speed resolution of shock (by increasing the sensitivity of **α-adrenergic receptors** on vascular smooth muscle). A corticotropin (Synacthen) stimulation test was previously advocated to identify patients with impaired pituitary–adrenal axis function; this is no longer recommended for identifying patients who may benefit from steroid therapy. Survival benefits are unclear and steroid use remains controversial; however, in extremely sick patients with high vasopressor requirements, many advocate administering a therapeutic trial with cessation if there is no clinical improvement.
- Complications: as for sepsis.

Rhodes A, Evans LE, Alhazzani W, et al (2017). Intensive Care Med; 43: 304–77

Septicaemia, *see Sepsis*

Sequential analysis, *see Statistical tests*

Serotonin, *see 5-Hydroxytryptamine*

Serotonin reuptake inhibitors, *see Selective serotonin reuptake inhibitors*

Serotonin syndrome. Impaired mental state, increased muscle activity and autonomic instability arising from excessive **5-HT** activity in the brainstem and spinal cord. Seen in **selective serotonin reuptake inhibitor** (SSRI) overdose, especially in combination with other **antidepressant drugs** (especially **monoamine oxidase inhibitors**). Has also been reported after intraoperative use of methylene blue (a potent inhibitor of **monoamine oxidase**) in a patient taking SSRIs. Also associated with the use of **tramadol**, **pethidine** and **cocaine**. Features include confusion, agitation, convulsions, myoclonus, rigidity, hyperreflexia, fever, diarrhoea, hyper- or hypotension and tachycardia. **DIC**, renal and cardiac failure may also occur. Treatment is supportive; 5-HT antagonists, e.g. methysergide, cyproheptadine, have been used. Usually lasts for <24 h but deaths have been reported.

A washout period of several weeks has been suggested between **monoamine oxidase inhibitor** and SSRI therapy.

Serratus anterior plane block. Regional anaesthetic technique used to provide analgesia to the sternum and thoracic wall, e.g. for breast, shoulder and thoracic surgery, and for rib fractures.

With the patient supine, the serratus anterior muscle is identified between the fourth and fifth rib in the mid-axillary line, using **ultrasound**, and ~20 ml local anaesthetic agent placed either deep or superficial to serratus anterior.

The anatomical basis for the block is uncertain, but blockade of the lateral cutaneous branches of the intercostal nerves has been suggested. The block has been suggested as an alternative to **paravertebral block**, although likely to be more limited in its extent.

Tighe SQ, Karmakar MK (2013). Anaesthesia; 68: 1103–6

Severe acute respiratory syndrome (SARS). Infectious respiratory condition caused by a new coronavirus originating in China and thought to have spread via air travellers to Europe and North America, causing a pandemic in 2002–2003 that resulted in >8000 cases and 774 deaths. Has mostly affected previously healthy adults, with an incubation period of 2–11 days. Spread mainly via airborne droplets, with most cases of transmission thought to involve close exposure to an infectious individual. Features include high fever initially with malaise, myalgia and headache; after 3–7 days dry cough and dyspnoea may occur, leading to acute respiratory failure in 10%–20% of cases and a mortality ranging from 1% in patients <24 years to >50% in those >65 years. CXR, initially normal, may show focal interstitial infiltrates that may become generalised. Thrombocytopenia and leucopenia are common; raised liver function tests may occur but renal function usually remains normal. Treatment is largely supportive, although the following have been used empirically:

- **ribavirin** 8 mg/kg iv tds (N.B. not licensed for this use in UK) or 1.2 g orally bd after a loading dose of 4 g orally, for 7–14 days (caution in impaired renal function).
- **hydrocortisone** 2–4 mg/kg iv tds/qds, for ~7 days. Methylprednisolone 10 mg/kg/day iv has been used for 2 days before hydrocortisone.
- antibacterial prophylaxis.

Staff require protection from infection because several cases of transmission to healthcare workers have occurred. No cases have been reported worldwide since 2004.

Lai TS, Yu WC (2010). Clin Med; 10: 50–3

Severinghaus electrode, *see* *Carbon dioxide measurement*

Sevoflurane. 1,1,1,3,3,3-hexafluoroisopropyl fluoromethyl ether (Fig. 143). **Inhalational anaesthetic agent**, first synthesised in 1968 but not introduced in the UK until 1995 because of the development of **isoflurane** in preference.

- Properties:
  - colourless liquid with pleasant smelling vapour, 7.5 times heavier than air.
  - mw 200.
  - boiling point 58°C.
  - **SVP** at 20°C 21 kPa (160 mmHg).
  - **partition coefficients**:
    - blood/gas 0.69.
    - oil/gas 53.
  - **MAC** 1.4% (80 years) to 2.5% (children/young adults); up to 3.3% in neonates.
  - non-flammable, non-corrosive.
  - supplied in liquid form with no additive.
  - interacts with **soda lime** at temperature of 65°C to produce compounds A, B, C, D and E, the first two the only ones produced in clinical practice. Production is more likely at high temperatures, high concentrations of sevoflurane, use of **baralyme** and low gas flows. Compound A (pentafluoroisopropenyl fluoromethyl ether) is no longer thought to be significant, despite its toxicity in rats at high dosage; clinical experience has never implicated it in causing harm in humans, even with sevoflurane at low fresh gas flows (maximal concentrations of compound A around 30 ppm; minimal levels for human toxicity thought to be around 150–200 ppm).
- Effects:
  - CNS:
    - smooth, extremely rapid induction and recovery. Concentrations of 4%–8% produce anaesthesia within a few vital capacity breaths.
    - increases the risk of emergence agitation, compared with isoflurane, in children <5 years.
    - anticonvulsant properties as for isoflurane.
    - at concentration of <1 MAC has minimal effect on **ICP** in patients with normal ICP. Studies suggest that **autoregulation** is preserved in patients with cerebrovascular disease, in contrast to other inhalational agents.
    - reduces **CMRO$_2$** as for isoflurane, with about a 50% reduction at 2 MAC.
    - decreases **intraocular pressure.**
    - has poor analgesic properties.
  - RS:
    - well-tolerated vapour with minimal airway irritation.
    - respiratory depressant, with increased rate and decreased tidal volume.
    - causes bronchodilatation.
  - CVS:
    - vasodilatation and hypotension may occur, but less than with isoflurane and with little myocardial depression. Little compensatory tachycardia, unlike isoflurane.
    - myocardial O_2 demand decreases.
    - **arrhythmias** uncommon, as for isoflurane. Little myocardial sensitisation to **catecholamines.**
    - renal and hepatic blood flow generally preserved.
  - other:
    - dose-dependent uterine relaxation.
    - nausea/vomiting occurs in up to 25% of cases.
    - skeletal muscle relaxation; **non-depolarising neuromuscular blockade** may be potentiated.
    - may precipitate **MH.**

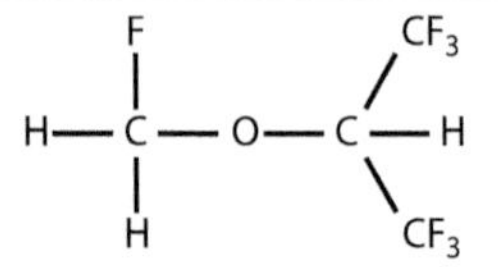

Under 5% metabolised in the liver to hexafluoroisopropanol and inorganic **fluoride ions**, the rest being excreted by the lungs. High levels of fluoride have never been reported, even after prolonged surgery, but avoidance in renal impairment has been suggested. Inducers of the particular cytochrome P_{450} enzyme involved (e.g. isoniazid, alcohol) increase metabolism of sevoflurane, but barbiturates do not.

0.5%–3.0% is usually adequate for maintenance of anaesthesia, with higher concentrations for induction. Tracheal intubation may be performed easily with

Fig. 143 Structure of sevoflurane

spontaneous respiration. Considered the agent of choice for inhalational induction in paediatrics because of its rapid and smooth induction characteristics. Has also been used for the difficult airway, including **airway obstruction**.
See also, Vaporisers

Shivering, postoperative. Tremors were first described after **barbiturate** administration, but they may occur following all types of general anaesthesia. Rarer in elderly patients due to decreased thermoregulatory control. May increase metabolic rate by up to six times and triple O_2 consumption. Can also aggravate postoperative pain, damage surgical wounds and increase intraocular and intracranial pressures. Damage to teeth may occur, especially in the presence of an oral airway.

EMG studies suggest that postoperative shivering differs from shivering due to cold. It has been suggested that anaesthetic agents suppress descending pathways that normally inhibit spinal reflexes; this may be more likely than a response to intraoperative hypothermia, although the latter may be of importance if severe.

- Suggested treatment:
  - O_2 administration.
  - **fentanyl** 25 μg iv or **pethidine** 10–25 mg iv may be effective. **Doxapram** 1 mg/kg, **ondansetron** or **dexmedetomidine** have also been used.

Shivering after **epidural anaesthesia** is common, and is thought to be caused by differential nerve blockade, either suppressing descending inhibition of spinal reflexes or allowing selective transmission of cold sensation. Shivering is rare in **spinal anaesthesia**, where blockade is more dense. Warming of epidural injectate has produced conflicting results. Epidural administration of **opioid analgesic drugs**, e.g. **sufentanil** 50 μg, fentanyl 25 μg, pethidine 25 mg, may be an effective remedy.

Shock. Syndrome, originally described by **Crile**, in which tissue perfusion is inadequate for the tissues' metabolic requirements. Sympathetic compensatory mechanisms may preserve organ perfusion initially, but subsequent organ dysfunction may lead to irreversible organ damage and death.

- Classically divided into:
  - hypovolaemic, e.g **haemorrhage, burns, dehydration.**
  - cardiogenic, following **MI, arrhythmia, cardiomyopathy**.
  - obstructive, e.g. **cardiac tamponade, PE**, tension **pneumothorax**.
  - distributive, e.g. **sepsis, anaphylaxis**, neurogenic (e.g. in high **spinal cord injury**).

Division into **hypovolaemia**, myocardial failure and peripheral vascular failure has been suggested as being more indicative of underlying mechanisms. Thus shock may arise from inadequate **cardiac output** or maldistribution of blood flow; the latter has been increasingly implicated by studies of **O_2 delivery** ($\dot{D}O_2$) and total body O_2 consumption ($\dot{V}O_2$). A decrease in $\dot{V}O_2$ is thought to represent maldistribution rather than an absolute decrease in blood flow. In cardiogenic shock both $\dot{V}O_2$ and cardiac output are reduced; in septic shock they may both increase initially. Features depend on the aetiology but include hypotension, tachycardia, oliguria and metabolic **acidosis. MODS** may follow, with **acute kidney injury** and **ALI**. Hepatic, gastrointestinal and pancreatic impairment, and **DIC** may occur.

- Management:
  - directed at the primary cause.
  - cardiovascular support: achieved with **iv fluids, blood products, inotropic drugs** and **vasodilator drugs.** Haemodynamic monitoring consists of measurement of BP, pulse rate, **CVP, urine** output, **cardiac output** and **fluid responsiveness; pulmonary capillary wedge pressure** is no longer recommended. **Lactate** and central venous oxygen saturations are also measured. $\dot{D}O_2$, $\dot{V}O_2$ and **gastric tonometry** have previously been used to guide therapy.
  - support of other organs: as for renal failure and ALI.

Mortality exceeds 50% for cardiogenic and septic shock.
Vincent JL, De Backer D (2013). N Engl J Med; 369: 1726–34

Shock index (SI). Ratio of heart rate to systolic blood pressure; has been used to identify and monitor **haemorrhage in trauma** patients. An elevated shock index (>0.9) has been suggested as an indication for admission to ICU.

Shock lung, *see Acute lung injury*

Shunt. One extreme form of **$\dot{V}/\dot{Q}$ mismatch**, causing **hypoxaemia**. Refers to the actual amount of venous blood bypassing ventilated alveoli and mixing with pulmonary end-capillary blood (cf. **venous admixture**, the calculated amount of shunt required to produce the observed arterial $P\text{O}_2$).

- May be:
  - intrapulmonary, e.g. **atelectasis, chest infection.**
  - extrapulmonary, e.g. **congenital heart disease.**

Physiological shunt (venous admixture) = shunt-like effect of $\dot{V}/\dot{Q}$ mismatch + anatomical shunt (actual shunt). The latter includes pathological shunt and normal mixing of bronchial and thebesian venous blood with oxygenated pulmonary venous blood.

Hypoxaemia due to shunt responds poorly to increased $F_I\text{O}_2$, because the O_2 content of pulmonary end-capillary blood is already near maximum, because of the shape of the **oxyhaemoglobin dissociation curve**. Some benefit is derived from increased dissolved O_2. Thus the amount of shunt may be estimated from the response to breathing high concentrations of O_2, assuming a haemoglobin concentration of 100–140 g/l, arterial $P\text{CO}_2$ of 3.3–5.3 kPa (25–40 mmHg) and arteriovenous O_2 difference of 5 ml/100 ml (Fig. 144). Amount of shunt may also be estimated from the **shunt equation.**
[Adam Thebesius (1686–1732), German physician]

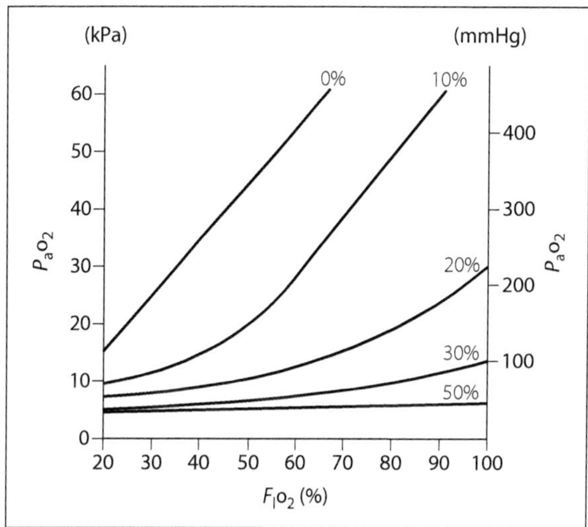

Fig. 144 P_aO_2 at varying F_IO_2 for different percentages of shunt

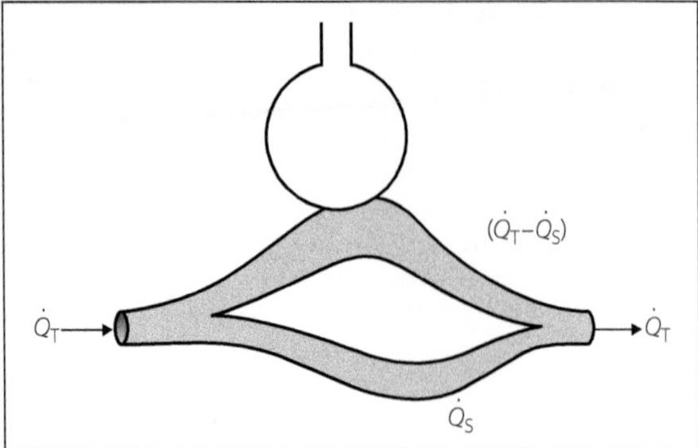

Fig. 145 Calculation of shunt equation

Shunt equation.

$$\frac{\dot{Q}_S}{\dot{Q}_T}=\frac{(C_cO_2-C_aO_2)}{(C_cO_2-C_{\bar{v}}O_2)}$$

Allows calculation of **shunt**. Derived as follows. Total pulmonary blood flow equals $\dot{Q}_T$, made up of blood flow to unventilated alveoli ($\dot{Q}_S$) and blood flow to ventilated alveoli ($\dot{Q}_T - \dot{Q}_S$; Fig. 145).

In unit time, the volume of O_2 leaving the lungs equals the volume of O_2 in blood draining ventilated alveoli plus the volume of O_2 in shunted blood. Or:

$$\dot{Q}_T \times C_aO_2 = [(\dot{Q}_T-\dot{Q}_S)\times C_cO_2]+[\dot{Q}_S\times C_{\bar{v}}O_2],$$

where C_aO_2 = arterial O_2 content
C_cO_2 = end-capillary O_2 content
$C_{\bar{v}}O_2$ = mixed venous O_2 content

Thus $\dot{Q}_T \times C_aO_2 = (\dot{Q}_T\times C_cO_2)-(\dot{Q}_S\times C_cO_2)+(\dot{Q}_S\times C_{\bar{v}}O_2)$

or $(\dot{Q}_S\times C_cO_2)-(\dot{Q}_S\times C_{\bar{v}}O_2)=(\dot{Q}_T\times C_cO_2)-(\dot{Q}_T\times C_aO_2)$

or $\dot{Q}_S(C_cO_2-C_{\bar{v}}O_2)=\dot{Q}_T(C_cO_2-C_aO_2)$

Therefore

$$\frac{\dot{Q}_S}{\dot{Q}_T}=\frac{(C_cO_2-C_aO_2)}{(C_cO_2-C_{\bar{v}}O_2)}=\text{shunt fraction.}$$

Arterial and venous O_2 contents may be estimated thus:

$$C_aO_2=(P_aO_2\times S)+(Hb\times 1.34\times S_aO_2)$$
$$C_vO_2=(P_{\bar{v}}O_2\times S)+(Hb\times 1.34\times S_{\bar{v}}O_2)$$

where P_aO_2 and S_aO_2 = arterial PO_2 and haemoglobin saturation, respectively,
$P_{\bar{v}}O_2$ and $S_{\bar{v}}O_2$ = mixed venous PO_2 and haemoglobin saturation, respectively,
S = volume of O_2 dissolved in 100 ml blood per kPa applied O_2 tension (0.0225) or mmHg (0.003),
Hb = haemoglobin content in g/100 ml.
1.34 = **Hüfner constant**.

End-capillary O_2 content cannot be measured directly, but is estimated from calculation of the **alveolar air equation**:

$$C_cO_2=(P_AO_2\times S)+(Hb\times 1.34)$$

where P_AO_2 = 'ideal' alveolar PO_2, and saturation is assumed to be 100%.

Shunt procedures. Performed to provide access to the circulation for **haemodialysis** and related procedures, thus requiring the capacity for high flow rates of blood both out of and back into the circulation. May involve:

- temporary cannulation of vessel(s), e.g. **central venous cannulation** with a double-lumen catheter (or two single ones). Choice of vessel and technique is as for placement of any central line, although the catheter is usually required for a longer time. Venous stenosis or thrombosis may be more common if the subclavian vein is used. Most double-lumen dialysis catheters are designed with one channel for withdrawal and one for return of blood; the latter opens proximal to the former to reduce the withdrawal of freshly dialysed blood from the return channel via the withdrawal channel, and thus inefficiency.
- surgical creation of a permanent arteriovenous shunt between adjacent vessels, e.g. radial artery/cephalic vein, using either direct anastomosis of the vessels (fistula) or insertion of a Silastic catheter (Scribner shunt). Venous wall thickening allows repeated cannulation, although thrombosis and venous stenosis may occur. Other complications include infection, pseudoaneurysm and arm ischaemia. Surgical shunts may be performed under local infiltration anaesthesia, regional anaesthesia (e.g. **brachial plexus block**) or general anaesthesia. Anaesthetic considerations are as for **renal failure**.

[Belding H Scribner (1921–2003), Seattle nephrologist]

Shy–Drager syndrome, *see Autonomic neuropathy*

SI units, Units of the Système International d'Unités, *see Units, SI*

SIADH, *see Syndrome of inappropriate antidiuretic hormone secretion*

Siamese twins, *see Conjoined twins*

Sick Doctor Scheme. Scheme set up in 1981 in the UK by the **Association of Anaesthetists** and Royal College of Psychiatrists, to encourage voluntary reporting of sick doctors practising anaesthesia. The anonymous reporter, having contacted the Association, is given the name and telephone number of a referee. The latter contacts an appointed psychiatrist from another region, who in turn contacts the sick doctor. Has led to similar schemes for doctors from all specialties. Intended as an alternative to the more formal scheme available via the Department of Health (previously involving appropriate action taken via a subcommittee; more recently replaced by a framework involving the National Clinical Assessment Service) and General Medical Council (assesses doctors on health and performance as well as conduct).

A scheme of the same name exists in Ireland, to help doctors affected by **substance abuse**.

Sick euthyroid syndrome (Non-thyroidal illness syndrome). Abnormal thyroid function tests occurring in critically ill patients. The most common pattern is low triiodothyronine (T_3) and thyroxine (T_4) and normal or mildly reduced thyroid stimulating hormone (TSH). Low T_3 and T_4 are generally associated with more severe critical illness and worse prognosis. Most patients are clinically euthyroid. Thought to result from **cytokine** release as part of the acute phase reaction, impaired pulsatile secretion of TSH, reduced peripheral conversion of T_4 to T_3, reduced plasma protein binding and poor nutrition.

It is not clear if the changes seen are an appropriate response to severe illness or a maladaptive response that should be treated; correction of deficits with thyroid hormone replacement has not shown consistent survival benefit.

Fliers E, Bianco AC, Langouche L, Boelen A (2015). Lancet Diabetes Endocrin; 10: 816–25

Sick sinus syndrome. Syndrome caused by impaired sinoatrial node activity or conduction; may lead to periods of severe bradycardia with intermittent loss of **P waves** or sinus arrest, and may alternate with periods of **SVT** or **AF** (bradycardia–tachycardia syndrome; bradytachy syndrome). Although it usually occurs in elderly patients with **ischaemic heart disease**, it is also a major cause of sudden death in children and young adults. May be precipitated by anaesthesia and result in refractory bradycardia or even asystole. Requires **cardiac pacing** if diagnosed preoperatively or if it occurs perioperatively.

Staikou C, Chondrogiannis K, Mani A (2012). Br J Anaesth; 108: 730–44

See also, Heart, conducting system

Sickle cell anaemia. Haemoglobinopathy, first described in 1910 in Chicago. Caused by substitution of glutamic acid by valine in the sixth amino acid from the N-terminal of **haemoglobin** β chains. Inherited as an autosomal gene; heterozygotes (genotype HbAS; sickle cell trait) possess both normal (HbA) and abnormal (HbS) haemoglobins (though they may also possess other abnormal haemoglobin combinations [e.g. HbSC]) or **β-thalassaemia** (Sβ); homozygotes (HbSS) possess only abnormal haemoglobin. Thought to have originated from spontaneous genetic mutation, with subsequent selection owing to the relative resistance against falciparum **malaria** conferred by sickle cell trait. Most common in West Central Africa, North-East Saudi Arabia and East Central India, but has been described in Southern Mediterranean populations. In the US, 1:13 Black/African-American babies is born with HbAS, and 1:365 with HbSS. In the UK, an estimated 12 500–15 000 have HbSS, mostly in London.

Deoxygenated HbS polymerises and precipitates within red blood cells, with distortion and increased rigidity. Sickle-shaped red cells are characteristic. The distorted cells increase blood **viscosity**, impair **blood flow** and cause capillary and venous thrombosis and organ infarction. They have shortened survival time. O_2 affinity of dissolved HbS is normal, but overall affinity is reduced if some of the HbS is polymerised. HbS polymerises at $P\text{O}_2$ of 5–6 kPa (40–50 mmHg); thus HbSS patients are continuously sickling. HbAS patients' red cells contain both HbS and HbA and sickle at 2.5–4.0 kPa (20–30 mmHg).

- Features:
  - HbSS:
    - **haemolysis** causing **anaemia** and hyperbilirubinaemia. Gallstones may occur. Enlargement of the skull and long bones is common, due to compensatory bone marrow hyperplasia. Acute aplastic crises may occur, and sequestration crises in children.
    - impaired tissue blood flow may result in **stroke**, papillary necrosis of the kidney, ulcers, pulmonary infarcts, priapism and avascular necrosis of bone. Crises are caused by acute vascular occlusion, and may feature neurological lesions and severe pain, e.g. abdominal, back, chest (the sickle chest syndrome is a common cause of death and includes cough, fever and severe **hypoxaemia**). They may be precipitated by **hypothermia**, **dehydration**, infection, exertion and hypoxaemia.
    - increased susceptibility to infection (especially pneumococcal infections) due to splenic infarction. Osteomyelitis is typically caused by unusual organisms, e.g. salmonella.
  - HbAS: usually asymptomatic, because arterial $P\text{O}_2$ is unlikely to reach the level required to induce sickling.
  - combinations of HbS with other haemoglobins usually produce mild disease. In heterozygotes for HbS and haemoglobin C (HbC), red cells may sickle at around 4 kPa (30 mmHg) because HbC is less soluble than HbA, and makes red cells more rigid.

Diagnosis is by detection of HbS in the blood. The Sickledex test involves addition of reagent to blood, with observation for turbidity. It detects HbS but provides no information about other haemoglobins. A sodium metabisulfite test induces sickling in susceptible cells, which are then counted. Haemoglobin electrophoresis is the definitive method of determining the nature of the haemoglobinopathy. Sickle cells are usually present in peripheral blood in HbSS.

Management is supportive, avoiding risk factors where possible and early treatment of infection; prophylactic daily antibiotic is often recommended. Hydroxycarbamide (hydroxyurea) may be used to boost fetal haemoglobin production; it may suppress white blood cell and platelet production. Treatment of crises may require opioids, e.g. by **PCA**, O_2 and rehydration. Exchange **blood transfusion** may be required. **Bone marrow transplantation** is the only definitive treatment.

- Anaesthetic considerations:
  - preoperatively:
    - all races at risk should be screened for HbS, ideally by electrophoresis. In the UK, Sickledex testing is usual initially, with progression to electrophoresis if positive. In emergencies, if the Sickledex test is positive, diagnosis may be aided by blood counts and peripheral film. If the history does not suggest HbSS, and haemoglobin/reticulocyte count and peripheral film are normal with no red cell fragments, HbAS is likely, although HbSC and other heterozygous variants may still be present. Management ultimately depends on the nature of the surgery and availability of blood.
    - **preoperative assessment** is directed towards the above complications, especially impairment of pulmonary and renal function. Preoperative folic acid has been suggested. Exchange transfusion is often used in HbSS patients before major surgery, aiming to reduce HbS concentrations to <30%. A less aggressive transfusion strategy is to aim for a haematocrit of >30%; both approaches have similar efficacy.
    - hypoxaemia, dehydration, hypothermia and **acidosis** should be prevented at all times perioperatively. Prophylactic antibiotics are often administered.
  - intraoperatively:
    - standard techniques may be used, apart from **tourniquets**, which cause tissue ischaemia (**IVRA** is contraindicated). **Heat loss** should be prevented and cardiovascular stability maintained. **Preoxygenation** and F_IO_2 of 50% reduces the risk of hypoxaemia by increasing arterial $P\text{O}_2$ and

pulmonary O_2 reserve. IV hydration should be maintained. Frequent analysis of acid–base status is required in HbSS patients. Prophylactic **bicarbonate** administration has been suggested, but administration according to acid–base analysis is usually preferred.
- intraoperative crises may present with changes in breathing pattern or BP, acidosis and hypoxaemia. Detection may be difficult.

- postoperatively: the precautions already instituted should continue, because complications may occur postoperatively. Patients have traditionally been considered unsuitable for most **day-case surgery** but this would depend on the planned procedure and the state of the patient. O_2 administration for at least 24 h is usually advocated after all but minor surgery.

Narjeet Khurmi N, Gorlin A, Misra L (2017). Can J Anesthesiol; 64: 860–9

SID, *see Strong ion difference*

Siggaard-Andersen nomogram. Diagram derived from analysis of many blood samples, showing the plot of log arterial $P\text{CO}_2$ against plasma **pH**, with **base excess**, **standard bicarbonate** and **buffer base** illustrated as additional lines (Fig. 146). Allows determination of arterial $P\text{CO}_2$ by equilibrating a blood sample with two known concentrations of CO_2, and measuring the sample pH at each concentration. The points are plotted on the diagram and joined by a line, and the $P\text{CO}_2$ read from the vertical scale according to the pH of the original sample. Alternatively, if arterial $P\text{CO}_2$ can be measured directly, a single measurement of pH and $P\text{CO}_2$, together with **haemoglobin** concentration (because haemoglobin is a major blood **buffer**), allows determination of the derived data. Modern blood-gas machines automatically perform the required calculations, making such plotting unnecessary.
[Ole Siggaard-Andersen, Danish biochemist]

Sigh, *see Intermittent positive pressure ventilation*

Significance, *see Statistical significance*

Sildenafil (Viagra). Orally active **phosphodiesterase inhibitor**, selective for cyclic guanine monophosphate (cGMP)-specific phosphodiesterases. Licensed for use in **pulmonary hypertension** and male erectile dysfunction. Catastrophic interactions with nitrates (e.g. **GTN**) have been reported, resulting in severe hypotension and death; thus a history must be obtained in suspected **ischaemic heart disease** before administering nitrates. Tadalafil and vardenafil are related drugs.

Simplified acute physiology score (SAPS). Scoring system used to assess severity of illness by determining the degree of deviation of physiological variables from normal values. Originally incorporating 14 variables and excluding pre-existing disease, a modified version (SAPS II) has been developed in which 12 variables are weighted according to age and underlying disease. SAPS III uses a new, improved model for risk adjustment. Used in a similar way to **APACHE**.

Capuzzo M, Moreno RP, Le Gall JR (2010). Curr Opin Crit Care; 16: 477–81

See also, Mortality/survival prediction on intensive care unit

Simpson, James Young (1811–1870). Scottish obstetrician; Professor of Midwifery at Edinburgh. The first to administer

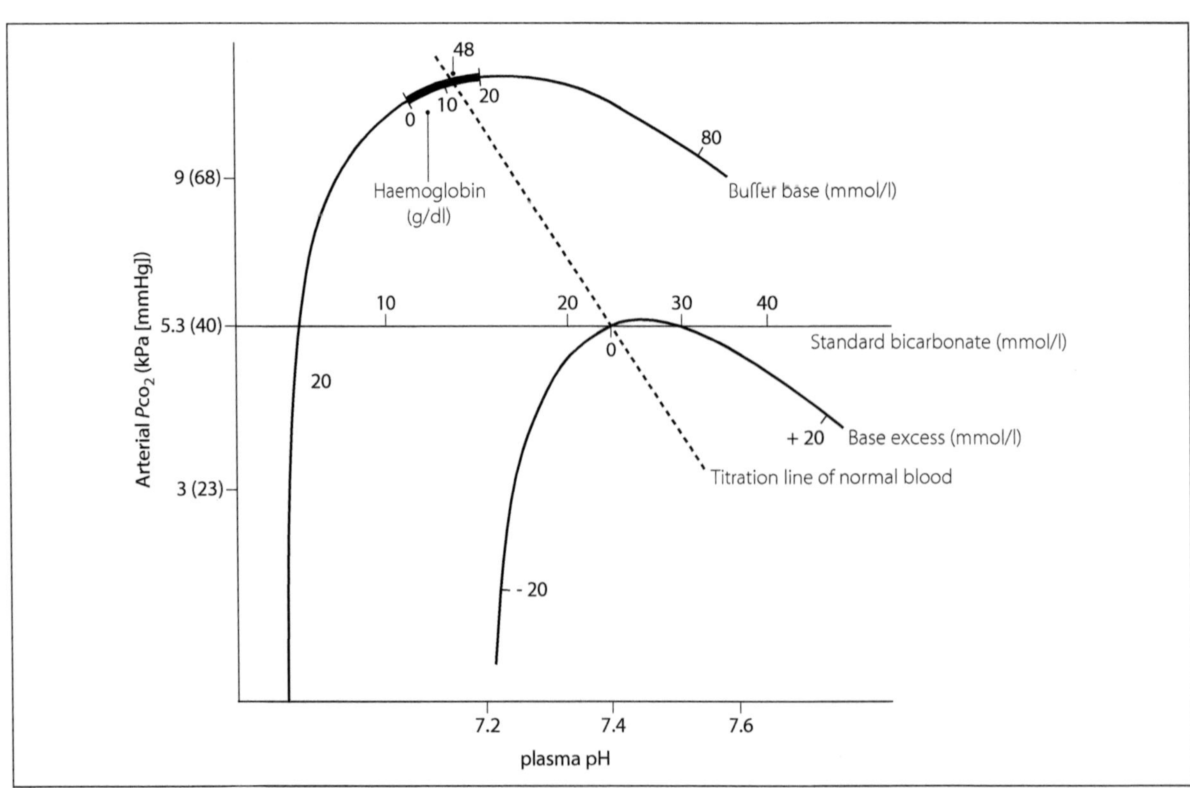

Fig. 146 Siggaard-Andersen nomogram

an anaesthetic for obstetrics in 1847, using **diethyl ether**. Following a suggestion by Waldie later that year, he used **chloroform** for the same purpose. Encountered stiff opposition from the clergy and others, who maintained that painful childbirth was either God's will, beneficial to the patient, or both; this continued until **Snow**'s administration of chloroform to Queen **Victoria** in 1853 ('*chloroform à la reine*'). Helped popularise chloroform as the replacement for ether. Was made baronet in 1866.
[David Waldie (1813–1889), Scottish-born Liverpool doctor and chemist]
McKenzie AG (2011). Anaesthesia; 66: 438–40

Simulators. Training devices that allow the recreation of specific clinical scenarios. Useful in the development of diagnostic and therapeutic skills, decision-making, team training, analysing tasks and errors and assessing risks. Allow prospective and repeated observation and analysis of actions rather than retrospective assessment. Individual components, e.g. manikins, may be used to teach specific skills (part-task trainers), or combined within the setting of an entire operating suite with monitoring equipment and controlled with computers (high-fidelity simulation), often interacting through a mathematical model.

Now widely used in areas other than anaesthesia, e.g. obstetrics, emergency medicine and surgery.

Despite best efforts, simulators may not always reflect real conditions accurately. For instance, some activities may be easier to perform on simulators than in the operating room; conversely, some may be more difficult. Reality is further impeded by the need to model average 'patients' who may not respond in the 'extreme' ways of some real patients; equally, subjects' responses may be different when they are aware that they are working with a simulator. The cost of sophisticated simulators and the labour-intensive staffing requirements are further disincentives. Nevertheless, simulation has become an established part of training programmes in many countries, and has also been studied as a means of assessing practitioners.
Naik VN, Brien SE (2013). Can J Anesth; 60: 192–200
See also, Crisis resource management

SIMV, Synchronised intermittent mandatory ventilation, *see Intermittent mandatory ventilation*

Simvastatin, *see Statins*

Single-pass albumin dialysis, *see Liver dialysis*

Sinoatrial node, *see Heart, conducting system*

Sinus arrhythmia. Normal phenomenon (especially in young people) characterised by alternating periods of slow and rapid **heart rates**. The **ECG** shows **sinus rhythm** with irregular spacing of normal complexes. Most commonly related to respiration, with a rapid rate at end-inspiration and a slower rate at end-expiration. A number of mechanisms have been proposed, including: activation of **pulmonary stretch receptors** during inspiration, causing inhibition of the **cardioinhibitory centre** via vagal afferents; changes in intrathoracic pressure causing stretching of the sinoatrial node, producing cardiac accelerations during inspiration; and lower intrathoracic pressure during inspiration, causing reduced cardiac output, leading to an increase in heart rate mediated by the **baroreceptor reflex**. May also involve direct impulse conduction between medullary respiratory and cardiac neurones. Also seen in patients treated with **digoxin**. Abolished by **atropine**.

Sinus bradycardia. Usually defined as **sinus rhythm** at less than 60 beats/min. The **ECG** shows normal P waves and QRS complexes occurring at a slow rate.

- Caused by:
  - physiological slowing, e.g. in athletes, or during **sleep**.
  - disease states, e.g. **hypothyroidism**, raised **ICP**, acute **MI**, **sick sinus syndrome**, **jaundice**.
  - activation of vagal reflexes, e.g. **carotid sinus massage**, **Valsalva manoeuvre**. During anaesthesia, it may follow skin incision, stretching or dilatation of the anus, cervix, mesentery and bladder (**Brewer–Luckhardt reflex**), and pulling on the ocular muscles (**oculocardiac reflex**). May occur in critically ill patients during **tracheobronchial suctioning**.
  - **hypoxaemia**, especially in children. Thought to be caused by central depression of the **vasomotor centre**.
  - blockade of the cardiac sympathetic innervation during high **spinal** or **epidural anaesthesia**.
  - drugs, e.g. **propofol**, **neostigmine**, **digoxin**, **opioid analgesic drugs**, **β-adrenergic receptor antagonists**.

If it occurs, the stimulus should be stopped. It may be treated with **anticholinergic drugs** (e.g. **atropine**), **β-adrenergic receptor agonists** or **cardiac pacing**, but treatment is usually only required if accompanied by symptoms, hypotension or **escape beats**.

Sinus rhythm. Normal heart rhythm in which each **P wave** is followed by a **QRS complex** on the **ECG**; i.e., each impulse originates in the sinoatrial node, which has the fastest inherent rhythmicity of all cardiac **pacemaker cells**. Normal **heart rate** is usually defined as 60–100 beats/min.
See also, Cardiac cycle; Heart, conducting system; Sinus arrhythmia; Sinus bradycardia; Sinus tachycardia

Sinus tachycardia. Usually defined as **sinus rhythm** at over 100 beats/min. The **ECG** shows regular normal P waves and QRS complexes at a rapid rate.

- Caused by:
  - increased sympathetic activity, e.g. fear, anxiety; during anaesthesia, it may represent **hypoxaemia**, **hypercapnia**, and inadequate anaesthesia or neuromuscular blockade. It may also occur as a compensatory mechanism, e.g. in **anaemia**, **hypovolaemia**, **gas embolism/PE**.
  - increased metabolic rate, e.g. **hyperthyroidism**, **pyrexia**, **pregnancy**, **MH**.
  - drugs, e.g. **sevoflurane**, **isoflurane**, **pancuronium**, **sympathomimetic drugs**, **cocaine**, **anticholinergic drugs**.

Reduces the time available for ventricular filling and **coronary blood flow**; it may precipitate **myocardial ischaemia** if severe. Treatment is usually directed at the cause; **β-adrenergic receptor antagonists** may be required if the patient is at risk of myocardial ischaemia.

Sinusitis. Infection of the nasal sinuses of the **skull**. May occur as a consequence of upper respiratory tract infection, trauma or, especially relevant to ICU, prolonged tracheal intubation; has been reported in 2%–40% of patients requiring IPPV. Up to 10 times more common if nasotracheal or nasogastric tubes are in place; thought to be related to obstruction of drainage through the sinus ostia (although in a third of cases the contralateral side is affected). Also more common in immunosuppressed and diabetic patients. Usually affects the maxillary or sphenoid sinuses, although ethmoid and frontal sinusitis may also occur (and may result in **cerebral abscess** and **cerebral venous thrombosis**).

May present with non-specific features of **sepsis**; diagnosed by CT scanning (although plain x-rays may be helpful), ± antral puncture and aspiration. Ultrasound examination may be useful, but requires specialised equipment. Organisms involved are usually gram-negative **bacteria**, staphylococci or anaerobes. Management includes extubation, **antibacterial drugs** ± surgical drainage. Antihistamines and decongestants have also been used. Usually resolves within a week of extubation.

See also, Intubation, complications of

SIRS, *see Systemic inflammatory response syndrome*

Skin diseases. Anaesthetic considerations may be related to:
- diseases with cutaneous and systemic manifestations, e.g. **connective tissue diseases, porphyria, polymyositis, neurofibromatosis**, severe skin disease with **anaemia** and **malnutrition.**
- scarring or fibrosis of tissues around the face, mouth or neck causing difficulty with tracheal intubation, e.g. **systemic sclerosis**, epidermolysis bullosa dystrophica. In the latter, bullous lesion formation may follow instrumentation (e.g. laryngoscopy), and may be followed by scarring.
- involvement of the immune system causing **airway obstruction** (e.g. **hereditary angio-oedema**) or severe manifestations of **histamine** release (e.g. urticaria pigmentosa). Histamine-releasing drugs should be avoided.
- increased **heat loss during anaesthesia** if large areas of erythema are present.
- susceptibility to skin trauma following handling, laryngoscopy, and use of sticking plaster or ECG electrodes.
- effect of drug therapy, e.g. **corticosteroids, immunosuppressive drugs.**

In addition, anaesthetic agents may precipitate cutaneous lesions (e.g. in **adverse drug reactions**, bullous eruption following **barbiturate poisoning**, porphyria).

Skull. The upper part contains the **brain**, while the lower anterior portion forms the facial skeleton:
- superior aspect: divided from left to right by the coronal suture, separating the frontal bone anteriorly and the parietal bones posteriorly. The sagittal suture separates the two parietal bones in the midline, and the lambdoid suture separates the parietal bones and occipital bone posteriorly. The anterior fontanelle closes at about 18 months of age.
- lateral aspect: consists of parietal and occipital bones posteriorly, temporal and sphenoid bones inferiorly, and frontal bone, with the zygomatic and maxillary bones below, anteriorly. The mandible articulates with the temporal bone at the **temporomandibular joint.**
- anterior aspect: consists of frontal bone superiorly, zygomatic bones at the inferolateral edges of the orbits, and maxilla centrally, with the mandible inferiorly. Nerves and vessels pass through the anterior foramina and the inferior and superior orbital fissures (Fig. 147a). In addition, the foramen rotundum (below and medial to the superior orbital fissure's medial end) transmits the maxillary division of the fifth **cranial nerve.**
- inferior aspect: especially important because of the structures transmitted by its foramina (Fig. 147b).

In addition, branches of the first cranial nerve pass through the cribriform plate's perforations.

See also, Mandibular nerve blocks; Maxillary nerve blocks; Ophthalmic nerve blocks; Orbital cavity

Skull x-ray. Useful investigation for the detection of linear and depressed **skull** fractures following **head injury**, for classifying **facial trauma** and planning of **maxillofacial surgery**. Although the presence of a fracture increases the likelihood of intracranial damage, significant injury may be present with a normal x-ray. May show basal skull fractures but these are better visualised by **CT scanning**. Pneumocephalus is easily evident on a plain skull x-ray as are foreign bodies in the scalp. 'Open mouth' views are useful for diagnosing fractures of C1/C2.

Sleep. Naturally occurring state of unconsciousness; the response to external stimuli is decreased, but the subject may usually be readily roused. Regulated by circadian rhythms controlled by the suprachiasmatic nucleus of the **hypothalamus.**
- Two patterns are described:
  - non-rapid eye movement (NREM) sleep, divided into four stages according to **EEG** activity:
    - stage 1: transition from wakefulness to sleep and follows a latency period of 10–20 min; characterised by low-amplitude, high-frequency theta waves (3–12 Hz). The lightest plane of sleep, it occupies 2%–5% of total sleep time (TST). An increase in stage 1 sleep suggests sleep fragmentation.
    - stage 2: lasts about 10 min but occupies 40%–55% of TST. Characterised by sleep spindles (12–14 Hz) and high-amplitude K complexes.
    - stages 3 and 4: known as slow-wave sleep or deep sleep with high-amplitude, low-frequency delta waves (0.5–2 Hz, 75 μV). Occupies 20% of TST; decreases with age.
  - rapid eye movement (REM) sleep (paradoxical sleep): rapid, irregular, low-amplitude waves occur, similar to those seen in awake subjects. Occurs every 90 min with duration increasing as night progresses and occupies 25% of TST. Dreaming occurs. The eyes make rapid movements, accompanied by tachycardia, tachypnoea, skeletal muscle relaxation and penile erection.

Sleep disruption is common in the ICU and consists of a decrease in TST, a predominance of light sleep (stages 1 and 2) and a decrease in restorative slow wave sleep (stages 3 and 4). Only 50% of sleep takes place at night.
- Effects of sleep deprivation:
  - immune dysfunction—decreases in phagocytic activity, **cytokine** levels and antioxidant activity result in increased susceptibility to infection.
  - hormonal and metabolic effects—sleep deprivation increases **insulin** resistance, **corticosteroid** secretion, catabolism and oxygen consumption.
  - respiratory mechanics—decreased ventilatory response to hypoxaemia and hypercapnia, reduced respiratory muscle stamina result in failure to wean from IPPV.
  - **confusion in the intensive care unit.**

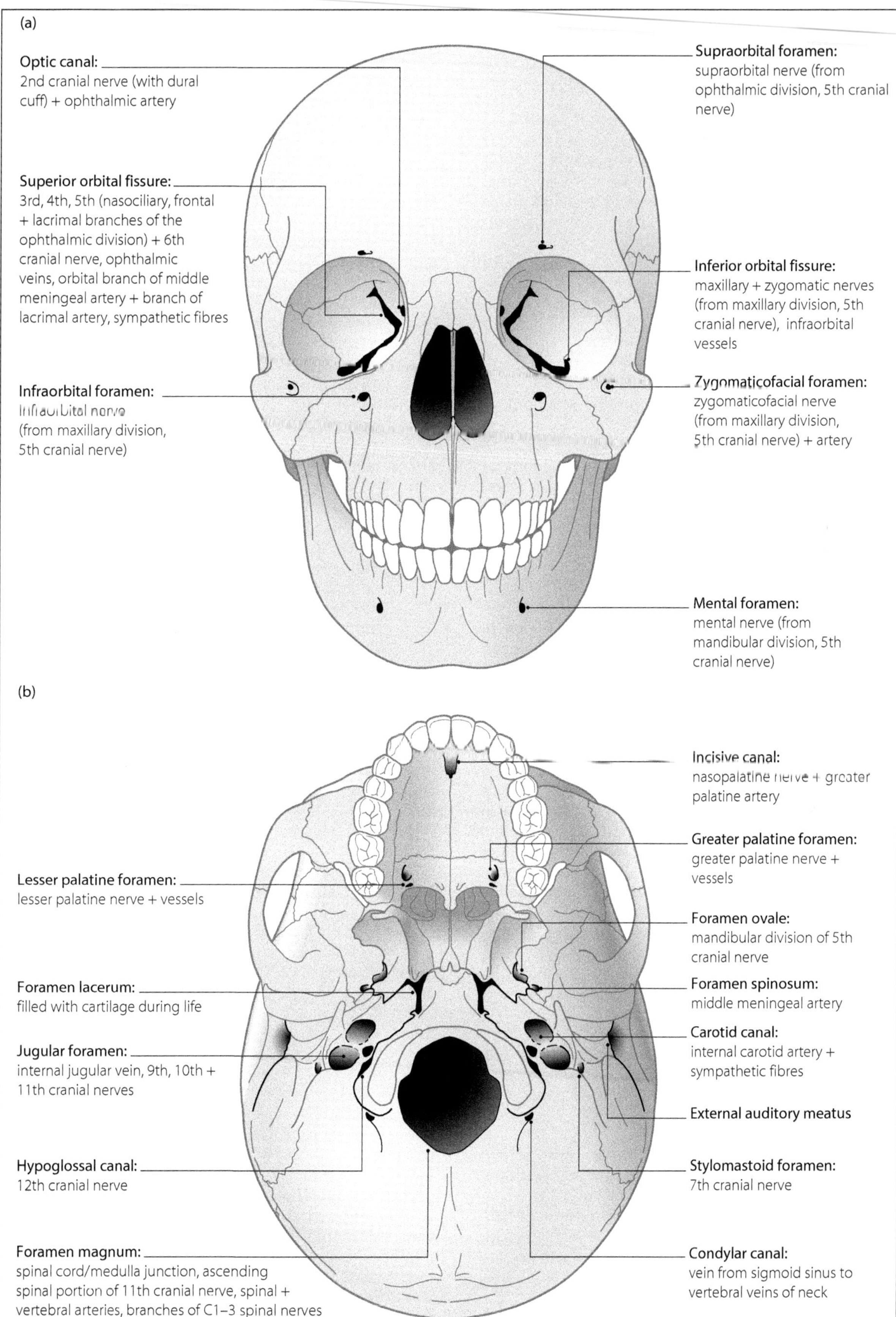

Fig. 147 Skull: (a) anterior aspect; (b) base, showing foramina

- Causes of sleep deprivation:
  - pre-existing disease: e.g. patients with **COPD** show decreased total sleep time and REM sleep with frequent arousals caused by hypoxaemia, hypercapnia and coughing.
  - mechanical ventilation especially if ventilator asynchrony, air leaks, etc., present.
  - drugs: e.g. **benzodiazepines** abolish stages 3 and 4 NREM sleep; **opioid analgesic drugs** increase arousal frequency; **tricyclic antidepressant drugs, barbiturates** and **amfetamines** inhibit REM sleep. **Catecholamines** increase wakefulness.
  - anaesthesia and surgery: the **stress response to surgery**, fever, pain, opioids, starvation and age decrease stages 3 and 4 NREM sleep and abolish REM sleep on subsequent nights.
  - environmental factors:
    - noise (e.g. telephones, conversations, alarms). Average noise level is 60 dB.
    - lighting levels too high and present at all times.
    - nursing, physiotherapy interventions occurring at night.

Reduction in noise levels, light levels and limiting nursing intervention to daylight hours have been shown to be beneficial. **Melatonin** may help restore normal sleep architecture.

Pulak LM, Jensen L (2016). J Intensive Care Med; 31: 14–23

See also, Sleep-disordered breathing

Sleep-disordered breathing. Group of conditions in which abnormal breathing occurs during **sleep**. Includes: **obstructive sleep apnoea** (OSA), the most common form; central sleep apnoea caused by lack of respiratory drive, e.g. **Ondine's curse**; and a mixed pattern. In OSA, there are typically repeating cycles of increasing **airway obstruction** that may become total, the resultant **hypoxaemia** and **hypercapnia** causing arousal, vigorous respiratory effort and noisy disruption of the normal sleep pattern. In central sleep apnoea, there are episodes of hypopnoea and apnoea without respiratory effort, and even **Cheyne–Stokes respiration**. All forms may result in chronic exposure to hypoxaemia and hypercapnia, with increased risk of cardiovascular disease including sudden death.

Slow-reacting substance-A, *see Leukotrienes*

Smallpox, *see Biological weapons*

Smoke inhalation. Occurs in up to 30% of patients presenting with flame burn injuries. Resultant pulmonary insufficiency is seen in ~75% and is the commonest cause of death in patients admitted to hospital with **burns**.

- Problems are related to:
  - low F_IO_2 of inspired gas, and inhalation of carbon monoxide, cyanide, nitrogen oxides and other substances. All may result in **hypoxaemia**.
  - inhaled carbon particles coated with irritant substances (e.g. aldehydes) that may cause **laryngospasm**, **bronchospasm** and inhibition of **ciliary activity**.
  - **$\dot{V}/\dot{Q}$ mismatch, shunt** and **pulmonary oedema** may occur.
  - thermal injury to the airway may be followed by upper **airway obstruction**, bronchospasm, tracheal and bronchial oedema and sloughing.

Further respiratory impairment may occur if infection and **ALI** supervene.

- Management: as for burns, **carbon monoxide poisoning, cyanide poisoning, respiratory failure**. Early fibreoptic **bronchoscopy** for assessment and clearance of particulate matter is advocated; an alternating regimen of aerosolised **heparin** and ***N*-acetylcysteine** has been shown to reduce mortality.

Sheridan RL (2016). N Engl J Med; 375: 464–9

See also, Nitrogen, higher oxides of

Smoking. Common cause of cardiovascular and respiratory pathology in surgical and non-surgical patients.

- Effects:
  - cardiovascular:
    - **nicotine** is an agonist at nicotinic **acetylcholine receptors** in sympathetic ganglia; it increases heart rate, SVR and thus BP. It also increases myocardial O_2 demand, and possibly decreases **coronary blood flow**.
    - carbon monoxide combines with up to 15% of **haemoglobin** to form carboxyhaemoglobin, reducing the O_2-carrying ability of blood. Causes shift of the **oxyhaemoglobin dissociation curve** to the left, further impeding release of O_2. Thus haemoglobin concentration and packed cell volume are often increased, increasing blood **viscosity** and hindering oxygen delivery further.
    - increased risk of **ischaemic heart disease** and frequency of ventricular arrhythmias.
    - increased risk of **DVT**.
  - pulmonary:
    - impaired **ciliary activity**.
    - impaired **leucocyte** activity.
    - increased risk of **bronchial carcinoma**.
    - increased bronchial reactivity and **COPD**.

Smokers are more likely to have increased sputum production and retention, **bronchospasm**, coughing, **atelectasis** and **chest infection** perioperatively. Poor wound and bone healing is also more common.

Stopping smoking is thought to be beneficial preoperatively, in order to minimise its acute adverse effects. Effects of carbon monoxide and nicotine are significantly reduced after 12–24 h abstinence; postoperative wound and respiratory complications are reduced after ~4 weeks' abstinence, although up to 6–8 weeks is thought to be necessary for restoration of ciliary and immunological activity.

Wong J, Chung F (2015). Anaesthesia; 70: 902–6

See also, Carbon monoxide poisoning

Snake bites, *see Bites and stings*

Snow, John (1813–1858). Pioneer of English anaesthesia, born in York. Moved to London in 1836. Developed the science and art of anaesthesia, describing five stages of anaesthesia in 1847. Designed inhalers for **diethyl ether** and **chloroform**, and wrote two famous textbooks on the use of these agents (his book on chloroform was published posthumously). Widely regarded as the expert in his field, he administered chloroform to Queen **Victoria** during childbirth in 1853 and 1857. Also famous for demonstrating that cholera was spread by contaminated drinking water, not by foul air, as previously believed. Removal of the Broad Street water pump handle on his suggestion is said to have stopped the London epidemic of 1854. One of the heraldic supporters of the **Royal College of Anaesthetists** (with **Clover**).

Society of Critical Care Medicine (SCCM). Founded in 1970 to support the specialty of critical care as a separate but interdisciplinary entity, with ***Critical Care Medicine*** as its official journal. Supports research, education and provision of resources.

Soda lime. Mixture used for **CO_2 absorption in anaesthetic breathing systems**, composed of calcium hydroxide (~90%), sodium hydroxide (4%–5%), potassium hydroxide (traditionally 1%; in the UK modern preparations do not contain potassium hydroxide), silicates (for binding; less than 1%) and indicators. Used with 14%–19% water content. CO_2 in solution reacts with sodium (± potassium) hydroxides to form the respective carbonates, which then react with calcium hydroxide to produce calcium carbonate, replenishing sodium and potassium hydroxides. Heat and water are also produced during the reaction. Exhaustion of its activity is indicated by dyes; several have been used. UK manufacturers voluntarily agreed to use the same colour change (white to violet) in 2013.

Provided in granules of size 4–8 mesh (will pass through a mesh of 4–8 strands per inch in each axis; i.e., pore size of 1/16–1/64 in^2). Canisters should be tightly packed to reduce channelling of gases through large gaps. The total volume of space between granules should equal the volume of the granules themselves. Dust may be inhaled using older systems, especially the 'to-and-fro' system. Large canisters containing up to 2 kg soda lime are commonly employed.

Known to react with **trichloroethylene**, with the risk of neurological damage. The modern **inhalational anaesthetic agents**, especially **sevoflurane**, may react with soda lime if the latter is warm and very dry. Compound A, **carbon monoxide**, formic acid and formaldehyde may be produced. Compound A is a particular product of sevoflurane, leading to fears over its use in circle systems, although evidence of toxic levels of compound A within such systems has not been found. Significant levels of carbon monoxide have been reported. Furthermore, the temperature in the absorber may increase to dangerous levels and there may be some absorption of the volatile agent itself. The minimal level of moisture that will prevent such reactions is 2% for sodium hydroxide and 4.7% for potassium hydroxide, leading to the latter's removal from modern preparations in the UK. Normal use of circle systems is not thought to result in such low levels of moisture, but they have been found after prolonged passage of dry gas through the absorber, e.g. at the start of a Monday morning operating session if gases are left running over the weekend.

Attempts to prevent the soda lime drying out include shutting off anaesthetic machines after use, changing the soda lime regularly and not relying on colour changes to indicate dehydration, checking for unusually hot absorption canisters or unexpectedly low concentrations of volatile agent, and addition of zeolites that can physically trap water, or inorganic chlorides that crystallise water within the soda lime. A new mixture (calcium hydroxide lime) consisting of calcium hydroxide with calcium chloride (plus calcium sulfate and polyvinylpyrrolidone to improve hardness and porosity) has been developed that does not contain sodium or potassium hydroxide and does not react with any of the currently used volatile agents.
See also, Baralyme

Sodium (Na^+). Principal cation in the **ECF**, accounting for 90% of the osmotically active solute in **plasma** and **interstitial fluid**. Thus the prime determinant of ECF volume. Total body content is about 4000 mmol, of which 50% is in bone, 40% in ECF, and 10% intracellular. About 70% is available for exchange. Normal plasma levels: 135–145 mmol/l. Of central importance in the function of excitable cells, e.g. concerning **membrane potentials** and **action potentials**.

Actively absorbed from the small intestine and colon, facilitated by **aldosterone** and the presence of **glucose** in the gut lumen. The kidney filters approximately 26000 mmol Na^+/day, of which 99.5% is reabsorbed by passage through the **nephron** (mostly at the proximal convoluted tubule). Reabsorption is influenced by renal tubular hydrostatic and oncotic gradients, aldosterone, adrenocortical hormones, **atrial natriuretic hormone** and the rate of secretion of hydrogen and potassium ions.

- Sodium balance:
  - daily losses: about 150 mmol in the urine, with 10 mmol via each of faeces, sweat and skin. Saliva contains 10 mmol/l, sweat 50 mmol/l, gastric secretions 60 mmol/l and the rest of the GIT about 130 mmol/l.
  - daily requirement: about 1 mmol/kg/day; a normal diet usually far exceeds this.
  - regulated via changes in:
    - ECF sodium concentration and **osmolality** via **osmoreceptors**, affecting the **renin/angiotensin system** and aldosterone secretion.
    - ECF volume: via **baroreceptors**, affecting atrial natriuretic peptide secretion in addition to the above hormones.

See also, Hypernatraemia; Hyponatraemia

Sodium bicarbonate, *see Bicarbonate*

Sodium calcium edetate. Chelating agent, used in the treatment of acute and chronic lead poisoning. Has also been used successfully in poisoning with copper and radioactive materials.

- Dosage: 40 mg/kg iv bd for 5 days; repeated if necessary after a 7-day break.
- Side effects: nephrotoxicity, nausea and vomiting, myalgia, hypotension, T wave abnormalities on the **ECG**.

Sodium citrate. Non-particulate **antacid**, used preoperatively to increase gastric pH in patients at risk of **aspiration of gastric contents**, e.g. before general anaesthesia in obstetrics. Thought to be less harmful than **magnesium trisilicate** if inhaled. Effective for 30–50 min following oral intake of 30 ml 0.3 molar solution.

Also used to relieve discomfort from urinary tract infection by raising urinary pH.

Sodium clodronate, *see Bisphosphonates*

Sodium cromoglicate (Cromoglycate). Drug used in the prophylaxis of **asthma**; of no value in acute attacks. Thought to stabilise **mast cells** by preventing **calcium** ion entry, thus preventing IgE-triggered release of inflammatory mediators. Particularly useful in allergic and exercise-induced asthma in children. Should be taken regularly as a powder, aerosol or nebulised solution, usually 10–20 mg 4–8 times daily. Generally less effective than **corticosteroids**.
See also, Bronchodilator drugs

Sodium dichloroacetate. Activator of pyruvate dehydrogenase, resulting in increased oxidation of **lactate** to acetylcoenzyme A and CO_2. Has been used to treat **lactic acidosis**, although randomised trials have not found an increase in survival.

Sodium nitrite, *see Cyanide poisoning*

Sodium nitroprusside (SNP). **Vasodilator drug**, used as an **antihypertensive drug**, e.g. in **hypotensive anaesthesia**. Also used in **cardiac failure**. Presented as a powder for reconstitution in 5% dextrose. Unstable in solution, with decomposition to highly coloured products. Solutions require protection from light and should be used within 24 h of preparation.

Reacts with thiol groups in vascular smooth muscle and converted to nitrite, which reacts with hydrogen ions to produce **nitric oxide**. Acts mainly on arteries, although veins are also affected. Thus reduces **SVR**, maintaining **cardiac output** and tissue perfusion. Also reduces myocardial O_2 consumption while increasing **coronary blood flow**, although **coronary steal** has been reported. Compensatory tachycardia is common. Hepatic blood flow remains constant, while **renal blood flow** and **cerebral blood flow** increase. Active within 30 s of administration. Broken down non-enzymatically within red blood cells (catalysed by **haemoglobin**) to produce five cyanide ions from each molecule, some of which combine with haemoglobin to form methaemoglobin; the remainder are converted to thiocyanate in the liver by rhodonase and then excreted in the urine. Plasma **half-life** of SNP is about 2 min.

- Dosage: initially 0.5–1.5 μg/kg/min iv, increased to a maximum of 8 μg/kg/min (maximal total dose of 1 mg/kg over 2–3 h). **Tachyphylaxis** may occur.
- Side effects:
  - may cause rapid and profound hypotension.
  - rebound hypertension following its abrupt withdrawal. Caused by activation of the **renin/angiotensin system** and increased plasma **catecholamine** levels.
  - raised **ICP** may occur.
  - **platelet** aggregation may be inhibited.
  - pulmonary **shunt** may be increased in normal lungs via impairment of **hypoxic pulmonary vasoconstriction**.
  - cyanide toxicity and **methaemaglobinaemia** (hence limitation of dose). More likely in **vitamin** B_{12} deficiency. May present with metabolic **acidosis**, and reduced **arteriovenous** O_2 **difference**. Treated as for **cyanide poisoning**. Combination of SNP with **trimetaphan** and prophylactic administration of thiosulfate have been suggested as methods for reducing risk of cyanide toxicity.
  - thiocyanate may accumulate after more than 3 days' infusion, with possible interference with thyroid function.

Sodium/potassium pump. Protein pump present in every cell **membrane**, responsible for **active transport** of **sodium** out of cells and **potassium** into cells. The protein is an **enzyme** that catalyses hydrolysis of **ATP** to ADP, providing the energy required for the transport. Consists of two α subunits (mw 95 000) that extend through the membrane and provide the binding site for ATP, and two β subunits (mw 40 000). Three sodium ions are transported for every two potassium ions, creating a net negative charge within the cell. Required for maintenance of cellular **membrane potential** and electrolyte composition. Inhibited by **cardiac glycosides**.

Sodium thiosulfate, *see Cyanide poisoning*

Sodium valproate. **Anticonvulsant drug** used for all forms of **epilepsy** but the first-line drug for tonic or atonic seizures. Acts mainly by blocking neuronal sodium channels but also by inhibiting calcium channels in thalamic neurones and enhancing **GABA** activity. Rapidly absorbed by mouth and largely protein-bound (90%), its **half-life** is approximately 12 h.

- Dosage:
  - 20–30 mg/kg/day orally, up to 2.5 g daily.
  - 400–800 mg (up to 10 mg/kg) iv over 3–5 min followed by iv infusion up to 2.5 g/day. Plasma levels are poor indicators of efficacy but are useful in monitoring toxicity at high doses.
- Side effects: GIT disturbances, transient hair loss, rarely **thrombocytopenia** and impaired **platelet** function, **pancreatitis** and severe **hepatitis**. A dose-dependent increase in plasma ammonia level occurs in 20% of patients but is usually transient.

SOFA, *see Sepsis-related organ failure assessment*

Solubility. Extent to which a substance dissolves in another substance.

- Examples of clinical relevance:
  - **inhalational anaesthetic agents**: speed of onset of anaesthesia depends on their solubility in blood, and **potency** depends on their solubility in lipids (**Meyer–Overton rule**). The ability of N_2O to expand gas-containing cavities depends on its greater blood solubility than nitrogen. For a gas dissolving in a liquid, solubility depends on the temperature (solubility decreases as temperature increases), and the properties of the gas and liquid (expressed by the **solubility coefficient**). Some volatile agents (e.g. **halothane**) may also dissolve in rubber anaesthetic tubing, producing significant concentrations even when the vaporiser is turned off.
  - non-gaseous drugs: solubility in water determines requirement for other solvents, e.g. **Cremophor EL** or propylene glycol for parenteral injection. Solubility in lipid **membranes** affects the extent to which a drug crosses membranes, e.g. GIT wall, **blood–brain barrier**.

See also, Partition coefficient

Solubility coefficients. Expression of **solubility**. Two coefficients are commonly used:

- Bunsen solubility coefficient: volume of gas measured at **STP** that dissolves in unit volume of liquid.
- Ostwald solubility coefficient: volume of gas dissolved in unit volume of liquid at the stated temperature and pressure, i.e., equals the **partition coefficient** between liquid and gas phases. If measured at 0°C and at 1 atm, it equals the Bunsen solubility coefficient.

For solubility of **inhalational anaesthetic agents**, the Ostwald solubility coefficient (at 37°C) is usually used as it is independent of pressure.
[Robert WE Bunsen (1811–1899) and Wilhelm Ostwald (1853–1932), German chemists]

Solvent abuse. Form of **substance abuse** involving the intake (usually by inhalation) of a variety of solvents used in glues, paints and similar products; include toluene, petroleum products and carbon tetrachloride. Acute problems may include depressed consciousness and **arrhythmias**, the latter probably related to myocardial sensitisation to endogenous **catecholamines**. Sudden death has occurred. Specific organ damage (renal, hepatic) may occur with specific substances, e.g. toluene after prolonged usage. Management is largely supportive.

Somatostatin (Growth hormone inhibiting hormone). Hormone secreted by the pancreas, GIT mucosa and hypothalamus. Exists in two forms, with either 14 or 28 amino acid residues. Also a **neurotransmitter** in the brain and spinal cord (especially substantia gelatinosa, where it is involved in **pain** transmission—somatostatin has been shown to produce analgesia when injected epidurally). Other actions include:
- inhibition of release of growth hormone and thyroid stimulating hormone.
- suppression of release of GIT hormones e.g. gastrin, cholecystokinin, **vasoactive intestinal peptide**.
- inhibition of release of **insulin** and **glucagon**.

Analogues (lanreotide and **octreotide**) have been used: to control diarrhoea and flushing in the **carcinoid syndrome**, possibly via inhibition of **5-HT** release; in the management of bleeding **oesophageal varices**; and in the management of **acromegaly**.

Sonoclot, *see Coagulation studies*

Sore throat, postoperative. Reported in up to 90% of cases in some studies, and in up to 25% of patients following spontaneous breathing via a **facemask**.
- May be related to:
  - **tracheal intubation**:
    - use of **suxamethonium**.
    - shape and type of **tracheal tube** and **cuff** (and inflation pressure of the latter); larger tubes are associated with a greater incidence of sore throat and hoarse voice than smaller ones.
    - trauma on laryngoscopy, intubation and extubation.
    - use of stylets or bougies.
    - pharyngeal suction.
    - use of throat packs.
    - use of lubricating/local anaesthetic gel or spray.
  - use of nasogastric tubes.
  - anticholinergic **premedication**.
  - use of a **SAD** (especially if the cuff is overinflated) or oro-/nasopharyngeal **airways**.
  - use of unhumidified gases.

Also common after tracheal intubation in the ICU, especially after prolonged IPPV.

El-Boghdadly K, Bailey CR, Wiles MD (2016). Anaesthesia; 71: 706–17

Sotalol hydrochloride. Water-soluble non-selective **β-adrenergic receptor antagonist** and class III **antiarrhythmic drug**, available for oral and iv administration. Used for prophylaxis and treatment of **SVT** and **VT**.
- Dosage: 80 mg orally daily in 1–2 doses (with ECG monitoring), increased up to 160–320 mg/day. Dosage is reduced in **renal failure**.
- Side effects: as for β-adrenergic receptor antagonists. **Prolonged Q–T interval** and **torsade de pointes** may occur, especially in the presence of **hypokalaemia** (electrolyte deficiencies should be corrected before starting treatment).

SPAD, Single-pass albumin dialysis, *see Liver dialysis*

SPEAR, Selective parenteral and enteral antisepsis regimen, *see Selective decontamination of the digestive tract*

Specific dynamic action. Energy required to assimilate food into the body, manifested as an increase in metabolic rate following intake. Thus the net total amount of energy obtained from food is reduced (by 30% for protein, 6% for carbohydrates and 4% for fats).
See also, Nutrition

Specific gravity (Relative density). The **density** of a substance divided by that of water. Still used to indicate urinary concentration because measurement is easy (using a hydrometer), although not as useful clinically as **osmolality**. Varies with temperature. Depends on the mass and number of solute particles, whereas osmolality depends only on number of particles. Thus heavy molecules (e.g. radiographic contrast media) greatly increase specific gravity with only small increases in osmolality. Normal values: for urine (at 20°C), 1.002–1.035; for plasma (at 20°C), 1.010; for **CSF** (at 37°C), 1.004–1.008.

Glucose 2.7 g/l and protein 4 g/l each increase specific gravity by 0.001.

For a gas, the ratio of substance to that of **air** is often used. Most anaesthetic-related gases and vapours are heavier than air, e.g. **isoflurane, enflurane, sevoflurane** and **desflurane** (×7.5), **halothane** (×6.8), **N_2O** (×1.53), **CO_2** (×1.5), **O_2** (×1.1).

Specific heat capacity, *see Heat capacity*

Specific latent heat, *see Latent heat*

Specificity. In **statistics**, the ability of a test to exclude false positives. Equals:

$$\frac{\text{the number correctly identified as negative}}{\text{total without the condition}}$$

See also, Errors; Predictive value; Sensitivity

SPECT, Single photon emission computed tomography, *see Positron emission tomography*

Spectroscopy. In anaesthesia, used for **gas analysis**, especially for estimation of **CO_2**, **N_2O** and volatile agent concentrations. Different types:
- infrared spectroscopy: depends on the ability of gases containing different atoms to absorb infrared light (thus O_2 and nitrogen cannot be analysed):
  - side stream: sample gas is drawn into a chamber through which half of a split infrared beam is passed, the other half passing through a reference chamber containing air. The amount of infrared light absorbed by the sample gas depends on the amount of gas present, and is determined by comparing the emergent beams from the sample and reference chambers. This is done with photoelectric cells behind each chamber, or by passing the beams through two further chambers containing, e.g. CO_2, separated by a diaphragm. The heating effect of the infrared light causes pressure to rise within these chambers; the difference in pressure between them depends on the amount of infrared light absorbed by the original gas sample. Some devices employ a single chamber instead of two, and some use a rotating perforated wheel to divide the beam(s) of light into pulses. The wheel may incorporate different filters to measure different

substances. The technique may be used for multiple simultaneous gas analysis.

Sources of error include overlap of absorption spectra by several gases (e.g. CO, CO_2 and N_2O all share some absorption range) and collision broadening, whereby the presence of one gas broadens the absorption spectrum of another. These may be compensated for with electronic correction factors and the use of a different (or more than one) wavelength for each gas.

- main stream: analysis takes place at the breathing system itself, by incorporating a special connector near the patient end of the tubing. An emitter/detector is attached to the connector and light is passed through small sapphire windows in the connector. Although more rapid and not requiring sample tubing, the device may be bulky and heavy.

- photoacoustic spectroscopy: relies on absorption of infrared light of different wavelengths by different molecules, with subsequent emission of sound at the wavelengths concerned for each molecule. Detection is with a microphone. Multiple simultaneous gas analysis may be performed.
- Raman spectroscopy: relies on Raman scattering, the absorption and immediate emission of light by gases in a pattern specific to the individual molecules. All gaseous molecules may be analysed in this way (but not single atoms). Powerful light sources (e.g. **lasers**) are required to give an adequate signal. Multiple simultaneous gas analysis may be performed.
- ultraviolet spectroscopy: has been used to measure halothane concentrations. Requires lengthy warming up and frequent calibration; now rarely used routinely.
- gas discharge meter: used to measure nitrogen concentration. 1500 V potential is passed across the gas sample in a tube. Intensity of purple light at a specific wavelength is measured.
- mass spectroscopy: now usually referred to as mass spectrometry (*see Mass spectrometer*).

[Chandrasekhara V Raman (1888–1970), Indian physicist]

See also, Carbon dioxide, end-tidal; Carbon dioxide measurement; Near infrared spectroscopy

Spider bites, *see Bites and stings*

Spinal anaesthesia (Subarachnoid/intrathecal anaesthesia). Probably first performed by **Corning** in 1885, but first performed for surgery by **Bier** in 1898. Initial use of **cocaine** was associated with tremor, headache and muscle spasms. The less toxic **procaine** was first used by **Braun** in 1905 and was soon used widely. Hyperbaric solutions were introduced by **Barker** in 1907. Further refinements were related to new **local anaesthetic agents**. Continuous spinal techniques were described in the 1940s, initially via rubber tubing connected to the **needle** left in situ.

Popularity waned in the late 1940s following reports of neurological damage and the introduction of **neuromuscular blocking drugs** for general anaesthesia (GA). In the classic Woolley and Roe case in the UK in 1947, two cases of paraplegia during the same operating list followed spinal anaesthesia. Phenol contamination via cracks in the cinchocaine ampoules was blamed at the time, although contamination of the syringes and needles with acidic descaler solution from the steriliser has since been suggested as being more likely.

Increasing popularity over the last 40–50 years has followed better understanding of the technique, and acceptance that the incidence of side effects is low when spinal anaesthesia is correctly performed.

- Indications: surgical procedures to the lower body, especially perineum and legs. Considered the method of choice by many anaesthetists for **TURP**, **caesarean section** and **orthopaedic surgery**, especially to the hip and knee. Has also been used for upper abdominal surgery. Deliberate high or total spinal anaesthesia was formerly used for **hypotensive anaesthesia**, and to provide abdominal muscle relaxation.
- Anatomy:
  - the **spinal cord** ends at L1–2 in adults, lower levels in children. The dura ends at S2; therefore lumbar puncture is usually performed at the L3–4, L4–5 or L5–S1 interspaces (N.B. the actual interspace used is commonly higher than that intended).
  - the L4 or L4–5 interspace is usually crossed by a line drawn between the iliac crests (Tuffier's line), although this is not very reliable. The spinous process of T12 has a notched lower edge.
  - the course taken by the needle is as for reaching the **epidural space**, plus the dura (*see also, Meninges; Vertebrae; Vertebral canal; Vertebral ligaments*).
- Technique:
  - **preoperative assessment**, preparation and **premedication** are as for GA. Facilities for resuscitation and progression to GA must be available.
  - **monitoring** is as for GA. An iv cannula must be placed. Preloading with fluid is controversial (*see later*).
  - the patient is placed in the lateral position, with chin on the chest and knees drawn up, or sitting on the edge of the trolley. Back flexion opens the intervertebral spaces. An assistant is required to steady the patient.
  - in the UK, facemasks, sterile drape, gown and gloves are considered mandatory. The back is cleaned, avoiding contamination of gloves, needles and other equipment with cleaning solution (implicated in causing **arachnoiditis** and **meningitis**), which must be allowed to dry thoroughly before touching the back. Chlorhexidine 0.5% in alcohol has been recommended as the most suitable cleansing agent, because stronger solutions—although possibly providing more effective antisepsis—may carry a greater risk of chemical-induced arachnoiditis/meningitis.
  - median approach:
    - the chosen interspace is infiltrated with local anaesthetic.
    - the spinal needle is inserted in the midline, aiming slightly cranially. Non-cutting needles, e.g. Sprotte (smooth-sided pointed tip, with wide lateral hole proximal to the tip), Whitacre (pencil tip-shaped, with a smaller hole just proximal to the tip) or Greene (oblique bevel, with bevel edges rounded) are associated with a lower incidence of **post-dural puncture headache** and are often used (Fig. 148). The **Quincke** needle point, with its short-bevelled cutting tip, is rarely used nowadays, except in patients at low risk of headache, e.g. the elderly. 22–27 G needles are commonly used; the larger are easier to use but increase the risk of headache. Thinner needles are often inserted through a 19 G iv needle or introducer (the latter are usually

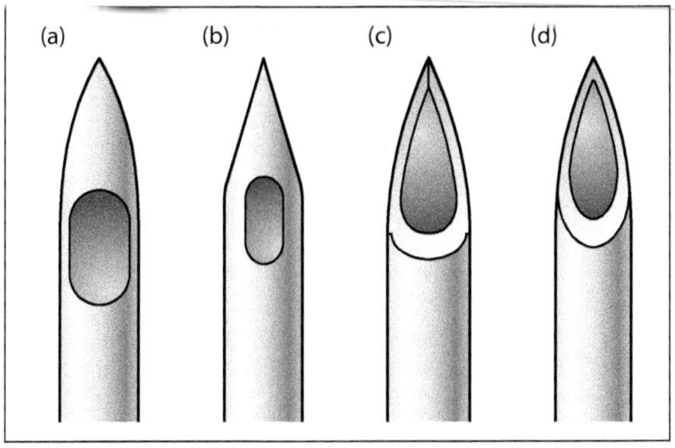

Fig. 148 Different types of spinal needles: (a) Sprotte; (b) Whitacre; (c) Greene: (d) Quincke

Table 47 Doses (mg) of local anaesthetics required for spinal blockade of different heights

Agent	L4	T10	T4–6	Duration (h)
Bupivacaine 0.5% (heavy)	5–10	10–15	15–20	1.5–2.5
Cinchocaine 0.5% (heavy)	4–6	6–8	10–12	2–3
Levobupivacaine 0.5% (plain)	2.5–7.5	7.5–12.5	12.5–15	1.5–2
Lidocaine 5% (heavy)	25–50	50–75	75–100	1–1.5
Prilocaine 2% (heavy)	20–40	40–60	60–80	1.5–2
Tetracaine 1% (heavy; mixed with equal volumes of CSF)	4–6	8–12	14–16	1.5–2.5

included in the sterile pack; formerly, separate devices were used, e.g. Sise introducer). The bevel (if present) is faced laterally to reduce the risk of headache.
- resistance increases as the ligamentum flavum is entered and when dura is encountered, with a sudden give as the dura is pierced. Correct location is confirmed by CSF at the needle hub; aspiration may be required with very fine needles. Rotation of the needle in 90-degree steps may produce CSF if none is obtained initially.

  Hanging drop and other techniques have been used to identify the epidural space before dural puncture.
- with one hand securing the needle against the patient's back to avoid dislodgement, the solution is injected, with aspiration before, during and after injection to confirm correct placement. Injection should cease if pain is experienced.
- non-**Luer connector** systems are now available to reduce the risk of wrong-route drug administration errors (i.e., intrathecal administration of an iv drug).

▸ paramedian approach: requires less back flexion, and is easier if the vertebral ligaments are calcified:
- infiltration is performed 1.5 cm lateral to the cranial border of the spinous process at the selected interspace.
- the needle is inserted, aiming medially and cranially until the resistance of the ligamentum flavum is felt. If the lamina is encountered, the needle is walked off its cranial edge.
- dural puncture and injection as before.

▸ a continuous catheter technique may be used as for epidural anaesthesia; it has been unpopular because of fears over infection and CSF leak, difficulty of handling the very fine catheters (28–32 G), and the occurrence of **cauda equina syndrome** following use of **lidocaine**, but allows incremental injection of solution and therefore greater cardiovascular stability during onset of block. Both catheter-through-needle and catheter-over-needle systems are available.

- Solutions used (Table 47):

▸ only hyperbaric **bupivacaine** 0.5%, hyperbaric **prilocaine** 0.5% and plain **levobupivacaine** 0.5% are available specifically for spinal anaesthesia in the UK. In the USA, hyperbaric bupivacaine 0.25%–0.75%, hyperbaric **tetracaine** (amethocaine) 1%, lidocaine 0.5%–2%, **mepivacaine** 1%–2%, **ropivacaine** 0.5%–1% and **chloroprocaine** 3% are used (the latter for dilution to 2.5% before administration because of risks of **transient radicular irritation syndrome** or damage).

▸ larger volumes are required for plain solutions than for heavy ones. Duration of block may be extended by addition of vasopressors; **adrenaline** 0.2–0.5 ml 1:1000 and **phenylephrine** 0.5–5 mg have been used, although rarely in the UK, and fears have been expressed concerning possible cord ischaemia provoked by their use. L5–S2 segments remain blocked for the longest.

▸ low-dose techniques may be used, e.g. 1 ml bupivacaine 0.25% with **fentanyl** 10–25 µg, or 3–4 ml of a bupivacaine 0.1%/fentanyl 2 µg/ml mixture, in obstetrics.

▸ spread of solution and extent of blockade are affected by many factors, including:
- dose: thought to be the most important; increased variability may occur with altered concentration and volume.
- site of injection.
- baricity of solution and position: thus hyperbaric solutions affect dependent parts, hypobaric solutions, e.g. tetracaine 0.1%, affect upper parts. Plain bupivacaine 0.5% is slightly hypobaric; tetracaine 1% is isobaric.

- Use of hyper- or hypobaric solutions relies on lateral/supine positioning and head-up/down tilt, combined with the normal curvature of the spine:
  - thoracic curve is concave anteriorly; T4 is traditionally held to be the most posterior part (most dependent in the supine position) but recent imaging studies suggest T8 instead.
  - lumbar curve is convex anteriorly; L3–4 is the most anterior part (uppermost in the supine position). This curve may be abolished by flexing the hips in the supine position.

  In addition, the greater width of females' hips compared with their shoulders tends to tip their spinal canal head-down, in the lateral position; in males, the opposite occurs.

  Thus slow injection of 1 ml hyperbaric solution at L5–S1 with the patient sitting produces saddle block suitable for perineal surgery, with minimal hypotension. Blocks may be restricted to one side by injection in the lateral position, although 'fixing' of local anaesthetic may require up to 40 min. Injection of hyperbaric solution in the lateral

position with immediate turning into the supine position usually produces blockade to T4–6.
  - patient factors, e.g. weight, height, sex, age, are not thought to be as critical as previously suspected, but they have a small influence. Large variability of blockade between patients is normally found. Recently, volume of CSF has been implicated at least partly in this variability. Reduced volumes of agent are required in **obstetric analgesia and anaesthesia**.
  - technical factors, e.g. speed of injection, barbotage (repeated aspiration of CSF into syringe, mixing it with local anaesthetic before re-injection) and direction of the needle, tend to affect variability of blocks; thus slow injection without barbotage produces the most reliable results.
- **spinal opioids** improve the quality and duration of analgesia but at the risk of specific side effects.
- other drugs have been studied, e.g. **ketamine, midazolam** and **clonidine**, but these are not licensed.

- Effects:
  - results in rapid onset of block (usually within 3–5 min), although maximal effect may take up to 30 min. Vasodilatation in the feet is usually seen first, with flushing and increased warmth.
  - thought to act mainly at **spinal nerve** roots, although some effect is possible at the **spinal cord** itself. Differential blockade of different motor and sensory modalities is thought to be related to the size and therefore sensitivity of different **neurones** to local anaesthetics. Thus the smaller sympathetic preganglionic fibres are more easily blocked than larger sensory and motor fibres, with the sympathetic 'level' higher than the sensory level. Assessment of the sympathetic level is difficult; the **galvanic skin response** has been used. The level of blockade for touch sensation is usually 1–2 segments below that for pinprick, whereas that for motor innervation is 1–2 segments lower than that for sensory innervation.
  - CVS:
    - sympathetic blockade causes vasodilatation below the level of block. Reductions in cardiac output and BP are thought to be caused mainly by reduced venous return consequent to venous dilatation, although the fall in SVR contributes. Increased or unaltered cardiac output has also been reported. Reflex vasoconstriction occurs above the level of block. Hypotension is particularly likely in **hypovolaemia**, because cardiac output in this case is dependent on resting vasoconstriction.

      Hypotension is also more likely in obstetrics, when **aortocaval compression** may occur. Hypotension may be exacerbated by bradycardia and sedative drugs (depressant effects of local anaesthetic are minimal). The drop in BP may be greater with higher levels of blockade, but this is not always so.
    - bradycardia may be due to block of sympathetic cardiac innervation (T1–4), vagal stimulation during surgery or a reflex response to decreased venous return. **Cardiac arrest** has been reported, possibly involving the **Bezold–Jarisch reflex**.
    - cardiac work and O_2 demand are reduced.
    - renal, hepatic, cerebral and coronary blood flows are maintained if marked hypotension does not occur.
    - reduction in perioperative bleeding is thought to be due to reduced BP, lack of venous hypertension due to venodilatation and pooling of blood in dependent vessels.
    - reduction of postoperative **DVT** is thought to be due to vasodilatation, **haemodilution** and reduced **viscosity** secondary to **iv fluid administration**, and increased **fibrinolysis**.
    - absorbed adrenaline may have systemic effects, if used.
  - RS: intercostal and abdominal weakness may impair active exhalation and coughing, although tidal volume and inspiratory pressure are maintained by intact diaphragmatic innervation (C3–5). **FRC** is reduced when supine, and hypoventilation may follow sedation; thus O_2 is usually administered via a **facemask** as a precaution, and to allow concurrent N_2O administration if required.
  - GIT: bowel contraction results from dominant parasympathetic tone following sympathetic blockade. Sphincters relax and peristalsis increases.
  - **urinary retention** may occur.
  - **stress response to surgery** is attenuated. Injected drug is eliminated via absorption by subarachnoid and epidural vessels.

- Management:
  - assessment: level of sensory blockade is usually determined by testing for temperature (e.g. using ice or **ethyl chloride** spray) or pinprick sensation, though touch is thought to be a more reliable predictor of intraoperative (dis)comfort. Knowledge of appropriate **dermatomes** is required. Motor block is assessed by testing muscle groups of appropriate **myotomes**; commonly expressed using the **Bromage scale** or variants thereof.
  - positioning of the patient may be used to extend or reduce spread of the block as required, until fixed.
  - a high level of block may produce feelings of impaired breathing and nasal stuffiness, plus impaired sensation or power in the arms. Total spinal blockade results in apnoea and loss of consciousness, with fixed dilated pupils. Treatment is as for hypotension, plus tracheal intubation and IPPV. Recovery is complete if BP and oxygenation are maintained.
  - preloading with iv fluid before performing spinal anaesthesia is controversial, with some authorities favouring the use of **vasopressor drugs** as being equally efficacious and more logical. In addition, fears have been expressed concerning fluid overload, especially in the elderly. In practice, many anaesthetists give a more modest volume of fluid as the spinal block develops ('coload') together with a small dose of prophylactic vasopressor.

    A drop in systolic BP by one-third normal value is often considered acceptable in young, healthy patients. Management of larger decreases or in elderly/less healthy patients:
    - positioning the patient head-down: increases venous return but risks a higher level of block unless the head is raised.
    - iv fluid administration, usually with **crystalloids** initially.
    - use of vasopressor drugs. May increase myocardial work and O_2 demand secondary to increases in SVR. **Ephedrine** (3–6 mg iv repeated as required) is commonly used; effects on venous tone may be greater than with other drugs, e.g. phenylephrine

(10–50-µg increments iv), **metaraminol** (0.5–1-mg increments iv).
  - **atropine** 0.3–0.6 mg or **glycopyrronium** 0.2–0.3 mg if bradycardia occurs.
- nausea: may be related to vagal stimulation, e.g. during handling of the bowel. Hypotension is an important cause.
- **sedation** may be used to reduce awareness and improve patient comfort. **Benzodiazepines** and **propofol** are commonly used; ketamine provides some analgesia, e.g. while positioning for injection in trauma cases. Disadvantages include respiratory and cardiovascular depression and confusion, especially if sedation is excessive. General and spinal anaesthesia may be combined, not necessarily with increased risk of hypotension.

- Complications:
  - hypotension and high blockade as above.
  - post-dural puncture headache.
  - neurological injury:
    - **transient radicular irritation syndrome** especially associated with lidocaine in concentrations >2.5%.
    - direct trauma is extremely rare. Injection should stop immediately if pain is felt.
    - haematoma formation with spinal cord compression is extremely rare with normal coagulation. It may be masked by regional blockade. Permanent neurological damage may occur if surgical decompression is delayed >8–12 h.
    - cord ischaemia, e.g. **anterior spinal artery syndrome**, thought usually to occur with severe hypotension. Vasopressor drugs have been implicated but their role is unclear.
    - infection/aseptic meningitis.
    - cauda equina syndrome.
    - arachnoiditis.

    Temporary and relatively minor injury (e.g. numbness/weakness in foot or toe) is thought to occur in ~1–2:2000 cases, with >90% recovering within 3–6 months. Severe permanent damage is thought to occur in <1:100 000 cases.
  - backache (the contribution of spinal anaesthesia itself is doubtful but muscular relaxation with possible stretching of ligaments has been suggested rather than direct trauma).
- Contraindications:
  - non-acceptance by the patient.
  - infection, both generalised and local.
  - hypovolaemia/shock.
  - neurological disease: raised **ICP** is an absolute contraindication because of the risk of **coning**. Other disease is controversial; there may be a fear of being blamed if a naturally progressive lesion becomes worse, but avoidance of general anaesthesia and/or postoperative opioids may be advantageous. Careful consideration of the potential risks/benefits, with clear documentation of the preoperative discussion(s) is vital.
  - abnormal coagulation: full anticoagulation and significant coagulopathy are considered absolute contraindications due to the risk of vertebral canal haematoma. The decision around prophylactic **heparin** therapy depends on consideration of individual risks and benefits, the timing, and **coagulation studies**. Widely accepted guidelines state that a spinal or epidural needle or catheter should not be inserted (or a catheter manipulated or removed) within 6 h of prophylactic unfractionated heparin or 12 h after low-molecular-weight heparin. Heparin should not be given until 2–4 h after an epidural or spinal. Although these guidelines are not based on strong evidence, they are widely followed (but may be overridden if the clinical circumstances suggest the benefit outweighs the risk).

    A platelet count of 80–100 × 10^9/l is usually taken as the lower safe limit, but the true safe value is unknown. Platelet dysfunction is clearly important, but the actual risks of **antiplatelet drugs** are unclear. Current guidance recommends against central neuraxial blockade in patients taking aspirin in combination with any other anticoagulant agent; aspirin in isolation is not a contraindication. For patients taking **clopidogrel**, a period of 7 days between discontinuation of therapy and neuraxial blockade is recommended by international consensus and the drug manufacturer.

    Spinal anaesthesia has been claimed to be safer than epidural anaesthesia, because the needles are finer and a catheter is not placed.
  - emergency abdominal surgery, especially intestinal obstruction: hypovolaemia may be present, and increased GIT activity following spinal anaesthesia may increase the risk of perforation.

[Albert Woolley (1891–?) and Cecil Roe (1902–?), English labourers; Theodore Tuffier (1857–1929), French surgeon; Nicholas Greene (1922–2005) and Lincoln F Sise (1874–1942), US anaesthetists; Günter Sprotte, German anaesthetist; Rolland J Whitacre (1909–1956), US anaesthetist]

Spinal cord. Cylindrical structure lying within the **vertebral canal**, beginning at the foramen magnum and terminating inferiorly level with L1–2 (L3 at birth, rising to the adult level by 20 years). May rarely end at T12 or L3. Continuous superiorly with the medulla oblongata, it tapers inferiorly to form the conus medullaris. The filum terminale, an extension of the pia mater, attaches the lower end to the back of the coccyx. Has cervical and lumbar enlargements corresponding to innervation of the upper and lower limbs, respectively. Surrounded by the **meninges** and bathed in **CSF**. The anterior median fissure is a deep longitudinal fissure and the posterior median sulcus is a shallow furrow. Gives off 31 pairs of **spinal nerves** throughout its length. On cross-section, consists of central H-shaped grey matter surrounded by white matter. The grey matter is composed of anterior and posterior horns, with lateral horns (sympathetic columns) in the thoracic region. The two halves are joined across the midline by the grey commissure, which contains the central canal (Fig. 149).

- Main ascending tracts:
  - posterior (dorsal) columns: convey ipsilateral touch and vibration/proprioception sensation, from the lower body via the fasciculus gracilis and upper body via the fasciculus cuneatus.
  - posterior and anterior spinocerebellar tracts: convey proprioception sensation to the cerebellum via inferior and superior cerebellar peduncles, respectively.
  - lateral and anterior spinothalamic tracts: the former conveys contralateral pain and temperature sensation; the latter conveys contralateral touch and pressure sensation.
  - spinotectal tract: conveys information to the brainstem involved in spinovisual reflexes.

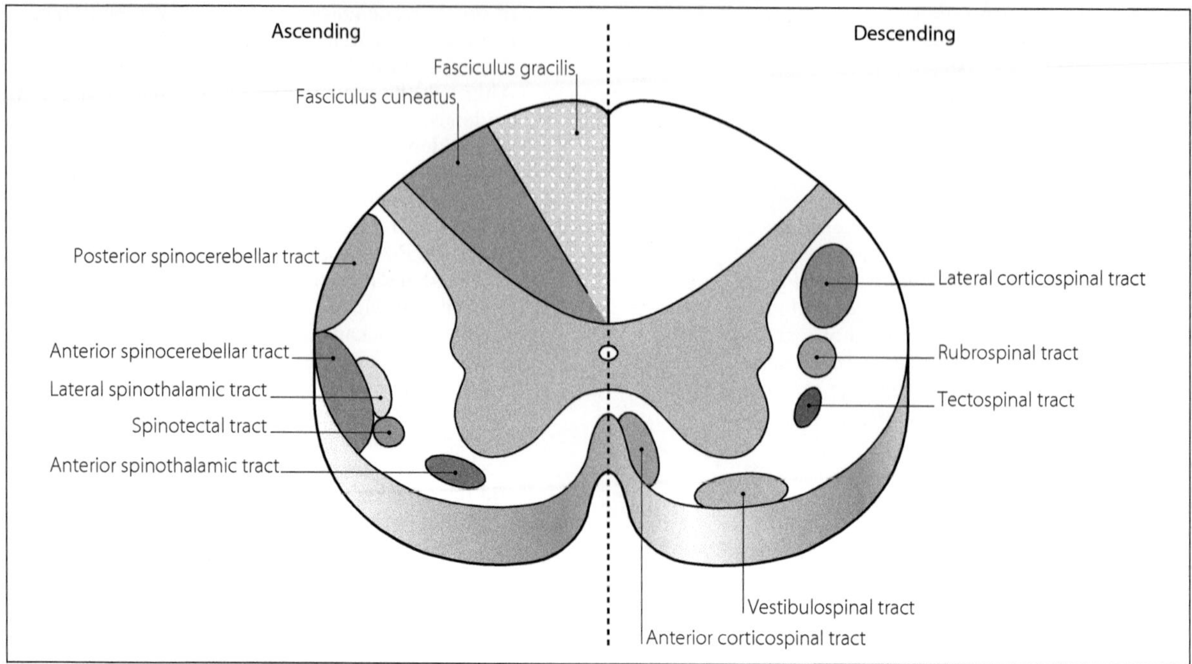

Fig. 149 Anatomy of spinal cord showing ascending and descending tracts

- Main descending tracts:
  - lateral and anterior corticospinal tracts: convey motor innervation from the cerebral cortex; the former via crossed (pyramidal) fibres and the latter via uncrossed (extrapyramidal) fibres.
  - rubrospinal, tectospinal and vestibulospinal tracts: contain extrapyramidal fibres passing from brainstem nuclei to lower motor neurones.
- Blood supply:
  - anterior spinal artery: formed from two branches of the vertebral arteries, and descends in the anterior median fissure from the brainstem to the conus medullaris. Supplies the anterior two-thirds of the cord.
  - posterior spinal arteries: arise from the vertebral arteries, each dividing into two branches that descend along the side of the cord, one anterior and one posterior to the dorsal nerve roots. Supply the posterior one-third of the cord.
  - radicular branches: arise from local arteries (e.g. intercostal, lumbar) and feed the spinal arteries. The most important are at T1 and the lower thoracic/upper lumbar level (artery of Adamkiewicz). The cord at T3–5 and T12–L1 is thought to be most at risk from ischaemia.

[Albert Adamkiewicz (1850–1921), Polish pathologist]

See also, Anterior spinal artery syndrome; Motor pathways; Sensory pathways; Spinal cord injury

Spinal cord injury (SCI). Damage to the **spinal cord** resulting in permanent or transient loss of usual spinal motor, sensory or autonomic function. Incidence is 13 per million population in the UK, 35 per million in the US. In the UK 80% occur in men with a mean age of 33 years. 40% are associated with motor vehicle accidents and 40% with falls (often at ground level in people with known degenerative spine disease). Penetrating SCI is increasing with increasing gun and knife violence. 30% of cases have associated major injuries, e.g. **TBI** or other **trauma**.

- Pathophysiology:
  - primary injury is caused by direct compression of the spinal cord, often caused by subluxation of the vertebrae; this can lead to complete transection of the cord. This may occur in the absence of a vertebral fracture. In addition, haemorrhage and impairment of the cord's vascular supply may exacerbate the injury.
  - secondary injury occurs minutes to days after the initial insult. Spinal cord **oedema** results in ischaemia, which leads to loss of spinal cord **autoregulation**; in high thoracic injuries, neurogenic shock produces hypotension, which further decreases cord perfusion. Further damage results from release of excitatory neurotransmitters (e.g. **glutamate**), release of **free radicals**, mitochondrial dysfunction and inflammatory responses.
  - lesions above T2–T5 abolish cardiac sympathetic outflow resulting in hypotension and bradycardia (neurogenic shock). **Spinal shock** refers to the acute loss of spinal reflexes below the level of the SCI and is accompanied by flaccid paralysis; it is followed by a spastic hyperreflexia after 2–3 weeks. **Autonomic hyperreflexia** may occur after 4–6 weeks if the lesion is above T5–6.
- Certain clinical syndromes may occur:
  - complete injury, with loss of motor or sensory function below a certain level.
  - incomplete injury syndromes:
    - central cord: arms paralysed more than legs, with bladder dysfunction and variable sensory loss.
    - anterior cord: paralysis below the level of lesion, with proprioception, touch and vibration sense preserved.
    - posterior cord: only touch and temperature sensation impaired.
    - hemisection of cord (Brown-Séquard): ipsilateral paralysis and loss of proprioception, touch and vibration sensation, with loss of contralateral pain and temperature sensation.

- Management:
  - as for any **trauma**, with particular emphasis on the **airway**, maintenance of cardiac output and oxygenation, and stabilisation of the spine. Manual in-line cervical spine stabilisation should be carried out during intubation, which should especially avoid flexion of the neck. Hypotension should be aggressively treated to maintain spinal cord perfusion pressure.
  - 80% of patients with cervical SCI will require IPPV within the first 48 h. Those with lesions at C3 and above will have a lifetime dependence on mechanical ventilation because of loss of **phrenic nerve** function.
  - urgent surgical stabilisation should be considered if neurological deterioration occurs.
  - high-dose methylprednisolone (30 mg/kg iv, followed by 5.4 mg/kg/h for 24–48 h) within 8 h of injury has been shown to reduce the level of injury slightly. However, worries about increased incidence of **sepsis** in those treated with steroids has stopped them being recommended.
  - prevention of **DVT**, **stress ulcers** and **decubitus ulcers**.

Mortality is highest in patients under 1 year and over 70 years. Pulmonary complications (e.g. **hypoventilation**, **aspiration pneumonitis**, **chest infection**, **PE**) are the commonest causes of death within the first 3 months of injury. Other complications are related to **nutrition**, urinary function and sepsis, osteoporosis, psychological problems and **pain** syndromes, the latter experienced by 70% of patients.

- Anaesthetic management is related to:
  - other injuries and cardiorespiratory impairment.
  - potential difficult intubation and risk of aspiration.
  - hyperkalaemic response to **suxamethonium** within 10 days–6 months of injury
  - **positioning of the patient.**
  - impaired **temperature regulation.**
  - requirement for postoperative IPPV.
  - impaired cardiovascular responses and autonomic hyperreflexia.

[Charles E Brown-Séquard (1818–1894), Mauritius-born US, English and French physician]

Stein DM, Pineda JA, Roddy V, Knight WA (2015). Neurocrit Care; 23 (suppl 2): S155–64

See also, Anterior spinal artery syndrome

Spinal cord stimulation (SCS). Technique used in chronic **pain management**. Exact mechanism is unclear but it modulates concentrations of **GABA** and **5-HT** in the dorsal horn of the **spinal cord**, potentially reducing the release of excitatory amino acids and the responsiveness of wide dynamic range neurones involved in the potentiation of chronic **pain**. Used primarily for treatment of neuropathic or ischaemic pain, e.g. failed back surgery syndrome, **complex regional pain syndrome** type 1 and refractory angina, when medical management has failed.

May be performed percutaneously using a wire electrode connected to an external power source, but an implantable system is usually employed. Electrodes may be placed at open laminectomy, or inserted into the epidural space through a needle. The electrodes are placed above the highest level of the pain, and connected either to a subcutaneous self-powered pulse generator, usually implanted in the lower abdomen or upper buttock, or to a subcutaneous radiofrequency receiver (if high power settings are required) that is activated by an external battery-operated transmitter. Various aspects of the pulse (voltage/current, duration, frequency, etc.) can be programmed and adjusted according to each patient's requirements.

If patients receiving SCS require surgery, the stimulator may be turned off perioperatively. The position of the pulse generator must be confirmed and marked, to avoid damage to it or the wires. Heating of the implanted electrodes by **diathermy** and MRI scanning has been described; if diathermy is required, the bipolar type is preferred. Spinal or epidural anaesthesia has been described but requires care to avoid damage to the electrodes; fluoroscopic or ultrasound guidance has been recommended.

Moore DM, McCrory C (2016). BJA Educ; 16: 258–63

Spinal headache, *see Post-dural puncture headache*

Spinal nerves. Consist of pairs of **nerves** (8 cervical, 12 thoracic, 5 lumbar, 5 sacral and 1 coccygeal). Formed within the **vertebral canal** from anterior (ventral) and posterior (dorsal) roots, themselves formed from rootlets that emerge from the antero- and posterolateral aspects of the **spinal cord**. The anterior roots convey efferent motor fibres from the cord, and the posterior roots convey afferent sensory fibres to the cord; thus they are mixed nerves. Each spinal nerve leaves the vertebral canal through an intervertebral foramen. The posterior (dorsal) root ganglia lie within the foramina, except for C1 and C2 (lie on the posterior vertebral arches) and the sacral and coccygeal ganglia (lie within the canal). The first cervical nerve emerges between the occiput and the arch of the atlas; C2–7 emerge above their respective **vertebrae** and C8 emerges between C7 and T1. Below this, each spinal nerve emerges below its corresponding vertebra. After giving off a small meningeal branch, each divides into a large anterior and smaller posterior primary ramus (Fig. 150).

- Anterior primary rami:
  - supply cutaneous and motor innervation of the limbs, and front and sides of the neck, thorax and abdomen.
  - cervical: C1–4 form the **cervical plexus**, C5–8 the **brachial plexus.**
  - thoracic: the **intercostal nerves**; T1 contributes to the brachial plexus.
  - lumbar: L1–4 form the **lumbar plexus.**
  - sacral and coccygeal: contribute to the **sacral plexus.**

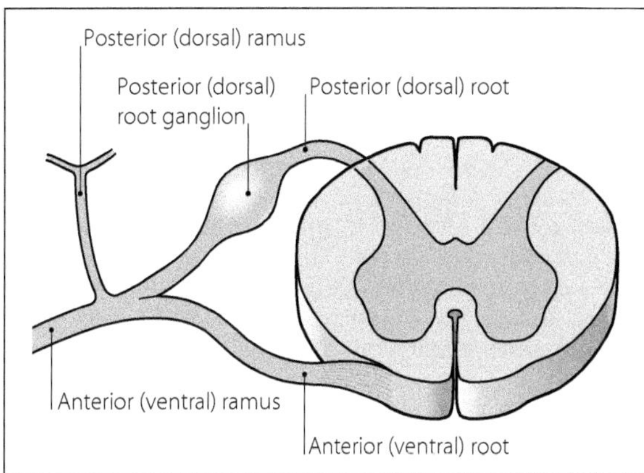

Fig. 150 Typical spinal nerve

- Posterior primary rami:
  - supply motor and sensory innervation to the muscles and skin of the back.
  - do not contribute to limb innervation or plexus formation.
  - divide into medial and lateral branches (except for C1, S4, S5 and coccygeal rami). Cutaneous innervation of T6 and above is contained in the medial branch, below this in the lateral branch.
  - cervical:
    - C1: entirely motor, supplying the muscles of the upper neck.
    - C2: supplies the skin of the back of the head via the greater occipital nerve; motor supply to the neck muscles.
    - C3–8: sensory supply to the lower occiput and neck; motor fibres to the neck muscles.
  - thoracic, lumbar, sacral and coccygeal: unremarkable.

Embryonic segmental distribution of nerves to the skin and muscles is represented by the segmental distribution of cutaneous and motor innervation (**dermatomes** and **myotomes**, respectively).

Spinal opioids. Spinal or epidural administration of **opioid analgesic drugs** has become widespread since the first report of epidural **morphine** administration in humans in 1979. Thought to bind to **opioid receptors** in the substantia gelatinosa of the **spinal cord**, modulating **pain pathways**. Although systemic absorption may contribute to analgesia, a spinal site of action is suggested by a high **CSF**:plasma drug ratio and the low doses required compared with iv administration.

The main advantage of spinal opioids over systemic opioids is profound, long-lasting analgesia. Advantages over spinal or epidural **local anaesthetic agents** are the lack of sympathetic, motor or sensory blockade, and the ability to provide analgesia distant to the level of injection.

A segmental effect has been reported, i.e., maximal analgesia corresponding to the level of injection, although lumbar administration has been used for analgesia after **thoracic surgery**. This may be related to the lipid solubility of the opioid used; thus morphine diffuses further in the CSF than more lipid-soluble drugs. Onset and duration of action are also determined by lipid solubility; e.g. highly lipid-soluble drugs (e.g. **fentanyl** and **methadone**) cross the CSF and bind to the spinal cord rapidly. Only a small amount is thus available to diffuse throughout the CSF. However, their duration of action is short because they are more rapidly absorbed into the bloodstream. They are more likely to act (at least partially) via systemic absorption. Poorly lipid-soluble drugs (e.g. morphine) have slower onset time (up to 1 h) and their actions last for up to 24 h (Table 48).

Opioids are often mixed with local anaesthetics because combination has been shown to be synergistic. Such mixtures may be given by bolus or by infusion; commonly used mixtures for the latter include 0.1%–0.2% **bupivacaine** plus fentanyl 2–4 µg/ml or **diamorphine** 50–100 µg/ml, infused at 5–15 ml/h for, e.g. **postoperative analgesia** and chronic pain management. In **obstetric analgesia and anaesthesia**, fentanyl is widely used in the UK for bolus and infusion in labour; in the USA **sufentanil** is commonly used. Epidural infusion of opioids alone is less commonly used:
- diamorphine 0.25–2.0 mg/h; morphine 0.5 mg/h.
- fentanyl 40–100 µg/h; sufentanil 20–50 µg/h.
- methadone 0.5 mg/h.
- **pethidine** 10–15 mg/h.

Table 48 Epidural and spinal doses of commonly used opioids

Drug	Epidural dose	Spinal dose	Duration (h)
Buprenorphine	60–300 µg	25–50 µg	8–10
Diamorphine	1–5 mg	100–300 µg	6–8
Fentanyl	50–150 µg	10–25 µg	2–4
Methadone	4–8 mg	0.5–2.0 mg	4–6
Morphine	1–8 mg	100–400 µg	12–18
Pethidine	25–100 mg	10–100 mg	6–8
Sufentanil	10–75 µg	5–20 µg	2–6

Pethidine is unique in that it has local anaesthetic properties and has thus been used as the sole agent e.g. for spinal anaesthesia and epidural infusion.

An extended-release preparation of morphine is available for epidural administration, consisting of morphine sulfate pentahydrate encapsulated within ~20-µm diameter liposomes, suspended in 0.9% saline. Onset of analgesia takes ~3 h, with duration of action up to 48 h after a single lumbar epidural injection of 10–15 mg.

- Side effects of spinal opioids:
  - respiratory depression:
    - early (within an hour of administration): due to systemic absorption; thus more common if highly lipid-soluble drugs are used and if sedative drugs are also given.
    - late (4–24 h after administration, depending on the drug): caused by rostral spread of the drug within the CSF to the medullary respiratory centre. Although uncommon (0.5%–3.0%), more likely with poorly lipid-soluble drugs (e.g. morphine), after intrathecal administration, in the elderly, and if systemic opioids are also given. Respiratory rate alone is a poor indicator of the degree of depression; arterial oxygen saturation and level of sedation may be more useful. **Naloxone** may reverse respiratory depression without affecting analgesia.
  - urinary retention: occurs in 30%–40% of cases, although its occurrence in up to 90% of males has been reported. Presence of vesical opioid receptors has been suggested.
  - **pruritus**: affects up to 70% of patients after morphine, 10% after fentanyl. More common after intrathecal administration. May be relieved by **antihistamine drugs**, naloxone and **ondansetron**. The cause is unknown.
  - nausea and vomiting: similar incidence to that after parenteral administration, although more common after intrathecal opioids.
  - herpes simplex virus reactivation has been described in obstetric patients.

Spinal shock. Syndrome following sudden **spinal cord injury**, characterised by hypotension (level of injury above T6) and bradycardia (level above T1), with flaccid paralysis. Hypotension arises from interrupted sympathetic vasoconstrictor tone, and is greatest in the upright position. Usually replaced by **autonomic hyperreflexia** after 4–6 weeks. Hypotension may be dramatic on **induction of anaesthesia** and institution of **IPPV**.

See also, Valsalva manoeuvre

Spinal surgery. May be required for degenerative disease (e.g. prolapse of intervertebral disc, spondylolisthesis, spinal stenosis), **kyphoscoliosis** (idiopathic or associated with neuromuscular disorders, e.g. cerebral palsy, **muscular dystrophies**), autoimmune diseases (e.g. **rheumatoid disease**, **ankylosing spondylitis**), trauma (e.g. **spinal cord injury**) and tumours.

- Anaesthetic management is as for kyphoscoliosis and **neurosurgery**; main points:
  - **preoperative assessment** for co-morbidity, ventilatory impairment or neurological deficits. If **vital capacity** is <30% of predicted, postoperative IPPV is likely. Assessment of the airway for associated **temperomandibular joint** stiffness, limited neck movement and **cervical spine** instability is essential.
  - severe **hyperkalaemia** may follow **suxamethonium** if **spinal cord injury** is present. Period of risk: 10 days–6 months.
  - **positioning of the patient**, often in the prone position, must be meticulously carried out.
  - surgery may be prolonged with major **blood loss** or **hypothermia**. Damage to inferior vena cava, aorta and iliac arteries may lead to rapid exsanguination without obvious bleeding from the operation site. **Cell salvage** is increasingly used for non-tumour surgery.
  - **hypotensive anaesthesia** reduces blood loss but may risk **spinal cord** ischaemia.
  - **epidural anaesthesia** has been used with good results, e.g. for laminectomy.
  - cord function may be assessed by the **wake-up test** or more commonly by monitoring **evoked potentials**.
  - **airway obstruction** may follow anterior cervical spine surgery if extensive. **Ondine's curse** may also occur.
  - postoperative analgesia often requires a multimodal approach including peroperative **ketamine**, continuous local anaesthetic agent infusion, regional anaesthesia, **opioid analgesic drugs** and epidural analgesia. **Gabapentin** may also be useful.

Admission to ICU/HDU may be required if there is a risk of airway obstruction, respiratory impairment or excessive bleeding and for pain management.

Spirometer. Device for measuring **lung volumes**. The wet spirometer consists of a lightweight cylinder suspended over a breathing chamber with a water seal (Fig. 151). Vertical movement of the cylinder corresponding to respiratory movements is recorded on a rotating drum via a pen attached to the cylinder.

May be used to measure volumes directly, or using **dilution techniques**. Also used to calculate flow rates and **basal metabolic rate**. Inaccuracies may arise from inertia of the system at high respiratory rates, and the dissolution of small amounts of gas into the water of the seal.

Dry spirometers (e.g. the Vitalograph) are more convenient for clinical use. It contains bellows attached to a pen, with a sheet of recording paper automatically moved by a motor during expiration. The best results from three attempts are usually recorded.

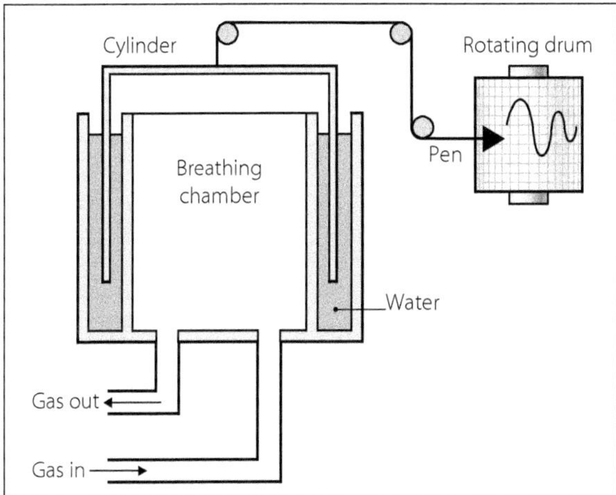

Fig. 151 Wet spirometer

Spironolactone. **Diuretic**, acting via competitive antagonism of **aldosterone**. Inhibits sodium/potassium exchange in the distal renal tubule, with retention of potassium and hydrogen ions. Also has anti-androgen and anti-progesterone effects. Used to treat oedema due to secondary **hyperaldosteronism**, e.g. associated with **hepatic failure** and **cardiac failure**, and in primary hyperaldosteronism. Diuresis occurs 2–3 h after oral administration. Also available in combination with hydroflumethiazide or **furosemide**. A related drug, eplerenone, is more selective for the mineralocorticoid receptor and is used as an adjunct in chronic cardiac failure or in cardiac failure after acute **MI**.

- Dosage: 100–400 mg orally od (25–50 mg daily for cardiac failure).
- Side effects: GIT disturbances, gynaecomastia, sexual dysfunction, hyperkalaemia.

Splitting ratio. Ratio of gas flow bypassing an anaesthetic **vaporiser** to the gas flow entering it. At a splitting ratio of zero, the total gas flow passes through the vaporiser; at a ratio of infinity, none passes through (i.e., the vaporiser is switched off).

Sprays. In anaesthesia, usually employed to deliver **local anaesthetic agent** (usually 4% **lidocaine**) to the **larynx** and trachea, e.g. for awake tracheal intubation, and to reduce stimulation during positioning and tracheal extubation. Spraying the cords at laryngoscopy does not attenuate the hypertensive response to laryngoscopy itself. Most commonly used sprays are now either single-use (e.g. prefilled syringes with long perforated nozzles) or have disposable, single-use nozzles for attachment to metered-dose aerosols (e.g. delivering 10 mg of 10% lidocaine per spray). Previously, reusable sprays consisted of metal nozzles with red rubber bulbs.

Sprays may also be used to apply **cocaine** to the nose, to produce anaesthesia and vasoconstriction. Other sprays used in anaesthesia include the **ethyl chloride** spray for **refrigeration anaesthesia** and testing **regional anaesthesia**, and disinfectant sprays and dressings.

SRS-A, Slow reacting substance-A, *see Leukotrienes*

SSRIs, *see Selective serotonin reuptake inhibitors*

S–T segment. Portion of the ECG between the end of the **QRS complex** and the beginning of the **T wave** (*see Fig. 60b;* **Electrocardiography**). Represents the depolarised plateau phase of the ventricular **action potential**. As there is no net current flow during this period, the S–T segment is normally within 1 mm of the isoelectric line (between the T wave and following P wave). Myocardial damage results in 'injury currents' that cause S–T elevation (e.g.

MI and **pericarditis**) or depression (e.g. **myocardial ischaemia**). S–T depression may also be caused by **hypokalaemia** and **digoxin** therapy, the latter typically producing a 'reverse tick' pattern. May also be depressed in reciprocal leads following S–T elevation MI.
See also, Acute coronary syndromes

Stages of anaesthesia, *see Anaesthesia, stages of*

Standard bicarbonate. Plasma concentration of **bicarbonate** when arterial $P\text{CO}_2$ has been corrected to 5.3 kPa (40 mmHg), with **haemoglobin** fully saturated and at a temperature of 37°C. Thus eliminates the respiratory component of **acidosis** or **alkalosis**. Normally 24–33 mmol/l.
See also, Acid–base balance

Standard deviation (SD). Expression of the variability of a **population** or **sample**. Equals the square root of **variance**, i.e.

$$\text{SD} = \sqrt{\frac{\Sigma(x-\bar{x})^2}{n-1}}$$

Squaring $(x-\bar{x})$ eliminates any minus signs, i.e., for those values of x less than $\bar{x}$.

In a sample of normal distribution, a range of 1 SD on either side of the **mean** includes about 68% of all observations, 2 SDs on either side include about 95%, and 3 SDs on either side include about 99.7%.
See also, Statistical frequency distributions; Statistics

Standard error of the mean (SE). Indication of how well the **mean** of a **sample** represents the true **population** mean.

$$\text{SE} = \frac{\textbf{standard deviation}\ (\text{SD})}{\sqrt{n}}$$

where n = number of values.

SE is large when n is small, i.e., the sample mean is less likely to represent the population mean. Often presented with the mean in statistical **data**, because the data appear tidier, and mean ± SE has a smaller spread than mean ± SD. Apart from this, SE has no advantage over SD.
See also, Statistical tests; Statistics

Staphylococcal infections. Caused by members of the staphylococcus genus of gram-positive **bacteria**. *Staphylococcus aureus* is the major pathogen, causing a spectrum of infections, including boils, abscesses, **cellulitis**, wound infection, osteomyelitis, **chest infection** and **septic shock**. Infection is especially problematic in **immunodeficiency**, e.g. in critically ill patients. Other conditions arise from **exotoxin** production, e.g. **toxic shock syndrome**, scalded skin syndrome and food poisoning.

S. aureus produces an **enzyme** (coagulase) that converts fibrinogen to fibrin and thus clots blood. Strains may be typed by viral bacteriophages; up to 65% of strains produce exotoxins. Nasal carriage of *S. aureus* occurs in about a third of normal subjects; the organism may also be present on the skin, especially perineum. Over 30 coagulase-negative staphylococcus species exist, mostly as skin commensals, although they may cause clinical infection, especially *S. epidermidis* (typically associated with prosthesis- and **catheter-related sepsis**) and *S. saprophyticus* (typically causing **urinary tract infection**).

Bacterial resistance is an increasing problem, with 90% of hospital staphylococci resistant to **benzylpenicillin** and related drugs via production of β-lactamase. Meticillin-resistant *S. aureus* (MRSA) is a particular problem in hospitals and increasingly in the community too. **Glycopeptides** are usually reserved for its treatment, although resistance has been reported. Strict **infection control** is required to reduce cross-contamination and spread of infection.

STaR, *see Safe transport and retrieval*

Starch solutions, *see Hydroxyethyl starch*

Starling forces. Factors determining the movement of fluid across the capillary wall endothelium. Movement into the interstitial space is normally encouraged by the hydrostatic pressure gradient (capillary hydrostatic pressure $[P_c]$ – interstitial fluid hydrostatic pressure $[P_i]$). This is opposed by the normal colloid osmotic gradient (capillary colloid osmotic pressure $[\pi_c]$ – interstitial fluid colloid osmotic pressure $[\pi_i]$):

$$\dot{Q} = K[(P_c - P_i) - \sigma(\pi_c - \pi_i)]$$

where $\dot{Q}$ = net flow of fluid for a given surface area
K = permeability or filtration coefficient (flow rate per unit pressure gradient across the endothelium)
σ = reflection coefficient (represents permeability of the endothelium to plasma proteins).

The equation does not account for **active transport** of solutes and effects of **surface tension** in the lung.

In a 'standard' systemic capillary: π_c ~25 mmHg; π_i ~5 mmHg; P_i ~0 mmHg. P_c falls from about 30 mmHg at the arteriolar end (favouring net flow of fluid out of the capillary) to 15 mmHg at the venous end (favouring net flow in). In health, the volume of fluid leaving the capillary exceeds that being reabsorbed by about 10%, the excess being absorbed by the lymphatic system. Greater imbalance may result in **oedema**.
[Ernest H Starling (1866–1927), London physiologist]

Starling resistor. Model consisting of a length of collapsible tubing passing through a rigid box (Fig. 152). The effects of different upstream pressures (P_1), pressures in the chamber (P_2) and downstream pressures (P_3) on flow through the tubing can be studied. Used to illustrate the effect of gravity on regional **pulmonary circulation**, P_1, P_2 and P_3 representing arterial, alveolar and venous pressures, respectively. Also used to model the interactions between **MAP**, **ICP** and **CVP**.
See also, Ventilation/perfusion mismatch; Cerebral perfusion pressure

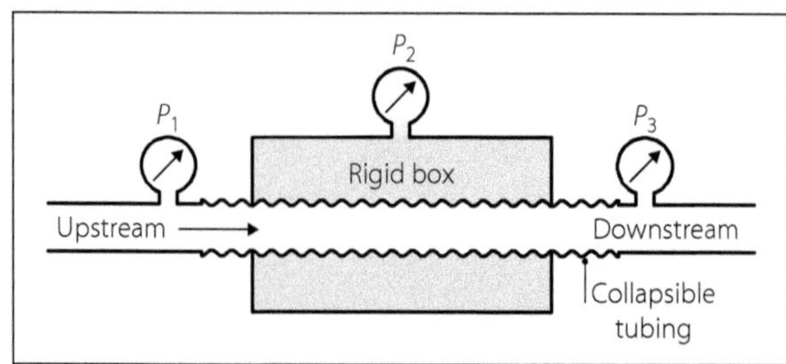

Fig. 152 Starling resistor (see text)

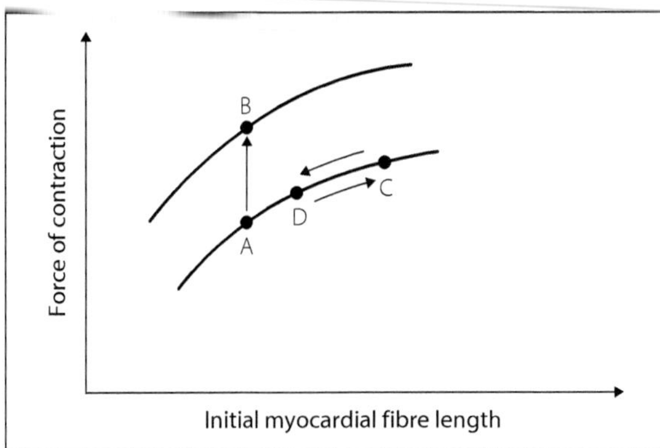

Fig. 153 Starling's law

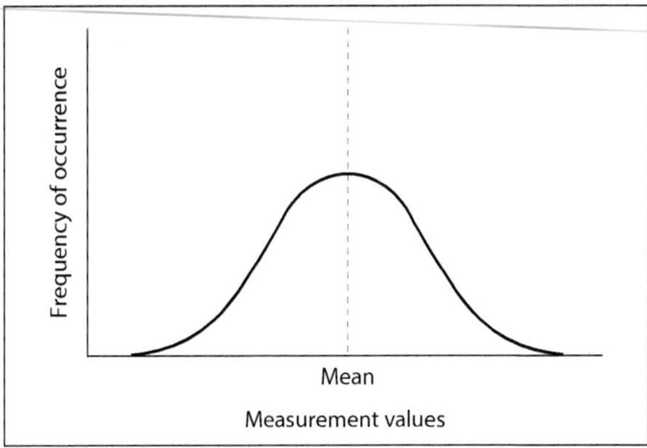

Fig. 154 Normal frequency distribution curve

Starling's law (Frank–Starling law). Intrinsic regulatory mechanism of the heart stating that force of myocardial contraction is proportional to initial fibre length, up to a point (Fig. 153). Neither variable is easily measured; hence myocardial contraction is often represented by **cardiac output, stroke volume, stroke index** or **stroke work** (y-axis) and initial fibre length is represented by **left ventricular end-diastolic volume, left ventricular end-diastolic pressure** or **pulmonary capillary wedge pressure** (x-axis). Increasing stretch is thought to facilitate greater actin–myosin cross-link formation; the optimum sarcomere length is 2.2 µm.

The law explains how right and left ventricular outputs remain matched, i.e., if right ventricular output increases, the increase in pulmonary venous pressure in turn increases left ventricular filling; the resultant increased stretch increases left ventricular output in line with that of the right ventricle.

Changes in **myocardial contractility** shift the curve's position; e.g. in **cardiac failure** and **MI** it is moved downwards and to the right (e.g. in Fig. 153, from the upper curve to the lower curve). Cardiac dilatation compensates initially, by moving along the curve to the right.

The (Starling) curves may be plotted for individual patients, and have been used to guide management of reduced output states. Therapeutic measures alter the heart's position on the curve (Fig. 153), e.g. use of **inotropic drugs** moves heart function from A to B, venodilators move it from C to D, and a fluid bolus challenge moves it from D to C.
[Otto Frank (1865–1944), German physiologist]
O'Rourke MF (1984). Aust N Z J Med; 14: 879–87

Starvation, *see Malnutrition*

Static electricity, *see Antistatic precautions; Explosions and fires*

Statins. Group of competitive inhibitors of 3-hydroxy-3-methylglutaryl coenzyme A (HMG CoA) reductase, an enzyme required for hepatic cholesterol synthesis. Because most cholesterol is endogenously synthesised, they significantly reduce plasma levels of total and low-density lipoprotein (LDL) cholesterol. Licensed for both treatment of primary/familial hypercholesterolaemia and prevention of cardiovascular events (e.g. **acute coronary syndromes**, ischaemic **stroke**). Reduce mortality and morbidity in all patients with symptomatic CVS disease (i.e., secondary prevention), regardless of baseline cholesterol level. Their use for primary prevention is advocated in those at high risk (e.g. 20% 10-year risk) of developing CVS disease; all patients over 40 years with **diabetes mellitus** should be considered for primary prevention. Although they also have anti-inflammatory properties, statin therapy has shown no benefit in the treatment of **ALI, ventilator-associated pneumonia, COPD** or **subarachnoid haemorrhage**. Prior statin use may improve mortality in **sepsis**. Examples include atorvastatin, simvastatin, pravastatin, rosuvastatin and fluvastatin. Dosages vary according to target LDL levels and indication (e.g. lower doses for primary prevention; higher doses after **acute coronary syndromes**).

- Side effects (more likely with higher doses): myopathy, myalgia, **rhabdomyolysis**, abnormal liver function (severe **hepatitis** rarely), depression, fatigue, skin reactions.

Statistical frequency distributions. In **statistics**, relationships between measured variables and the frequency with which each value occurs. For continuous **data**, the resultant curve may often be described by a mathematical equation, allowing **statistical tests** and other analyses to be performed. Many types of biological data have a 'normal' (Gaussian) distribution (Fig. 154). Such data are described by the **mean** and **standard deviation** (SD). The standard normal deviate (z) describes any individual value by relating it to the mean and SD, and can be used to calculate the **probability** that such a value lies within the 'normal' range. Parametric statistical tests may be used to test the hypothesis that different **samples** of normally distributed data are in fact taken from the same **population** (**null hypothesis**). They compare within-group variability with between-group differences; e.g. two samples are likely to represent different populations if the scatter (SD) of each is small and their means are very different.

Data that are not normally distributed (e.g. skewed) may often be 'normalised' (e.g. by logarithmic transformation), allowing application of parametric tests, which are more sensitive than non-parametric tests.

Other types of distribution include the binomial (in which there are two possibilities for each measurement, e.g. yes or no, dead or alive), multinomial and Poisson distribution (which describes random events where non-events cannot be counted, e.g. radioactive decay).
[Karl F Gauss (1777–1855), German mathematician; Simeon D Poisson (1781–1840), French mathematician]
See also, Samples, statistical

Statistical significance. Term denoting a **probability** of less than an arbitrary cut-off for a **statistical test** or a result of inferential **statistics**. By convention, usually taken as a value for P <0.05, though more stringent 'levels' of probability

Table 49 Examples of statistical tests used for different types of comparison

Type of data	*Two groups, different subjects*	*Same subjects, before + after intervention*	*More than two groups, different subjects*	*Serial measurements*
Continuous	Unpaired t test	Paired t test	ANOVA	Repeated measures ANOVA
Ordinal	Mann-Whitney rank-sum test	Wilcoxon signed-rank test	Kruskal-Wallis test	Friedman statistic
Nominal	Chi-square test	McNemar's test	Chi-squares test	Cochran's test

are sometimes used (e.g. P <0.01), e.g. to account for the increased likelihood of a significant result due to chance alone when large numbers of comparisons are made. The terms 'very' or 'highly' significant to describe very small P values should not be used when presenting results, but the P value itself should be provided.
See also, Errors

Statistical tests. Methods of comparing or extrapolating **data** in inferential **statistics**, e.g. in **clinical trials**. Involve mathematical calculations depending on the descriptive statistics of each **sample** group. Results are traditionally expressed as the **probability** that any observed differences between groups are due to chance alone, i.e., the likelihood that the samples are taken from the same **population** (**null hypothesis**). Increasingly, **confidence intervals** are used to indicate the range within which a real difference is likely to lie.

- Many different tests have been described, applicable to specific types of data and situations, e.g. (Table 49):
  - comparing groups consisting of:
    - different subjects with different treatments:
      - two groups:
        - parametric (for normally distributed continuous data): unpaired (Student's) t test. Compares the **mean** and **standard deviation** for each group. Two-tailed tests allow for either an increase or a decrease in the variable measured.
        - non-parametric:
          - ordinal data: Mann–Whitney rank sum test. Ranks all the results in ascending order and compares the group's distributions within the ranking.
          - nominal data: chi-squared test (contingency table) with Yates's correction for continuity. Compares the observed frequency of events with the expected frequency. Fisher's exact test is used if any expected frequency is less than 5.
        - all types of data: sequential analysis. Relies on the relationship between the size of difference between groups, and the number of subjects required to achieve **statistical significance** for that difference (as the size of difference increases, fewer subjects are required). A graph is drawn with pre-calculated 'significance' boundaries, with an indicator of sample size on the x-axis and an indicator of size of difference on the y-axis. Results are analysed at intervals as the study progresses, and points plotted on the graph; the study is stopped when a boundary is crossed, thus minimising the number of subjects required to achieve a significant result.
      - more than two groups:
        - parametric: analysis of **variance** (ANOVA). Similar basis to the t test. Only indicates that a significant difference exists, not between which groups it exists. Student–Neuman–Keuls, Tukey's and other tests are used to indicate which of the comparisons achieve statistical significance.
        - non-parametric:
          - ordinal data: Kruskal–Wallis test. Similar basis to the Mann–Whitney test.
          - nominal data: chi-square test as above (Yates's correction is not required).
    - same subjects before and after a treatment:
      - two groups:
        - parametric: paired t test. More powerful than the unpaired test because intersubject variability is reduced, because each subject acts as his or her own control.
        - non-parametric:
          - ordinal data: Wilcoxon signed-rank sum test. Ranks the differences between the paired results.
          - nominal data: McNemar's test.
    - serial measurements following a treatment:
      - parametric: repeated-measure ANOVA.
      - non-parametric:
        - ordinal data: Friedman statistic.
        - nominal data: Cochrane's test.
  - comparing two variables for association:
    - parametric: linear regression analysis and correlation. Regression analysis determines the magnitude of change of one variable produced by the other variable. Expressed as the slope of the line of best fit, the equation relating the two variables, indicators of scatter or statistical differences from the line of no association. Correlation indicates the degree of association only and is expressed as the Pearson correlation coefficient (r). An r of +1 or −1 indicates complete positive or negative association, respectively, whereas an r of 0 indicates no association. For comparison of two methods of measurement (e.g. invasive and non-invasive **arterial BP measurement**), the difference between the two values obtained at each measurement is calculated. Bias and precision (mean and standard deviation, respectively, of the differences) indicate the degree of agreement between the two methods (Bland and Altman plot).
    - non-parametric:
      - ordinal data: Spearman rank correlation.
      - nominal data: contingency coefficient.

Non-normally distributed interval data may be transformed and normalised before application of parametric tests; otherwise weaker non-parametric tests must be applied.

- Inappropriate study design or tests may result in **errors** and incorrect conclusions. Common examples include:
    - multiple testing without correction. With a probability (*P*) of 0.05 taken as representing statistical significance, one test in 20 would be expected to produce a 'significant' result by chance. The Bonferroni correction is commonly used to account for multiple comparisons between groups.
    - insufficient **power**.
    - application of the incorrect test, e.g. use of the t test to compare ordinal data.

The tests and modifications are usually named after the mathematicians who described or developed them (apart from Student's t test).

[Carlo Bonferroni (1892–1960), Italian mathematician; Student: pseudonym used by William S Gosset (1876–1937), English chemist, in order to publish his work (publication of papers on any subject was banned by his employers, Guinness, after trade secrets had been included in a paper published by another employee); Arthur Guinness (1725–1803), Irish brewer]

See also, Statistical frequency distributions

Statistics. Collection, analysis and interpretation of numerical **data**, used to describe and compare **samples** and **populations.** May be:

- descriptive; i.e., describes sample data without extrapolation to the whole population. Descriptive terms vary according to the type and distribution of data but include measures of:
    - central tendency, e.g. **mean, mode, median.**
    - scatter, e.g. **standard deviation, percentiles.**

  Thus normally distributed data are described by their mean and standard deviation, ordinal data by the median and percentiles (usually 25th–75th [i.e., interquartile range]) and range, and nominal by the mode and a list of possible categories.
- inferential (analytical); i.e., used to relate sample data to the whole population. Applications include the use of clinical or laboratory measurements to define disease, and determining whether different samples are from the same population (**null hypothesis**). The latter is commonly performed in **clinical trials**, using **statistical tests.**

See also, Confidence intervals; Meta-analysis; Predictive value; Sensitivity; Specificity; Standard error of the mean; Statistical frequency distributions; Statistical significance

Status asthmaticus. Obsolete term describing refractory, acute, severe **asthma.** Acute severe asthma is now the preferred term.

Status epilepticus (SE). A prolonged epileptic seizure or multiple seizures without regaining consciousness that last for ≥5 min. This operational definition replaces the mechanistic one that specifies seizures lasting >30 min. Generalised convulsive status epilepticus (GCSE) accounts for about 70% of SE and in 50% of cases it is the first presentation of **epilepsy**; non-convulsive forms, including partial SE, complex partial SE and absence attacks are less associated with systemic complications and are considered less of an emergency.

GCSE is the second commonest neurological emergency after stroke. Its incidence in Europe is 10–16 per 100 000 population with an overall mortality of 20%.

- Aetiology:
    - acute processes, e.g. **stroke** (22%), metabolic imbalance (15%), **cerebral hypoxic ischaemic injury** (13%), **sepsis, TBI** (3%), drug abuse (e.g. alcohol, **cocaine**) (3%), CNS infection (e.g. **encephalitis, meningitis**) (3%). Autoimmune encephalitis (e.g. anti-**NMDA** receptor encephalitis) is increasingly recognised as an important cause.
    - chronic disease, e.g. pre-existing epilepsy ± low **anticonvulsant drug** levels (34%), delayed effects of stroke, TBI, cerebral tumours (25%), chronic **alcoholism** (13%), idiopathic (3%).

After 30 min seizures, increased **ICP**, hypotension and failure of cerebral **autoregulation** result in decreased **cerebral perfusion pressure.** Failure of central control of breathing causes **hypoxaemia, pulmonary hypertension** and **cardiac failure.** At this stage, visible seizures may be absent despite continuing cerebral seizure activity (non-convulsive status). Neuronal injury in unchecked SE especially affects the hippocampus, thalamus and neocortex; mechanisms include excitotoxicity (e.g. through NMDA and **AMPA** receptors), a decrease in inhibitory trafficking (e.g. through **GABA receptors**), increases in neuropeptide expression (e.g. **substance-P**) and mitochondrial dysfunction.

- Management: success in treating SE depends on terminating seizures as rapidly as possible as mortality is related to duration; in addition, the longer SE continues, the more refractory to treatment it becomes:
    - prehospital treatment: although traditionally used, rectal **diazepam** is being replaced with buccal or intranasal **midazolam**, which is more effective.
    - general hospital management:
        - initial rapid assessment and **CPR.** O_2 and iv cannulation are mandatory as are monitoring of BP, ECG and temperature.
        - 50 ml of 50% glucose should be given iv if hypoglycaemia is the suspected aetiology; thiamine 100 mg iv should be given if alcoholism/**malnutrition** is present.
        - **acidosis** is neuroprotective and rarely requires **bicarbonate** therapy following resuscitation.
        - **hyperthermia** may require active cooling.
    - drug treatment:
        - first-line: im midazolam (10 mg) will terminate SE in 73% of patients and has been shown to be superior to **lorazepam** (4 mg). However, this is a lower dose than the recommended 0.1-mg/kg dose of lorazepam, which remains the drug of choice in emergency departments.
        - second-line: includes **phenytoin, fosphenytoin, sodium valproate, phenobarbital** and more recently **levetiracetam** and **lacosamide.** No good randomised controlled trials exist due to the heterogeneous nature of SE but it appears that sodium valproate is the preferred second-line drug.

      Failure to terminate SE following second-line drugs is termed refractory SE. Mortality is approximately 40%. Treatment:
        - requires admission to ICU, tracheal intubation and general anaesthesia. Anaesthetic agents used include **thiopental, propofol** and midazolam. No differences in efficacy exist between thiopental and propofol but most favour the latter despite the risk of **propofol infusion syndrome** because of its more suitable **pharmacokinetics.**

- anaesthetic agents are titrated against the **EEG** until burst suppression is obtained and maintained for 24–48 h. In the absence of EEG, a **bispectral index monitor** score of 40 correlates with burst suppression. During this period, patients are given long-term **anticonvulsant drugs** and their levels monitored.
- if seizures continue upon withdrawal of general anaesthesia, the patient is said to be in super-refractory SE. Additional treatment at this stage may include **ketamine** and ketogenic diet.

Betjemann JP, Lowenstein DH (2015). Lancet Neurol; 14: 615–24

Status lymphaticus. Obsolete term used to describe a 'syndrome' causing unexpected intraoperative death in children. Now thought not to exist, and merely an excuse for poor management.

Macintosh RR, Pratt FB (1995). Paediatr Anaesth; 5: 354, 388

Stellate ganglion block. Performed for painful arm conditions (e.g. **complex regional pain syndrome** type 1, herpes zoster, **phantom limb**, shoulder/hand syndrome) and to improve circulation, e.g. in Raynaud's syndrome, postembolectomy. Has formerly been performed in quinine poisoning, angina and asthma.

The ganglion represents the fused inferior cervical and first thoracic sympathetic ganglia, and is present in 80% of subjects. It usually lies on or above the neck of the first **rib**. Some sympathetic fibres may leave the sympathetic chain below the ganglion of T1, and run directly to the **brachial plexus**, bypassing the ganglion. The precise site of action of the block is controversial, because studies using dye have shown that the ganglion itself may not be affected by injected solution.

Usually performed under fluoroscopic guidance but ultrasound has also been used. With the patient supine and the neck extended, **Chassaignac's tubercle** (transverse process of C6) is palpated level with the cricoid cartilage. The carotid sheath is retracted laterally with the fingers, and a skin wheal raised over the tubercle. A 5-cm needle is inserted directly posteriorly to contact the tubercle, passing medial to the retracted carotid sheath. It is withdrawn 1–2 mm and correct positioning is confirmed by appropriate spread of injected **radiological contrast media**; 5–10 ml **local anaesthetic agent** is then injected after careful aspiration. A 2-ml test dose has been suggested before injection of the main dose. Successful block results in ipsilateral **Horner's syndrome**.

Complications include intravascular injection (including into the vertebral artery), recurrent laryngeal nerve and brachial plexus blocks, pneumothorax, subarachnoid and epidural injection, and haematoma formation.

[Maurice Raynaud (1834–1881), French physician]

See also, Sympathetic nerve blocks; Sympathetic nervous system

STEMI, S–T segment elevation myocardial infarction, *see Acute coronary syndromes*

Stents, coronary, *see Percutaneous coronary intervention*

Sterilisation of breathing equipment, *see Contamination of anaesthetic equipment*

Steroid therapy, *see Corticosteroids*

Stethoscope. Invented in its monaural form (as a wooden trumpet-shaped tube) by Laennec in 1819; Cammann's binaural model appeared in 1852. During anaesthesia, allows continuous auscultation of breath sounds and **heart sounds**. Two forms are commonly used in anaesthesia:

- precordial stethoscope: may be connected to a monoaural earpiece to allow the anaesthetist greater freedom.
- oesophageal stethoscope: a modified nasogastric tube. Addition of temperature probe, ECG electrodes and pacing wires has been described.

[René TH Laennec (1781–1826), French physician; George Cammann (1804–1863), US physician]

Stevens–Johnson syndrome. Immune complex-mediated hypersensitivity skin disorder resulting in the separation of the epidermis from the dermis. Erythema multiforme major and toxic epidermal necrolysis are, respectively, considered lesser and more severe forms of the same condition. Caused by drugs (most commonly allopurinol, carbamazepine, lamotrigine, phenobarbital, phenytoin and co-trimoxazole), viral infections (including **HIV**) and malignancy, although in 50% of cases the cause is unknown.

In its severe forms, may present with fever and widespread epidermal erythema, blistering and necrosis, including membranes (e.g. pharyngitis, conjunctivitis, and rarely involving the oesophagus, rest of the GIT, tracheobronchial tree and kidney). May result in significant fluid loss, altered **temperature regulation** and increased susceptibility to infection.

Treatment is mainly supportive but includes careful fluid and electrolyte replacement; skin lesions are treated as **burns**. Specific treatment with **cyclophosphamide**, **plasma exchange** and intravenous **immunoglobulins** has been used. Mortality is up to 50% depending on the body surface area involved.

[Albert M Stevens (1884–1945), Frank C Johnson (1894–1934), New York paediatricians]

Yau F, Emerson B (2016). BJA Educ; 16: 79–86

Stewart–Hamilton equation. Formula used in **cardiac output measurement** when using thermodilution techniques:

$$\dot{Q} = \frac{V(T_B - T_1)K_1K_2}{T_B(t)dt}$$

where $\dot{Q}$ = cardiac output
V = volume of injectate
T_B = blood temperature
T_1 = injectate temperature
K_1 and K_2 = computer constants
$T_B(t)dt$ = change in blood temperature over time.

[GN Stewart (1860–1930), Canadian-born US scientist; WF Hamilton (1893–1964), US physiologist]

Stings, *see Bites and stings*

Stoichiometric mixture. Mixture of reactants in such proportions that none remains at the end of the reaction. Stoichiometric mixtures often react violently, and are thus more likely to be involved in **explosions and fires**.

Stokes–Adams attack. Syncope secondary to cardiac **arrhythmias**. Occurs without warning, and may progress to **convulsions**. Recovery is typically rapid. Originally described in complete **heart block**, but is also used in reference to syncope due to other arrhythmias (e.g.

tachybrady syndrome, paroxysmal **VT/VF**). The term is now less frequently used in favour of more precise diagnostic classifications. Differential diagnosis includes postural hypotension, **vasovagal syncope**, transient ischaemic attack, micturition and cough syncope. Treatment may involve **antiarrhythmic drugs**, electrophysiological ablation, **cardiac pacing** or insertion of an implantable **defibrillator** as appropriate.
[William Stokes (1804–1878), Irish physician; Robert Adams (1791–1875), Irish surgeon]

STOP-BANG score. Validated screening test used to identify patients at high risk of **obstructive sleep apnoea**. One point is scored for each of the following that is present:
- Loud snoring (e.g. heard through a closed door).
- Tiredness or sleepiness during the day.
- Observation of breathing cessation, choking or gasping during sleep.
- Raised blood pressure requiring treatment.
- BMI >35 kg/m^2
- Age >50 years.
- Neck circumference >43 cm (17 in) for males, >41 cm (16 in) for females.
- Male gender.

A score ≥5 suggests a high probability of OSA and the need for specialist referral, although a score <4 does not exclude OSA, especially if there is a history of severe exertional dyspnoea, morning headaches and evidence of right atrial hypertrophy.
See also, Sleep-disordered breathing

Stovaine. **Local anaesthetic drug**, introduced in 1904, as a less toxic alternative to **cocaine**. Slightly irritant, and replaced in turn by **procaine**.
[Ernest Forneau (1872–1949), French chemist; *fourneau* is French for stove]

STP/STPD. Standard temperature and pressure (0°C; 101.3 kPa [760 mmHg]) and STP dry. Used for standardising gas volume measurements.

Streptococcal infections. Caused by members of the streptococcus genus of gram-positive **bacteria**. Several species exist, usually as normal commensals in the upper respiratory tract, but they may cause a wide range of clinical infections. Classified according to the type of haemolysis they cause on blood agar (none, α and β), the latter also subclassified according to cell wall antigens into groups A–H and K–V.
- Important pathogenic streptococci:
  - *Streptococcus pyogenes* (group A β-haemolytic): the major pathogen, causing pharyngitis, **cellulitis**, **necrotising fasciitis**, erysipelas, scarlet fever and **septic shock**. The organism is further subdivided into strains and types according to surface antigens. The M antigen confers particular virulence. Several **exotoxins** may contribute to the clinical features of infection, e.g. scarlet fever, **toxic shock syndrome**. In addition, cross-reactivity between anti-streptococcal antibodies and host tissue may result in disease, e.g. **rheumatic fever** and **glomerulonephritis**.
  - *S. agalactiae* (Group B β-haemolytic): especially important in neonates/infants (arthritis, **meningitis**, **peritonitis**) and obstetrics/gynaecology (septic abortion, chorioamnionitis). May also cause adult meningitis, **endocarditis** or osteomyelitis.
  - Groups C and G β-haemolytic: similar to group A organisms; group D are different and have been renamed enterococci (e.g. *Enterococcus faecalis*; may cause **nosocomial infection**).
  - *S. viridans*: a group of partial α- or non-haemolytic streptococci; may cause endocarditis and abscesses, especially in **immunodeficiency**, e.g. on the ICU and in the elderly. Includes *S. mitis, S. sanguis, S. mutans* and *S. milleri*.
  - *S. pneumoniae* (pneumococcus): α-haemolytic organism present in up to 70% of the population's oropharynx. May cause pneumonia (the most common cause in the community; in hospital it is especially common in impaired protective reflexes, e.g. the elderly and frail, CNS depression), otitis media, meningitis and septic shock. Prophylactic pneumococcal vaccine is recommended for those at risk, e.g. those with immunodeficiency or diabetes, following splenectomy and in the elderly.

Usually sensitive to **penicillins** among other **antibacterial drugs**.

Streptokinase. **Enzyme** obtained from group C β-haemolytic streptococci; used as a **fibrinolytic drug** in life-threatening arterial or venous thromboembolism, e.g. acute **PE** and **MI**. Binds to plasminogen to form an activator complex, resulting in breakdown of plasminogen to form plasmin, which causes **fibrinolysis**. Because most individuals have antibodies to streptokinase, a loading dose is required to overcome this natural resistance. Resultant immune complexes are rapidly cleared from the bloodstream; subsequent streptokinase is split into fragments during its action and cleared.
- Dosage: MI: 1 500 000 units iv over 60 min, within 12 h of symptoms; for other indications 250 000 iv over 30 min, then 100 000/h for up to 24–72 h.
- Side effects: nausea, vomiting, bleeding (including **stroke**), embolic complications from break-up of thrombi, allergic reactions (including **anaphylaxis**). Contraindicated in conditions where bleeding is likely.

Streptomycin. **Aminoglycoside** and **antibacterial drug**; now used as an **antituberculous drug** in drug-resistant TB or in brucellosis. **Half-life** is about 2.5 h with normal renal function.
- Dosage: 15 mg/kg daily (up to 1 g) by deep im injection.
- Side effects: as for aminoglycosides. Hypersensitivity may occur. Plasma concentrations should be monitored, especially in renal impairment; peak and trough levels should not exceed 40 µg/ml and 5 µg/ml, respectively.

Stress response to surgery. Term used to encompass the metabolic and hormonal changes following surgery, although the same may occur after **trauma**, **burns** or **haemorrhage**. The response has been suggested as being necessary for survival and recovery after trauma.

Tissue trauma, **hypovolaemia** and **pain** initiate a neuroendocrine reflex involving secretion of **ACTH**, **endorphins**, **growth hormone**, **vasopressin** and prolactin. Stimulation of the **sympathetic nervous system** increases plasma **catecholamines**. Plasma cortisol and **aldosterone** increase, with increased **renin/angiotensin system** activity. These changes induce a state of **catabolism**, the magnitude and duration of which are proportional to the extent of injury. Fatty acids are mobilised and utilised, **amino acids** are converted to **carbohydrate** and negative **nitrogen balance** occurs. Plasma **glucose** is raised, with reduced **insulin** secretion. Metabolic rate, body temperature, O_2 consumption and CO_2 production increase. Water and sodium retention occurs, with increased urinary potassium loss. Immunological and haematological changes include increased **cytokine** production, acute-phase reactions, leucocytosis and lymphocytosis.

- Effects of anaesthesia:
  - **inhalational anaesthetic agents** have little effect.
  - **opioid analgesic drugs** in high dosage (e.g. 50–100 µg/kg **fentanyl**, 2–4 mg/kg **morphine**) attenuate the response to abdominal and pelvic surgery, but do not abolish the response to initiation of **cardiopulmonary bypass.**
  - **etomidate** infusion prevents the cortisol response, but with little other effect.
  - **spinal** and **epidural anaesthesia** with **local anaesthetic agents** abolish the response to surgery on the lower part of the body. The effect on upper abdominal and thoracic surgery is less clear, with suppression of the glucose response but not of the cortisol response. Block of autonomic and somatic afferent pathways is thought to be required for complete prevention. **Spinal opioids** do not prevent the response despite good analgesia, although slight modification may occur.

  To be effective, the above require administration before the surgical stimulus; their effects last for several hours after single dosage.

The benefit of attenuating the stress response is controversial, although improved outcome has been claimed in critically ill patients.

Stress ulcers. Acute gastric ulceration secondary to any severe medical or surgical illness, e.g. classically burns (**Curling ulcers**) and head injury (**Cushing's ulcers**). Usually involve the fundus and may be multiple. Associated with **hypovolaemia**, reduced cardiac output and splanchnic hypoperfusion. Gastric mucosal ischaemia and acid production are thought to be involved, although the aetiology is unclear. Routine prophylaxis with **proton pump inhibitors** or **H_2 receptor antagonists** is no longer advocated for ICU patients as they increase the incidence of **nosocomial infection**. Early enteral feeding reduces the incidence of GIT ulceration.

See also, Peptic ulcer disease

Stridor. Harsh high-pitched sound occurring in upper **airway obstruction.** Inspiratory stridor suggests obstruction at or above the upper trachea (e.g. **epiglottitis**), because extrathoracic obstruction is exacerbated by the negative intrathoracic pressures generated during inspiration. Expiratory stridor suggests obstruction of the lower trachea or bronchi with exacerbation as the airways are compressed during forced expiration. Typically present on exertion initially, progressing to stridor at rest as obstruction worsens.

More common in children because of the smaller diameter of their airways. Slight narrowing thus has a proportionately greater effect.

Treatment is as for airway obstruction. **Helium/O_2** mixtures (which are less dense than air/O_2 mixtures) may decrease work of breathing and improve oxygenation.

Stroke (CVA). Third commonest cause of death in developed countries.

- Caused by:
  - infarction (85%–90%), e.g. caused by atheroma, embolism, arteritis/arterial spasm or hypotension. If symptoms resolve within 24 h defined as a transient ischaemic attack, although **CT scanning** may reveal evidence of permanent damage. Recurrent multiple small emboli may cause vascular dementia.
  - haemorrhage (10%–15%). Primary (spontaneous) intracranial haemorrhage (ICH) accounts for 85% and is due to rupture of small arteries/arterioles due to **hypertension** or amyloid angiopathy. More common in patients taking **anticoagulant drugs**. Secondary ICH causes include trauma, rupture of aneurysms (resulting in **subarachnoid haemorrhage**) or arteriovenous malformations, **cocaine poisoning** and haemorrhagic transformation of ischaemic infarcts.
- Features include:
  - upper and lower **motor neurone** lesions; distribution depends on the site and extent of the lesion, e.g. lesions may cause contralateral hemiplegia/paresis, hemisensory loss and homonymous hemianopia. Single limbs and the face may be affected. Speech disorders are common if the dominant hemisphere is affected.
  - signs of raised ICP (more likely in haemorrhagic stroke): headache, vomiting, impaired consciousness.
- Management depends on whether the stroke is ischaemic or haemorrhagic:
  - ischaemic stroke:
    - emergency department assessment:
      - immediate resuscitation as necessary.
      - full history regarding symptom onset (to identify eligibility for thrombolysis), examination of neurological deficits, exclusion of conditions mimicking stroke (e.g. migrainous hemiplegia, seizures, **hypoglycaemia**, drug toxicity).
      - baseline blood tests including glucose, renal function, **coagulation studies**, troponins, etc.
      - non-contrast CT scan to exclude haemorrhagic stroke, subdural haematoma, etc. Angiography should be considered if carotid dissection/occlusion is suspected.
    - stroke unit management:
      - stroke unit protocols reduce morbidity and mortality by >20%.
      - regular monitoring and O_2 administration to keep arterial saturation >95%. Hypertension is only treated if BP >220/120 mmHg. If thrombolysis is performed, BP should be kept <185/110 mmHg for 24 h after the procedure.
      - blood glucose must be kept within normal limits as abnormalities are associated with worse outcomes.
      - **aspirin** should be started within 48 h of stroke onset to reduce the incidence of recurrent stroke.
    - thrombolysis:
      - iv thrombolysis with tissue plasminogen activator (r-tPa) **alteplase** is effective treatment if given <4.5 h from symptom onset. If given within 1.5 h it doubles the odds of complete recovery. Intracerebral haemorrhage is the major risk. Intra-arterial thrombolysis, in which the agent is injected directly into the thrombus, may have a role in middle cerebral artery and basilar artery thrombotic strokes and for patients in whom iv thrombolysis is contraindicated.

- contraindications for thrombolysis include previous stroke within the last 3 months, any history of intracranial haemorrhage, GIT bleeding within the last 21 days and **MI** in the previous 3 months.
- endovascular mechanical removal of clot (thrombectomy) is now supported by **NICE** for patients with a high degree of neurological impairment following the stroke, a large arterial occlusion and arrival in hospital within 6 hours of onset of symptoms. Has been shown to be superior to thrombolysis alone in anterior circulation stroke.
- decompressive craniectomy: patients with a middle cerebral artery (MCA) stroke and accompanying oedema may develop an acute and catastrophic rise in ICP (malignant MCA syndrome); mortality is >80% if untreated. Decompressive craniectomy performed within 48 h increases survival but with markedly increased risk of severe neurological disability. Indications for craniectomy include age <60 years, clinical evidence of infarction in the MCA territory with severe neurological deficit, decreased level of consciousness and signs on CT scanning that >50% of the MCA territory is infarcted.

- Management of haemorrhagic stroke:
  - emergency department assessment: as for ischaemic stroke. The ICH score (based on the **Glasgow coma scale** score on presentation, ICH volume on CT scan, presence of infratentorial or intraventricular haemorrhage and age) may be used to indicate the risk of mortality.
  - stroke unit management:
    - monitoring and O_2 administration as for ischaemic stroke.
    - **anticoagulant drugs** should be reversed and pneumatic calf compression instituted to prevent **DVT**.
    - 30% of patients will have haematoma expansion during the first 24 h. Studies suggest that for patients with a systolic BP 150–220 mmHg, rapid reduction in BP to 110–140 mmHg, e.g. with **nicardipine**, decreases the incidence of expansion and improves functional outcome.
    - trials of recombinant factor VIIa have shown reduction in haematoma volume expansion but no effect on outcome.
    - continuing pre-haemorrhage use of **statins** appears to improve mortality and functional outcome.
    - seizures occur in 8% of patients with ICH and should be aggressively treated.
  - surgery and removal of clot is indicated if neurological deterioration or brainstem compression occurs or for treatment of **hydrocephalus**.

- Anaesthetic considerations for patients with established strokes:
  - assessment for predisposing conditions, e.g. hypertension, **coagulation disorders**, embolic conditions, trauma, arteritis due to **connective tissue diseases**, infections.
  - immobility, contractures: may affect drip sites. Risk of DVT.
  - bulbar lesions and laryngeal incompetence, and autonomic disturbances.
  - communication difficulties.
  - severe hyperkalaemia after **suxamethonium** has been reported up to 6 months after stroke.
  - **hyperventilation** and reduction of **cerebral blood flow**, and hypotension, should be avoided during anaesthesia. **Cerebral steal** may occur.
  - **confusion** is common postoperatively.

Risk of stroke during anaesthesia is increased in **cardiac surgery**, **carotid endarterectomy** and **neurosurgery**. Perioperative ischaemic stroke occurs with an incidence of 0.1%–0.6% in non-cardiac surgery; its incidence is increased in patients with previous stroke, and an interval of at least 6 months between stroke and elective surgery is suggested.

Hankey GJ (2017). Lancet; 389: 641–54

See also, Brain; Cerebral circulation; Cerebral hypoxic ischaemic injury

Stroke index. **Stroke volume** divided by body **surface area**, thus accounting for the effect of body size. Normally 30–50 ml/m^2.

Stroke volume (SV). Volume of blood ejected by the ventricle per contraction; i.e.:

$$SV = \frac{\textbf{cardiac output}}{\textbf{heart rate}}$$

Also equals end-diastolic volume − end-systolic volume. Normally 70–80 ml for a 70-kg man at rest.

Affected by: ventricular filling and **preload; myocardial contractility**; and outflow resistance and **SVR**.

See also, Starling's law

Stroke work. The ventricular work done per cardiac cycle, usually with reference to the left ventricle. Correlates with **stroke volume** multiplied by the change in ventricular pressure. Described using several **units** of measurement (e.g. g, g/m, g m). Strictly correct expression is in terms of work (e.g. **joule**, N m, mmHg ml):

$$\text{Stroke work (J)} = \textbf{stroke volume}\text{ (ml)} \times (\text{MAP} - \text{PCWP [mmHg]})$$

where PCWP = **pulmonary capillary wedge pressure**

Stroke work index = stroke work divided by body **surface area.**

Increased in **hypertension** and hypervolaemia, and decreased in **shock**, **cardiac failure** and **aortic stenosis**.

Strong ion difference (SID). Difference between the concentrations of the strong cations (those that dissociate almost totally at the pH of interest, e.g. in blood, Na^+, K^+, Ca^{2+}, Mg^{2+}) and strong anions (e.g. Cl^-, lactate, SO_4^{2-}) in a solution. Based on the concept of electroneutrality, proposed in the 1980s by Stewart as part of his 'alternative approach' to **acid–base balance**, in which the number of positive ions in a solution equals the number of negative ones. A SID >0 represents the presence of unmeasured anions; the normal value is 40–44 mmol/l in plasma, this value representing the contribution made by weak acids (mostly albumin) and carbon dioxide. As SID falls it results in increased dissociation of water to maintain electroneutrality, leading to increased H^+ and therefore reduced pH, i.e., metabolic **acidosis**. As SID increases, plasma pH rises.

The strong ion gap (SIG) accounts for the effect of other anions not included in the SID equation; i.e., SIG = SID − [HCO_3^-] − [albumin$^-$].

[Peter A Stewart (1921–1993), Canadian-born US physiologist]

Stump pressure, *see Carotid endarterectomy*

Subarachnoid block, *see Spinal anaesthesia*

Subarachnoid haemorrhage (SAH). Bleeding into the subarachnoid space. Non-traumatic SAH accounts for about 5% of all **strokes** and affects 10 per 100 000 population/year. Most frequent at 40–60 years of age. 30-day mortality ranges from 35% to 45% and permanent disability occurs in 50% of survivors. Most common cause of non-traumatic SAH is rupture of an intracranial (Berry) aneurysm, which accounts for 75%–85%; arteriovenous malformations account for 5%. Risk factors for the development of aneurysms include a familial tendency among first-degree relatives, **hypertension**, smoking and alcohol abuse. Other disorders associated with the condition include autosomal dominant polycystic kidney disease, **Marfan's syndrome**, Ehlers-Danlos syndrome type IV and **neurofibromatosis**.

- Clinical features:
  - most aneurysms remain asymptomatic until rupture but may be an incidental finding during intracranial imaging for other conditions. Risk factors for rupture include female sex, smoking, hypertension, posterior circulation aneurysms and **cocaine** use.
  - sudden severe headache preceded in 30%–40% by headaches in the preceding weeks (sentinel headaches).These probably represent small leaks from the aneurysm.
  - nausea, vomiting, neck stiffness, photophobia.
  - drowsiness, confusion, coma according to the severity of the SAH.
  - neurological deficit depends on location of aneurysm:
    - bitemporal hemianopia and leg weakness: anterior communicating artery aneurysm.
    - unilateral **cranial nerve** III palsy: posterior communicating artery aneurysm.
    - facial/orbital pain, visual loss, ophthalmoplegia: internal carotid artery aneurysm (in the cavernous sinus).
    - **brainstem** dysfunction: posterior cerebral circulation aneurysm.
- Diagnosis and assessment:
  - non-contrast CT scanning is the initial investigation of choice; if SAH is seen, it should be followed by CT angiography, which will delineate aneurysmal anatomy if present in 99% of cases. Lumbar puncture (revealing xanthochromic CSF) is only necessary if CT does not detect SAH. The anterior (30%) and posterior (25%) communicating arteries, middle cerebral (20%) and basilar (10%) arteries are most commonly affected by aneurysmal disease (*see Cerebral circulation*).
  - assessment of severity: the most frequently used grading systems are the Hunt and Hess and the World Federation of Neurosurgeons Scale (WFNS), which are based on clinical findings (Table 50). Although prone to observer variability, they are useful as prognostic tools, a higher score indicating worse outcome.
- Acute management of SAH:
  - **CPR** as necessary.
  - tracheal intubation is indicated for a **Glasgow coma score** <8 or a reduction ≥2 following stabilisation, to protect the airway, to optimise P_{aO_2} and P_{aCO_2} and to control seizures.
  - arterial BP should be controlled to <140 mmHg (MAP <100 mmHg) to reduce risk of rebleeding. Hypotension (systolic BP <100 mmHg) should be corrected to ensure adequate **cerebral perfusion pressure**.
  - adequate analgesia and maintenance of normal glycaemic control and body temperature are essential.

Table 50 Hunt and Hess scale for classifying subarachnoid haemorrhage

Grade	Features	Mortality
0	Unruptured aneurysm	
1	Asymptomatic or mild headache and neck stiffness	0%–5%
2	Severe headache, neck stiffness, cranial nerve palsy	2%–10%
3	Mild focal deficit, lethargy, confusion	8%–15%
4	Stupor, hemiparesis, early decerebrate rigidity	60%–70%
5	Deep coma, decerebrate posture	70%–100%

Following the initial aneurysmal SAH, there is up to a 10% risk of re-bleeding during the next 48 hours; this is more likely in poorer grade SAH, large aneurysms and in women. The risk can be lessened by avoiding surges in BP, coughing, and vomiting (i.e., by the use of antihypertensive, analgesic and antiemetic agents). Definitive management involves either surgical clipping or endovascular coiling of the aneurysm. Initial findings of the International Subarachnoid Aneurysm Trial (ISAT) favoured coiling over clipping when looking at death or dependence at 1 year. However, follow-up shows coiling presents a slightly increased risk of requiring retreatment or rebleeding longer term. Despite this, at present, coiling is favoured unless the morphology or position of the aneurysm does not allow it.

Once the aneurysm has been secured, management is directed at the prevention and treatment of delayed neurological deficit (DND), which is the major cause of death and disability following initial stabilisation. Causes of DND include:

- delayed cerebral ischaemia (DCI): often due to vasospasm but sometimes involving more than one vascular territory. Other mechanisms include microthrombi, vascular dysregulation and a generalised neuronal depolarisation (cortical spreading depolarisation). Affects >60% of patients usually between 4–10 days after the SAH and is more common in poor grade patients, those with large volumes of blood in the subarachnoid space, and smokers. Characterised by neurological deterioration lasting >1 h related to ischaemia. Vasospasm may be diagnosed using **transcranial Doppler ultrasound**, CT angiography or conventional angiography. Prevention and treatment of vasospasm:
  - **nimodipine**: significantly reduces the incidence of cerebral ischaemia and improves outcome. It should be started on diagnosis and continued for 21 days.
  - 'triple H therapy': hypertension, hypervolaemia and haemodilution have traditionally been used to improve **cerebral blood flow** and cerebral oxygen delivery, despite a lack of evidence. Induction of hypertension is currently only used if DCI occurs; hypervolaemia has been replaced with euvolaemia

and although the optimum haemoglobin level is unknown, most aim for 80–100 g/l.
  - endovascular treatment of vasospasm has been used.
  - magnesium reduces the incidence of DCI but does not affect outcome.
  - statins have shown no benefit.
- **hydrocephalus**: occurs in 20%–30% of patients following SAH and should be considered if neurological deterioration occurs.
- seizures: occur in only 5% of patients but should be treated aggressively. Prophylactic use of phenytoin is associated with worse outcome and is avoided.

- Systemic complications of SAH:
  - cardiac: SAH significantly increases sympathetic outflow; the resultant tachycardia and hypertension often result in myocardial ischaemia. ECG changes (S T segment changes, T wave abnormalities and arrhythmias) are common and usually self-limiting.
  - pulmonary: impaired oxygenation is seen in most patients and may be due to aspiration pneumonia, neurogenic or cardiac pulmonary oedema, pneumonia or **ALI**.
  - electrolyte imbalance: **hyponatraemia** is commonly seen and may be due to excessive fluid resuscitation, **cerebral salt-wasting syndrome** or **syndrome of inappropriate antidiuretic hormone secretion**. Hyperglycaemia is common but 'tight' glycaemic control may result in cerebral hypoglycaemia; current recommended levels are 4.5–11 mmol/l.
- Anaesthetic considerations:
  - as for **neurosurgery** and **neuroradiology**.
  - **hypotensive anaesthesia** has previously been employed but normotension is now recommended to maintain cerebral perfusion pressure.

[Sir James Berry (1860–1946), Canadian surgeon; Robert M Hess and William Hunt (1921–1999), US neurosurgeons]

Mcdonald RL, Schweizer TA (2017). Lancet; 389: 655–66

See also, Neuroradiology

Subclavian venous cannulation. The subclavian vein is the continuation of the axillary vein and arises at the lateral border of the first **rib** (*see Fig. 90;* **Internal jugular venous cannulation**). It passes over the first rib anterior to the subclavian artery, separated from it by scalenus anterior, to join with the internal **jugular vein** at the medial end of the clavicle. It receives the external jugular vein at the clavicle's midpoint. The right **phrenic nerve** lies between the vein and scalenus anterior, the left phrenic nerve between the vein and artery.

- Technique:
  - head-down position distends the vein and reduces risk of **gas embolism**. The head is turned to the contralateral side. Aseptic technique is used.
  - a finger is run medially in the subclavian groove until an 'obstruction' is felt (subclavius muscle), also marked by a notch on the undersurface of the clavicle. This point lies between the midpoint of the clavicle and a point dividing its middle and medial thirds.
  - after local anaesthetic infiltration, a needle is introduced under the clavicle and directed towards the sternal notch, aspirating during advancement. When the vein has been entered, the cannula is advanced or a wire inserted (**Seldinger technique**).

The approach is contraindicated in patients with coagulopathy, because direct pressure cannot be applied to the bleeding vessel. Use of **ultrasound** may reduce complications and increase the rate of successful cannulation, although the evidence is weaker than that for **internal jugular cannulation**.

See also, Central venous cannulation, for complications and comparison with other techniques

Subdural haemorrhage. Haemorrhage between the pia and arachnoid layers of the **meninges**. May be:

- acute: usually caused by acceleration–deceleration **TBI** resulting in tearing of veins connecting the cortical surface to dural sinuses (bridging veins). May also occur in elderly patients with relatively insignificant head injuries especially if they are taking **anticoagulant drugs**. Risk factors include:
  - **alcoholism**.
  - **coagulation disorders** including anticoagulant drug therapy (e.g. with **warfarin, aspirin**).
  - **thrombocytopenia**.
  - intracranial hypotension e.g. following **lumbar puncture, spinal anaesthesia** and accidental **dural tap**. The associated headache may be confused with **post-dural puncture headache**.
  - postoperative e.g. following craniotomy, **CSF** shunting procedures.
  - spontaneous (rare).

  Patients usually present with confusion or loss of consciousness following a **lucid interval** (occurs in 40%). Unchecked, **coning** may occur. CT scanning shows a hyperdense (white) crescentic mass, often with surrounding oedema. Mortality ranges from 60% to 90% depending on the underlying parenchymal brain injury, **Glasgow coma scale** on admission, patient's age and concurrent anticoagulant therapy. Treatment consists of emergency evacuation of the clot either through burr holes or craniotomy.
- chronic: usually seen in elderly patients and may follow mild trauma, acute subdural haemorrhage or may be spontaneous. Characterised by cerebral atrophy and presents with reduced level of consciousness, headache, gait disturbance and memory loss. CT shows a hypodense lesion most easily seen on non-contrast scan. Treatment consists of surgical decompression if mass effect is present; if not, patients are managed with serial scans.

See also, Neurosurgery

Substance abuse. Difficult to define, because society tolerates intake of certain substances (e.g. alcohol, tobacco) but not others (illicit drugs); in addition, excessive intake of otherwise acceptable substances (e.g. alcohol) is generally considered abuse. Addiction is a state of compulsive use associated with physical, psychological or social harm and despite evidence of that harm; dependence is a physiological adaptation associated with withdrawal symptoms when ingestion ceases.

- Potential problems for anaesthesia or intensive care:
  - **alcohol poisoning** and **alcoholism** commonly accompany abuse of other substances. **Solvent abuse** is more common in young patients.
  - **malnutrition** may accompany chronic substance abuse.
  - effects of iv/sc/im administration, often with non-sterile needles (e.g. **opioid analgesic drugs, barbiturates**):
    - high risk of **sepsis**, thrombophlebitis, **cellulitis**, bacterial **endocarditis** and septic systemic and pulmonary embolism.

  - veins are often difficult to find and cannulate.
  - high-risk group for **hepatitis** and **HIV infection**.
- chronic effects of the substance, e.g. hepatic impairment/**enzyme induction** (e.g. opioids, barbiturates); **cardiomyopathy** (**cocaine**). **Thrombocytopenia** may occur in cocaine and opioid abuse.
- acute effects:
  - depressant, e.g. opioids, barbiturates: respiratory depression, hypotension.
  - excitatory, e.g. **amfetamines**, cocaine, lysergic acid diethylamide (LSD): tachycardia, hypertension, arrhythmias, pyrexia. Hallucinations may occur postoperatively. **Anticholinergic drugs**, drugs that sensitise the myocardium to **catecholamines** and indirectly acting **sympathomimetic drugs** should be avoided. LSD may impair plasma **cholinesterase**.
- effects of withdrawal:
  - opioids: tachycardia, tremor, acute anxiety, GIT symptoms, piloerection and sweating ('cold turkey'). Unpleasant but rarely life-threatening.
  - barbiturates: anxiety, tremor, hallucinations and convulsions. May be life-threatening.

- Conduct of anaesthesia:
  - patients may be resistant to iv anaesthetic agents, with rapid recovery.
  - surgical cut-down, central venous cannulation or inhalational induction may be required if peripheral venous cannulation is impossible.
  - estimation of appropriate doses of opioids may be difficult, especially in opioid addicts. Inhalational and regional techniques are often preferred. **Opioid antagonists** may provoke acute withdrawal and should be avoided.
  - withdrawal states may occur postoperatively.

Wong GT, Irwin MG (2013). Anaesthesia; 68 (Suppl 1): 117–24

See also, Abuse of anaesthetic agents; Barbiturate poisoning; Misuse of Drugs Act; Opioid poisoning; Rapid opioid detoxification; Solvent abuse

Substance P. 11-amino-acid **tachykinin** neuropeptide, involved in pain pathways (*see Gate control theory of pain*). High levels are found in axons and cell bodies of primary afferent fibres in the dorsal root ganglia, also in the superficial levels of the dorsal horn of the **spinal cord**.

- Evidence for its involvement in pain transmission includes:
  - distribution in the regions of pain pathways.
  - depletion by **capsaicin**, a red pepper extract, reduces sensitivity to noxious thermal and chemical stimuli, without affecting other sensory modalities.

Also involved in the regulation of the respiratory rhythm, nausea and vomiting, and mood.

Substantia gelatinosa, *see Pain pathways; Sensory pathways; Spinal cord*

Sub-Tenon's block. Used in **ophthalmic surgery** as an alternative to **retrobulbar block** and **peribulbar block**. Tenon's capsule is a connective tissue layer surrounding the eye and extraocular muscles. The posterior part separates the globe from the retrobulbar space; injection of local anaesthetic between the capsule and sclera posteriorly results in spread along the extraocular muscles and diffusion into the retrobulbar space.

Topical anaesthesia is applied first. With the patient looking up, the conjunctiva and anterior Tenon's capsule are picked up with toothed forceps, 5–6 mm inferomedial to the limbus (the junction of the cornea and sclera). A small incision is made with scissors, which are then passed backwards around the globe underneath Tenon's capsule to reach the posterior part. A curved, blunt cannula is then passed into this space and 3–4 ml solution slowly injected. Gentle external pressure is applied to the eye and further injections made if required. Suitable solutions include a mixture of **lidocaine** 2% and **bupivacaine** 0.5%–0.75% in equal volumes with or without **adrenaline** 1:400 000 and **hyaluronidase** 5 U/ml.

Provides rapid anaesthesia and akinesia with less risk of globe perforation or retrobulbar haemorrhage than retrobulbar block; the block is also usually more comfortable than alternatives.

Complications include: pain on injection; subconjunctival oedema (chemosis); subconjunctival or retrobulbar haemorrhage; globe perforation (rarely).

[Jacques R Tenon (1724–1816), French ophthalmologist]

Guise P (2012). Local Reg Anesth; 5: 35–46

Succinylcholine, *see Suxamethonium*

Sucralfate. Complex of aluminium hydroxide and sulfated sucrose. Provides mucosal protection from gastric acid and promotes ulcer healing. Has no antacid effect. Used in **peptic ulcer disease**, and has been used on **ICU** as prophylaxis against peptic ulceration; thought to be associated with fewer nosocomial infections than the **H_2 receptor antagonists**.

- Dosage: 1 g orally/nasogastrically 4–6-hourly.
- Side effects are rare; include constipation, nausea, vomiting, rash.

Suction equipment. Consists of:

- pump to generate a vacuum. Effectiveness of the system is related to the degree of subatmospheric pressure generated, and the volume of air that can be moved in unit time (displacement). Pumps may employ pistons (usually low displacement), rotating fans (high displacement), foot-operated bellows and compressed gases using the **Venturi principle**. Piped suction systems use a high displacement pump connected to a large central reservoir, with traps to prevent contamination.
- reservoir: must be large enough to enable aspiration of large volumes, but not so large that the desired vacuum takes too long to achieve. A filter and float valve prevent contamination of the pump with aspirated liquid.
- delivery tubing; usually disposable, attached to rigid (Yankauer) or flexible catheters. Smooth-tipped catheters may reduce mucosal damage following endotracheal suctioning. Prolonged **tracheobronchial suctioning** may cause lung collapse and hypoxaemia; bradycardia is common in critically ill patients. Preoxygenation should thus precede tracheal suction. Enclosed suction catheters that do not require detachment of the patient from the breathing system are available; the catheter is handled through a plastic sleeve, maintaining sterility. Hypoxaemia and dispersal of infectious droplets are thus reduced.

A minimal flow rate of 35 l/min air, and generation of at least 80 kPa (600 mmHg) negative pressure, have been suggested for apparatus for anaesthetic use. For tracheobronchial suctioning, limiting the negative pressure to –20 kPa (–150 mmHg), applying suction for less than 15 s,

and restricting the diameter of the suction catheter (e.g. to <2/3 of the internal diameter of the tracheal tube) have been suggested.
[Sidney Yankauer (1872–1932), US surgeon]

Sudeck's atrophy, *see Complex regional pain syndrome*

Sufentanil citrate. Synthetic **opioid analgesic drug**, introduced in the USA in 1984. An analogue of **fentanyl**, with 5–7 times the latter's potency. Of shorter elimination **half-life** (about 2–3 h) than fentanyl, with similar clearance and slightly smaller volume of distribution. Has similar clinical effects to fentanyl, including cardiovascular stability and lack of **histamine** release. Usual dose is 0.1–0.5 µg/kg for minor surgery, up to 8 µg/kg for longer procedures and up to 30 µg/kg as the sole agent for, e.g. **cardiac surgery**. May be given epidurally (10–75 µg) and spinally (5–20 µg), effects lasting 2–6 h. In the UK, only licensed for sublingual use (15 µg bolus; lockout 20 min) for up to 72 h in acute moderate-to-severe postoperative pain in adults, via a patient-specific, electronic dispenser PCA device.

Sugammadex sodium. Modified **γ-cyclodextrin** licensed for reversal of **non-depolarising neuromuscular blockade** caused by **rocuronium** or **vecuronium**. Has a ring-shaped structure that forms a water-soluble complex with rocuronium/vecuronium, thus favouring removal from the neuromuscular junction into the plasma.

- Dosage:
  - routine reversal: 2 mg/kg if spontaneous recovery of >1 twitch has occurred on train-of-four nerve stimulation; 4 mg/kg if >1–2 post-tetanic counts are present. Recovery of T4:T1 ratio to 0.9 occurs within 2–3 min. Recovery is slightly slower with vecuronium than rocuronium.
  - immediate reversal of rocuronium-induced blockade (e.g. after **failed intubation** during **rapid sequence induction**): 16 mg/kg; if administered 3 min after a bolus dose of 1.2 mg/kg rocuronium, produces recovery of T4:T1 ratio to 0.9 after 1.5 min.
  - recurrence of neuromuscular blockade: additional dose of 4 mg/kg.
  - in **obesity**, dosing based on both total and adjusted **body weight** has been recommended.
- Side effects: bronchospasm, **anaphylaxis** (rarely), taste disturbance. May interfere with the oral contraceptive pill.

Due to high cost, its use is often confined to the emergency setting.
See also, Neuromuscular blockade monitoring

Sulfhaemoglobinaemia. Presence of an abnormal **haemoglobin** of uncertain chemical structure, but which may be produced by adding hydrogen sulfide in vitro. Often coexists with **methaemoglobinaemia.** Reduces O_2-carrying capacity of blood and shifts the **oxyhaemoglobin dissociation curve** to the left, decreasing O_2 delivery to the tissues. Usually due to ingestion of phenacetin, sulfonamides, primaquine or **metoclopramide**. Treatment includes O_2 therapy; normal haemoglobin cannot be regenerated from sulfhaemoglobin.

Sulfonamides. Group of broad-spectrum **antibacterial drugs**, less commonly used now because of **bacterial resistance** and side effects. Also active against certain protozoa, e.g. toxoplasma and **pneumocystis.** Act by inhibiting bacterial dihydrofolate synthesis; their action is enhanced by **trimethoprim**, which inhibits tetrahydrofolate production from dihydrofolate. Toxic effects include renal impairment, blood dyscrasias and allergic reactions.

Sulfonylureas. Group of oral **hypoglycaemic drugs**, used in non–insulin-dependent **diabetes mellitus.** Act by stimulating secretion of **insulin** by surviving pancreatic β cells, and possibly by increasing peripheral uptake of glucose. Several have been used; the following are available in the UK:

- glibenclamide, gliclazide: half-life 8–12 h.
- tolbutamide, glimepiride: half-life 5–8 h.
- glipizide: half-life 2–4 h.

All of the above are excreted by the liver.

The shorter-acting drugs may be stopped on the day of surgery; perioperative **hypoglycaemia** is most likely in the elderly and with longer-acting drugs.

Sumatriptan, *see Triptans*

Superior vena caval obstruction (Superior vena caval syndrome). 80%–90% of cases are caused by malignancy, especially **bronchial carcinoma** and lymphoma. Other causes include mediastinal fibrosis and thrombosis. Results in distended veins, oedema and cyanosis in the arm, head and neck, with prominent collateral vessels in the chest wall. Visual disturbances and headache may occur. Most patients have dyspnoea and orthopnoea. Emergency radiotherapy may be required if malignancy is the cause. Steroids have also been used to reduce oedema.

- Anaesthetic considerations:
  - patients should be nursed sitting up preoperatively, to minimise facial and neck swelling.
  - induction of anaesthesia with iv agents may be prolonged if an arm vein is used.
  - tracheal intubation may be difficult. Laryngeal oedema may be present.
  - bleeding may be torrential, especially during median sternotomy.

Supine hypotension syndrome, *see Aortocaval compression*

Supraglottic airway device (SAD). Used for maintaining a patent airway in the unconscious patient without tracheal intubation; the terms 'extraglottic' or 'periglottic' have also been used to distinguish from oropharyngeal/nasopharyngeal **airways**. The **LM** was the first type of SAD, and remains the most widely used (Fig. 155), with dozens of variants since introduction of the original LMA in 1988. Used for spontaneous or controlled ventilation, the latter limited by the effective seal pressure of the particular device.

- Features common to all devices:
  - inflatable cuff (e.g. LM) or sculpted 'bowl' (e.g. i-gel) that is positioned over the larynx.
  - wide bore airway tube with an ISO 15-mm male connector for connection to an angle piece or **breathing system.**
  - ability to insert 'blindly' without the need for laryngoscopy.

May be divided into first- and second-generation SADs with the latter distinguished by features designed to reduce the risk of regurgitation and **aspiration of gastric contents.** First generation devices include the original LMA Classic, LMA Fastrach (originally called intubating LMA) and Cobra. Examples of second-generation SADs include: the i-gel, LMA Proseal, LMA Supreme, laryngeal tube and Streamlined Liner of the Pharyngeal Airway (SLIPA).

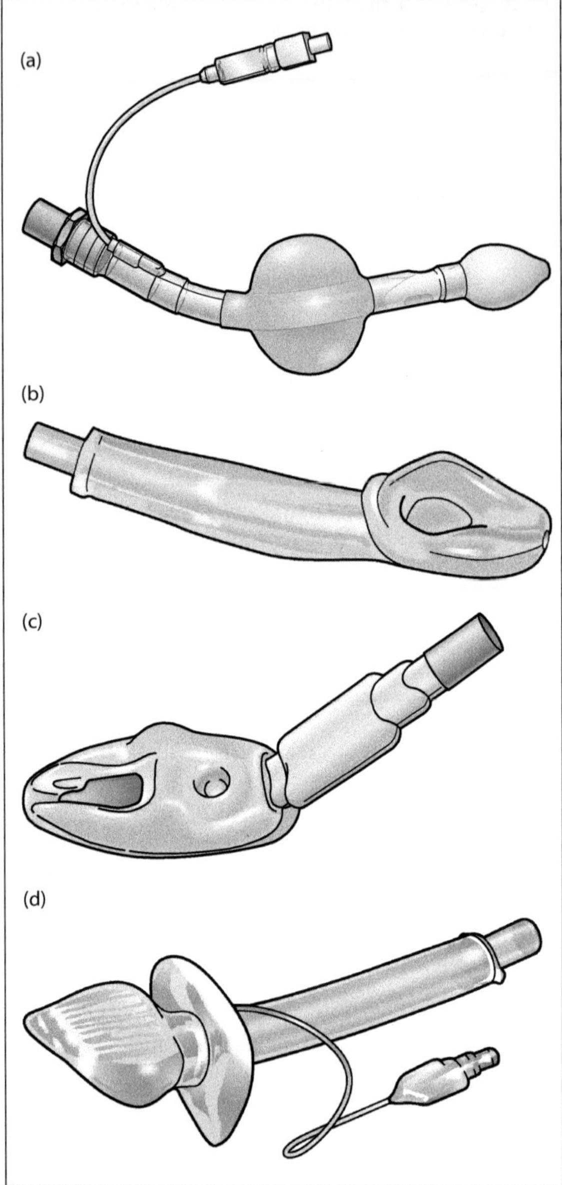

Fig. 155 Examples of supraglottic airways: (a) laryngeal tube; (b) i-gel; (c) SLIPA; (d) Cobra

Second generation devices have higher effective seal pressures than the LMA Classic, and either a gastric drainage channel or, in the case of the SLIPA, a hollow pharyngeal portion for collecting regurgitant fluid.

- Indications for use include:
  - providing a reliable airway during routine anaesthesia.
  - maintenance of ventilation in difficult facemask ventilation/tracheal intubation.
  - management of failed intubation (e.g. as a conduit for tracheal intubation).
  - SAD/**tracheal tube** exchange during **extubation** (the SAD is less likely to elicit coughing and straining than a tracheal tube during emergence).
  - **CPR.**
- Insertion technique:
  - the head and neck are placed in the 'sniffing position'; cradling the occiput in the non-dominant hand can achieve this while causing the mouth to open.

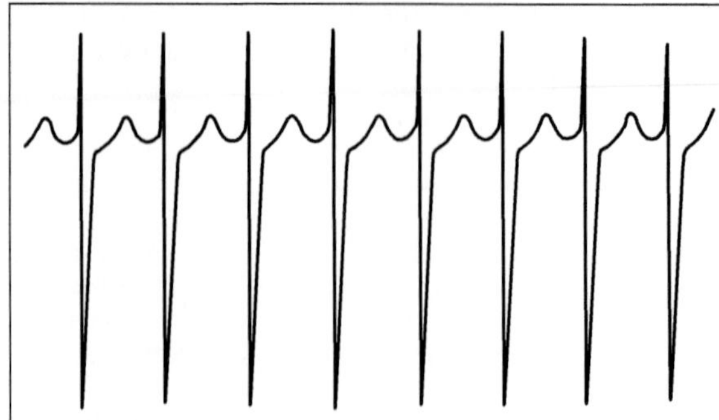

Fig. 156 SVT

  - the cuff (or bowl) is inserted blindly into the pharynx to lie against the back of the larynx. Several insertion methods have been described; the original recommended technique for the LMA Classic was to place the index finger at the junction of the cuff and tube and to press backward and upward against the palate; alternatively, the cuff may be inserted facing upwards and rotated 180 degrees once at the soft palate (this avoids blind insertion of the hand into the patient's mouth).
  - the cuff (if present) is inflated to form a seal. As with a tracheal tube, air should be injected slowly until no audible leak is present; maximum cuff volumes stated by the manufacturer should not be exceeded.

Insertion is smoother following induction with **propofol** than **thiopental**, because of the former's greater suppression of laryngeal reflexes. Inadequate depth of anaesthesia during insertion is a common cause of difficulty, and may provoke **laryngospasm**. Other complications of SAD use include aspiration of gastric contents, sore throat and nerve palsies (rarely).

(N.B. 'LMA' refers to one manufacturer's products [The Laryngeal Mask Company Ltd]; similar devices are made by other manufacturers but strictly should be referred to as 'laryngeal masks', not LMAs.)

Supraorbital nerve block, *see Ophthalmic nerve blocks*

Suprascapular nerve block. Performed for analgesia in painful shoulders. A needle is inserted 1–2 cm cranial to the scapular spine, on a line bisecting the inferior scapular angle. 5 ml **local anaesthetic agent** is injected when the scapular notch is identified.

Supraventricular tachycardia (SVT). Paroxysmal tachycardia with a rate of 140–250 beats/min, caused by a rapidly firing ectopic focus in the atria or atrioventricular node. Circular conduction of impulses via abnormal anatomical pathways or within the node itself results in re-entry and perpetuation of the **arrhythmia**. Occurs in otherwise healthy individuals, although it may be associated with heart disease, **Wolff–Parkinson–White** and **Lown–Ganong–Levine syndromes, hyperthyroidism**, and excessive consumption of **caffeine, nicotine** or alcohol. Typically sudden in onset. May cause palpitations, dyspnoea, dizziness and polyuria if prolonged.

- Features: regular narrow **QRS complexes** on the **ECG** (Fig. 156), unless **bundle branch block** is also present (causing widened QRS complexes). A degree of atrioventricular block may be present, especially when associated with **digoxin** toxicity. It may be difficult to distinguish SVT from **VT**.

- Treatment: **Resuscitation Council (UK)** guidelines (N.B. based around peri-arrest SVT):
  - O_2 therapy, iv cannulation.
  - if there are no adverse signs (**shock**, **myocardial ischaemia**, **cardiac failure** or syncope), options include vagal stimulation manoeuvres (e.g. **carotid sinus massage**, **Valsalva manoeuvre**).
  - if there are adverse signs: synchronised electrical **cardioversion** (70–120 J, up to three attempts) with sedation/general anaesthesia if required, followed by **amiodarone** 300 mg over 10–20 min then 900 mg over 24 h.
  - **antiarrhythmic drugs**:
    - **adenosine** 6 mg iv initially; if unsuccessful, two further doses of 12 mg may be given at 1–2-min intervals.
    - if heart rate is still above 200 beats/min, one or more of the following may be used:
      - amiodarone 300 mg iv over 10–15 min.
      - digoxin up to two iv doses of 0.5 mg over 30 min (not in Wolff–Parkinson–White syndrome).
      - verapamil 2.5–5 mg iv over 2 min.
  - overdrive **cardiac pacing** (not in atrial fibrillation).
  - **hypokalaemia** and **hypomagnesaemia** should be corrected if present.

Other drugs, e.g. **β-adrenergic receptor antagonists**, **disopyramide**, **diltiazem**, have also been used. Ablation therapy or surgery may be required.

Soar J, Nolan JP, Böttiger BW, et al (2015). Resuscitation; 95: 100–47

See also, Atrial flutter

Sural nerve block, *see Ankle, nerve blocks*

Surface area, body. Used in physiological calculations (e.g. **cardiac index**, **basal metabolic rate**), because it reflects body requirements and activity more accurately than weight and height; however, use of basal metabolic rate has been suggested as being more logical. Also used to estimate drug doses (e.g. chemotherapy, maintenance **glucocorticoid** therapy), although drug administration according to **body weight** is more common.

The **rule of nines** is used to estimate surface area of parts of the body. Nomograms for total surface area are based on the formula:

$$\text{surface area (m}^2) = \text{weight}^{0.425}\ \text{(kg)} \times \text{height}^{0.725}\ \text{(cm)} \times 0.007184$$

Surface tension. Tangential **force** in the surface of a liquid, defined in terms of the force acting perpendicularly across a line of unit length. Caused by attraction between the liquid molecules; whereas molecules in the main body of the liquid are attracted in all directions, those at the surface are only attracted inwards and along the surface. Thus the surface tends to contract to the smallest possible area, e.g. a free drop tends to be spherical. Has important implications in lung mechanics; normally reduced by pulmonary **surfactant**. Measured in N/m.

See also, Laplace's law

Surfactant. Complex material composed of dipalmitoyl phosphatidyl choline (DPPC), protein and carbohydrate that prevents alveolar collapse at lower lung volumes by reducing alveolar **surface tension**. Thought to do this by alignment of the hydrophilic parts of the DPPC molecules on the surface of the alveolar fluid lining, with repulsion between adjacent molecules. Repulsion increases as the molecules are pressed together at low volumes. **Compliance** is increased, **alveoli** are held open and alveolar fluid is reduced.

Produced by type II pneumocytes, partly under control of the hypothalamic–pituitary–adrenal axis. Appears at about 24 weeks' gestation. Deficiency due to immaturity causes the **respiratory distress syndrome** (RDS). It may also be deficient in areas of lung affected by **PE**, bronchial obstruction, and in heavy smokers.

Bovine/porcine surfactant is licensed for prophylaxis and treatment of neonatal RDS; it has no proven benefit in adult **ALI**.

Surviving Sepsis Campaign. Global initiative of the **European Society of Intensive Care Medicine**, **Society of Critical Care Medicine** and International Sepsis Forum (the latter no longer involved), with the aim of improving the management, diagnosis and treatment of **sepsis** through increasing awareness, educating healthcare professionals, developing guidelines/**care bundles** and facilitating data collection.

Suxamethonium chloride (Succinylcholine). Depolarising **neuromuscular blocking drug**, introduced in 1951. Structurally composed of two **acetylcholine** molecules joined together (Fig. 157). Stored at 4°C to prevent hydrolysis. Incompatible with **thiopental** (causes crystallisation).

- Dosage:
  - 0.5–1.5 mg/kg iv depending on the relaxation required. Usual initial dose is 1 mg/kg iv, producing paralysis within 30–90 s that lasts 2–5 min. Subsequent doses: 0.2–0.5 mg/kg. Low doses (5–10 mg) may be effective for treatment of **laryngospasm**.
  - has been given by infusion of 0.1% solution with 5% dextrose or 0.9% saline at 2–5 mg/min, for short cases (rarely employed nowadays).
  - may also be given im (2–4 mg/kg) or sc, or even into the tongue in emergency situations when iv access is not available.

Rapidly hydrolysed by plasma **cholinesterase** to succinyl monocholine and choline, then to succinic acid and choline. Succinyl monocholine has weak blocking properties.

Hexafluorenium and **tetrahydroaminacrine** have been used to prolong the action of suxamethonium.

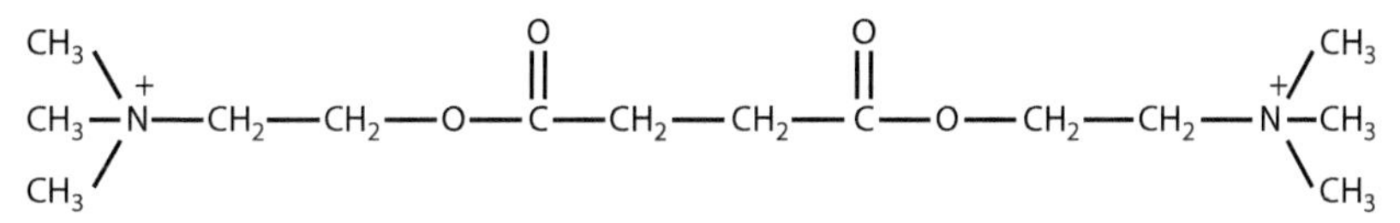

Fig. 157 Structure of suxamethonium

- Side effects:
  - prolonged paralysis. May be caused by:
    - reduced cholinesterase activity (*see Cholinesterase, plasma*) due to:
      - inherited atypical cholinesterase.
      - reduced amount of cholinesterase.
      - inhibition of cholinesterase by drugs.
    - excessive dosage and production of **dual block**. The latter may occur after 200–500 mg in adults. Dual block may also develop with reduced enzyme activity. Management of prolonged paralysis:
      - maintenance of anaesthesia and oxygenation.
      - diagnosis of the nature of block using **neuromuscular blockade monitoring**. **Edrophonium** has been suggested to distinguish non-depolarising from depolarising blockade, but is less commonly used.
      - **neostigmine** may be used to reverse dual block.
      - in prolonged depolarising blockade ('suxamethonium or Scoline apnoea'), recovery usually occurs within 4 h. It may be speeded by administering fresh frozen plasma, but spontaneous recovery is usually preferable.
      - blood may be analysed for cholinesterase activity, and screening of relatives performed.
  - muscle **fasciculations**, coinciding with initial depolarisation of muscle fibres. They are painful if the patient is awake. Thought to contribute to:
    - postoperative muscle pains, typically around the neck, back and upper arms, lasting 2–3 days. Most common in young fit women and after early ambulation.
    - increased **intraocular pressure**. Suxamethonium causes contraction of the extraocular muscles, but may also cause choroidal vasodilatation; the response may still occur if the extrinsic muscles are cut. The increase usually lasts for under 10 min. Suxamethonium is usually avoided in penetrating eye injuries but this is controversial (*see Eye, penetrating injury*).
    - increased intragastric pressure. Formerly thought to increase risk of **aspiration of gastric contents**, but an accompanying increase in **lower oesophageal sphincter** tone maintains barrier pressure.
    - increased plasma **potassium**. Although this arises mainly from depolarisation (*see later*), leakage of potassium from damaged muscle fibres may contribute. Plasma **myoglobin** and creatine phosphokinase (normally intracellular) are increased after injection of suxamethonium.

    Fasciculations and the resulting complications may be reduced by pretreatment with other drugs, although not consistently. Adverse effects may also still occur despite lack of fasciculations. Drugs that have been described include:
    - non-depolarising neuromuscular blocking drugs (usually 1/10 usual intubating dose), given 2–3 min before suxamethonium, which may be required in increased dosage. **Tubocurarine** is the best studied, although others have been used. The possibility of aspiration pneumonitis precludes this technique in rapid sequence induction.
    - **lidocaine** 1–2 mg/kg iv, given 2–3 min before suxamethonium.
    - **diazepam** 10 mg iv.
    - **dantrolene** 100–200 mg orally, 2 h preoperatively.
    - suxamethonium 0.1 mg/kg iv 1–2 min before the main dose.
    - **calcium** 10 mmol iv. Arrhythmias may occur.
    - **magnesium** sulfate 1–2 g iv.
    - chlorpromazine 0.1 mg/kg.
    - hexafluorenium.
  - **hyperkalaemia**. Plasma potassium increases usually by 0.5 mmol/l in normal patients, and lasts for 3–5 min. This follows normal movement of potassium out of myocytes during depolarisation at the **neuromuscular junction**, with some leakage due to trauma following fasciculations, as above. The increase may be dangerous in patients whose plasma potassium levels are already high (typically **renal failure**, although the response is of normal magnitude unless neuropathy is present). Increases of several mmol/l may occur if the **acetylcholine receptors** are not confined to the neuromuscular junction, but have spread along the whole length of the muscle fibres, as occurs in **denervation hypersensitivity**. This process is also thought to occur in other conditions in which massive hyperkalaemia may follow administration of suxamethonium for certain periods after the lesion:
    - **burns**: 9 days–2 months.
    - **spinal cord injury**, intracranial lesions (e.g. **stroke**, **subarachnoid haemorrhage**, **head injury**) and muscle trauma: 10 days–6–7 months.
    - peripheral nerve injury: 4 days–6–7 months.
    - peripheral neuropathy, **tetanus** and severe infection: uncertain period of risk.

    Maximal risk occurs at 14–28 days. Severe arrhythmias and **cardiac arrest** may occur, usually responding well to iv calcium and **CPR**. The same drugs used to attenuate the fasciculations have been used to reduce the hyperkalaemic response, with varying success. **Salbutamol** has also been used.

    The risk of hyperkalaemia in **disseminated sclerosis** and **Parkinson's disease** is unclear. It has been described in **muscular dystrophies** (related to massive rhabdomyolysis and possibly **MH**), but not in **motor neurone disease**.
  - bradycardia: common after the second dose, but may occur after the first dose, especially in children. Other muscarinic effects may occur, e.g. increased GIT motility and secretion.
  - **adverse drug reactions**: although rare, they may be severe, e.g. **anaphylaxis**.
  - MH.
  - **masseter spasm**.
  - abnormal sustained contraction in **dystrophia myotonica**.

Resistance occurs in **myasthenia gravis** due to reduced receptor density, and increased sensitivity is seen in the **myasthenic syndrome**.

Its use has declined because of its many disadvantages and the introduction of alternative drugs, e.g. **atracurium**, **vecuronium**, **rocuronium** and **mivacurium**. In particular, the use of large doses of rocuronium with **sugammadex** immediately available offers an alternative method of producing fast-onset, easily reversible paralysis, that does not rely on the sometimes variable offset of action of suxamethonium.

See also, Depolarising neuromuscular blockade

Suxethonium bromide/iodide. Depolarising **neuromuscular blocking drug**, introduced with **suxamethonium** in 1951. Similar to suxamethonium, but the quaternary ammonium group at each end of the molecule contains two methyl and one ethyl group instead of three methyl groups.

SVP, *see Saturated vapour pressure*

SVR, *see Systemic vascular resistance*

SVT, *see Supraventricular tachycardia*

Swallowing (Deglutition). Active passage of liquid or food bolus from mouth to stomach. Initiated voluntarily by the **tongue** pressing against the palate from the tip back, pushing food into the oropharynx. Continues by reflex activity, with afferent fibres in the 9th and 10th **cranial nerves**; impulses pass to the tractus solitarius and nucleus ambiguus of the medulla, with efferent fibres to pharyngeal and tongue muscles via 9th, 10th and 12th nerves. The nasopharynx is sealed by soft palate elevation and superior constrictor contraction, and the **larynx** by elevation and glottic closure. The epiglottis moves posteriorly but does not seal the glottic opening, as formerly suspected. Respiration ceases. Food is propelled by the inferior constrictor into the upper oesophagus, where it initiates peristalsis (*see Oesophageal contractility*).

Suppressed in plane 1 of surgical anaesthesia; its reappearance may herald the onset of **vomiting**.

Difficulty with swallowing (dysphagia) may be caused by anatomical (e.g. local tumours, inflammation, **achalasia**) or neurological (e.g. **myasthenia gravis**, bulbar palsies) factors; pulmonary aspiration of food and saliva may lead to repeated **chest infection**.

Swan–Ganz catheter, *see Pulmonary artery catheterisation*

Sympathetic nerve blocks. Although blockade of sympathetic nerves commonly accompanies various regional techniques (e.g. **epidural** or **spinal anaesthesia**, **brachial plexus block**), selective blockade of sympathetic fibres is used for:

- **pain management**: certain pain syndromes are thought to involve abnormal sympathetic activity, e.g. **complex regional pain syndrome**, **phantom limb** pain. The underlying mechanism is unknown but may involve abnormal linkage between mechanoreceptors and sympathetic neurones. Recent evidence suggests that sympathetic blocks may not actually improve outcome, as traditionally believed.
- improvement of blood flow, e.g. in peripheral ischaemia, Raynaud's disease, accidental intra-arterial injection of **thiopental**.
- treatment of excessive sweating.

Sympathetic ganglia may be blocked at three levels: the cervicothoracic ganglia (**stellate ganglion block**), coeliac plexus (**coeliac plexus block**) and lumbar ganglia (**lumbar sympathetic block**). Blockade may be short-term (using local anaesthetic agents) or permanent (chemical sympathectomy), when neurolytic agents such as **phenol** or alcohol are used. **IVRA** using **guanethidine** is also used.

[Maurice Raynaud (1834–1881), French physician]

Bantel C, Trapp S (2011). Anaesthesia; 66: 541–4

Sympathetic nervous system. Part of the **autonomic nervous system**. Myelinated preganglionic efferent fibres emerge from spinal segments T1–L2 into the corresponding primary ramus at each level, and pass via a white ramus communicans into the sympathetic trunk (*see Fig. 20;* **Autonomic nervous system**). They may then:

- synapse in the corresponding ganglion and pass via a grey ramus communicans to the corresponding **spinal nerve** for distribution.
- ascend or descend in the sympathetic chain, and synapse at a distant ganglion.
- pass without synapsing to a peripheral ganglion, to synapse there.

The sympathetic trunk is a ganglionated nerve chain extending from the base of the skull to the coccyx, and lying about 2–3 cm lateral to the vertebral column. The portion above T1 does not receive any rami communicantes; i.e., the cervical sympathetic outflow must descend to T1, then into the sympathetic trunk and ascend to the cervical ganglia. The trunk descends in the neck behind the carotid sheath and enters the thorax anterior to the neck of the first rib. It passes over the heads of the upper ribs and overlies the sides of the lower four thoracic vertebrae. It enters the abdomen behind the medial arcuate ligament (*see Diaphragm*) and lies between the lumbar vertebral bodies and psoas major, passing into the pelvis anterior to the sacral ala. The two chains meet and terminate on the anterior surface of the coccyx.

- Ganglia:
  - cervical:
    - superior:
      - lies opposite C2–3.
      - branches: superior cardiac nerve, and branches to the upper four cervical nerves, internal carotid plexus and **cranial nerves** VII, IX, X and XII.
    - middle:
      - lies opposite C6.
      - branches: middle cardiac nerve, and branches to C5 and C6.
    - inferior:
      - lies opposite C7; often fused with the first thoracic ganglion to form the stellate ganglion on the neck of the first rib.
      - branches: inferior cardiac nerve, and branches to C7 and C8.
  - thoracic:
    - usually 12, although variable.
    - branches: to splanchnic and **intercostal nerves**.
  - lumbar: usually four ganglia.
  - sacral: usually four ganglia.
- Sympathetic innervation of viscera is via the cardiac, coeliac and hypogastric plexuses. The sympathetic nervous system is concerned with the 'flight or fight' response to stress. Stimulation causes:
  - pupillary dilatation and ciliary muscle relaxation.
  - tachycardia and increased **myocardial contractility**.
  - α-**adrenergic receptor**-mediated vasoconstriction (β_2-receptor-mediated vasodilatation in skeletal muscle, abdominal viscera, and coronary, pulmonary and renal circulations).
  - bronchodilatation and reduced bronchial secretion.
  - decreased GIT motility, contraction of sphincters and reduction of secretions (thick viscous secretion from salivary glands). Mixed effects on **insulin** and **glucagon** secretion (decreased by α-receptor stimulation, increased by β_2-receptor stimulation).
  - bladder relaxation and sphincteric contraction. Increased **renin** secretion.
  - variable effect on the **uterus**.
  - ejaculation of semen.
  - piloerection and sweating of palms.
  - hepatic glycogenolysis and adipose lipolysis.

Table 51 Actions of sympathomimetic drugs

Drug	Direct stimulation α	β	Indirect activity
Adrenaline	+	++	–
Noradrenaline	++	+	–
Isoprenaline	–	++	–
Phenylephrine	++	–	–
Methoxamine	++	–	–
Salbutamol	–	++	–
Ephedrine	+	+	++
Metaraminol	++	+	++
Amfetamine	+	+	++

Acetylcholine is the **neurotransmitter** at ganglia and the adrenal medulla; **noradrenaline** is the neurotransmitter at postganglionic nerve endings (except for sweat glands, where acetylcholine is the transmitter). The adrenal medulla is effectively a sympathetic ganglion that secretes directly into the bloodstream.

Central control of sympathetic activity is from the medulla, pons and ventromedial hypothalamus.

See also, Acetylcholine receptors; Sympathetic nerve blocks

Sympathomimetic drugs. Drugs that stimulate **adrenergic receptors**. Actions of individual drugs vary depending on whether they affect predominantly α- or β-receptors, or both. Some stimulate receptors directly; others act indirectly via release of endogenous **catecholamines** (Table 51).

Used clinically as **vasopressor, inotropic** and **bronchodilator drugs**. Amfetamine is used in narcolepsy for its CNS stimulant action.

See also, individual drugs

Synapse. Specialised junction between a **neurone** (presynaptic cell) and another (postsynaptic) cell, usually another neurone but also **muscle** or glandular cells. Allows unidirectional transmission of **action potentials** between cells (**synaptic transmission**), via **neurotransmitter** release (although electrical transmission across gap junctions also occurs). One presynaptic neurone may contribute to over 1000 synapses. Most presynaptic nerve endings bear terminal buttons (synaptic knobs), with up to several thousand from different cells contacting each postsynaptic neurone. The terminal buttons contain many mitochondria and vesicles containing neurotransmitter, and are separated from the postsynaptic membrane by the synaptic cleft (30–50-nm wide). Neurotransmitter receptors are present in high concentrations in the postsynaptic membrane opposite the terminal buttons.

See also, Neuromuscular junction

Synaptic transmission. Usually involves release from presynaptic cells of a **neurotransmitter** that passes across the synaptic cleft and binds to specific receptors in the postsynaptic membrane. This elicits a response in the postsynaptic cell (e.g. change in **membrane potential**, activation of a **second messenger**); the neurotransmitter is then broken down by a specific **enzyme** (e.g. **acetylcholinesterase**), diffuses into surrounding tissues or is taken up by the presynaptic nerve ending (e.g. **noradrenaline**).

Initiation of an **action potential** in the postsynaptic cell depends on the number and frequency of impulses arriving from different presynaptic cells; impulses may be excitatory or inhibitory, depending on the neurotransmitter/receptor complex. In addition, presynaptic inhibition and facilitation may occur, via neurones forming synapses at the presynaptic nerve ending.

Some **synapses** are electrical, with transmission across gap junctions; some are both electrical and chemical. A synaptic delay of at least 0.5 ms occurs at chemical synapses, but not at electrical ones.

See also, Neuromuscular transmission

Synchronised intermittent mandatory ventilation, *see Intermittent mandatory ventilation*

Syndrome of inappropriate antidiuretic hormone secretion (SIADH). Increased plasma **vasopressin** levels and water retention despite plasma hypo-osmolality and expanded or normal **ECF**.

- Caused by:
  - ectopic production of vasopressin, e.g. by carcinoma of bronchus, pancreas, prostate, colon and other tissue, or lymphoma.
  - pulmonary disease, e.g. **chest infection, TB**, abscess.
  - CNS disorders, e.g. brain tumour, **stroke, TBI, encephalitis, meningitis**, neurosurgery (e.g. on the **pituitary gland**).
  - stress, e.g. **pain**, severe illness, **trauma**.
  - acute intermittent **porphyria**.
  - drugs, e.g. vasopressin overtreatment, **oxytocin**, indometacin, antidepressants, chlorpropamide, carbamazepine.
- Features: those of euvolaemic **hyponatraemia**. Urinary sodium exceeds 20 mmol/l (often 50–150 mmol/l), plasma osmolality is low (<280 mosmol/kg), and urinary/plasma osmolality ratio exceeds 1.
- Treatment:
  - of primary cause.
  - traditionally, the mainstay of treatment has been with fluid restriction (e.g. with 1–1.5 l/day of isotonic saline) and remains appropriate for mild hyponatraemia. More recently, it has been shown that treatment with hypertonic saline and vasopressin receptor antagonists (e.g. tolvaptan) results in faster and more permanent resolution of SIADH.
  - **demeclocycline** 600 mg daily in divided doses if persistent (thought to block the renal effects of vasopressin). **Furosemide** and **phenytoin** have been used.

Verbalis J, Greenberg A, Burst V, et al (2016). Am J Med; 129: e9–23

See also, Cerebral salt-wasting syndrome

Syphilis. Sexually transmitted infection caused by the spirochaete *Treponema pallidum*.

- Divided clinically into:
  - primary stage: appearance of chancre at site of infection, 10 days–10 weeks after inoculation.
  - secondary stage: faint macular rash, condylomata and lymphadenopathy.
  - tertiary stage: lesions in skin, subcutaneous tissue, bone, tongue, testes, liver and CNS (meningovascular syphilis, tabes dorsalis, general paralysis of the insane).

Carditis and aortitis may occur, leading to ascending or arch **aortic aneurysm** and **aortic regurgitation**. Angina may occur in 50% of patients with aortitis.

Serological tests are strongly positive after 3 months in untreated cases. Treatment is usually with penicillin. Anaesthetic considerations are mainly related to the CVS effects. Blood donors are screened for syphilis before donation.
Hook EW (2017). Lancet; 389: 1550–7

Syringe labels. The system of colour-coded labels widely used in the UK differed from that in use in the USA, Canada, Australia and New Zealand, until in 2003 the Royal College of Anaesthetists, Association of Anaesthetists, Faculty of Accident and Emergency Medicine, and Intensive Care Society agreed to recommend the international system, updated in 2004:

- sedatives/tranquillisers: orange.
- induction agents: yellow.
- neuromuscular blocking drugs: red.
- opioids: blue.
- vasopressors: violet.
- local anaesthetics: grey.
- anticholinergics: green.
- antiemetics: salmon.
- others: white. Antagonists are marked by appropriately coloured oblique stripes on the label's upper and side edges.

Because of the importance of recognising **suxamethonium** and **adrenaline** rapidly, these two drugs are highlighted by their labels bearing a black upper half with the drug's name in reverse colour. Combinations of drugs bear both relevant colours.

Syringes. First use is attributed to both Wood and Pravaz in 1855, although parenteral administration of drugs had been described earlier (e.g. by Wren in 1656). Disposable polystyrene or polypropylene syringes are now widely used. Glass syringes are used for injecting drugs that are incompatible with plastic (e.g. **paraldehyde**) and for location of the **epidural space**. Plastic 'loss of resistance devices' resemble syringes but do not meet the required standards to be termed as such.
[Alexander Wood (1817–1884), Scottish physician; Charles Gabriel Pravaz (1791–1853), French surgeon; Sir Christopher Wren (1632–1723), English architect, mathematician and physicist]
Ball C, Westhorpe R (2000). Anaesth Intensive Care; 28: 125

Systemic inflammatory response syndrome (SIRS). Clinical state resulting from many different disease processes (e.g. **trauma, pancreatitis, burns**, infection) but which are all thought to involve activation of the cytokine cascade. Defined as two or more of:

- hypothermia (<36°C) or hyperthermia (>38°C).
- heart rate >90 beats/min.
- tachypnoea (>20 breaths/min.)
- leucopenia (<4000/mm^3), leucocytosis (>12 000/mm^3), or the presence of greater than 10% immature neutrophils.

Sepsis has previously been defined as SIRS due to infection, but SIRS is no longer included in the definition as it is both common and too non-specific to be of use clinically.

Systemic lupus erythematosus (SLE). **Connective tissue disease** most commonly affecting women aged 15–55, with a prevalence of up to 250 per 100 000. More common in Afro-Caribbeans. Its aetiology is unknown; both genetic and environmental factors have been implicated. May also be drug-induced; classic causes include **methyldopa, procainamide** and **hydralazine**. Involves many abnormalities of the immune system, with autoantibodies a central feature; they may affect tissues directly or via immune complex deposition. General features and anaesthetic considerations are as for connective tissue diseases; the most common features of SLE are fatigue, fever, arthralgia and myalgia, skin rashes, psychological involvement and haematological abnormalities (**thrombocytopenia** and **anaemia** in about 50% and lupus anticoagulant in about 10%; the latter may prolong **coagulation**, especially the intrinsic pathway. Risk of bleeding is not increased if other factors and **platelets** are normal, but risk of thrombosis is increased, possibly via inhibition of **prostacyclin** production and platelet aggregation).

Renal, cardiac and pulmonary complications (e.g. nephritis, peri- or **myocarditis**, pneumonitis) each occur in about 50% of cases. Patients may present with acute organ failure requiring admission to the ICU. Laryngeal oedema, epiglottitis and cricoarytenoiditis requiring emergency intubation have been reported.

Diagnosed by clinical features and results of investigations, especially autoantibody titres (e.g. antinuclear and anti-double-stranded DNA antibodies), although these may be elevated in other connective tissue diseases and other conditions.

Treatment includes **corticosteroids, NSAIDs, immunosuppressive drugs** and **antimalarial drugs**. Prognosis is generally good, although long-term treatment is usually required; prognosis is worse with CNS involvement, hypertension and early onset.

Systemic sclerosis (SS; Scleroderma). Rare **connective tissue disease** most commonly affecting women in their 40s. Its aetiology is unknown. Involves increased deposition of connective tissue components and fibrosis affecting small vessels, skin and other tissues. General features and anaesthetic considerations are as for connective tissue diseases; the disease may be limited to the skin or be truly systemic, involving:

- peripheral vasculature and skin: calluses, ulceration or ischaemia of the extremities may occur. The tight skin may make iv cannulation or mouth opening difficult.
- **oesophagus**: impaired motility occurs in about 90% of cases, with potential risk of **aspiration of gastric contents.**
- lungs: pleurisy, effusions, fibrosis and **pulmonary hypertension** are common.
- kidneys: affected to some degree in most patients with diffuse SS. Hypertension may signal life-threatening renal impairment (scleroderma renal crisis) and the need for **angiotensin converting enzyme inhibitor** therapy; **dialysis** is required in 25% of patients. Function may recover after many years' dysfunction.
- heart: involved in over 90% of cases, usually pericardial effusion.
- others: joints, muscle peripheral nerves.

The CREST syndrome comprises calcinosis, Raynaud's phenomenon, (o)esophagitis, sclerodactyly and telangiectasia.

Treatment includes **penicillamine**, colchicine and **immunosuppressive drugs**, including corticosteroids.
[Maurice Raynaud (1834–1881), French physician]
Denton CP, Khanna D (2017). Lancet; 390: 1685–99

Systemic vascular resistance (SVR; Peripheral vascular resistance, PVR; Total peripheral resistance, TPR). **Resistance** against which the heart pumps. May be calculated using the principle of **Ohm's law**:

$$\text{SVR (dyne s/cm}^5) = \frac{\text{MAP} - \text{CVP (mmHg)}}{\text{cardiac output (1/min)}} \times 80 \text{ (correction factor)}$$

Normally 1000–1500 dyne s/cm^5 (N.B. 1 dyne s/cm^5 = 100 N s/m^5).

The above equation ignores the effects of blood **viscosity**, pulsatile **flow** and the different results of pressure changes on different vascular beds.

- SVR is mainly determined by the diameter of the arterioles, small changes in their calibre producing large changes in resistance. Arteriolar calibre may be affected by:
  - intrinsic contractile response of vascular smooth muscle to increased intravascular pressure (myogenic theory of **autoregulation**).
  - locally produced substances causing vasodilatation (e.g. CO_2, **potassium** and **hydrogen ions**, **lactic acid**, **histamine**, **nitric oxide**, **adenosine**, **prostaglandins** and **kinins**; metabolic theory of autoregulation), or vasoconstriction, e.g. **5-HT**. **Hypoxia** causes vasodilatation peripherally and vasoconstriction in the lungs. Increased temperature causes vasodilatation, whereas cold causes vasoconstriction.
  - neural innervation:
    - **α-adrenergic receptors**: the most important type, affecting most vessels. Stimulation causes vasoconstriction.
    - β_2-adrenergic receptors: stimulation causes vasodilatation of arterioles to muscle and viscera.
    - **dopamine receptors**: stimulation causes vasodilatation of renal and splanchnic vessels.
    - sympathetic cholinergic receptors: stimulation causes vasodilatation in skeletal muscle.
    - other **neurotransmitters** may be involved, e.g. **substance P**, **vasoactive intestinal peptide**.
  - circulating substances, e.g. **noradrenaline**, angiotensin II, **vasopressin**, **vasopressor drugs** (causing vasoconstriction); **vasodilator drugs**, **atrial natriuretic peptide** (causing vasodilatation). **Adrenaline** causes vasodilatation in skeletal muscle and the liver. Toxins released in **septic shock** may cause vasodilatation. The locally produced substances above may also cause systemic effects.

SVR increases progressively with age. Chronically increased SVR is the hallmark of essential **hypertension**.

SVR ÷ body surface area (SVR index; SVRI) adjusts for differences in body size between individuals.

See also, Arterial blood pressure; Renin/angiotensin system

Systole, *see Cardiac cycle*

Systolic time intervals. Measurements derived from the systolic phase of the **cardiac cycle**, obtained from simultaneous **phonocardiography** and recording of **ECG** and carotid artery tracing. Allow evaluation of left ventricular function.

- Include:
  - QS_2 (qA_2): interval between the ECG **QRS complex** and the aortic component of the second **heart sound**.
  - left ventricular ejection time (LVET): period from the beginning of the carotid upstroke to the dicrotic notch.
  - pre-ejection period (PEP): QS_2 – LVET. Represents the rate of ventricular isometric pressure change, i.e., dp/dt.
  - others, e.g. duration of mechanical systole, are less commonly measured. Ratios of the intervals have been calculated, e.g. PEP ÷ LVET.

T

t$_{1/2}$, *see Half-life*

T-piece breathing systems, *see Anaesthetic breathing systems*

t tests, *see Statistical tests*

T wave. Wave on the ECG representing ventricular repolarisation (*see Fig. 60b;* **Electrocardiography**). Normally upright in leads I, II and V_{3-6}; the upper height limit is 5 mm in the standard leads and 10 mm in the chest leads.

- Abnormalities:
  - may be inverted in **myocardial ischaemia**, ventricular hypertrophy, **mitral valve prolapse**, **bundle branch block** and **digoxin** toxicity.
  - may be notched in **pericarditis**.
  - tall peaked waves may occur in **hyperkalaemia**.

Tachycardias, *see Sinus tachycardia; Supraventricular tachycardia; Ventricular tachycardia*

Tachykinins. Group of neuropeptides involved in cardiovascular, respiratory, endocrine and behavioural responses. Include **substance P**, neurokinin A and neurokinin B, which are natural agonists at NK1, NK2 and NK3 **G protein coupled receptors**, respectively. Particular interest has focused on NK1 and NK2 receptor activation, which results in bronchoconstriction, and on development of **neurokinin-1 receptor antagonists** as antiemetic drugs.

Steinhoff MS, von Mentzer B, Geppetti P (2014). Physiol Rev; 94: 265–301

Tachyphylaxis. Term usually referring to acute drug **tolerance**, usually due to depletion of receptors (or for indirectly acting drugs, depletion of neurotransmitter/signalling molecule) following repeated exposure.

TACO, *see Blood transfusion*

Tacrine, *see Tetrahydroaminacrine*

Tacrolimus. **Immunosuppressive drug**; acts by inhibiting cytotoxic lymphocyte proliferation and cytokine expression. Used to prevent graft rejection after heart, lung, liver and renal **transplantation**. A topical preparation is available for treatment of eczema. Extensively bound to red blood cells and plasma proteins. Achieves steady-state concentrations after about 3 days' administration; **half-life** varies from 3 to 40 h with mainly hepatic metabolism and biliary excretion. Toxicity and rejection have occurred when switching between different oral brands.

- Dosage varies widely according to preparation and organ transplanted. May be given 1-2 oral doses or iv infusion over 24 h.
- Side effects: renal impairment, central and peripheral neurological disturbances, cardiomyopathy, diabetes.

Tamponade, *see Cardiac tamponade*

TAP block, *see Transversus abdominis plane block*

Tapentadol hydrochloride. **Opioid analgesic drug**, similar in structure to **tramadol**, used to treat moderate-to-severe pain. Acts centrally via agonism at mu **opioid receptors** (50 times less affinity than **morphine**) and peripherally via inhibition of reuptake of **noradrenaline**. Rapidly absorbed via the oral route; undergoes extensive **first-pass metabolism**. Available in immediate-release and prolonged-release forms. Cleared by hepatic metabolism to inactive metabolites, followed by renal excretion; used with caution in patients with **hepatic failure**.

- Dosage: 50 mg orally 4–6-hourly, adjusted to response, maximum 600 mg daily.
- Side effects: nausea, vomiting, dizziness, dry mouth, sweating, confusion, hallucinations, seizures, respiratory depression, sedation (the latter two less commonly than with morphine). Drug dependence and withdrawal have been reported, especially following prolonged treatment.

Ramaswamy S, Chang S, Mehta V (2015). Anaesthesia; 70: 518–22

Target-controlled infusion (TCI). Technique utilising a computer-controlled intravenous infusion device to achieve and maintain a desired target drug concentration (in plasma, or at the 'effect site'). May be used for **sedation** or **total intravenous anaesthesia**.

- Requires:
  - an accurate infusion pump.
  - a computer programmed with an algorithm based on a model of the drug's **pharmacokinetics**. Familiarity with the specific model incorporated into the TCI system being used is important; the clinical effect associated with a given target concentration for one model may be different for another.
  - an interface for the anaesthetist to select the appropriate drug, target concentration and patient-specific variables (e.g. weight, sex, age).
  - a second microprocessor that calculates the expected plasma concentration from the amount of drug actually given, and shuts down the pump if there is a discrepancy with that predicted by the first.

The first licensed TCI system was for **propofol**, using a proprietary microprocessor that could only be used with electronically tagged prefilled syringes. Since the expiry of the patent on propofol, several 'open-label' pharmacokinetic protocols have been developed and incorporated into a range of TCI devices. The two models most commonly used for propofol TCI are the Marsh and the Schnider models:

- Marsh:
  - older model (1991; modified in 2000).
  - higher effect site elimination rate constant (k_{e0}) i.e. more rapid equilibration.

- includes total body weight but not age in the calculation.
- calculates a larger central compartment, a slower time to peak effect and a slower fall in concentration when the infusion is stopped.

- Schnider:
  - more recent model (1998).
  - includes age, height, lean body mass (calculated from total body weight) and gender in the calculation.
  - calculates k_{e0} for each patient.
  - uses a fixed (smaller) central compartment, and calculates a faster time to peak effect and a faster fall in concentration when the infusion is stopped.

TCI systems for other drugs (e.g. **remifentanil** and **sufentanil**) are also available and widely used. The Minto model was described for remifentanil in 1997, and is a three-compartment model using lean body mass (calculated from total body weight), height, age and gender, with k_{e0} adjusted for age.

The TCI models are based largely on healthy volunteers and several assumptions that may not apply to physiologically challenged patients undergoing surgery. It is therefore important to monitor the clinical effect of any drug given using TCI systems.

[Brian Marsh, Irish intensivist; Thomas W. Schnider, Swiss anaesthetist/intensivist; Charles Minto, Australian anaesthetist]

Targeted temperature management (TTM). Therapeutic **hypothermia** (to 32°–36°C) to provide **cerebral protection**. Mechanisms include reduction of: **cerebral metabolism**; release of excitatory amino acids (e.g. **glutamate**); intracellular **calcium** levels; and **free radicals**. Also helps maintain integrity of the **blood–brain barrier**.

Induction of TTM is usually performed with infusion of cold saline (e.g. 2 l at 4°C), that is safe and effective without causing pulmonary oedema. Maintenance of desired temperature is with circulating cold-water blankets/suits, ice packs, external central venous catheter heat exchange devices or via extracorporeal circuits. Rewarming must be slow (e.g. 0.1°–0.25°C/h) to minimise complications (*see later*).

- Clinical applications:
  - cardiac arrest: two randomised controlled trials in 2002 showed improved neurological outcome in comatose patients who had suffered out-of-hospital cardiac arrest with a 'shockable' rhythm treated with TTM (32°–34°C) within two hours of return of spontaneous circulation (ROSC) and maintained for 12–24 h. A subsequent trial showed similar benefit of cooling to 36°C. Standard of **post-resuscitation care** is now to cool cardiac arrest patients to 36°C irrespective of the cardiac rhythm preceding the ROSC.
  - neonatal hypoxic ischaemic encephalopathy: TTM (to 34°–35°C) improves survival and reduces neurological disability. Treatment should be started within 6 hours of birth and continued for up to 72 h.
  - **TBI**: although TTM reduces raised **ICP** following TBI, trials in both adults and children have failed to show benefit, with some showing increased mortality and morbidity.
  - **stroke**: although TTM may reduce infarct size in ischaemic stroke, trials are ongoing. Intraoperative cooling during aneurysm surgery following **subarachnoid haemorrhage** does not improve outcome and increases complications.
- Complications:
  - cardiac dysfunction: includes reduced myocardial contractility, HR, arterial BP and cardiac output. Temperatures <32°C are associated with AF, VT and VF.
  - electrolyte disturbances: **hypokalaemia** and **hypophosphataemia** occur during cooling and levels rise during rewarming; the latter must be controlled to avoid severe **hyperkalaemia**.
  - acid–base abnormalities and **hyperglycaemia** due to insulin resistance. Rewarming may result in **hypoglycaemia**.
  - immune dysfunction resulting in increased incidence of bacterial infection, especially pneumonia.
  - coagulation disturbance is unusual if temperature is maintained >35°C.

Perman SM, Goyal M, Neumar RW, et al (2014). Chest; 145: 386–93

TB, *see Tuberculosis*

TBI, *see Traumatic brain injury*

TCD, *see Transcranial Doppler ultrasound*

TEE, Transesophageal echocardiography, *see Transoesophageal echocardiography*

Teeth. Composed of the crown (consisting of enamel, dentine and pulp from outside inwards) and root. All parts may be damaged during anaesthesia; the deeper the damage, the more extensive is the treatment required. Traumatic damage is involved in about 30% of malpractice claims against anaesthetists, with a rough incidence of 1:1000 general anaesthetics and, because of its frequency, claims are rarely contested. Damage most commonly occurs during intubation or postoperatively when the patient bites on an oral airway. **Preoperative assessment** of the teeth is essential, recording any loose, chipped or false teeth. Patients with caries, prostheses and periodontal disease, and those in whom tracheal intubation is difficult, are at particular risk. Appropriate warnings should be given and noted on the anaesthetic chart preoperatively.

Dentures and removable bridges are traditionally removed before anaesthesia, in case they become dislodged and obstruct or pass into the airway. However, the need for routine preoperative removal of dentures has been questioned because this may cause distress to patients. If damage to teeth does occur, avulsed or broken teeth should be retrieved and stored in saline for possible reimplantation (up to 90% success rate if performed within 30 min); the extent of damage should be documented and the patient referred as soon as possible to a dentist (ideally in the same hospital) who can carry out necessary emergency treatment.

Yasny JS (2009). Anesth Analg; 108: 1564–73

See also, Dental surgery; Mandibular nerve blocks; Maxillary nerve blocks

Teicoplanin. Glycopeptide and **antibacterial drug**, related to **vancomycin** but longer acting, allowing once-daily dosing. Active against most gram-positive organisms, as for vancomycin. 90% protein-bound, with a **half-life** of 7 days. Excreted unchanged in urine.

- Dosage: 400 mg (10 mg/kg in endocarditis, 12 mg/kg in bone/joint infections) bd for three doses, od thereafter. 400 mg may also be given up to 30 min before surgery

Table 52 Corresponding points on different temperature scales

	Kelvin (K)	Celsius (°C)	Fahrenheit (°F)
Absolute zero	0	−273	−459
Melting point of ice	273	0	32
Boiling point of water	373	100	212

for prophylaxis (800 mg in open fractures). Has also been used orally (100–200 mg bd for 10–14 days) in **pseudomembranous colitis**.
- Side effects: GIT disturbance, allergic reactions, blood dyscrasias, hepatic and renal impairment, erythema.

Temazepam. **Benzodiazepine** used for insomnia, and commonly used for **premedication**. Shorter acting than **diazepam**, with faster onset of action. **Half-life** is 8 h.

10–30 mg orally, 45–60 min preoperatively, is usually an effective anxiolytic. For children, 0.5 mg/kg may be given. Gel-filled capsules were withdrawn from NHS use in 1995 because of abuse by iv drug users, the liquefied gel causing marked vascular damage on injection. Temazepam became a Schedule 3 **Controlled Drug** in 1996, although without special prescription requirements; this exemption was removed in 2015 and prescriptions for temazepam are now required to meet the same requirements as for other Schedule 3 controlled drugs.
See also, Misuse of Drugs Act

Temperature. Property of a system that determines whether **heat** is transferred to or from other systems. Related to the mean kinetic energy of its constituent particles. Three temperature scales are recognised: **Kelvin** (formerly Absolute) scale, Celsius (formerly Centigrade) scale and Fahrenheit scale (Table 52). The SI **unit** of temperature is the kelvin.
[Anders Celsius (1701–1744), Swedish scientist; Gabriel D Fahrenheit (1686–1736), German scientist]

Temperature measurement. Performed routinely as part of basic clinical monitoring including wards, ICUs, and perioperatively to monitor **heat loss during anaesthesia** and detect **hyperthermia**.
- Methods used:
  - electrical:
    - thermocouple: relies on the Seebeck effect; i.e., the production of voltage at the junction of two different conductors joined in a loop; the magnitude of the voltage generated is proportional to the **temperature** difference between the two junctions. The circuit thus consists of a measuring junction and a reference junction, with measurement of the voltage difference between the two. Because voltage is also produced at the reference junction, electrical manipulation is required to compensate for changes in temperature at the latter.
    - thermistor: semiconductor whose resistance changes predictably with temperature; a commonly used type consists of a metal oxide bead with resistance that falls exponentially as temperature rises. Small enough to be placed within body cavities. Calibration may be difficult.
    - platinum resistance wire: resistance increases proportionately with temperature. Very accurate but fragile.
  - non-electrical:
    - liquid thermometers: the liquid (usually mercury) expands as temperature increases, and moves out of its glass bulb and up the barrel of the instrument. Temperature is read from a scale along its length. A constriction just above the bulb prevents the mercury from withdrawing back into the bulb. Alcohol is used for very low temperatures.
    - gas expansion thermometers, e.g. an anaeroid gauge used for **pressure measurement** is calibrated in units of temperature. Accuracy is poor and calibration may be difficult.
    - bimetallic strip, arranged in a coil. A pointer is moved by coiling or uncoiling of the strip as temperature changes.
    - infrared thermometry: relies on the principle that the maximal amount of radiation (black box radiation) emitted by a body depends only on that body's temperature. The radiation emitted by a surface is less than that emitted by a black body at the same temperature; the ratio is defined as emissivity of the surface. Measurement of radiation emitted by a surface plus knowledge of its emissivity allows calculation of the surface's temperature. Infrared thermometers detect infrared radiation emitted by the tympanic membrane and calculate its temperature in under a second, allowing for heat loss in the ear canal. They may also be used to measure surface temperature at other sites (e.g. skin) or to estimate temperature at these sites from tympanic membrane temperature.
    - chemical thermometers: consist of a plastic strip containing a number of cells, each holding liquid crystals that melt and change colour according to temperature. Accurate to 0.5°C.
- Sites of measurement:
  - tympanic membrane: correlates most closely with hypothalamic temperature, and has a rapid response time. Carries risk of tympanic perforation if direct contact techniques are used.
  - oesophageal: accurate if the lower third is used, otherwise measured temperature is influenced by the temperature of inspired gases.
  - nasopharyngeal and bladder: similar to oesophageal.
  - rectal: usually 0.5°–1.0°C higher than core temperature, because of bacterial fermentation. Response time is slow because of insulation by faeces.
  - blood: thermistors incorporated into pulmonary artery catheters allow continuous measurement.
  - skin: does not reflect core temperature. The difference between core and skin temperatures gives some indication of peripheral perfusion, and may be used in the ICU.

[Thomas J Seebeck (1770–1831), Russian-born German physicist]

Temperature regulation. Humans are homeothermic, maintaining body core **temperature** at 37° ± 1°C. The core usually includes cranial, thoracic, abdominal and pelvic contents, and variable amounts of the deep portions of the limbs. Temperature is lowest at night and highest in mid-afternoon, also varying with the menstrual cycle.

Constant temperature is required for optimal **enzyme** activity. Denaturation of proteins occurs at 42°C. Loss of consciousness occurs at **hypothermia** below 30°C.

- Mechanisms of heat loss/gain:
  - heat gain:
    - from the environment.
    - from **metabolism** (mainly in the brain, liver and kidneys): approximately 80 W is produced in an average man under resting conditions. This would raise body temperature by about 1°C/h if totally insulated. Vigorous muscular activity may increase heat production by up to 20 times. In babies, **brown fat** produces significant heat.
  - heat loss:
    - radiation from the skin. May account for 40% of total loss.
    - convection: related to airflow (e.g. 'wind chill'). Accounts for up to 40% of total loss.
    - evaporation from the respiratory tract and skin: the latter is increased by sweating, which normally accounts for 20% of total loss, but this figure may increase markedly.
    - conduction: of little importance in air, but significant in water.

Temperature-sensitive cells are present in the anterior **hypothalamus** (thought to be the most important site), **brainstem, spinal cord**, skin, skeletal muscle and abdominal viscera. Peripheral temperature receptors are primary afferent nerve endings and respond to cold and hot stimuli via Aδ and C fibres, respectively. Central control of thermoregulation is by the hypothalamus. Efferents pass via the **sympathetic nervous system** to blood vessels, sweat glands and piloerector muscles. Local reflexes are also involved. Efferents also pass to somatic motor centres in the lower brainstem to cause shivering, and to higher centres.

- Regulatory mechanisms:
  - behavioural, e.g. curling up in the cold, wearing appropriate clothing.
  - skin blood flow: may be altered by vasodilatation or vasoconstriction of skin vessels, and by opening or closing of arteriovenous anastomoses in the skin. Affects all routes of heat loss. Alteration alone is sufficient to maintain constant body temperature in environments of 20°–28°C in adults and 35°–37°C in **neonates** (**thermoneutral range**).
  - shivering and piloerection (reduced or absent in babies, brown fat metabolism occurring instead). Reflex shivering can hinder induced hypothermia; measures to inhibit shivering include use of **neuromuscular blocking drugs**, **α_2-adrenergic receptor agonists** and skin surface warming (with core cooling).
  - sweating.

Pitoni S, Sinclair HL, Andrews PJD (2011). Curr Opin Crit Care; 17: 115–21

See also, Heat loss during anaesthesia

Temporomandibular joint (TMJ). Synovial joint between the mandibular condyle and the articular surface of the squamous temporal bone. Protrusion, retraction and grinding movements of the lower jaw occur by a gliding mechanism whereas mouth opening and closing involve gliding and hinging movements. Joint stability is least when the mouth is fully open (e.g. during laryngoscopy) and forward dislocation may occur. Affected by **rheumatoid arthritis**, degenerative disease, **ankylosing spondylitis** and **systemic sclerosis**; in addition, TMJ disorders (e.g. caused by prolonged mouth opening during dental treatment or by joint degeneration) are the commonest cause of facial pain. Mouth opening may be severely limited, hindering laryngoscopy.

See also, Intubation, difficult; Trismus

Tenecteplase. **Fibrinolytic drug**, used in acute management of **acute coronary syndromes**. Binds to fibrin, the resultant complex converting plasminogen to plasmin, which dissolves the fibrin. Has a lower rate of bleeding complications than **alteplase**.

- Dosage: 0.3–0.5 mg/kg (to a maximum of 50 mg) iv over 10 s.
- Side effects: as for fibrinolytic drugs.

TENS, *see Transcutaneous electrical nerve stimulation*

Tensilon test, *see Edrophonium*

Tension. In physics, another word for **force**, implying stretching (cf. compression). Also refers to the **partial pressure** of a **gas** in solution.

Tension time index. Area between tracings of left ventricular pressure and aortic root pressure during systole, multiplied by heart rate (*see Fig. 62;* **Endocardial viability ratio**). Represents myocardial workload and hence O_2 demand; when taken in conjunction with **diastolic pressure time index**, it may indicate the myocardial O_2 supply/demand ratio and the likelihood of **myocardial ischaemia**.

Terbutaline sulfate. **β-Adrenergic receptor agonist**, used as a **bronchodilator drug** and **tocolytic drug**. Has similar effects to **salbutamol**, but possibly has less cardiac effect.

- Dosage:
  - 2.5–5 mg orally bd/tds.
  - 250–500 μg im/sc qds as required.
  - 250–500 μg iv slowly, repeated as required. 1–5 μg/min infusion may be used (containing 3–5 μg/ml). Up to 20 μg/min may be required in premature labour.
  - 1–2 puffs by aerosol (250–500 μg) tds/qds.
  - 5–10 mg by nebulised solution qds as required.
- Side effects: as for salbutamol.

Terlipressin, *see Vasopressin*

Terminal care, *see Palliative care; Withdrawal of treatment in ICU*

Test dose, epidural. In **epidural anaesthesia**, injection of a small amount of **local anaesthetic agent** through the catheter before injection of the main dose, in order to identify accidental subarachnoid or iv placement of the catheter. Less commonly performed before 'through the needle' epidural block, because leakage of CSF or blood should be more easily noticeable.

Controversial, because it is not always reliable. The volume and strength of the test solution are also controversial. 3 ml 2% **lidocaine** with **adrenaline** 1:200 000 has been suggested as the ideal solution; subarachnoid injection should produce **spinal anaesthesia** within 2–3 min, and iv injection produces tachycardia within 90 s. Injection of **fentanyl** 50–100 μg or 1 ml air (with **Doppler** monitoring) has also been used. In modern 'low-dose' techniques (e.g. epidural analgesia for labour), each dose 'acts as its own test' because a standard dose of, e.g. 10 ml bupivacaine 0.1% with 20 μg fentanyl would be expected to produce noticeable effects were it to be injected subarachnoid or

iv without causing a dangerously high block or severe systemic toxicity.
Camorcia M (2009). Curr Opin Anesthesiol; 22: 336–40

Tetanic contraction. Sustained **muscle contraction** caused by repetitive electrical stimulation of a motor nerve. About 25 Hz stimulation is required for frequent enough **action potentials** to produce it, although the necessary rate varies according to the muscle studied. The force produced exceeds that of single muscle twitches. During tetanic contraction, **acetylcholine** is mobilised from reserve stores to the readily available pool.

Produced during **neuromuscular blockade monitoring**. *See also, Neuromuscular junction; Neuromuscular transmission; Post-tetanic potentiation*

Tetanus. Disease caused by infection with *Clostridium tetani*, a prevalent spore-forming gram-positive bacillus found in soil, dust and faeces. Inoculation may be via minor injury. Rare in developed countries following immunisation programmes, but a consistent cause of deaths worldwide. Has sporadically been reported in drug abusers 'skin-popping' contaminated heroin.

Clinical features are caused by a potent **exotoxin**, tetanospasmin, which moves retrogradely along peripheral nerves to the **spinal cord**, where it blocks release of neurotransmitters at inhibitory neurons, causing muscle spasm and autonomic disturbance. Incubation period is 3–21 days (average 7 days). Local infection may cause muscle spasm around the site of injury; generalised tetanus is characterised by **trismus**, irritability, rigidity and opisthotonos. Cardiac **arrhythmias**/arrest and **hypertension** may occur due to sympathetic hyperactivity. As binding of tetanospasmin is irreversible, recovery depends on formation of new nerve terminals. The diagnosis is based on clinical findings but the spatula test (touching the oropharynx with a wooden spatula; in tetanus this results in spasm of the masseter muscles causing biting of the spatula) is highly sensitive and specific for tetanus.

- Treatment:
  - human antitetanus **immunoglobulin** (5000–10 000 units): neutralises circulating toxin.
  - surgical excision and debridement of the wound.
  - **metronidazole** to eradicate existing organisms.
  - **sedation, neuromuscular blocking drugs** and **IPPV** may be required. **Dantrolene** and **magnesium sulfate** have been used. The latter reduces sympathetic overactivity and reduces spasm by decreasing presynaptic activity.
  - of cardiovascular complications.

Mortality is 15% in those treated in modern ICUs (greater in previously unvaccinated individuals, if age exceeds 50, and if generalised spasms rapidly follow initial symptoms).

Active immunisation with tetanus vaccine should always be performed in **trauma** and **burns** unless within 5–10 years of previous administration. Antitetanus immunoglobulin is given to non-immune patients with heavily contaminated or old wounds.
Rodrigo C, Fernando D, Rajapakse S (2014). Crit Care; 18: 217
See also, Clostridial infections

Tetany. Increased sensitivity of excitable cells, manifested as peripheral muscle spasm. Usually facial and carpopedal, the shape of the hand in the latter termed *main d'accoucheur* (French: obstetrician's hand). Usually caused by **hypocalcaemia**; it also occurs in **hypomagnesaemia** and may be hereditary.

Tetracaine hydrochloride (Amethocaine). Ester **local anaesthetic agent**, introduced in 1931. Widely used in the USA for **spinal anaesthesia**; in the UK, used only for topical anaesthesia, e.g. in ophthalmology. More potent and longer lasting than **lidocaine**, but more toxic. Toxicity resembles that of **cocaine**. Weak base with a **p*K*** of 8.5. Rapidly absorbed from mucous membranes. Hydrolysed completely by plasma **cholinesterase** to form butylaminobenzoic acid and dimethylaminoethanol. Administration: 0.5%–1% solution for spinal anaesthesia; 0.4%–0.5% for **epidural anaesthesia**; 0.1%–0.2% solution for infiltration, usually with adrenaline; 0.5%–1% solutions for surface analgesia.

Available in a 4% gel for topical anaesthesia of the skin, e.g. before venepuncture. The melting point of the drug is lowered by the formation of specific hydrates within the gel. The resultant oil globules penetrate the skin readily with onset of action about 30–45 min; effects last 4–6 h. Skin blistering may occur. Has been combined with **lidocaine** (7% concentration of each), either in a cream or in a patch including a heating compound, for topical anaesthesia before venepuncture and minor skin procedures.

Maximal safe dose: 1.5 mg/kg.

Tetracyclines. Broad-spectrum **antibacterial drugs**, used mainly for chlamydia, rickettsia, spirochaete and brucella infections, certain **mycoplasma infections**, acne, acute exacerbations of **COPD** and **leptospirosis**. Several exist, with **tigecycline** the only one available for iv administration in the UK. Tetracycline has also been instilled into the pleural cavity to treat recurrent pleural effusions.

- Side effects: stained teeth (if given to children), renal impairment, GIT upset, benign intracranial hypertension, hepatic impairment.

Tetrahydroaminacrine hydrochloride (Tetrahydroaminoacridine; Tacrine). **Acetylcholinesterase inhibitor** formerly used to prolong the action of, and prevent muscle pains following, **suxamethonium**, and as a central stimulant. Was reintroduced as a treatment for Alzheimer's disease in 2005 but withdrawn in 2013 because of side effects.
[Alois Alzheimer (1864–1915), German neurologist and pathologist]

Tetrodotoxin. Toxin, obtained from puffer fish that selectively blocks neuronal voltage-gated fast sodium channels. Used experimentally, e.g. for investigating **neuromuscular transmission**.

TEVAR, Thoracic endovascular aneurysm repair, *see Aortic aneurysm, thoracic*

Thalassaemia. Group of autosomally inherited disorders involving decreased production of the α or β chains of **haemoglobin** (Hb). More common in Mediterranean, African and Asian areas. Severity is related to the pattern of inheritance of the Hb genes (normally, one β gene and two α genes are inherited from each parent).

- Divided into:
  - β thalassaemia:
    - not apparent immediately as **fetal haemoglobin** does not contain β chains.
    - heterozygous β thalassaemia (thalassaemia minor) produces mild (often asymptomatic) **anaemia**, but

may be associated with other types of Hb (e.g. HbC, HbE, HbS); resultant anaemia may vary from mild to severe.
- homozygous β thalassaemia (Cooley's anaemia; thalassaemia major) results in severe anaemia in infancy, with no production of HbA. Features include craniofacial bone hyperplasia, hepatosplenomegaly and **cardiac failure**. Haemosiderosis may occur due to repeated **blood transfusion**. Usually fatal before adulthood, although bone marrow transplantation may offer a cure. Some genetic subtypes are associated with a milder clinical course (thalassaemia intermedia).
- α thalassaemia: severity varies, depending on the number of gene deletions. Usually causes mild anaemia; deletion of all four α genes is incompatible with life.

[Thomas B Cooley (1871–1945), US paediatrician]

Taher AT, Weatherall DJ, Cappellini MD (2018). Lancet; 391: 155–67

THAM, tris-(hydroxymethyl)-aminomethane, *see 2-Amino-2-hydroxymethyl-1,3-propanediol*

Theophylline. **Bronchodilator drug**, used alone or in combination with ethylenediamine as **aminophylline**. Actions and effects are as for aminophylline.
- Dosage: slow-release preparations, 200–500 mg bd depending on preparation.

Therapeutic intervention scoring system (TISS). Scoring system for assessing the severity of critical illness according to the number of interventions a patient receives. Originally comprising over 70 interventions that were scored 1–4 according to complexity and invasiveness; more recent modifications have reduced this number to 28. Although of value in an individual clinician's practice, the score for a particular patient may vary between clinicians and units according to differences in treatment strategies. Has been used as a means of assessing the need and cost of ICU resources.

Miranda DR (1997). Intensive Care Med; 23: 615–17

Therapeutic ratio/index. Relationship between the doses of a drug required to produce toxic and therapeutic effects. A drug with a high therapeutic ratio has a greater margin of safety than one with low therapeutic ratio. Defined experimentally as the ratio of median lethal dose to median effective dose:

$$\frac{LD_{50}}{ED_{50}}$$

Thermal conductivity detector, *see Katharometer*

Thermistor, *see Temperature measurement*

Thermocouple, *see Temperature measurement*

Thermodilution cardiac output measurement, *see Cardiac output measurement*

Thermoneutral range. Temperature range in which **temperature regulation** may be maintained by changes in skin blood flow alone. Corresponds to the temperature that feels 'comfortable'. About 20°–28°C in adults and 35°–37°C in **neonates**. Neonatal metabolic rate and mortality are reduced if body temperature is kept within the thermoneutral range.

Thiamylal sodium. **Intravenous anaesthetic agent**, with similar properties to **thiopental**. Unavailable in the UK.

Thiazide diuretics. Group of **diuretics** used to treat mild **hypertension**, **oedema** caused by **cardiac failure** and nephrogenic **diabetes insipidus**. Chlorothiazide was the first to be studied but many now exist, e.g. bendroflumethiazide (bendrofluazide). Act mainly at the proximal part of the distal convoluted tubule of the **nephron**, where they inhibit **sodium** reabsorption. They also act at the proximal tubule, causing weak inhibition of **carbonic anhydrase** and increasing **bicarbonate** and **potassium** excretion, and have a direct vasodilator action. Their antihypertensive action increases only slightly as dosage is increased. Rapidly absorbed from the GIT with onset of action within 1–2 h, lasting 12–24 h. Some non-thiazide drugs have thiazide-like properties (e.g. chlortalidone, metolazone).

Side effects include **hypokalaemia**, **hyponatraemia**, hyperuricaemia, **hypomagnesaemia**, hypochloraemic **alkalosis**, **hyperglycaemia**, hypercholesterolaemia, exacerbation of renal and hepatic impairment, impotence, and, rarely, rashes and **thrombocytopenia**.

Thiazolidinediones. Oral **hypoglycaemic drugs** used in management of type 2 **diabetes mellitus**. Bind to a nuclear receptor, peroxisome proliferator-activated receptor (PPAR)γ in adipose cells, liver and skeletal muscle, increasing sensitivity to **insulin** among other actions. Not indicated for monotherapy; usually used in combination with a **biguanide** or **sulfonylurea**. Agents include pioglitazone (restricted in some countries because of the risk of bladder cancer), rosiglitazone (restricted in the USA and unavailable in Europe because of the risk of cardiovascular events) and troglitazone (withdrawn because of the risk of hepatitis).

Thigh, lateral cutaneous nerve block. Provides analgesia of the anterolateral thigh/knee, e.g. for leg surgery (especially skin graft harvesting) and diagnosis of meralgia paraesthetica (numbness and paraesthesia caused by lateral cutaneous nerve compression by the inguinal ligament, under which it passes).

With the patient supine, a needle is introduced perpendicular to the skin, 2 cm medial and caudal to the anterior superior iliac spine. A click is felt as the fascia lata is pierced. 10–15 ml **local anaesthetic agent** is injected in a fan shape laterally.

Thiopental sodium (Thiopentone; 5-ethyl-5-(1-methylbutyl)-2-thiobarbiturate). **Intravenous anaesthetic agent**, synthesised in 1932 and first used in 1934 by **Lundy** and **Waters**. Also used in refractory **status epilepticus**. The sulfur analogue of pentobarbitone (Fig. 158). Stored as the sodium salt, a yellow powder with a faint garlic smell, with 6% anhydrous sodium carbonate added to prevent formation of (insoluble) free acid when exposed to atmospheric CO_2 and presented in an atmosphere of nitrogen. Most commonly used as a 2.5% solution, with pH of 10.5. pK_a is 7.6; at a pH of 7.4 about 60% is unionised. The solution is stable for 24–36 h after mixing, although the manufacturers recommend discarding after 7 h.

About 85% bound to plasma proteins after injection. Follows a multicompartmental pharmacokinetic model after a single iv injection, with redistribution from

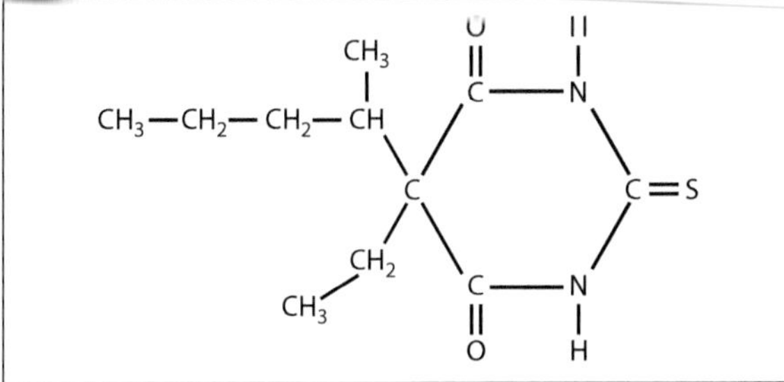

Fig. 158 Structure of thiopental

vessel-rich tissues (e.g. brain) to lean body tissues (e.g. muscle), with return of consciousness. Slower redistribution then occurs to vessel-poor tissues (e.g. fat: *see Fig. 92;* **Intravenous anaesthetic agents**).

- Effects:
  - induction:
    - smooth, occurring within one **arm–brain circulation time**. Involuntary movements and painful injection are rare.
    - recovery within 5–10 min after a single dose.
  - CVS:
    - causes dose-related direct myocardial depression, decreasing cardiac output and causing compensatory tachycardia with increased myocardial O_2 demand. Cardiovascular depression is related to speed of injection and is exacerbated by **hypovolaemia.**
    - has little effect on SVR but may decrease venous vascular tone, reducing venous return.
  - RS:
    - causes dose-related depression of the respiratory centre, decreasing the responsiveness to CO_2 and **hypoxia. Apnoea** is common after induction.
    - **laryngospasm** readily occurs following laryngeal stimulation.
    - has been implicated in causing **bronchospasm**, but this is disputed.
  - CNS:
    - anticonvulsant.
    - decreases pain threshold (**antanalgesia**).
    - reduces **cerebral perfusion pressure, ICP** and **cerebral metabolism.**
  - other:
    - causes brief skeletal muscle relaxation at peak CNS effect.
    - reduces renal and hepatic blood flow secondary to reduced cardiac output. Causes hepatic **enzyme induction.**
    - reduces **intraocular pressure.**
    - has no effect on uterine tone.

Metabolised by oxidation in the liver (10%–15% per hour), with <1% appearing unchanged in the urine. Desulfuration to pentobarbitone may also occur following prolonged administration. Elimination **half-life** is 5–10 h. Up to 30% may remain in the body after 24 h. Accumulation may occur on repeated dosage.

- Complications:
  - extravenous injection causes pain and erythema.
  - intra-arterial injection causes intense pain, and may cause distal blistering, oedema and gangrene, attributed to crystallisation of thiopental within arterioles and capillaries, with local **noradrenaline** release and vasospasm. Endothelial damage and subsequent inflammatory reaction have been suggested as being more likely. Particularly hazardous with the 5% solution, now rarely used. Treatment: leaving the needle/cannula in the artery, the following may be injected:
    - saline, to dilute the drug.
    - vasodilators, traditionally **papaverine** 40 mg, **tolazoline** 40 mg, **phentolamine** 2–5 mg, to reduce arterial spasm.
    - local anaesthetic, traditionally **procaine** 50–100 mg (also a vasodilator), to reduce pain.
    - **heparin**, to reduce subsequent thrombosis.

    Brachial plexus block and **stellate ganglion block** have been used to encourage vasodilatation (before heparinisation). Postponement of surgery has been suggested.
  - respiratory/cardiovascular depression as above.
  - **adverse drug reactions.** Severe **anaphylaxis** is rare (1:14 000–35 000), typically occurring after several previous exposures.

Contraindicated in **porphyria.**

- Dosage:
  - 3–6 mg/kg iv. Requirements are reduced in **hypoproteinaemia**, hypovolaemia, the elderly and critically ill patients. Injection should be over 10–15 s, with a pause after the expected adequate dose before further administration.
  - has also been given rectally: 40–50 mg/kg as 5%–10% solution.
  - by infusion for convulsions: 2–3 mg/kg/h.

Has largely been replaced by **propofol** as the standard iv induction agent as the price of the latter has fallen relative to that of thiopental, and because of propofol's superior recovery characteristics. In 2011, the sole US manufacturer ceased production in its Italian plant because of objections from the Italian government that the thiopental produced there might be used for lethal injection in the USA, capital punishment being banned in the Italian constitution. It has therefore been unavailable in the USA since then, and there have been intermittent shortages worldwide. In the UK, thiopental's place in the traditional 'rapid sequence induction', especially in obstetrics, has been questioned, partly because of reduced familiarity with the drug.

See also, Induction, rapid sequence

Thiosulfate, *see Cyanide poisoning*

Third gas effect, *see Fink effect*

Third space. 'Non-functional' **interstitial fluid** compartment, to which fluid is transferred following **trauma, burns,** surgery and other conditions, including infection, **pancreatitis.** Most of the fluid originates from the **ECF,** but some movement from **intracellular fluid** also occurs. Includes fluid lost to the transcellular fluid compartment, e.g. ascites, bowel contents. Although not lost from the body, fluid shifts to the third space are equivalent to functional ECF losses and must be accounted for when estimating **fluid balance.** Losses may exceed 10 ml/kg/h during abdominal surgery, and should be replaced initially with 0.9% **saline** or **Hartmann's solution.**

See also, Stress response to surgery

Thoracic inlet. Kidney-shaped superior (cranial) opening of the thorax, bounded by the superior border of the manubrium sternum anteriorly, first thoracic vertebra posteriorly, and the first ribs laterally. Anteroposterior diameter is about 5 cm; transverse diameter about 10 cm. Its plane slopes downward (60 degrees to the horizontal) and forward.

- Contents (*see Fig. 26*; **Brachial plexus** *and Fig. 107;* **Mediastinum**):
  - median plane (from anterior to posterior): sternohyoid and sternothyroid muscles; remains of thymus; inferior thyroid ± braciocephalic veins; trachea; **oesophagus**; recurrent laryngeal nerve; thoracic duct.
  - laterally:
    - both sides: upper pleura/apex of lung; sympathetic trunk, superior intercostal artery and ventral ramus of T1 (from medial to lateral) between the pleura and neck of the first rib; internal thoracic artery anteriorly.
    - right side: brachiocephalic vessels; vagus; phrenic nerve.
    - left side: common carotid/subclavian arteries; vagus; brachiocephalic vein; phrenic nerve.

Thoracic inlet x-ray views may be useful if tracheal compression or displacement is suspected.

Thoracic surgery. The first pneumonectomy was performed in 1895 by **Macewen**. Surgical and anaesthetic techniques improved with experience of treating chest injuries during World War II. The commonest indication for thoracic surgery was formerly **TB** and empyema but is now **malignancy**, especially **bronchial carcinoma**.

- Main anaesthetic principles:
  - preoperatively:
    - **preoperative assessment** of exercise tolerance, cough and haemoptysis. **Ischaemic heart disease** secondary to **smoking** is common. **Cyanosis**, tracheal deviation, **stridor**, abnormal chest wall movement, **pleural effusion** and systemic features of malignancy may be present.
    - investigations include **CXR**, **CT scanning** and **MRI**. Distortion of the **trachea**/bronchi should be noted as this may hinder endobronchial intubation. Rarely, bronchography is performed, e.g. in **bronchiectasis**. Arterial **blood gas interpretation** and **lung function tests** are routinely performed, e.g. spirometry, **flow–volume loops**. A poor postoperative course following pneumonectomy is suggested if any of **FVC**, **FEV$_1$**, **maximal voluntary ventilation**, **residual volume**:total lung capacity ratio or **diffusing capacity** is <50% of predicted. **Pulmonary hypertension** is also associated with poor outcome.
    - **cardiopulmonary exercise testing** may be employed; a maximum O_2 uptake of <15 ml/kg/min is cited as predictive of poorer outcomes.
    - preparation includes antibiotic therapy, **physiotherapy** and use of **bronchodilator drugs** as appropriate.
    - **premedication** commonly includes **anticholinergic drugs** to reduce secretions.
  - perioperatively:
    - specific diagnostic procedures include **bronchoscopy**, mediastinoscopy, bronchography and oesophagoscopy.
    - **preoxygenation** is usually employed. Intravenous **induction of anaesthesia** is usually suitable; difficulties may include cardiovascular instability, **airway obstruction**, difficult tracheal intubation, risk of **aspiration of gastric contents** in oesophageal disease and problems of lesions affecting the **mediastinum**.
    - **endobronchial tubes** are often used, although standard **tracheal tubes** are usually acceptable unless isolation of lung segments is required. **Endobronchial blockers** may also be used.
    - large-bore iv cannulae are vital, because blood loss may be severe.
    - standard **monitoring** is used; **arterial** and **central venous cannulation** is often employed.
    - maintenance of anaesthesia is usually with standard agents and techniques. **Pendelluft**, **$\dot{V}/\dot{Q}$ mismatch** and decreased venous return secondary to mediastinal shift may also occur. **Hypoxaemia** is common during **one-lung anaesthesia. Injector techniques** and **high-frequency ventilation** have been used for tracheal resection.
    - **positioning of the patient**: the lateral position with the operative lung uppermost is usual. The arm is placed over the head, displacing the scapula upwards. Drainage of secretions from the affected lung without soiling the unaffected lung may be achieved using the Parry Brown position (prone, with a pillow under the pelvis and a 10-cm rest under the chest; the arm on the operated side overhangs the table's edge with the head turned to the opposite side, and the table is tipped head-down so that the trachea slopes downwards).
    - at closure of the chest, the lung is re-expanded after endobronchial suction. Up to 40 cmH_2O airway pressure may be requested by the surgeon to test bronchial sutures. Tubes are placed for **chest drainage**. After pneumonectomy, chest drains are often not used; air is introduced or removed to equalise the intrapleural pressures on both sides and centralise the mediastinum. The pleural space slowly fills with fluid postoperatively, with eventual fibrosis.
  - postoperatively:
    - IPPV is usually avoided if possible, as it risks leakage from the bronchial stump with possible fistula formation.
    - postoperative analgesia is vital to ensure adequate ventilation. Standard techniques are used, including patient-controlled analgesia, paravertebral blocks, thoracic epidural anaesthesia and use of spinal opioids. Cryoanalgesia and intercostal nerve block may be performed by the surgeon while the chest is open.
    - physiotherapy is important postoperatively.

Specific procedures and conditions include removal of inhaled **foreign body**, repair of **bronchopleural fistula**, **chest trauma** and **bronchopulmonary lavage**.

Similar considerations apply to oesophageal surgery. Ivor Lewis oesophagectomy (performed for carcinoma of the middle third of the **oesophagus**) involves laparotomy to mobilise the stomach and duodenum, followed by turning of the patient and right thoracotomy. Patients are often malnourished.

[Arthur I Parry Brown (1908–2007), London anaesthetist; Ivor Lewis (1895–1982), London surgeon]

See also, Pneumothorax

Thoracocardiography, *see Inductance cardiography*

Three-in-one block, *see Femoral nerve block; Lumbar plexus*

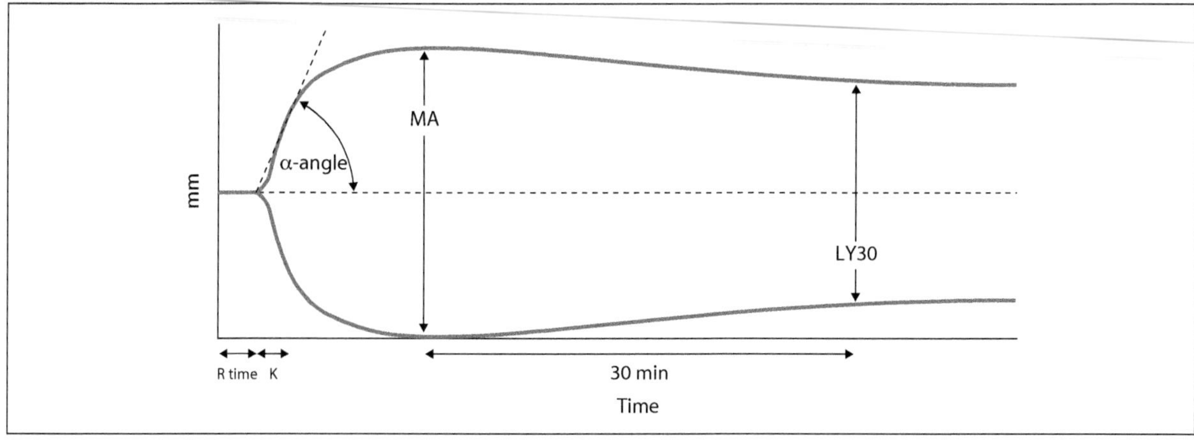

Fig. 159 Thromboelastography (TEG) trace (*see text for explanation of symbols*)

THRIVE, *see Transnasal humidified rapid-insufflation ventilatory exchange*

Thrombin inhibitors. Group of compounds that bind to various sites on the thrombin molecule, investigated as alternatives to **heparin**. Divided into: bivalent (bind to the active site and exosite 1 of the thrombin molecule), e.g. **hirudin** and related substances; and monovalent (bind to the active site only), e.g. **argatroban** and **dabigatran**.
Lee CJ, Ansell JE (2011). Br J Clin Pharmacol; 72: 581–92

Thrombin time, *see Coagulation studies*

Thrombocytopenia. Defined as a **platelet** count below 150 × 10^9/l.

- Caused by:
  - decreased production: e.g. bone marrow depression (by drugs, infection, aplastic anaemia, etc.), **vitamin B_{12}**/folate deficiency, **malignancy** and its treatments, hereditary defects, **paroxysmal nocturnal haemoglobinuria**, **thiazide diuretics**, **alcoholism**.
  - shortened survival:
    - immune: autoantibodies (e.g. idiopathic thrombocytopaenic purpura, **SLE**, **rheumatoid arthritis**, **malignancy**), drugs (e.g. **heparin-induced thrombocytopenia**, **α-methyldopa**), infection (e.g. **HIV**, **sepsis**), alloantibodies (e.g. post-transfusion).
    - non-immune: **DIC**, **thrombotic thrombocytopenic purpura**, **cardiopulmonary bypass**, **haemolytic–uraemic syndrome**.
  - abnormal distribution, e.g. hypersplenism, **hypothermia**.

Patients with platelet counts above 50 × 10^9/l are usually asymptomatic. Bleeding time increases progressively as the count falls below 100 × 10^9/l. Counts below 20–30 × 10^9/l may be associated with spontaneous bleeding, e.g. mucocutaneous, gastrointestinal, cerebral. Diagnosis of the underlying condition requires examination of the blood film and bone marrow and **coagulation studies**. Common in critically ill patients, in whom there may be multiple causative factors.

- Treatment: according to the underlying cause. Platelet transfusion is required for counts below 20–30 × 10^9/l or if bleeding occurs; transfusion may be ineffective if antibody-mediated platelet destruction is responsible.

Regional anaesthesia in the presence of thrombocytopenia (e.g. in **obstetric analgesia and anaesthesia**) is controversial, with any benefits weighed against the potential risk of spinal haematoma. Many anaesthetists would consider a platelet count above 70–80 × 10^9/l acceptable if there is no clinical evidence of impaired function (e.g. bruising or noticeably prolonged bleeding), coagulation studies are normal, the count has been stable for at least several days and regional anaesthesia would be particularly advantageous.

Thromboelastography (TEG). Point-of-care coagulation monitoring technique that assesses the speed and quality of clot formation (and resolution). A pin is suspended via a torsion wire in a sample of whole fresh blood held in a rotating cuvette (usually combined with a coagulation activator); as the clot forms, the rotation of the cuvette is transmitted to the pin, the movement of which thus reflects the viscoelastic properties of the clot as it forms and resolves. This movement is transduced to an electrical signal and displayed, giving the characteristic TEG trace (Fig. 159). The latest TEG system assesses clot viscoelasticity by measuring (using LED illumination) the vertical motion of the blood meniscus induced by exposure of the blood sample to vibration at fixed frequencies, stronger clots having higher resonant frequencies.

A related technique uses an optical detector system to measure the movement of the pin (termed ROTEM or rotational thromboelastometry). Initially used mainly during **liver transplantation** and **cardiac surgery**, it is increasingly being used to guide administration of **blood products** in other situations involving major haemorrhage, e.g. obstetrics and **trauma**.

- TEG parameters and normal ranges:
  - reaction/'R' time (time until initial fibrin formation): 4–8 min. Prolonged by anticoagulants and low levels of clotting factors/fibrinogen.
  - clot formation/'K' time (time for clot firmness to reach 20 mm): 1–4 min. Prolonged by **thrombocytopenia**, hypofibrinogenaemia and anticoagulants.
  - α-angle (a tangent to the TEG trace drawn at the end of the K interval): 47–74 degrees. Reduced by thrombocytopenia, hypofibrinogenaemia and anticoagulants.
  - maximum amplitude (MA; maximum clot strength): 55–73 mm. Parameter most influenced by platelet

number and function; reduced by thrombocytopenia and **antiplatelet drugs**.
  - LY30 (percent clot lysis at 30 s): <7.5%. Increased in early **DIC**.
  - may incorporate a number of additional tests through addition of activators/inhibitors (e.g. heparinise) to the sample cuvette.
- Advantages over standard laboratory studies:
  - faster acquisition of results.
  - incorporates assessment of **platelet** function.
  - analysis can be performed at the patient's body temperature (thus taking into account the effect of **hypothermia** if present).
  - ability to add activators/inhibitors to analyse specific aspects of coagulation (e.g. heparinase to assess the effect of administered **heparin**)

Hans GA, Besser MW (2016). Br J Haematol; 173: 37–48

Thromboembolism, *see Coagulation; Deep vein thrombosis*

Thrombolytic drugs, *see Fibrinolytic drugs*

Thrombophlebitis, *see Intravenous fluid administration*

Thromboplastin time, *see Coagulation studies*

Thrombotic thrombocytopenic purpura (TTP). Rare disorder characterised by intravascular thrombosis, consumptive **thrombocytopenia** and haemolytic **anaemia** (due to mechanical damage to red cells). May be difficult to distinguish from **haemolytic–uraemic syndrome** (with which it is thought to overlap) and **DIC**. Often associated with increased plasma levels of large **von Willebrand** factor multimers and a congenital deficiency of a specific metalloprotease that cleaves it, ADAMTS13. Clinical episodes are often preceded by triggering events (e.g. surgery, infection, pregnancy) in susceptible individuals.

Typically presents with abdominal pain, nausea/vomiting and weakness. Neurological symptoms (e.g. **stroke**, **convulsions**) may also occur. Diagnosed largely clinically.

First line treatment is **plasma exchange**, for which there is good evidence of efficacy. **Immunosuppressive drugs** have also been used, e.g. **corticosteroids**, rituximab. Refractory disease has been treated with intravenous **immunoglobulins**. Untreated, may rapidly progress to death in ~80% of cases; mortality with treatment is ~20%.

Blombery P, Scully M (2014). J Blood Med; 5: 15–23

Thromboxanes. Substances related to **prostaglandins**, synthesised by the action of **cyclo-oxygenase** on **arachidonic acid**. Thromboxane A_2 is released by platelets at sites of injury, causing vasoconstriction and platelet aggregation, and is opposed by **prostacyclin**. It is metabolised to thromboxane B_2, which has little activity.

Thymol. Aromatic hydrocarbon used as an antioxidant in **halothane** and **trichloroethylene**. May build up inside vaporisers unless cleaned regularly. Also used as a disinfectant and deodorant, e.g. in mouthwashes.

Thyroid crisis (Thyroid storm). Rare manifestation of severe **hyperthyroidism**. May be triggered by stress, including surgery and infection. Features include tachycardia, **arrhythmias** (including **VT**, **VF** and **AF**), **cardiac failure**, fever, diarrhoea, sweating, hyperventilation, confusion and coma.
- Treatment:
  - supportive, e.g. cooling, sedation, rehydration, treatment of arrhythmias (**β-adrenergic receptor antagonists** are usually employed). **IPPV** may be required in **respiratory failure**.
  - **hydrocortisone** 100 mg iv qds.
  - antithyroid drugs:
    - 200 mg potassium iodide orally/iv qds.
    - 60–120 mg carbimazole or 600–1200 mg propylthiouracil orally/day.
  - **plasma exchange** and exchange transfusion have been used in severe cases.

Chiha M, Samarasinghe S, Kabaker AS (2015). J Intensive Care Med; 30: 131–40

Thyroid gland. Largest endocrine gland, extending from the attachment of sternothyroid muscle to the thyroid cartilage superiorly, to the sixth tracheal ring inferiorly. The two lateral lobes lie lateral to the **oesophagus** and pharynx, with the isthmus overlying the second to fourth tracheal rings anteriorly. Arterial supply is via the superior and inferior thyroid arteries (branches of the external **carotid arteries** and thyrocervical trunk of the subclavian artery, respectively). The external and recurrent **laryngeal nerves** are closely related to the superior and inferior thyroid arteries, respectively.

Produces thyroxine (T_4) and triiodothyronine (T_3), which increase tissue metabolism and growth. They also increase the effects of **catecholamines** by increasing the number and sensitivity of **β-adrenergic receptors**. Iodine is absorbed from the GIT as iodide and actively transported into the thyroid gland, where it is oxidised by a peroxidase and bound to thyroglobulin. Iodination of tyrosine residues of thyroglobulin produces T_3 and T_4, which are cleaved from the parent molecule. Both hormones are more than 99% bound to plasma proteins, including thyroxine binding globulin (TBG) and albumin. T_3 is secreted in smaller amounts than T_4, is 3–5 times as potent, is faster acting, and has a shorter **half-life**. T_4 is converted to T_3 peripherally.

Control of T_3 and T_4 production is by thyroid stimulating hormone (TSH), secreted by the **pituitary gland**. Secretion is inhibited by T_3, T_4 and stress, and stimulated by thryotropin releasing hormone (TRH), secreted by the **hypothalamus**. TRH secretion is also inhibited by T_3 and T_4.
- Tests of thyroid function:
  - radioactive iodine uptake.
  - total plasma T_3 and T_4 (normally 1–3 nmol/l and 60–150 nmol/l, respectively). Increased in **hyperthyroidism**, and when TBG levels are raised, e.g. in **pregnancy**, **hepatitis**. Decreased in **hypothyroidism** and when TBG levels are reduced, e.g. **corticosteroid** therapy, or when binding of T_3 and T_4 is inhibited, e.g. by **phenytoin** and **salicylates**.
  - free T_3 or T_4 index: obtained by adding radioactive T_3/T_4 to plasma, then adding a hormone-binding resin. Any radioactive T_3/T_4 not bound to TBG is taken up by the resin. Free T_3/T_4 index is the product of the resin uptake and plasma T_3/T_4 levels.
  - plasma TSH: indicates the level of hypersecretion in hyperthyroidism (usually depressed, due to negative feedback by T_3 and T_4). High in primary hypothyroidism. May be measured after injection of TRH.

The gland also secretes **calcitonin**, important in **calcium** homeostasis, from parafollicular (C) cells.

Anaesthetic considerations of thyroid surgery: as for hyper-/hypothyroidism.

See also, Neck, cross-sectional anatomy; Sick euthyroid syndrome

Thyroidectomy, *see Hyperthyroidism; Thyroid gland*

Thyrotoxicosis, *see Hyperthyroidism; Thyroid crisis*

Tibial nerve block, *see Ankle, nerve blocks; Knee, nerve blocks*

Ticagrelor. Nucleoside analogue **antiplatelet drug**, used in combination with **aspirin** in patients with **acute coronary syndromes**. More effective than **clopidogrel** at reducing ischaemic events and all-cause mortality, but with a higher risk of minor bleeding.

Antagonises platelet $P2Y_{12}$ ADP receptors, thereby inhibiting ADP-mediated platelet aggregation by blocking the glycoprotein IIb/IIIa pathway. Oral **bioavailability** is 35%, with peak clinical effect occurring within 2–4 h. Eliminated via hepatic metabolism, with a **half-life** of 7–8 h. As with clopidogrel, cessation 7 days before surgery is recommended.

- Dosage: 180 mg orally initially, followed by 90 mg bd.
- Side effects: bleeding, GI upset, dyspnoea, rash.

Ticarcillin. Carboxypenicillin **antibacterial drug**, used primarily for pseudomonas infections, although also active against other gram-negative organisms. Available in the UK only in combination with **clavulanic acid.**

- Dosage: 3.2 g 4–8-hourly (depending on severity), iv 3.2 g contains 3 g ticarcillin and 200 mg clavulanic acid.
- Side effects: as for **benzylpenicillin.**

Tick-borne diseases. Common worldwide, although uncommon in the UK; soft ticks cause a variety of skin lesions and transmit spirochaetal relapsing fevers whereas hard ticks are the vectors for arboviral haemorrhagic fevers, **encephalitis**, typhus and **Lyme disease**. Rarely, tick bites may result in ascending flaccid paralysis, leading to respiratory and bulbar involvement within a few days unless the tick is removed. The causative agent is unknown. Treatment is supportive, with appropriate **antibacterial drugs** (e.g. **tetracyclines** or **aminoglycosides**).

Tidal volume. Volume of gas inspired and expired with each breath. Normally 7 ml/kg. Measured using **spirometers** or **respirometers.** 'Effective' tidal volume equals tidal volume minus **dead space** volume. Typically set at 10–12 ml/kg for **IPPV** during anaesthesia, with lower volumes (5–6 ml/kg) thought to be associated with less **barotrauma**, especially in patients with lung disease, including **ALI.** Reduced tidal volumes are therefore commonly used as part of **lung protection strategies** in the ICU.

See also, Lung volumes

Tigecycline. Broad-spectrum glycylcycline **antibacterial drug** related to **tetracycline.** Active against several gram-positive (including multiresistant staphylococci) and -negative organisms and some anaerobic bacteria, though not pseudomonas or proteus species. Reserved for complicated soft tissue and abdominal infections, especially involving resistant organisms.

- Dosage: 100 mg iv initially, then 50 mg bd.
- Side effects: as for tetracyclines; also GIT upset, blood dyscrasias, rash.

Time constant (τ). Expression used to describe an **exponential process**; its reciprocal is the rate constant (k). Equals the time in which the process would be completed if the rate of change were maintained at its initial value. May also be described as the ratio of quantity present to the rate of change of quantity at that moment. At 1τ the process is 63% complete (i.e., 37% of the initial quantity remains), at 2τ it is 86.5% complete, and at 3τ it is 95% complete. After 6τ the process is 99.75% complete. For a negative exponential process, the **half-life** equals 0.69τ.

When used to refer to passive expiration of air from the lungs, τ equals **compliance** × **resistance**; thus stiff alveoli served by narrow airways empty at similar rates to compliant alveoli served by wide airways. May also be applied to the **washout** of nitrogen from the lungs during **preoxygenation**; τ equals **FRC** divided by **alveolar ventilation.**

Time to sustained respiration. Time for adequate regular respiration to occur in the **neonate** after delivery, without stimulation. Related to fetal well-being and respiratory depression caused by drugs administered to the mother before delivery.

See also, Fetus, effects of anaesthetic drugs on; Obstetric analgesia and anaesthesia

Tinzaparin sodium, *see Heparin*

Tirofiban. Antiplatelet drug, used in **acute coronary syndromes** in combination with other anticoagulant agents, within 12 h of the last episode of chest pain. Acts by reversibly inhibiting activation of the glycoprotein IIb/IIIa complex on the surface of **platelets.**

- Dosage: 400 ng/kg/min iv for 30 min, followed by 100 ng/kg/min for at least 48 h (and during and 12–24 h after **percutaneous coronary intervention** if performed). If angiography <4 h after diagnosis, 25 µg/kg iv over 3 min at start of procedure, followed by 150 ng/kg/min for 12–24 h up to 48 h.
- Side effects are related to increased bleeding. Platelet function takes up to 2–4 h to return to normal after discontinuation of therapy.

TISS, *see Therapeutic intervention scoring system*

Tissue oxygen tension, *see Oxygen, tissue tension*

TIVA, *see Total intravenous anaesthesia*

TMJ, *see Temporomandibular joint*

TNS, Transcutaneous nerve stimulation, *see Transcutaneous electrical nerve stimulation*

Tobramycin. Aminoglycoside and **antibacterial drug** with similar activity to **gentamicin** but more active against pseudomonas, although less active against other gram-negative organisms.

- Dosage:
  - 1 mg/kg im/slowly iv tds; increased to up to 5 mg/kg/day in severe infections (decreased again as soon as possible). For urinary tract infection,

2–3 mg/kg/day as a single im dose. Blood concentrations: 1 h post-dose <10 mg/l; predose <2 mg/l.
- in chronic pseudomonas infection associated with cystic fibrosis: 300 mg inhaled nebulised solution or 112 mg powder bd for 28 days.
- Side effects: as for aminoglycosides.

Tocainide hydrochloride. Class Ib **antiarrhythmic drug** previously used for life-threatening ventricular arrhythmias. Withdrawn from use in the UK and USA due to severely toxic side effects, including life-threatening agranulocytosis, thrombocytopenia, hepatitis, pneumonitis and an SLE-like syndrome.

Tocolytic drugs. Used to inhibit uterine contractions when premature delivery of the fetus is threatened, to prevent uterine activity during/after incidental maternal surgery or fetal surgery, and to relax the uterus acutely, e.g. in fetal distress, obstructed delivery or uterine inversion. Drugs traditionally used are **β_2-adrenergic receptor agonists** and include **salbutamol** and **terbutaline**, usually by infusion because the evidence for benefit from oral treatment is weak. Side effects may persist after discontinuation of the infusion; these include tachycardia, arrhythmias, hypotension and occasionally **myocardial infarction** and **pulmonary oedema** (unclear mechanism, but thought to involve increased pulmonary hydrostatic pressure; fluid administration and concomitant **corticosteroids** may also contribute). Treatment should therefore be limited to 48 h, and oral therapy avoided altogether.

Other tocolytic drugs include atosiban (an **oxytocin** antagonist), which is more expensive but has fewer side effects than β_2-agonists in preterm labour (although it may cause nausea, vomiting, tachycardia and hypotension). **Nifedipine**, **magnesium sulfate** and inhibitors of **prostaglandin** synthesis (e.g. **indometacin**) also cause tocolysis but are not widely used in the UK. **GTN** patches have also been used. Acutely, GTN 100–400 μg iv or sublingually may also be used.

See also, Obstetric analgesia and anaesthesia

TOE, *see Transoesophageal echocardiography*

Tolazoline hydrochloride. **α-Adrenergic receptor antagonist**, structurally related to **phentolamine**. Traditionally used by iv infusion to relieve arterial spasm following accidental intra-arterial injection of **thiopental**. Also used to reduce **pulmonary vascular resistance**, e.g. in congenital **diaphragmatic hernia**.
- Dosage: 1 mg/kg.

Tolerance. Progressively decreasing response to repeated administration of a drug. May result from altered number of receptors, altered response to receptor activation, altered **pharmacokinetics** (e.g. **enzyme induction**) or development of physiological compensatory mechanisms. Classically occurs with **morphine**.

See also, Tachyphylaxis

Tongue. Muscular organ attached to the hyoid bone and mandible. Covered by mucous membrane and divided into anterior two-thirds and posterior one-third by a V-shaped groove, the sulcus terminalis. At the latter's apex is a small depression, the foramen caecum. The lower surface is attached to the floor of the mouth by the frenulum.
- Muscles of the tongue:
  - genioglossus: fibres fan back from the superior genial spine of the mandible to the tip and whole length of the dorsum of the tongue. The lowest fibres attach to the hyoid bone.
  - hyoglossus: attached to the body and greater horns of the hyoid bone, passing upwards and forwards into the sides of the tongue.
  - palatoglossus and styloglossus: pass from the palate and styloid process, respectively.
  - intrinsic muscles: include vertical, longitudinal and transverse fibres.
- Nerve supply:
  - sensory: glossopharyngeal nerve to the posterior one-third and lingual branch of mandibular division of the trigeminal nerve (V_3) to the anterior two-thirds. Gustatory fibres pass from the anterior two-thirds of the tongue via the chorda tympani to the facial nerve.
  - motor: hypoglossal nerve.

The tone of genioglossus is important in preventing approximation of the tongue and posterior pharyngeal wall, which results in **airway obstruction**. Genioglossus tone varies with respiration and is maximal in inspiration. It also decreases during **sleep**; this may contribute to the development of **sleep-disordered breathing**. Anaesthetic and sedative agents decrease this tone and thus predispose to obstruction, which may be relieved by elevating the jaw, placing the patient in the lateral position, and use of pharyngeal **airways**.

Macroglossia predisposes to respiratory obstruction and may hinder tracheal intubation, e.g. in **acromegaly**, **Down's syndrome** and light chain amyloidosis. It may also occur after posterior fossa **neurosurgery**. Tongue piercing studs should be removed preoperatively.

Tongue forceps, *see Forceps*

Tonicity. Refers to the effective **osmotic pressure** of solutions in relation to that of **plasma**. Thus a urea solution may be isosmotic with plasma but its effective osmotic pressure (and thus tonicity) falls after infusion because urea distributes evenly across cell membranes. Similarly, 5% dextrose solution is isosmotic with plasma but hypotonic when infused because the dextrose is metabolised by red blood cells leaving water.

See also, Intravenous fluids

Tonometry, gastric, *see Gastric tonometry*

Tonsil, bleeding. Haemorrhage usually occurs within a few hours postoperatively, but may be delayed.
- Problems include:
  - hidden blood loss if the patient (usually a child) swallows it; **hypovolaemia** may thus be severe before diagnosis is made.
  - risk of **aspiration of gastric contents** (mostly altered blood).
  - airway management and tracheal intubation may be difficult if bleeding is torrential.
  - significant amounts of the anaesthetic agents used previously may still be present.
  - possibility of an undiagnosed **coagulation disorder**.
- Management:
  - preoperative assessment of coagulation and cardiovascular status, with iv resuscitation. Nasogastric aspiration is controversial, because it may exacerbate bleeding.

- experienced assistance is required. Each of the following techniques has its advocates:
  - inhalational induction in the left lateral position (with suction available), traditionally using **halothane** (superseded by **sevoflurane**) in O_2, and tracheal intubation during spontaneous ventilation. The main advantage is the maintenance of spontaneous ventilation if intubation is difficult. However, induction may be prolonged and hindered by bleeding and gagging, and the high concentrations of volatile agent required plus hypovolaemia may cause significant hypotension.
  - rapid sequence induction using a small dose of iv agent, e.g. **thiopental** followed by **suxamethonium** and intubation. Advantages of this technique include rapidity of intubation and the greater familiarity of most anaesthetists with it. However, it should only be attempted if intubation was easy at the initial operation. Hypotension may follow induction, and laryngoscopy may be difficult in torrential haemorrhage.
- nasogastric aspiration is performed before extubation, which should be performed when the patient is awake and laryngeal reflexes have returned.

See also, Ear, nose and throat surgery; Induction, rapid sequence

Topical anaesthesia. Application of **local anaesthetic agent** (e.g. **cocaine, lidocaine, tetracaine**) to skin or mucous membranes to produce anaesthesia. Used on the skin, conjunctiva, nasal passages, larynx and pharynx, tracheobronchial tree, rectum and urethra. Local anaesthetic has also been instilled into the bladder, pleural cavity, peritoneal cavity and synovial fluid of joints.

May be applied via direct instillation, soaked swabs, pastes/ointments or **sprays**. Systemic absorption may be rapid and the maximal safe doses should not be exceeded.

See also, EMLA cream; Iontophoresis

Topiramate. Anticonvulsant drug, licensed for monotherapy and adjunctive therapy for primary generalised tonic–clonic and partial seizures. Also licensed for **migraine** prophylaxis. Mechanism of action is unknown, although it potentiates neuronal **GABA** transmission and decreases excitatory **glutamate** transmission in vitro. Has possible **cerebral protection** properties. Plasma level monitoring is not required, with dosage titrated to clinical effect. Largely (>80%) excreted unchanged via the kidney.

- Dosage: initially 25 mg orally od titrated to a maximum of 500 mg/day in two divided doses for seizures, 100 mg/day for migraine prophylaxis. Dose escalation should be cautious in patients with renal impairment.
- Side effects: nasopharyngitis, anorexia, depression, drowsiness, fatigue, hyperchloraemic metabolic acidosis, GI upset.

Torr. Non-SI **unit** of pressure; 1 torr = 1/760 atmosphere = 1 mmHg.

[Evangelista Torricelli (1608–1647), Italian physicist]

Torsade de pointes. Atypical **VT** characterised by polymorphic **QRS complexes** with repeated fluctuations of QRS axis, the complexes appearing to twist about the baseline (Fig. 160). Often associated with a prolonged **Q–T interval**. Initiated by a **ventricular ectopic beat** occurring during a prolonged pause after a previous ectopic.

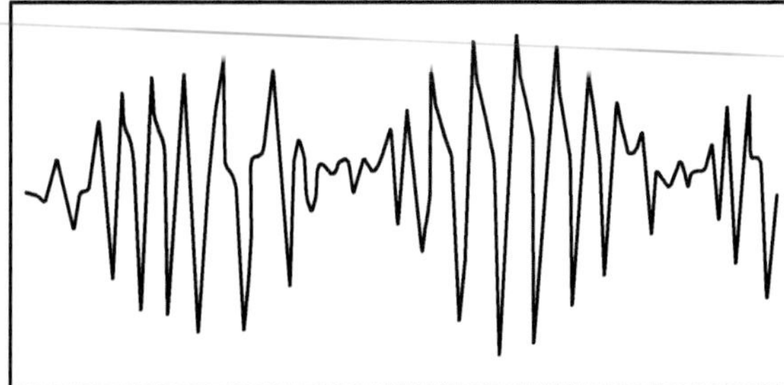

Fig. 160 Torsade de pointes

- Causes include:
  - electrolyte abnormalities, e.g. **hypokalaemia, hypomagnesaemia, hypocalcaemia.**
  - drugs, e.g. class I **antiarrhythmic drugs**, **tricyclic antidepressant drugs, phenothiazines.**
  - **ischaemic heart disease.**
  - congenital **prolonged Q–T syndromes.**
- Treatment:
  - of predisposing condition.
  - **cardioversion.**
  - **magnesium sulfate.**
  - increasing the heart rate, e.g. **isoprenaline**, **cardiac pacing.**

Class I antiarrhythmic drugs should be avoided.

Total intravenous anaesthesia (TIVA). Anaesthetic technique employing iv agents alone, and avoiding the use of inhalational agents. The patient breathes O_2, air, or a mixture of the two. Drugs are given usually by infusion to achieve anaesthesia and appropriate analgesia. The drugs chosen are usually of short action and **half-life** to prevent accumulation and prolonged recovery. Examples include **propofol**, together with **alfentanil, fentanyl** or **remifentanil. Ketamine** has been used for its analgesic properties, e.g. together with **midazolam. Neuroleptanaesthesia** has also been used. Current recommendations are that **depth of anaesthesia monitoring** should be used if **neuromuscular blocking drugs** are used alongside TIVA.

- Advantages:
  - avoids unwanted effects of **inhalational anaesthetic agents.**
  - avoids pollution by gases and vapours.
  - may be used without complex apparatus such as anaesthetic machines, cylinders and vaporisers, e.g. in war zones.
- Disadvantages:
  - requires repeated injections or infusion devices.
  - accurate prediction of plasma levels of anaesthetic agents is more difficult than with inhalational agents, because of the more complicated **pharmacokinetics** and the absence of actual measurements of drug concentration. Thus **awareness** or excessive dosage may occur unless one is familiar with the technique. **Target-controlled infusion** (TCI) devices employ pharmacokinetic models derived from real data to run a special syringe driver according to patients' characteristics (entered by the anaesthetist) and the desired plasma or 'effect-site' drug concentration. The various models perform differently and the patient must be carefully observed for clinical effects.
  - obstruction or misplacement of the iv cannula may go undetected, e.g. if the cannula site is covered by drapes, etc., and may result in awareness.

- once a drug has been infused, it cannot be removed from the body other than by metabolism and excretion. Thus, there is less control than with inhalational agents, which may be removed by ventilation.

Meta-analysis of comparisons of TIVA and anaesthesia with newer inhalational agents (e.g. isoflurane and sevoflurane) shows a slightly decreased incidence of PONV and faster recovery times with the former; no significant differences in unplanned readmission to hospital have been demonstrated. TIVA is more expensive.

Total lung capacity. Volume of gas in the lungs after maximal inspiration. Normally approximately 6 l. Determined by helium dilution (does not measure gas in poorly ventilated regions) or with the **body plethysmograph**.
See also, Lung volumes

Total parenteral nutrition, *see Nutrition, total parenteral*

Tourniquets. Used to reduce bleeding during limb surgery, and to allow **IVRA**. Inflated following exsanguination of the limb, e.g. by raising it for 2–3 min with the artery compressed, or by using a rubber Esmarch bandage. The latter increases CVP and may provoke cardiac failure in susceptible patients. It may also dislodge emboli from **DVTs**. Complications from tourniquets include: direct skin, muscle, nerve or vascular injury; reperfusion hyperaemia and limb oedema; and hypertension and tachycardia due to pain.

- Measures suggested to reduce compression and ischaemic injury:
  - inflation pressures:
    - arm: systolic BP + 75 to 100 mmHg (+100 mmHg for IVRA).
    - leg: systolic BP × 2.

    Suggested values vary, and depend partly on age, weight, etc.
  - inflation time: 2 h maximum is the most common recommendation, although 60 min for the arm and 90 min for the leg are often quoted. Periodic deflation and reinflation may allow longer use.

Equipment should be checked before use. Tourniquets should not be used in **sickle cell anaemia** (avoidance in sickle trait has also been suggested). Protective padding is required under the tourniquet. Skin preparation solutions may cause chemical burns if allowed to soak into the padding.

[Johann FA von Esmarch (1823–1908), German surgeon]

Estebe JP, Davies JM, Richebe P (2011). Eur J Anaesthesiol; 28: 404–11

See also, Compartment syndromes

Toxic epidermal necrolysis, *see Stevens–Johnson syndrome*

Toxic shock syndrome. Systemic illness associated with certain *Staphylococcus aureus* strains and *Streptococcus pyogenes*, thought to be caused by **exotoxins** (possibly with concurrent gram-negative **endotoxin** production).

First described in 1978; the reported incidence increased around 1980, especially associated with menstruation and use of tampons. Features typically occur rapidly and include fever, hypotension, GIT upset, headache and myalgia. Generalised rash and/or oedema leads to desquamation 10–20 days later. **MODS** may occur. Treatment is supportive, with **antibacterial drug** therapy.

TPN, Total parenteral nutrition, *see Nutrition, total parenteral*

TPR, Total peripheral resistance, *see Systemic vascular resistance*

Trachea, *see Tracheobronchial tree*

Tracheal administration of drugs. Previously used when iv administration was not possible, e.g. **cardiac arrest**. Superseded by the intraosseous route in the emergency setting. Previously advocated at 2–3 times the iv dose, diluted in 10 ml saline; **atropine**, **adrenaline** and **lidocaine** were the drugs most commonly administered in this way. Many respiratory drugs are administered using inhalers and nebulisers.

Tracheal extubation, *see Extubation, tracheal*

Tracheal intubation, *see Intubation, tracheal*

Tracheal tubes. Developed along with techniques for tracheal intubation. **O'Dwyer** described his intubating tube in 1885, although various tubes had been used previously, e.g. for **CPR**. The modern wide-bore tracheal tube was developed by **Magill** and **Rowbotham** after World War I, following the use of thin gum-elastic tubes for **insufflation techniques**. Separate tubes were placed into the trachea for delivery and removal of gases; these were eventually replaced by a single rubber ('Magill') tube. **Cuffs** were introduced by Guedel in 1928. Red rubber tracheal tubes have largely been replaced by sterile disposable polyvinyl chloride tubes, because the former deteriorate on repeated sterilisation, are costlier to use, and are irritant to the respiratory mucosa. Plastic tubes soften as they warm, e.g. in the trachea, and may be vulnerable to kinking.

Size 8–9 mm and 7–8 mm internal diameter orotracheal tubes are often employed for men and women, respectively; smaller tubes (e.g. 7 mm and 6 mm) are often used in the elective surgical setting because they are associated with a lower incidence of sore throat and hoarse voice. However, for emergency intubation and ICU admission, larger-bore tubes are often preferred to facilitate **tracheobronchial suctioning** and fibreoptic **bronchoscopy**. Average suitable length is 22–25 cm for oral tubes, and 25–28 cm for nasal tubes (*for sizes of tubes for children, see Paediatric anaesthesia*).

- Features of 'typical' modern tracheal tubes (Fig. 161a):
  - marked with the following information:
    - size (internal diameter in mm; the external diameter may be marked in smaller lettering).
    - the letters IT or Z79-IT (for plastic tubes) denote that the material has been implantation tested in rabbit muscle for tissue compatibility, according to the American National Standards Committee, which met in committee room no. Z79 in 1956.
    - the distance from the tip of the tube is marked at intervals along the tube's length. Most plastic tubes are longer than is usually required, and may be cut to size.
    - other markings may refer to the manufacturer, the trade name of the type of tube, and whether it is intended for oral or nasal use.

    A radio-opaque line is incorporated in most modern tubes, to aid detection on **CXR**.
  - curved with a left-facing bevel at the distal end. There may be a hole in the wall opposite the bevel (Murphy

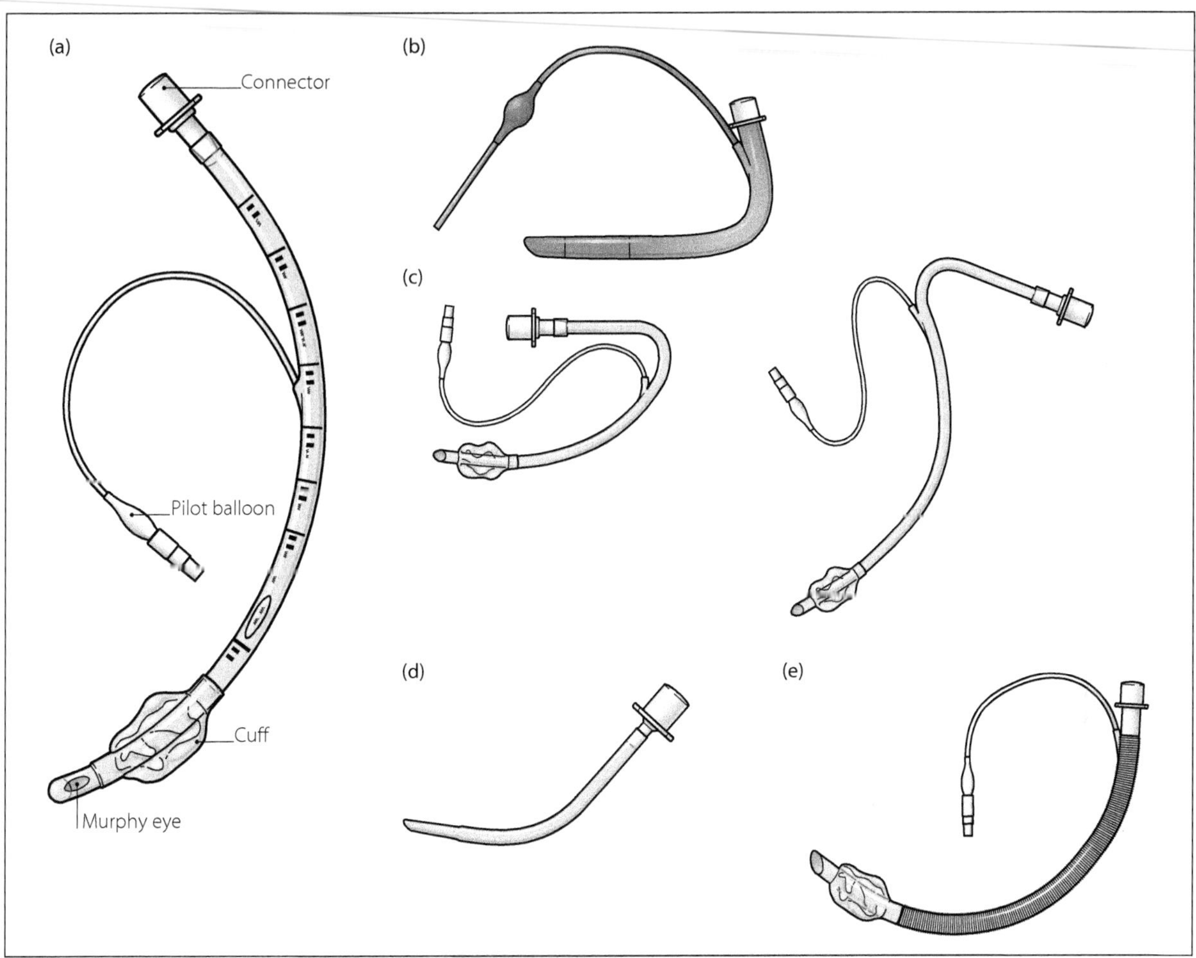

Fig. 161 Tracheal tubes: (a) 'typical'; (b) Oxford; (c) oral and nasal RAE; (d) Cole; (e) reinforced (not to scale)

eye) to allow ventilation should the end become obstructed by the tracheal wall or mucus.
 - attached to a tracheal tube **connector** at the proximal end.
 - may bear a cuff near the distal end, with a pilot balloon running towards the proximal end.
- Other shapes and types of tubes (Fig. 161b–e):
 - Oxford tube: conforms more closely with the shape of the mouth and pharynx; thus less liable to kink. The bevel faces posteriorly; insertion of the tube is aided by a gum-elastic bougie protruding a short distance from the distal end. Traditionally made of red rubber, they are thicker-walled than traditional red rubber tubes. Available with or without cuffs.
 - RAE tube: plastic; designed to be even more 'anatomically' shaped than the Oxford tube. Nasal RAE tubes are also available, as are other manufacturers' versions. Available with or without cuffs.
 - Cole tube: used in **neonates**. Shouldered, with thickened walls to prevent kinking. Designed to minimise **resistance** to **flow** of gas by virtue of their wide proximal portion; however, they increase resistance by causing turbulence at the junction with the narrow portion. They also may cause damage to the **larynx** and trachea if the shoulder is forced too far distally. Their avoidance has therefore been repeatedly suggested.
 - reinforced tubes: resemble standard tubes but contain a spiral of metal or nylon in the tube wall. Used where kinking of the tube may otherwise occur, e.g. **neurosurgery, maxillofacial surgery**. Originally made of latex rubber, they are now commonly made of plastic. They cannot be cut to size. Available with or without cuffs. The silicone tube supplied with the LMA (Fastrach [*see Laryngeal mask*]) is reinforced and has a tapered tip, making it easier to pass through the device without catching on the vocal cords or arytenoids. This tube is also easier to railroad over a fibreoptic scope than standard tracheal tubes.

Tubes may bear an extra channel for sampling of distal gases or for jet ventilation. A directional tube has also been described, in which traction on a ring at the proximal end flexes the distal end, aiding placement during tracheal intubation. **Laser**-protected tubes include tubes made totally out of metal and those coated with 'laser-proof' substances. Other specialised tubes include those incorporating stimulating electrodes for monitoring nerve function during neck surgery, or optical fibres to allow placement of the tube under direct vision.

[Francis J Murphy (1900–1972), Detroit anaesthetist; Frank Cole (1918–1977), US anaesthetist; RAE: Wallace H Ring, John C Adair, Richard A Elwyn (1930–2004), Salt Lake City anaesthetists]

See also, Endobronchial tubes; Intubation, tracheal; Tracheostomy

Tracheobronchial suctioning. Required in patients who have a tracheal tube in place because of inability to mobilise secretions effectively. Also useful for diagnostic purposes, e.g. for obtaining sputum samples. The catheter should be inserted gently until resistance is felt, withdrawn slightly and suction applied while withdrawing. 'Closed' suction systems are used in the ICU setting to reduce the risk of bacterial contamination of the airway.

- Complications:
  - **hypoxaemia**: may be related to rapid removal of airway gases, causing **atelectasis**, **bronchospasm**/coughing or disconnection from the ventilator. Particularly likely if the patient is **PEEP**-dependent. Reduced by preoxygenation before and after suctioning, limitation of catheter size (e.g. appropriate size [FG] = 1.5 × tracheal tube internal diameter), avoiding negative pressures greater than −20 kPa (−150 mmHg) and limiting suction to ≤15 s, and use of self-contained suction catheters within the breathing system that avoid the need for disconnection.
  - trauma, haemorrhage and oedema: reduced by careful technique, avoidance of excessive negative pressure, use of rounded-tipped catheters and intermittent rather than continuous suction. Special care should be taken in the presence of coagulopathy.
  - cross-infection/dispersal of infected material: reduced by sterile technique and self-contained **suction equipment** incorporating a catheter within the breathing tubing.
  - **arrhythmias**: may be related to hypoxaemia. **Sinus bradycardia** is especially common, via vagal stimulation.
  - increased **ICP**: especially detrimental in patients with pre-existing raised ICP. May be reduced by increased **sedation**.

See also, Ciliary activity

Tracheobronchial tree. Branching system consisting of 23 generations of passages from trachea to alveoli, comprising:

- conducting airways: make up anatomical **dead space**:
  - trachea (generation 0): 10 cm long and 2 cm wide in the adult. Descends from the **larynx** level with C6, passing through the neck and thorax to its bifurcation level with T4–5 (at the level of the angle of Louis). Its walls are formed of fibrous tissue reinforced by 15–20 U-shaped cartilaginous rings (deficient posteriorly), united behind by fibrous tissue and smooth muscle. Lined with ciliated epithelium.

    Relations: lies anterior to the **oesophagus**, with the left and right recurrent **laryngeal nerves** in the grooves between them. In the neck (*see Fig. 116;* **Neck, cross-sectional anatomy**) it is crossed anteriorly by the isthmus of the **thyroid gland**. Laterally lie the lateral lobes of the thyroid, the inferior thyroid artery and carotid sheath (containing the internal **jugular vein**, common **carotid artery** and **vagus nerve**). In the thorax (*see Fig. 107b;* **Mediastinum**) it is crossed anteriorly by the brachiocephalic artery and left brachiocephalic vein. On the left lie the common carotid and subclavian arteries above, and the aorta below. On the right lie the mediastinal pleura, right vagus nerve and azygous vein.
  - right and left main bronchi (generation 1): arise at T4–5:
    - right:
      - 3 cm long, and wider and more vertical than the left, and therefore likelier to receive inhaled foreign bodies. The right upper main bronchus arises about 2.5 cm from its origin.
      - relations: separated from the pericardium and superior vena cava by the right pulmonary artery. The azygous vein lies above.
    - left:
      - about 5 cm long.
      - relations: separated from the left atrium by the left pulmonary artery. The aortic arch lies above, and the bronchial vessels posteriorly (separating it from the oesophagus and descending thoracic aorta).
  - lobar and segmental bronchi (generations 2–4) (Fig. 162).
  - small bronchi to terminal bronchioles (generations 5–16).
- respiratory airways:
  - respiratory bronchioles (generations 17–19): bear occasional alveoli.
  - alveolar ducts (generations 20–22): lined with alveoli.
  - alveoli (generation 23).

[Pierre CA Louis (1787–1872), French physician]

See also, Alveolus; Ciliary activity; Lung

Tracheo-oesophageal fistula (TOF). Oesophageal atresia occurs in 1:3000 births, with TOF in 25% of cases. Different forms exist (Fig. 163). Babies may be premature and have other congenital abnormalities. TOF may present with choking during feeds, production of copious frothy mucus from the mouth or repeated chest infections following pulmonary aspiration. It is diagnosed by passing a radio-opaque nasogastric tube into the blind pouch; contrast medium is avoided because of risk of aspiration. Treated by surgery, performed thorascopically or via right thoracotomy. Primary anastomosis of the **oesophagus** is performed if possible, otherwise an oesophagostomy is performed.

- Anaesthesia is as for **paediatric anaesthesia**. In particular:
  - preoperatively:
    - the baby is nursed head-up, with continuous suction to the blind pouch to prevent pulmonary aspiration.
    - correction of electrolyte abnormalities.
  - perioperatively:
    - historically, tracheal intubation was performed awake, avoiding IPPV by **facemask** to prevent gastric inflation. Inhalational induction with gentle lung ventilation is now standard practice. Intubation of the fistula may occur; if this happens the tracheal tube may be withdrawn and reinserted with the bevel direction altered. Positioning of the tip of the tube distal to the fistula reduces gastric inflation; this may be achieved by deliberate endobronchial intubation, followed by careful withdrawal of the tracheal tube until breath sounds are heard on both sides of the chest.
    - surgical manipulation may cause sudden increases in airway pressures or reductions in cardiac output; close communication between surgeon and anaesthetist is essential.
  - postoperatively: IPPV is often continued, especially if the oesophageal anastomosis is under tension.

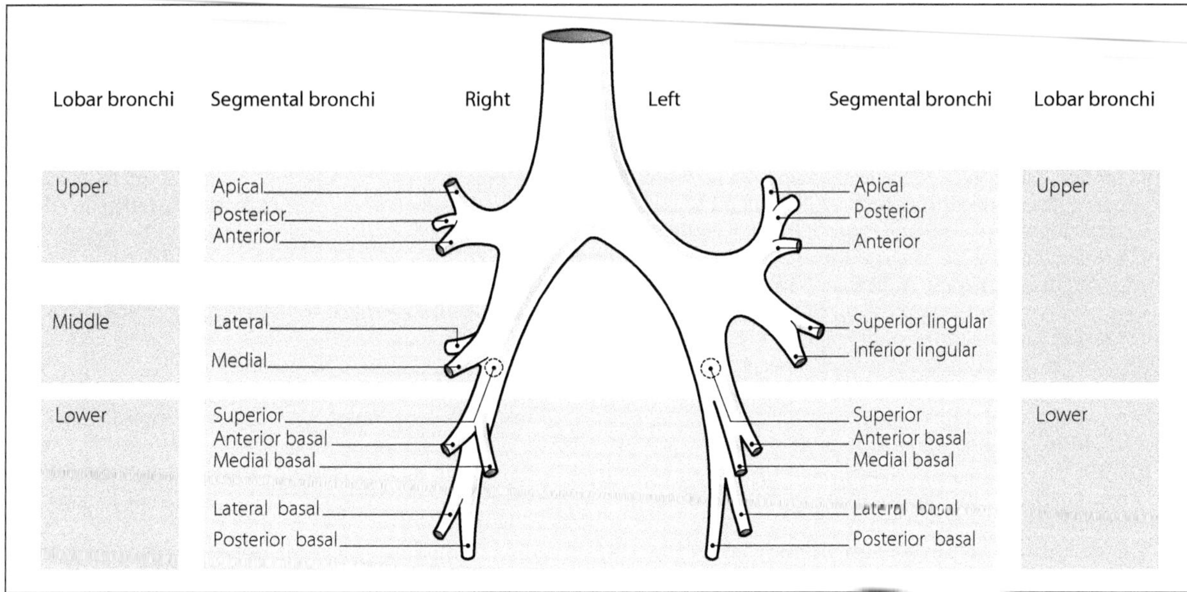

Fig. 162 Lobar and segmental bronchi

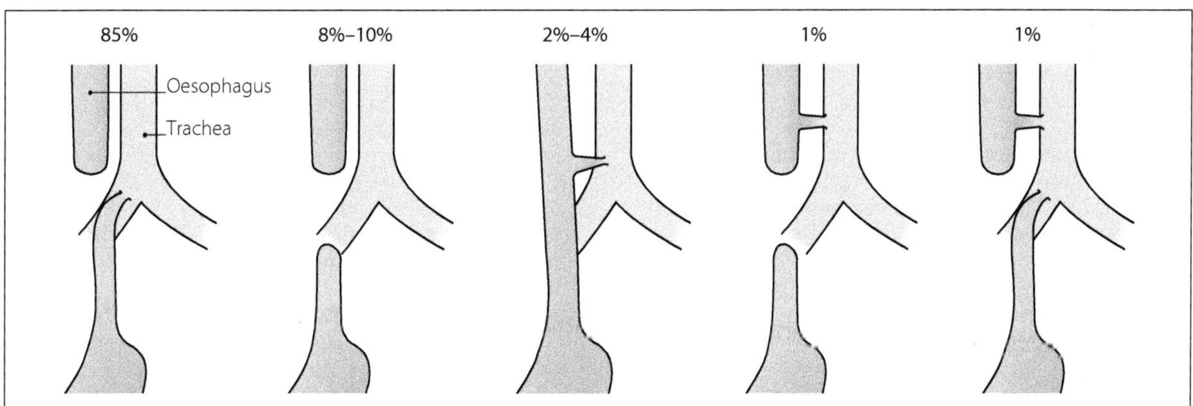

Fig. 163 Different forms of tracheo-oesophageal fistulae and their incidence

After repair, a blind passage may remain at the site of the fistula, making subsequent tracheal intubation difficult. Tracheomalacia may also occur.

Broemling N, Campbell F (2011). Paediatr Anaesth; 21: 1092–9

Tracheostomy. First performed in the 1700s for upper **airway obstruction**. Modern indications:

- prophylactic or therapeutic relief of airway obstruction.
- to protect the **tracheobronchial tree** against aspiration of food, saliva, etc., when pharyngeal and laryngeal reflexes are obtunded, e.g. neurological disease.
- to allow suction and removal of secretions.
- **IPPV** in ICU. If a prolonged period of ventilation is needed, early (<10 days) rather than late tracheostomy is performed although the timing does not significantly reduce ICU or hospital stay. Advantages over conventional tracheal intubation include easier nursing management and oral hygiene care, improved patient comfort (and therefore reduced **sedation** requirements), potential for eating and speaking, decreased incidence of **sinusitis**, and possibly assistance of **weaning** by a 30% reduction in **dead space**.

The traditional open procedure may be performed under general or local anaesthesia. The patient lies supine with the neck hyperextended, and a horizontal incision is made 1.5 cm below the level of the cricoid cartilage. After location of the trachea, a vertical incision is made through the second, third and fourth tracheal rings. A slit or circular opening is made in the trachea (creation of a tracheal flap has been implicated in causing tracheal stenosis). During general anaesthesia, ventilation with 100% O_2 should precede withdrawal of the tracheal tube (which is withdrawn into the larynx only, in case re-advancement is required). The tracheostomy tube is then inserted. Stay sutures may be brought out on to the skin from the trachea, to aid subsequent tube reinsertion.

Increasingly, surgical tracheostomy is being replaced by the percutaneous procedure, especially in critically ill patients receiving IPPV (*see Tracheostomy, percutaneous*).

- Tracheostomy tubes may be:
  - uncuffed: plastic or metal (usually silver). They may allow speech if a one-way valve is used; air is drawn into the lungs through the tracheostomy and exhaled

through the larynx and mouth. A fenestration in the tube improves the strength of the voice.
- cuffed: plastic, with low-pressure, high-volume **cuffs** to minimise tracheal mucosal damage. The cuff may be deflated and the tube occluded with a finger during expiration, to allow speech. Cuffed tubes may also be fenestrated. Some incorporate a separate catheter opening just above the cuff, through which O_2 may be diverted using a manual control to allow speech. The catheter may also be used for suction.

Most modern tracheostomy tubes are double cannula tubes that consist of outer and inner cannulae, the latter being removable for cleaning, reducing the risk of blockage with encrusted secretions. If longer tubes are needed (e.g. in the obese patient), adjustable flange models are available.

- Complications may be early or late:
  - early:
    - haemorrhage, especially from branches of the anterior jugular veins or thyroid isthmus.
    - displacement of the tube: extrusion or endobronchial intubation. The 4th **National Audit Project** identified displaced tracheostomy tubes as a major cause of tracheostomy-related morbidity and mortality in inpatients, and stressed the importance of an emergency reintubation protocol.
    - blockage, e.g. by secretions, compression by the cuff or occlusion against the tracheal wall.
    - **pneumothorax**.
  - late:
    - infection, including superficial wound infection, tracheitis and **chest infection**.
    - tracheal erosion and ulceration, e.g. into blood vessels, **oesophagus**.
    - tracheal stenosis; usually occurs level with the stoma or the tube's cuff, although subglottic stenosis may also occur. Surgical resection may be required.
    - tracheal dilatation may occur.
- Tracheostomy care is increasingly performed by multidisciplinary tracheostomy teams, often including speech therapists, which have been shown to reduce complications and decrease time to decannulation. Care includes:
  - **humidification**: vital to reduce risk of obstruction by viscous secretions.
  - **tracheobronchial suctioning**: sterile technique is mandatory. The suction catheter's diameter should not exceed half that of the tracheostomy tube. Suction is applied on withdrawal, not insertion, of the catheter.
  - daily cleaning and dressing to reduce risk of obstruction and infection.
  - secure fixation, e.g. with double tapes.
  - the adherence to the National Tracheostomy Safety Project guidelines for the management of displacement/blockage of tracheostomy tubes including availability of all necessary airway equipment.
  - provision of a means of communication, e.g. pen and paper.

The initial tube is usually left in situ for at least a week, to allow formation of a tract. Thereafter, single-lumen tubes should be changed every 10–14 days and double-lumen tubes monthly. The tube may be changed over a thin catheter or guide-wire. Tracheostomy weaning protocols start with increasing the frequency and length of cuff deflation followed by 'capping off' of the tracheostomy tube. If successful, the tracheostomy tube is removed. Once decannulated, the stoma usually closes spontaneously within a few days, but surgical closure may be required.

McGrath BA, Bates L, Atkinson D, Moore JA (2012). Anaesthesia; 68: 1025–41

See also, Minitracheotomy

Tracheostomy, percutaneous. Used in up to 70% of critically ill patients requiring **tracheostomy** instead of the traditional open procedure because of the following advantages:
- may be performed in the ICU or other clinical area, thus avoiding transfer of critically ill patients to the operating suite.
- does not require a surgeon.
- is quicker in skilled hands.
- may be associated with fewer complications, e.g. wound infection.
- provides an opportunity for teaching emergency access to the airway (i.e., percutaneous location of the trachea).

Avoided in children and in the presence of coagulopathy, localised infection and difficult anatomy.

- Methods:
  - neck ultrasound may be performed before the procedure to exclude thyroid enlargement over the planned entry site.
  - initial preparation and positioning as for the open procedure.
  - following infiltration with local anaesthetic, a small horizontal incision is made over the space between the first/second tracheal rings and the trachea located with a syringe and cannula (the tracheal tube is withdrawn into the larynx under direct vision to avoid damage). Fibreoptic endoscopy is usually used to confirm correct needle placement but may result in damage to the 'scope.
  - the cannula is left in the trachea, a wire advanced through it and the cannula withdrawn.
  - blunt dissection of the superficial tissues is performed using artery forceps. Some operators would regard blunt dissection down to the trachea, before location of the tracheal lumen with the needle and subsequent cannulation, as being a safer technique. Once the wire is in place in the trachea, different methods of passing the tracheostomy tube have been described:
    - serial dilatation method (original Ciaglia technique): special dilators are slid over the wire, starting with 12 FG and proceeding up to 36 FG, depending on the size of tracheostomy tube, which is finally passed into the trachea mounted on the appropriate dilator.
    - single dilatation method: a specially tapered smooth dilator (Ciaglia Blue Rhino), with a progressively larger diameter along its length, is slid over the wire. After a single-pass dilatation, the tracheostomy tube is passed into the trachea mounted on the same dilator. A related method involves a conical threaded dilator that is 'screwed' into place over a guide-wire akin to a self-tapping screw.
    - balloon dilatation (Blue Dolphin): a balloon dilatation catheter is introduced over the guide-wire; inflation of the balloon dilates the tracheal wall and soft tissues. Removes the need for application of downwards force with a rigid dilator, theoretically reducing the risk of injury to the posterior tracheal wall.

- dilating forceps (Griggs) method: a special pair of curved forceps, incorporating a groove in the opposing surfaces of its jaws, is slid over the wire with the jaws closed. The forceps are then opened outside the trachea to dilate the soft tissues before being closed and passed into the trachea. They are then opened forcibly within the trachea and removed while still open; the tracheostomy tube is then passed over the wire into the trachea.
- translaryngeal tracheostomy method: a guide-wire is passed retrogradely into the mouth via a percutaneous needle in the trachea, under bronchoscopic control. A reinforced flexible tube with a cuff at its proximal end and a cone-shaped dilator fixed to its distal end are then passed over the guide-wire from the mouth and pulled out through the front of the neck; the cone portion is then removed and the tube manipulated so that the intratracheal portion (bearing the cuff) passes caudally to lie in the standard tracheostomy tube position.

Complications are as for open surgery; initial studies suggest their incidence is low. Tracheal tears and oesophageal perforation may occur with all the above methods. The 2014 NCEPOD study into ICU tracheostomy care highlighted poor **consent** documentation and WHO checklist adherence and often inadequate availability of difficult airway equipment including fibreoptic devices.

[Pasquale Ciaglia (1912–2000), US thoracic surgeon; Bill Griggs, Australian intensivist]

Cheung NH, Napolitano LM (2014). Resp Care; 59: 895–915

Train-of-four nerve stimulation, *see Neuromuscular blockade monitoring*

TRALI, *see Transfusion-related acute lung injury*

Tramadol hydrochloride. **Opioid analgesic drug**, introduced in the UK in 1994. A pure agonist at mu **opioid receptors**, it is also a delta and kappa receptor agonist; it also inhibits **noradrenaline** uptake and enhances **5-HT** release. Undergoes hepatic and renal elimination; contraindicated in patients with end-stage **renal failure**. **Half-life** is about 6 h. Administration with **morphine** was previously suggested to reduce the efficacy of both (i.e., an infra-additive effect); however, this is disputed, and several studies demonstrate that tramadol improves analgesia and reduces morphine requirements after major surgery.

- Dosage:
  - 50–100 mg orally 4–6-hourly up to 400 mg/day. A slow-release formulation is available: 50–200 mg od/bd. A combined preparation with **paracetamol** is also available (37.5 mg tramadol with 325 mg paracetamol): 1–2 tablets qds.
  - 50–100 mg im/slowly iv 4–6-hourly (up to 250 mg in divided doses as initial dose for postoperative pain, up to 600 mg/day). Dosage interval should be increased in the elderly and those with liver and/or renal impairment.
- Side effects: nausea, vomiting, dizziness, dry mouth, sweating, confusion and hallucinations, respiratory depression, sedation (the latter two less commonly than with **morphine**). Drug dependence and withdrawal have been reported, especially following prolonged treatment. **Convulsions** have been reported, especially in combination with other drugs known to reduce seizure threshold, e.g. tricyclic antidepressants and selective serotonin reuptake inhibitors. Contraindicated in patients receiving **monoamine oxidase inhibitors**. Analgesic efficacy is reduced by concurrent administration of **5-HT$_3$ receptor antagonists** (e.g. **ondansetron**). Became a Schedule 3 Controlled Drug in 2014.

Miotto K, Cho AK, Khalil MA, et al (2017). Anesth Analg; 124: 44–51

See also, Misuse of Drugs Act

Tranexamic acid. **Antifibrinolytic drug**, used to reduce bleeding, e.g. in **trauma**, **cardiac surgery**, menorrhagia or dental extraction in haemophiliacs; it has also been used in **streptokinase** overdose and **hereditary angioneurotic oedema**. Decreases mortality by 30% in trauma patients; the CRASH-2 trial reported a significant reduction in MI and no increase in thromboembolic events after its use in this group. Also reduces perioperative bleeding and requirement for blood transfusion, e.g. in knee/hip arthroplasty and prostatectomy, and in the treatment of obstetric haemorrhage. The CRASH-3 trial will study its effects in **TBI**.

- Dosage: 1.0 g orally tds/qds; 0.5–1.0 g slowly iv bd/tds.
- Side effects: GIT disturbances, dizziness. Seizures may occur with higher doses. Contraindicated in thromboembolic disease.

Hunt BJ (2015). Anaesthesia; 70 (Suppl 1): 50–3

Transcranial Doppler ultrasound (TCD). Application of **ultrasound** to demonstrate cerebral vessels. A low-frequency (2 MHz) pulse range-gated ultrasound beam is directed through the thin-boned transtemporal acoustic window (present in 80%–90% of people); this allows assessment of the middle and anterior cerebral arteries of the **cerebral circulation**. Using the **Doppler effect**, flow velocities within these vessels can be determined. Uses include: detection of cerebral vasospasm following **subarachnoid haemorrhage** and in **sickle cell disease**; assessment of **cerebral blood flow** (e.g. in **TBI**, **carotid endarterectomy**, **stroke**); detection of **gas embolism**; and assessment of right-to-left shunts through patent foramen ovale. Has also been used to assess cerebral **autoregulation**. The technique is highly operator-dependent.

Naqvi J, Yap KH, Ahmad G, Ghosh J (2013). Int J Vasc Med: 629378

Transcutaneous electrical nerve stimulation (TENS). Stimulation of peripheral nerves via cutaneous electrodes, to relieve **pain**. Based on the **gate control theory of pain** transmission; i.e., stimulation of Aβ fibres (by high-frequency TENS) and Aδ fibres (by low-frequency TENS) inhibits pain transmission by C fibres. Current is provided by a battery-powered pulse generator, which typically delivers a range of currents (0–50 mA), frequencies (0–200 Hz) and pulse widths (0.1–0.5 ms). Rectangular pulses are usually employed. Surface electrodes are usually carbon-impregnated silicone rubber.

The electrodes are placed either side of the painful area or its supplying nerves, and the current increased until tingling is felt. Experimentation with timing and duration is usually required to achieve maximal effects.

Has been used successfully in acute pain (e.g. for fractured ribs, labour, postoperatively), but is usually employed for chronic **pain management** (peripheral nerve disorders, spinal cord and root disorders, muscle pain and joint pain). Efficacy is difficult to assess as there is significant placebo effect, but TENS may reduce analgesic requirements.

Allergic dermatitis at electrode sites may occur. Contraindicated in patients with pacemakers.

Vance CGT, Dailey DL, Rakel BA, Sluka KA (2014). Pain Manag; 4: 197–209

Transducers. Devices that convert one form of energy to another, usually to electricity in **monitoring** systems.

- May be:
  - passive: involving changes in:
    - **resistance**, e.g. strain gauge, thermistor, photoresistor.
    - **inductance**, e.g. pressure transducers.
    - **capacitance**, e.g. condenser microphone.
  - active, i.e., involving generation of potentials:
    - piezoelectric effect: generation of voltage across the faces of a quartz crystal when deformed.
    - photoelectric cell.
    - thermocouple.
    - radiation counters.
    - electrode potentials, e.g. pH electrode.
    - electromagnetic induction.

See also, Arterial blood pressure measurement; Damping; pH measurement; Pressure measurement; Temperature measurement

Transfer factor, *see Diffusing capacity*

Transfusion, *see Blood transfusion*

Transfusion-associated circulatory overload, *see Blood transfusion*

Transfusion-related acute lung injury (TRALI). **ALI** occurring within 6 h of **blood transfusion** in the absence of any other risk factor for ALI (defined as 'suspected TRALI'; with another risk factor present for ALI defined as 'possible TRALI', and possible TRALI occurring 6–72 h after transfusion defined as 'delayed TRALI'). Has been described after all plasma-containing blood products.

Thought to arise from capillary leakage and **pulmonary oedema** resulting from activation of primed neutrophils that adhere to the pulmonary endothelium, by mediators present within the blood transfusion. The initial step of neutrophil priming and adherence is thought to be **cytokine**-mediated and secondary to the underlying clinical condition. The second step, direct or indirect activation of adherent neutrophils, is thought to involve either infused antibodies against recipient antigens, or infused inflammatory mediators.

Has been reported in up to 15% of patients receiving blood transfusion, although study criteria have varied and the true incidence is thought to be lower than this. Critically ill patients and those undergoing **cardiac surgery** are thought to be at increased risk, possibly because of greater baseline activation of inflammatory mediator pathways. Clinical presentation varies but is primarily pulmonary; there is no specific diagnostic test, although leukopenia is common. Treatment is supportive and as for ALI. Mortality is reported as 5%–10%.

Methods to reduce TRALI include restrictive blood transfusion policies. Exclusion of female donors (especially those previously pregnant) has been implemented in some countries for high-volume plasma products because of a possible association with blood products derived from this group. Treatment of donated blood to remove plasma and/or screen for anti-HLA antibodies has also been suggested.

Kenz H, Van der Linden P (2014). Eur J Anaesthesiol; 31: 345–50

Transient radicular irritation syndrome (Transient neurologic syndrome). Pain and dysaesthesia in the buttocks, thighs or calves following **spinal anaesthesia**; usually occurs within 24 h of the block and typically resolves within 72 h. Particularly associated with the use of **lidocaine** in hyperbaric solutions of higher concentrations (2.5%–5%), and very narrow-gauge needles or microcatheters, which result in pooling of the drug around nerve roots (leading to the withdrawal of spinal microcatheters and lidocaine for spinal anaesthesia in the late 1990s/early 2000s). The lithotomy position has also been implicated, via stretching of the lumbosacral nerve roots and increasing their vulnerability. The syndrome may reflect a transient form of **cauda equina syndrome** following continuous spinal anaesthesia.

Zaric D, Pace NL (2009). Cochrane Database Syst Rev; 2: CD003006

Transnasal humidified rapid-insufflation ventilatory exchange (THRIVE). The delivery of transnasal high-flow (e.g. 70 l/min) humidified oxygen during **preoxygenation** and **laryngoscopy**. Uses a similar principle to **apnoeic oxygenation**, but the higher flow and consequent **CPAP** are thought to allow improved **CO_2** clearance. Thus, has been shown to significantly increase time to desaturation during **apnoea** in obese adults with anticipated difficult airways, while maintaining CO_2 levels within acceptable limits. Has also been applied successfully for emergency tracheal intubation in the ICU. Requires the maintenance of a patent airway, and its use in patients with known or suspected skull base fractures is not recommended.

Patel A, Nouraei SAR (2015). Anaesthesia; 70: 323–9

Transoesophageal echocardiography (TOE). Form of **echocardiography** allowing imaging of the heart in a variety of different planes without requiring access to the chest. Increasingly used to assess cardiac function in awake, anaesthetised and critically ill patients. Basic principles are as for echocardiography and **ultrasound**, combined with the ability to manipulate the probe's tip and place it under the heart within the stomach, behind the heart in the **oesophagus** or anywhere in between. Views may be obtained of the left and right atria and ventricles (both transversely and longitudinally), all valves and outflow tracts, and proximal aorta and pulmonary vessels.

Can be used to detect structural abnormalities, **myocardial ischaemia** or **MI** (manifest by changes in segmental wall motion), valve vegetations, **pericarditis** and aortic abnormalities. **Doppler** analysis allows estimation of blood flows and **cardiac output**. Commonly used perioperatively during **cardiac surgery**, especially for:

- assessment of valves pre- and post-repair.
- detecting perivalvular leaks after valve replacement.
- determining the position/extent of aortic atheromatous plaques or dissection.
- detection and removal of intracardiac air before coming off **cardiopulmonary bypass**.
- guiding fluid therapy and assessing fluid responsiveness, **preload** and **myocardial contractility**.

- guiding the position of an intra-arterial balloon pump distal to the left subclavian artery.

May also be useful in high-risk patients undergoing non-cardiac surgery, especially those with haemodynamic instability, and in ICU and emergency departments.

Complications include dental, pharyngeal and oesophageal trauma and cardiovascular disturbances. Contra-indicated in oesophageal disease and upper GIT bleeding.

Barber RL, Fletcher SN (2014). Anaesthesia; 69: 764–76 & 919–27

Transplantation. Transfer of tissue from one site to another in the same person (autograft), from one body to another (allograft if non-identical, isograft if identical e.g. twins), or between species (xenograft). Use of cadaveric or live donor tissues has increased with improved techniques and introduction of **immunosuppressive drugs** such as **ciclosporin.**

- Main points:
  - identification of donors and matching with recipients. There may be underutilisation of potential donor organs following **brainstem death** in some ICUs.
  - **organ donation.**
  - preoperative state of the recipient, surgical procedure and postoperative course.
  - chronic physical and psychological effects of transplantation, drug therapy and possible organ rejection.

See also, Graft-versus-host disease; Heart–lung transplantation; Heart transplantation; Liver transplantation; Lung transplantation; Renal transplantation

Transportation of critically ill patients. May refer to transfer of patients between departments in a single hospital, e.g. from ICU to the radiology department, or to transfer of patients to a treating hospital. The latter may be primary (from site of injury or illness to hospital, e.g. by ambulance) or secondary (from one ICU to another). Up to 10000 interhospital transfers of critically ill patients occur per year in the UK.

- Reasons include:
  - upgrade in the level of care required (e.g. for specialist surgery, dialysis).
  - to obtain a specialised investigation unavailable in the base hospital.
  - local lack of ICU resources (no bed available).
  - repatriation to a unit closer to the patient's home.

Ideally, transfer and retrieval systems should be planned and co-ordinated at local, regional and national levels, with adequate funding, clear guidelines and communication channels, and a transport co-ordinator (consultant) identified in each hospital. Considerable stabilisation may be required before transfer, avoiding transfer of unstable patients. All relevant notes and radiographs should accompany the patient.

- Requirements:
  - vehicle: standard ambulance or a specifically designed mobile ICU. Dedicated aircraft have been used.
  - team: should be experienced in transporting critically ill patients. Includes a suitably senior doctor, assistant (ICU nurse, **ODP**, nurse) and driver/pilot ± other staff for ongoing training.
  - equipment: should be robust, lightweight and portable, including a **ventilator** (allowing synchronised intermittent mandatory ventilation and PEEP), monitors (as for any anaesthetic/ICU), O_2, defibrillator, infusion pumps/syringe drivers, anaesthetic/resuscitation drugs and all necessary disposables. All equipment should be battery-operated with sufficient charge. Other equipment includes a mobile telephone. A mobile ICU stretcher makes transfer easier.

Other aspects include **audit** of transfers (there should be documentation of patient observations, transfer events and any critical incidents) and team insurance. Although, in general, patients' relatives should not travel with the patient, arrangements should be made for them to travel and be received at the receiving hospital.

Transfer of patients between departments in a single hospital involves similar considerations to those above.

Handy JM (2011). Anaesthesia; 66: 337–40

See also, Safe transport and retrieval

Transposition of the great arteries. The second commonest congenital cardiac lesion (after **VSD**), accounts for 5% of **congenital heart disease.** Caused by failure of the truncus arteriosus to rotate during embryological development. The aorta arises from the right ventricle and the pulmonary artery from the left ventricle; the pulmonary and systemic circulations exist in parallel (rather than the usual series arrangement). Survival is only possible if a connection exists between the two circulations, e.g. **ASD**, VSD or **patent ductus arteriosus.** Other malpositions of the great arteries may occur.

Features include **cyanosis,** early **cardiac failure** and right ventricular hypertrophy, with normal pulmonary and systemic pressures. 85%–90% of infants die within a year without treatment. Fetal **echocardiography** allows antenatal diagnosis; immediate postnatal management includes intubation/ventilation and maintenance of ductal patency with iv **prostaglandin.**

- Treatment:
  - palliation: **shunt** procedures, e.g. creation of an ASD by balloon septostomy or surgery.
  - correction: early techniques used intracardiac baffles to redirect vena caval flow into the left atrium and pulmonary venous blood into the right atrium, such that the right ventricle supplied the systemic circulation, e.g. Mustard procedure (or 'atrial switch'). However, poor long-term outcomes with eventual failure of the systemic right ventricle has seen this approach replaced by the arterial switch procedure, in which the great arteries are disconnected from their anomalous positions and reconnected to the opposite root.

[William T Mustard (1914–1987), Toronto surgeon]

Transpulmonary thermodilution cardiac output measurement, *see Cardiac output measurement*

Transurethral resection of the prostate (TURP). Cystoscopic procedure for the removal of hypertrophied prostatic tissue.

- Anaesthetic considerations:
  - **preoperative assessment:** most patients are elderly, with coexisting disease. Some may have prostatic **malignancy** with systemic manifestations; oestrogen therapy may cause fluid retention. Renal impairment may be present.
  - use of irrigating solution (traditionally 1.5% **glycine,** because it is non-haemolytic and non-ionic and has a refractive index close to that of water, leading to good visibility properties) may result in the **TURP syndrome,** caused by fluid overload and dilutional

hyponatraemia. Use of saline is possible with bipolar **diathermy** and reduces the risk of dilutional hyponatraemia, though fluid (saline) overload may still occur.

- **positioning of the patient** in the lithotomy position, with restricted ventilation and increased venous return. Hypotension due to venous pooling in the legs may occur when the legs are brought down at the end of the procedure.
- **blood loss** may be major but is difficult to assess clinically. Devices for bedside measurement of capillary blood **haemoglobin** concentration may be useful. Portable photometric devices may be used to estimate haemoglobin concentration in the irrigating fluid. **Tranexamic acid** reduces blood loss.
- **hypothermia** may contribute to the features of the TURP syndrome. Irrigating fluid should be warmed because this may be a major route of heat loss.
- postoperative complications are common and include urinary and chest **sepsis**, and haemorrhage.
- mortality from the procedure is now less than 1:1000, usually due to perioperative **acute coronary syndromes** or infection.

General or regional techniques may be used. The postoperative course is generally considered to be better with the latter (**spinal** or **epidural anaesthesia**), which also allows monitoring of CNS function during the procedure.

Transversus abdominis plane block (TAP block). Block of the nerves supplying the anterior abdominal wall by deposition of **local anaesthetic agent** in the fascial plane between the internal oblique and transversus abdominis muscles. Useful as part of a multimodal **postoperative analgesia** strategy, reducing requirements for **opioid analgesic drugs** after major abdominal surgery.

A landmark method was described initially: with the patient supine, a blunt needle is inserted perpendicular to the skin just cranial to the iliac crest and just anterior to the edge of the latissimus dorsi muscle. A resistance is felt as the external oblique aponeurosis is encountered, followed by a 'give' as it is pierced and a second 'give' as the needle passes through the internal oblique aponeurosis. After aspiration, 20 ml solution (e.g. 0.25%–0.5% **bupivacaine**) is injected.

An in-plane **ultrasound**-guided technique is usually preferred, allowing visual confirmation of accurate placement of local anaesthetic; the ultrasound probe is placed in the mid-axillary line midway between the iliac crest and the costal margin. A subcostal approach has also been described, in which the needle is passed under the rectus abdominis muscle from near the xiphisternum. A posterior approach, in which the needle tip is positioned under ultrasound guidance at the antero- or posterolateral aspect of the quadratus lumborum muscle (quadratus lumborum block type 1 and 2, respectively), or through the quadratus lumborum to lie between the quadratus lumborum and the psoas muscle (transmuscular quadratus lumborum block), has also been described, and may offer more reliable spread from T4/5 to L1/2 with a single injection.

Abdallah FW, Chan VW, Brull R (2012). Reg Anesth Pain Med; 37: 193–209

See also, Abdominal field block; Rectus sheath block

Trauma. Major trauma is defined by an **injury severity score** >15 and is the most common cause of death in those <40 years old in the UK and USA, third commonest cause overall. Accounts for ~20 000 cases/year in England, most due to road traffic accidents; may also occur after relatively minor trauma in the elderly (e.g. following a fall).

Previously considered inadequate, trauma care has improved recently with lessons taken from the battlefield and, in 2010, the establishment of a network of major trauma centres in England that serve as hubs linked with local trauma units.

- Criteria for transfer to a major trauma centre include:
  - traumatic event with S_pO_2 <90%, systolic BP <90 mmHg, respiratory rate <9 or >30/min.
  - penetrating injury to head, neck, chest, abdomen, pelvis.
  - all gunshot wounds.
  - skull fractures, pelvic fracture, two or more proximal long bone fractures.
  - traumatic amputations.
  - major **burns**.
  - road traffic accidents: high-speed crash (>30 mph), motorcycle accident, falls from >3 m height.
- Organisational measures to improve outcomes include:
  - prehospital care with rapid **triage** and use of **trauma scales** to assess severity of injury. Most deaths occur within 4 hours of injury (*see 'Golden hour'*) and seriously injured patients are transported rapidly (e.g. via helicopter if available) to a major trauma centre, bypassing other hospitals that may be closer. Airway management remains controversial and although a small percentage of patients require drug-assisted rapid sequence intubation, basic airway management may be more appropriate at the scene if experienced airway practitioners are not available.
  - on arrival at the trauma centre, the patient should be managed by a designated multidisciplinary trauma team, consisting of: the team leader (e.g. an emergency department [ED] consultant); a primary survey doctor (e.g. an ED trainee); an anaesthetist; a recorder (trauma nurse co-ordinator); nursing staff; orthopaedic and general surgeons; and a radiographer. Each member has a designated role and contributes to the simultaneous assessment and management of the patient. Such teams have been shown to expedite assessment/stabilisation and reduce the time to surgery, and to improve survival. Handover from prehospital team usually follows the AT-MIST acronym (Age, Time of injury, Mechanism of injury, Injuries sustained, Signs present and Treatment given).
- Management:
  - initial management follows the <C>ABC scheme:
    - catastrophic haemorrhage control, using compression bandages and tourniquets.
    - airway with cervical spine stabilisation. Tracheal intubation is often required for **airway obstruction** or compromise and to enable safe transport of the patient to CT, etc. Trauma intubations are more likely to fail because of the need for cervical spine neutrality, local neck trauma, operator stress, etc.
    - breathing: may be inadequate due to decreased level of **consciousness**, **rib fractures**, **flail chest**, **pneumothorax**, etc. Ventilatory support should be given as required.
    - circulation: 30% of trauma deaths are due to exsanguination. Causes include injury to the aorta (25%), **chest trauma** (25%), **pelvic trauma** (25%) and **abdominal trauma** (10%). Activation of the

Bezold-Jarisch reflex in some patients results in an absence of tachycardia. Haemorrhage is exacerbated by acute coagulopathy of trauma (*see Coagulation disorders*). **Damage control resuscitation** and surgery involves titration of **blood** and **blood products** to correct coagulopathy and maintain a radial pulse, with surgery restricted to the immediate control of haemorrhage and limitation of contamination. Activation of a massive **blood transfusion** protocol should be by predetermined criteria (*see Blood transfusion, massive*). **Tranexamic acid** is given within 3 h of the injury as it reduces mortality from haemorrhage by a third.
  - imaging for major haemorrhage includes: CT scanning for patients with multiple injuries if haemodynamically stable or responding to resuscitation; and chest and pelvis x-rays or focused assessment with ultrasonography for trauma (FAST) in those not responding to resuscitation. Intra-abdominal bleeding may be revealed by **peritoneal lavage**.
  - specific management as for **haemorrhage, head injury**, chest trauma, **spinal cord injury**, abdominal trauma, pelvic trauma; coexistent conditions, e.g. **smoke inhalation, aspiration of gastric contents, hypothermia, eye injury** may be present.
  - monitoring of **oxygen saturation**, pulse, BP, **urine** output, neurological signs and **CVP**.
  - analgesia, e.g. **Entonox**, local blocks, iv opioids.
- Late problems:
  - **fat embolism**: classically occurs on the second day; its incidence may be reduced if fractures are fixed early.
  - **DVT**.
  - wound infection: **tetanus** prophylaxis and antibiotics are given as appropriate; staphylococcal, streptococcal and anaerobic infections are most common.
  - **chest infection/ALI**.
  - those associated with massive blood transfusion.
  - **acute kidney injury**, e.g. associated with hypotension, **crush syndrome**.
  - **catabolism** may be marked after multiple trauma.
- Anaesthesia may be required for fixation of fractures, removal of foreign bodies, cleaning/debridement/suturing of wounds, evacuation of clot, control of internal haemorrhage and skin grafting. Problems:
  - nature of injury.
  - presence of alcohol or other drugs.
  - **gastric emptying** is reduced by trauma; the time between last oral intake and injury is more important than the time between intake and surgery.
  - hypovolaemia.
  - risk of massive **hyperkalaemia** following **suxamethonium** (e.g. in the context of burns or spinal cord injury).

Adequate resuscitation is required first unless surgery is life-saving. For surgery, regional techniques may be useful if no contraindications exist. Sedation should be avoided in head injury. Postoperative care should be on ICU/HDU unless injury is minor.

Recommendations now exist for the uniform reporting of data following major trauma using an **Utstein style** system.

Advances in trauma care (2014). Br J Anaesth; 113: 201–94

See also, Emergency surgery; Transportation of critically ill patients

Trauma revised injury severity score (TRISS). **Trauma scale** combining the **revised trauma score** (RTS), **injury severity score** (ISS), age and type of injury in an attempt to improve the individual scoring systems' usefulness. Used primarily in **audit** because it provides a probability of survival and thus comparison against actual survival rates. Revised trauma and injury severity scores are each weighted by a coefficient depending on whether injury was blunt or penetrating, and the result adjusted again by a factor accounting for the patient's age.

Trauma scales. Scoring systems developed to aid assessment and **triage** of **trauma** cases, prediction of outcome, comparison between centres/countries. Several have been described:
  - primarily used for triage: simple and quick to perform; examples include:
    - **Glasgow coma scale.**
    - **trauma score** and **revised trauma score**.
    - **circulation, respiration, abdomen, motor and speech scale.**
    - **prehospital index.**
    - **AVPU.**
    - **paediatric trauma score.**
  - primarily used for outcome prediction: more detailed; examples include:
    - **injury severity score.**
    - **trauma revised injury severity score.**
    - **abbreviated injury scale.**
    - **a severity characterisation of trauma.**
    - **international classification injury severity score.**

Lecky F, Woodford M, Edwards A, et al (2014). Br J Anaesth; 113: 286–94

See also, Audit; Mortality/survival prediction on intensive care unit

Trauma score. Scoring system based on the **Glasgow coma score**, systolic BP, respiratory rate and effort, and capillary refill. Each is awarded points between 0–1 and 1–5, giving a total of 1–16, with 16 the best possible. Originally presented as a means of **triage**, with transfer of patients scoring under 12 to a trauma centre. Because capillary refill and respiratory effort may be difficult to assess in the field, they have been removed in the **revised trauma score**.

Traumatic brain injury (TBI). Leading cause of morbidity and mortality in young individuals. Incidence is increasing globally due to rising motor vehicle use in developing countries. In developed countries, TBI due to vehicle accidents is decreasing, but its incidence due to falls is increasing as the population ages. Violence accounts for about 10% of closed head injuries; the rise in firearm use has increased the incidence of penetrating head injuries. Incidence of TBI in Europe is approximately 250 per 100,000 of which 10%–15% have serious injuries requiring specialist care.
- Classification of TBI:
  - mechanistic—closed, penetrating, blast injuries.
  - level of consciousness assessed by **Glasgow coma scale** after resuscitation, although the true level of consciousness may be obscured by intoxication, paralysis or sedative drugs:
    - mild TBI—GCS 15–13.
    - moderate TBI—GCS 13–9.
    - severe TBI—GCS <8.

- the **FOUR score** is increasingly used for patients whose tracheas are intubated.
- CT findings and prognostic risk have also been used.

- Brain injury can be divided into:
  - that occurring at the time of injury (primary): includes direct impact, penetrating and acceleration/deceleration injuries. Results in focal contusions, haematomas (in 25%–35% of patients) and shearing of white matter tracts. Diffuse axonal injury is characterised by multiple small white matter tract lesions and profound coma, often without highly raised **ICP**; it carries a poor prognosis.
  - that occurring hours to days after the initial injury (secondary) resulting from release of excitatory neurotransmitters (e.g. **glutamate**) and **free radicals**, mitochondrial dysfunction and inflammatory responses. Further astrocytic swelling and increased vasogenic **cerebral oedema** result in raised ICP, cerebral hypoperfusion and **cerebral ischaemia**. **Hypoxaemia, hyper**- or **hypocapnia, hypotension** and **hyper**- or **hypoglycaemia** may all cause further injury. Intervention to prevent secondary injury can profoundly affect outcome.
- Diagnosis:
  - not all head injuries result in TBI. Risk of intracranial lesions in patients with a GCS of 15 on admission is low unless risk factors are present (e.g. basal skull fracture, **CSF** leak, post-traumatic seizures, vomiting, age >65, continuing amnesia, neurological deficit or anticoagulant therapy).
  - 14% of patients with a GCS of 14 will have intracranial lesions. Therefore, all patients with GCS ≤14 should undergo **CT scanning**. Repeat CT should be performed if any clinical deterioration occurs.

Prehospital management involves assessment, resuscitation and stabilisation. **Cervical spine** injuries frequently coexist with severe TBI and cervical immobilisation is required until clearance is performed. Tracheal intubation should be performed if patients cannot maintain their own airway or S_pO_2 <90% on supplemental oxygen. Hypotension should be treated aggressively as a single episode is associated with a doubling of mortality. Similarly, hypoxaemia is associated with worse outcome.

- Emergency department management:
  - assessment and resuscitation as for all **trauma** patients. Severe TBI is associated with major extracranial injuries in 50%.
  - regular assessment of conscious level using GCS.
  - tracheal intubation should be performed if GCS ≤8. P_aO_2 should be maintained above 10 kPa and P_aCO_2 at 4.5–5.0 kPa.
  - mean arterial BP should be maintained at 80–90 mmHg. Fluid resuscitation should be carried out with isotonic saline. Colloids should be avoided (albumin use increases mortality in TBI). Hypertonic saline use is under investigation.
  - hyperglycaemia is common following TBI and should be closely controlled as it exacerbates cerebral ischaemia. A target of 6–10 mmol/l is currently suggested.
  - **anticoagulant drugs** should be reversed.
- Transfer of patients to a neurosurgical unit:
  - ideally, all patients with severe TBI should be treated in dedicated neurosurgical centres, that increases the likelihood of survival. However, paucity of beds makes this unfeasible.
  - 30% of patients with severe TBI will require neurosurgical intervention e.g. evacuation of acute **extradural** or **subdural haematoma**. The latter requires urgent treatment as delay of >4 h increases mortality to >90%.
  - transfer requires an experienced escorting doctor, monitoring and recording of respiration (including end-tidal CO_2), invasive monitoring of arterial BP, neurological observations (e.g. GCS, pupillary responses), etc. (*see Transportation of critically ill patients*).
- ICU management:
  - aims to reduce brain swelling by controlling raised ICP while providing optimum levels of oxygenation, **cerebral perfusion pressure** (CPP), temperature homeostasis, glycaemic control and **nutrition.**
  - **intracranial pressure monitoring** allows early detection of developing intracerebral mass lesions as well as allowing calculation of cerebral perfusion pressure. At present, a CPP target of 60 mmHg is considered optimum; higher levels are associated with pulmonary complications. Despite its widespread adoption, measurement of ICP has not been shown to influence outcome from TBI.
  - treatment of raised ICP (>25 mmHg) includes ensuring:
    - head-up tilt of 15 degrees and no evidence of neck vein obstruction (e.g. no ties from tracheal tube, neck in neutral position).
    - adequate sedation and neuromuscular blockade if necessary. **Thiopental** may be effective if **propofol** has failed to control ICP but there is little evidence that barbiturates per se improve outcome.
    - prevention of pyrexia (e.g. with **paracetamol**, active cooling). Hypothermia using **targeted temperature management** decreases ICP but has not been shown to reduce mortality.
    - treatment of seizures. Prophylactic **anticonvulsant drugs** are not routinely administered.

    No neuroprotective agents have been shown to be effective yet.
  - if raised ICP persists, osmotherapy with **mannitol** or hypertonic saline should be considered. Neurosurgical interventions to reduce ICP include drainage of CSF via a ventricular drain and decompressive craniectomy.
  - other methods of monitoring the injured brain include **jugular bulb catheterisation, transcranial Doppler ultrasound, EEG** and related monitoring, **cerebral microdialysis** and **near infrared oximetry**.
  - other complications:
    - infection.
    - **Cushing's ulcers.**
    - disturbance of CSF dynamics, causing CSF leak (rhinorrhoea or otorrhoea) or **hydrocephalus.**
    - respiratory, e.g. **aspiration pneumonitis**, infection, **PE, pulmonary oedema, ALI.**
    - **diabetes insipidus** or **syndrome of inappropriate antidiuretic hormone secretion, cerebral salt-wasting syndrome.**
    - **DIC.**
- Prognosis:
  - prognosis varies from complete recovery via mild, moderate and severe disability to **vegetative states** and **death.**
  - 85% of recovery occurs within the first 6 months following the injury but further recovery can occur later.

- the most powerful prognostic indicators include age, GCS motor score, pupillary response and CT characteristics; others include hypoxaemia, hypotension and eye and verbal GCS responses.

Kolias AG, Guilfoyle MR, Helmy A, et al (2013). Pract Neurol; 13: 228–35

See also, Brainstem death; Cerebral metabolic rate for oxygen; Coning; Emergency surgery; Neurosurgery

Traumatic neurotic syndrome. Obsolete psychological diagnosis applied to patients whose claims of **awareness** during anaesthesia were met with professional denial, before the possibility of awareness was fully appreciated by anaesthetists. Sharing features with a general **post-traumatic stress disorder**, it was characterised by recurrent nightmares, anxiety, irritability, preoccupation with death and fear of insanity. An excellent prognosis was possible once the patient's experience was accepted by health workers.

Treacher Collins syndrome, *see Facial deformities, congenital*

TREM-1 (Triggering receptor expressed on myeloid cells-1). Immunoglobulin molecule thought to be involved in, and to amplify, the inflammatory pathway that is activated in **sepsis**.

Triage. Sorting of patients according to severity of injury in order to maximise total number of survivors. Usually refers to **trauma** cases in battles or major **incidents**, although similar approaches have been used in other fields of acute medicine, e.g. chest pain. First used during Napoleon's Russian campaign by **Larrey**, who scored soldiers according to their need for medical treatment, treating the most severely injured first. Modern triage systems give first priority to those patients who might survive only if treated, leaving until later those expected to die even if treated, and those expected to survive even without treatment.

- Many systems exist, but most divide survivors into:
  - first priority: immediate treatment/transfer required.
  - second priority: treatment urgent, but with stabilisation first.
  - third priority: minor injury, e.g. 'walking wounded'.
  - fourth priority: expected to die, therefore low priority.

Assisted by **trauma scales**, with attention also paid to the mechanism of injury. Some systems include colour-coded labels with details of injuries and treatments, to be attached to patients. Triage may be repeated at different stages of retrieval and treatment, e.g. at the scene of accident, at the receiving hospital, on wards. Thus patients may change in priority as circumstances change.

Trials, clinical, *see Clinical trials*

Tribavirin, *see Ribavirin*

Tricarboxylic acid cycle (Citric acid cycle; Krebs cycle). Final common pathway for oxidation of **carbohydrate, fat** and some **amino acids** to CO_2 and water. Consists of a sequence of reactions that occur within mitochondria and require O_2. Acetyl coenzyme A (containing two carbon atoms) enters the cycle, having been formed from fat **metabolism** or **glycolysis** via pyruvate (Fig. 164). At each step where a carbon atom is lost, CO_2 is produced. For each turn of the cycle, 15 ATP molecules are formed via transfer of hydrogen atoms to the **cytochrome oxidase system** or formation of guanosine triphosphate (including the two ATP molecules generated by conversion of pyruvate to acetyl coenzyme A).

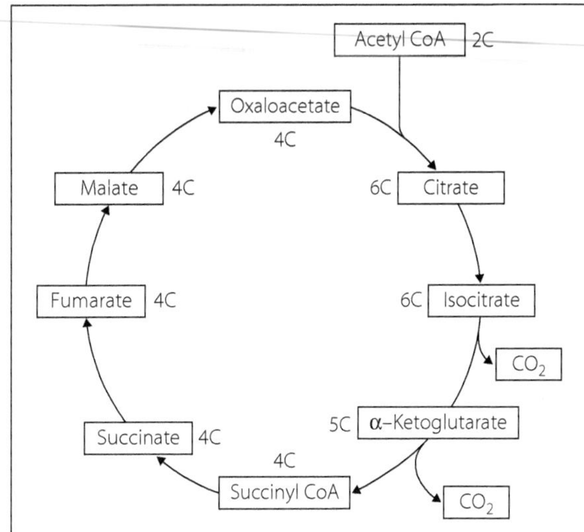

Fig. 164 Tricarboxylic acid cycle

[Hans A Krebs (1900–1981), German-born English biochemist]

Trichloroethylene. CCl_2CHCl. **Inhalational anaesthetic agent**, synthesised in 1864 and used clinically in 1935; withdrawn from use in the UK in 1988. Similar smell and properties to **chloroform** (hence coloured with waxoline blue to distinguish them). Decomposed by light, and stabilised by thymol 0.01%. Interacts with **soda lime** at 60°C to form dichloroacetylene (C_2Cl_2), a potent neurotoxin that may cause temporary or permanent damage to the **cranial nerves**, especially V and VII. Very soluble in blood (blood/gas **partition coefficient** of 9); induction and recovery are thus slow. Extremely potent (**MAC** 0.17) and a powerful analgesic. Previously popular in obstetrics as an analgesic agent, and for providing analgesia during IPPV; traditionally used instead of N_2O by the Armed Forces (e.g. in the **triservice apparatus**).

Triclofos. Related drug to **chloral hydrate** but with fewer GIT side effects. Metabolised to trichloroethanol, as is chloral hydrate. Discontinued in the UK in 2010.

Tricuspid valve lesions. Tricuspid stenosis is usually associated with **mitral stenosis** and aortic valve disease resulting from **rheumatic fever**; may also coexist with pulmonary stenosis in the **carcinoid syndrome**. Isolated tricuspid stenosis is very rare.

- Features:
  - increased right atrial pressure with peripheral oedema and hepatomegaly.
  - prominent 'a' wave in the jugular **venous waveform**.
  - mid and late diastolic **heart murmur**, heard best in inspiration at the left lower sternal edge.
  - right atrial enlargement may be shown on **CXR** and **ECG**.

Tricuspid regurgitation usually results from right ventricular enlargement, e.g. in right-sided **cardiac failure**. Usually causes little functional impairment.

- Features:
  - large systolic wave in the jugular venous waveform.
  - pansystolic murmur at the left lower sternal edge.

Anaesthetic considerations are related more to the accompanying mitral and aortic lesions than to the tricuspid lesion itself.

Rodés-Cabau J, Taramasso M, O'Gara PT (2016). Lancet; 388: 2431–42

See also, Ebstein's anomaly

Tricyclic antidepressant drug poisoning. Accounts for about 10% of cases of poisoning. Newer drugs (e.g. **selective serotonin reuptake inhibitors**) have better safety profiles.
- Features:
  - tachycardia, hypotension; impaired myocardial contractility and conduction may cause **AF**, widening of the **QRS complex**, **heart block**, **VT** and **VF**.
  - severe metabolic **acidosis** may occur.
  - agitation, hyperreflexia, hallucinations, convulsions, coma, blurred vision, urinary retention, pyrexia.
- Management:
  - ICU admission has been suggested at plasma levels >1 mg/ml or when QRS complex duration exceeds 100 ms.
  - as for general **poisoning and overdoses**, including measures to prevent gastric absorption.
  - ECG monitoring is usually recommended for at least 12–24 h. **Lipid emulsion** has been used successfully in refractory cardiovascular collapse.
  - induction of **alkalaemia** (pH >7.5) is used to reduce the amount of free drug, e.g. with **bicarbonate** or **hyperventilation**. **β-Adrenergic receptor antagonists** have been used in ventricular tachyarrhythmias; **cardiac pacing** may be required for bradyarrhythmias. **Physostigmine** has been used to restore consciousness and slow the heart rate, although this is controversial and convulsions have occurred following its use.

See also, Tricyclic antidepressant drugs

Tricyclic antidepressant drugs. Group of **antidepressant drugs**; the term includes several newer one-, two- and four-ring structured drugs with similar actions. Competitively block neuronal reuptake of **noradrenaline** and **5-HT**. Also have CNS anticholinergic properties. Used in depression and **pain management**; analgesic properties are thought to be associated with impairment of 5-HT reuptake (e.g. especially by **amitriptyline** and clomipramine). Many cause sedation, e.g. amitriptyline, **dosulepin** (dothiepin), mianserin, trazodone and trimipramine. Sedation is less likely with clomipramine, nortriptyline, imipramine and desipramine.

2–4 weeks' therapy is required before their effect is apparent. **Half-lives** may be up to 48 h. Metabolised in the liver and excreted renally.
- Anaesthetic considerations: increased sensitivity to **catecholamines** may result in hypertension and **arrhythmias** following administration of **sympathomimetic drugs**. Ventricular arrhythmias may occur with high concentrations of volatile anaesthetic agents.

See also, Tricyclic antidepressant drug poisoning

Trigeminal nerve blocks, *see Gasserian ganglion block; Mandibular nerve blocks; Maxillary nerve blocks; Nose; Ophthalmic nerve blocks*

Trigeminal neuralgia (Tic douloureux). Chronic facial **pain** characterised by brief, severe lancinating pain involving the trigeminal nerve distribution. Incidence is 25:100,000 population with a peak age of 50–60 years; twice as common in women. Usually involves the mandibular division; glossopharyngeal neuralgia can also occur. Pain tends to be unilateral during the acute attack, which may be triggered by non-noxious stimulation of the ipsilateral nasal or perioral region (sometimes restricted to one specific zone). There is minimal or no sensory loss in the trigeminal distribution. Pain-free intervals typically separate attacks, which may be so severe as to lead to suicide. Most cases are related to vascular compression of the nerve root near its entry to the pons by an aberrant vascular loop. Other causes include multiple sclerosis and amyloidosis. Similar symptoms may occur in posterior fossa tumours.
- Treatment includes:
  - drugs: **carbamazepine** is the first-line treatment; others include **topiramate**, oxcarbazepine, lamotrigine, **gabapentin**, **pregabalin** and **baclofen**.
  - trigeminal nerve blocks.
  - surgical microvascular decompression of the trigeminal nerve root.
  - destructive lesions, e.g. radiofrequency coagulation, surgical destruction or gamma knife stereotactic radiosurgery. **Anaesthesia dolorosa** may ensue.
  - neurostimulation.

Zakrzewska JM, Linskey ME (2014). BMJ; 348: g474

See also, Gasserian ganglion block

Trigger points. Areas in muscle or fascia in which mechanical stimulation may cause muscle pain, weakness and/or local twitching. May be latent (tender when palpated) or active (painful at rest or on exertion or stretching). Pain is often referred, giving rise to **myofascial pain syndromes**. Examination may reveal tender nodules within taut bands of muscle, felt especially if the fingertips are moved perpendicular to the direction of muscle fibres. May be numerous, and may correspond to traditional **acupuncture** points. Local anaesthetic injection and acupuncture may relieve symptoms.

Trimeprazine, *see Alimemazine*

Trimetaphan camsilate. Obsolete **ganglion blocking drug**, infused iv to lower BP during **hypotensive anaesthesia**.

Trimethoprim. Antibacterial drug used especially in **urinary tract infections**, exacerbations of **COPD** and in combination with the **sulfonamide** sulfamethoxazole (**co-trimoxazole**). Reversibly inhibits bacterial dihydrofolate dehydrogenase.
- Dosage: 200 mg orally bd.
- Side effects: GIT upset, pruritus.

Triple point. Temperature and pressure at which the solid, liquid and gas phases of a substance exist in equilibrium. The **kelvin** is defined according to the triple point of water (273.16 K at 611.2 Pa).

Triptans. 5-HT$_{1D}$ receptor agonists, used to treat acute **migraine** and cluster headache. Should not be used for prophylaxis. Have also been used in **post-dural puncture headache**, although evidence is anecdotal only. Sumatriptan was the first developed; almotriptan, eletriptan, frovatriptan, naratriptan, rizatriptan and zolmitriptan are newer drugs.

All except sumatriptan are prescription-only; sumatriptan became available over the counter in the UK in 2006.

- Side effects: tingling, heaviness or tightness of any part of the body, nausea, dizziness, dry mouth, chest pain, flushing, drowsiness, hypotension. Contraindicated in ischaemic heart disease and concurrent therapy with related drugs or ergotamine. Coronary vasospasm may follow iv injection. Not licensed for use in the elderly.

Triservice apparatus. Anaesthetic apparatus adopted by the Armed Forces for battle use. Consists of (in order, starting at the patient):
- **facemask** with **non-rebreathing valve** fitted.
- short length of ordinary tubing connected to a **self-inflating bag**.
- another length of tubing.
- two Oxford miniature **vaporisers** in series.
- an O_2 cylinder may be attached, between the vaporisers and a further length of tubing that acts as a reservoir.

For spontaneous ventilation, a **draw-over technique** is employed. Controlled ventilation may be performed by squeezing the bag, or replacing it with a suitable ventilator. A variety of volatile agents may be used in the vaporisers, the calibration scales of which may be changed accordingly. They are specially adapted to contain more liquid (50 ml), and are fitted with extendable feet. **Halothane**, **enflurane** or **isoflurane** is traditionally used in the upstream vaporiser, and **trichloroethylene** (to compensate for the absence of N_2O) in the downstream one.

Trismus. Spasm of the masseter muscles, resulting in impaired mouth opening (lockjaw).
- Causes may be:
  - local:
    - abscess/infection around jaw, teeth, etc.
    - mandibular fractures.
    - parotitis.
    - **temporomandibular joint** disease.
  - systemic:
    - **tetanus**.
    - strychnine poisoning.
    - **phenothiazines**.
    - **stroke**.
    - hysteria.

May occur after administration of **suxamethonium** (e.g. **masseter spasm** or in **dystrophia myotonica**).

Anaesthesia in the presence of trismus is as for **airway obstruction** and difficult intubation. Injection of local anaesthetic into the masseter muscle may relieve the spasm. *See also, Intubation, difficult*

Trisodium edetate. **Chelating agent** used in severe hypercalcaemia. Rarely used because of the risk of renal damage.
- Dosage: up to 70 mg/kg iv over 2–3 h, daily.
- Side effects: hypocalcaemia, nausea, diarrhoea, pain on injection, renal impairment.

TRISS, *see Trauma revised injury severity score*

Tropical diseases. Many diseases are restricted to tropical and subtropical regions. Several are considered ‘tropical’ because they have been largely eradicated in developed countries, but may be imported by travellers. **Anaemia** and **malnutrition** are common features. Anaesthetic involvement may be related to ICU management or perioperative care.
- Examples include:
  - **malaria**.
  - diarrhoeal illness (e.g. typhoid, giardiasis, amoebic dysentery, cholera): cause electrolyte imbalance and **dehydration**.
  - amoebiasis: may cause systemic illness, diarrhoea, bowel perforation and hepatic abscesses. Treatment may include surgery.
  - hydatid disease: parasites may form cysts, usually in the liver but occasionally in the lungs, heart, kidneys or brain. Spillage of hydatid fluid intraoperatively may cause **anaphylaxis**.
  - leprosy: chronic infective granulomatous disease affecting peripheral nerves, skin and upper respiratory tract mucosa. Patients may be taking corticosteroids. Areas of skin may be anaesthetic.
  - trypanosomiasis:
    - African (sleeping sickness): parasitic CNS invasion with confusion, coma and death. **Myocarditis** and hepatitis may occur.
    - American (Chagas’ disease): meningoencephalitis, **hepatic failure**, **cardiomyopathy** and **achalasia** of the cardia may occur.
- Other diseases much more common in developing countries include:
  - **syphilis**.
  - **tetanus**.
  - **hepatitis**.
  - **HIV infection**.
  - **TB**.
  - **poliomyelitis**.
  - **rabies**.

[Carlos Chagas (1879–1934), Brazilian physician]

Tropisetron hydrochloride. **5-HT$_3$ receptor antagonist**, used as an **antiemetic drug** but unavailable in the UK. Similar to **ondansetron** but with longer duration of action.

Trypanosomiasis, *see Tropical diseases*

TS, *see Trauma score*

TSR, *see Time to sustained respiration*

TT, Thrombin time, *see Coagulation studies*

TTP, *see Thrombotic thrombocytopenic purpura*

Tuberculosis (TB). Infection with the acid- and alcohol-fast bacillus *Mycobacterium tuberculosis* that most commonly affects the lungs and lymph nodes, although any tissues may be affected. Declined in incidence through much of the twentieth century until an increase in the 1980s/1990s, thought to be related to increases in world population, population movement, resistance to **antituberculous drugs** (itself related to poor compliance with treatment) and **HIV infection**, with which it is often associated. It has been estimated that one-third of the world’s population is infected with TB. In the UK, it is still largely restricted to migrants from developing countries, immunosuppressed patients and the homeless.
- Classified into:
  - primary TB: occurs in patients not previously infected (i.e., tuberculin-negative). Following a mild inflammatory reaction at the site of infection (e.g. lung or

GIT), infection spreads to the regional lymph nodes. The lesions usually heal and calcify without further sequelae, but occasionally active organisms enter the bloodstream. This may cause 'haematogenous lesions', especially involving the lungs, bones, joints and kidneys. Rarely, a tuberculous focus ruptures into a vein, causing acute dissemination (acute miliary TB).

Patients may be asymptomatic, with evidence of infection provided by routine **CXR** or conversion of the tuberculin test from negative to positive. Primary infection may be accompanied by a febrile illness. Occasionally primary TB is progressive and may cause pleurisy, pleural effusions and **meningitis**.

- post-primary pulmonary TB: occurs in patients previously infected (i.e., tuberculin-positive). Usually affects the upper lobes. Reactivation (or reinfection) causes a brisk inflammatory response; resultant fibrosis tends to limit the spread of infection. Regional lymph node involvement is therefore unusual. Again the lesion usually heals, but it may rupture into a bronchus, causing cavitation. It may then spread throughout the lung, or rarely via the bloodstream, causing miliary TB.

  Usually insidious in onset, features include productive cough, haemoptysis (early) and dyspnoea (late). Pleuritic pain may be caused by pleurisy or **pneumothorax**.

Diagnosis includes history and examination, CXR, examination and culture of sputum for acid-fast bacilli (poor **sensitivity**), tuberculin test (poor **specificity**), and interferon-gamma release assays (e.g. T-SPOT).

- Management includes isolation, testing of contacts and antituberculous drug therapy (**isoniazid**, **rifampicin**, **pyrazinamide**, **ethambutol**, **streptomycin**, **capreomycin**, **cycloserine**, **azithromycin**, **clarithromycin** and **4-quinolones**). Programmes of supervised drug administration have been instituted in many countries to improve compliance. Multidrug resistance occurs in about 25% of cases in China, India and Russia. 'Extensively resistant' and completely drug-resistant strains of TB are now emerging.

Ideally, single-use anaesthetic and respiratory equipment should be used for patients with active TB. Cases of spread to other patients have been reported in the ICUs of UK hospitals.

Horsburgh CR, Barry CE, Lange C (2015). N Engl J Med; 373: 2149–60

See also, Contamination of anaesthetic equipment

Tubocurarine chloride (D-tubocurarine chloride). Non-depolarising **neuromuscular blocking drug**, isolated from **curare** in 1935. Its name is derived from the early classification of curare according to the means of storage ('tubes' refers to tubular bamboo canes). Commonly caused **histamine** release and ganglion blockade, with vasodilatation and hypotension. Severe **anaphylaxis** is rare. Excreted mainly in the urine, but 30% via the liver. Discontinued in the UK since 1996.

Tuffier's line, *see Spinal anaesthesia*

Tumescent anaesthesia. Method of infiltrating large volumes of dilute **local anaesthetic agent** into tissues until they become swollen, used mainly for **plastic surgery**, e.g. liposuction. Typical solutions contain 0.05%–0.1% **lidocaine** ± 1:1 000 000–1:2 000 000 **adrenaline**; bicarbonate, steroids and antibiotics have also been added. The volumes may exceed several litres, leading to the risk of local anaesthetic toxicity and fluid overload. **PE** and surgical complications have also been reported. May be used alone or in combination with sedation or general anaesthesia.

Tumour lysis syndrome. Condition in which medical treatment of an aggressive **malignancy** (typically haematological) causes sudden release of intracellular contents, resulting in severe and potentially life-threatening **hyperkalaemia**, **hypocalcaemia**, **hyperphosphataemia**, **lactic acidosis** and hyperuricaemia. May occasionally occur spontaneously. Individual electrolyte abnormalities are managed along standard lines. Good hydration and prevention of renal uric acid precipitation by alkalisation of the urine (e.g. with **bicarbonate** or **acetazolamide**) and allopurinol administration may prevent **acute kidney injury** from developing.

Tumour necrosis factor, *see Cytokines*

Turbulence, *see Flow*

Turner's syndrome (Gonadal dysgenesis). Congenital absence of the second X chromosome. Sufferers are female in appearance, but with primary amenorrhoea and immature genitalia. Other features include short stature, short webbed neck and high palate; tracheal intubation may be difficult. Renal abnormalities, **hypertension** and **coarctation of the aorta** may occur.

[Henry H Turner (1892–1970), US physician]

TURP, *see Transurethral resection of the prostate*

TURP syndrome. Syndrome following **TURP**, thought to occur in a mild form in up to 8% of cases but severe in only 1%–2%. Caused by absorption of irrigating fluid (usually hypotonic **glycine** 1.5%) through open prostatic vessels or from the extraprostatic tissues. Has also been reported following other procedures involving irrigation with electrolyte-free solutions, e.g. percutaneous lithotripsy and hysteroscopic endometrial resection.

Symptoms are caused by intravascular volume overload, dilutional **hyponatraemia** and intracellular oedema. Additional effects are caused by glycine and its metabolites, e.g. **ammonia** (produced by deamination of serine, itself produced by transamination of glycine).

Features include bradycardia, hypotension (often preceded by hypertension), angina, dyspnoea, visual and mental changes, convulsions and coma. Severity depends on the volume of irrigant absorbed (e.g. lethargy and nausea after 1–2 l glycine; severe symptoms after >2 l) and the rate of absorption (faster onset if absorbed via prostatic veins; slower if absorbed from the extravascular tissues. Absorption rates of irrigating solution of up to 240 ml/min have been reported). Features may occur during surgery, or postoperatively.

- Preventive measures:
  - using saline instead of glycine solution for irrigation (requires bipolar diathermy, and may still result in fluid overload if not hyponatraemia).
  - limiting the height of the reservoir bag of irrigant to 60 cm, and using low-pressure irrigation systems.
  - limiting the volume of irrigant infused, and measuring the volume deficit intraoperatively (volume

in – volume out). Measuring the patient's weight may also indicate the amount of fluid retained but is usually impractical.
  - restriction of resection time to 60 min.
  - resection by experienced surgeons.
  - avoidance of hypotonic iv fluids.
- Measures to aid its detection:
  - use of **spinal** or **epidural anaesthesia**, allowing respiratory monitoring and detection of mental changes.
  - **CVP** measurement for patients at risk.
  - monitoring of plasma sodium concentration (more than a 10-mmol/l drop indicates >2 l irrigating fluid absorbed) or **osmolality** gap.
  - monitoring of tracer substances, e.g. ethanol 10% added to the irrigating fluid and measured in the blood or using a breath analyser (over 0.6 mg/ml indicating >2 l fluid absorbed).
- Management: as for hyponatraemia, convulsions, raised **ICP**, **acidosis**. Diuretics (e.g. **furosemide**) are used if **pulmonary oedema** is present. Hypertonic saline solutions have been used to expand circulating volume. **Vasopressor drugs** may be required.

Twilight sleep. Obsolete technique developed in Freiburg, Germany (as Dämmerschlaf), formerly popular in obstetrics as a means of easing labour pain and reducing subsequent recall. Injection of **morphine** and **hyoscine** was followed by hyoscine alone. Apart from causing maternal restlessness, it often caused neonatal respiratory depression.
See also, Obstetric analgesia and anaesthesia

U

U wave. Low-amplitude positive deflection following the **T wave** of the **ECG**, possibly representing slow repolarisation of papillary muscle. Seen best in the right chest leads and at slow heart rates but not always present. Made more prominent by **hypokalaemia**, **hypocalcaemia**, **hypomagnesaemia**, **hypothermia** and raised **ICP**. Reversed polarity may indicate **myocardial ischaemia**.

U–D interval. During **caesarean section**, the time between incision of the uterus and delivery of the baby. As the interval increases, so fetal well-being is compromised, probably due to disruption of placental blood flow. Fetal acidosis is thought to be unlikely at U–D intervals of 1.5–3 min.
See also, I–D interval

UEMS, European Union of Medical Specialties (Union Européenne des Médecins Spécialistes; UEMS), *see European Board of Anaesthesiology*

Ulcerative colitis, *see Inflammatory bowel disease*

Ulnar artery. A terminal branch of the brachial artery, arising at the apex of the **antecubital fossa**. Lies superficial to flexor digitorum profundus and deep to the superficial flexors in the forearm. Then passes deep to flexor carpi ulnaris, lateral to the **ulnar nerve**. At the wrist, it lies between flexor carpi ulnaris and flexor digitorum profundus tendons. Passes anterior to the flexor retinaculum to end lateral to the pisiform bone. Branches supply the deep extensor and ulnar muscles of the forearm, the wrist and elbow joints and the deep and superficial palmar arches. May be cannulated for **arterial BP measurement** but the **radial artery** is preferred because it is thought to be associated with a lower risk of digital ischaemia.
See also, Allen's test

Ulnar nerve (C7–T1). A terminal branch of the medial cord of the **brachial plexus**. Descends on the medial side of the upper arm, first in the anterior, and later in the posterior compartment. Passes behind the medial epicondyle to enter the forearm; descends on the medial side deep to flexor carpi ulnaris, medial to the **ulnar artery**. Divides into cutaneous branches 5 cm above the wrist. Dorsal and palmar cutaneous sensory branches supply the skin of the ulnar half of the hand and palm, and the medial 1½ fingers. Also supplies the elbow joint, flexor carpi ulnaris and the ulnar side of flexor digitorum profundus. In the hand, it supplies the hypothenar muscles, interossei, medial two lumbricals and adductor pollicis.

The nerve may be damaged by trauma to the elbow, or if the elbows rest on unpadded surfaces during prolonged anaesthesia in the supine position. Injury results in loss of cutaneous sensation on the ulnar 1½ fingers and the ulnar side of the hand. Paralysis of the small muscles of the hand results in clawing.

May be blocked at various sites.
See also, Brachial plexus block; Elbow, nerve blocks; Wrist, nerve blocks

Ultrafiltration. Process by which water is removed from the blood during various forms of **dialysis**. Water passes across the semipermeable membrane as a result of positive pressure on the blood side of the membrane (e.g. the patient's BP or use of a pump), negative pressure on the other side, or an osmotic gradient from use of dialysate fluid. Rates of up to 1.5 l/h may be removed by intermittent isolated ultrafiltration (IIUF) in which a **haemodialysis** circuit is used but without dialysate, but more controlled removal of fluid (100–150 ml/h) may be achieved in slow continuous ultrafiltration (SCUF), with greater haemodynamic stability and without the need for fluid replacement. Effective for treatment of decompensated **cardiac failure**. Combination with dialysis may also be employed (SCUF-D) but removal of larger molecules is less efficient than with continuous **haemofiltration**.

Ultra-rapid opioid detoxification, *see Rapid opioid detoxification*

Ultrasound (u/s). Sound waves of frequency above the normal upper limit of human hearing (>20 kHz). Originally developed for use in industry, now has a wide range of medical applications including: soft tissue imaging; assessment of blood flow; tumour ablation; and fragmentation of renal and biliary calculi (lithotripsy).

- Principles of u/s imaging:
  - a **transducer** uses a piezoelectric material to convert electrical energy into intermittent pulses of high frequency (3–15 MHz) sound waves.
  - as the pulses travel through the tissues they are partially reflected at tissue interfaces; these 'echoes' are detected by the transducer (which alternates between emitting and receiving modes). The degree of reflection depends on the difference in acoustic impedance between tissues; acoustic gel must therefore be applied to the transducer to ensure that there is no air (which has high acoustic impedance) between the transducer and the skin.
  - the intensity and time delay of reflected signals are interpreted and displayed. The simplest system uses a single 'beam' and displays the amplitude of reflected echoes as a function of depth, either as a series of lines or shaded spots (amplitude or A mode). If pulses are emitted in rapid succession, detailed assessment of movement at tissue interfaces (e.g. a heart valve) can be made (movement or M mode). If an array of piezoelectric elements is used to produce a series of pulses along a plane, a two-dimensional real-time image may be produced (brightness or B mode); this is the mode utilised most commonly for soft-tissue imaging.
  - transducer probes may have linear, curvilinear or phased arrays. Linear arrays tend to emit at a higher

frequency than curvilinear arrays (e.g. 10 vs. 3 MHz), delivering greater resolution, but poorer tissue penetration; they are therefore suitable for imaging superficial structures, e.g. for **internal jugular venous cannulation.** Curvilinear arrays produce a signal that spreads out within the body, allowing imaging of deeper and larger structures (e.g. fetus). Phased arrays deliver electronically angulated beams that can be 'swept' through the body, providing relatively large sector images from a small probe 'footprint' (e.g. allowing passage of the beam between ribs for **echocardiography**).

- Clinical applications:
  - diagnostic and fetal imaging.
  - echocardiography.
  - assessment of blood flow (using the **Doppler effect**): e.g. in **cardiac output measurement**; **transcranial Doppler ultrasound**; assessing patency of peripheral vessels.
  - regional anaesthesia:
    - real-time guided needle placement for blockade of peripheral nerves and nerve plexuses. Evidence suggests that u/s-guided nerve block is associated with faster sensory onset and greater success than landmark-based blocks.
    - identification of vertebral anatomy and estimation of the depth of the **epidural space** during central neuraxial blockade.
  - confirmation of normal anatomy and/or real-time guided needle placement during **central venous cannulation** (recommended by **NICE**).
  - thoracic imaging, e.g. to detect pleural or lung pathology and guide thoracocentesis.
  - assessment of the airway and guidance of instrumentation.

When used to guide needle placement, the needle may either be viewed 'in-plane' (needle shaft parallel to the long axis of the transducer) or 'out-of-plane' (needle perpendicular to the long axis of the transducer); the former allows continuous viewing of the entire needle shaft and tip, while the latter allows only the portion of the shaft crossing the beam to be seen. The preferred approach depends on the structures being imaged and related anatomy.

Marhofer P, Harrop-Griffiths W, Willschke H, Kirchmair L (2010). Br J Anaesth; 104: 673–83

See also, Doppler effect; Imaging in intensive care; Transoesophageal echocardiography

Unconsciousness, *see Coma*

Units, SI. System of units (Système Internationale d'Unités) introduced in 1960 by the General Conference of Weights and Measures (Conférence Générale des Poids et Mesures) and based on the metric system. There are seven base (or fundamental) units: **metre, second, kilogram, ampere, kelvin, candela** and **mole.** Derived units include the **newton, pascal, joule, watt** and **hertz.** Standard terms denote multiples and divisions of units, e.g. kilo- ($\times 10^3$), mega- ($\times 10^6$), giga- ($\times 10^9$), tera- ($\times 10^{12}$) and peta- ($\times 10^{15}$); and milli- ($\times 10^{-3}$), micro- ($\times 10^{-6}$), nano- ($\times 10^{-9}$), pico- ($\times 10^{-12}$) and femto- ($\times 10^{-15}$), respectively.

Manohin A, Manohin M (2003). Eur J Anaesth; 20: 259–81

Universal gas constant. Constant (symbol R) in the **ideal gas law** equation $PV = nRT$, where P = pressure, V = volume, n = number of moles of gas and T = temperature of a perfect gas. Equals 8.3144 J/K/mol (1.987 cal/K/mol).

Uraemia. Strictly, a plasma **urea** exceeding 7.0 mmol/l; the term was formerly used to describe the clinical picture in **renal failure.**

Urapidil. **α_1-Adrenergic receptor antagonist** with central **5-HT$_{1A}$** receptor agonist activity. Causes reduction in **preload** and **afterload** by causing arteriovenous vasodilatation with little reflex tachycardia. Has little effect on the coronary vessels. Available commercially as an **antihypertensive drug** in several countries including Germany, Switzerland, France, Japan and China, but unavailable in the UK and USA.

Urea (NH_2CONH_2). A product of hepatic **amino acid** breakdown to **ammonia.** Produced in the urea cycle from hydrolysis of arginine; ornithine is also produced and reacts with carbamoyl phosphate and then aspartate to reform arginine. Ammonia and CO_2 are introduced into the cycle by 'carrier' molecules. Freely filtered at the glomerulus of the **nephron**; about 50% is reabsorbed in the proximal tubule. Excretion in the **urine** accounts for 85% of daily nitrogen excretion. Normal plasma levels: 2.5–7.0 mmol/l. Increased production (e.g. from increased **protein** intake or **catabolism**) or dehydration may increase plasma urea slightly, but levels above 13 mmol/l usually represent impaired renal function. **Creatinine** measurement or **clearance** studies may aid diagnosis.

See also, Nitrogen balance

Urinalysis, *see Urine*

Urinary retention. Inability to pass urine. May be either acute or chronic (the latter often leading to retention with overflow). May occur with prostatic enlargement, urethral stricture, **spinal** or **epidural anaesthesia** (including use of **spinal opioids**), after abdominal or pelvic surgery and following administration of drugs with anticholinergic effects. Neurological causes are rarer but include **spinal cord injury, cauda equina syndrome, Guillain–Barré syndrome** and **autonomic neuropathies,** e.g. diabetic. Signs include a full bladder, tender to palpation and dull to percussion. Can be confirmed with bladder ultrasound. May cause agitation and **confusion** postoperatively; can cause **hypertension,** tachycardia and raised **ICP** in unconscious patients. May cause acute pyelonephritis.

Urinary catheterisation (either urethral or, occasionally, suprapubic) may be required if encouragement is unsuccessful.

See also, Oliguria

Urinary tract infection (UTI). Most common **nosocomial infection** seen in critically ill patients and a common cause of generalised **sepsis.** In hospitals, almost always associated with urinary catheterisation, with the risk increasing the longer the catheter is in place. Gram-negative organisms (e.g. *Escherichia coli*, **pseudomonas**) are commonly involved, gaining entry to the bladder either through the catheter's lumen or along its surface. Diagnosis is confirmed by the presence of white blood cells and >100 000 organisms/mm^3 on urine microscopy. Urinary catheterisation should only be performed when necessary, aseptic technique used (often accompanied by a single prophylactic dose of **gentamicin**) and the catheter removed as soon as possible. Treatment of established UTI is with **antibacterial drugs** according to the results of urine culture.

Urine. Liquid containing **urea** and other waste products, excreted by the **kidneys.** Normal output in temperate climates is 800–2500 ml/day. Coloured yellowish by the pigments urochrome and uroerythrin, it darkens on standing by oxidation of urobilinogen to urobilin (colour does not necessarily reflect urine's concentration). Coloured red by **haemoglobin** or **myoglobin** and purple in **porphyria. Specific gravity** is normally 1.002–1.035. **Osmolality** may range between 30 and 1400 mosmol/kg, depending on fluid and hormonal status. **pH** is usually below 5.3. Normally contains under 150 mg protein/24 h. Abnormal constituents include **glucose**, ketones, bilirubin, erythrocytes, large numbers of leucocytes and casts.

Urinalysis is usually performed using reagent sticks; the reagents change colour according to the presence and amount of various normal and abnormal constituents in the sample. Specific gravity, electrolyte and solute content and pH can also be quantified.

Despite the kidneys' ability to concentrate the urine, a minimum of 500 ml/day is required to eliminate urea and other electrolytes. **Oliguria** is usually defined as less than 0.5 ml/kg/h and may indicate **hypovolaemia** or **renal failure**; anuria is complete cessation of urine flow and may indicate obstruction or urinary retention in addition. Polyuria occurs in **diabetes insipidus**, renal failure, diuretic therapy, **diabetes mellitus** (because of the osmotically active glucose load) and excessive water intake (**water diuresis**).

Urine output is routinely measured during critical illness and major surgery, because it reflects tissue perfusion and volume status of the circulation (assuming normal renal and cardiac function). Although **renal blood flow** is often reduced and circulating levels of **vasopressin** are high during surgery, urine output is usually maintained. An hourly urine output of >0.5 ml/kg/h is regarded as the minimum acceptable during critical illness or surgery by most anaesthetists.

See also, Nephron

Urokinase. Enzyme extracted from male human urine, used as a **fibrinolytic drug** in thromboembolic occlusive disease e.g. **DVT**, **PE**, blocked intravascular shunts/cannulae and occlusive peripheral arterial disease. Acts via activation of plasminogen.

- Dosage:
  - PE/DVT: 4400 IU/kg iv over 10–20 min, then 4400 IU/kg/h or 100 000 IU/h for 2–3 days.
  - 5000–25 500 IU instilled into the shunt/cannula and left for 20–60 min.
- Side effects: nausea, vomiting, back pain. Allergic reactions are rare.

Urotensin II. Peptide hormone found in fish and discovered in human tissues in 1999, with specific receptors in the heart and arterial vessels and CNS. Has extremely potent vasoconstrictive properties that vary according to vessel type. Its role as a major mediator in metabolic and cardiovascular regulation and a potential role for urotensin II antagonists have been suggested.

Uterus. Pear-shaped pelvic organ, 7.5 cm long, 5 cm wide and 2.5 cm thick when non-gravid. Divided into the upper body and lower cervix, separated by the isthmus. Separated from the bladder anteriorly by the uterovesical pouch, and from the rectum posteriorly by the uterorectal pouch. The broad ligaments lie laterally.

Blood supply is from the uterine artery, a branch of the internal iliac artery. The uterine vein drains into the internal iliac vein.

- Nerve supply:
  - sympathetic motor preganglionic fibres from T1–L2 and parasympathetic motor preganglionic fibres from S2–4 via the paracervical plexus. Actions are variable, depending on the stage of the menstrual cycle and **pregnancy**.
  - sensory fibres via sympathetic pathways, emerging in the paracervical tissues and passing through the hypogastric plexus to T11–12, sometimes also to T10 and L1.
- Actions of drugs on the pregnant uterus:
  - **α-adrenergic receptor agonists**, e.g. **noradrenaline**: increase uterine tone and strength of contraction.
  - **β-adrenergic receptor agonists**, e.g. **adrenaline, salbutamol**: decrease uterine tone and strength of contraction. Agonists specific for β_2-receptors are used as **tocolytic drugs** to delay premature labour.
  - **oxytocin** and **ergometrine**: produce powerful contraction. Atosiban (oxytocin antagonist) causes uterine relaxation.
  - **prostaglandins** PGE_2 and $PGF_2\alpha$: stimulate uterine contraction.
  - volatile **inhalational anaesthetic agents**: cause dose-related reduction of uterine tone.
  - iv anaesthetic agents, sedative and analgesic drugs, neuromuscular blocking drugs, acetylcholinesterase inhibitors: no effect on uterine tone.
  - others: **acetylcholine**, bradykinin, **histamine** and **5-HT** increase contraction. Smooth muscle relaxants (e.g. amyl nitrite, **GTN** and **papaverine**) cause relaxation. Alcohol has a direct relaxant action and suppresses oxytocin secretion from the **pituitary gland.**

See also, Obstetric analgesia and anaesthesia

UTI, *see Urinary tract infection*

Utstein style. Uniform system of reporting data for out-of-hospital **cardiac arrests**, arising from a meeting of representatives of international Resuscitation Councils in Utstein Abbey on the Norwegian Island of Mosterøy in June 1990. A second meeting (the Utstein II conference) in London the same year resulted in the publication of recommended guidelines for uniform reporting of such data, the 'Utstein style'. This 'style' has been recommended for in-hospital **CPR** attempts, paediatric CPR, laboratory CPR research and trauma.

Idris AH, Bierens JLM, Perkins GD et al. (2017). Circ Cardiovasc Qual Outcomes; 10: e000024

Vacuum insulated evaporator (VIE). Container for storage of liquid O_2 and maintenance of **piped gas supply**. An outer carbon steel shell is separated by a vacuum from an inner stainless steel shell that contains O_2. The inner temperature varies between –160°C and –180°C, at a pressure of 7–10 **bar**. Gaseous O_2 is withdrawn and heated to ambient temperature (and thus expanded) as required (Fig. 165); a pressure regulator distal to the superheater prevents pipeline pressure from exceeding 4.1 bar. If pressure within the container falls due to high demand, liquid O_2 may be withdrawn, vaporised in an evaporator and returned to the system, restoring working pressure. If passage of heat across the insulation causes vaporisation of liquid O_2 and a rise in pressure, gas can escape through a safety valve. The contents are indicated by a weighing device incorporated into the chamber's supports. The VIE must be kept outside, away from possible sources of ignition or combustion. Similar systems are used for storage of other gases, e.g. for industrial processes.

Howells RS (1980). Anaesthesia; 35: 676–98

Vagus nerve. Tenth **cranial nerve**. Arises in the medulla from the:
- dorsal nucleus of the vagus (parasympathetic).
- nucleus ambiguus (motor fibres to laryngeal, pharyngeal and palatal muscles).
- nucleus of the tractus solitarius (sensory fibres from the **larynx**, **pharynx**, GIT, **heart** and **lungs**, including taste fibres from the valleculae).

Leaves the medulla between the olive and inferior cerebellar peduncle, and passes through the jugular foramen of the **skull**. Descends in the neck within the carotid sheath between the internal **jugular vein** and internal/common **carotid arteries** (*see Fig. 116;* **Neck, cross-sectional anatomy**, *and Fig. 107a;* **Mediastinum**). Passes behind the root of the lung to form the pulmonary plexus, then on to the **oesophagus** to form the oesophageal plexus with the vagus from the other side. Both pass through the oesophageal opening of the **diaphragm** to supply the abdominal contents and GIT as far as the splenic flexure (*see Fig. 20;* **Autonomic nervous system**)
- Branches:
  - to the external auditory meatus and tympanic membrane.
  - to muscles of the pharynx and soft palate.
  - **laryngeal nerves**.
  - to cardiac, pulmonary and oesophageal plexuses.
  - to intra-abdominal organs.

The vagi form a major part of the **parasympathetic nervous system**. Vagal reflexes causing bradycardia, **laryngospasm** and **bronchospasm** may occur during anaesthesia. Intense stimulation may result in partial or complete **heart block** or even **asystole**. Anal and cervical stretching (e.g. **Brewer–Luckhardt reflex**) and traction on the extraocular muscles (**oculocardiac reflex**) are particularly intense stimuli, but it may also follow skin incision and stimulation (e.g. surgical) of the mesentery, biliary tract, uterus, bladder, urethra, testes, larynx, glottis, bronchial tree and carotid sinus. Also involved in the **diving reflex**.

Anticholinergic drugs antagonise vagal reflexes during surgery. Should they occur, surgical activity should cease, and **atropine** or **glycopyrronium** be administered if necessary.

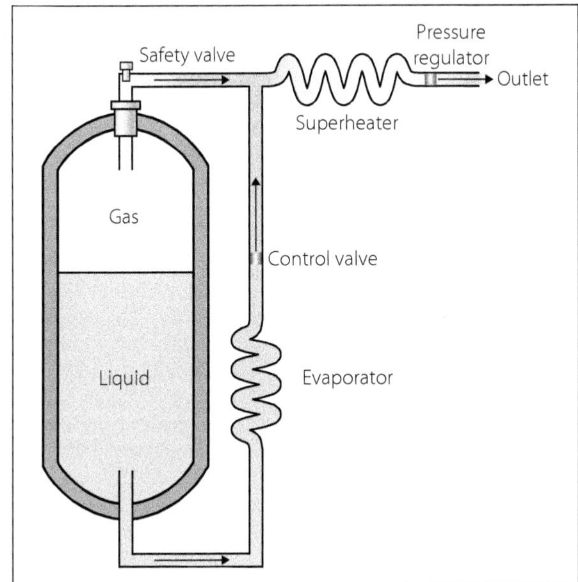

Fig. 165 Vacuum insulated evaporator

Valence. Capacity of an atom to combine with others in definite proportions; compared with that of hydrogen (value of 1). Dependent on the number of electrons in the outer shell of the atom; covalent bonds are formed when electrons are shared between different atoms, e.g. water: H–O–H.

VALI, *see Ventilator-associated lung injury*

Valproate/valproic acid, *see Sodium valproate*

Valsalva manoeuvre. Forced expiration against a closed glottis after a full inspiration, originally described as a technique for expelling pus from the middle ear. In its standardised form, 40 mmHg pressure is held for 10 s.
- Direct arterial BP tracings in normal subjects show four phases (Fig. 166):
  - phase I: increase in intrathoracic pressure expels blood from thoracic vessels.
  - phase II: decrease in BP due to reduction of venous return; activation of the **baroreceptor reflex** causes tachycardia and vasoconstriction, raising BP towards normal.
  - phase III: second drop in BP as intrathoracic pressure suddenly drops, with pooling of blood in the pulmonary vessels.

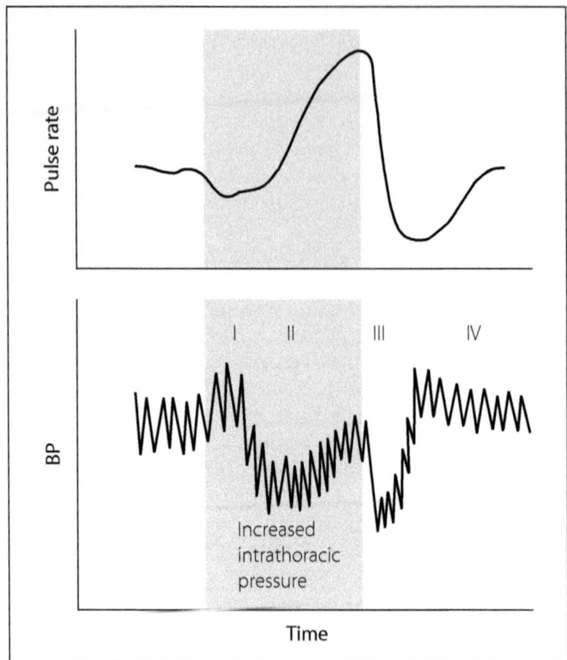

Fig. 166 Normal Valsalva response (*see text*)

- phase IV: overshoot, as compensatory mechanisms continue to operate with venous return restored. Increased BP causes bradycardia.

- Abnormal responses:
  - 'square wave' response, seen in **cardiac failure**, constrictive **pericarditis**, **cardiac tamponade** and valvular heart disease, when **CVP** is markedly raised. BP rises, remains high throughout the manoeuvre and returns to its previous level at the end.
  - autonomic dysfunction, e.g. **autonomic neuropathy**, drugs. BP falls and stays low until intrathoracic pressure is released. Pulse rate changes and overshoot are absent. The Valsalva ratio is the ratio of the longest R–R interval on the **ECG** (i.e., the slowest heart rate) to the shortest R–R interval (fastest heart rate). The normal value is >15 beats/min; <10 beats/min indicates parasympathetic autonomic dysfunction.
  - an exaggerated reduction in BP may be seen in **hypovolaemia**, e.g. during **IPPV**.

Useful as a bedside test of autonomic function. Concurrent ECG tracing allows accurate measurement of changes in heart rate. The manoeuvre may be useful in evaluating **heart murmurs**, and may be successful in terminating **SVT** (because of increased vagal tone in phase IV).
[Antonio Valsalva (1666–1723), Italian anatomist]

Valtis–Kennedy effect. Shift to the left of the **oxyhaemoglobin dissociation curve** during **blood storage**, originally described in 1954 for acid–citrate–dextrose storage. The shift reflects progressive depletion of **2,3-DPG**.
[Dimitrios J Valtis, Greek physician; Arthur C Kennedy (1922–2009), Glasgow physician]

Valveless anaesthetic breathing systems. Anaesthetic breathing systems designed to eliminate resistance due to **adjustable pressure-limiting valves**. In the Samson system, the valve is replaced by an adjustable orifice; in the Hafnia systems, expired gases pass through a port, assisted by an **ejector flowmeter**.
[Heyman H Samson (1911–1990), South African anaesthetist; *Hafnia*: Latin name for Copenhagen]

Valves, *see Adjustable pressure-limiting valves; Demand valves; Non-rebreathing valves*

Valvular heart disease. Causes, features and anaesthetic management: as for **congenital heart disease** and individual lesions. Valve replacement: as for **cardiac surgery**. Many prosthetic valves are available in different sizes, e.g. Silastic ball-and-cage, metal flaps and porcine valves. Thrombosis may form on prostheses, hence the requirement for long-term anticoagulation. Patients with prosthetic valves may also require prophylactic antibiotics as for congenital heart disease.

van der Waals equation of state. Modification of the **ideal gas law**, accounting for the forces of attraction between gas molecules, and the volume of the molecules:

$$RT = (P + a/V^2)(V - b)$$

where R = **universal gas constant**
T = temperature
P = pressure exerted by the gas
V = molar volume of gas
a and b = correction terms.
[Johannes van der Waals (1837–1923), Dutch physicist]

van der Waals forces. Weak attractive forces between neutral molecules and atoms, caused by electric polarisation of the particles induced by the presence of other particles.
See also, van der Waals equation of state

van Slyke apparatus. Device used to measure blood gas partial pressures. O_2 and CO_2 are released into a burette from the blood by addition of a liberating solution. Each gas in turn is converted to a non-gaseous substance by chemical reaction, and the pressure drop in the burette measured for each. The same reagents may be used as in the **Haldane apparatus**.
[Donald D van Slyke (1883–1971), US chemist]
See also, Carbon dioxide measurement; Gas analysis; Oxygen measurement

Vancomycin. Glycopeptide and **antibacterial drug** with bactericidal activity against aerobic and anaerobic gram-positive **bacteria** (including multiresistant staphylococci). Usually reserved for severe infections, resistant organisms or **penicillin** allergy. Despite this restriction in use, resistant species of vancomycin-resistant *Staphylococcus aureus* and entercocci are increasingly seen. Not absorbed orally.

- Dosage:
  - 1–1.5 g iv bd, subsequently adjusted according to plasma levels; the predose ('trough') level should be 10–15 mg/l (15–20 mg/l in **endocarditis** or severe infections/less sensitive *S. aureus*). May also be given by continuous 24-h infusion, delivering more consistent plasma levels; dosing is then guided by a 'random' plasma level.
  - 125–500 mg orally qds, in pseudomembranous colitis (for 7–10 days).
- Side effects: renal impairment, ototoxicity, blood dyscrasias, nausea, fever, allergic reactions, phlebitis. Rapid infusion may cause hypotension, urticaria, pruritus, flushing ('red man syndrome'), dyspnoea and cardiac arrest.

See also, Clostridial infections; Infection control

Vancomycin-resistant enterococci, *see Infection control; Vancomycin*

VAP, *see Ventilator-associated pneumonia*

Vaporisers. Devices for delivering accurate and safe concentrations of volatile **inhalational anaesthetic agents** to the patient.

- Classified into:
  - plenum vaporisers (*plenum* = chamber): widely used in modern anaesthesia despite their cost and complexity, because of their reliability, safety features and accuracy:
    - gas passes through the vaporiser under pressure at the back bar of the **anaesthetic machine**.
    - in most modern types (e.g. 'Tec' [temperature-compensated] vaporisers) fresh gas is divided by the control dial into two streams, one of which enters the vaporisation chamber, becomes fully saturated with agent and rejoins the other stream at the outlet (Fig. 167a). The ratio of the two streams (**splitting ratio**) determines the final delivered concentration (N.B. a different mechanism exists for the Tec 6 **desflurane** vaporiser: *see later*). In older vaporisers the delivered concentration was also affected by other factors (*see later*). In the obsolete 'copper kettle' type, a separate supply of O_2 was passed through the vaporiser, becoming fully saturated. It was then added to the main fresh gas flow, at a rate calculated according to desired final concentration and vaporiser temperature. The original design included a large mass of copper as a heat sink, hence its name.
    - have high resistance, so unsuitable for positioning in a **circle system.**
    - performance is not affected by whether ventilation is spontaneous or controlled.
    - include the Tec series of vaporisers. Features of the newer models include:
      - flow of liquid agent into the delivery line is prevented if the vaporiser is inverted.
      - interlock system prevents use of more than one vaporiser at a time, if mounted side by side.
      - **key filling system** prevents filling with the wrong agent.

      The Mark 6 is specific for desflurane and differs from those for other modern agents (Fig. 167b):
      - cannot use the above mechanism because desflurane's boiling point is very close to room temperature and therefore small variations in the latter result in large changes in SVP.
      - requires an electrical power supply for the heating elements and control mechanisms.
      - the fresh gas does not enter the vaporising chamber, but passes along a separate path to mix with pure desflurane vapour, leaving the chamber at the outlet (produced by heating the vaporising chamber to 39°C, thus ensuring complete vaporisation).
      - fresh gas encounters a flow restriction within the vaporiser, causing back pressure that varies according to fresh gas flow.
      - a system of pressure transducers and internal circuitry is used to monitor and adjust the performance to produce a consistent output even if fresh gas flow alters (detected by a change in back pressure). Internal switches cut out the system if temperature increases above 57°C or if the vaporiser is tilted or becomes empty.

      The current Tec model, the Mark 7 (Fig. 167c), is suitable for all modern agents except desflurane. It has improved accuracy of output over different flow ranges and protection against spillage and contamination compared with previous models.
  - draw-over vaporisers: despite their variable output, often preferred in the battlefield (e.g. **triservice apparatus**) and developing countries because they are cheap, simple and portable:
    - gas is drawn into the vaporising chamber by the patient's inspiratory effort.
    - resistance must be low.
    - performance is affected by minute ventilation, the output falling as ventilation increases.
    - may be suitable for use within **circle systems**, e.g. Goldman vaporiser (Fig. 167b), a small, light, uncompensated device with a glass container (originally adapted from a motor vehicle fuel pump). Similar vaporisers were designed by **McKesson** and **Rowbotham**, the latter's containing a wire gauze wick.
    - also used for **draw-over techniques**, e.g. (Fig. 167b):
      - EMO (Epstein and **Macintosh** of Oxford) **diethyl ether** inhaler: large vaporiser, incorporating a large vaporisation chamber, a water jacket for a heat sink and a temperature-compensating fluid-filled bellows at the outlet.
      - OMV (Oxford miniature vaporiser): small, uncompensated device, containing a water-filled heat sink (with antifreeze). Contains wire wicks; may thus be emptied of one agent, flushed and refilled with another. Different calibration scales may be fixed to the control valve for the various agents. A modified form is used in the triservice apparatus.
      - obsolete types, used formerly for obstetric analgesia:
        - Emotril (Epstein and Macintosh of Oxford/Trilene) **trichloroethylene** apparatus: incorporated within a metal box.
        - Cardiff **methoxyflurane** inhaler: free-standing on a base.
  - systems involving addition of liquid volatile agent directly to the fresh gas stream:
    - require delivery of liquid agent at a rate calculated automatically to produce the desired concentration.
    - incorporated into computerised anaesthetic machines.
    - combined with a carbon filter/evaporator system that fits into the patient's breathing system, conserving and recycling ~90% of the administered agent. Have been used for **sedation** on ICU without the need for anaesthetic machines.
- Factors affecting the delivered concentration:
  - splitting ratio (plenum vaporisers).
  - SVP of the volatile agent: equals the partial pressure of the agent within the vaporiser. Agents with high SVP (e.g. diethyl ether) vaporise more readily than those with low SVPs, e.g. methoxyflurane.
  - temperature of the liquid: affects the SVP. As liquid vaporises, **latent heat** of vaporisation is lost, and temperature and thus SVP fall. Delivered concentration of agent would therefore fall if not for temperature compensation devices, e.g.:

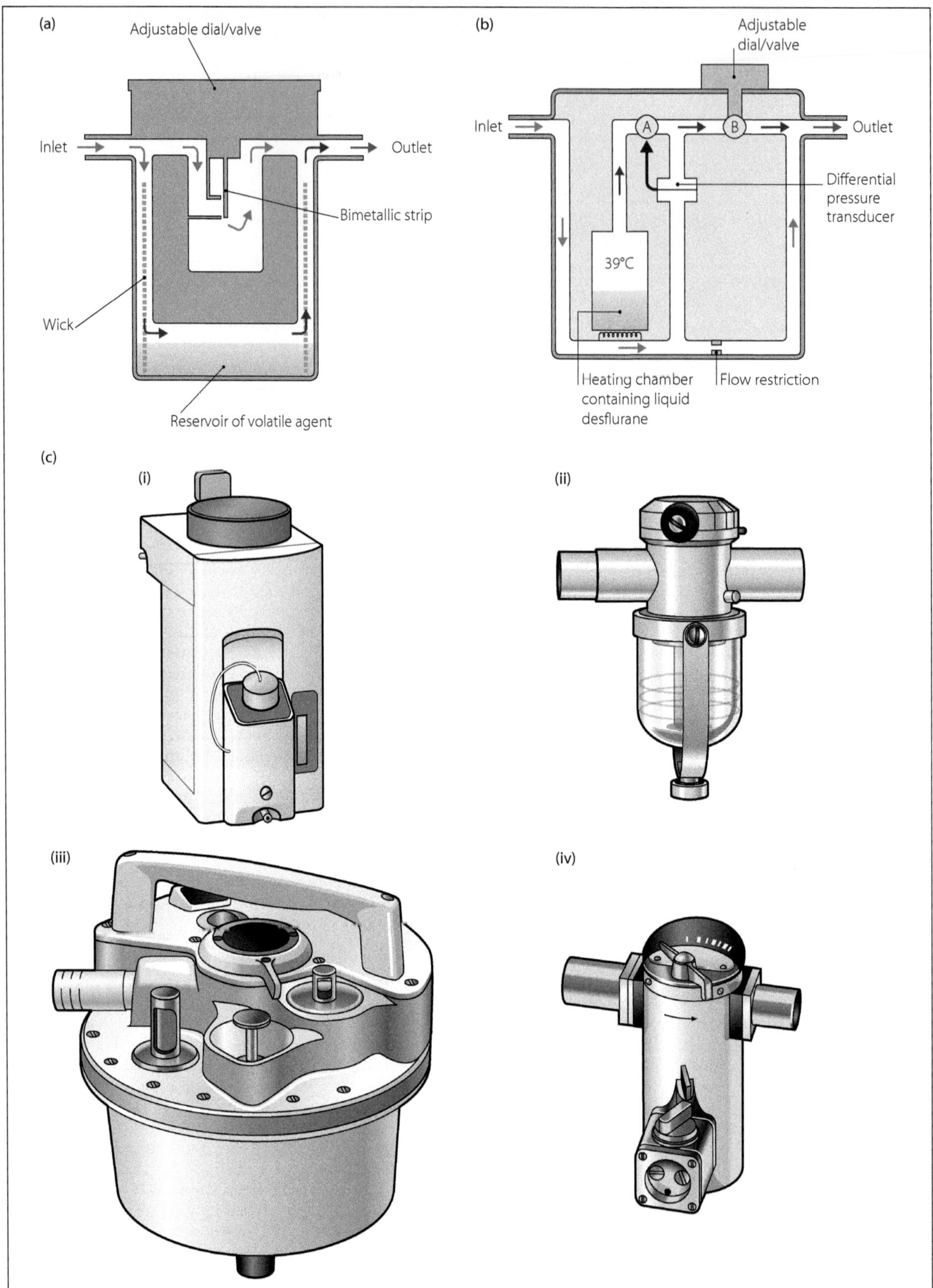

Fig. 167 (a) Principles of modern Tec vaporiser. When the dial/valve is adjusted, it alters the 'splitting ratio' of the gas that passes through the two paths shown. When it is in the 'off' position, all the gas passes via an additional route through the top (not shown) that bypasses these two paths completely. (b) Principles of Tec 6 desflurane vaporisor. The flow of pure desflurane vapour from heating liquid desflurane is controlled by valve A, which is adjusted automatically according to the differential pressures across a transducer. A second valve, B, is adjusted manually by the operator, altering the degree of mixing of gas streams and final output. *Pale purple arrows,* no volatile agent vapour; *dark arrows,* containing vapour. (c) 'Classic' types of vaporiser: (i) Tec Mark 7; (ii) Goldman; (iii) EMO; (iv) OMV (*see text*).

- bimetallic strip at the outlet (Tec Mark 2) or inlet (subsequent Tec models) of the vaporisation chamber.
- fluid-filled bellows at the gas outlet, e.g. EMO inhaler (*see later*); expands as temperature rises.
- longitudinally expanding metal rod at the gas outlet, e.g. Dräger models.

Temperature loss is reduced by providing heat sinks of metal (e.g. Tec) or water (EMO). Older vaporisers incorporated heating devices or thermometers to allow adjustment as temperature changed.

- surface area of the gas/liquid interface: increased with:
  - wicks and baffles, e.g. most plenum vaporisers (*see later*). Wicks maintain surface area despite gradual emptying of the vaporiser (level compensation).
  - a cowl to direct gas flow on to or into the liquid (e.g. the original **Boyle's** bottle).
  - production of many tiny bubbles with a sintered brass or glass diffuser, e.g. copper kettle-type vaporisers.
- fresh gas flow: the output of older devices varied considerably with gas flow (e.g. the Tec Mark 2 was supplied with charts showing the delivered versus the set concentrations at various flow rates); modern plenum vaporisers perform more consistently. Draw-over vaporisers are more efficient at lower gas flows.
- **pumping effect**.

For vaporisers in series: contamination of the second with vapour from the first may occur if both are turned on simultaneously. Although this cannot occur with modern vaporisers, for other types the one containing the less volatile agent (i.e., with lower SVP) should be placed upstream, because:

- it requires proportionally more of the fresh gas flow than the vaporiser containing the more volatile agent, and would thus receive more contaminant if placed downstream.
- the more volatile agent, being easier to vaporise, would attain higher (and thus potentially dangerous) concentrations than those set if it contaminated the vaporiser designed for a less volatile agent.

Vaporisers have been associated with many hazards, and require regular servicing.

[Heinrich Dräger (1847–1917), German engineer; Victor Goldman (1903–1993), London anaesthetist; Hans G Epstein (1909–2002), Berlin-born Oxford physicist]

See also, Altitude, high

Vapour. Matter in the gaseous state below its **critical temperature**; i.e., its constituent particles may enter the liquid state. As liquid vaporises, heat is required (**latent heat** of vaporisation); as vapour condenses, an equal amount of heat is produced. These processes occur continuously above the surface of a liquid at equilibrium.

See also, Vapour pressure

Vapour pressure. **Pressure** exerted by molecules escaping from the surface of a liquid to enter the gaseous phase. When equilibrium is reached at any temperature, the number of molecules leaving the liquid phase equals the number entering it; the vapour pressure now equals **SVP**. Raising the temperature of the liquid increases the kinetic energy of the molecules, allowing more of them to escape and raising the vapour pressure. When SVP equals atmospheric pressure, the liquid boils.

Vaptans, *see Vasopressin receptor antagonists*

Variance. **Standard deviation** squared. Thus an indicator of spread of values within a **sample**. Although standard deviation is commonly used when describing data, many statistical calculations employ its square; hence the use of variance as a meaningful term (e.g. analysis of variance, ANOVA).

See also, Statistics

VAS, Visual analogue scale, *see Linear analogue scale*

Vascular access, *see Central venous cannulation; Intravenous fluid administration*

Vascular resistance, *see Pulmonary vascular resistance; Systemic vascular resistance*

Vasculitides. Group of conditions characterised by inflammation of blood vessels. All except giant cell arteritis are uncommon and associated with **connective tissue diseases** or drug hypersensitivity. Diagnosis requires biopsy, which often shows granuloma formation associated with vessel inflammation.

- Classification:
  - large vessel vasculitis:
    - Takayasu's arteritis: rare large vessel arteritis affecting young women. Affects the aorta and its branches, causing inflammation and then stenosis of affected vessels. Features include cerebrovascular insufficiency (fainting, dizziness) and reduced peripheral pulses. Treatment depends on the underlying condition but usually includes **immunosuppressive drugs**.
    - giant cell arteritis (temporal arteritis): usually affects the elderly and often associated with polymyalgia rheumatica. Predominantly involves branches of the external carotid artery. Headache, often localised, is the predominant symptom. Blindness may result if **corticosteroids** are not given promptly.
  - medium vessel vasculitis:
    - **polyarteritis nodosa**.
    - **Kawasaki disease**.
  - small vessel vasculitis:
    - anti-neutrophil cytoplasmic antibody (ANCA) associated vasculitis:
      - **Wegener's granulomatosis**.
      - eosinophil granulomatosis with polyangiitis (Churg-Strauss disease).
    - immune complex small vessel vasculitis:
      - antiglomerular basement membrane disease.
      - IgA vasculitis—Henoch–Schönlein purpura: usually occurs in childhood following an upper respiratory tract infection. Features include fever, headache, macular/urticarial rash becoming purpuric, over the buttocks and limbs. Inflammatory synovitis is common. Focal **glomerulonephritis** may lead to **nephrotic syndrome** and, rarely, **renal failure**.
  - vasculitis associated with systemic disease, e.g. **rheumatoid arthritis, sarcoidosis, SLE**.
  - others: associated with **hepatitis** B and C, **syphilis** (aortitis), malignancy.

[Jacob Churg (1910–2005); Lotte Strauss (1913–1985), US pathologists; Eduard H Henoch (1820–1910), German physician; Johann L Schönlein (1793–1864), German

paediatrician; Michishige Takayasu (1860–1938), Japanese ophthalmologist]
Jennette JC (2013). Clin Exp Nephrol; 17: 603–6

Vasoactive intestinal peptide (VIP). GIT hormone, also found in the hypothalamus, cortex, primary afferent neurones, spinal cord, retina and bloodstream. Causes oesophageal relaxation preceding a peristaltic wave, relaxation of sphincters, stimulation of intestinal electrolyte and water secretion and inhibition of gastric secretion. Dilates peripheral blood vessels and causes bronchodilatation. Has positive inotropic and chronotropic action on the heart and causes coronary vasodilatation. Has an important role in the regulation of circadian rhythms. Tumours secreting VIP (VIPomas) may cause severe diarrhoea and hypotension.

Vasoconstrictor drugs, *see Vasopressor drugs*

Vasodilator drugs. Drugs causing vasodilatation as their primary effect (cf. **isoflurane**, **morphine**). The term is sometimes reserved for drugs acting directly at vascular smooth muscle. **Nitric oxide** is thought to be a common end pathway for many drugs.

- May be divided according to their main site of action, although considerable overlap occurs:
  - venous system: **GTN**, **isosorbide**.
  - arterial system: **hydralazine**, **calcium channel blocking drugs**, **salbutamol**, **diazoxide**, **minoxidil**, **adenosine**.
  - venous and arterial systems: **sodium nitroprusside**, **α-adrenergic receptor antagonists**, **angiotensin converting enzyme inhibitors**, **ganglion blocking drugs**, **potassium channel activators**.
- Used to reduce **SVR** and thus:
  - systemic BP, e.g. in **hypotensive anaesthesia**, **hypertensive crisis**, **pre-eclampsia**. Their effect is sometimes offset by reflex tachycardia.
  - **afterload** and ventricular work, e.g. in **cardiac failure**, **shock**. Increase **stroke volume** and reduce myocardial O_2 demand.

Also reduce **preload** via venous dilatation. Also used to reduce **pulmonary vascular resistance** in **pulmonary hypertension**, although the systemic circulation is usually affected too.
See also, Antihypertensive drugs; Inotropic drugs

Vasomotor centre. Group of neurones in the ventrolateral medulla, involved in the control of **arterial BP**. Projects to sympathetic preganglionic neurones in the **spinal cord**. Normal continuous discharge causes partial contraction of vascular smooth muscle (vasomotor tone) and resting sympathetic stimulation of the heart.

- Discharge is increased by:
  - **chemoreceptor** discharge.
  - pain, emotion.
  - **hypoxia** (causes direct stimulation initially, but depression follows).
- Discharge is decreased by:
  - **baroreceptor** discharge.
  - lung inflation.
  - prolonged pain, emotion.

Thus responds to hypotension (reduced baroreceptor discharge) by increasing sympathetic activity.

Dorsal and medial neurones functionally constitute the **cardioinhibitory centre**, stimulation of which inhibits the vasomotor centre and increases vagal activity.

Vasopressin (Arginine vasopressin, AVP; Antidiuretic hormone, ADH). Neuropeptide synthesised in the cell bodies of the supraoptic and paraventricular nuclei of the hypothalamus. Transported down their axons to the posterior lobe of the **pituitary gland**, from where it is secreted. Metabolised in the kidney and liver, it has a circulatory **half-life** of 10–30 min. There are at least three types of vasopressin receptor, all of which are **G protein-coupled receptors**: V_1 receptors are G_q-coupled and located primarily on vascular smooth muscle and platelets; V_2 receptors (G_s-coupled) mediate vasopressin's antidiuretic actions on the kidney; and V_3 receptors (coupled to multiple G proteins) are located centrally and involved in vasopressin's **neurotransmitter** actions.

- Main effects:
  - water retention by the kidney, acting via V_2 vasopressin receptors. These increase adenylate cyclase activity and **cAMP** levels, triggering transcription and insertion of aquaporin 2 water channels into the luminal membranes of cells in the distal convoluted tubules and collecting ducts. This results in water reabsorption from the renal tubules. Urine volume decreases; its concentration increases. Conversely, plasma volume increases; its concentration decreases.
  - vasoconstriction, acting via V_1 vasopressin receptors on vascular smooth muscle. Thought to have a minor role in normal BP regulation.
  - has a role in **temperature regulation**, control of circadian rhythm and memory function.
  - increased plasma levels of **coagulation** factor VIII.
- Release is increased by:
  - increased plasma **osmolality**; detected by **osmoreceptors** in the anterior hypothalamus.
  - decreased **ECF** volume and hypotension (e.g. in **haemorrhage**); detected by **baroreceptors**.
  - pain, nausea, hypoxaemia, emotional and physical stress.
  - drugs, e.g. **morphine**, **barbiturates**.
  - angiotensin II.
- Release is inhibited by:
  - decreased plasma osmolality.
  - increased ECF volume.
  - drugs, e.g. alcohol, **butorphanol**.
- Used therapeutically in various forms:
  - argipressin: synthetic vasopressin; used in pituitary **diabetes insipidus** (DI; 5–20 U sc/im, 4-hourly) and for control of bleeding **oesophageal varices** (20 U iv over 15 min). Side effects include pallor, nausea, abdominal cramps and myocardial ischaemia. **GTN** (patch or iv) has been used to reduce the incidence and severity of side effects.
  - terlipressin: a **prodrug**, it is enzymatically cleaved to release vasopressin. Dosage: 1–2 mg iv, repeated 4–6-hourly for up to 72 h. Side effects are milder than after argipressin.
  - lypressin: used as a nasal spray in pituitary DI: 5–10 U 6–8-hourly. Side effects are milder than after argipressin.
  - **desmopressin**: may be given nasally, orally or by im/sc/iv injection. Minimal vasoconstrictor activity; used in pituitary DI and to boost factor VIII levels in **haemophilia** and **von Willebrand's disease**.
  - **felypressin**: used as a vasoconstrictor in local anaesthesia.

Vasopressin has been used as an alternative to **adrenaline** in the treatment of **cardiac arrest** and **septic shock**, and as a means of preserving organ function in brainstem-dead

donors. Has been used in **anaphylaxis** resistant to adrenaline treatment (5 U repeated as necessary). **Vasopressin receptor antagonists** have been studied for use in **cardiac failure** and **hyponatraemia**.
See also, Syndrome of inappropriate antidiuretic hormone secretion

Vasopressin receptor antagonists (Vaptans). Competitive antagonists at V_2 **vasopressin** receptors, used for the treatment of hyper- and euvolaemic **hyponatraemia**, e.g. in **cardiac failure, hepatic failure** and **syndrome of inappropriate antidiuretic hormone secretion** (SIADH), respectively. Cause increased free water excretion, leading to an increase in plasma **sodium** concentration and reduced total body water.

Increased water intake due to increased thirst may reduce their efficacy. Other side effects include **dehydration**, nausea, skin rashes and orthostatic hypotension. Contraindicated in hypovolaemic hyponatraemia. All vaptans are substrates and inhibitors of the CYP3A4 isoenzyme of the **cytochrome oxidase system**; caution is therefore required when co-administered with drugs causing **enzyme induction/inhibition**. Tolvaptan is the only agent available in the UK and is licensed for the treatment of hyponatraemia secondary to SIADH. It has also been recommended for the treatment of autosomal dominant polycystic kidney disease.
Berl T (2015). N Engl J Med; 372: 2207–16

Vasopressor drugs. Drugs causing vasoconstriction; used to increase arterial BP, e.g. during anaesthesia, intensive care or **CPR**, or to prolong the action of **local anaesthetic agents** by preventing their systemic absorption. Formerly used rather indiscriminately to increase BP, they are now reserved for situations where vasodilatation is a specific problem, e.g. **anaphylaxis, spinal anaesthesia**.

- Mostly sympathomimetic drugs:
  - **catecholamines**, e.g. **adrenaline**, **noradrenaline**, dopamine.
  - non-catecholamines, e.g. **ephedrine**, **metaraminol**, **phenylephrine**.
- Directly acting vasopressor hormones and their analogues have also been used, e.g. in hypotension refractory to other potent vasopressors:
  - **vasopressin** and its synthetic analogues.
  - angiotensin (*see Renin/angiotensin system*).

Convincing data now exist supporting the use of noradrenaline as the preferred first-line drug in the treatment of **septic shock**; vasopressin may be added for those patients not responding to noradrenaline or to allow reduction of the dose of noradrenaline. Dopamine use is associated with increased mortality and the development of arrhythmias.
See also, Inotropic drugs

Vasovagal syncope. Fainting, often caused by emotion or pain. May occur in patients undergoing venous cannulation or regional anaesthesia. Vasodilatation in muscle (sympathetic discharge) and bradycardia (vagal discharge) cause hypotension and loss of consciousness, usually short-lived.

vCJD, *see Creutzfeldt–Jakob disease*

Vecuronium bromide. Non-depolarising **neuromuscular blocking drug**, introduced in the UK in 1983. A monoquaternary aminosteroid, similar in structure to **pancuronium**. Initial dose is 80–100 μg/kg; good intubating conditions occur within 90–120 s. Relaxation lasts for 20–30 min; duration is increased to 50 min if 150 μg/kg is used, and 80 min if 250 μg/kg is used. Supplementary dose: 20–30 μg/kg (30–50 μg/kg initial dose after administration of **suxamethonium** for intubation). May also be given by infusion, at 50–80 μg/kg/h.

Causes minimal **histamine** release, ganglion or vagal blockade, even at several times the usual doses. Thus has minimal effects on BP and pulse, but may allow unopposed vagal stimulation to cause bradycardia. Metabolised in the liver to the active 3-desacetylvecuronium. Excreted mainly in bile, but also in urine. Reversal of action is fast, and **acetylcholinesterase inhibitors** may not always be required. Cumulation is unlikely. Has been in short supply for 5–10 years.

Vegetative state. Disorder of **consciousness** in which the patient appears to be awake but is unaware of him-/herself or the surrounding environment; differs from **coma** (patient is neither awake nor aware) or the minimally conscious state (patient is awake and appears to be intermittently aware). Due to injury to cortical, subcortical and thalamic structures.

- May be:
  - acute: **TBI**, **cerebral hypoxic ischaemic injury**, infection (**meningitis, encephalitis**), **stroke**.
  - subacute: during a neurodegenerative process e.g. Alzheimer's disease.

Clinical features include complete non-responsiveness with preservation of hypothalamic/brainstem function and cycles of eye opening/closing suggestive of sleep–wake cycles. Diagnosis is based on the lack of reproducible response to visual, olfactory, auditory, tactile or noxious stimuli. Recent functional MRI and EEG studies suggest that some patients formerly diagnosed as being in a vegetative state are, in fact, in a minimally conscious state but are unable to respond to stimuli due to their disability.

The vegetative state is called continuous (in the UK) or persistent (in the US) when it lasts >1 month and permanent after 6–12 months. The abbreviation PVS refers to persistent rather than permanent vegetative state.

- Prognosis depends on:
  - time spent in vegetative state (only 3% of patients regain independence after 6 months).
  - age (best prognosis is in those <20 years old).
  - type of brain injury: 50% of patients in a vegetative state for one month following TBI will regain consciousness compared with 13% of those in a vegetative state following stroke.

[Alois Alzheimer (1864–1915), German neurologist and pathologist]
Brogan ME, Provencio JJ (2014). J Crit Care; 29: 679–82

Venous admixture. Refers to lowering of arterial $P\text{O}_2$ from the 'ideal' level that would occur if there were no **shunt** or $\dot{V}/\dot{Q}$ **mismatch**, either of which may lower $P\text{O}_2$. Defined as the amount of true shunt that would give the observed $P\text{O}_2$. May be calculated from the **shunt equation**.

Venous cannulation, *see Central venous cannulation; Intravenous fluid administration*

Venous drainage of arm. Deep veins accompany the arteries (deep venae comitantes). Superficial veins on the

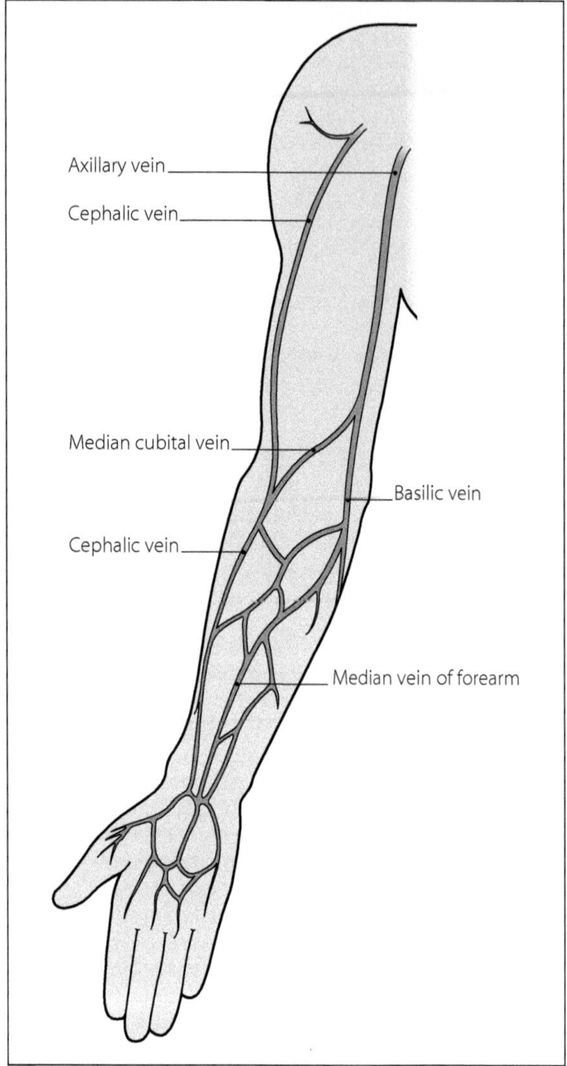

Fig. 168 Superficial venous drainage of the arm

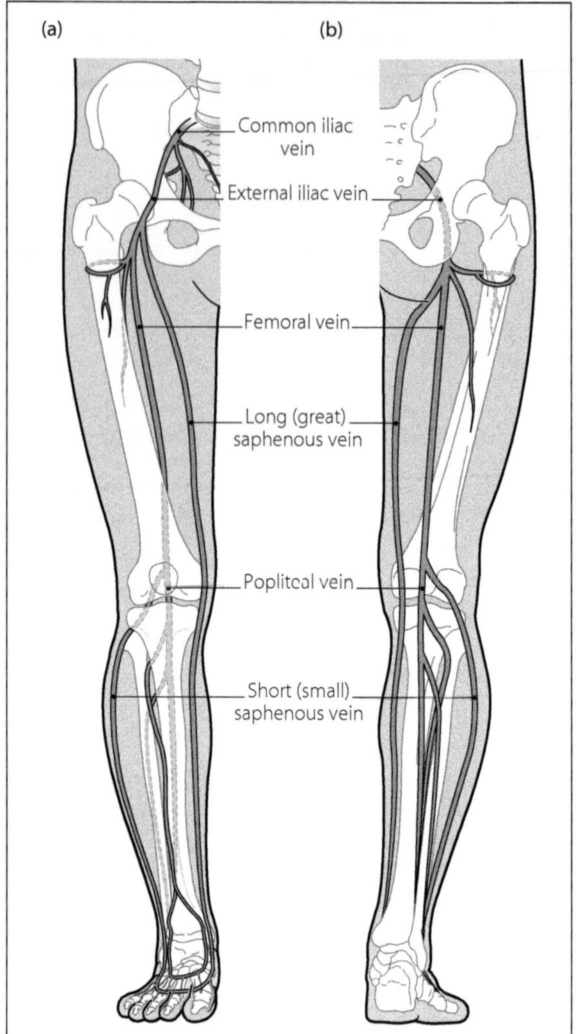

Fig. 169 Venous drainage of the leg: (a) anterior; (b) posterior

back of the hand form the dorsal venous arch, from which the basilic and cephalic veins arise. Smaller veins arise from the anterior aspect of the arm (Fig. 168). The anatomy of the veins may vary considerably, especially that of the cephalic vein.

- Main veins of the forearm:
  - basilic vein: ascends on the posteromedial side of the forearm, passing to the anterior side below the elbow. Passes along the medial side of the biceps muscle and pierces the deep fascia. At the axilla it joins the deep venae comitantes of the brachial artery to form the axillary vein.
  - cephalic vein: ascends on the lateral side of the forearm, passing anterior to the elbow. Runs on the lateral aspect of biceps, along the groove between deltoid and biceps, and pierces the clavipectoral fascia at the lower border of pectoralis major, to join the axillary vein. The angle at which the vessels meet, and the presence of valves at the junction, may cause difficulty in passing an iv catheter past this point.

See also, Antecubital fossa

Venous drainage of head and neck, *see Cerebral circulation; Jugular veins*

Venous drainage of leg. Comprises superficial and deep veins (Fig. 169):

- the important superficial veins arise at the ankle:
  - long (great) saphenous vein: passes anterior to the medial malleolus behind the saphenous nerve. Ascends behind the medial condyles of the tibia and femur, passing into the thigh and through the saphenous opening in the deep fascia to end in the femoral vein.
  - short (small) saphenous vein: passes behind the lateral malleolus, piercing the deep fascia to join the popliteal vein.
- deep veins start as digital and metatarsal veins in the sole, forming the lateral and medial plantar veins. These form the posterior tibial veins. The anterior tibial veins pass through the interosseus membrane, joining the posterior tibial veins to form the popliteal vein. This ascends through the popliteal fossa to form the femoral vein, which becomes the external iliac vein deep to the inguinal ligament.

Venous pressure, *see Central venous pressure; Jugular venous pressure; Venous waveform*

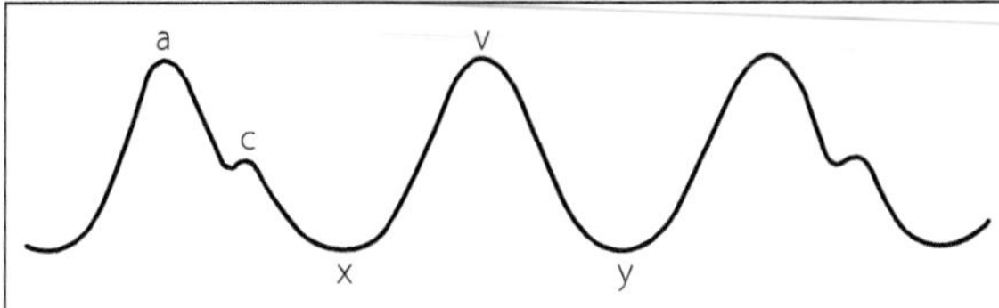

Fig. 170 Venous waveform (*see text*)

Venous return. Refers to the volume of blood entering the right atrium per minute. A major determinant of **cardiac output**, as described by **Starling's law**.
- Depends on:
  - venous tone.
  - intrathoracic pressure.
  - intra-abdominal pressure.
  - blood volume.
  - right and left ventricular function.
  - skeletal muscle activity (muscle pump).
  - posture.
  - vasodilator/vasopressor drug therapy.

See also, Preload

Venous waveform. Obtained from the tracing of **CVP**. Can be seen but not felt in the neck as the **JVP**. Consists of named waves and descents (Fig. 170):
  - 'a' wave is due to atrial contraction.
  - 'c' wave is thought to be due to transmitted pulsation from the carotid arteries, or to bulging of the tricuspid valve into the right atrium.
  - 'v' wave is due to atrial filling.
  - 'x' descent is due to atrial relaxation.
  - 'y' descent is due to atrial emptying as the tricuspid valve opens and blood drains into the ventricle.
- Abnormalities seen in the JVP wave may assist diagnosis of certain valve and rhythm disorders:
  - no 'a' wave: **AF**.
  - enlarged 'a' wave:
    - tricuspid stenosis.
    - stiff right ventricle, e.g. pulmonary stenosis, **pulmonary hypertension**.
  - enlarged 'v' wave: tricuspid regurgitation, e.g. due to **cardiac failure**.
  - cannon waves (large waves, not corresponding to 'a', 'v' or 'c' waves):
    - complete **heart block** (irregular).
    - **junctional arrhythmias** (regular).

A similar waveform is seen in the left atrial pressure tracing.
See also, Cardiac cycle

Ventilation, controlled, *see Airway pressure release ventilation; Assisted ventilation; High-frequency ventilation; Inspiratory pressure support; Inspiratory volume support; Intermittent mandatory ventilation; Intermittent negative pressure ventilation; Intermittent positive pressure ventilation; Inverse ratio ventilation; Mandatory minute ventilation; Non-invasive positive pressure ventilation; Pressure-regulated volume control ventilation; Proportional assist ventilation; Synchronised intermittent mandatory ventilation*

Ventilation, liquid, *see Liquid ventilation*

Ventilation, spontaneous, *see Breathing, control of; Breathing, work of; Respiratory muscles*

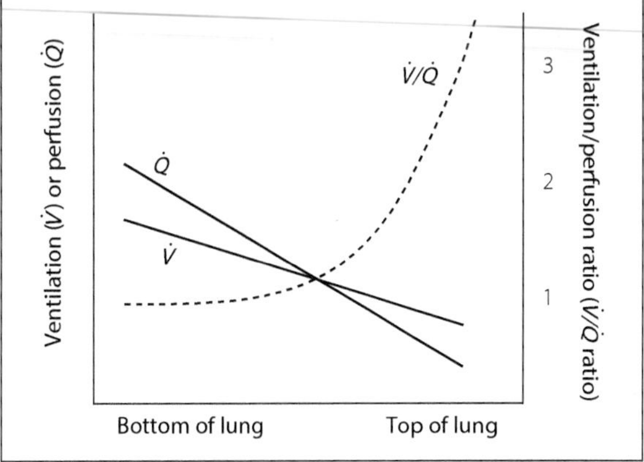

Fig. 171 $\dot{V}/\dot{Q}$ mismatch graph

Ventilation/perfusion mismatch ($\dot{V}/\dot{Q}$ mismatch). Imbalance between **alveolar ventilation** ($\dot{V}$) and pulmonary capillary blood flow ($\dot{Q}$). In the ideal lung model, ventilation would be distributed uniformly to all parts of the lung and would be matched by uniform distribution of blood flow (i.e., $\dot{V}/\dot{Q} = 1$). However, even in a healthy 70-kg male, alveolar ventilation and blood flow are unequal (4 l/min and 5 l/min, respectively), giving a $\dot{V}/\dot{Q}$ ratio of 0.8.

In addition, gravitational forces result in a gradient of $\dot{V}/\dot{Q}$ ratios in the lung as one travels from the base to the apex in the upright position (Fig. 171). Both ventilation and perfusion decrease from base to apex, but perfusion to a greater extent than ventilation. Thus the $\dot{V}/\dot{Q}$ ratio is higher at the apex ($\dot{V}/\dot{Q} = 3.3$) than at the base ($\dot{V}/\dot{Q} = 0.63$). Similar but smaller changes occur across the lung in the supine position.

$\dot{V}/\dot{Q}$ mismatch may result in $\dot{V}/\dot{Q}$ ratios ranging from zero (perfusion but no ventilation) to infinity (ventilation but no perfusion). Its effects on gas exchange are those of **shunt** and **dead space**, respectively, and can be assessed by determining **venous admixture** and physiological dead space. $\dot{V}/\dot{Q}$ mismatch is a common cause of **hypoxaemia** in pulmonary disease, e.g. **COPD**, **asthma**, **chest infection** and **pulmonary oedema** and circulatory disorders, e.g. **PE**.

Mismatch may be measured using **radioisotope** scanning of ventilation and perfusion separately, e.g. with xenon and technetium.
See also, Pulmonary circulation

Ventilator-associated lung injury (VALI). **ALI** associated with mechanical **IPPV**; may occur in previously normal lungs or worsen pre-existing lung pathology. Attributed to: the use of high inspiratory plateau pressures; high tidal volumes; and repeated recruitment and derecruitment of airways and associated lung units. These result in **barotrauma**, volutrauma and atelectrauma, respectively, that in turn lead to biotrauma (local and systemic inflammation with activation of neutrophils and release of chemokines and **cytokines**). **Oxygen toxicity** may also contribute. **Lung protection strategies** aim to mitigate these effects.
Slutsky AS, Ranieri VM (2013). N Engl J Med; 369: 2126–36
See also, Barotrauma; Intermittent positive pressure ventilation

Ventilator-associated pneumonia (VAP). **Nosocomial pneumonia** occurring after 48–72 h following tracheal intubation and **IPPV**. Accounts for approximately 50% of nosocomial pneumonia and occurs in ~30% of patients requiring IPPV. It is the most common ICU infection and accounts for 50% of antibacterial drug treatment in the ICU. It increases ICU stay and patient ventilator days and increases the mortality of the underlying disease by ~30%. Risk of VAP is highest during the first 5 days of IPPV with a mean duration between intubation and the development of VAP of 3.3 days. Attributable mortality of VAP is ~10% and this has decreased due to the adoption of **lung protection strategies**. Early VAP is most often due to common, antibiotic-sensitive organisms (e.g. *Streptococcus pneumonia, Haemophilus influenzae, Escherichia coli, Klebsiella pneumoniae*, etc.) whereas later infection is often due to multidrug-resistant organisms (e.g. methicillin-resistant *Streptococcus aureus*, *Acinetobacter*, *Pseudomonas aeruginosa* etc.). Viruses and fungi may also be causal agents.

- Risk factors:
  - patient-related: age, cardiorespiratory disease, **immunodeficiency**, **ALI**, **coma**, **MODS**.
  - ventilator-related: duration of IPPV, tracheal cuff pressure <20 cmH_2O, reintubation.
  - general ICU care: supine position, invasive devices, aspiration, **H_2 receptor antagonists**, recent antibiotic therapy.

Diagnostic criteria include: CXR infiltrates; fever; leucocytosis; purulent sputum; and positive microbiological cultures of sputum samples. Sputum may be obtained from tracheal tube suction, bronchoalveolar lavage (BAL) or protected brush specimens (PSB) (where a brush at the tip of the aspiration catheter is rubbed against the bronchial wall). Recent trials show no advantages of BAL or PSB over conventional tracheal aspiration sampling.

Differential diagnosis includes **pulmonary oedema**, **atelectasis**, **PE**, ALI and pulmonary haemorrhage.

Treatment includes chest **physiotherapy** and appropriate antibacterial drug therapy, guided either by positive cultures and sensitivities, or empirical selection based on the most likely organisms.

Preventive measures, often delivered as a **care bundle**, include: good oral care; avoidance of nasotracheal intubation, use of silver or antibiotic coated tracheal tubes, early **tracheostomy**, subglottic drainage devices, elevation of the bed-head to 30–45 degrees; **rotational therapy**; prevention of over-**sedation**; protocol-driven **weaning from ventilators**; and monitoring of tracheal cuff pressures.

Nair GB, Niederman MS (2015). Intensive Care Med; 41: 34–48

See also Chest infection; Intubation, tracheal; Nosocomial infections; Sepsis

Ventilators. Mechanical devices for ventilating the lungs. First described in the early 1900s as an alternative to resuscitation equipment incorporating **bellows**. The polio epidemic in Denmark in 1952 was a major impetus to the development of reliable positive pressure ventilators.

- Divided into:
  - negative pressure devices used for **intermittent negative pressure ventilation**: the negative pressure around the thorax causes chest expansion and draws in air:
    - tank ventilators ('iron lungs'):
      - enclose the whole body (apart from the head and neck) within an airtight casing.
      - efficient, but access to the patient is very restricted.
    - cuirass ventilators:
      - enclose the thorax and upper abdomen. Inflatable jacket versions have been described.
      - less restrictive but less efficient.

    Do not protect against **aspiration of gastric contents**. Their effectiveness may be reduced by indrawing of the soft tissues of the upper airway during inspiration. **Tracheostomy** may be required if this occurs.
  - positive pressure devices used for **IPPV**: deliver positive pressure to the lungs either invasively via a **tracheal tube**, tracheostomy, or injector device, or non-invasively via **facemask** or nasal mask (**non-invasive positive pressure ventilation**).

    Positive pressure ventilators are widely used during anaesthesia and in ICU. They may be powered:
    - electrically, e.g. employing a crankshaft (e.g. Cape ventilator) or solenoid (e.g. Siemens or Engström ventilators).
    - by a separate supply of compressed air or O_2, employing **fluidics** or pneumatics (e.g. Penlon Nuffield ventilator).
    - by anaesthetic gases (e.g. Manley ventilator). These types are 'minute volume dividers' (*see later*).
- Classification of positive pressure ventilators: many different classifications have been suggested, e.g. according to the mechanism of action:
  - 'mechanical thumbs': intermittent occlusion of the open limb of a T-piece, e.g. by a solenoid, e.g. the Sheffield infant ventilator. 'Intermittent blowers' may be used to achieve a similar effect by moving a column of driving gas forwards and backwards along a length of tubing connecting the ventilator with the T-piece, e.g. the Penlon Nuffield ventilator attached to the Bain **coaxial anaesthetic breathing system**. Anaesthetic gases are delivered separately through the other limb of the T-piece. A similar technique may be used with a **circle system**.
  - 'minute volume dividers': supply only the minute volume of anaesthetic gas delivered to them, by dividing the preset minute volume into equally sized breaths, e.g. Manley ventilators and (obsolete) 'vents' (e.g. Minivent, East–Freeman automatic vent: small devices, placed at the patient end of an **anaesthetic breathing system**, that intermittently allow gas flow when upstream pressure is sufficient to overcome the resistance offered by a magnetised bobbin within them). Delivered minute volume may be read directly from the **anaesthetic machine** flowmeters.
  - 'bag-squeezers': employ mechanical or pneumatic force to compress the bag or bellows intermittently, e.g. Air-shields ventilator, Oxford ventilator (pneumatic), Cape ventilator (mechanical). Widely used with modern circle systems. Bellows that ascend during filling are preferable to those that descend during filling, because the former will not fill if there is a disconnection or leak, whereas the latter will still descend.
  - 'intermittent blowers': produce intermittent flow from a high-pressure source, e.g. **cylinders**. Include the Bird ventilators used on ICU, and small devices used for transport of ventilated patients, e.g. Pneupac ventilator. The Penlon Nuffield ventilator is suitable for use with the Bain and circle systems; it may also be used for children (with a paediatric pressure release valve) using the T-piece.
  - jet ventilators: include those used for **injector techniques** and **high-frequency ventilation**.

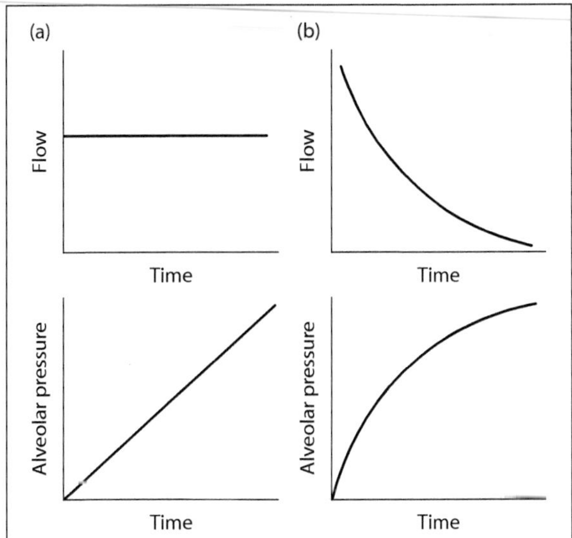

Fig. 172 Inspiratory characteristics of (a) constant flow and (b) constant pressure generators

- Another widely used classification is that suggested by Mapleson in 1969, according to the characteristics during the inspiratory phase and inspiratory to expiratory (I-to-E) cycling:
  - inspiratory characteristics:
    - flow generators: produce a high generating pressure (e.g. 400 kPa) and are thus able to deliver flow that is unaffected by patient characteristics. The flow produced may be constant or non-constant (usually the former). Non-constant flow generators include the Cape ventilator, in which flow is sinusoidal because of the crank mechanism employed. Most ICU ventilators are flow generators (Fig. 172a), as they are able to produce the high inflation pressures required to achieve the preset flow in non-compliant lungs, e.g. in **bronchospasm. Barotrauma** may occur if high **airway pressures** are reached.
    - pressure generators: produce low generating pressure (e.g. 1.5 kPa); thus the flow delivered is affected by patient characteristics (Fig. 172b). Because the airway pressure attainable is preset, the risk of barotrauma is reduced. However, the **tidal volume** delivered depends on the resistance of the tubing and the patient's respiratory mechanics, e.g. **compliance, airway resistance**. Pressure generators are usually employed in **paediatric anaesthesia**, to reduce the risk of barotrauma. Examples of constant pressure generators are the Manley and East Radcliffe ventilators.
  - I-to-E cycling:
    - time-cycled: the duration of inspiration is preset, e.g. Manley MP2, Penlon Nuffield, Siemens Servo 900 series.
    - pressure-cycled: expiration begins when a preset airway pressure is reached, e.g. Bird ventilator.
    - volume-cycled: expiration begins when a preset tidal volume has been delivered, e.g. Manley Pulmovent ventilator.
    - flow-cycled (pressure generators only): expiration begins when a preset inspiratory flow is reached, e.g. Bennett PR-2 ventilator. Rarely used as a method of cycling.

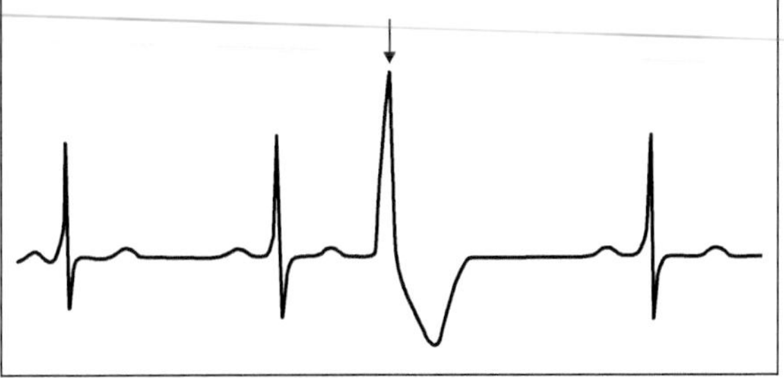

Fig. 173 Ventricular ectopic beat *(arrowed)*

Most of the above have been superseded by modern ventilators, which may be employed as either flow generators or pressure generators, with a choice of cycling methods. Thus they may be used both for anaesthesia and (with more complex features) for different clinical situations, e.g. on ICU.

During expiration, airway pressure may be allowed to fall to atmospheric pressure; most ventilators also allow application of **PEEP. Negative end-expiratory pressure** is no longer used. The switch from expiratory to inspiratory phases is usually time-cycled, although it may be triggered by the patient in some modes.

The ideal ventilator for use on ICU should: be flexible in flow or pressure generation and cycling as above; allow PEEP and special modes (e.g. for **weaning**); allow **humidification** and administration of nebulised drugs; be easy to sterilise; and incorporate monitors and alarms. Specific advanced ventilator modes used in ICU include **airway pressure release ventilation, inspiratory pressure support, inspiratory volume support, intermittent mandatory ventilation, inverse ratio ventilation, mandatory minute ventilation, pressure-regulated volume control ventilation, proportional assist ventilation** and **synchronised intermittent mandatory ventilation.** Many permit alteration of the I:E ratio, inspiratory waveform and PEEP.

[Ernst W von Siemens (1816–1892), German engineer; Carl-Gunnar Engström (1912–1987), Swedish physician; Roger EW Manley (1930–1991), UK anaesthetist and engineer; William W Mapleson, Cardiff physicist; Forrest M Bird (1921–2015), US aviator and engineer]

Smallwood RW (1988). Anaesth Intensive Care; 14: 251–7

See also, Monitoring

Ventile, *see Scavenging*

Ventricular ectopic beats (VEs, VEBs; Premature ventricular contractions/beats, PVCs/PCBs). Contraction of ventricular muscle caused by an ectopic focus instead of normal impulse conduction. The ventricles discharge early; the next sinus impulse finds the ventricular muscle refractory, causing a pause before the next beat. VEs typically appear as wide bizarre complexes on the **ECG** (Fig. 173); VEs arising from different sites (i.e., multifocal) may have different configurations.

They may occur in normal hearts, but may also indicate organic heart disease. Other causes include drugs (e.g. **halothane, digoxin, antiarrhythmic drugs**), electrolyte and acid–base disturbances, **hypoxaemia, hypercapnia** and pain. May occur at regular intervals, e.g. every second or third beat. Usually do not require treatment, apart from correction of the cause. Antiarrhythmic drugs (usually **lidocaine**) are usually recommended for VEs more frequent

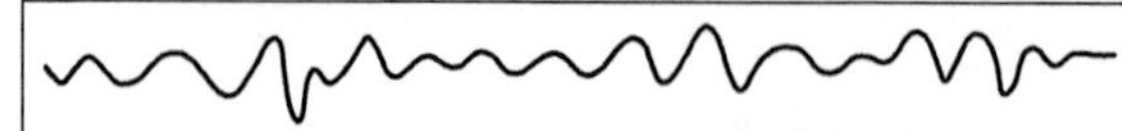

Fig. 174 Ventricular fibrillation

than 5 per minute, or if multifocal or close to the preceding **T wave** with risk of the **R on T phenomenon.**
See also, Arrhythmias

Ventricular fibrillation (VF). Uncoordinated and ineffective ventricular contraction caused by completely irregular ventricular depolarisation. May follow the **R on T phenomenon.** Causes include **myocardial ischaemia, MI, hypoxaemia, electrocution,** electrolyte imbalance, **hypothermia** and drug toxicity (e.g. **adrenaline, digoxin**). There is no cardiac output; **asystole** therefore follows unless treated. VF is the most common cause of **cardiac arrest** in adults. The **ECG** shows continuous random electrical activity without **QRS complexes** (Fig. 174).

Treated by **defibrillation**, although a single precordial thump is advocated for monitored arrests.

Soar J, Nolan JP, Böttiger BW, et al (2015). Resuscitation; 95: 100–47

Ventricular septal defect (VSD). The commonest congenital heart defect, occurring in 50% of all children with **congenital heart disease**, either in isolation or in combination with other defects. May also follow **MI** or **trauma.** The commonest congenital form (accounting for 80% of VSDs) involves the membranous septum immediately below the tricuspid valve; bulbar or muscular septal involvement is rarer. Blood flows across the defect from left to right during systole. As right ventricular pressures decrease after birth, **shunt** increases. May cause **cardiac failure** in infancy, manifesting as feeding difficulty and failure to thrive. Small defects with normal **pulmonary artery pressures** are often asymptomatic (*maladie de Roger*) and may close spontaneously. Large defects may lead to **pulmonary hypertension** and **Eisenmenger's syndrome.**

- Features:
  - harsh pansystolic murmur, heard best in the left fourth intercostal space (louder with small defects). Splitting of the second **heart sound.**
  - of Eisenmenger's syndrome if present.
  - of left and right ventricular hypertrophy on **ECG** and **CXR.**

May be complicated by bacterial **endocarditis.**

Treated by surgery or placement of a septal occluder using a percutaneous technique. Anaesthesia is as for congenital heart disease and **cardiac surgery.**

[Henri L Roger (1809–1891), French physician]

Ventricular stretch receptors, *see Baroreceptors*

Ventricular tachycardia (VT). Rapid series of **ventricular ectopic beats** (usually defined as more than three in succession). The rate usually lies between 130 and 250 beats/min. Normal atrial activity may continue independently, or the ventricular impulses may pass retrogradely to the atria.

- Distinguished from **SVT** by the following features (Fig. 175):
  - **QRS complexes** are usually wide and bizarre.
  - retrograde conduction to the atria may result in inverted **P waves** (which may be hidden by the QRS complexes).

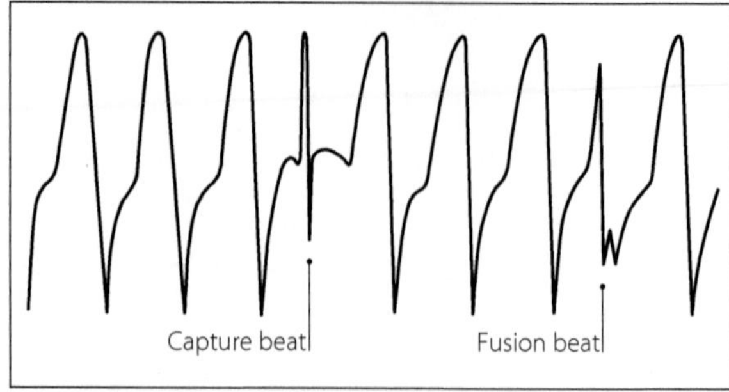

Fig. 175 Ventricular tachycardia, showing capture and fusion beats

  - independent atrial activity may be suggested by:
    - occasional P waves.
    - capture beats (normal QRS complexes following occasional normal atrioventricular conduction).
    - fusion beats (with combined features of normal and ectopic QRS complexes, representing simultaneous atrially conducted and ectopic ventricular activity).
  - marked left axis deviation, with all of the chest leads either negative or positive.

  Both VT and SVT may be regular, and associated with normotension or hypotension. Differentiation between broad-complex VT and SVT with aberrant conduction may be particularly difficult. The response to **adenosine** may aid diagnosis. Causes are as for ventricular ectopic beats.
- Treatment (following **CPR** if necessary):
  - **antiarrhythmic drugs,** e.g. **amiodarone.**
  - **cardioversion** if there are adverse signs (e.g. hypotension) or drugs are contraindicated/ineffective.
  - **cardiac pacing** has also been used.
  - management of recurrent VT includes antiarrhythmic drugs, catheter ablation of the ectopic focus and implantable defibrillators.

Soar J, Nolan JP, Böttiger BW, et al (2015). Resuscitation; 95: 100–47
See also, Torsade de pointes

Venturi principle. Entrainment of a fluid into an area of low pressure caused by a constriction in a tube (**Bernoulli effect**). Entrainment depends on appropriate positioning of the side-arm or entrainment port, a suitably shaped constriction and the gradual increase in diameter of the limb distal to the constriction.

The principle is employed in gas-mixing devices (including fixed performance **oxygen therapy** devices), **suction equipment, ejector flowmeters, scavenging** equipment and devices used to circulate gases around breathing systems.

[Giovanni Venturi (1746–1822), Italian physicist]

Verapamil hydrochloride. Calcium channel blocking drug, mainly used as an **antiarrhythmic drug** to treat **SVT.** Acts by prolonging conduction through the atrioventricular node. Also used in angina, hypertension and (off-licence) the prevention of cluster headache. Undergoes extensive **first-pass metabolism** when given orally. Excreted renally.

- Dosage:
  - SVT: 5–10 mg over 2–3 min iv, with a further 5 mg after 5–10 min if required. Orally, 40–120 mg tds.
  - angina: 80–120 mg orally tds.
  - hypertension: 240–480 mg orally per day, in 2–4 divided doses.

- Side effects: hypotension, bradycardia, complete heart block and asystole, especially if the patient has received **β-adrenergic receptor antagonists**. Contraindicated in **Wolff–Parkinson–White syndrome**, because atrioventricular block may promote conduction through accessory pathways with resultant arrhythmia. Also contraindicated in infants in whom it may cause life-threatening bradycardia and hypotension. Its action may be potentiated by **inhalational anaesthetic agents**, especially **halothane**.

Vertebrae. Bony components of the vertebral column, which is about 70 cm long in the adult male and is flexed throughout its length in the fetus; after birth two secondary curves appear so that the cervical and lumbar regions are convex forwards and the thoracic and sacral regions are concave. There are 7 cervical vertebrae, 12 thoracic, 5 lumbar, 5 fused sacral and 3–5 fused coccygeal. Vertebral bodies of C2 to L5 are separated by fibrocartilaginous vertebral discs, accounting for about 25% of the spine's total length. Each has an outer fibrous annulus fibrosus, and the more fluid inner nucleus pulposus. The latter may prolapse through the former, impinging upon the **spinal cord** or spinal nerves. Discs thin with age, resulting in reduced height. Vertebrae and discs are united by the **vertebral ligaments**.

- Structure of a typical vertebra:
  - body: short and cylindrical and lies anteriorly.
  - arch: encloses the **vertebral canal** and lies posteriorly. Composed of the rounded pedicles anteriorly and the flattened laminae posteriorly. The laminae are united in the midline by the spinous process. They also bear transverse processes and superior and inferior articular processes that bear facets for articulation with adjacent vertebrae.
- Regional differences:
  - cervical (Fig. 176a):
    - each has the foramen transversarium passing through its transverse processes, through which pass the **vertebral arteries**.
    - C1 (atlas):
      - has neither body nor spine.
      - articular facets articulate superiorly with the base of the skull.
      - facet on the anterior edge of the vertebral canal articulates with the odontoid peg.
    - C2 (axis): odontoid peg projects from the superior surface of the body, held against the body of the atlas by the transverse ligament. The gap between the peg and atlas is normally less than 3 mm on neck flexion (5 mm in children).
    - C2–6: bifid spinous processes.
    - C7 (vertebra prominens): non-bifid spine (the first easily palpable spine encountered, feeling from the skull downwards; T1 below it has a more prominent spine).
  - thoracic (Fig. 176b):
    - body: heart-shaped, articulating with the **ribs** via superior and inferior costal facets at the rear of the body.
    - transverse processes: large, passing backwards and laterally, and bearing facets that articulate with the ribs' tubercles (except the last two thoracic vertebrae).
    - spinous processes: long, inclined at about 60 degrees to the horizontal.
    - anatomical variations:
      - T1: has a longer upper facet for the first rib and a smaller lower facet for the second rib.
      - T10–12: usually bear single costal facets on their bodies.
      - T12: spinous process has notched lower edge.
  - lumbar (Fig. 176c):
    - body: kidney-shaped.
    - transverse processes: thick, passing laterally. Bear the accessory processes posteriorly at their bases.
    - spines: project horizontally backwards.
    - L5: short but massive transverse processes, arising from the sides of the body and pedicles. The body is deeper anteriorly than posteriorly.
  - sacral: fused to form the sacrum, enclosing the **sacral canal**.
  - coccygeal: fused to form the triangular coccyx, the base of which articulates with the sacrum.

Vertebral arteries. Arise from the subclavian arteries, passing upwards through the foramina transversaria of the upper six cervical **vertebrae** and passing medially behind the lateral mass of the atlas. They enter the **skull** through the foramen magnum, uniting to form the basilar artery after piercing the dura. Vertebrobasilar insufficiency typically results in dizziness, vertigo, diplopia and hemiparesis.

May be punctured during central venous cannulation and brachial plexus block.

See also, Cerebral circulation

Vertebral canal. Triangular canal within the **vertebrae**, with its base posteriorly. Contains:

- **epidural space** and contents.
- **spinal cord** and **spinal nerves**/roots.

Vertebral ligaments. Individual **vertebrae** are linked by a number of ligaments (Fig. 177):

- anterior longitudinal ligament: runs from C2 to the sacrum, attached to the anterior aspects of the vertebral bodies. Continues superiorly to form the anterior atlanto-occipital membrane.
- posterior longitudinal ligament: as for the anterior, but attached to the posterior vertebral aspects. Continues superiorly to form the membrana tectoria between the axis and occiput.
- ligamenta flava (yellow ligaments): run between the laminae of adjacent vertebrae. More developed in the lumbar than thoracic regions. Continue superiorly as the posterior atlanto-occipital membrane.
- interspinous ligaments: run between the spines of adjacent vertebrae.
- supraspinous ligament: runs from C7 to the sacrum, attached to the tips of the spines.

- Additional ligaments at the atlanto-occipito-axial complex:
  - transverse ligament of the atlas: runs between medial aspects of the lateral masses of the atlas, securing the odontoid peg.
  - alar ligaments: pass from the sides of the odontoid peg to the occipital condyles.
  - apical ligament: thin band, connecting the odontoid's tip to the anterior aspect of the foramen magnum.
- Sacrococcygeal ligaments:
  - posterior: overlies the sacral hiatus.
  - anterior: passes over the anterior aspect of the sacrum and coccyx.
  - lateral: joins the lateral angle of the sacrum to the transverse processes of the coccyx.

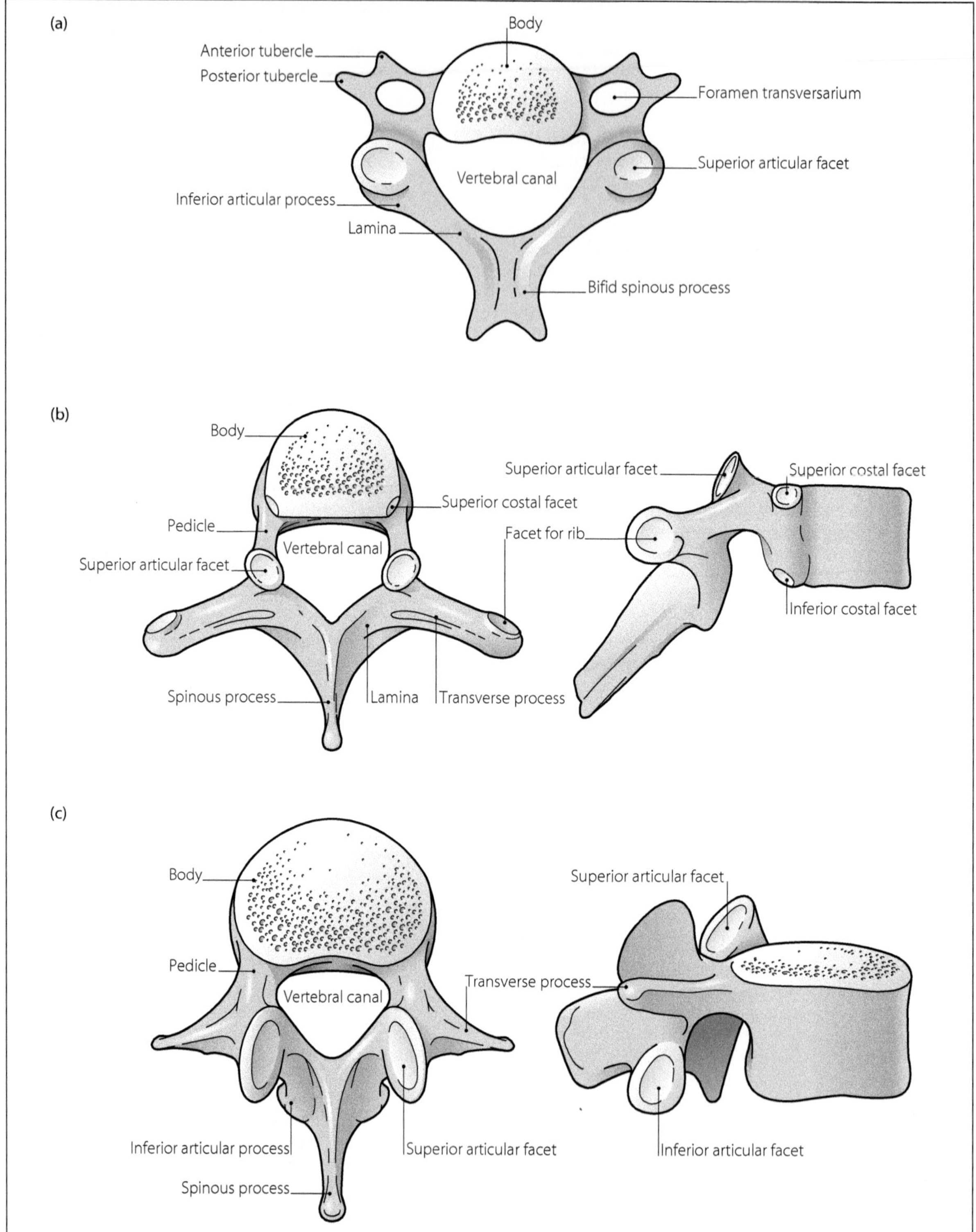

Fig. 176 Typical vertebrae: (a) cervical, superior view; (b) thoracic, superior and lateral views; (c) lumbar, superior and lateral views

VF, *see Ventricular fibrillation*

Viagra, *see Sildenafil*

Victoria, Queen (1819–1901). British monarch, given **chloroform** by **Snow** during the births of her eighth and ninth children: Prince Leopold in 1853, and Princess Beatrice in 1857 (on the latter occasion, Prince Albert administered chloroform himself before Snow's arrival). This gave respectability to pain relief during labour, which had been criticised as being against God's will.
[Leopold (1853–1884), Beatrice (1857–1944), Albert (1819–1861)]
See also, Obstetric analgesia and anaesthesia

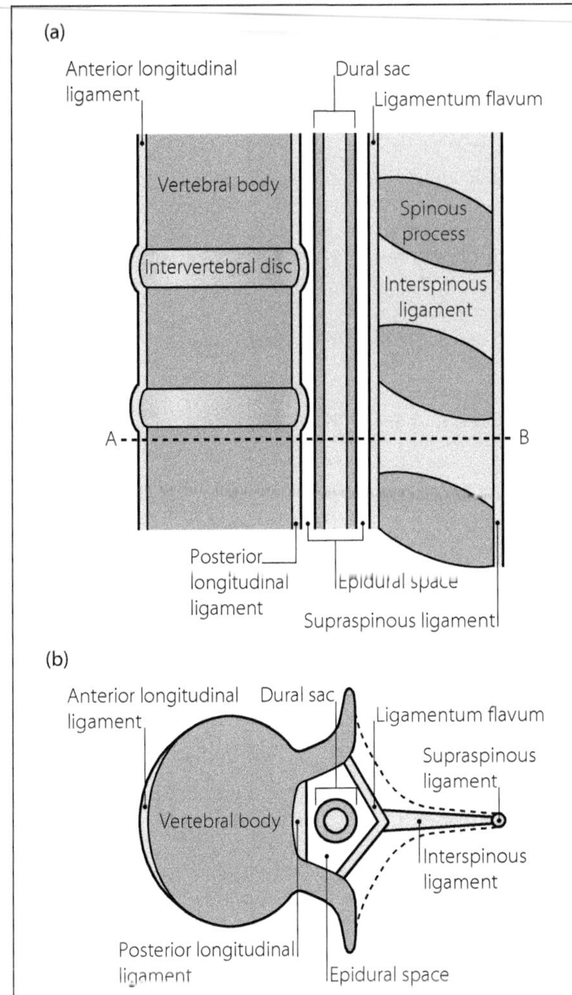

Fig. 177 Vertebral ligaments: (a) longitudinal section of vertebral column; (b) transverse section through A–B

Videolaryngoscope. Device used for indirect **laryngoscopy** to enable tracheal **intubation**. Based on the general principles of the direct **laryngoscope**, but the intubator views the glottis via a camera incorporated into the blade. (Other, including earlier, attempts to improve the view at laryngoscopy include the use of rigid **fibreoptic instruments** (e.g. Airtraq) that may be used with a camera at the eyepiece, whereas early precursors of videolaryngoscopes incorporated a camera in the handle but retained fibreoptic components). Cameras of modern videolaryngoscopes are very small and have a wide-angle, heated lens (to avoid fogging), and display an image on a screen that may be attached to the handle of the device itself (e.g. McGrath, Airway Scope) or mounted separately (e.g. Glidescope, C-MAC and variants). Some blades include channels to guide the tube during placement.

- Main advantages over traditional, rigid laryngoscopes:
  - improved intubation success, especially with less experienced practitioners.
  - may require less mouth opening (especially without tube channels).
  - may show the glottis when a direct view is difficult to obtain; thus may be useful in difficult intubation.
  - allow others to see the image, e.g. for teaching.

They have been suggested as a replacement for rigid laryngoscopes in routine intubation, and an alternative to awake fibreoptic intubation in known difficult cases; however, comparisons of different models suggest differing performance.

[Matt McGrath, Scottish designer]

See also, Intubation, awake; Intubation, difficult

VIE, *see Vacuum insulated evaporator*

Vigabatrin. Anticonvulsant drug used as an adjuvant treatment for partial and secondary generalised seizures. Its efficacy in tonic–clonic seizures is less well documented. Irreversibly inhibits **γ-aminobutyric acid** transaminase (GABA-T), the enzyme responsible for breakdown of GABA. Duration of action approximately 24 h with elimination **half-life** of 7 h. Excreted unchanged in the urine.

- Dosage: 1 g orally initially, increased up to 2–3 g/day (15–20 mg/kg to 75 mg/kg twice daily in children).
- Side effects: sedation, dizziness, headache, agitation, psychosis, visual disturbances.

VIP, *see Vasoactive intestinal peptide*

Viscosity (η). Tendency of **fluids** to resist **flow**. Measured in **poise**. Equal to shear **force** (force per unit surface area) divided by velocity gradient between adjacent fluid layers. Dependent on intermolecular attractive forces (e.g. **van der Waals forces**) and entanglement of bulky molecules. Decreased at high temperatures; particles have more kinetic energy and may escape from their neighbours more easily. Laminar flow is inversely proportional to viscosity.

Blood viscosity depends largely on **haematocrit** (increasing exponentially as haematocrit increases), red cell characteristics and blood protein concentration. It rises with age and smoking. It is increased slightly by volatile anaesthetic agents. Blood viscosity alters with different flow rates; i.e., blood is a non-Newtonian fluid. At vessel diameters of less than 0.3 mm, it drops markedly, resulting in greater flow than with a Newtonian fluid. The reason is unclear, but may involve 'plasma skimming' (the tendency of cellular components of blood to remain in the middle of vessels while plasma passes into branches arising from the vessel wall). Blood cell deformability may also be important. At very low **blood flow**, viscosity increases as the cells clump together.

Relative viscosity (compared with water) of normal plasma is 1.5; that of normal whole blood is 3.5.

Viscosity may be derived by measuring the time taken for a liquid to drain through a narrow tube. Alternatively, the torque on an inner drum may be measured when an outer drum is rotated, the specimen liquid filling the space between the drums.

[Sir Isaac Newton (1642–1727), English scientist]

Vishnevskiy technique (Transverse injection anaesthesia). Injection of local anaesthetic agent into a transverse 'slice' of a limb; originally described using **procaine**. Infiltration is performed from skin to bone, using large volumes of agent. Has been called the 'squirt and cut' technique.

[Aleksandr V Vishnevskiy (1874–1948), Russian surgeon]

Visual analogue scale, *see Linear analogue scale*

Vital capacity. The maximum volume of gas that can be expired slowly after maximal inspiration; measured by a

spirometer. Reduced in the supine position. Also reduced in the elderly, and in patients with restrictive lung disease, muscle weakness, abdominal swelling and pain.
See also, Forced vital capacity; Lung function tests; Lung volumes

Vitamin B_{12} (Cobalamin). Water-soluble **vitamin** present in many animal tissues, especially eggs and liver. Exists as various related compounds, e.g. hydroxo- or cyanocobalamin. Combines with gastric intrinsic factor, enabling its absorption from the terminal ileum. Required for red blood cell maturation and as a cofactor for **methionine synthase**. Deficiency may be caused by failure of intrinsic factor production due to atrophic gastritis (pernicious anaemia) or gastric resection, or by disease/resection of the ileum. Dietary deficiency is rare. Inhibited by **N_2O**. Deficiency results in macrocytic megaloblastic **anaemia** and subacute combined degeneration of the **spinal cord**.

Administered im 3-monthly as hydroxocobalamin; cyanocobalamin requires more frequent administration. Also used in the treatment of **cyanide poisoning**.

Romain M, Sviri S, Linton DM, et al (2016). Anaesth Intensive Care; 44: 447–52

Vitamin deficiency. May occur in:
- inadequate intake relative to requirements, e.g. **malnutrition** (including inadequate provision during **TPN**).
- malabsorption, e.g. due to gastric disease (**vitamin B_{12}**), pancreatic disease (fat-soluble vitamins: A, D, E and K).
- impaired metabolism of precursors, e.g. osteomalacia in renal failure.
- antagonism by drugs, e.g. **warfarin** (vitamin K), **N_2O** (folate and vitamin B_{12}).

- Specific deficiency states of possible anaesthetic importance:
  - vitamin A: night blindness, dry skin.
  - vitamin B_1 (thiamine): **peripheral neuropathy**, Wernicke's syndrome (ataxia, nystagmus, ophthalmoplegia and **encephalopathy**), **cardiomyopathy** (beriberi). May accompany chronic **alcoholism**. Vitamin B_1 is used in **ethylene glycol poisoning**.
  - vitamin B_2 (riboflavin): **anaemia**, mouth lesions.
  - vitamin B_6 (pyridoxine): **convulsions**, anaemia. May accompany chronic alcoholism. Vitamin B_6 is used in ethylene glycol poisoning and **isoniazid** therapy.
  - niacin: dermatitis, diarrhoea, dementia (pellagra).
  - vitamin B_{12}: anaemia, subacute combined degeneration of the cord.
  - vitamin C: generalised bleeding (especially gums), anaemia, weakness, poor wound healing (scurvy).
  - vitamin D: **hypocalcaemia**, hyperphosphataemia, muscle weakness, rickets (in children), osteomalacia (in adults). Deficiency in ICU patients is associated with increased mortality but correction appears not to influence outcomes.
  - vitamin E: **haemolysis**, oedema.
  - vitamin K: bleeding tendency.

[Karl Wernicke (1848–1904), German neurologist]

Vitamin K. Fat-soluble group of **vitamins** that catalyse the carboxylation of glutamic acid residues to activate **coagulation** factors II, VII, IX and X. Deficiency results in increased tendency to bleed and may result from:
- inadequate intake: rare in adults, common in the newborn.
- inadequate absorption, e.g. malabsorption syndromes, biliary obstruction.
- inadequate utilisation, e.g. liver disease.
- drug therapy: especially **warfarin** and similar drugs, which act as vitamin K antagonists.

May be given orally, iv or im to help correct deficiency or as an antidote to excessive anticoagulation with warfarin; takes up to 12 h to work. May cause several weeks' upset to coagulation control in patients on long-term warfarin therapy. Available as a synthetic analogue (menadiol sodium phosphate) or as phytomenadione (vitamin K_1).
- Dosage: 5 mg, orally or by slow iv injection, depending on severity of bleeding, repeated after 24 h if necessary. Prothrombin time should be monitored.

Anaphylaxis has been reported.
See also, Coagulation studies

Vitamins. Term derived from 'vital amines'. Group of dietary compounds necessary for health and growth but which do not supply energy (Table 53). Lack of one or more produces **vitamin deficiency** states. Vitamins A, D, E and K are fat-soluble; the rest are water-soluble.

Vocal cords, *see Larynx*

Volatile anaesthetic agents, *see Inhalational anaesthetic agents*

Table 53 Functions, sources and adult daily requirements of vitamins

Vitamin	*Function*	*Sources*	*Daily requirements*
A	Retinal pigmentation, fetal development	Yellow vegetables and fruit	15–20 µg/kg
B_1 (thiamine)	Cofactor in decarboxylation	Liver, cereals	20 µg/kg
B_2 (riboflavin)	Flavoproteins	Liver, milk	20 µg/kg
Niacin	Constituent of NAD and NADP	Yeast and lean meat	0.4 mg/kg
B_6 (pyridoxine)	Decarboxylases and transaminases	Yeast, wheat and liver	20 µg/kg
Pantothenic acid	Constituent of coenzyme A	Eggs, liver	0.3–0.8 mg/kg
Biotin	Fatty acid synthesis	Egg yolk, liver	2–3 µg/kg
Folic acid	Methylating reactions	Green vegetables	2–3 µg/kg
Vitamin B_{12}	Amino acid metabolism, erythropoiesis	Liver, meat, eggs	0.04–0.1 µg/kg
Vitamin C (ascorbic acid)	Collagen synthesis	Citrus fruits	1.0 mg/kg
Vitamin D	Intestinal absorption of calcium and phosphate	Fish, liver	0.1–0.2 µg/kg
Vitamin E	Antioxidants	Milk, eggs, meat	0.1–0.2 µg/kg
Vitamin K	Blood coagulation	Green vegetables	1.0 µg/kg

Volt. Unit of electrical potential. One volt is the potential difference between two points when 1 **joule** of **work** is done per **coulomb** of electricity passing from one point to the other.
[Alessandro Volta (1745–1827), Italian physicist]

Volume of distribution (V_d). Theoretical term indicating the degree to which a drug redistributes and/or accumulates in body tissues. Equals the ratio of the amount of drug present in the body at a given time, to the concentration of the drug in plasma at that time. Alternatively described as the volume of plasma throughout which an injected dose would have to be distributed in order to give the measured plasma concentration. May be used to estimate the loading dose required to achieve a desired plasma concentration, e.g. in a **target-controlled infusion**.

Initial volume of distribution (V_{dI} or V_c) refers to the V_d immediately after injection, when the drug is distributed throughout the central compartment, but before any elimination or redistribution to the tissues has occurred. However, commonly cited values for different drugs usually refer to V_d at equilibrium or steady state (V_{dss}):
- for a drug confined to the intravascular compartment (e.g. large, highly plasma protein-bound molecules), V_{dss} equals blood volume.
- for a drug that can leave the intravascular space but cannot freely enter cells (e.g. highly ionised molecules), V_{dss} equals the ECF volume.
- for a drug that can easily penetrate cell membranes (and distributes equally throughout the body), it equals total body water volume.
- for a drug that concentrates preferentially in the tissues (e.g. lipophilic drugs accumulating in adipose), V_{dss} may greatly exceed total body water volume.

- Examples (approximate values for a 70-kg man):
  - **propofol**: 700–1200 l.
  - **morphine**: 210–280 l.
  - **insulin**: 50 l.
  - **atracurium**: 12 l.
  - **warfarin**: 9 l.

Drugs or poisons with a small V_d are more readily cleared from the plasma by **haemodialysis** or **haemoperfusion**; those with large V_d may be cleared from the plasma but levels tend to rise again (with possible recurrence of toxic effects) following cessation of dialysis.
See also, Pharmacokinetics

Volume support, *see Inspiratory volume support*

Volutrauma, *see Ventilator-associated lung injury*

Vomiting. Reflex involving retrograde passage of **gastric contents** through the mouth. The vomiting centre in the lateral medullary reticular formation receives afferent impulses from the:
- GIT, abdominal organs and peritoneum via the vagus and sympathetic nerves.
- heart mainly via the **vagus nerve**.
- vestibular apparatus.
- **chemoreceptor trigger zone** (CTZ).
- higher centres.

Chemical irritants stimulate the vomiting centre via receptors in the GIT. Drugs (e.g. **apomorphine**) and **neurotransmitters** (e.g. **dopamine, noradrenaline, acetylcholine, 5-HT**) stimulate the CTZ. Raised **ICP** is thought to cause vomiting via increased pressure on the floor of the fourth ventricle.

Motor impulses travel through **cranial nerves** V, VII, IX, X and XII to the facial muscles and upper GIT and through spinal nerves to the diaphragm and abdominal muscles.
- Sequence of events:
  - salivation increases.
  - breathing deepens.
  - glottis closes.
  - breath is held in mid-inspiration.
  - abdominal muscles contract.
  - oesophageal sphincters relax.
  - gastric contents are expelled.

Nausea is a sensation that may or may not be associated with the act of vomiting itself, although the two are usually considered together because the neurological pathways are similar. The incidence of **PONV** has been found to vary from 15% to 90%. Usually distressing, it is particularly undesirable in ear and **ophthalmic surgery**, and **neurosurgery**.
- Effects of prolonged vomiting:
  - loss of water and hydrogen, chloride, potassium and sodium ions, causing metabolic **alkalosis**.
  - renal bicarbonate loss to restore pH, causing alkaline urine.
  - fall in sodium and ECF causing **aldosterone** release, which causes renal sodium and fluid retention, in exchange for potassium and hydrogen ions. If **hypokalaemia** is severe, hydrogen ion loss predominates, with paradoxical acid urine.
  - thus **dehydration**, metabolic alkalosis and total body potassium depletion may occur.

von Recklinghausen's disease, *see Neurofibromatosis*

von Willebrand's disease. Commonest inherited **coagulation disorder** (affects ~1:100–1000 people but may be very mild); first described in 1926, with mostly autosomal dominant transmission, depending on the subtype. Abnormality of von Willebrand factor (VWF), the major protein involved in **platelet** adhesion and carriage of **coagulation** factor VIII, leads to factor VIII deficiency, abnormal platelet adhesiveness and abnormal vascular endothelium. Epistaxis and bruising are more common than haemarthrosis and haematoma, although there is marked variation in clinical severity.
- Classified into three main types:
  - type 1: quantitative reduction in VWF; accounts for ~90% of cases.
  - type 2: qualitative abnormality of VWF structure and function, resulting in decreased (2A) or increased (2B) activity; accounts for ~10% of cases. Rarer additional subtypes also exist (2N, 2M).
  - type 3: similar to type 1 but a severe autosomal recessive form; accounts for <1% of cases.

  A 'pseudo' or 'platelet' form also exists, in which the defect is in platelet function rather than VWF.

Definitive diagnosis is made via VWF activity assay, VWF antigen testing and factor VIII assay; in combination, these have high **sensitivity** and **specificity** but may not be readily available, e.g. for emergency surgery. Routine **coagulation studies** are more accessible, but less useful for diagnosis:
- platelet count: low or normal.
- prothrombin time: normal.
- bleeding and activated partial thromboplastin times: prolonged.

Desmopressin boosts levels of factor VIII and VWF, and may be used preoperatively (0.3 μg/kg iv, effects lasting

6–8 h) for treatment of mild type 1 and 2A disease. Severe disease is treated with fresh frozen plasma, cryoprecipitate or specific factor concentrates before surgery. **Tranexamic acid** 1 g orally may be useful. **Antiplatelet drugs** must be avoided.

During pregnancy, levels of factor VIII and VWF increase, but they may fall rapidly after delivery.

[Erik von Willebrand (1870–1949), Swedish physician]

Mensah PK, Gooding R (2015). Anaesthesia; 70 Suppl 1: 112–20

See also, Blood products

Voriconazole. Broad-spectrum triazole **antifungal drug**, related to **fluconazole** and used for severe fungal infections.

- Dosage: 200–400 mg orally bd for 2 doses, then 100–300 mg bd. Alternatively 6 mg/kg iv bd for 2 doses, then 4 mg/kg bd.
- Side effects: as for fluconazole, though most organ systems can be affected.

$\dot{V}/\dot{Q}$ mismatch, *see Ventilation/perfusion mismatch*

VRE, Vancomycin-resistant enterococci, *see Infection control; Vancomycin*

VSD, *see Ventricular septal defect*

VT, *see Ventricular tachycardia*

W

Wakefulness, *see Awareness*

Wake-up test. Intraoperative awakening to allow assessment of spinal cord function during **spinal surgery**. Has also been used to assess cerebral function during basilar artery clipping.

Warfarin sodium. Oral **anticoagulant drug**, first synthesised in 1944. Rapidly absorbed by mouth and almost totally protein-bound. Competes with **vitamin K** in the synthesis of **coagulation** factors II, VII, IX and X in the liver; hence requires 1–2 days for its effect to develop. Also inhibits **protein** C and S. Metabolised in the liver and excreted in urine and faeces. **Half-life** is about 30 h. Dosage is adjusted according to results of **coagulation studies**: the International Normalised Ratio (INR) is maintained at about 2–3 for prophylaxis and treatment of **DVT**, **PE**, transient ischaemic attacks and in patients with atrial fibrillation at high risk of embolisation; 3–4.5 for recurrent DVT/PE, cardiac and arterial prostheses. The usual maintenance dose is 3–9 mg/day. The INR is usually checked daily or on alternate days initially, but thereafter up to every 2 months, depending on the response. Home self-monitoring may be used in selected cases.

Drugs causing hepatic **enzyme induction** (e.g. **rifampicin**, **phenytoin**) reduce its effect. If the second drug is withdrawn without reducing the dose of warfarin, haemorrhage may occur. Effects may be enhanced by drugs that displace it from protein-binding sites, e.g. sulfonamides, **NSAIDs**. Emergency treatment of haemorrhage due to excessive warfarin effect involves use of vitamin K injection (up to 5 mg iv) and the administration of factors II, VII, IX and X (**prothrombin complex concentrate**, or fresh frozen plasma).

Teratogenic; thus avoided in the first trimester of pregnancy, although there is evidence it may be more effective than heparin at preventing valve thrombosis and thus safer for pregnant women with prosthetic heart valves. Warfarin crosses the placenta, risking placental or fetal haemorrhage if given in the third trimester.

Patients taking warfarin who present for surgery may pose problems with perioperative coagulation. Units will have their own local guidelines but in general they tend to follow the following:

- heart valves: warfarin therapy maintained for short (under 30 min) surgery, with fresh frozen plasma available. Otherwise, warfarin is stopped 3 days preoperatively, and low-molecular-weight **heparin** twice daily (dose depending on the drug used) started 24 h later. Heparin is stopped 24 h preoperatively, and INR checked preoperatively. Surgery may be delayed, or plasma or vitamin K administered, if INR exceeds 1.5–2. Heparin is restarted 6–8 h postoperatively, and warfarin the day after surgery; the heparin is stopped when the INR reaches 2.
- other conditions: preoperative management is as for heart valves, above. Postoperatively, the risk of bleeding is increased if low-molecular-weight heparin is started within 12–24 h of surgery so this is usually delayed for 24 h, with warfarin restarted on the evening of surgery or the next day. The heparin is stopped when INR reaches 1.5.
- emergency surgery: vitamin K may be given if there is time to wait for synthesis of new clotting factors (about 6–12 h); this may interfere with subsequent anticoagulation for weeks afterwards. Alternatively, fresh frozen plasma or prothrombin complex concentrate may be given. The INR is monitored throughout.

[Wisconsin Alumni Research Foundation, where warfarin was developed]

Warren, John C (1778–1856). Professor of Surgery and Anatomy at Harvard Medical School. It was at Warren's invitation that **Wells** gave his demonstration of N_2O anaesthesia, which ended in failure. Later, at **Morton**'s first public demonstration of **diethyl ether**, Warren performed the surgery.

Cooper DKC (2012). Br Med J; 345: 42–3

Washout curves. Graphs displaying the exponential decline in concentration of a substance that is continuously being removed from a system. The substance may be 'washed out' by blood flow, in the case of dye dilution **cardiac output measurement**, or by ventilation of the lungs, in the case of **nitrogen washout**. The term is sometimes used to describe any negative **exponential process**.

Water, *see Fluid balance; Fluids, body*

Water balance, *see Fluid balance*

Water diuresis. Diuresis occurring about 15 min after the intake of a large volume of hypotonic fluid. Absorption of the fluid is followed by inhibition of **vasopressin** secretion and by increased urinary water loss.

Water intoxication, *see Hyponatraemia*

Waterhouse–Friderichsen syndrome, *see Adrenocortical insufficiency*

Waters bag, *see Anaesthetic breathing systems*

Waters canister, *see Carbon dioxide absorption in anaesthetic breathing systems*

Waters, Ralph Milton (1883–1979). US anaesthetist; became Assistant Professor of Surgery in charge of anaesthetics at the University of Wisconsin, leading to his appointment as the first university Professor of Anaesthesia in the USA (1933). Was the first to establish a resident training programme in anaesthesia and the first to use **cyclopropane** clinically (1930). Re-examined **chloroform**

toxicity, advocated the use of inflatable **cuffs** on tracheal tubes, and was involved in many aspects of anaesthesia, including the use of **thiopental** and **endobronchial intubation**. Designed his 'to-and-fro' canister for **CO_2 absorption in anaesthetic breathing systems**, and the Waters airway, a metal oropharyngeal airway with a side-arm for attachment to a gas supply.

Waterton, Charles (1783–1865). Squire of Walton Hall, Yorkshire; made his first voyage to South America in 1812. Described the preparation of **curare** and the blowpipes, darts, bows and arrows used by the Indians of the Amazon and Orinoco basins. Experimented with the drug on his return to England, and maintained life in a paralysed donkey by employing **IPPV**. Published details of his work and travels in *Wanderings in South America* (1825).

Watt. **Unit** of **power**. One watt (W) = 1 **joule** per second (J/s).
[James Watt (1736–1819), Scottish engineer]

Waveforms. Repetitive patterns plotted against time produce waveforms that may be complex (e.g. **ECG**) or simple, as in the sine wave. All complex waveforms may be mathematically deconstructed into component sine waves (**Fourier analysis**). For any sine wave, there is oscillation about a mean value, the maximal displacement from which is the amplitude. The number of complete oscillations per second is the frequency, and the distance between successive points at the same stage of the cycle is the wavelength (Fig. 178). Waveform monitoring is very common in anaesthesia and intensive care, e.g. cardiovascular (ECG, intravascular pressures, plethysmography), respiratory (rate, depth, pattern), ventilatory (gas flow, pressure), neurological (intracranial pressure, EEG, nerve conduction studies).

Weaning from ventilators. Process of gradual withdrawal of mechanical ventilatory support. Usually presents no problems after less than a few days' ventilation; following longer periods or poor baseline respiratory function, rapid weaning is less likely. Protocol-driven weaning programmes have been shown to significantly reduce total duration of mechanical ventilation, the time taken to wean and ITU stay.

- Criteria for beginning weaning vary considerably; the following have been suggested:
  - absence of major organ or system failure, particularly CVS.
  - precipitating illness is successfully treated.
  - absence of severe infection or fever.
  - adequate **nutrition**.
  - low intra-abdominal pressure.
  - absence of severe fluid, acid–base, endocrine or electrolyte disturbance, e.g. of potassium, magnesium, calcium or phosphate.
  - minimal **sedation** with absence of severe pain.
  - respiratory function:
    - arterial blood gases are near premorbid values.
    - respiratory rate <35 breaths/min.
    - maximal negative inspiratory airway pressure attainable exceeds –25 cmH_2O.
    - airway occlusion pressure greater than 6 cmH_2O below atmospheric.
    - **tidal volume** >5 ml/kg.
    - minute ventilation <10 l.
    - **vital capacity** >10–15 ml/kg.
    - **FRC** >50% of predicted value.
    - ratio of breaths/min to tidal volume in l <100.

After long-term ventilation, scoring systems have been proposed to predict difficult weaning, reflecting F_IO_2 and level of **PEEP** required, lung compliance, work of breathing, temperature, pulse rate and arterial BP. Other risk factors for difficult weaning include: increased airway resistance (e.g. **COPD**, tracheal stenosis); **respiratory muscle fatigue**; hypoxia and **acidosis**; **cardiac failure**; **confusion**; sleep deprivation; prolonged illness; and **critical illness polyneuropathy/myopathy**.

- Techniques of weaning:
  - **humidification** of inspired air.
  - sitting the patient up increases FRC and diaphragmatic efficiency.
  - the lowest F_IO_2 necessary to maintain adequate oxygenation should be used, to decrease the risk of absorption **atelectasis**, and possibly promote **hypoxic pulmonary vasoconstriction**. Inappropriately high F_IO_2 should be avoided in CO_2-retaining patients with COPD.
  - a simple T-piece is often used when **IPPV** has been for a short duration. A 30-cm expiratory limb and fresh gas flow of twice minute volume will prevent indrawing of room air with lowering of F_IO_2, and rebreathing. Use should be limited in duration as the loss of physiological PEEP may increase the risk of atelectasis.
  - **CPAP** is often preferred, especially following high PEEP, in **ALI** and in left ventricular dysfunction.
  - specific ventilatory modes:
    - **IMV** and variants: the set mandatory ventilator rate is decreased as patient spontaneous rate increases. Spontaneous breaths are usually augmented with inspiratory pressure support (*see later*). Allows closer monitoring of recovery and reduces complications of IPPV.
    - **airway pressure release ventilation**, inspiratory **pressure support**, **pressure-regulated volume control ventilation, mandatory minute ventilation, inspiratory volume support, high-frequency ventilation** and variants and **negative pressure ventilation** have also been used.
  - **non-invasive positive pressure ventilation.**
  - overall time for completion of weaning may not be reduced by the above methods, but sedation and complications of IPPV may be reduced, and patient morale may benefit from 'coming off' the ventilator sooner. Assessment is also made easier.
  - short periods of spontaneous or assisted ventilation may be introduced and gradually increased, with clinical monitoring, assessment of S_pO_2 and frequent arterial blood gas measurements. Inspiratory muscle resistance training may be incorporated. Re-introduction of IPPV should be considered if tachypnoea (>30 breaths/min), tachycardia (>110

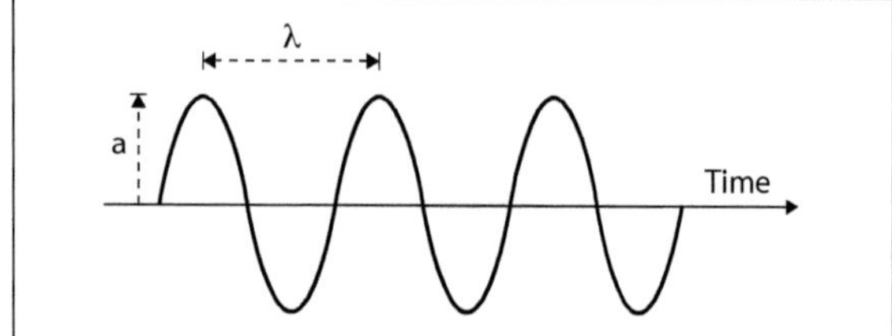

Fig. 178 Sine wave: a, amplitude; λ, wavelength

beats/min), fatigue, restlessness, distress or falling S_pO_2 occur.

- **extubation** may be performed when the patient is stable and able to protect the airway. Excessive secretions may be removed via **minitracheotomy**. Elective formation of a **tracheostomy** may assist in weaning by reducing dead space, allowing easy access for tracheobronchial toilet and permitting a reduction in sedation.

Work of breathing is increased by demand and expiratory valves and tubing, especially using CPAP and IMV circuits through certain **ventilators**. Modern ventilators provide circuits of low resistance, with minimal exertion required to open demand valves.

Peñuelas Ó, Thille AW, Esteban A (2015). Curr Opin Crit Care; 21: 74–81

Wedge pressure, *see Pulmonary capillary wedge pressure*

Wegener's granulomatosis (Granulomatosis with polyangiitis). Anti-neutrophil cytoplasmic antibody (ANCA)-associated small vessel vasculitis with inflammatory granulomatosis, particularly involving pulmonary and renal vessels. Features include non-specific symptoms (malaise, weight loss, fever, night sweats), nasal discharge and ulceration, pleurisy, haemoptysis, myalgia, arthralgia and **renal failure**. Subglottic stenosis may result in difficult airway management. Progression is variable but some cases rapidly develop **MODS** requiring ICU admission for **IPPV** and **haemofiltration**/dialysis. The diagnosis may be suspected clinically if both lungs and kidneys are involved, supported by detecting ANCA in plasma. Tissue biopsies are frequently unhelpful as granulomatous deposits are difficult to locate in life, even in the kidney.

Treatment of organ failure is supportive; Wegener's itself is treated with **cyclophosphamide** and **corticosteroids**, or other **immunosuppressive drugs**. Eventual remission is complete in approximately 75% of cases.

[Friedrich Wegener (1907–1990); German pathologist]

Comarmond C, Cacoub P (2014). Autoimmun Rev; 13: 1121–5

See also, Vasculitides

Weight. The **force** exerted upon a body due to gravity. Equals the product of the mass of the body and local acceleration due to gravity. The weight of a body of **mass** 1 **kilogram** is 1 **kilogram weight** (kilogram force).

Weil's disease, *see Leptospirosis*

Wells, Horace (1815–1848). US dentist, present at **Colton**'s demonstration of N_2O in Hartford, Connecticut on 10 December 1844. Noticing that a member of the audience (Samuel Cooley) had knocked his shin under the influence and felt no pain, he suggested its use for dental extraction. Wells had one of his own teeth pulled out by John Riggs the following day, while breathing N_2O prepared by Colton. Performed successful painless extractions in several patients over subsequent days, before his ill-fated demonstration of N_2O before **Warren** at Harvard Medical School, Boston, at which the patient complained of pain and Wells was denounced as a fraud. Continued to practise dentistry, but became increasingly disillusioned as acceptance of N_2O was overshadowed by **Morton**'s discovery of **diethyl ether**. Later a chloroform addict, he committed suicide by cutting his femoral artery while in prison.

[Samuel Cooley (1809–?), druggist's assistant; John Riggs (1810–1885), US dentist]

Haridas RP (2013). Anesthesiology; 119: 1014–22

Wenckebach phenomenon, *see Heart block*

Wernicke's encephalopathy, *see Vitamin deficiency*

WFSA, *see World Federation of Societies of Anesthesiologists*

Wheezing. Sustained, polyphonic whistling **respiratory sound** usually produced during expiration, indicating narrowing of the natural or artificial airway. Distinguished from **stridor** by being lower pitched and composed of a wider range of frequencies, and usually represents obstruction of smaller airways. May be generalised or localised.

- Caused by:
  - narrowed bronchi: **bronchospasm**, **bronchiolitis**, **pulmonary oedema**, **aspiration of gastric contents**, inhaled **foreign body**, airway tumour, **pneumothorax**, coughing or straining (causing airway collapse via increased intrathoracic pressure).
  - narrowed artificial airway: kinked tracheal tube, overinflated tracheal/tracheostomy tube cuff, placement of the tracheal tube's bevel against the posterior wall of the trachea, endobronchial intubation, kinked/obstructed respiratory tubing, malfunction of breathing system or ventilator valves.

Bronchospasm should be diagnosed only when other causes have been excluded.

Whistle discriminator. Obsolete device used to confirm correct attachment of N_2O and O_2 supplies to an **anaesthetic machine** by virtue of the differently pitched sounds produced when the gases flow through it, because of their different densities.

WHO Surgical Safety Checklist, *see World Health Organization Surgical Safety Checklist*

Whole bowel irrigation. Technique of GIT decontamination used in the treatment of **poisoning and overdoses**, especially with metals and delayed-release drug preparations, although convincing evidence for its efficacy is lacking. Employs large volumes (up to 2 l/h in adults) of polyethylene glycol administered via mouth or nasogastric tube until the rectal effluent is clear. Should not be used in obtunded patients or in the presence of gastrointestinal **ileus**, **intestinal obstruction**, perforation or haemorrhage. Electrolyte disturbances have not been reported with polyethylene glycol, unlike preoperative bowel preparations, which were studied initially. Also used before endoscopy or imaging of the GIT.

Wilcoxon signed rank test, *see Statistical tests*

Willis, circle of, *see Cerebral circulation*

'Wind-up'. Phenomenon in which the electrophysiological response of central pain-carrying neurones (e.g. those in the dorsal horn of the **spinal cord**) increases in the short-term with repetitive stimulation of peripheral nociceptors (C fibres); in addition the receptive fields of the individual neurones expand. The stimuli that cause wind-up may also contribute to the development of central sensitisation, the process by which painful input may alter the connections and activity of central neurones. Excitatory amino acids (e.g. **glutamate**) are thought to be involved, acting especially via **NMDA receptors**. Other receptor types including neurokinin-1 receptors (*see Tachykinins*) are also thought to be involved, as are other modulating substances such as **substance P** and calcitonin gene-related peptide. Prevention of wind-up is a central tenet of preventive and **pre-emptive analgesia**.

Withdrawal of treatment in ICU. Cessation of all or individual components of treatment is a frequent mode of **death** in the ICU and occurs in ~70% of deaths. In general, life-sustaining therapy is withheld or withdrawn when it has ceased or failed to achieve the benefits for which it was employed. It usually takes place when there is confirmed **brainstem death** or the patient's prognosis is poor with no prospect of returning to a reasonable quality of life. Occasionally, even a treatment that might produce benefit may be withheld or withdrawn if the patient is suffering from a terminal illness. Withdrawal of each medical treatment should be considered from the patient's perspective in the context of benefit. Withdrawal of treatment should be regarded as permitting the dying process to continue, rather than 'causing' death.

Factors considered in the decision to withdraw treatment include the patient's physiological reserve, diagnosis, severity of disease, co-morbidity, prognosis, response to treatment, anticipated quality of life and wishes, if known.

- Ethical issues include:
  - the wishes (often unknown) of an unconscious patient.
  - the validity and legality of decisions made by a surrogate.
  - the diversion of limited resources from patients with a good chance of survival to those who are unlikely to benefit.
  - the definition of futility.
  - the definition of a good quality of life.
  - the nature of medical treatment, e.g. feeding, hydration.
  - consideration of religious beliefs.
- Before withdrawal of treatment, the following should be undertaken/sought:
  - full discussion among all medical, nursing and paramedical staff treating the patient during which consensus should be obtained that the patient is dying. **Palliative care** physicians are increasingly involved in discussions.
  - the views of the family, the legal status of any appointed representative and **advance decision** of the patient.
  - consensus on the mode, extent and timing of treatment withdrawal by clinical staff and patient's family.

If brainstem death is diagnosed and **organ donation** is intended, withdrawal of support takes place after organ removal (beating heart donation). Otherwise, observations, monitoring, drugs, procedures and routine care (apart from symptom palliation) can be withdrawn once clinical staff and the patient's family have reached a consensus. IPPV may continue unchanged during this period or the technique of 'terminal weaning' of ventilation may be employed, in which inspired oxygen concentration is reduced to a F_IO_2 of 0.21. Feeding/antibiotics are stopped and inotropic support terminated. Sedation and analgesia are maintained, or increased if the patient becomes distressed, to ensure a peaceful, humane, comfortable and dignified death for the patient and to diminish distress for the family. Privacy is important for the patient and family during the dying process. Organ donation after death is known as non-beating heart donation.

Where the condition that precipitated the patient's admission to ICU involves suspicious circumstances (e.g. poisoning, assault), contact with the **coroner** is advised before treatment withdrawal. Whatever the circumstances, good clinical records of all discussions and actions should be kept.

Delaney JW, Downar J (2016). J Crit Care; 35: 12–18

See also, Ethics; Euthanasia; Mental Capacity Act

Wolff–Parkinson–White syndrome. Condition in which a congenital accessory connection between the atria and ventricles conducts more rapidly than the atrioventricular (AV) node, but has a longer refractory period. An atrial extrasystole finds the accessory bundle still refractory, but when the impulse passes via the AV node to the ventricles, the accessory bundle has recovered, and can conduct the impulse back to the atria. Circular conduction can continue with resultant **SVT**. **AF** and **atrial flutter** may also occur, but less commonly.

The **ECG** classically shows a short **P–R interval** and wide **QRS complexes** with δ waves (Fig. 179). A positive QRS complex in lead V_1 denotes type A (accessory bundle on the left side of the heart); if negative, type B (right side of heart).

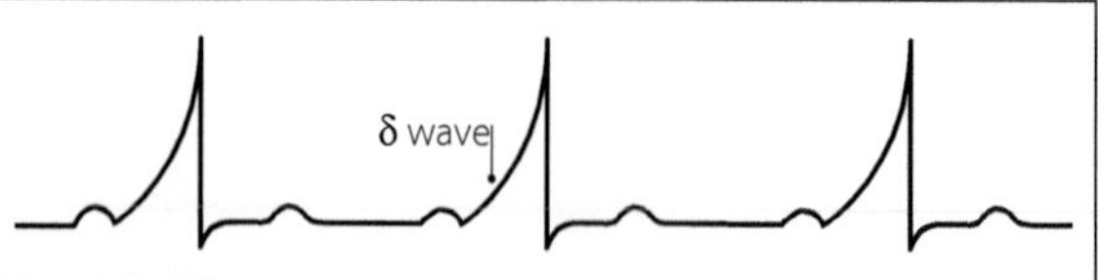

Fig. 179 ECG showing δ waves

Anaesthetic management of known cases should be directed at avoiding increased sympathetic activity, including that due to anxiety. **Antiarrhythmic drugs** should be continued perioperatively. Drugs causing tachycardia (e.g. **atropine**, **ketamine**, **pancuronium**) should be avoided. **Isoflurane**, **desflurane** and **sevoflurane** are all considered safe to use, as is **propofol**, as they have no clinical effect on conduction.

Treatment of arrhythmias (including perioperatively) follows standard measures. **Digoxin** and **verapamil** may increase impulse conduction through accessory pathways by blocking conduction through the AV node, and should be avoided. Management of established cases includes electrophysiological assessment (accessory pathway mapping), long-term prophylactic therapy (e.g. with **flecainide**, **sotalol**) and radiofrequency ablation of the accessory pathway.

[Sir John Parkinson (1885–1976), London cardiologist; Louis Wolff (1898–1972) and Paul White (1886–1973), US cardiologists]

Bengali R, Wellens HJ, Jiang Y (2014). J Cardiothorac Vasc Anesth; 28: 1375–86

Wood units. Unit of vascular **resistance**, derived by dividing the vascular pressure gradient (in mmHg) by the blood flow through the system (in l/min). Often used to express **pulmonary vascular resistance** in the context of **pulmonary hypertension** or **congenital heart disease**. Multiplying by 80 converts Wood units to dyne.s/cm^5.

[Earl H Wood (1912–2009), American physiologist]

Work. Product of **force** and the distance through which it acts. Work is done whenever the point of application of a force moves in the direction of that force. Also expressed as the product of the change in volume of a system and the pressure against which this change occurs (e.g. **stroke work**). SI **unit** is the **joule**.

Work of breathing, *see Breathing, work of*

World Federation of Societies of Anaesthesiologists (WFSA). Founded in 1955 at the first World Congress of Anaesthesiologists in the Hague, Holland, to promote anaesthetic education, research, training and safety standards throughout the world. World Congresses are held every 4 years (since 1960). Membership is via 120 anaesthetic societies from over 140 countries. Has several regional sections: African; Asian/Australian; European; Latin American; Pan-Arab; and South Asian.

World Health Organization Surgical Safety Checklist. Tool introduced by the World Health Organization (WHO) in 2008 to improve patient safety during surgery, and implemented within the NHS in 2010. Consists of a series of questions confirming the main issues that may hinder safe operating or result in adverse outcomes, arranged in three phases:

- Before anaesthesia ('sign in'): patient's identity, site (marked) and type of procedure and consent; presence of allergies; expected blood loss; anaesthetic equipment/drugs checked; risk of aspiration or difficult airway.
- Before the surgical procedure ('time out'): introduction of all team members; patient's identity, site and type of procedure; **ASA physical status**, expected blood loss; any anticipated critical events; need for antibiotics or imaging/specialised equipment (including monitoring); sterility of instruments.
- Before the patient leaves the operating theatre ('sign out'): correct record of procedure and labelling of specimens; correct instrument, sponge and needle counts; any equipment issues addressed; any key concerns for recovery.

Supported by evidence in many hospital settings, with the biggest reductions in morbidity and mortality seen in (but not restricted to) developing countries. Has been modified according to local needs, e.g. in obstetric and other specialised units.

Bergs J, Hellings J, Cleemput I, et al (2014). Br J Surg; 101: 150–8

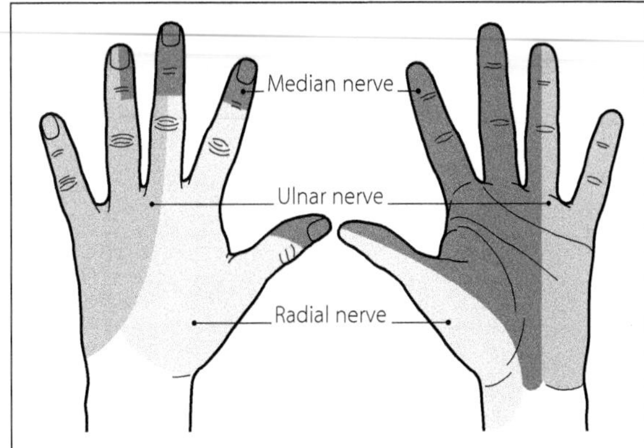

Fig. 180 Cutaneous innervation of the hand

Wrist, nerve blocks. Used for minor surgery to the hand.

- The following nerves are blocked (Fig. 180):
  - **median nerve** (C6–T1): at the level of the proximal skin crease, it lies between flexor carpi radialis tendon laterally and palmaris longus tendon medially. With the wrist dorsiflexed, 2–5 ml **local anaesthetic agent** is injected just lateral to the palmaris longus tendon, at a depth of 0.5–1 cm.
  - **ulnar nerve** (C7–T1): lies under flexor carpi ulnaris tendon proximal to the pisiform bone, medial and deep to the **ulnar artery**. At the level of the ulnar styloid process, a needle is inserted between flexor carpi ulnaris tendon and the ulnar artery, and 2–5 ml solution injected. The two cutaneous branches of the nerve may be blocked by subcutaneous infiltration around the ulnar side of the wrist from the flexor carpi ulnaris tendon.
  - **radial nerve** (C5–T1): its branches pass along the radial and dorsal aspects of the wrist. At the level of the proximal skin crease, a needle is inserted lateral to the **radial artery**, and 3 ml solution injected. Infiltration around the radial border of the wrist blocks superficial branches.

X

Xanthines (**Methylxanthines**). Derivatives of dioxypurine; they include **caffeine** and **theophylline. Phosphodiesterase inhibitors**, with wide spectra of activity, including CNS stimulation, diuresis, increased **myocardial contractility** and smooth muscle relaxation. May also inhibit **adenosine** and reduce **noradrenaline** release.

Xenon. Inert gas, making up less than 0.00001% of **air**. Shown to have analgesic and anaesthetic properties with a blood/gas **partition coefficient** of 0.14, resulting in extremely rapid uptake and excretion regardless of duration of use. Oil/gas partition coefficient is 1.9, with a **MAC** of 71%. Has respiratory depressant effects but provides greater cardiovascular stability and faster emergence from anaesthesia than volatile or **propofol** anaesthesia, though with a greater incidence of **PONV**. Increases **cerebral blood flow** and **intracranial pressure** but may have neuroprotective properties through its inhibition of **NMDA receptors**. Its features, plus the lack of adverse environmental properties (unlike N_2O), have led to investigations into its use as an anaesthetic agent, although it is too expensive for routine use.

Its radioactive isotope ^{133}Xe is used in estimations of organ blood flow (e.g. Xe CT for assessment of **cerebral blood flow**) and in analysis of distribution of ventilation in lung perfusion/ventilation scans.

Law LSC, Lo EA, Gan TJ (2016). Anesth Analg; 122: 678–97

Xylometazoline. Vasoconstrictor **sympathomimetic drug**, acting via α-adrenergic receptor agonism. Used as a nasal decongestant and to reduce bleeding during nasal intubation, including awake intubation. Instilled into each nostril as either drops or a spray of a 0.1% solution. Hypertension may rarely occur in susceptible patients, e.g. those taking **monoamine oxidase inhibitors**. Should be avoided in closed-angle glaucoma.

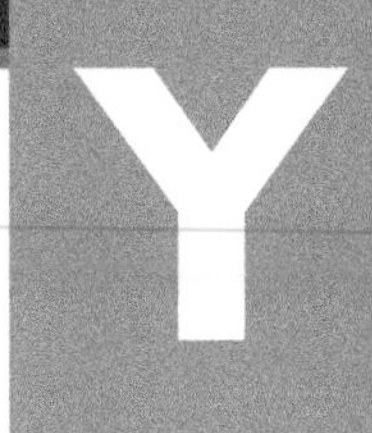

Yates's correction, *see Statistical tests*

Yohimbine, *see α-Adrenergic receptor antagonists*

Z

Zeolite. Hydrous silicate, used for ion or molecule trapping. An artificial zeolite is used in **O_2 concentrators**, to retain nitrogen from compressed air. Has also been added to **soda lime** to retain water and prevent drying out. Also used in many industrial processes, agriculture and water purification.

Zero, absolute. The lowest possible **temperature** that can be attained: 0 **kelvin** (corresponds to –273.15°C).

Zero-order kinetics, *see Pharmacokinetics*

Ziconotide acetate. Synthetic form of a peptide derived from the venomous sea snail *Conus magus*, introduced in 2006 for the treatment of chronic **pain.** Acts as a neurone-specific N-type **calcium channel blocking drug** and thought to interrupt ascending **pain pathways** in the **spinal cord.** Not available in the UK.

- Dosage: 2.4 µg/day by continuous intrathecal infusion, increased up to 19.2 µg/day.
- Side effects: confusion, dizziness, headache, visual disturbances, nausea/vomiting, agitation and psychiatric symptoms.

Pope JE, Deer TR (2013). Expert Opin Pharmacother; 14: 957–66

Zidovudine (**Azidothymidine**; **AZT**). Nucleoside reverse transcriptase inhibitor; a thymidine derivative, it inhibits DNA synthesis via incorporation into DNA. The first anti-HIV drug used; other similar drugs are now available but zidovudine is still used for prevention and treatment of **HIV infection** and AIDS. Traditionally used in cases of needlestick injury to medical/nursing staff.

- Dosage:
  - 250–300 mg orally bd.
  - 0.8–1 mg/kg iv over an hour, 4-hourly.
- Side effects include bone marrow depression, nausea and vomiting, anorexia, GIT disturbance, neuropathy, convulsions, myopathy, hepatic impairment.

Zinc deficiency. May occur in patients with inadequate diets, malabsorption, catabolism and during **TPN.** Essential for normal immune function, oxidative stress response, glycaemic control and wound healing; deficiency causes angular stomatitis, eczematous eruptions and impaired wound healing. Despite this, there is no good evidence that zinc supplementation alters outcome in critically ill patients. Normal plasma zinc level (assuming normal serum albumin) is 12–20 µmol/l; daily requirement is 2.5–6.4 mg/day.

Replacement therapy dosage: 125 mg zinc sulfate monohydrate od–tds. Side effects of therapy include abdominal pain and dyspepsia.

Zoledronic acid, *see Bisphosphonates*

Zone of risk, *see Explosions and fires*

Zopiclone. Non-benzodiazepine hypnotic agent used for the short-term (<4 weeks) treatment of insomnia. Acts at **$GABA_A$ receptors**, potentiating the action of endogenous **GABA**. Rapidly absorbed, with minimal 'hangover'. Undergoes hepatic metabolism with minimal renal excretion of the unchanged drug; dosage should therefore be reduced in **hepatic failure.**

- Dosage: 3.75–7.5 mg at night.
- Side effects: taste disturbance, nausea, dry mouth, headache, rebound insomnia upon cessation.